MENTAL HEALTH NURSING
A Holistic Approach

ELAINE ANNE PASQUALI, R.N., Ph.D.

Professor of Nursing, School of Nursing,
Adelphi University, Garden City, New York;
volunteer therapist in a community mental health
day treatment program; consultant; anthropologist

HELEN MARGARET ARNOLD, R.N., Ph.D.

Holder of postdoctoral certificate in psychoanalysis and
psychotherapy, Institute of Advanced Psychological Studies, and
Professor of Nursing, School of Nursing, Adelphi University,
Garden City, New York

NANCY DeBASIO, R.N., M.A.

Doctoral candidate in human sexuality education,
Graduate School of Education, University of Pennsylvania,
Philadelphia, Pennsylvania; Assistant Professor of Nursing,
School of Nursing, Seton Hall University, South Orange, New Jersey

ELEANORE GORTHEY ALESI, R.N., M.S.

Formerly Professor of Nursing, School of Nursing,
Adelphi University, Garden City, New York

SECOND EDITION

The C. V. Mosby Company

ST. LOUIS • TORONTO • PRINCETON   1985

MOSBY

A TRADITION OF PUBLISHING EXCELLENCE

Editor: Alison Miller
Assistant editor: Susan Epstein
Manuscript editor: Stephen C. Hetager
Book design: Gail Morey Hudson
Cover design: Kathleen A. Johnson
Production: Gail Morey Hudson, Barbara Merritt
Cover photo: Photofile International, Ltd.

SECOND EDITION

The C.V. Mosby Company
11830 Westline Industrial Drive, St. Louis, Missouri 63146

Library of Congress Cataloging in Publication Data

Pasquali, Elaine Anne, 1940-
  Mental health nursing.

  Rev. ed. of: Mental health nursing / Elaine Anne
Pasquali . . . [et al.]. 1981.
  Includes bibliographies and index.
  1. Psychiatric nursing.   I. Arnold, Helen Margaret.
II. DeBasio, Nancy. III. Mental health nursing.
IV. Title. [DNLM: 1. Mental Health—nurses' instruction.
2. Psychiatric Nursing. WY 160 P284m]
RC440.P36   1985   610.73'68   84-1128
ISBN 0-8016-3825-9

AC/VH/VH 9 8 7 6 5 4 3   01/A/077

Preface

What is mental health? What is mental illness? When is a person ill enough to require treatment? These questions have long concerned society in general and mental health practitioners in particular. Of all mental health workers, nurses are in the best position to become actively involved in a broad range of mental health care activities. In primary prevention roles, nurses provide health education and perform health promotion activities. In secondary prevention roles, nurses play an important and integral part in identifying health care needs and providing therapeutic care. In tertiary prevention roles, nurses assist in reducing the severity and limitations of disabilities and are actively involved in rehabilitation.

The concepts and skills of mental health nursing are not limited to any particular practice setting. Staff nurses, individual practitioners, community health nurses, industrial nurses, and nursing instructors may all actively participate in the promotion of mental health. The health education and emotional support that nurses offer to persons facing maturational and situational stress help these persons to mobilize resources, to resolve crises, and to maintain emotional stability. When mental illness does develop, it is often these same nurses who recognize the early signs of maladaptive behavior or emotional distress and help the individuals involved to obtain early treatment. At this point, these clients may come into contact with psychiatric nurses, who may then assume a vital role in all aspects of treatment. Later, community mental health nurses may help the clients to reestablish family and social networks and to reassume social roles. Regardless of whether nurses function in psychiatric settings or other health care settings, they may be engaged in a variety of activities that serve to promote and restore mental health.

Philosophical approach

This book advocates an eclectic and holistic approach to mental health nursing. It is our belief that no one theory or model can provide a complete basis for understanding all aspects of human functioning or the complexities of human behavior. We believe further that anyone practicing mental health nursing must acknowledge, identify, and explore the many interrelationships among biological, psychological, intellectual, spiritual, and sociocultural dimensions of behavior.

While many nurses conceptually agree with this approach, most textbooks as well as many nurses in practice tend to emphasize a particular dimension to the minimization or exclusion of others. To fail to recognize all the dimensions of behavior and their interrelationships, however, is to fail to address the primary objectives of mental health nursing: (1) promotion of mental health, (2) intervention in mental illness, and (3) restoration of mental health. Drawing on a variety of theories and concepts from a number of sources, this book develops a theoretical framework that examines and integrates concepts and skills involving all the dimensions of behavior.

Rather than emphasizing only theory, however, this holistic approach focuses on *people* and on the myriad of interrelated factors that both affect and are affected by them. Nursing should not be hospital oriented or community oriented but *people oriented*. Because people—their behavior and the reasons for their behavior—are the focus of mental health nursing, nurses must learn to view and understand the ways in which people interrelate within a wide social field. By using the nursing process, nurses can endeavor to promote healthy behavior, to sustain people during stress-producing situations, to intervene during maladaptive behavior, and to restore adaptive behavior.

The major objectives of this book are to provide a theoretical background for the understanding of human coping with stress and crisis and to present a basis for therapeutic intervention designed to promote, maintain, or restore mental health. In keeping with the holistic, humanistic philosophy of nursing and the belief that mental health nursing is an integral part of all nursing as well as a specialized area of professional practice, this book emphasizes nursing interventions both for persons who are coping with physical illness and injury and for individuals with psychiatric disorders. Attention is also given to the functions of the nurse as a collaborative member of the mental health team and to the social forces of power and politics as they relate to mental health nursing.

New organization and coverage

The second edition of this book has been logically and cohesively reorganized to provide:

1. A theoretical framework for understanding human behavior
2. A historical perspective on mental health nursing
3. An understanding of political and other forms of power inherent in the health care system and the nursing profession
4. A theoretical foundation for understanding and practicing psychiatric nursing
5. An understanding of how people cope with stress
6. A framework and methods for the implementation of the nursing process in primary, secondary, and tertiary prevention

In addition to this reorganization, nine new chapters have been added to expand the book's coverage and provide for a more in-depth exploration of pertinent issues and topics in mental health nursing. The following is a brief description of the new organization and the new chapters.

Unit I, "The Domain of Mental Health Nursing," consists of three chapters that provide the reader with an orientation to mental health nursing. Chapter 1, "Framework for Mental Health Nursing Practice," defines mental health, mental illness, and mental health nursing and presents the holistic and eclectic theoretical framework used and further developed throughout the book. The concepts of primary, secondary, and tertiary prevention are also presented—as part of a systems-theory approach—along with a discussion of how these concepts can be used as an organizing framework for nursing intervention. Chapter 2, "Historical Overview of Psychiatric Nursing," new to this edition, examines historical aspects of psychiatry and psychiatric nursing and considers their influence on contemporary nursing practice. Focusing on contemporary nursing practice, Chapter 3, "Power, Politics, and Psychiatric Nursing," provides both a theoretical and a practical basis for understanding the political forces that are inherent in any situation in which groups of people work together. Describing strategies for utilizing power and political action to promote mental health, this chapter also discusses the roles of the nurse as client advocate and change agent.

Unit II, "Concepts Basic to Understanding Behavior and to Nursing Intervention," explores in depth the fundamental concepts of mental health nursing. Because the ways in which people perceive and respond to stress and to health problems are culturally influenced, Chapter 4, ''The Sociocultural Context of Behavior,'' introduces theories that provide a foundation for understanding enculturation and acculturation. Sociocultural influences related to stress and coping are explored, as are theories that provide approaches to understanding and assessing ethnic or cultural factors in relation to health care. The discrepancies that may exist between the cultural values of a client and those of a health care provider are also discussed. A section on attitude clarification explores how a professional nurse's own cultural and ethnic values may inhibit the nursing process and discusses techniques for avoiding this dilemma. This section also explores the function of self-awareness and self-understanding in the therapeutic interpersonal process between nurse and client.

New to this edition, Chapter 5, ''The Family,'' investigates the many factors that influence the composition, form, and dynamics of the family. The family is viewed as a social system whose effective functioning depends not only on internal variables but also on the family's relationship with the social, cultural, emotional, and physical environment.

Experiences early in life have a major influence on the ways in which each of us perceives and copes with the stress caused by anxiety, fear, frustration, loss, and other threats to emotional and mental well-being. Chapter 5, ''Human Development,'' discusses the processes of human development from biological, psychological, and sociocultural perspectives. A variety of theories are presented and integrated to provide a comprehensive understanding of this important topic, which continues as a conceptual strand throughout the book. This chapter provides the theoretical basis for nursing interventions for clients at all stages of the life cycle and aids in understanding behavioral responses that may have their origins in early developmental experiences.

Because dealing with stress is an ongoing process throughout life, it is a theme that recurs throughout the book. However, this theme serves as the focus for Chapter 7, ''Adaptation and Stress.'' Concepts such as biological, psychological, spiritual, intellectual, and sociocultural responses to stress are discussed in relationship to mechanisms for adaptation in mental health and mental illness. In addition, the stressors commonly encountered in association with physical health problems, such as pain, threats to body image, loss, and immobilization, are described and explored. Primary, secondary, and tertiary prevention in cases involving these threats to mental health are discussed in terms of the nurse-client interpersonal process as a tool of nursing practice.

The therapeutic interpersonal process is fundamental to all areas of practice in mental health nursing. A knowledge of communication theory and the ability to use therapeutic communication processes with individuals and groups are at the heart of psychiatric nursing. We have expanded the coverage of this important topic to two chapters in this edition. Chapter 8, ''Basic Concepts of Communication,'' provides a theoretical basis for understanding communication in relation to cultural and mental processes. Theories of verbal, kinesic, and proxemic communication are discussed. Communication theory and the relationships among different levels of communication are discussed to promote an understanding of the use of the therapeutic interpersonal process with clients from various ethnic backgrounds. Chapter 9, ''Therapeutic Communication and the Nursing Process,'' specifically addresses the nurse-client relationship and the application of the nursing process to mental health nursing.

Unit III, ''Therapeutic Settings and Modalities,'' focuses on the application of theory and explores a variety of treatment settings and the more common forms of treatment in conjunction with the many roles of the psychiatric nurse. The material in this unit, virtually all of which is new to this edition, provides the reader with an opportunity to examine and explore new and expanding roles and responsibilities in mental health nursing. Chapter 10, ''The Therapeutic Milieu,'' introduces a wide range of therapeutic modalities and the concept and realities of the therapeutic milieu. The client is considered an integral part of the health care team. The role of the nurse is emphasized, and levels of psychiatric nursing practice are discussed in relation to mental health team functions.

Chapters 11, 12, and 13, all of which are new to this edition, focus on nursing functions in relation to group therapy, crisis intervention, and family therapy. Chapter 11, "Group Therapy," explores group processes and dynamics, along with a variety of approaches to group therapy. Chapter 12, "Family Dysfunction and Family Therapy," discusses the stressors that may contribute to family dysfunction and the implications of these factors for the dynamics of the family and the role of the nurse. Chapter 13, "Crisis Intervention," defines and describes both maturational and situational crises and examines the role of the nurse in this important short-term form of therapy.

Chapter 14, "Community Mental Health," focuses upon mental health services that are oriented toward defined communities or catchment areas. Characteristics of the community mental health movement are described as well as the scope of mental health problems and the current status of community mental health services. The organization of community mental health services is considered in terms of primary, secondary, and tertiary prevention, and in relation to the roles and functions of community mental health nurses.

Unit IV, "Client Behavior and the Nursing Practice," identifies and discusses major psychogenic and psychiatric conditions of children, adolescents, and adults. Although most of these chapters consider the development and implications of particular disorders throughout the life cycle, a new chapter, Chapter 15, "Coping with the Conflicts and Stressors of Childhood and Adolescence," explores in depth and within a family context selected disorders specific to children or adolescents. In Chapters 16 through 22, patterns of coping with stress are discussed. The earlier chapters concern conditions that involve relatively little interference with psychosocial functioning, such as the psychosomatic and neurotic disorders. The later chapters concern conditions, such as schizophrenia and organic brain disorders, in which there may be great interference with psychosocial functioning. Chapter 20, "Coping with Emotional Turbulence through Primitive Defenses," a new chapter, unique to this book, explores disruptive, "borderline" personality disorders and the role of the nurse in helping affected clients to maintain psychological equilibrium.

Pedagogy

Each unit opens with a brief introduction, and each chapter begins with an outline of its contents and a brief statement of chapter focus. These tools should help orient the reader to the logical progression in subject matter as well as the purposes and coverages of individual chapters. Many new case studies have been added to help the reader understand and apply the theoretical concepts to practical situations.

New to this edition is the inclusion of sensitivity-awareness exercises at the ends of most chapters. These exercises are designed to help the reader to become a more active participant in the learning process. As in the first edition, references, annotated suggested readings, and further readings are included for all chapters to provide the reader with a basis for further exploration of the topics presented.

Unlike the first edition, the second edition has two supplements—an instructor's manual and a QUESTBANK. The instructor's manual contains learning objectives, lists of terms and concepts introduced in each chapter, chapter outlines, multiple-choice, fill-in-the-blank, and true-false questions with answer keys, classroom discussion/essay questions, and lists of audiovisual aids. The QUEST-BANK, a computerized testbank, includes approximately 200 multiple-choice questions correlated with the chapters in the book. The software is available for Apple II+, Apple IIe, and IBM-PC microcomputers.

• • •

We believe that people should be actively involved in their own health care. Since the term "client" denotes such a participatory role, this term is used predominantly in this book. However, there are times in the delivery of health care when people are (or have historically been) acted upon, when they are forced by illness or other circumstances to assume a submissive, dependent role—the role of patient. Thus, in appropriate instances we have used the term "patient" instead.

The terminology in many of the chapter titles in Unit IV reflects patterns of coping with stress rather than psychiatric diagnostic categories. Psychiatric terminology is used in the text, however, when it is appropriate to learning objectives and when it facilitates communication.

We would like to take this opportunity to thank a number of people who have contributed in various ways to the development of this book. We are indebted to the hundreds of students who have taken our courses. Their learning needs have motivated us to write the book, and their learning experiences have formed the basis for much that appears in it.

We would also like to acknowledge the original contributions of the late Eleanore Alesi. Much of what she developed for the first edition has been retained in this second edition, and we remember Eleanore with love, affection, and admiration.

Valuable assistance in typing and duplicating was given by Rosemary Frey, Kathleen Becker, and Margaret Wilder.

Finally, we want to thank our friends and families, who have patiently lived with the development of the book and who have offered constant encouragement. Without their support this book might never have been written.

Elaine Anne Pasquali
Helen Margaret Arnold
Nancy DeBasio

Contents

17 Coping through socially deviant behavior, 462

18 Coping through inwardly directed aggression, 524

22 Coping with impaired brain function, 700

Glossary, 733

Appendixes

UNIT I

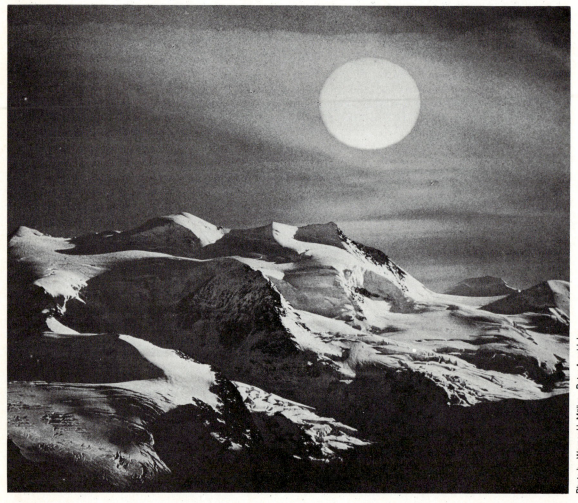

The domain of mental health nursing

Mental health nursing concepts and principles are an integral part of professional nursing practice today. By nature, nursing is a people-oriented profession, and every contact or interaction provides an opportunity for the nurse to observe and intervene on behalf of people who have emotional needs. In order to enhance such interactions, it is important to have an understanding of the various ways to view behavior, the evolution of those theories and approaches, and their implications for contemporary nursing practice. This unit provides such an orientation to the practice and profession of psychiatric nursing.

Chapter 1 defines mental health nursing and describes a number of the more influential and dominant theories of behavior. The holistic approach is explored and endorsed as the theoretical framework used throughout this book. The three levels of prevention—primary, secondary, and tertiary—are defined as an organizing structure for nursing intervention. The five-step nursing process is described in relationship to the three levels of prevention.

In order to know where we are and where we are going, it is important to have an understanding of where we have been. Chapter 2 provides a historical overview of psychiatric nursing and briefly discusses how events in the past have had an impact on contemporary nursing practice.

Focusing on contemporary issues, Chapter 3 describes strategies for utilizing power and political action to promote mental health and to meet such professional objectives as client advocacy and improvement of mental health facilities and services.

CHAPTER 1

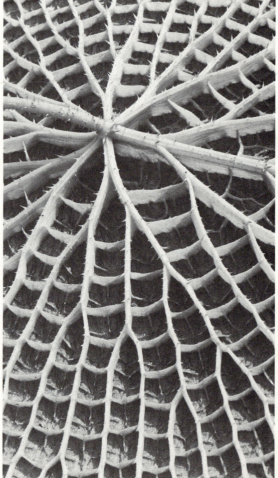

Photo by W.H. Hodge—Peter Arnold, Inc.

Framework for mental health nursing practice

CHAPTER FOCUS

Professional nursing is essentially an interpersonal process. Professional nursing acknowledges the complexities of human nature and promotes a holistic view—the person as a biological, psychological, intellectual, spiritual, and sociocultural being. Mental health, or psychiatric, nursing is that aspect of professional nursing which is concerned with people's emotional responses to stress and crisis and with the interplay of the many health factors that enhance and/or inhibit the ability to cope with stress. Psychiatric nursing is both an integral part of all professional nursing and a specialized area of nursing practice. There are two levels of preparation for psychiatric nursing—the generalist and the psychiatric nursing specialist.

The concepts of wellness and holistic health stress an evolving rather than an absolute state of mental health. Wellness is a process of ongoing growth toward self-actualization. Stress disrupts this process. People participate in the process of becoming mentally ill, and they should also participate in the process of getting well and staying well. Thus, crisis can be an opportunity to grow toward one's fullest potential. In their roles as counselors, teachers, and advocates, mental health nurses help clients to make life-style changes directed toward high-level wellness. Because a systems-theory approach explores how a myriad of factors interrelate and contribute to human behavior, systems theory can be effectively applied to wellness and holistic health and to nursing intervention. Since it incorporates the concepts of stress, coping, and levels of prevention that are set forth in this book, Neuman's systems-theory model is compatible with the orientation of this book.

Nursing intervention is based on the nursing process and is organized according to the concepts of primary, secondary, and tertiary prevention. These concepts offer a framework for providing holistic mental health care to clients.

PHILOSOPHY OF PROFESSIONAL NURSING

The activities of the health professions are predicated upon certain beliefs about the nature of human beings, the nature of society, and the role of the professions within that society. These fundamental beliefs provide a philosophical foundation for the attitudes, ideals, and theoretical concepts underlying professional education and practice. Professional philosophy also recognizes the dynamic nature of society and of the health professions and incorporates the ideals toward which the professions strive.

Professional nursing is essentially an *interpersonal process,* and psychiatric nursing is an integral part of that process (Travelbee, 1971). The primary concern and central focus of nursing is people coping with present and potential health problems. People and the interactions between them are a central component of the nursing process (Peplau, 1952).

Nursing is a *humanistic* profession. It shares with other health professions the responsibility for meeting the health needs of society. These needs include the maintenance and promotion of health, the prevention and treatment of health problems, and the rehabilitation of clients after treatment. Inherent in the concept of humanism is a belief in the worth, dignity, and human rights of every individual. Among the rights that are of concern to the nursing profession are the right to an optimum level of health and the right to comprehensive health services. The protection of human rights and civil rights, including the right to privacy and the right to participate in health care processes, has a high priority in professional nursing practice.

Professional nursing acknowledges the complexities of human nature and promotes a *holistic* view—the person as a biological, psychological, intellectual, spiritual, and sociocultural being. Knowledge and understanding of the complex interactions and interrelationships between these dimensions of behavior, as each individual continually adapts and adjusts to his or her internal and external environments, are essential to the practice of nursing. Inherent in the holistic concept is an awareness that many aspects of human nature are universal and that others are unique to the individual. Sullivan's statement (1953) that ''we are all more simply human than otherwise'' expresses the common humanity that each of us shares with all other people on our planet. The uniqueness can be observed in so basic a biological phenomenon as fingerprints, which are so individual that they are used to distinguish one person from every other. Each personality is even more complex and unique. Each individual is more than a bio-psychosocial being. Each has needs and aspirations as a part of the self, which may be referred to as spiritual being. Recognition of the uniqueness of each personality and of the cultural and ethnic variations in our society is a basic precept of professional nursing practice.

Because nursing is a profession, nurses are responsible for the quality of practice and accountable to the public. A professional level of practice is maintained through a continuing process of formal and informal study. Formal education for professional nursing is a blend of liberal arts and professional education.

Definition of mental health nursing

Mental health, or psychiatric,* nursing is that aspect of professional nursing which is concerned with a person's emotional responses to stress and crisis and with the interplay of the many factors that enhance and/or inhibit the ability to cope with stress. The therapeutic interpersonal process is central to the practice of mental health nursing. Nursing intervention emphasizes interpersonal in-

---

*We use the terms ''mental health nursing'' and ''psychiatric nursing'' interchangeably throughout this book, since both terms describe the same area of nursing practice.

teractions with individuals and groups coping with present or potential mental health problems. The objectives of nursing intervention are as follows: maintenance and promotion of mental health (primary prevention), early identification and intervention in maladaptive disorders (secondary prevention), and rehabilitation in chronic disorders (tertiary prevention). Psychiatric nursing practice extends across the spectrum of human behavior, from the most adaptive to the least adaptive levels of coping with stress, and involves persons of all stages of the life cycle.

To meet their objectives, psychiatric nursing professionals collaborate with other health professionals and community groups in social, political, and educational activities that promote the mental health of individuals, families, and communities. Psychiatric nursing is both an integral part of all professional nursing and a specialized area of nursing practice (Travelbee, 1971).

As in all other areas of professional nursing, the level of psychiatric nursing practice varies with the educational preparation and clinical expertise of the practitioners. There are two levels of preparation for psychiatric nursing. The *generalist* has educational preparation at the undergraduate level and has demonstrated clinical ability in psychiatric nursing. The *psychiatric nursing specialist* has educational preparation at the master's or doctoral level, has supervised clinical experience, and has evidenced in-depth knowledge, ability, and skill in psychiatric nursing (American Nurses' Association, 1982).

Clinical expertise is assessed through a formal review process. Professional nurses who meet the criteria for either of the levels of preparation are prepared to function as members of mental health teams in any clinical setting that provides mental health services. The psychiatric nursing specialist must, in addition, be prepared in research, teaching, clinical supervision, and independent practice. The term ''psychiatric nurse'' is applied to persons working at either of the two levels of practice.

Relevance of psychiatric nursing to all areas of professional nursing practice

The professional nurse practitioner with basic preparation in nursing, including bio-psycho-social theory and therapeutic interpersonal skills, views the psychiatric nursing component as an integral part of nursing practice to meet the comprehensive health needs of clients.

There is general consensus in the profession that the theories of human behavior and interpersonal skills encompassed in psychiatric nursing are essential aspects of basic nursing education and professional practice. In 1950, the National League for Nursing, the organization responsible for accrediting nursing education programs, required that psychiatric nursing be included in all nursing curricula. Sometime thereafter, the federal government, through the National Institute for Mental Health, provided grant funds for faculty in baccalaureate programs in nursing for the purpose of integrating psychiatric nursing concepts and skills into the curricula.

The practice of mental health nursing is not limited to any particular health care setting or to any one age group of clients. Rather, it is an integral part of nursing in all areas of professional practice and for clients throughout the life span. The nursing profession has long been committed to the concepts of health maintenance and prevention of physical and psychological disorders. Providing emotional support to adults and children who are coping with physical illness and injury has long been part of the nursing process in hospitals, clinics, and the home. Health teaching, supervision, and anticipatory guidance practiced by parent-child nurses are forms of primary prevention in physical and mental health that are accepted aspects of professional practice. Nurses working in community health programs, schools, and industry engage in a variety of activities that promote mental and physical health.

Recent developments in health care have placed

increased emphasis upon the need for the integration of mental health concepts. Among these developments are the public criticism of the health care delivery systems for failure to meet the health needs of many segments of society, particularly the elderly, the poor, and ethnic groups in inner-city ghettos. The demand for comprehensive health care and the focus upon physical and mental health maintenance—in addition to treatment and rehabilitation—place a responsibility upon professional nursing and other health professions for meeting these needs.

THE MENTAL HEALTH TEAM

Professional nurses work with other health professionals in the delivery of comprehensive mental health care. The nurse and the other health professionals are collectively referred to as the mental health team. The roles, educational preparation, and some of the professional backgrounds of the members of the mental health team are discussed below.

The nurse

Nursing actions are many and varied. According to the American Nurses' Association's Statement on Psychiatric and Mental Health Nursing Practice,'' the functions of a psychiatric nurse include the following:

1. Responsibility for maintaining a therapeutic milieu
2. Working with clients to help resolve some of their problems in living
3. Acceptance of the surrogate parent role
4. Supervision of the physical aspects of the client's health needs, including responses to medications and treatments
5. Health education, particularly in the area of emotional health
6. Helping to improve the client's recreational, occupational, and social competence
7. Providing supervision and clinical assistance to other health workers, including other nurses
8. Psychotherapy
9. Involvement in social action related to the mental health of the community

The social worker

Social workers function in many settings—for example, medical services, public welfare programs, family and adoption agencies, prisons, community health clinics, and psychiatric facilities. While the largest portion of social workers work in psychiatric settings, the term ''psychiatric social worker'' is considered obsolete. Most professional social workers are prepared at the master's level (M.S.W.); a smaller number are graduates of baccalaureate programs with a major in social welfare. Some social workers have doctorates in social work (D.S.W. or Ph.D.) or in related fields. Some states have licensing or certification laws for social workers (C.S.W.). The national professional organization is the National Association of Social Workers (N.A.S.W.). A social worker who has a master's degree, who has completed 2 years of supervised practice, and who has passed a qualifying examination administered by the N.A.S.W. may be admitted to the Academy of Certified Social Workers. The worker is then entitled to use the designation A.C.S.W.

Social workers are particularly concerned with the family, community, and social networks of clients, and they have a good deal of expertise in carrying out appropriate referrals. At the master's level, social workers are trained in individual, group, and family treatment. At this level there seems to be a good deal of overlapping with the functions of the master's-trained clinical specialist in psychiatric nursing. Social workers and clinical specialists work cooperatively in many settings. Some social workers and clinical specialists are enrolled in postdoctoral programs that provide training in psychoanalysis.

The clinical psychologist

The clinical psychologist is educated at the Ph.D. level. Four to five years of graduate school and one year of clinical internship are usually required. Clinical psychologists are trained in individual, group, and family psychotherapy. In several states they are licensed through qualifying examinations and other criteria. Some psychologists also receive several years of postdoctoral training in psychoanalysis. A unique facet of the psychologist's education is preparation in the area of psychological testing. Tests are used for diagnostic purposes, modification of treatment plans, and research projects. The professional organization is the American Psychological Association, which maintains standards and sponsors various professional activities.

The psychiatrist

The psychiatrist is a medical doctor who has specialized in psychiatry. Some psychiatrists are "board certified," a designation that involves meeting clinical requirements and passing written examinations administered by the American Board of Psychiatry and Neurology. Like psychologists, some psychiatrists seek additional training as psychoanalysts. The professional organization for psychiatrists is the American Psychiatric Association. Psychiatrists make diagnoses; they are usually the professionals who admit or discharge clients from hospitals, and they prescribe and supervise the administration of medication and other somatic treatments, such as electroconvulsive therapy.

The physician

The client is a bio-psycho-social organism, a *whole person*. Too often in psychiatric settings, however, there is a tendency to focus only on the psychosocial aspects of a client and to neglect the physical aspects. Most general hospital psychiatric units therefore include a medical internist or general practitioner as an active team member. Another important role that such a physician plays is in the area of referral. Indeed, many referrals of clients to psychiatric care originate with family doctors.

The occupational therapist

Occupational therapists have been educated and trained to promote the recovery and rehabilitation of clients through manual creative and self-help activities. After assessing clients and participating in conferences with other team members, occupational therapists may prescribe activities that involve learning new job skills or relearning old ones, learning crafts and hobbies, and mastering the activities of daily living. There are two entry levels for the occupational therapist—the B.A. degree and the M.S. degree. Certification is granted by the Occupational Therapist Association, which is the professional organization for occupational therapists.

The recreational therapist

Recreational therapists assess the needs of clients in the areas of recreation, sports, and cultural enrichment, and they plan programs that will enhance the treatment plans for individuals and groups. Being involved in leisure-time pursuits can increase individuals' self-esteem, encourage them to interact with others, and help them gain ego strength as a result of increased competence in dealing with the environment. Most recreational and occupational therapists have majored in their areas in colleges, and some have advanced degrees (M.A. or Ph.D.). In addition to their specialties, they are educated in counseling and other social sciences. Recreational therapists often utilize volunteer services in order to maintain the necessary link between client and community. They also plan and supervise trips from the agencies to such places as shopping centers, theaters, beaches, and cultural and sports events. Registration for recreational therapists is, at present, on a voluntary basis, it is administered by the National Recreation and Parks Association (N.R.P.A.). Within the N.R.P.A., the Division of Therapeutic Recreation provides the professional organization for recreational therapists.

The psychiatric aide or clinical assistant

In traditional state hospital settings, an aide works under the direction of a nurse and is often the person who spends most time in direct client care. Thus, adequate and extensive in-service training programs for aides are essential in order to maximize effective and therapeutic interaction with clients.

The preparation of psychiatric aides varies greatly. Many are high school graduates, but an increasing number of people with additional education—including persons who have master's degrees in psychology and are either working toward a doctoral degree or awaiting admission to a doctoral program—are functioning as psychiatric aides in order to increase their clinical experience and competence.

In many psychiatric facilities these people are referred to as psychiatric technicians; they are given more responsibility and greater remuneration than the less-educated aide, but there is little upward mobility.

• • •

Since mental health services are provided through a system of cooperating health, welfare, and social systems in a geographically defined community, the mental health team may function in any one of a variety of settings. The therapeutic services offered in any setting depend upon whether the major focus is primary, secondary, or tertiary prevention, although some treatment modalities may be utilized in all three levels of prevention.

DEFINITIONS OF MENTAL HEALTH AND MENTAL ILLNESS

The terms "mental health" and "mental illness" are used in a very broad, general sense to imply some optimum level of psychosocial functioning or some level of deviation from such a state. Although these terms are widely used in the literature, they have not been clearly defined.

Peplau (1952), one of the outstanding leaders in psychiatric nursing, has written: "Health has not been clearly defined; it is a word symbol that implies forward movement of personality and other ongoing processes in the direction of creative, constructive, productive personal and community living." Leighton (1959) suggests that there are "numerous patterns of psychiatric wellness . . . or many mental healths." Doona (1979) observes: "The problem in defining mental health (and health in general) derives from the fact that health is not a scientific term." Science is concerned with particular, or specific and discrete, aspects that can be clearly defined and measured, while concepts such as "health" and "illness" relate to very general, nonspecific characteristics of an individual or a group or class of a population.

Problems arise when one attempts to apply concepts of health and illness to human behavior—to the complex ways in which people think, feel, and behave in relation to the joys and troubles of life. The ways in which an individual or a group perceives, interprets, and responds to health problems are culturally determined, as are attitudes about which types of treatments are effective. Mental health and mental illness are culturally defined. Each culture sanctions some types of defensive behavior that provides culturally acceptable means of coping with stress, anxiety, and other noxious feelings. Definitions of mental health and illness tend to be based upon particular cultural or ethnic orientations, a situation that may lead to subjective or judgmental attitudes and values being used to assess mental health status.

Kellam and Schiff (1967) observe that "concepts of health and normality tend to reflect the particular orientation or values of the investigator." The term "mental health" also has a static quality: it fails to convey a sense of the dynamic process through which each personality and environment mutually interact.

Mental health

Such terms as "normal" or "well adjusted," which are sometimes used in preference to "mental health," are vague and subject to cultural bias. "Normal," for example, suggests the existence of a universal standard of mental functioning and a constancy that are inconsistent with the broad range of human experience and the multiplicity of cultural mores and values.

Despite the difficulties involved in finding a satisfactory definition of mental health, there remains a need for some objective standard based on a general concept of mental health or psychological maturity. Cox (1974) has identified "trends or themes of a mature person" that she believes are "most nearly universal and timeless." These include a firm grasp of reality, a value system, a sense of self, and the ability to care for others, to work productively, and to cope with stress. Travelbee (Doona, 1979) views mental health not as something one has but as "something one is." She incorporates themes similar to those listed above into "the ability to love," which includes the love of self, "the ability to face reality," and "the ability to find meaning." Concepts of mental health will be discussed further in Chapter 6.

Mental illness

Mental illness may be defined as psychosocial responses to stress that interfere with or inhibit a person's ability to comfortably or effectively meet human needs and function within a culture. It may be viewed more simply as "problems in living set in motion by stress" (Kolb, 1973). Other terms frequently used include psychiatric or mental disorder, psychopathology, and abnormal or maladaptive behavior.

The use of the term "mental illness" to define or refer to emotional pain and behavioral responses to stress is subject to criticisms beyond those of the ambiguity and imprecision discussed in relation to mental health. Many social scientists and health professionals have raised serious objections to such use. Medical terms such as "illness" or "pathology" suggest the presence of a disease process, which cannot be substantiated in the majority of psychiatric conditions. Of even greater concern is the use of diagnostic categories inherent in the medical model. Diagnostic labeling can have "some very unfortunate effects" (Baron, Byrne, and Kantowitz, 1978). One such effect is that it tends to "assign the person to the dependent patient status" (Mendel and Greene, 1967).

In addition, labeling clients by means of psychiatric nomenclature subjects them to public and professional attitudes toward mental illness in general and toward certain diagnostic categories in particular. For example, labeling a person "schizophrenic" in childhood or adolescence may have a profound and lasting impact upon the person's life, especially if the label becomes known to school systems, employers, law enforcement agents, and the like.

Questions have also been raised about attempts to fit people of various ethnic backgrounds, and with innumerable behavioral responses to stress, into specific diagnostic categories. Such an effort may lead to a focus upon the diagnostic category rather than upon the person who is suffering. Mendel and Greene (1967) observe that a diagnosis serves the purpose of the physician rather than the client.

Defenders of the medical model point out the need for standards and definitions as a basis for assessment, therapeutic intervention, and prognosis. The American Psychiatric Association, which publishes the *Diagnostic and Statistical Manual of Psychiatric Disorders,* has recently revised the manual to bring it more into line with current needs.

We have attempted to avoid diagnostic labeling in relation to understanding behavior and nursing intervention. Diagnostic categories are, however, utilized in many agencies. It is therefore important for the student of nursing to become familiar with the terminology used in the mental health field and to become aware of both the limitations and the advantages of this form of short-hand communication. Diagnostic terminology is used to facilitate communication and to avoid repetition, and it provides reference points for the study of pertinent literature.

Although mental illness or maladaptive behavior is found in all societies (Murphy and Leighton, 1965; Wittkower and Prince, 1974), the definition, explanation, expression, and treatment of mental illness vary from culture to culture. Culture may in fact contribute to the development of mental illness through child-rearing practices, culture strain, and acculturation pressures. Syndromes or symptoms unique to a particular culture are said to be ''culture bound.'' (Culture and adaptation will be discussed in Chapter 4.)

Mindful of the influence of culture on adaptation, we can best understand abnormal or maladaptive behavior if we think of it as a way of coping with stress (Baron, Byrne, and Kantowitz, 1978). As a basis for nursing intervention, we have utilized the concept of *levels of adaptation to psychosocial stress* across the mental health continuum. (This will be discussed further in Chapter 7.)

Psychosocial threat and stress are inherent in the human condition. Threats or stressors may include any perceived threat to the physical or psychosocial self, any loss or threat of loss, and so on. Adaptation to stress is an ongoing process throughout the life cycle. It includes all of the ways in which we cope with anxiety, guilt, fear, frustration, anger, rejection, loss, and so on. Coping processes are strategies for dealing with stress (Lazarus, 1966) and for mastering noxious feelings. They are the processes of adaptation; they include mechanisms of which we are aware and mechanisms of which

we are not conscious. Just as physiological adaptation serves the purpose of physiological homeostasis, coping processes serve the purpose of psychological equilibrium. Behavioral responses to psychosocial stress may be expressed through the emotions, through motor behavior, and through thought processes, including language.

Responses to stress become maladaptive (we prefer ''least adaptive'') when coping processes are unable to control noxious feelings or when the coping mechanisms themselves result in symptoms. For example, in an acute anxiety attack, the defensive or coping mechanisms have failed to contain or master the emotion of anxiety. In obsessive-compulsive behavior, the coping processes result in the behavior. However, all coping processes, regardless of whether they are socially acceptable, are adaptive in the sense that they help a person maintain some level of psychological equilibrium. An individual's ability to cope effectively with stress is influenced by a combination of factors, which include the degree of stress perceived, the current psychosocial situation, and the individual's holistic health status.

THEORETICAL FRAMEWORK

Wellness–holistic health orientation

Human behavior can be studied from several perspectives, any one of which can be useful in understanding various aspects of human functioning. The psychologist may study the forces within the individual (the psychodynamic forces), and the anthropologist may study child-rearing practices within a particular culture (sociocultural aspects). Each may extrapolate some general principles that may be used to enhance our understanding of behavior. No single one of these perspectives, however, will provide a complete basis for understanding the complexities of human responses to stress. We believe that the practice of mental health nursing requires knowledge of the biological, psychological, intellectual, spiritual, and sociocultural dimensions of behavior and of their interrelationships in human responses to stress. In this book we have therefore adopted a wellness–holistic health orientation to human behavior and mental health. However, in the discussions of human behavior and mental health, we have often synthesized these concepts into a three-faceted approach, in which the intellectual dimension is considered part of the psychological dimension and the spiritual dimension is considered part of the sociocultural dimension.

The concepts of wellness and holistic health stress an evolving process rather than an absolute state of mental health. A state of wellness or well-being evolves from the integration of the five dimensions of a person. Wellness is therefore a process of ongoing growth toward self-actualization. One's goals become not merely the avoidance of disorders and premature death but progress toward self-actualization and the optimum enjoyment of life.

A wellness-holistic health orientation toward human behavior rests on the following premises (Flynn, 1980; Goldway, 1979; Tulloch and Healy, 1982):

1. Wellness evolves out of the integration and balance of a person's five dimensions—biological, psychological, intellectual, spiritual, and sociocultural.
2. Stress disrupts a person's inner balance or wellness.
3. Unhealthy life-styles (for example, value conflicts, acculturative pressures, substance abuse, noise pollution, compulsive working) produce stress. People respond to stress with biochemical, physiological and psychological changes. Prolonged or multiple stressors may precipitate psychophysiological or psychopathological disorders (see Chapter 7).
4. Once a psychophysiological or psychopathological disorder develops, a person needs assistance to relieve symptoms and to prevent a relapse or recurrence.
5. A person participates in (contributes to) the process of becoming mentally ill and should also participate in the processes of getting well and staying well.

6. All therapies are temporary expedients until a person can be helped to understand how life-style influences mental health.
7. A crisis can be an opportunity to grow toward one's fullest potential.

People should actively participate in the changes that are necessary to achieve high-level wellness. By increasing self-awareness and by clarifying values and establishing realistic and attainable goals, people can begin to develop positive approaches to their lives. Self-esteem then begins to improve and feelings of hopelessness and helplessness (a victim orientation) begin to diminish. The locus of decision making for achieving high-level wellness rests ideally with the client. Clients who agree to changes or who make decisions in order to please the nurse or other care givers usually do not integrate these changes into their life-styles. Such changes are usually short lived. Clients should be encouraged to explore and to utilize both traditional and nontraditional approaches that support the life-style changes toward high-level wellness that they desire.

The roles of nurses and other care givers in facilitating change* toward high-level wellness consist primarily in (1) counseling (viewing and accepting clients as whole people, assessing their health statuses, supporting them, and guiding them toward high-level wellness), (2) teaching (educating clients about the processes of problem solving and change so that they can increase their self-awareness and learn to appreciate and integrate the five dimensions of the self), and (3) advocacy (ensuring clients' rights and the quality of care) (Goldwag, 1979; Flynn, 1980; Tulloch and Healy, 1982).

Wellness–holistic health assessment guide

The following assessment guide has been developed to assist clients in assessing their levels of

---

*Refer to Chapter 3 for discussions of the process of change and client advocacy.

wellness and to enable students to assess their own levels of wellness. The five major areas of assessment correspond with the five interrelated dimensions of a ''whole'' person. Assessments should be made within the context of a person's family, social networks, and community, since it is within this context that a person's ideology, values, and behavior are developed and reinforced.

I. Biological dimension
  A. Physical activity
    1. Frequency, duration, and types of planned exercise (for example, brisk walking, jogging, aerobics)
    2. Frequency and types of activity required by social roles (for example, sedentary versus physically active job)
  B. Health habits
    1. Personal habits (for example, smoking versus nonsmoking; number of hours of sleep required versus number obtained)
    2. Personal and family history of physical illness and/or organ weakness
  C. Nutritional status
    1. Daily food intake (for example, amount of fiber in diet; consumption of foods from basic four food groups)
    2. Types of food preparation: broiled, boiled, fried, baked
    3. Frequency and types of food additives (for example, preservatives, sugars, salt), processed foods, and ''empty calorie'' foods (for example, soda, candy, alcoholic beverages) ingested
    4. Adherence to special dietary practices: cultural, religious, or social (for example, fad diets, fast foods)
    5. Frequency and types of dietary supplements consumed (for example, vitamins, lecithin)
    6. Frequency of snacking and types of foods eaten (for example, candy versus fruit)
  D. Environmental input
    1. Frequency and types of sensory stimulation, sensory deprivation, and/or perceptual monotony (for example, noise level, intensity of lights)
    2. Degree of exposure to atmospheric pollutants (for example, smog, smoke, vinyl chloride)
    3. Types of territorial imperatives*
      a. Built territories (for example, rooms that afford much or little privacy; architecture that facilitates accessibility [ramps, elevators] or impedes accessibility [stairs, curbs])
      b. Personal spacing (for example, clearly defined and acknowledged claims to space versus ambiguous or disputed claims; adequate space versus overcrowding)
    4. Frequency and degree of exposure to pathogens (for example, exposure to bacteria and viruses; level of immunity)
    5. Degree of relatedness to nature (exhibited through nature walks, gardening, ecological activities, and so on)
II. Intellectual dimension
  A. Formal idea stimulation
    1. Frequency and types of activity (for example, formal schooling, seminars, adult education courses)
    2. Valuation of and committment to education
  B. Informal idea stimulation
    1. Frequency and types of activity (for example, reading, educational television programs, discussion groups)

---

*See Chapter 8 for a discussion of territoriality.

2. Frequency and effectiveness of use of a problem-solving approach to life situations and difficulties

III. Sociocultural dimension
   A. Support systems
      1. Types of help offered (for example, emotional, economic)
      2. Constituents of support system (for example, family, friends, colleagues)
      3. Degree of availability of support systems (for example, available in crisis; must be asked for help; volunteer help)
   B. Sensitivity to others
      1. Degree of ability to listen to and empathize with others
      2. Degree of ability to reach out to help others
      3. Degree of ability to ask for help from others
   C. Cultural orientation
      1. Nature of the family (for example, members composing family unit; sense of obligation among family members)
      2. Nature of role relationships (for example, rigid vs. flexible sex-defined roles; egalitarian male-female relationships vs. unequal statuses; long-established vs. disrupted role relationships)
      3. Verbal, kinesic, and proxemic communication patterns
      4. Relationship to time (for example, past oriented, present oriented, or future oriented)

IV. Psychological dimension
   A. Personal insight
      1. Degree of awareness of own attitudes, feelings, beliefs, goals, and plans
      2. Degree of awareness of sources of and/or influences on own attitudes, feelings, beliefs, goals, and plans
      3. Degree of awareness of own strengths and weaknesses and modes of interaction with the social and physical environment
      4. Degree of awareness of own locus of control (for example, autonomous, fatalistic, victim oriented)
      5. Frequency, types, and outcomes of own risk-taking behaviors
   B. Concept of happiness or well-being
      1. Description of happiness or well-being (for example, characteristics; how it is obtained; who deserves it)
      2. Degree to which attainment of happiness or well-being depends on oneself; degree to which it depends on others
   C. Stressors*
      1. Identification of perceived positive stressors (for example, challenges, excitements) and of perceived negative stressors (for example, threats, problems) and of their sources
      2. Perception of probable durations of stressors (for example, short-lived, long-term, chronic)
      3. Identification of types of coping behavior that are adaptive (for example, sublimation, verbalization, problem-solving) and those that are maladaptive (for example, substance abuse, compulsive eating, hypochondriasis)
      4. Personal and family history of maladaptive coping behavior

V. Spiritual dimension
   A. Ideology
      1. Nature of belief in a supernatural being and/or supernormal energy
      2. Nature of belief in communion between a supernatural being or supernormal energy and people alive and dead

---

*See Chapter 7 for a discussion of stress.

3. Conceptualizations about the quality of life and the quality of death
4. Nature of belief about life after death
5. Effectiveness or ineffectiveness of ideology as a coping mechanism
B. Inner life
   1. Frequency and type of inner-life activity (for example, meditation, yoga, prayer)
   2. Interrelationship between one's spiritual life and the other parts of one's life (for example, meditate when under stress; pray when in trouble)
   3. Effectiveness or ineffectiveness of inner-life activity as a coping mechanism

After they have assessed their levels of wellness, clients and/or students should decide whether they want to make changes in their lifestyles and in what areas they want to make these changes. Tulloch and Healy (1982) suggest that only one behavior be modified at a time, that a concrete, measurable, and attainable goal be set, and that a time frame be established for achieving the goal. Support systems, such as self-help groups, families, and friends, may be helpful to clients or students who are attempting to make changes toward high-level wellness.

Locus of decision making

Since we are basing the nurse-client relationship on a wellness–holistic health model of care, the *locus of decision making* ideally rests with clients. These are clients who are able to assume responsibility for meeting their own mental health needs and who require nursing assistance for health education and health promotion and for guidance in establishing an environment that will support high-level wellness. However, some clients may be only partially able to assume responsibility for meeting their mental health needs, and they may require a therapeutic regimen to meet those needs.

In these situations, the locus of decision making is shared by the client and the nurse. Other clients may have such severely impaired reality-testing ability or such severe emotional problems that therapeutic intervention is necessary to improve their mental health before they can assume self-responsibility. In these situations, the locus of decision making rests primarily with the nurse (National Council of State Boards of Nursing, Inc., 1980).

Dorothy Orem's (1971) self-care model is pertinent to any discussion of the locus of decision-making. According to Orem, self-care actions or systems of self-care can be considered therapeutic when they contribute to the following outcomes:

1. Maintenance and promotion of life processes and functioning
2. Promotion of normal growth and development, both physical and social
3. Prevention, treatment, or cure of disease conditions and injuries
4. Prevention of disability or rehabilitation after a disabling injury or disease

The first two outcomes are pertinent to everyone, while the last two are pertinent only to people who are at risk for, or who are suffering from, disease or injury.

Because self-care is goal- or outcome-seeking activity, it may be characterized as deliberate action. A client appraises a situation, weighs the anticipated results of alternative courses of action, determines which result he or she desires, makes a thoughtful and deliberate choice of one appropriate course of action, and then follows through on the selected course of action. Therefore, according to Orem, deliberate action is a process that is "self-initiated, self-directed, controlled," and based on informed judgment.

In order to have informed judgment, a client needs (1) to be knowledgeable about the demands of self-care, the actions necessary to accomplish self-care, and factors in the environment (such as social values and rules and availability of resources) that may facilitate or impede self-care and (2) to be skillful in performing tasks, making judgments, and validating judgments. Any deficiencies in these areas of knowledge or skill may limit a client's ability to assume responsibility for self-care and may shift the locus of decision making partially or totally from the client to the nurse.

Because the locus of decision making is not always centered in clients, in this book, both long- and short-term goals are stated without reference to a locus of control. Goals can then be modified to reflect a client's status. For example, the goal "Select activities that provide an outlet for angry feelings" can be modified as follows:

Locus of decision making	*Goal*
Client	Client will select activities that provide an outlet for angry feelings.
Client and nurse	With assistance from the nurse, client will select activities that provide an outlet for angry feelings.
Nurse	Nurse will select activities that provide an outlet for client's angry feelings.

In a situation in which the locus of decision making is not centered in the client, changing this situation should be the objective toward which the client and the nurse work.

Since we believe that people should be actively involved in their health care, and that the term "client" denotes such a participatory role, this term is predominantly used in this book. However, we recognize that there are times when, in the delivery of health care, people are (or have historically been) acted upon, when they are placed in a submissive, dependent role—the role of patient. Therefore, in appropriate instances, we depart from the term "client" and use the term "patient."

Major theories

The complex nature of human mental functioning, the large quantity of ongoing research, and the extensive literature available in relation to human behavior make it impossible for a single book to cover the field fully. The mental health practitioner is responsible for continued study in order to keep abreast of developments. Selected theories are introduced in this section to provide a historical perspective and some background for the discussions in the various chapters of this book.

BIOLOGICAL THEORIES

A recent report of the National Institute of Mental Health task force on research observed that "more has been learned about the brain and behavior in the last quarter-century than in all previous history" (Segal and Boomer, 1975). Research in neurophysiology has increased our knowledge of the complex processes through which messages or impulses are transmitted in the brain and the central nervous system. This has led to theories about alterations in neurochemical processes that may contribute to such mental disorders as schizophrenia and the depressions. Research in genetics, particularly the discovery by Watson and Crick of the chromosomal structure, and developments in research methodology, such as the electron microscope, have increased the ability to identify genetic abnormalities responsible for some forms of mental retardation and other hereditary disorders. But despite the impressive advances that have been made, knowledge of the complex processes involved in human thought, memory, and emotions, and their interrelationships, is limited.

▶ Genetic theories

At the present time, no single gene aberration has been found that can be cited as a factor in the etiology of schizophrenia (Kety, 1978) or in other functional mental disorders. Genetic defects have, however, been identified in some forms of mental retardation. Phenylketonuria, or PKU, for example, is known to be caused by an "inability to convert the amino acid phenylalanine into tyrosine" (Segal and Boomer, 1975) because of a defect in a single gene that controls the ability to produce the enzyme necessary for the conversion. Phenylketonuria thus is an example of the way in which a genetic defect can alter biochemistry to produce mental retardation.

The observation that such psychiatric disorders as the schizophrenias and the depressions tend to run in families has led naturally to an assumption that these disorders may be hereditary. Research studies of the incidence of schizophrenia in children of schizophrenic parents, and particularly the study of monozygotic and dizygotic twins of schizophrenic parents, have provided statistical evidence to support this theory. Many studies have found that there is a higher incidence of schizophrenia in the children of schizophrenic parents than in children whose parents are not schizophrenic, and an even higher incidence among monozygotic twins of schizophrenic parents. (Studies involving twins will be discussed further in Chapter 21.) In order to avoid the psychological and sociocultural influences that can result from growing up in a family in which the parents are schizophrenic, studies of children and twins raised by adoptive parents who were not schizophrenic have also been conducted. These studies, too, have found the incidence of schizophrenia to be higher in children of schizophrenic parents than in children whose biological parents are not schizophrenic.

▶ Neurophysiological theories

Neurophysiological research has been going on for more than a quarter of a century, during which time many theories about the biological nature of mental disorders have been studied. Fairly recent developments in neurophysiological research have contributed to our knowledge of the complex processes by which messages, or impulses, are transmitted from one nerve cell, or neuron, to another. Several chemicals called neurotransmitters have been identified, among them dopamine, norepinephrine, and serotonin. Because of their chemical structure, neurotransmitters are also referred to as biogenic amines and as monoamines. In the transmission of messages or impulses from the axon, or nerve ending, of one neuron to a receptor site in an adjacent neuron, a chemical neurotransmitter,

dopamine for example, is released into the synaptic space between the neurons. Following transmission, the neurotransmitter in the synaptic space is either taken back into the axon of the transmitter neuron through the cell membrane (re-uptake) or metabolized by enzymes or other chemical substances. An enzyme, monoamine oxidase, is believed to be essential to the neutralization of the neurotransmitter and possibly to the re-uptake process (Schildkraut, 1978). Nerve cells are highly specialized in the neurotransmitters that they produce and respond to and in their locations and functions in relation to other neurons (Segal and Boomer, 1975).

Research in neurochemistry has been stimulated and influenced by study of the action and side effects of the psychopharmaceuticals that are effective in the treatment of psychoses and depressions. The dopamine hypothesis, for example, which posits some disturbance in the neurotransmitter dopamine, was stimulated by the observation that parkinsonism was a prominent side effect of treatment with the phenothiazines and other antipsychotic drugs. Since it was known that in Parkinson's disease there is a deficiency of dopamine or a disturbance in dopamine transmission, the assumption was made that the antipsychotic drugs acted by blocking dopamine receptors (see Chapter 21). Other studies have focused upon the group of antidepressant drugs that are monoamine oxidase inhibitors. Such drugs are effective in treating certain forms of depression (see Chapter 18).

▶ Developmental theories

The relationship between experience and psychological development, particularly in the early years of life and personality development, has been a major concern in psychological theories since the works of Freud, early in this century. Biological research in recent years has focused upon the importance of adequate nutrition and environmental stimulation to brain cell development. Nutritional deficiencies during the prenatal period and during infancy, when the brain is undergoing the most rapid development, have been found to have a direct impact upon brain cell development. Studies in mice have demonstrated that malnutrition during these critical periods "permanently reduces the number of neurons in the brains of mice" (Segal and Boomer, 1975). Lack of environmental stimulation during the early developmental years also has a negative impact upon brain cell development and function (Segal and Boomer, 1975). (See Chapter 6.)

▶ Theories related to brain cell changes

Recent research in relation to Alzheimer's disease has identified changes in the neurons of the cerebral cortex. Alzheimer's disease, a condition occurring in some older people, involves a progressive deterioration in intellectual functioning. Originally described as a condition associated with premature aging, Alzheimer's disease is now believed to be the major cause of severe organic brain dysfunction in older people (National Institutes of Health, 1979). The results of neuronal changes that occur in this condition are of two types, often referred to as neurofibrillary tangles and senile plaques. Viewed under the electron microscope, neuronal cell proteins appear as threadlike filaments—hence the term neurofibrillary tangles. The change that produces plaques in the cerebral cortex has been identified as the degeneration of groups of nerve endings. (National Institutes of Health, 1979). The cause of the degeneration of nerve cell bodies and terminals is not known. Similar changes have been found in persons with Down's syndrome who survive "beyond 35 to 40 years of age" (Wells, 1978). Further research promises to provide an understanding of the etiology, treatment, and prevention of Alzheimer's disease.

PSYCHOLOGICAL THEORIES

A variety of psychological theories or schools of psychological thought have developed during the last century. Two major schools of psychological theory began at about the same time with the works of Freud in Austria and Pavlov in Russia. Freud introduced the psychodynamic or intrapsychic theory, which has led to a variety of additional theories of intrapsychic functioning. In his studies of animals, Pavlov introduced behavior theory, which has also been expanded upon and applied to human behavior.

Some of the basic concepts of each of these two schools of thought will be presented here. Additional theoretical formulations will be discussed in the chapters in which they are relevant.

▶ Freudian, or classical, theory

Freud's work spanned more than half a century, during which time he developed several interrelated theoretical formulations of mental functioning. He also developed the psychoanalytic method of psychotherapy. Freud's work aroused controversy in that it challenged accepted beliefs and doctrines. Some of the controversy continues to the present time, although many of the terms and concepts Freud introduced have become part of our language and important to the understanding of human behavior.

Psychodynamic or intrapsychic theory, upon which psychoanalysis is based, is a conceptual framework that aids in the understanding of the complex forces and functions related to human behavior and personality. Several aspects of this theory will be discussed.

Levels of awareness or consciousness. The concept of levels of consciousness, often referred to as the topographical theory, is important in psychodynamic theory. According to this concept, there are three levels of awareness, or consciousness, which influence behavior—the conscious level, the preconscious level, and the unconscious level.

The conscious level is that part of experience which is in awareness. This level encompasses the broad range of intellectual, emotional, and interpersonal aspects of behavior, among others, over which we have conscious control. The preconscious level includes those areas of mental functioning that, although not in immediate awareness, can be recalled with some effort. Anyone who has had some difficulty in recalling information necessary to answer a question on an examination, even when the information has been reviewed the night before, has had experience with this level of awareness. The preconscious level serves an important function in screening out extraneous data and incoming stimuli when one is trying to concentrate on a particular matter.

The unconscious level is characterized by mental functioning that is out of awareness and that cannot be recalled. Inherent in Freud's view of the unconscious is the idea that the level of mental functioning in early life, prior to the development of language and logical thought processes, still exists within the psyche and must be maintained on the unconscious level in order to protect one's ability to function as a mature adult. This is accomplished, after the ability for logical thought has developed, through the process of repression. Repression is one of the counterforces or ego-defense mechanisms that maintain a hypothetical boundary between conscious and unconscious levels of functioning. Thoughts, wishes, ideas, and so on that are in conflict with one's internalized stadards and ideals are also maintained in the unconscious level through repression and other counterforces.

An important aspect of the unconscious level of functioning is that such forces as drives and wishes that are kept out of awareness are dynamic forces that seek expression, even in a disguised form—hence the need for counterforces. Therefore, in topographical theory the unconscious level of functioning is viewed as one of the motivating forces of behavior. Some of the forms through which unconscious forces may be expressed are dreams, slips of the tongue, and impulsive acts. Expression may also seen in disturbances in thinking and behavior that appear in symptoms of psychoses and neuroses.

The idea of a dynamic unconscious process as one of the motivating forces of human behavior—the idea of unconscious motivation—is one of the freudian views that aroused controversy. The idea that all of our thinking, feeling, and acting is not under fully conscious control is threatening to our view of ourselves as fully rational people. This concept has, however, become a part of our language and can be useful in understanding otherwise inexplicable behavior, such as that often displayed in symptoms of mental disorder.

Structural theory. Freud's development of a theory of personality—which holds that the personality consists of three parts: id, ego, and superego—occurred after his development of the levels-of-consciousness theory (Fine, 1962). Although often referred to as constituting the structural theory, the id, the ego, and the superego can more accurately be viewed as interacting systems of the personality.

The id is the part of the personality with which one is born and from which the ego and the superego, the more mature parts of the personality, develop as the individual progresses through the stages of psychosexual development from infancy to adulthood (see Chapter 6). The infant is born with the potential for such development and with innate or inborn drives for the survival of the self and the survival of the species. Survival of the self requires that such basic biological needs as those for food, sleep, and shelter be met; since the infant is helpless, these needs must be met by the mother or by others in the environment. The sexual and aggressive drives are also viewed as inborn tendencies or instincts present in the id. The id is therefore often referred to as the seat of the passions.

Freud introduced the term "pleasure principle" to describe one aspect of functioning at the id level of personality. The pleasure principle means that internal needs, experienced by the infant as tension, demand immediate gratification—that is, relief of tension. This principle is in accord with Cannon's theory of homeostasis, which holds that an organism always seeks a return to a steady state. There is no ability to discriminate, at this early level of development, between an object that will satisfy a need and one that will not. Any available vehicle will be utilized to reduce tension. For example, to reduce hunger tension, the young infant will suck upon anything near the mouth. In later life, similar indiscriminate behavior can often be observed as psychiatric symptoms. Compulsive hand washing, for example, may be utilized to reduce the tension of anxiety and conflict.

Primary process thinking is another aspect of the id level of functioning that can be helpful in understanding behavior. Primary process thinking is a form of mental functioning that precedes the ability to use logical thought processes. It is the form of thought believed to occur in early life, before the development of language. Dreams are one example of primary process thinking, and it is, perhaps, through dreams that this level of mental functioning can best be understood. One feature of dreams is their incomprehensibility. Dreams are highly symbolic, and much of the symbolism is of the earlier or more primitive level of mental functioning. One symbol may represent more than one unconscious wish, thought, emotion, or object. Put another way, many forces that are seeking expression may be condensed into a single symbolic expression. Another aspect of dreams is the lack of logic. Contradictory or mutually exclusive wishes, thoughts, and so on can occur together.

Dreams serve an important function in mental life in that they provide expression, in a disguised form, of some of the unconscious forces of the personality and thus help to maintain mental health. Primary process thinking can also be seen in some of the behavioral symptoms in mental disorders. For example, the compulsive hand washing mentioned earlier makes no sense from the logical point of view. But in relation to the symbolism of primary process, this symptoms becomes more comprehensible when it is viewed as a means of reducing the tension of anxiety, conflict, and guilt.

The ego is the part of the personality that interacts with both the external environment and the somatic and psychic aspects of the individual's internal environment. The ego is, of course, a highly complex system of functions that is sometimes referred to as the execuve part of the personality and the site of reason. The ego develops over time as an individual matures physically, psychologically, and socially. Since the ego is involved with learn-

ing, reason, and creativity, ego development continues over a lifetime. Ego functions encompass all of the intellectual and social abilities that we think of as being particularly human. Imagination, creativity, and the ability to use spoken and written language, logic, and abstract thought are but a few of these complex human functions. The ego is also the system that experiences emotions, which range from joy to fear, anxiety, and depression. Another major function of the ego that is of special importance to mental health is that of maintaining the integrity of the personality when it is coping with stress. The noxious feelings often aroused by internal and external stress threaten the integrity of the personality by upsetting the balance between unconscious forces seeking expression and counterforces preventing a breakthrough of the unconscious forces into awareness. The ego maintains the delicate balance between the conscious and unconscious aspects of the personality through such mental mechanisms as repression, denial, and projection. Stress and the anxiety that accompanies it can bring about the need for additional, often more primitive, mental mechanisms, or ego-defense mechanisms, to cope with it. When stress is severe, such mechanisms may result in symptoms of mental illness. (Ego-defense mechanisms and concepts of anxiety will be discussed further in Chapter 7.)

The superego represents the internalization of the ethical precepts, standards, prohibitions, and taboos of parents and other authority figures responsible for the acculturation of the child. This complex system develops in childhood through a process of rewards and punishments, approval and disapproval, and through identification with parents, peers, and others in one's culture. The superego provides an individual with a system of internal controls over thoughts, feelings, and actions that is essential to independent, adult functioning in the culture. The ego ideal, a part of the superego system, is an internalized ideal image of the self toward which the ego strives and against which ego functioning is measured. Striving to realize the idealized image provides some of the motivation for achievement of a person's higher aspirations. However, when the idealized image is too far removed from the real self, the struggle to achieve unrealistic ideals can lead to frustration and feelings of hopelessness.

The conscience is another aspect of the complex superego system. The conscience monitors thoughts, feelings, and actions and measures them against internalized values and standards. When one's internalized values are not adhered to in a particular sphere of behavior, feelings of guilt and shame are aroused. A person who has a strict, inflexible superego is highly susceptible to experiencing guilt and other painful emotions. Since portions of ego and superego functioning are unconscious, the person who is unduly susceptible to experiencing guilt is often unaware that the feelings arises from within the self. In such instances, the feeling is perceived as coming from a punitive environment. In contrast, people in whom the superego is weak or nonexistent do not experience feelings of guilt or shame, even when behavior grossly violates cultural norms. Such individuals lack the internal controls needed to function responsibly in society.

Developmental theory. One of Freud's major contributions to the understanding of human behavior was the introduction of the theory of personality development, or psychosexual development, as he termed it. Although Freud's ideas about infantile sexuality remain controversial, the concept that there are predictable developmental stages has been generally accepted. The importance of personality development to mental health is implicit in all of the schools of psychoanalytic thought. Since theories of personality development will be the focus of Chapter 6, they will not be discussed here. It is important to note, however, that the degree to which one masters the sequential, developmental tasks of one stage can have an impact upon mastery of the tasks of succeeding stages. For example, difficulty in developing trust in self and others can inhibit the ability to develop autonomy.

The theoretical formulations of Freud have been expanded and given new focus by many theorists during the years following his work. Anna Freud, for example, further developed the concept of the ego and the mental mechanisms utilized in coping with stress. Erik Erikson expanded Freud's theory of personality development to cover the entire life span. Erikson also refocused developmental theory to incorporate social science concepts concerning the interaction of the individual with the environment. Others have advanced different aspects of freudian theory.

▶ Interpersonal theories

The interpersonal theorists, sometimes referred to as neo-Freudians, placed emphasis upon the interaction between the individual and society in relation to mental health and mental illness. Karen Horney, Harry Stack Sullivan, and Erich Fromm utilized modern concepts from such disciplines as sociology and anthropology, to a greater extent that Freud had, in developing their theories.

Horney's theory of neuroses emphasizes the importance of interpersonal interactions in the origin and perpetuation of neurotic behavior. Sullivan also views the individual as primarily a socially interacting organism. Sullivan developed a comprehensive theory to explain human behavior in mental health and mental illness. His theory of personality development and functioning is often considered to be couched more in operational terms than in concepts. Sullivan's terms are often utilized by nurses and other health professionals. Fromm's theory has focused more broadly upon social forces and their impact upon the individual. (The interpersonal theories will be discussed more fully in later chapters.)

▶ Behavior theory

Behavior theory, which was developed in the laboratory through experimental research with animals, had its origins in the work of Ivan Pavlov, in Russia. Interest in this field has steadily expanded, and it is now one of the major branches of psychology in Europe and America. The best known contemporary American in this field is B.F. Skinner, whose *Beyond Freedom and Dignity* (1971) applies some of the behavioral concepts to aspects of society. More recent research in behavior, or learning, theory has also focused upon human, rather than animal, behavior, and advances have been made in the study of human motivation and biological rhythms.

One basic premise of behavior is that all behavior is learned—that is, conditioned by events in the development of the organism that arouse the behavior or perpetuate it. From this point of view, psychiatric symptoms are also learned—or, to use the behavioral term, conditioned. Learning occurs in one of two ways—either by respondent conditioning or by operant conditioning.

In respondent conditioning, an event occurs that serves as a stimulus to which the organism responds. A simple type of such stimulus-response conditioning occurs when a child puts a hand on a hot stove. The hot stove causes pain, and the hand is quickly withdrawn. Once an association has been made between the hot stove and the pain in the hand, the response becomes automatic. The child learns to avoid the hot stove.

Emotional responses may also be the result of this stimulus-response conditioning. For example, a young child who becomes separated from his or her mother in a department store may become terrified. Subsequent visits to the store may elicit the terror response automatically. Theoretically, many emotional or affectual responses have their origins in such chance occurrences. Once such an emotional response, like the terror response in this example, has been acquired, it may become associated with or extended to other events or situations in the environment, which then arouse the same emotion. For example, the child who experiences terror in a department store may later experience terror in any large space in which many strangers are present. In theory, at least, this could result in a school phobia, one of the more common phobias of childhood.

In operant conditioning, the organism acts upon the environment to produce a response. Or, to put it another way, the organism emits, or exhibits, a type of behavior that produces a response from the environment that may tend to reinforce the behavior. For example, a laboratory animal presses on a bar of its cage, and a food pellet is emitted. Once the animal makes an association between pressing the bar and receiving the food pellet, it quickly learns to press the bar to get the food, even when the bar must be pressed a given number of times to receive the food pellet. The food pellet serves as a reinforcement for the pressing behavior. The learned behavior continues as long as the reinforcement continues. The behavioral pattern may be extinguished, or unlearned, if the pellet, the reinforcement, is withheld when the bar is pressed. Learned behavior also may be extinguished by the substitution of an aversive stimulus (punishment) for the reinforcement—for example, the administration of a small electric shock instead of a food pellet when the bar is pressed. Although stimuli and responses may be somewhat more complex in human behavior, the principles are the same.

Wolpe (1974) and others have applied behavior, or learning, theory to the treatment of some of the symptoms of mental disorders. Many neurotic and psychotic symptoms are regarded by behaviorists as learned but unadaptive behavioral patterns that are maintained by their consequences—that is, by their reinforcements. Behavior therapy, sometimes referred to as behavior modification, focuses upon the overt behavior or symptom that is unadaptive rather than upon the underlying dynamics or subjective experience, which is the focus of the intrapsychic therapists.

The methods that are employed in behavior therapy for humans include the operant conditioning techniques of positive and negative reinforcement, extinction, and aversive control. Behavior is positively reinforced by the provision of attention, approval, praise, or other forms of reward by people in the environment. Behavior is negatively reinforced by avoidance of an aversive reinforcer. For example, client A leaves the day room when clients B and C try to involve him in their argument and he thereby avoids a confrontation. Client A will be likely in the future to leave the room whenever clients B and C begin to argue. Extinction is accomplished when reinforcing stimuli (both negative or positive) are omitted. The "token economy," in which tokens can be exchanged for candy, cigarettes, and so on as a reward for desired behavior, is often used in the treatment of chronically ill clients in mental hospitals (see Chapter 21). Aversive control is achieved through some form of aversive stimulus when clearly identified undesirable behavior occurs. Negative reinforcement and aversive control are quite often used in adolescent treatment centers, the former by the ignoring of unacceptable behavior that has been identified as attention-seeking and the latter through a system of demerits for undesirable behavior.

Other forms of behavior therapy include desensitization techniques (which are combined with forms of deep muscle relaxation, to enable the individual to cope with anxiety and other noxious feelings), assertiveness training, persuasion, and advice giving. Desensitization techniques have been used extensively in the treatment of phobias. In such a method, the phobic person is repeatedly exposed in a limited way, to the stimulus that induces anxiety. The therapy is combined with deep muscle relaxation. When the client is completely relaxed, the suggestion is made by the therapist that the person imagine being in the situation that produces the phobic response. An elevator or a bus, for example, may be the object of the abnormal fear. The treatment may be repeated several times until the anxiety response is reduced. Then another step is taken—for example, the client walks toward the elevator with the therapist. This gradual approach is continued until the client is able to overcome the phobia.

Any behavior therapy should be designed and carried out, or directed, by a skilled behavioral therapist, or by a person who has extensive knowledge of theory and techniques. Prior to any attempt to institute behavior therapy, the particular behavior to be modified must be clearly identified. The contingencies, or events that reinforce the behavior, must also be understood. Then a program can be developed that can be followed consistently by everyone who will participate in the therapy. The client who is the object of the behavior modification techniques should be included in decisions about the behavior to be modified and the techniques to be used and should agree to participate in the program.

SOCIOCULTURAL THEORIES

A sociocultural perspective on mental health focuses on the influence of social definitions, social norms, and social values on human behavior. Sociocultural theory explores social processes in an attempt to better understand mental illnesses and to promote mental health. The sociocultural theories used in this book may be divided into three categories: functionalism model, psychocultural model, and communication model.

▶ Functionalism model

The functionalism model holds that society is an organismic whole. The various parts of society (that is, institutions and groups) articulate smoothly with one another and thereby maintain equilibrium. New ideas and practices that maintain the existing social order are readily accepted by members of society. Ideas and practices that seriously disrupt the existing social order tend to be resisted. Disjunctions in society may produce social strain.

Functionalists like Durkheim, Merton, Srole, and Parsons use social strain theory to explain social deviance and psychopathology. Society stresses certain values, roles, and standards, but the social structure may make it difficult to act in accordance with them. There may be a disjunction between socially sanctioned goals and access to legitimized ways of achieving those goals, or the social system may make the rules contradictory and meaningless. Leighton and Yablonsky suggest that sociocultural disjunctions may result in inadequate socialization of children. Family patterns, kinship obligations, child-rearing practices, and economic activities may be disrupted. Value systems and role relationships may become confused, fragmented, or conflicting. Children may fail to learn socially sanctioned values, standards, and roles. The resultant frustration, alienation, and tension may produce socially deviant or maladaptive behavior.

▶ Psychocultural model

The psychocultural model focuses upon the relationship between the individual psyche and the social field. Society is viewed as having a profound impact upon the development of an individual's personality. Society provides an individual with opportunities for role development, independence, and socially acceptable emotional expression.

Children are born into a family unit. The family unit becomes the first socializing agent. Later in life, children encounter other socializing agents, such as teachers, clergymen, and peers. A socializing agent serves as a cultural ideal. Children identify with socializing agents, emulate their behavior, and thereby inculcate the norms, standards, and values of society. Through the process of socialization, individuals eventually want to act the way society demands and desire what society needs.

Since family units are never identical, what a child learns at home may later come into conflict with what is learned from other socializing agents. The manner of resolving such conflict, as well as the inherent conflict between the desires of the individual and the demands of society, varies from one society to another. While every society defines what is acceptable and unacceptable behavior, each society offers a range of acceptable alternatives from which an individual may choose.

Social scientists like Fromm, Wallace, Whiting, and Child look at the sociocultural context in which individuals develop and at the mechanisms individuals use to adjust to society. While the majority of a society's members are usually able to use socially sanctioned techniques for keeping stress within tolerable limits, some persons may find socially sanctioned stress-reduction behavior ineffective and may try alternative techniques. Some of these alternative types of behavior may be defined by society as social deviance or mental illness.

▶ Communication model

The communication model focuses upon the cultural specificity of communication. Communication is a process of regulating relationships and exchanging ideas, information, values, and feelings with others. Communication occurs on both verbal and nonverbal levels. Verbal communication is the use of spoken language. Nonverbal communication embraces kinesics (the way people use body parts to communicate) and proxemics (the way people use space to communicate). These different types of communication are systematically interrelated to reinforce, supplement, or contradict one another.

Communication specialists like Birdwhistle, Hall, Scheflen, and Ashcraft maintain that kinesic and proxemic communication are as culturally specific as verbal communication. The form and meaning of linguistic, kinesic, and proxemic behavior are dependent upon the sociocultural context in which they occur. Ethnicity, age, sex, social class, institutional membership, and geographic locale are only a few of the factors that influence the form and meaning of verbal and nonverbal communication.

People from different cultures inhabit different sensory worlds. Selective screening of sensory data results in some information being admitted and other information being filtered out. An experience that is perceived through one set of culturally patterned sensory screens is quite different from the same experience perceived through another set of screens. An encounter or interaction is one type of experience. When persons from different cultural backgrounds interact, using dissimilar linguistic, kinesic, or proxemic cues and having different assumptions and orientations, communication is impaired and role relationships may be disrupted. A sense of nonrelatedness to persons with a different cultural heritage may develop. In addition, culturally determined and culturally acceptable behavior that is foreign to members of a dominant culture may be misinterpreted and labeled as deviant or pathological. (Sociocultural theories will be discussed further in Chapter 4 and in other chapters in which they are relevant.)

GENERAL SYSTEMS THEORY

A system is a set of interacting and interrelated parts that constitute a whole. General systems theory is an approach to conceptualizing and analyzing relationships between interacting units. It allows us to explore problems beyond the level of the individual person and to see how myriad relationships—biological, physiological, social, economic, and psychological—are involved.

Social scientists such as Moynihan, Janchill, and Hazzard describe systems as being either open or closed. An open system has a permeable boundary, and it is characterized by active interaction with the outside environment. An example of an open system is a family that has many social relationships, that utilizes such social institutions as church, school, and health facilities, and that buys consumer goods from both local and nonlocal merchants. A closed system is self-contained; it has a definite boundary, and interaction with the outside environment is nonexistent. Few families represent such a system, but we may find families whose networks are restricted or limited. For example, an elderly couple living in a depressed urban area may have lost contact with relatives and may be hesitant to make new friends and afraid to venture outside an apartment. The man and the woman in such a couple rely upon each other for support and may have little social interaction with others. However, even such a seemingly closed system has some avenues of interaction with the outside environ-

ment. Food must be purchased at the market. Health problems require the services of physicians or nurses. A clergyman may attend to religious needs. Nevertheless, such a family is very vulnerable during crisis periods because of the large expenditure of energy needed to defend its boundaries and the paucity of support resources.

In contrast, a family that is an open system has more access to outside resources and social networks that can provide support and assistance when they are needed. In addition, more energy is available for problem solving and life pursuits, since it is not being expended on maintaining boundaries.

Systems therapy takes into consideration all factors that may contribute to a problem. The illness of one member of a family often indicates that a pervasive, stress-producing problem may exist within the family unit. Treatment may involve all members of the family and may even include other relatives, as well as friends. During a period of hospitalization, other clients may also be included in this social network. Through the inclusion of many vital linkages in a social system, there is increased opportunity for feedbak and exploration of alternative avenues of problem solving. Change in any one of the component linkages in a system ultimately affects, and is affected by, the other linkages in the system.

A nurse can become a linkage in the social system of an emotionally ill person. The nurse thus can focus on the person's relationships with other people and with the environment. The actions of either the nurse or the client may affect the entire system. Concentrating on making the system open and adaptable facilitates the evaluation of health care strategems, the development of a holistic approach to health care, and an understanding of mentally disturbed individuals and their place in society. To work on improving people's feelings of self-worth, only to discharge them back into families that scapegoat and derogate them and into communities that are fearful of them and reluctant to employ them is self-defeating. The hospital, the family, and the community are component linkages in the emotionally disturbed person's social field. Negative feedback from one will undermine the efforts of the other linkages.

Neuman's systems-theory model (1982) incorporates the concepts of stress, coping, and levels of prevention that are set forth in this book. Neuman's model is based upon a person's dynamic relationship to stress. Neuman views systems theory as "a unifying force for scientific exploration," one that can provide nurses a fresh perspective for understanding and intervening in people's responses to stress.

Neuman defines a systerm as a set of component parts in dynamic interaction. The "pervasive order" of the system is maintained through regulatory mechanisms that evolve from the dynamics of the open system.

Neuman applies such a systems approach to health. People, whether they are well or ill, are dynamic systems having four component parts—physiological, psychological, developmental, and sociocultural. Wellness exists when all component parts or subparts are "in harmony with the whole of man." Disharmony thus contributes to various degrees of nonwellness. *Environment* (both internal and external) affects and is affected by human needs, drives, perceptions, and goals. People are open systems, constantly interacting with their environments, and this interaction contributes to their states of wellness or illness.

Any system strives for a dynamic state of balance. Forces (harmful or beneficial) that tend to disrupt this state of balance, or *normal line of defense,* Neuman labels *stressors.* Stressors are characterized by their nature, timing, duration, and intensity, and they can affect more than one human component part. In addition, not only do stressors influence people's behavior, but they are influenced by people's responses to them.

A *flexible line of defense,* consisting of coping mechanisms that can be mobilized to deal with stressors, acts as a buffer between a person's normal line of defense and the stressors in the environment. When the flexible line of defense is ineffective in protecting a person from stressors, the stressors penetrate the normal line of defense and the person experiences a state of disequilibrium. Such a state of imbalance is accompanied by a "violent energy flow," as the person tries to cope with the stressors and the resultant disorganization. At this point, the person's internal resistance factors, or *lines of resistance,* try to stem the disorganization and to reinstate the normal line of defense (a state of homeodynamics).

If the lines of resistance are effective in stabilizing the system, the energy flow is arrested and the person may begin to move toward a state of wellness (negentropy). If the lines of resistance are ineffective in stabilizing the system, large amounts of energy continue to be expended. As more energy is expended than is stored or produced, illness (entropy) and, eventually, death may occur. The function of nursing is to help clients conserve energy.

Applying this systems approach to nursing intervention, Neuman looks at the three levels of preventive intervention—primary, secondary, and tertiary.

1. Primary prevention. Stressors are primarily covert, and nursing actions are designed to *promote* or *retain* system stability by strengthening the flexible line of defense. Nursing actions include the identification and modification of risk factors associated with stressors, through education, desensitization, and the strengthening of coping behaviors.
2. Secondary prevention. Stressors are primarily overt, and nursing actions are designed to *reinstate* system stability. Such nursing actions as early case finding, establishing intervention priorities, and instituting appropriate treatment are aimed at decreasing the severity of reactions to stressors.
3. Tertiary prevention. Stressors are primarily overt or residual, and nursing actions are designed to *attain* or *maintain* system stability. Such nursing measures as progressive goal

setting, reeducation, and optimum utilization of health services support internal and external resources for reconstitution.

ORGANIZATION OF NURSING INTERVENTION

Health maintenance and prevention of disease have long been basic goals of professional nursing. Thus psychiatric nursing, as a part of the nursing profession, has a commitment to mental health promotion and maintenance, as well as to treatment of the mentally ill. In addition, the public and many health professionals have been encouraging the health professions to place more emphasis upon maintenance and promotion of health. The chapters on maladaptive disorders therefore include discussion of the nurse's role in primary, secondary, and tertiary prevention in each mental health problem.

"Preventive psychiatry" is a term used by Caplan (1964) to describe a body of theoretical and practical knowledge that can be used to plan and implement programs whose goals are the improvement of the mental health of the community and its residents. Prevention, as defined by Caplan, consists of primary, secondary, and tertiary levels. Primary prevention seeks to reduce the incidence of mental illness in a community, secondary prevention attempts to reduce the duration of mental illness and to prevent sequelae, and tertiary prevention seeks to reduce residual effects of mental disorders through rehabilitation. This concept of prevention has been widely utilized in the community mental health movement in the planning and implementation of treatment and prevention programs to serve the mental health needs of individuals and communities with a variety of sociocultural characteristics.

We have found the concept of preventive psychiatry to be an effective approach in professional nursing. It is an approach that can be used in any area of professional practice to meet the compre-hensive health needs of clients. Applying the concepts of primary, secondary, and tertiary prevention to the nursing process, on the basis of a holistic philosophy of the nature of human beings, offers a theoretical framework for meeting a client's health needs in the biological, psychological, spiritual, intellectual, and sociocultural spheres. The level of prevention and the priority of needs in each sphere vary from one individual to another and depend on the nature of the health problem and other factors related to it.

Primary prevention

Primary prevention is oriented toward limiting or reducing the incidence of psychiatric disorders in a community. This type of prevention involves an epidemiological, public health approach, which has achieved marked success in eliminating communicable diseases. It places emphasis on the community as well as on the individual or family coping with stress. The focus is upon diminishing or removing sources of stress in the community and upon early identification of, and intervention for, persons in crisis situations, with the goal being to prevent the development of psychiatric disorders. Primary prevention of mental health problems is an aspect of many health and social welfare activities that involve cooperation with community groups in the planning and implementation of preventive services. These services include providing consultation and education programs to increase understanding of psychiatric problems, identifying potential threats to mental health, and providing assistance to community groups and residents who may be at risk of developing psychiatric disorders. Preventive measures may also include efforts to strengthen or increase support systems for groups who may be isolated or alienated and participation in social and political action to reduce such sources of stress as poverty, joblessness, and poor or inadequate housing.

Activities aimed at reducing the incidence of alcoholism, a mental health problem found in many communities or catchment areas, are examples of primary prevention. Nurses and other health professionals may:

1. Collaborate with community groups in assessing the level of potential alcohol abuse and the resources available for intervention and in disseminating information about alcoholism to the community through mass media and other means.
2. Provide consultation and education services to special groups, such as teachers, grammar and high school students, and police officers, who may be serving the population at risk or who may be a part of such a population.
3. Provide crisis-intervention and other supportive services to groups and individuals at risk. The population at risk may include anyone who uses alcohol to cope with loss, or the threat of loss, of love, security, esteem, and other basic elements of human existence.

Additional examples of primary prevention will be found in the chapters dealing with the major mental health problems.

Secondary prevention

Secondary prevention is oriented toward reducing the disability rate from psychiatric disturbances in a community through early identification and effective treatment. The underlying theory is that, in many disorders, early and effective treatment will reduce the duration of illness. Measures to accomplish secondary prevention include screening programs in schools, golden age centers, and other places where groups of residents gather, case finding by public and community health workers, and education programs oriented toward members of the population who may be at risk. Inherent in the concept of secondary prevention is the availability in the community of referral resources for diagnosis and treatment.

Therapeutic modalities utilized in secondary prevention may include any of those used in the treatment of psychiatric disorders. Individual therapy, group and family therapy, brief hospitalization, and chemotherapy may be employed, depending upon the nature of the mental health problem. Brief psychotherapy, crisis intervention, and short-term hospitalization in a psychiatric unit of a general hospital are often employed in secondary intervention.

If we again use alcoholism for the purpose of illustration, examples of secondary prevention may be found in industrial programs for early identification and treatment of the alcoholic. Industrial nurses and community health nurses are often involved in such programs. Nurses in any area of practice may also be involved in case finding. For example, clients admitted to general hospitals for treatment of physical disorders may develop withdrawal symptoms, which may be an early indication of physical addiction to alcohol.

Once identified, the client has the right to accept treatment or to reject treatment. Early intervention may, therefore, include the development of a supportive, therapeutic nurse-client relationship oriented toward helping the client in this decision-making process.

Tertiary prevention

Tertiary prevention is concerned with preventing or reducing the duration of the long-term disability that is often a residual effect of such major psychiatric disorders as schizophrenia, organic brain dysfunction, and some of the psychiatric disorders of childhood. The treatment and rehabilitative objectives are to restore the person to an optimum level of functioning.

Treatment in tertiary prevention depends upon the particular psychiatric disorder. Treatment may include any of the somatic therapies, the individual and group psychotherapies, and other measures employed to ameliorate psychological distress and maladaptive coping processes. In addition, rehabilitative measures, which are designed to prevent or to shorten the period of long-term disability, are important aspects of tertiary prevention.

The nursing process

The nursing process* is the framework for nursing intervention. Although the nursing process is used in primary, secondary, and tertiary prevention of mental illness, in this book we have delineated the nursing process only for the secondary level of preventive intervention.

The nursing process is a form of the scientific method. Although the steps in the nursing process have been described in various ways, in this book we are using a five-step process: assessment, analysis, planning, implementation, and evaluation. *Assessment* refers to collecting and verifying data about clients, whether they be individuals, aggregates, or communities. The aims of assessment are to systematically gather information, to confirm it through consensual validation or additional information, and to communicate it to other health team members, verbally and through charting. *Analysis* refers to the making of inferences based on the collected data. The aim of this step of the nursing process is to understand the meaning of a client's behavior patterns. During the analysis phase a *nursing diagnosis* of the client's actual or potential behavior problem is made. Step three of the nursing process, *planning,* refers to establishing goals and developing intervention for client care. The aims of planning are twofold: (1) to develop a plan of action for initiating change or for enabling a client to better cope with an existing situation and (2) to design and modify a client care plan that is based on psychiatric nursing principles, psychiatric literature, and nurses' own experiences with effective approaches to specific behavior problems. *Implementation,* step four of the nursing process, refers to instituting and completing nursing actions that are necessary for the achievement of established goals and the facilitation of growth-promoting behavior. The aims of implementation are to counsel a client and to provide care that will facilitate the accomplishment of therapeutic goals.

---

*Refer to Chapter 9 for an in-depth discussion of the nursing process.

The last step of the nursing process, *evaluation,* refers to determining the degree of goal achievement. One aim of this step is to have the client participate in the estimation of his or her progress toward the attainment of goals.

Thus, the nursing process provides a framework for nursing intervention, guiding nurses as they assess and analyze client behavior, develop plans for client care, implement those care plans, and evaluate the outcomes.

CHAPTER SUMMARY

Professional nursing acknowledges and promotes the view that people are multidimensional beings. Mental health nursing is the aspect of professional nursing that deals with human responses to stress and crisis and with the relationships between the many factors that influence a person's ability to cope with stress.

A wellness–holistic health approach to mental health and mental illness stresses an evolving rather than an absolute state of mental health. Wellness, a process of ongoing growth toward self-actualization, can be disrupted by stress. Mental health nurses, in their roles as change facilitators, help clients to make life-style changes toward high-level wellness. Therefore, a crisis may provide a client with an opportunity to grow to his or her fullest potential. Because a systems-theory approach facilitates the exploration of how various interrelated factors contribute to human behavior, systems theory can effectively be applied to nursing intervention. Neuman's systems-theory model, which incorporates the concepts of stress, coping, and levels of prevention, is compatible with the orientation of this book.

Nursing intervention is based on the nursing process. The concepts of primary, secondary, and tertiary prevention provide a framework for organizing nursing intervention and for providing holistic mental health care to clients.

REFERENCES

American Nurses' Association Division on Psychiatric–Mental Health Nursing Practices
1982 Standards of Psychiatric and Mental Health Nursing Practice. Kansas City, Mo.: ANA Publications.

Baron, R., D. Byrne, and B. Kantowitz
1978 Psychology: Understanding Behavior. Philadelphia: W.B. Saunders Co.

Caplan, G.
1964 Principles of Preventive Psychiatry. New York: Basic Books, Inc., Publishers.

Cox, R.D.
1974 "The concept of psychological maturity." In American Handbook of Psychiatry (ed. 2), vol. 1. Sylvano Arieti (ed. and ed.-in-chief). New York: Basic Books, Inc., Publishers, Ch. 9.

Doona, M.E.
1979 Travelbee's Intervention in Psychiatric Nursing (ed. 2). Philadelphia: F.A. Davis Co.

Fine, R.
1962 Freud: A Critical Re-Evaluation of His Theories. New York: David McKay Co., Inc.

Flynn, P.
1980 Holistic Health: The Art and Science of Care. Bowie, Md.: Robert J. Brady Co.

Goldwag, E.M. (ed.)
1979 Inner Balance: The Power of Holistic Healing. Englewood Cliffs, N.J.: Prentice-Hall, Inc.

Kellam, S.G., and S.K. Schiff
1967 "The origins and early evaluations of an urban community mental health center in Woodlawn." In Casebook on Community Psychiatry. S.G. Kellam and S.K. Shiff (eds.). New York: Basic Books, Inc., Publishers.

Kety, S.S.
1978 "Genetic and biochemical aspects of schizophrenia." In The Harvard Guide to Modern Psychiatry. Armand M. Nicholi, Jr. (ed.). Cambridge, Mass.: The Belknap Press of Harvard University Press.

Lazarus, R.S.
1966 Psychological Stress and the Coping Process. New York: McGraw-Hill Book Co.

Leighton, A.H.
1959 My Name Is Legion. New York: Basic Books, Inc., Publishers.

Mendel, W.M., and G.A. Green
1967 The Therapeutic Management of Psychological Illness. New York: Basic Books, Inc., Publishers.

Murphy, J.M., and A.H. Leighton (eds.)
1965 Approaches to Cross-Cultural Psychiatry. Ithaca, N.Y.: Cornell University Press.

National Council of State Boards of Nursing, Inc.
1980 Test Plan for the National Council Licensure Examination for Registered Nurses. Chicago: The Council.

National Institutes of Health
1979 "Alzheimer's disease." Department of Health, Education and Welfare Publication No. 79-6146. Washinton, D.C.: U.S. Government Printing Office.

Neuman, B.
1982 The Neuman Systems Model. New York: Appleton-Century-Crofts.

Orem, D.E.
1971 Nursing: Concepts of Practice. New York: McGraw-Hill Book Co.

Peplau, H.
1952 Interpersonal Relations in Nursing. New York: G.P. Putnam's Sons.

Schildkraut, J.J.
1978 "The biochemistry of affective disorders." In The Harvard Guide to Modern Psychiatry. Armand M. Nicholi, Jr. (ed). Cambridge, Mass.: The Bellknap Press of Harvard University Press.

Segal, J., and D. Boomer (eds.)
1975 Research in the Service of Mental Health: Summary Report of the Research Task Force of the National Institute of Mental Health. Department of Health, Euducation and Welfare Publication No. (ADM) 75-237. Washington, D.C.: U.S. Government Printing Office.

Sullivan, H.S.
1953 Conceptions of Modern Psychiatry. New York: W.W. Norton & Co., Inc.

Travelbee, J.
1971 Interpersonal Aspects of Nursing (ed. 2). Philadelphia: F.A. Davis Co.

Tulloch, J., and C. Healy
1982 "Changing lifestyles: a wellness approach." Occupational Health Nursing, pp. 13-21, 45.

Wells, C.E.
1978 "Chronic brain disease: an overview." American Journal of Psychiatry 135:1.

Wittkower, E.D., and R. Prince
1974 "A review of transcultural psychiatry." In American Handbook of Psychiatry (ed. 2), vol. 2. Gerald Caplan (ed.). Sylvano Arieti (ed.-in-chief). New York: Basic Books, Inc., Publishers, Ch. 35.

Wolpe, J.
1974 "The behavior therapy approach." In The American Handbook of Psychiatry (ed. 2), vol. 1. Sylvano Arieti (ed. and ed.-in-chief). New York: Basic Books, Inc., Publishers, Ch. 43.

ANNOTATED SUGGESTED READINGS

Goldwag, E.M. (ed.)
  1979 Inner Balance: The Power of Holistic Healing. Englewood Cliffs, N.J.: Prentice-Hall, Inc.
  This is a book of readings. The readings can essentially be categorized under one of two headings: (1) stress as a basis for illness and (2) self-regulation as a response to stress. The themes recurring throughout the book are the maintenance of health and the prevention of illness.

Neuman, B.
  1982 The Neuman Systems Model. New York: Appleton-Century-Crofts.
  Neuman views systems theory as "a unifying force for scientific exploration," one that can provide nursing with a fresh perspective for understanding and intervening in people's responses to stress. Utilizing the three levels of preventive intervention (primary, secondary, and tertiary), Neuman applies a systems approach to nursing intervention into clients' responses to stress.

Tulloch, J., and C. Healy
  1982 "Changing lifestyles: a wellness approach." Occupational Health Nursing, pp. 13-21, 45.
  The authors discuss the concept of a wellness approach to health and set forth areas to be included in a wellness assessment. Tulloch and Healy then discuss factors that influence change toward high-level wellness and the role of the nurse as a change facilitator.

FURTHER READINGS

Blaney, P.H.
  1975 "Implications of the medical model and its alternatives." American Journal of Psychiatry 132:9.

Erikson, E.
  1963 Childhood and Society (ed. 2). New York: W.W. Norton & Co., Inc.
  1968 Identity and Youth in Crisis. New York: W.W. Norton & Co., Inc.

Fromm, E.
  1962 The Art of Loving. New York: Harper & Row, Publishers, Inc.

Horney, K.
  1945 Our Inner Conflicts. New York: W.W. Norton & Co., Inc.

Jahoda, M.
  1958 Current concepts of Positive Mental Health. New York: Basic Books, Inc., Publishers.

Kolb, L.D.
  1973 Modern Clinical Psychiatry (ed. 8). Philadelphia: W.B. Saunders Co.

Leighton, A.H.
  1974 "Social disintegration and mental disorder." In American Handbook of Psychiatry (ed. 2), vol. 2. Gerald Caplan (ed.). Sylvano Arieti (ed.-in-chief). New York: Basic Books, Inc., Publishers, Ch. 28.

May, R.
  1974 Love and Will. New York: Dell Publishing Co., Inc.

Mullahy, P.
   1955 Oedipus Myth and Complex: A Review of Psycho-analytic Theory. New York: Grove Press, Inc.
Offer, D., and M. Sabshin
   1974 "The concept of normality." In American Handbook of Psychiatry (ed. 2), vol. 1, Sylvano Arieti (ed. and ed.-in-chief). New York: Basic Books, Inc., Publishers, Ch. 8.
Portnoy, I.
   1974 "The school of Karen Horney." In American Handbook of Psychiatry, (ed. 2), vol. 1. Sylvano Arieti (ed. and ed-in-chief). New York: Basic Books, Inc., Publishers, Ch. 40B.
   1978 Report to the President of the President's Commission on Mental Health. Washington, D.C.: U.S. Government Printing Office.
Rickelman, B.
   1979 "Brain bio-amines and schizophrenia: a summary of research findings and implications for nursing." Journal of Psychiatric Nursing and Mental Health Services 17: 9.
Riehl, J.B., and R. Callistra
   1974 Conceptual Models for Nursing Practice. New York: Appleton-Century-Crofts.
Schildkraut, J.J.
   1974 "Depressions and biogenic amines." In American Handbook of Psychiatry (ed. 2), vol. 6. David Hamburg and Keith H. Brodie (eds.). Sylvano Arieti (ed.-in-chief). New York: Basic Books, Inc., Publishers.

Seltzer, B., and S.H. Frazier
   1978 "Organic mental disorders." In The Harvard Guide to Modern Psychiatry. Armand M. Nicholi, Jr. (ed.). Cambridge, Mass.: The Belknap Press of Harvard University Press, Ch. 15.
Seltzer, B., and I. Sherwin
   1978 "Organic brain syndromes: an empirical study and critical review." American Journal of Psychiatry 135:1.
Skinner, B.F.
   1971 Beyond Freedom and Dignity. New York: Alfred A. Knopf, Inc.
Spector, R.E.
   1979 Cultural Diversity in Health and Illness. New York: Appleton-Century-Crofts.
Szasz, T.
   1961 The Myth of Mental Illness. New York: Harper & Row, Publishers, Inc.
   1970 Ideology and Insanity. New York: Doubleday & Co., Inc.
Werner, H.D.
   1970 New Understandings of Human Behavior: Non-Freud Readings from Professional Journals, 1960-1968. New York: Associated Press.
Wolpe, J.
   1973 The Practice of Behavior Therapy (ed. 2). New York: Pergamon Press, Inc.

CHAPTER 2

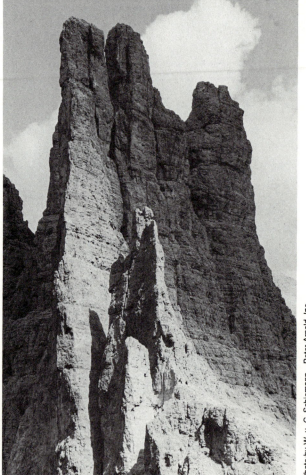

Photo by W. u. C. Schiemann—Peter Arnold, Inc.

Historical overview of psychiatric nursing

CHAPTER FOCUS

This chapter explores some of the important developments in mental health care in general, and psychiatric nursing in particular, during several eras. The effects of scientific and clinical discoveries in the medical and behavioral fields, as well as the profound influences of social and political change, are noted.

HISTORICAL ASPECTS OF MENTAL HEALTH CARE

Mental disorders are believed to have been a part of human experience throughout history. The *Nei Ching* (also known as the *Yellow Emperor's Classic of Internal Medicine*), written in China as early as the twenty-seventh century BC, states:

When the minds of the people are closed and wisdom is locked out they remain tied to disease. Yet their feelings and desires should be investigated and made known, their wishes and ideas should be followed; and then it becomes apparent that those who have attained spirit and energy are flourishing . . . . (Veith, 1965)

Insanity was mentioned by Homer in the *Iliad*. Plato distinguished between "divine madness," the madness given by the gods, and "natural madness." Hippocrates, a Greek physician who lived from 460 to 370 BC, described depressed states. Claudius Galen, a Roman physician who lived from 138 to 250 AD, wrote a treatise on melan-

cholia that remained an important work on the subject for many centuries (Manfreda and Krampitz, 1977). Justinian, an emperor of the Eastern or Byzantine Empire, in the sixth century AD, established many charitable institutions, including some for the care of the mentally ill (Ellenberger, 1974).

As early as the thirteenth century, the people of Gheel, in what is now Belgium, had pioneered in community psychiatry to meet the needs of the mentally ill, many of whom made pilgrimages to the Shrine of St. Dymphna, the patron saint of the mentally ill. Some of the pilgrims to St. Dymphna's shrine stayed on in Gheel, and a practice of foster family care evolved that has continued to the present time.

Attitudes toward mental illness and the treatment of people regarded as being mentally ill have not always been so enlightened. During the Middle Ages, a theory of demonology, or possession by the devil or evil spirits, was prevalent in some areas of Western Europe. Such views persisted at

33

least into the seventeenth century—for example, in the town of Salem, Massachusetts. In some cases, people who may have been mentally ill were regarded as witches and at times, burned at the stake. In other instances, rites of exorcism were practiced as a means of driving out evil spirits.

Developments in mental health care have always been influenced by cultural attitudes, the level of knowledge available, and the religious beliefs and sociopolitical events of particular eras. Johan Weier (1515-1588) a Dutch physician and humanist, was moved by the plight of the many women who were being tortured and executed as witches. Weier believed that these women were mentally ill—melancholic and prone to believing that their fantasies were true. He spoke out for treatment rather than torture, and did so at no small peril to himself (Swales, 1982).

Phillipe Pinel, who has been credited with liberating mental patients from their chains in Salpetrière hospital in France in 1795, was also influenced by the problems of his time. His work received public support as a result of the spirit of "liberté, égalité, and fraternité" that prevailed in France around the period of the French Revolution. The spirit of humanism and concern for humane treatment of the mentally ill was greatly influenced by Pinel's philosophy that mental illness was caused by an individual's experiences in life rather than by some lesion in the brain or by demons or devils. The humanistic philosophy and the enlightened treatment of the mentally ill embraced by Pinel could also be found in the work of Vincenzo Chiarugi in Italy and William and Samuel Tuke in England.

Benjamin Rush (1745-1813), an American physician who is sometimes described as the "father of American psychiatry," provided humane treatment for the mentally ill in the late eighteenth and early nineteenth centuries (Greenblatt, 1977; Manfreda and Krampitz, 1977). During this time the people of the United States were fairly homogeneous in cultural background, and they often were highly dependent upon one another for survival because they lived predominantly in

small, largely agricultural, communities. The shared sense of responsibility was reinforced by the Christian ethic. These factors influenced Rush and others to provide humanistic treatment and care for the mentally ill. The humanistic movement lasted until about the middle of the nineteenth century (Greenblatt, 1977).

In the latter half of the nineteenth century there was a decline in public interest in mentally ill persons in the United States and a concurrent decline in the number and quality of facilities available for their care. This change in public attitude was related to the wave of poor immigrants from Europe. Many of the immigrants suffered from poverty and culture shock, which increased the incidence of mental disorders and the need for mental health services but also taxed the nation's ability to provide humanistic care. In addition, the nation's growing preoccupation with the Industrial Revolution tended to reduce the importance placed on the individual.

Dorothea Lynde Dix (1802-1887), a retired Boston schoolteacher, became alarmed by the condition of the mentally ill and the prevailing practice of incarcerating mentally ill persons in filthy almshouses and jails. She traveled thousands of miles in the United States and abroad, urging state legislatures and other governmental agencies to assume responsibility and to establish hospitals for the care of mental patients. Miss Dix's reform effort was successful in that the individual states assumed responsibility for mental health care and built state hospitals to care for persons with emotional disorders. The state hospitals, often large, understaffed, and built in locations remote from population centers, served primarily to provide custodial care. These hospitals were a major mental health resource until the community mental health movement of the 1960s.

In 1903, a book by Clifford Beers entitled *The Mind That Found Itself,* in which he described his experiences in a custodial institution, attracted the attention of several prominent people. Among them were William James, the great American psychologist, Adolph Meyer, a leading

American psychiatrist, and William Welch, the father of American pathology. They joined with Beers and others to form the National Committee for Mental Hygiene. Under the leadership of Adolph Meyer, the movement took a preventive approach to mental illness similar to that of the community mental health movement of the 1960s. The movement failed, however, to attract public and governmental support.

The work of Freud, in the late nineteenth and early twentieth centuries, and that of his contemporaries and of the neo-Freudians who followed, dominated psychiatric thought in the first half of the twentieth century. Although Freud's work markedly increased our knowledge of human behavior, it had a limited effect upon the treatment of patients in the large state hospitals, where canvas restraints and locked doors often replaced the chains of Salpetrière.

World War II, which brought universal conscription of young men for military service in the United States, focused national attention upon the extent of the nation's mental health problems. Levenson (1974) notes that "approximately 40% of the 5,000,000 men rejected for military service for medical reasons, during this time, were rejected because of some neuro-psychiatric defect." Levenson also notes that such disturbances were responsible for the greatest number of medical discharges from the armed services during the war. In addition, the success of military psychiatry in returning soldiers to active duty following brief crisis-intervention treatment near the front lines served to alert the nation to the possibility of more effective treatment of mental disorders.

World War II focused attention upon the scope of the nation's mental health problems, but it was not until the 1950s that several important developments in the therapeutic measures available for treating the mentally ill occurred. These developments improved the quality of health care and changed the attitudes of both the general public and health professionals about psychiatric disorders. Among the developments were group therapy, which was adaptable to meeting a variety of

treatment goals; crisis intervention; the therapeutic community concept, developed by Maxwell Jones in England; and chemotherapy, which was in wide use by the mid-1950s. In addition to improving the treatment of people with psychiatric disorders, these advances spurred research into etiology and treatment modalities for such disorders.

The 1960s and 1970s saw the growth and development of the community mental health movement (see Chapter 14), which focuses on the delivery of health care to the mentally ill population and makes a strong effort in the direction of prevention of mental illness. The emergence of advocacy roles for clients and their families was also taking place during this time.

THE DEVELOPMENT OF MODERN PSYCHIATRIC NURSING

The roots of nursing care of the mentally ill can, of course, be traced back to very early times. The ancient Greeks cared for their emotionally ill citizens in the enlightened and humanistic way described in the following quotation from an ancient writing found in the temple of Aesculapius:

As often as they had phrenetic patients or such as were unhinged they did make use of nothing so much for the cure and restoration of their health as symphony, sweet harmony and concert voices." (Manfreda and Krampitz, 1977)

The power of suggestion, human kindness, music and dance, and something called "temple sleep" were all incorporated into the nursing care or milieu therapy of the time (Ducey and Simon, 1975; Howells and Osborn, 1975). The Greek Pythagorus traveled to Egypt to observe the treatment modalities commonly practiced in nursing the mentally ill back to health. He found that cold baths, amusements, and reading were all in vogue (Manfreda and Krampitz, 1977).

Even earlier—roughly 1400 BC—an ancient Hindu writing contained in the Ayur-Veda classified mental illnesses, while another of the Vedas set down functions and qualifications for nurses who cared for the mentally disturbed. Such a nurse was instructed to be

Cool headed, pleasant, kind-spoken, strong and attentive to the needs of the sick and indefatigable in following the physician's orders. (Manfreda and Krampitz, 1977)

Certainly psychiatric nursing has grown in complexity since these early descriptions were written (see Appendix B, ''ANA Standards of psychiatric and Mental Health Nursing Practice''), but one can definitely see the beginnings of *interpersonal relationship* and *management of the milieu* as tools for psychiatric nursing.

1882 to 1930

Psychiatric nursing in the United States is a little over 100 years old. It had its beginning in 1882, at McLean Hospital in Belmont, Massachusetts. This private facility (known then as the McLean Asylum) was the setting for the first training school for psychiatric nurses in this country. *Linda Richards,* famous as America's ''first trained nurse,'' was instrumental in the establishment of the school.

Linda Richards had graduated in 1873 from the New England Hospital for Women and Children, in Boston. She was profoundly influenced by the work of *Florence Nightingale,* who had established her own St. Thomas School of Nursing in 1860. In England, before the work of Nightingale, the care of patients in hospitals was carried out by family members, servants, religious orders, and sometimes even by convicts from the local prisons. After her graduation in 1873, Linda Richards traveled to England to meet with Florence Nightingale.

When she returned to this country, Richards was able to establish several hospitals for the mentally ill and also to help establish the school at McLean. The value of this school was quickly appreciated, and within the short period of 10 years there were 19 American institutions providing training pro-

grams for psychiatric nurses.

In 1886, four years after it opened, the training school at the McLean Asylum pioneered in nursing education by becoming affiliated with the Massachusetts General Hospital. Nurses-in-training from Massachusetts General could complete the senior year at McLean. As early as 1906, nurse educators began to work toward establishing similar affiliations for *all* students enrolled in general hospital schools of nursing. By 1935, one half of the existing schools of nursing offered a single course in psychiatric nursing. The goal of incorporating psychiatric nursing theory and practice into the curriculum of all professional nursing programs in the country was not reached until the 1950s, when completion of a course in psychiatric nursing became a requirement for eligibility for state licensure as a registered nurse.

As stated earlier, nursing care of the mentally ill in ancient times had much in common with some of the modern trends in psychiatric nursing. But there is a dramatic contrast between psychiatric nursing as it is practiced today and the roles and functions of psychiatric nurses during the period of 1882 to approximately 1930. Santos and Stainbrook, in their article ''A History of Psychiatric Nursing in the Nineteenth Century'' (1949) describe the functions of the psychiatric nurse as follows:

Her duties included carrying out or assisting the physician with the psychiatric procedures of the day; administering such as whiskey, chloroform, and paraldehyde; and therapeutic measures such as hot and cold douches, showers, continuous baths and wet sheet packs. Various methods of inducing patients to take food also played an important part in the therapeutic measures practiced by physicians and nurses. However, the nineteenth century psychiatric nurse had very few psychological nursing skills at her command.''

Custodial care was the main focus, and ''habit training'' was part of the required course content in psychiatric nursing. Habit training was aimed at assisting patients toward greater conformity or ''acceptable'' behavior (Peplau, 1981). Hildegarde Peplau notes that many of the routine nursing activities, such as "sharp counts," "bed counts," "belt counts," and periodic "body counts," were effective in reinforcing an atmosphere of mistrust between patients and their nurses (Peplau, 1981). In the years from 1882 to 1930, this custodial role for psychiatric nurses did not change greatly. Substantial changes did not occur until the 1950s, when the importance of the therapeutic nurse-patient relationship was finally realized (Lego, 1980). In 1920, one psychiatric nursing text had been published—*Nursing Mental Disease,* by Harriet Bailey—but psychiatric nursing in the period was mainly concentrated on providing for the patients' physical needs and safety through *control* of the patients. Hydrotherapy, tube feedings, and restraint procedures were part of the usual nursing measures. Some psychological interventions on the part of nurses existed, but they consisted primarily in the expectation that nurses should be kind and tolerant toward their patients. Few psychodynamic techniques were available to nurses, and they were often discouraged by the prevalent view in psychiatry that almost all mental illness was incurable—all that could be done was to "classify" the various conditions and provide custodial care. In addition, there was the stress associated with caring for very large numbers of patients. Individualized care was all but impossible. Peplau has pointed out that psychiatric nursing from the 1890s to the 1950s was not a particularly attractive field in which to work. In spite of this, the number of registered nurses employed in psychiatric settings grew from 471 in 1891 to 12,000 in 1951 (Peplau, 1981).

1930 to the 1950s

As descriptive, Kraepelinian psychiatry was gradually replaced by the new psychodynamic concepts, roles of psychiatric nurses also began to change. In private psychiatric facilities such as the well-known Chestnut Lodge in Maryland, nurses were actively involved in the treatment of mentally ill patients. Through their experiences in these settings, they became more aware of the value of healing relationships and therapeutic communication techniques. An effort was made to incorporate these concepts into the body of knowledge for education and clinical practice.

In the 1930s and 1940s, the somatic treatments for mental illness became prevalent, and the participation of nurses was crucial. Deep sleep therapy, psychosurgery, and insulin and Metrazol shock therapy all had their eras. The rapid growth in the use of these modalities contributed to the development of psychiatric nursing. These therapies all involved intensive nursing care, and Florence Nightingale had long since shown, through her hospital mortality statistics, the necessity of skilled nursing services in carrying out any somatic therapy.

The somatic therapies added another element to the evolution of psychiatric nursing. Patients were helped by these therapies and thus became more amenable to psychological intervention. This increased the demand for mental health workers, including psychiatric nurses, who could use their skills and knowledge of psychodynamic concepts to interact therapeutically with their patients. The psychodynamic concepts that had the greatest impact on psychiatric nursing were psychoanalytic theory, interpersonal theory, communication theory, and systems theory.

World War II was also an important influence. Since 43% of all army discharges were attributed to psychiatric disorder, the country became aware that mental illness was a major health problem (Kalkman and Davis, 1974). The *National Mental Health Act* (passed in 1946) authorized, among other things, a program for training professional psychiatric personnel. Psychiatric nursing was one of the four specific professions included in this training program, and this stimulated the growth and development of several undergraduate and graduate programs in colleges throughout the country. In 1950, a study by the National League for Nursing concluded that special training was required for psychiatric nurses. Psychologists, psychiatric residents, social workers, and psychiatric nurses (the four groups singled out for

National Insitute of Mental Health [N.I.M.H.] training) often took classes together during this period, and nurses began to work on a collegial basis with their fellow team members. The graduate-level programs in psychiatric nursing served to produce qualified teachers in psychiatric nursing for programs at all levels—practical nursing, diploma schools, and associate degree, baccalaureate, and graduate programs. Funds from the N.I.M.H. and the Bolton Act (the first federal program to subsidize nursing education for school and student) continued to support psychiatric nursing from 1946 until approximately 1979, when most of the funds were used up.

Also in the 1950s, psychiatric nursing began to focus on the importance of the nurse's "therapeutic use of self" in the nurse-patient relationship. Hildegarde Peplau's *Interpersonal Relations in Nursing*, published in 1952, helped to revolutionize the teaching and practice of psychiatric nursing by providing the theoretical basis for the therapeutic role that is practiced today. Another important event that occurred during this period, and one that greatly affected the care of the mentally ill population, was the discovery of the antipsychotic, major tranquilizers. By alleviating acute symptoms, these drugs enabled the patient to participate actively in psychological treatments of all kinds, including psychiatric nursing therapy and milieu therapy.

In the 1950s, just prior to the widespread use of these medications, a typical listing of psychiatric nursing procedures might include the following:

1. Nursing care of the lobotomized patient
2. Supervision of the admission of a patient, with a cataloguing of all clothing and belongings. Since most patients came into the hospital to stay for a long time, there were numerous belongings to store and keep track of.
3. Safe transportation of large groups of patients from one building to another.
4. Proper procedure for conducting utensil counts after every meal
5. Intensive nursing care of the patient under-

going insulin coma therapy
6. Correct procedure for continuous tub baths, wet sheet packs, showers, and other forms of hydrotherapy
7. Surveillance and supervision of patients at dances and religious services
8. Tube feeding or intravenous feeding and complete bed care for withdrawn, chronically schizophrenic patients, who lay in the dormitories of the "back wards." These patients were often ankylosed into fetal positions after many years of withdrawal and inadequate nursing care.
9. Preparation of patients for "shock therapy." This procedure was quite different from the electroconvulsive therapy procedure that is presently practiced; nursing care often involved joining a "posse" that searched for a frightened patient who was hiding to avoid the treatment.
10. The correct and safe way to enter and leave a seclusion room. There was not just one "quiet room," as is the custom in today's psychiatric facilities. Each ward had several seclusion rooms, and patients did not go into them for a few hours of therapeutically reduced stimuli, but spent months or even years living in them.

1960s and 1970s

The 1960s and the 1970s constituted a golden age for psychiatric nursing. Graduate education expanded, and the incorporation of psychiatric nursing principles into the undergraduate curriculum was well established. The community mental health movement flourished, and progressive psychiatric inpatient units were opened in several general hospitals. A liaison role for psychiatric nurses evolved—clinical specialists became consultants to nurses in other areas of the hospital. Maternity, pediatric, and medical and surgical units all sought the expertise of the psychiatric clinical nurse specialist to help them deal with nursing care problems. Maxwell Jones' therapeutic community concept influenced the nurse's role in milieu therapy. The prestigious psychiatric nursing journal *Perspectives in Psychiatric Care* began to be published in 1963. Psychiatric nurses published clinically focused articles in *Perspectives* and in several other professional journals. Many excellent textbooks became available. In the 1970s an increasing number of psychiatric nurses began to be involved in their own private practices.

The role of the psychiatric nurse was becoming increasingly interesting and challenging. Group dynamics, family therapy, and systems theory were some of the concepts that were added to the graduate-level curriculum and, later, to the undergraduate level. Clinical specialists, prepared at the master's level, became proficient in the treatment modalities of group therapy, couples therapy, and family therapy. Some clinical nurses specialists focused their education and practice on the field of child psychiatry. The number of psychiatric nurses with earned doctorates increased dramatically in this period—from approximately 200 in the 1960s to over 2000 in 1983.*

The role of the clinical specialist in psychiatric nursing became more clearly defined. Standards and functions were described by the American Nurses' Association for both the professional nurse working in a psychiatric setting and for the master's-level clinical specialist.

Another important development occurred in the middle to late 1970s—a certification process became available. Psychiatric nurses who wished to achieve certification could do so, either on a generalist level or as a clinical specialist, through the American Nurses' Association. The two levels have different educational standards and requirements; both involve written examinations, documented experience, and supervised practice. The ANA publishes a directory of all nurses who have been certified through this process.

Also in the 1970s, the ANA's *Division on Psychiatric–Mental Health Nursing Practice* established the *Council of Specialists in Psychiatric–Mental Health Nursing*. The council defined practice for such nurses as follows:

Psychiatric and mental health nursing is a specialized area of nursing practice directed toward prevention, treatment, and rehabilitative aspects of mental health care. Nursing treatments are based on assessment of need, diagnosis and evaluation of progress. They include individual and group psychotherapy, family therapy, screening and evaluation, making house calls, conducting health teaching activities, providing support and medication surveillance and responding to clients' needs through community action, if appropriate.'' (American Nurses' Association, 1981)

The Council also noted that specialists work in a variety of settings, such as acute care and long-term care institutions, outpatient clinics, community mental health centers, offices, schools, courts, and industrial surroundings. In 1983, 675 nurses were listed as members of the Council.

The 1980s

What are some of the current issues in psychiatric nursing? In Chapter 3, ''Power, Politics, and Psychiatric Nursing,'' current issues are discussed in depth. The following brief list indicates some of the possible future directions for psychiatric nursing:

1. The problems associated with applying the primary nursing model to psychiatric nursing practice need to be resolved. There is some conflict between the principles of milieu therapy and those of primary nursing. (For further discussion of this topic, see Ronoff and Kane, 1982.)
2. Nursing research must continue to develop. The number of nurses with earned doctorates is still relatively small, but it is increasing. An example of an appropriate and timely topic for research in psychiatric nursing is the effectiveness of therapy provided by psychiatric clinical nurse specialists (Smoyak, 1982).

---

*Figures from the research departments of the American Nurses' Association and the National League for Nursing.

3. Third-party payments for psychiatric nurses is an important issue. In December, 1981, a third-party reimbursement plan was approved by one large health insurance plan, CHAMPUS (Civilian Health and Medical Programs for Uniformed Services). After an experimental program providing for such reimbursement was authorized and carried out in fiscal 1980, the Defense Appropriations Conference Committee of the U.S. Senate adopted a proposal to make the program permanent. It provided that state-licensed nurse practitioners and certified psychiatric clinical nurse specialists be considered regular CHAMPUS authorized providers. The sponsor of the amendment was Senator Daniel Inoye of Hawaii (*The American Nurse,* 1982). This is an encouraging start toward promoting the autonomy of psychiatric nurse practitioners.

4. Networking, as a support system and as a communication facilitator for the psychiatric nurse practitioner, is becoming an important reality (*Pacesetter,* 1982).

CHAPTER SUMMARY

The roots of mental health can be traced to ancient times. Modern American psychiatric nursing however, is considered to have begun in 1882, when the first training school for psychiatric nurses was established. From that time to the 1950s, the role of the psychiatric nurse did not change very much; it consisted primarily of "custodial care giver." The impetus for change in the profession came from outside forces: the widespread acceptance of psychodynamic concepts; World War II; the National Health Act; the development of psychotropic drugs; the community mental health movement. At the present time the profession continues to grow—to increase its body of theoretical knowledge, to improve its scope of clinical experience,

and to develop network systems for mutual support and exchange of information. Psychiatric nursing is coming of age in that the stimulation for growth is coming from within the profession itself.

REFERENCES

The American Nurse
  1982 American Nurses' Association, vol. 14, no. 2, p. 19.
American Nurses' Association
  1981 Fact Sheet of the American Nurses' Association Division on Psychiatric–Mental Health Nursing Practice, Council of Specialists in Psychiatric–Mental Health Nursing. Kansas City, Mo.: ANA Publications.
Ducey, C., and B. Simon
  1975 "Ancient Greece and Rome." In World History of Psychiatry. John G. Howells (ed.). New York: Brunner/Mazel, Inc., pp. 1-38.
Ellenberger, H.F.
  1974 "Psychiatry from ancient to modern times." In American Handbook of Psychiatry (ed. 2), vol. 1. S. Arieti (ed.). New York: Basic Books, Inc., Publishers.
Greenblatt, M.
  1977a "Introduction to psychiatry and the third revolution." Psychiatric Annals 7(10):7-9.
Howells, J.G., and M.L.Osborn
  1975 "Great Britain." In World History of Psychiatry. J.G. Howells (ed.). New York: Brunner/Mazel, Inc., pp. 172-173.
Kalkman, M.E., and A.J. Davis
  1974 New Dimensions in Mental Health–Psychiatric Nursing (ed. 4). New York: McGraw-Hill Book Co., p. 10.
Lego, S.M.
  1980 "The one-to-one nurse-patient relationship." Perspectives in Psychiatric Care 18(2):67-89.
Levenson, A.I.
  1974 "A review of the federal community mental health centers programs." In American Handbook of Psychiatry (ed.2), vol. 2. G. Caplan (ed.). S. Arieti (ed.-in-chief). New York: Basic Books, Inc., Publishers.
Manfreda, M., and S. D. Krampitz
  1977 Psychiatric Nursing, ed. 10. Philadelphia: F.A. Davis Co., Ch. 4.
Pacesetter
  1982 Newsletter of the American Nurses' Association Council of Specialists in Psychiatric–Mental Health Nursing, vol. 7, no. 1, pp. 2 and 5.
Peplau, H.
  1981 "Reflections on earlier days in psychiatric nursing." Paper presented at the Elizabeth Palmieri Memorial Lecture, Adelphi University, Oct. 12, 1981.
Ronoff, V., and I. Kane
  1982 "Primary nursing in psychiatry: an effective and functional model." Perspectives in Psychiatric Care 20(2): 73-78.

Santos, E., and E. Stainbrook
1949 ''A history of psychiatric nursing in the nineteenth century.'' Journal of the History of Medicine and Allied Sciences, Winter, pp. 40-74.

Smoyak, S.
1982 ''Psychiatric/mental-health nursing research: what difference does a psychiatric nurse make?'' Pacesetter 7 (1):4-5.

Swales, P.J.
1982 ''A fascination with witches.'' The Sciences 22(8):21-23.

Veith, I. (trans.)
1965 The Yellow Emperor's Classic of Internal Medicine. Berkeley: University of California Press, p. 151.

CHAPTER 3

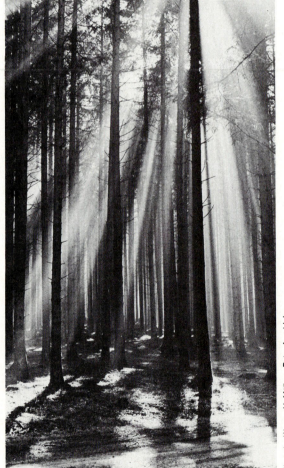

Photo by Werner H. Müller—Peter Arnold, Inc.

Power, politics, and psychiatric nursing

CHAPTER FOCUS

Power is a dynamic of interpersonal relationships. Power arises from many sources, has many forms, and comprises many strategies. To influence the nature and direction of mental health care and professional nursing, nurses must understand the interrelationship between power, politics, and planned change. Institutions, consumers, and nurses are major components of the contemporary mental health delivery system. Within this system, power strategies and power struggles sometimes arise around such issues as quality of care, client rights, and allocation of resources. Trends in mental health often portend the issues around which future power strategies and power struggles may revolve. In the United States today some major trends in mental health are consumerism, a questioning of the insanity defense, decreased funding for mental health research, and independent nursing practice.

Power is the ability to act, to do, and/or to control others. Everyone needs to experience some form of power. Peplau (1953) states that the need for power enters into every nursing situation. Whether a nursing situation involves clients, families of clients, health team members, or agency administrators, interacting participants are usually striving for, relinquishing, exerting, or submitting to power. Certain basic assumptions underlie this concept of power:

1. Power is a resource. It is neither innately good nor innately evil. Power may be used constructively to solve social problems or destructively for corrupt and selfish purposes.

2. Power is an essential dynamic of human interaction. In order for power to operate in an interaction, it must be acknowledged through "empowering responses."

3. Power is dynamic. Its supply is constantly being increased, decreased, and redistributed (Votaw, 1979).

There are many different types of power. Power may be exerted covertly or overtly. People may be subtly influenced (covert power) or coerced (overt power) into complying with the wishes of others (Ashley, 1975; Leininger, 1978, 1979). Power may be used either rationally or irrationally. Rational power structures behavior in a manner that allows people to act in accordance with their thoughts and feelings. Irrational power structures behavior in such a way that people's actions conceal their thoughts and feelings (Peplau, 1953).

Power arises from various sources. Power derived from one's role, status, or position is called legitimate power. Power based on one's expertise and knowledge is called expert power. Power founded on one's intimate relationship with a powerful person or persons is referred to as associative power. Power arising from one's admired personal attributes is known as referent power (McFarland and Shiflett, 1979; Zaleznik, 1979). An individual's power may originate from one source or from a combination of sources. For example, the power base of a nurse administrator who is a charismatic leader may be largely founded on referent power, while the power source of another nurse administrator may arise from legitimate and expert power.

Power may be used either constructively or destructively (Ashley, 1975; Leininger, 1978, 1979). The constructive use of power facilitates the functioning of those subject to it. For instance, a nursing care coordinator may use power to enable nurses to work toward specific goals of nursing care or to achieve desired results of nursing actions. The destructive use of power inhibits the functioning of those who must submit to it. For example, a director of nurses may decide, in collaboration with a medical director, that only psychiatrists, psychologists, and social workers should hold therapy groups. Nurses prepared in group therapy would not be permitted to function as group therapists. Such destructive use of power may be repressive, suppressive, and demoralizing.

Martin and Sims (1956) identify the following power strategies:

1. Formation of alliances
2. Development of maneuvers
3. Control of information
4. Utilization of self-dramatization
5. Employment of compromise
6. Use of decisiveness
7. Utilization of inaction (deciding not to act or make a decision)

The right to use power to command behavior, enforce rules, and make decisions is referred to as *authority* (Leininger, 1979; McFarland and Shiflett, 1979). Authority is often based on rank or position in a social hierarchy. Authority may be either of two types—line authority or staff authority. Line authority is based on job status. People with line authority have a position of power that enables them to hire, fire, and command. Overt use of power tends to predominate. Staff authority is based on interpersonal relationships. People with staff authority do not have the power to hire, fire, or command. A relatively nonthreatening environment is created, and the covert use of power tends to predominate.

Power is a complex concept; it has many sources and forms. There are various types of power strategies and various ways in which power can be used. To influence the nature and direction of mental health care and professional nursing, nurses need to understand that power, politics, and planned change are interrelated. We will explore this interrelationship.

POWER, POLITICS, AND THE PROCESS OF PLANNED CHANGE

Politics is the process of achieving and using power for the purpose of influencing decisions and resolving disputes between factions. A political system is a network of ideas and interpersonal relationships that effectively influences the thoughts, decisions, and behavior of people within formal, organized institutions (Leach, 1954; Ashley, 1975; Leininger, 1978). Each political system contains ideologies, goals, loyalties, interests, norms, and rules that foster cohesion within the political system and differentiate it from other political systems (Scheflen and Scheflen, 1972). For example, a neighborhood drug rehabilitation program will have a political system that is different from that of a neighborhood crisis center. The political system of a federal psychiatric hospital will differ from that of a state psychiatric hospital. An agency operated by a board of directors composed of community residents will have a political system that is different from that of an agency operated by a board of directors composed of mental health professionals.

To apply knowledge about power processes and strategies and to influence the nature and direction of mental health care and professional nursing, nurses must understand the process of planned change. Planned change involves the formulation of a program or scheme for altering the status quo. There are three basic types of planned change—collaborative, coercive, and emulative. Collaborative change involves mutual goal setting and planning. Interactions are characterized by the covert use of power. In contrast, coercive change involves the overt use of power to impose goals and plans on others. Emulative change is characterized by people identifying with an authority figure and adopting the goals and plans of the authority figure. The authority figure usually uses power covertly and serves as a role model.

Planned change is characterized by four phases:

1. Unfreezing the present situation
   a. Development of need for change
   b. Identification of need for change
2. Establishing a change relationship
   a. Clarification of problems and situations requiring change
   b. Examination of alternative procedures
3. Moving to a new level
   a. Establishment of goals and a plan of action
   b. Transformation of the plan of action into actual change efforts
   c. Incorporation of change efforts into the system
4. Freezing at the new situation
   a. Achievement of the desired goals
   b. Establishment of a state of equilibrium (Lippitt et al., 1958; Lewin, 1974)

Essential to the success or failure of planned change are motivational and resistive factors. *Motivational factors* include desire for alleviation of an intolerable situation, disparity between a hoped-for situation and an actual situation, external demands for change, and internal demands for change. *Resistive factors* include reluctance to accept any change, refusal to accept a particular change, satisfaction with the status quo, conflict in the relationship between an agent for change and a health delivery system, and transformation of initially obscure factors into major obstacles to change (Lippitt et al., 1958; Gerrard, Boniface, and Love, 1980).

When planned change is contemplated, it is essential that the people who will be affected by the change be involved in all aspects of the process of change. Whenever responsibility is given for effecting change, it is necessary that the authority to implement change also be delegated. Otherwise the persons trying to effect change will be powerless, and their efforts will be frustrated.

In an understaffed unit where there were many chronically ill clients who had been hospitalized for more than 12 months, a clinical nurse specialist was given the responsibility of instituting milieu therapy (see Chapter 10 for a discussion of milieu therapy). However, he was not empowered to fire staff members who were committed to a custodial care approach or to hire new staff members who would implement milieu therapy. In addition, he was not empowered to spend money for renovating the unit or for purchasing supplies.

Although the clinical nurse specialist was initially enthusiastic about establishing a therapeutic milieu on the unit, his lack of power thwarted all his efforts to implement change. After 6 months in this situation, he became so frustrated that he resigned from his position.

When faced with a need for change, a person can either adapt to a situation, leave a situation, or change a situation. If either of the first two options is selected, the status quo is maintained. If the last option is selected, change occurs. People who try to influence the making and implementing of decisions in a way that fosters change are referred to as change agents.

Change agents act as resource people, as catalysts for change, and as educators in techniques of planned change. To fulfill these roles, change agents need to be skilled in the following areas:

1. Identifying and helping others recognize a need for change
2. Assessing factors that may facilitate or impede change
3. Helping people view themselves as a group that can effect change
4. Helping a group explore its mode of interaction and correct disruptive interaction patterns
5. Helping a group establish goals for change
6. Selecting appropriate roles and techniques to assist a group in achieving goals
7. Helping a group develop methods for achieving goals
8. Supporting and guiding a group through the phases of change
9. Maintaining channels of communication within the health delivery system
10. Helping a group evaluate change efforts and results (Lippitt et al., 1958; Bennis, 1969; Argyris, 1972; Gerrard, Boniface, and Love, 1980).

Argyris (1972) believes that people who are committed to effecting change need to possess high degrees of candor and trust and that they must be willing to take risks. These personal attributes are especially important when change requires the adoption of deviant behavior (for example, promoting a policy that differs markedly from previous agency policy) or self-corrective behavior (self-evaluation or self-improvement), the unfreezing of present behavior, or a high degree of interdependence among participants in a group or situation.

Power, politics, and planned change are complex and interrelated processes. We will now look at the utilization of these processes in mental health care.

POWER, POLITICS, PLANNED CHANGE, AND PSYCHIATRIC CARE

Institutions

Institutions* are organizations that fulfill normative functions and purposes in society. An institution is a subsystem of a larger system (Blase, 1973). Federal, state, and local psychiatric hospitals and community mental health agencies are examples of institutions.

Institutions are often characterized by bureaucracy and hierarchy. The aim of a bureaucracy is efficiency. In a bureaucracy rules are established by authority figures, work is impersonally defined in terms of job descriptions, and activities are recorded and monitored by means of such written documents as timesheets, data cards, and monthly reports. Authority is vested in a hierarchy that can be displayed as an organizational chart. At the top of the hierarchy is a board of directors, which establishes rules. These rules are interpreted and applied by administrators. Division heads and supervisors enforce the rules, and staff members are expected to comply with the rules.

Establishment, interpretation, application, and enforcement of rules, and compliance with them, are facilitated by an institution's communication system. A communication system also serves two important political functions: regulation of vertical mobility and behavior and indoctrination of staff members into the ideology of the institution (Scheflen and Scheflen, 1972).

Regulation of vertical mobility is facilitated by a hierarchy. Even though an institution may have a philosophy of egalitarianism, in practice a hierarchy may be present, and upward mobility may be limited to persons who demonstrate loyalty to the institution, who possess certain educational qualifications, or who belong to the "right" social class or ethnic group (Scheflen and Scheflen, 1972).

---

*Refer to Chapter 4 for a discussion of institutions and culture shock.

Regulation of behavior can be accomplished nonverbally,* through the use of symbols and kinesic monitors (Scheflen and Scheflen, 1972). An institution usually officially communicates its philosophy of health care in verbal and written statements. However, an institution's unofficial philosophy may be reflected in symbols (for example, use or nonuse of uniforms, locked or unlocked psychiatric units). Institutions also officially and unofficially state expectations about members' performance. These expectations define acceptable behavior for all members (both staff members and clients). Members are then evaluated on the basis of their desire and ability to fulfill these expectations. Staff members who satisfy these expectations may be promoted or given salary increases. Clients who fulfill the expectations may be judged mentally healthy and discharged from the institution. Scheflen and Scheflen (1972) emphasize that kinesic monitors, especially those that convey negative feedback, are very effective in evaluating and controlling behavior.

A clinical nurse specialist thought that the wearing of uniforms in a psychiatric setting conveyed messages of control and authority, reinforced the passive client role, and contributed to an interaction theme of dominance (nurse)–submission (client). When she discussed this issue with the director of nurses, the director took a deep breath and rolled her eyes upward toward the ceiling. The director's kinesic monitor conveyed the message: "Here we go again. I've heard this before. I don't approve of the idea." The clinical nurse specialist felt intimidated and did not pursue the idea any further.

Because staff members and clients, to differing degrees, depend on an institution for gratification of security needs, negative kinesic monitors tend to be very effective in controlling behavior.

---

*Refer to Chapter 8 for a discussion of nonverbal communication.

Often there is incongruity between the verbal and kinesic levels of institutional communication. For instance, an administrator's verbal philosophy of care may emphasize client participation in the setting of treatment goals, while his kinesic behavior may severely restrict client input into the treatment program. Such inconsistency between verbal and kinesic messages tends to confuse staff members and to render them powerless to change the system. Kinesic monitors derive much of their power from the incongruity produced in the communication system (Scheflen and Scheflen, 1972).

A system of reinforcement that includes both kinesic monitors and negative and positive sanctions helps regulate the behavior of an institution's members. For instance, staff members who display institutionally approved behavior may be rewarded with job security, job advancement, and salary increments. Staff members who deviate markedly from institutionally approved behavior may be threatened with demotion, firing, and negative references for future jobs, or they may actually be demoted or fired.

Members of an institution may be, to varying degrees, indoctrinated into institutional *ideology*. An ideology projects an institution's ideas and purpose for existing outward onto its social environment. Indoctrination into institutional ideology promotes cohesion and commitment among members and minimizes the need for overt use of power in the implementation of programs and services. The more controversial an institution's programs and services, the greater the importance of ideology in defending and supporting its activities (Downs, 1967; Zentner, 1973).

Members who are fully indoctrinated into institutional ideology tend to believe and think along institutional lines—to engage in "institutional think." When institutional think occurs, members are apt not to recognize discrepancies, problems, or alternatives. At this point, members may so closely identify with the institution that an attack on it becomes an attack on them (Scheflen and Scheflen 1972).

The graduate students felt overwhelmed by course requirements. In addition, they felt that there was a degree of overlap and redundancy in such course requirements as process recordings, supervisory conferences, log entries, and sharing of clinical experiences in seminar. When the students complained to the faculty and asked that the assignments be reevaluated and streamlined, the faculty became very defensive. Not only had the faculty required these assignments for a number of years, but particular faculty members had designed particular assignments. The rationale for the assignments reflected the philosophy of the program. The faculty's identification with the program and the assignments made the faculty members resistant to any suggestions for change. They were unable to hear the students' complaints or to see any value in the students' suggestions for change. The faculty members were victims of "institutional think."

Any discussion of planned change in institutions must include three elements—institutional variables, networks, and transactions.

Institutional variables include leadership, ideology, programs, resources, and internal structure. Leadership must be displayed by the people who are actively involved in making policies and decisions and in directing institutional operations. Ideology consists of an institution's stated philosophy and its purpose for existing. Programs are methods for translating institutional ideology into actions and for allocating resources for accomplishing those actions. Resources include money, materials, labor, and political support, all of which may be necessary for implementation of programs. Internal structure, the organizing and channeling of power, authority, and decision making within an institution, may be either lateral or hierarchical* (Perrow, 1970; Argyris, 1972; Bumgardner et al.,

---

*Lateral structure involves a dispersed locus of authority, with all members presumably enjoying equal power and authority. Hierarchical structure involves a centralized locus of authority and a chain of command.

1972; Blase, 1973; Zaltman, Duncan, and Holbeck, 1973).

Networks are interrelationships between an institution and its social environment that influence and maintain the institution and provide it with a capacity for change. Blase (1973) and Bumgardner et al. (1972) describe several types of networks:

1. Enabling network—composed of organizations that give an institution both legal authority and resources for its existence. For example, the Community Mental Health Centers Act of 1963 authorized establishment of community mental health centers, and Title II provided funds for their establishment.
2. Normative network—composed of interrelationships between an institution and an organized body of people who determine norms and standards for the operation of the institution. For example, the Community Mental Health Centers Act amendments of 1975 established standards and guidelines for the operation of community mental health centers.
3. Diffuse network—composed of interrelationships between an institution and the public. For example, the National Association of Mental Health and organized consumer groups may be component linkages in a normative network.
4. Functional network—composed of interrelationships between an institution and a body of people who provide the institution with such resources as clients and professional staff.

Transactions are the actual interactions between an institution and the component linkages in its network, which both influence and are influenced by the institution. Transactions involve planning and strategy decisions. These plans and strategies comprise the matrix of planned change in institutions (Bumgardner et al., 1972; Scheflen and Scheflen, 1972; Blase, 1973).

Institutional variables, networks, and transactions can interrelate to produce planned change within an institution. When institutional ideology is not viable, impetus for change tends to develop from forces outside the institution (from component linkages in the institution's networks). The internal structure of the institution will then either respond to or resist pressure for change. If institutional structure is of a lateral type, all members will presumably be equally involved in the process of change and will respond to pressure for change. However, if institutional structure is of a hierarchical type, pressure from outside the institution for change will usually be met by resistance (Perrow, 1970; Argyris, 1972; Bumgardner et al., 1972; Blase, 1973).

When institutional ideology is variable, impetus for planned change tends to develop from forces within the institution. For instance, professional staff may realize that mental health services do not meet the needs of the catchment population. If commitment to institutional ideology is weak, then a hierarchical structure will be most effective in mandating and effecting planned change. If commitment to institutional ideology is strong, a lateral structure will be most effective in initiating and implementing planned change (Bumgardner et al., 1972; Blase, 1973).

Consumers

A consumer is an individual, a group, or a community that utilizes a product or service. In the area of mental health, consumerism refers to the utilization of all levels of mental health services (services designed for primary, secondary, and tertiary prevention of mental illness). Gonzalez (1976) points out that consumer groups have been organized on all levels—local, state, national, and international. These groups, which may operate either independently or corporately, often grow out of special interest movements in schools, health agencies, government, and industry. The Mental Patients' Liberation Movement—composed of people who have at some time in their lives been treated for mental illness—and the Federation of Parents' Organization—composed of parents of people who are mentally ill, as well as other concerned relatives and citizens—are examples of consumer groups that are actively involved in client advocacy and in upgrading the quality of mental health care.

Consumers, individually and organized as groups, serve two functions—to monitor and to regulate. In their function as monitors, consumers ascertain the need for and the accessibility, availability, and effectiveness of health care services; check into the cost effectiveness of health care activities; and watch for unethical behavior on the part of mental health professionals. In their function as regulators, consumers are concerned with the credentials and competence of mental health professionals and with standards of professional practice (Gonzalez, 1976).

To carry out these functions, consumers assume roles as planners, advisors, and educators. Consumers are actively involved in the following areas:

1. Lobbying for legislation that will upgrade mental health care
2. Lobbying for adequate funding of mental health programs
3. Reordering of local, state, and national priorities
4. Utilizing community resources for the planning and implementation of programs that will meet the mental health needs of the community
5. Contributing to the preparation of mental health workers by acquainting them with the needs, values, and goals of the community that the workers are servicing (National Commission on Community Health Services, 1966; Health Task Force of the Urban Coalition, 1970; National Association for Mental Health, 1974)

Consumers, individually or in groups, tend to have certain basic concerns. Fundamental to these concerns is the idea that mental health professionals have too much power over clients. Consumer groups point out that the courts usually accept a psychiatrist's observations or predictions of dangerous behavior over a client's request for discharge from a psychiatric institution. Consumers also express concern that, once a person is labeled mentally ill, the focus of mental health professionals is on abnormal rather than normal behavior. In addition, consumers are concerned that some psychiatric institutions do not provide adequate treatment and that transitional and aftercare facilities are insufficient.

Consumers of mental health services do not have the vested interest in protecting a mental health agency or program that mental health professionals may have. Moreover, consumers are the people who experience the health delivery system. For these reasons, it is often easier for consumers to identify areas where change is needed than it is for mental health professionals. Some mental health professionals may become accustomed to the status quo and may not be aware of a need to change practices. Other mental health professionals may fear the effect change will have on their role status and functioning and may therefore deny a need for change.

Consumers often have a better understanding of their mental health needs or of the mental health needs of their community than do mental health professionals. Epstein (1974) observes that the social class and life-style of mental health professionals often differ from those of their clients. Epstein suggests that even mental health professionals who originally came from backgrounds similar to those of the majority of their clients usually drastically alter their life-styles once they achieve the position of mental health professional. It becomes the function of indigenous workers, who still share the same life-styles as the clients, to serve as liaisons between clients and professionals. Indigenous workers may help professionals view clients within the sociocultural context of the community, facilitate communication between clients and practitioners, and articulate needs for change from the perspective of the client (Ruiz and Behrens, 1973; Epstein, 1974).

If change is to occur in the mental health delivery system, consumers must be involved in the decision-making process. To effectively participate in decision making, consumers are demanding information about mental health care. They want to know about the efficacy of various therapeutic approaches, the comparative costs of therapies, and the anticipated therapeutic results and side effects of various treatment modalities (Gonzalez, 1976).

Comprehensive health care programs operated by boards of directors composed of consumers have demonstrated that consumers are able to

1. make decisions and policies based on an intimate knowledge of a community's health needs.
2. identify areas that require professional expertise and seek consultation in those areas.
3. evaluate services and staff behavior from the perspective of the client.
4. identify areas that need change and effectively use power to achieve change in a mental health program (Ruiz and Behrens, 1973; Epstein, 1974).

The consumer movement has successfully used power to effect changes in the field of mental health that range from research to delivery of care. For example, in one year, consumers

1. initiated a lawsuit that resulted in release of $126 million for research, alcoholism, and manpower programs.
2. influenced the amending of a health maintenance organization bill to include basic mental health coverage.
3. helped amend a rehabilitation act so that affirmative action in hiring would include the "mentally handicapped."
4. succeeded in getting the United States Civil Service Commission to remove a question about previous treatment for mental illness from employment applications.
5. instituted and awarded National Association for Mental Health Research Fellowships.
6. successfully lobbied so that the Federal Edu-

cation Act would allocate funds to states for the establishment of programs for mentally ill children.

7. sponsored a conference, under the auspices of the National Association for Mental Health, on critical issues related to mental health research (National Association for Mental Health, 1974).

Nurses

Nurses are important members of the interdisciplinary mental health team. Many nurses work in psychiatric agencies. Some clinical specialists work independently or in group practice situations. Chapters 1 and 10 emphasize the role and functions of nurses as care providers in an interdisciplinary mental health setting and defines the various levels of practice in psychiatric nursing. In this section, we will focus on the nursing role of client advocacy.

NURSES AS CLIENT ADVOCATES

Because nurse-advocates have to be able to offer information objectively to clients and to support clients in their decisions, even when those decisions may not be the ones the nurses would have chosen, it is essential for nurse-advocates to be open minded. Kohnke (1982) suggests that to develop the open-mindedness essential to the advocate rule, nurses should be able to inform and support clients, analyze systems, utilize ethics, identify the effects of social issues on advocacy, understand the role of the medical-industrial complex, and recognize the impact of laws on advocacy. The following advocate self-assessment guide is based on these abilities.

Ability to inform and support a client
1. Do I have the facts necessary to thoroughly inform the client?
2. If I do not have the necessary facts, do I know where to get the information?
3. Do I believe the client should have this information?
4. Do I present this information to the client in a meaningful manner and in an appropriate context?

5. What people (other staff members, family) might object to the client having this information? How can I cope with these objections?
6. Do I allow the client to make a decision, or do I try to influence the client's decision? Do I play the role of rescuer when the decision does not work out?

Ability to analyze a system
1. What is an institution's official philosophy? What is its unofficial philosophy?
2. What are the stated and unstated expectations of myself and others?
3. What factors in a system, including vested interests of participants, constitute risks to informing and supporting clients? For example, an institution's official philosophy may be to encourage client participation in treatment planning, but the vested interests of staff members may operate to ensure their own power and status within the institution. A hierarchy is thereby created, with the client at the bottom. This situation might present a problem to a nurse-advocate who is supporting a client's right to accept or refuse a course of treatment.
4. What strategies might I utilize for dealing with these risks?

Ability to use ethics* to analyze a situation
1. Am I familiar with the ethics that should guide the conduct of psychiatric nurses?
2. How do these ethical positions guide my conduct and affect the decisions that I make?
3. How might differing ethical positions of the client and others (family, staff members) affect my ability to inform and support the client?

Ability to identify the effects of social issues on advocacy
1. What issues (racism, sexism, ageism) are operative in a situation?
2. What risks do these issues present for client advocacy? For example, if mental health professionals believe that Hispanics are volatile, emotional people, the staff may try to withhold information from an Hispanic client so as not to "upset" the client and cause the client to become "irrational" or to "overreact." This prejudicial attitude of staff members may present a problem to a nurse-advocate who is trying to ensure the right of Hispanic clients to in-

---

*Ethics is discussed in more depth in subsequent pages of this chapter.

formation about their psychiatric conditions and treatment plans.
3. What strategies are needed for dealing with these risks?

Ability to understand the role of the medical-industrial complex
1. What vested interest groups (pharmaceutical companies, mental health boards, consumer groups) might affect client care?
2. How might these groups affect my advocate role? For example, an agency's concern about liability suits may interfere with a nurse-advocate's responsibility to ensure that a client has the least restrictive conditions that will meet the aims of retention.

Ability to recognize how laws affect advocacy
1. How do laws affect the care of mentally ill clients?
2. How do these laws affect my advocate role? For example, the right of clients to confidentiality affects the information about the therapeutic relationship that a nurse can and cannot give the parents of an emotionally ill child.
3. What are the risks that might be encountered when, as an advocate, I ensure a client's rights? For example, if a nurse, in the advocacy role, gives a client information about the right to refuse treatment, will the client's family or the staff retaliate? Who will they retaliate against—the client? the advocate? the system?

As nurses develop the aforementioned abilities, they will be better able to carry out their responsibilities as advocates. As client advocates, nurses are responsible for the following functions:
1. Ensuring ethical practice. Nurses need to be committed to basic human rights, able to assess possible consequences of actions, and sensitive to situations that may influence the application of principles pertinent to accountable nursing practice (Nations, 1973; Annas and Healey, 1974; Curtin, 1978a, 1978b).
2. Ensuring client rights. Nurses assist clients to learn about, protect, and assert their rights. Nurses may explain civil rights, retention status, and institutional procedures to clients and may help them to obtain legal counsel. In addition, nurses act as monitors to assure that client rights are not violated.

3. Acting as liaisons. Nurses help clients and staff members develop effective interpersonal relationships, investigate clients' complaints, and assist clients in using institutional resources for problem solving (refer to Chapter 10).
4. Ensuring high-quality care. Nurses participate in and cooperate with quality assurance programs. Data are collected, analyzed, and utilized for planning, assessing, and improving the quality of mental health care.

▶ Ensuring ethical practice

Nursing is a ''moral art.'' Nursing combines a concern for a person's well-being with the technical skills needed to achieve that end. Basic ethical dilemmas encountered by nurses center around two major areas: institutional policies and/or physicians' orders that affect quality of client care and the appropriation of nurses' legitimate authority to make decisions about nursing care (Curtin, 1978a, 1978b). Rouslin (1976) states that mental health nurses should be guided by two rules: (1) optimal behavior concerning client welfare and (2) optimal professional conduct.

Nurses should use a *code of ethics* to direct their professional conduct. The International Code of Nursing Ethics (Grand Council, 1953) and the American Nurses' Association Code for Nurses (1968) state that the need for nursing care is universal and should not be denied because of a person's race, color, creed, politics, nationality, or social status. These codes emphasize that the primary responsibilities of nurses are the preservation of life, the relief of suffering, and the promotion and maintenance of health. These codes also stress the responsibilities that nurses have as citizens to follow laws, to carry out the duties of citizenship, and to work with other citizens to improve and preserve the health of communities on local, state, national, and international levels.

Some nurses' associations have adopted *codes of ethics for psychiatric nurses*. Such codes of ethics usually include the following provisions:
1. The promotion of mental health is a primary responsibility of psychiatric nursing.

2. Through continuing education, psychiatric nurses must increase their professional knowledge and competencies.
3. Maintenance and utilization of professional competencies are essential to the provision of optimal mental health care.
4. Regardless of the color, race, religion, or gender of clients, clients should be respected as individuals and should be the focus of nursing concern both during and after therapy.
5. Client-nurse interaction should be confidential except when there is a possibility of harm to self or others.
6. Psychiatric nurses are accountable for their own psychiatric nursing decisions and actions.
7. Psychiatric nurses work with and sustain confidence in other health professionals.
8. Psychiatric nurses should report incompetence or unethical conduct of health team members to appropriate authorities.
9. Psychiatric nurses assume responsibility as concerned citizens for promoting efforts to meet the mental health needs of a community.
10. Psychiatric nurses collaborate with other health professionals in informing clients of treatment plans and of the anticipated outcomes and side effects of treatment procedures.
11. Psychiatric nurses follow laws that relate to the practice of mental health nursing.
12. Psychiatric nurses should not engage in a nursing practice that violates the code of ethics (Psychiatric Nurses Association of Canada, 1977; American Nurses' Association, 1982).

In making use of mental health nursing codes of ethics, psychiatric nurses must learn to critically analyze situations. Curtin (1978a, 1978b) has developed a model for critical ethical analysis. Using Curtin's model, we can extrapolate the following steps:

1. Obtain an adequate data base of relevant information. This information should pertain to the situation, circumstances, and factors that directly influence the situation.
2. Identify ethical constituents. Sort out ethical from nonethical issues. Ethical issues may include alleviation of aggressive behavior vs. loss of ability to generate and express ideas (as with psychosurgery) and freedom vs. restriction of rights (as in the treatment of mental illness).
3. Identify ethical agents and their role in the situation. Ethical agents include people who are engaged in or will engage in or be affected by a decision. Clients, families, clergymen, court judges, and health team members are examples of ethical agents. The rights, responsibilities, and duties of ethical agents, as well as factors that may facilitate or impede their freedom to make and carry out a decision, should be explored.
4. Explore alternative actions. The possible consequences of each action should be considered. Instances in which duty or responsibility conflict with consequences of an action are especially difficult to resolve. For example, a nurse may be confronted with the following dilemma: "If I intervene to prevent a client from committing suicide (my responsibility as a nurse), I am denying the client's right to self-determination (the right to take his or her own life)."
5. Develop an approach based on ethical principles. Ethical principles include ideas about the nature of human beings and self-determination and the manner of ethical thinking and decision making. For example, nurses who rely on the authority of the Scriptures may hold that the taking of life is always wrong and therefore may view suicide as wrong. On the other hand, nurses who hold that actions that deny human freedom are wrong may view suicide as an act of self-determination and therefore as a rightful act.
6. Resolve the dilemma. After engaging in the process of obtaining pertinent information, identifying ethical agents and components, exploring alternative courses of action, and

developing an approach based on ethical principles, a nurse may more readily arrive at a decision or assist the client and/or the client's family to decide on a course of action. Utilization of these steps can help psychiatric nurses analyze and resolve client-care situations that present ethical dilemmas.

▶ Ensuring client rights

Ensuring client rights is a primary responsibility of nurses. To fulfill this responsibility, nurses should be knowledgeable about the legal aspects of mental health nursing practice. Nurses need to be aware of retention procedures, client rights, and client advocacy services.

There are three reasons for retaining a person in an institution: danger to self, danger to others, and need for psychiatric treatment. Each state in the United States has its own statutes or mental health code on which retention procedures are based. The purpose of legally defined retention procedures is to protect against retention abuses. A person may be retained in a psychiatric hospital or in a psychiatric unit of a general hospital. Retention procedures generally involve three steps: application, assessment and evaluation, and commitment to an institution. Most states recognize four types of retention: informal, voluntary, emergency, and involuntary.

To be informally retained, a person verbally requests admission to an institution for psychiatric treatment. In most states, a person who is being informally retained may leave the institution simply by notifying the director of the institution (through the professional mental health staff) of a plan to leave. If the mental health professionals think a client needs to remain in the institution, then application must be made to convert the client's status from informal to involuntary.

Voluntary retention has two components: a written request for admission to an institution and a voluntary seeking of psychiatric treatment. People who are voluntarily retained usually do not relinquish their civil rights and may vote, manage property, and conduct business (Lindman and Mc-

Intyre, 1961). If a client wants to leave the institution before he or she has been discharged, the client must make a written request to the director of the institution. The director must either honor the client's request or get a court order authorizing involuntary retention. Each state specifies the length of time a voluntary client may be retained after requesting discharge. For example, in New York and Pennsylvania, the director of an institution has 72 hours to either honor a client's request for discharge or obtain a court order converting the client's status to involuntary.

A person who is acutely mentally ill may be admitted to an institution on an emergency status. This type of admission is time limited. For example, in New York, emergency retention is valid for only 48 hours. If at the end of the time period it is felt that a client is not ready to be discharged, the client can agree to voluntary retention or the director of the institution can petition the court to convert the client's status to involuntary.

There are two avenues to involuntary retention:
1. Medical certification. A specified number of physicians certify that a person is mentally ill and *potentially dangerous to self or others*. The number of physicians required for certification is established by state statute and varies from state to state. In many states the assessment of two physicians is necessary for certification. The director of the institution then presents this assessment to the court and requests a court order for involuntary retention.
2. Status conversion. By court order, retention status is converted from informal, voluntary, or emergency to involuntary.

A court order for involuntary retention is time limited. The time period may vary from state to state. If at the expiration of the first court order it is felt that a client still needs to be retained in the institution, the director of the institution can petition the court for an extension of the involuntary retention order. Each time the order for involuntary retention is extended the time period may be increased. For example, in New York the first court order is valid for 60 days, the second for 6 months, and the third for 1 year. In many states, when the court is considering a retention order of 1 year or more, the client must be physically present in court. At any time, by using a habeas corpus procedure, a client or a client's family can petition the court for repeal of the retention order and discharge from the institution.

Ensuring client rights encompasses more than knowledge about retention procedures. A person with mental illness is the only "patient" who has to be granted, by state statutes, rights previously guaranteed to him or her as a citizen. These rights include the right to vote (by absentee ballot, if necessary), the right to personal freedom unless convicted of a crime, the right to a court hearing (in cases of involuntary retention), and the right of appeal and review by a higher court (Szasz, 1963; Ennis, 1978; Offir, 1974). Even persons certified as insane retain the civil rights of citizenship. In addition, no institutional regulation may deprive mentally ill clients of rights guaranteed them by state mental health statutes or codes (Lindman and McIntyre, 1961). Although state statutes vary, most state mental hygiene codes guarantee the following rights of mentally ill adults:

1. Right to know one's retention status
2. Right to the least restrictive conditions that will meet the aims of retention
3. Right to periodic review of one's mental health status if one is involuntarily retained
4. Right to an explanation of one's psychiatric condition and treatment plan and of any untoward reactions that may occur as a result of treatment
5. Right to treatment (An individualized treatment plan must be established by a qualified mental health professional within a specified period after admission—for example, 5 days. There must be prompt and adequate treatment of any physical illness. A discharge plan must be developed by a qualified mental health professional, and, when needed, transitional care after discharge must be provided.)
6. Right to accept or refuse a course of treatment
7. Right to judicious use of medication (Medications must be prescribed in writing, have a maximum termination date, and be reviewed periodically. Medications cannot be administered as a form of punishment, for staff convenience, in lieu of a treatment program, or in dosages that conflict with a treatment program.)
8. Right to judicious use of physical restraints and seclusion (Physical restraints and seclusion may only be used in a situation in which a client is deemed dangerous to self or others. Physical restraints and seclusion can only be ordered by a physician who has personally seen the client. The order must be in writing and cannot exceed a specified time period—for example, 24 hours. The client's physical and psychiatric status must be closely monitored and recorded—for example, every hour. Bathroom privileges must be allowed, and the client must be bathed regularly—for example, every 12 hours.)
9. Right to privacy and to be treated with dignity
10. Right to communicate with people outside the institution (Mentally ill clients have the same rights of access to telephones and visitors as clients in general hospitals. This right can be denied only by written order from a qualified mental health professional who is responsible for the client's therapeutic regimen. The order must be reviewed at regular intervals. Mentally ill clients have the right to visits from lawyers, private physicians, and other health professionals. Mentally ill clients have the right to receive sealed mail from attorneys, health professionals, courts, and government officials. The right to receive mail from other persons may be restricted or denied only by written order from a qualified mental health professional responsible for the client's treatment.)

11. Right to informed consent (Clients must give informed consent or have legal counsel prior to administration of such potentially dangerous treatment modalities as electroconvulsive therapy, psychosurgery, and aversion therapy or prior to experimental research. Research must be reviewed and approved by a human subjects committee. If a client is incompetent to consent, a judge or lawyer may become a proxy consenter.)

12. Right to confidentiality (Clients have the right to confidentiality about their diagnoses, types of treatment, and the fact that they are receiving treatment. "Privileged communication" is a legal term referring to a client's right not to have information gained through psychiatric therapy divulged in court. A client may waive, in writing, the right of privileged communication.)

13. Right to be adequately clothed (Unless such a right is denied or restricted in writing by a qualified mental health professional, clients have the right to wear their own clothes and keep personal belongings. If clients do not have adequate clothing, they have the right to be clothed by the institution.)

14. Right to regular physical exercise (The institution must supply facilities and equipment for exercising. Unless physically ill, a client has the right to go out of doors on a regular basis.)

15. Right to be paid the minimum wage for any work that contributes to the operation and maintenance of the institution

16. Right to engage in religious worship (Lindman and McIntyre, 1961; Shapiro, 1974; Miller et al., 1976; Stone, 1979)

Explicitly stated rights represent the strides that have been made in guaranteeing the civil rights of mentally ill clients. Yet, as Shindul and Snyder (1981) point out, such advances in the civil rights of clients may also pose dilemmas for mental health professionals.

Doris Peters had been admitted to the psychiatric unit of a general hospital following a suicide attempt. She was severely depressed and she was experiencing self-accusatory delusions. When the client's depression was not helped by antidepressants, the psychiatrist decided to try electroconvulsive therapy. The client consented. As electroconvulsive therapy progressed, the client showed marked mood elevation. Then, midway through the treatments, the client decided she did not wish to continue with electroconvulsive therapy.

Although the client's noncompliance could have led to deterioration in her condition and to possible harm to herself, the staff was unable to prevail upon her to continue electroconvulsive therapy.

Shindul and Snyder (1981) point out that similar dilemmas can occur in situations in which nurses are constrained from giving medications to potentially violent clients who refuse psychotropic medications. They suggest that, to safeguard clients' rights while protecting clients and others from potential harm, nurses should become more skilled in verbal and physical techniques for intervening with aggressively acting-out clients, that nurses become assertive in addressing the effects of social policies and mental health legislation on client care, and that nurses actively support or engage in research designed to predict violent behavior so that preventive intervention can be instituted.

Nurses also are responsible for ensuring the *rights of mentally ill children and adolescents*. Although these rights vary from state to state, most state mental health statutes guarantee the following:

1. Right to free educational services
2. Right to be free from involuntary sterilization (Parents cannot authorize the sterilization of their child.)
3. Right to have legal counsel for any retention procedures
4. Right to the least restrictive conditions that will meet the aims of retention

5. Right to treatment (A child or an adolescent has the right to an individualized treatment plan that considers the developmental stage of the child or adolescent and to treatment by a qualified mental health professional who is a specialist in child or adolescent mental health. There should be interaction between mental health personnel and the child or adolescent's family. When parents deny treatment for a child or an adolescent, the court may act as an advocate and make a decision on the child's or adolescent's behalf.)

6. Right to informed consent (Whenever possible, informed consent should be obtained from a child or an adolescent.)

7. Right to confidentiality (A child of any age has the right not to have detailed information derived from therapeutic relationships disclosed to parents. An adolescent over 16 years of age usually can decide what information he or she wants disclosed. When a child is unable to give consent, because of age or for other reasons, parents have the right to know the type of treatment their child is receiving and their child's progress in treatment and the right to decide about releasing information to a third party [Lindman and McIntyre, 1961; Burgdorf, 1979].)

Nurses can function as formal or informal child advocates. Formal advocacy involves appearing in court as a witness or being primary initiator of a lawsuit on a child's behalf. Informal advocacy involves educating parents, administrators, and health team members about the rights of mentally ill children and adolescents and guaranteeing these rights (Burgdorf, 1979).

State statutes usually provide a client advocacy service that is under the jurisdiction of the state courts. The purpose of a client advocacy service is to safeguard the rights of child and adult clients. For example, in New York State, the Mental Health Information Service informs clients of their retention status and rights, including their right to counsel from the Service. It reviews annually the status of involuntarily retained clients. If there is any doubt about the need for retention, the Mental Health Information Service must request a court hearing to resolve the issue.

Nurses are responsible for guaranteeing client rights, for educating others about the rights of mentally ill individuals, and for acting as liaisons between clients and a state-established client advocacy service. Nurses may be directly or indirectly involved in safeguarding client rights. For instance, when a nurse performs a nursing procedure (for example, administers a medication), he or she must explain the purpose, anticipated results, and possible side effects of the procedure to the client. If the client then allows the nurse to perform the procedure, the client is implicitly giving consent. If the client refuses the procedure, the nurse should comply with the client's refusal and should then inform the psychiatrist. For nonnursing procedures (such as aversion therapy), nurses are responsible for ascertaining that clients are giving informed and voluntary consent. Occasionally, nurses are asked to ensure that a client's consent is voluntary and informed. This entails detailed recording of the discussion with the client. The questions and responses of both nurse and client and the client's mental status should be included. These are instances of direct involvement of nurses in the safeguarding of client rights (Creighton, 1970; Willeg, 1970).

Sometimes nurses are indirectly involved in the protection of client rights. Education of nonprofessional staff about the rights of clients is an example of indirect protection of client rights. If a staff member does not believe in a particular right, he or she probably will not be vigilant in guaranteeing it. In a study of psychiatric aides, Daugherty (1978) found that aides supported rights that concerned abstract concepts or basic human needs (for example, adequate nutrition and treatment of medical problems) but had reservations about rights that might affect ward management or give increased responsibility to clients (for example, the right to be paid for work necessary to the operation of a psychiatric center and the right to judicious use of physical restraints and medications).

Nurses, as client advocates, are responsible for ensuring client rights. To fulfill this responsibility, they should be aware of retention procedures, the nature of client rights, client advocacy services, and the attitudes of the mental health staff members with whom they work.

▶ Ensuring high-quality care

As client advocates, nurses should be concerned with the quality of care provided, and they should be active participants in quality assurance programs. *Quality assurance* refers to activities designed to indicate the quality of health care and efforts aimed at improving the quality of health care (Towery and Windle, 1978; Standards of Psychiatric and Mental Health Nursing Practice, 1982).

In 1975, the Community Mental Health Centers Amendment (Public Law 94-63) made three stipulations concerning quality assurance in community mental health centers:

1. Development of national standards for community mental health centers
2. Development of quality assurance programs
3. Collection of data for the evaluation of quality assurance programs including operating costs and patterns of service utilization (acceptability of services, accessibility of services, and responsiveness of services to the needs of the catchment population)

A minimum of 2% of the previous year's operating expenses of a center must be allocated and used for implementation and evaluation of quality assurance programs (Towery and Windle, 1978).

Depending on the level of program development, either a formative or a summative evaluation may be used. Scriven (1967) explains that a formative evaluation involves the collection of empirical data for the purpose of developing a program. To date, designs for formative evaluation have not been well developed. A summative evaluation involves the collection of data for the purpose of assessing the effectiveness of an already existing

program. A summative evaluation may be conducted internally by the personnel responsible for the program, or it may be conducted externally by individuals or groups outside the program. Whether a summative evaluation is internal or external, it has the following objectives:

1. To establish outcome criteria for specific populations of clients. Comparing results of health care with outcome criteria gives an indication of the effectiveness of services.
2. To determine the least number of cost-effective activities and resources required to accomplish outcome criteria. Relating the expense incurred for required activities and resources to outcomes services as a measure of efficiency.
3. To ascertain the degree to which a health delivery program meets the needs of the catchment population. Identifying factors that facilitate or inhibit the use of program services provides a measurement of accessibility of services (Zimmer, 1974; Towery and Windle, 1978).

Nurses may participate in formative and summative evaluations of mental health programs. The collection and analysis of data for the purpose of planning, assessing, and improving the quality of mental health care is a vital component of client advocacy.

NURSES AND PLANNED CHANGE

The effectiveness of nurses as client advocates is often hampered by inadequate knowledge about the process of change and the use of power. Nursing education may not adequately prepare nurses to understand change and provides them with limited experience with power strategies.

Within an agency or institution, the power structure usually comprises three groups: administrative personnel, medical personnel, and nursing personnel. Power tends to shift continuously, through negotiation, among these three groups and among the individuals within these groups. It is not unusual for a given person (for example, a director of nurses) to belong to more than one group. The intergroup power system creates a balance of power. To participate effectively within this balance of power, nurses, especially nurse-leaders, should learn to negotiate for power. When power is controlled by one group or when one group has little power, there may be diminished morale, ineffective functioning of the group having little power, or abuse of power by the group controlling power (McFarland and Shiflett, 1979).

Conflicts in the vested interests of the individuals and groups that make up the health delivery system may result in a *power struggle* (Ashley, 1975). A power struggle often occurs between nurses and other professionals within the health delivery system. In mental health settings, power struggles often are related to such advocacy functions as ensuring ethical practice and quality care. Struggles may be centered around issues such as the following:

1. Agency or institutional philosophy and delivery of mental health care
2. Negotiation for limited strategic resources (human and material)
3. Autonomy in mental health nursing practice
4. Roles and functions of nurses within the mental health delivery system

In a broader social context, power struggles sometimes exist between nurses, special interest groups, and legislators, on local, state, or federal levels. Such power struggles often center around client advocacy issues such as the following:

1. Allocation of money for mental health research and preventive intervention
2. Legislation concerning client rights and affirmative action programs for children and adults with a history of mental illness
3. Legislation forbidding discrimination against children and adults because of a history of mental illness
4. Insurance coverage for the treatment of mental illness (including third-party payment)

Political nursing is the use of knowledge about power processes and strategies to influence the nature and direction of health care and professional nursing (Ashley, 1975; Leininger, 1978). To be effective client advocates, nurses need to learn how to use power for planned change. The goals of political nursing are the same as the goals of the mental health care system: the availability, quality, accessibility, and funding of mental health care (Brown et al., 1978; McFarland and Shiflett, 1979). The constituency of political nursing is clients: communities, groups, and individuals—both identified and potential.

Through political nursing, nurses attempt to provide input into power systems and to establish power strategies that can be used to regulate information and influence people in power. Methods for regulating information include rapid acquisition and distribution of accurate information by organizations to members; verification of information so that people do not have to act on the basis of rumor; and dissemination of knowledge about who to contact, how to initiate contact, and methods for conveying ideas to people in power. Involvement in local government, participation in public hearings, and lobbying are ways of influencing people in power (Ver Steeg, 1979).

Knowing how to regulate information and influence people in power is important in effecting change. Nurses can be instrumental in effecting change in their own mental health agencies or in the broader social contexts of community, state, and nation. To effect change, nurses should explore the following avenues for expanding their bases of power and authority:

1. Increase nursing knowledge and clinical expertise to provide a base for expert power.
2. Develop strong, creative, and knowledgeable nursing leadership. Such leadership serves as a source for role models, gives novices an opportunity to develop power strategies and to be socialized into leadership roles, and provides a foundation for assertive and effective action.
3. Recognize that power is a component of interpersonal relationships. Identify the source of one's own power, and learn to use power strategies effectively.
4. Develop alliances that will increase support

and power. Such alliances tend to diminish power struggles and to increase associative power.

5. Understand the channels of communication and authority. Nurses need to know about people who can serve as intermediaries in expediting change (Leininger, 1979; McFarland and Shiflett, 1979).

Because of the risks to personal security (for example, job security), nurses are sometimes hesitant to initiate change in their own agencies or institutions. However, these risks can be minimized. Epstein (1974) suggests that nurses minimize risks to personal security by identifying with like-minded colleagues, by expanding their power bases, and, whenever possible, by utilizing supportive agency policy. Identification with people who view the need for change in a similar way creates a network of support and action. Within this network, nurses can develop power strategies, evaluate progress, revise plans for change, and support one another in both success and failure. By talking with other members of the mental health team and with administrators, nurses can broaden their support bases both quantitatively and qualitatively. In addition, if an agency has a clearly and concisely written policy that supports a proposed change, nurses should use the policy in effecting change. If the policy is violated, violators may be confronted with the written policy. Whenever possible, such confrontation should be done by a group of people who are committed to the change. Confrontation by a group reduces the risk of retaliation against an individual.

Effecting change in the broader social contexts of community, state, and nation involves the use of many of the same strategies that are used in effecting change in an individual mental health agency. Burke (1979) suggests that nurses apply the interpersonal skills utilized in nurse-client relationships to relationships with community leaders and legislators. She suggests that a nurse should first establish a working relationship and then should identify appropriate contact people. Often local community leaders and their staffs can act as liaisons with other people and agencies. Maintaining an ongoing relationship is important. Even when a nurse is not lobbying for change, he or she should keep in touch with community leaders and legislative staff. Nurses must be knowledgeable: They should learn the names and functions of leaders who are involved with health issues, and they should be well informed about those issues. They should support lobbies and special interest groups that share their concerns. A nurse should provide community leaders and legislators with the local perspective—the way people in the community feel about an issue. Community leaders and legislators tend to be politically sensitive to this type of feedback (Burke, 1979; Donley, 1979).

Through political nursing, nurses use power processes and strategies to influence the nature and direction of health care and professional nursing. Political nursing is an essential element in client advocacy. McFarland and Shiflett (1979) caution nurses to consider the ethical implications of power strategies, not to use power solely for self-serving ends, and to be mindful of the responsibilities and obligations associated with the use of power.

Institutions, consumers, and nurses are the major components of the contemporary mental health delivery system. Within this delivery system, power strategies and power struggles sometimes arise around such issues as quality of care, client rights, affirmative action, and allocation of resources. We will now examine some major issues and trends in mental health that may indicate the areas in which future power strategies and struggles will occur.

ISSUES AND TRENDS IN MENTAL HEALTH

Issues* and trends in mental health develop within a social context and need to be examined

---

*Other mental health issues, such as family violence and abuse (Chapters 12 and 15), are discussed elsewhere in this book.

within that social context. Consumerism, questioning of the insanity defense, decreases in funding for mental health research, and independent nursing practice are trends that affect and are affected by such social factors as inflation, political activism, and community attitudes. As these trends evolve and ramify, implications for the future are suggested.

Consumerism

CONSUMER POWER

A philosophy is emerging that encourages equal participation in decision making between consumers and providers of mental health care. The trend toward increased involvement of and power for consumers is moving ahead on two levels—individual and community.

On the first level, individuals are being given knowledge that will make them educated consumers of and effective participants in the therapeutic process. Clients have a right to, and are being given, explanations about their psychiatric conditions, treatment plans, alternative types of treatment and their costs, and any untoward reactions that might occur as a consequence of treatment. Within the therapeutic relationship, mutuality between clients and nurses (or other mental health professionals) is also being encouraged. Stone (1979) notes that the introduction of mutuality between client and therapist restructures the therapeutic relationship from a status relationship (a relationship based on hierarchical positions) to a contract relationship (a relationship based on voluntary individual arrangements). Clients have an opportunity for more autonomy in contractual than in status relationships (Maine, 1907; Durkheim, 1933; Barth, 1959).

Many clients are turning for assistance to self-help groups composed of people who have recovered from specific psychosocial problems. Alcoholics Anonymous, Gamblers Anonymous, and Overeaters Anonymous are examples of such groups. In many instances, these self-help groups constitute the major treatment modality. In other instances, self-help groups are used in conjunction with other therapies or to prevent the development of psychosocial problems (for example, Compassionate Friends is a support group for bereaved parents). Client decisions to utilize the therapeutic properties of self-help groups and the assumption of care-provider roles by some recovered clients exemplify the increasing autonomy of consumers in the mental health delivery system.

The second level of the trend in consumerism is characterized by collaboration between the community and nurses and other professionals in community mental health centers. Increasingly, community representatives are sitting on the boards of community mental health centers. Community mental health boards thereby become a point of articulation between community residents and care providers. Such collaboration between community representatives and mental health professionals is a potentially educational experience. Community representatives may learn firsthand about the community mental health movement—its philosophy, goals, and problems. This educational process helps to demystify mental health and mental illness, to teach consumers (and potential consumers) about treatment modalities and the roles and functions of members of the mental health team, and to sensitize residents to the mental health problems in their community.

Community residents may become aware of the influence their involvement and support can have on a community mental health program. Community representatives may develop an increased understanding of their sources of power and of how power relationships affect budgeting, service priorities, and programing.*

Nurses and other mental health professionals can better view clients within the sociocultural context of the community. The values, ideologies, and traditions of subgroups (such as ethnic groups and classes) within the community may be better identified and understood. Nurses and other mental

---

*Chapter 14 discusses the effect of recent governmental budget cutbacks on community mental health centers.

health professionals can also increase their awareness of the perceptions that subgroups within the community have about the definition, cause, and treatment of mental illness (Borus, 1976; Ruiz and Behrens, 1973; Borus and Klerman, 1976; Landsberg and Hammer, 1978).

IMPLICATIONS FOR THE FUTURE

The role of consumers (actual and potential) in the mental health delivery system will probably continue to expand. Presently, people who have recovered from specific psychosocial problems (such as alcoholism, drug abuse, and compulsive eating) are effectively intervening in the treament of people who have not yet recovered. Gonzalez (1976) suggests that this trend may grow to include other psychosocial problems (for example, depression, phobias, and compulsive working).

In addition, consumers are becoming more vocal about their perceptions of effective treatment for mental illness, and nurses and other mental health professionals are becoming more responsive to the ideas of consumers. Gonzalez (1976) and Warner (1977) note that many consumers rely on the native healers and folk medicines of their cultures. Client belief in folk medicine and confidence in native healers need not rule out treatment by nurses and other mental health professionals. Torrey (1973), a psychiatrist who is associated with the National Institute of Mental Health, explains that both native healers and mental health professionals function as therapists in the treatment of mental illness and that both achieve therapeutic results. Native healers are important mental health resources and should be actively integrated into mental health programs.

Questioning of the insanity defense

CURRENT ATTITUDES

An increase of violence in the United States, underscored by the recent history of violent acts against public figures, has precipitated an outcry against the verdict ''not guilty by reason of insanity.'' Although the insanity defense has recently become the focus of much attention, it should be noted that most violent people are not mentally ill and most mentally ill people are not violent. People with a history of mental illness who commit violent acts usually have a history of criminal activity that predates their mental illness (Babich, 1981; Schell-King and Finneran, 1982; Steadman, 1982).

Forensic psychiatry is that specialty in psychiatry that deals with the legal facets of mental illness (Sadoff, 1975). People accused of crimes can be found incompetent to stand trial because of a mental condition, or they can plead not guilty on the basis of insanity and be so found by a jury.

A determination that a person is incompetent to stand trial is based upon his or her inability to understand the charges and to participate with a lawyer in his or her own defense because of mental disorder (Stone, 1975).

Many of our laws and legal procedures have developed from English common law. This is true of one of the more frequently invoked rules in cases involving the insanity plea—the *McNaughton Rule*. This rule, which was handed down in England in 1843, holds that a person is not guilty of a crime if the person did not understand the nature and quality of the act or did not know that the act was wrong (Stone, 1975). Although the McNaughton Rule has been criticized by legal scholars and members of the psychiatric profession, it has remained an important aspect of the insanity defense in many jurisdictions in the United States.

Another defense that is valid in some states is the *Irresistible Impulse Test,* which was introduced in Alabama in 1887 and has since been adopted by many states. The Irresistible Impulse Test expanded upon the McNaughton Rule by adding criteria for determining people's ability to control their behavior (Stone, 1975). Then, in 1954, the *Durham Rule,* which is still used in the District of Columbia, stated that accused people are not responsible for their unlawful behavior if that behavior is the result of mental illness or mental defect (Hallick, 1967).

Both the McNaughton Rule and the Irresistible

Impulse Test have been criticized by legal scholars and members of the psychiatric profession because of their moralistic quality and because they do not reflect current knowledge of human psychology. A recent attempt to develop a test or rule governing responsibility for criminal acts in relation to mental disorders resulted in the *American Law Institute Test*. According to this test, a person is not responsible for criminal behavior if at the time of committing a crime the person lacked substantial capacity either to appreciate the criminality of the act or to control his or her behavior so that it conformed to the law (Stone, 1975).

Those who would retain the insanity defense argue as follows:

1. If the insanity defense were eliminated, both the criminal law and the public conscience would no longer distinguish between mental illness and evil.
2. People who are charged with crimes should have defense choices available to them.
3. The decision to convict and punish or detain and treat should be arrived at democratically by a jury rather than by a panel of experts in forensic psychiatry.
4. The public's perception that people who benefit from the insanity defense are murderers and rapists is very inaccurate (Steadman, 1982; Schell-King and Finneran, 1982).

Those who would abolish the insanity defense argue as follows:

1. The questions asked of psychiatrists and psychologists by the law are beyond their scope of knowledge.
2. In practice, the insanity defense is a wealthy person's defense.
3. The ambiguous and confusing wording of the various insanity tests results in intuitive moral judgments rather than in objective determinations.
4. Insanity acquitees usually are incarcerated in correctional institutions for periods of time comparable to periods for criminals, but insanity acquitees detained in mental health facilities usually serve approximately six months less time than do comparable felons.

5. The legal system should not function in one manner for a ''normal'' defendant and in another manner for an ''abnormal'' defendant (Steadman, 1982; Schell-King and Finneran, 1982).

IMPLICATIONS FOR THE FUTURE

Central to any discussion of the insanity defense is concern about the lack of criteria for assessing—and, in effect, predicting—whether individuals will be dangerous to themselves or others because of mental disease or disorder. In many, if not in most, instances, a prediction of violence* is very difficult to make. Although such situational and environmental factors as poorly functioning family, peer, or occupational support systems seem to contribute to violent behavior, the common denominator among people who are violent appears to be simply a history of violent behavior (Babich, 1981).

Among others, Clarke (1982) wonders why the American public becomes outraged when someone who commits a violent act is found not guilty by reason of insanity but similar outrage is not expressed at the failure of psychiatry to more accurately predict violent behavior and to institute preventive therapy. Shindul and Snyder (1981) stress the fact that research into the predictability of violent behavior is necessary for preventive intervention. This is an area in which nurses and other mental health professionals should develop proposals, write grants, and otherwise engage in research.

Decreases in funding for research

In the United States, the National Institute of Mental Health (NIMH) is the major source of funding for mental health research. Over the past decade, the combination of budgetary cuts and inflation has resulted in a 50% decrease in the purchasing power of monies invested in mental health research (Brown, 1976).

---

*Refer to Chapter 17 for an in-depth discussion of violence.

STATUS OF MENTAL HEALTH RESEARCH

Because trained researchers are having difficulty obtaining research grants, many researchers are entering other fields of mental health, such as practice or teaching. Brown (1976) predicts that not only will the scarcity of research grants affect the current level of mental health research, but, because young scientists have limited research opportunities, there will be a dearth of prepared researchers for the next 10 or 20 years.

There is also a trend in American society toward evaluating the worth of a program in terms of its cost effectiveness. Mental health researchers have difficulty translating their results into a dollar amount. While dollar savings can be attached to decreases in the number of people hospitalized for mental illness, similar cost effectiveness cannot as readily be demonstrated for such improvements in human functioning as increased sense of well-being or more effective coping behavior. The difficulty of translating research results into cost-effectiveness formulae plus the stigma that much of the general public still attaches to mental illness result in a lack of public support for mental health research (Brown, 1976).

IMPLICATIONS FOR THE FUTURE

Nurses and other mental health professionals will need to become more politically active and politically effective in educating legislators and the general public about the importance of mental health research. Brown (1976) suggests that such an educational program should encompass the crisis in mental health research, as well as the process, purpose, and importance of mental health research. Public support will be essential if mental health professionals are to successfully compete for scarce research resources. The National Association for Mental Health, a consumer citizen group that in the past used its political influence to engender support for mental health services, is beginning to use its political influence to engender support for mental health research.

Nurses and other mental health professionals are becoming politically active. They will need to direct some of their political activity toward influencing legislation concerning mental health research. Such political activity should involve more than lobbying and contacting legislators. Ver Steeg (1979) believes that mental health professionals who are experts in their fields and who are also politically active are more apt to be asked to serve on advisory committees. Serving on advisory committees may increase the opportunities for mental health professionals to influence legislation concerning research in mental health.

Moreover, nurses and other mental health professionals will need to learn the art of grantsmanship. Donley (1979) stresses that it is not enough to write a grant; an application for a grant must be followed up with telephone calls and visits to regional offices in order to clarify the purpose and the importance of the proposal.

In addition to becoming politically active in advancing the cause of mental health research, nurses also will need to actively engage in research. One area of nursing research that is often overlooked is the evaluation of outcome effectiveness. Connolly (1982) suggests that the resistance of nurses and other mental health professionals to conducting outcome research studies can be explained in several ways. First, there are few reliable and valid instruments available with which to evaluate mental health outcomes. For instance, who should determine that the mental health of a client has improved—the client, the mental health professional, or both? The difficulty in finding adequate research tools can often serve as an excuse for not conducting outcome research.

The reluctance of nurse-researchers to report their findings when no statistical significance is found may also contribute to the paucity of published outcome research studies. Nurse-researchers sometimes associate statistical significance with valuable research. Nurses will need to recognize that human behavior cannot be reduced to a unifactorial, cause-and-effect explanation. Because many factors interrelate and contribute to human behavior, nurse-researchers should report both their positive *and* negative findings and they should discuss the many possible reasons why statistical significance was not found.

Finally, because quality assurance programs are operative in mental health agencies, nurses may assume that their work is already being evaluated and that there is no further need or professional responsibility for reporting or documenting outcome effectiveness. Thus, nurses will need to recognize that they have a professional responsibility for conducting outcome research studies that are separate from the evaluations done by quality assurance programs.

The American Nurses' Association, in its Standards of Psychiatric and Mental Health Nursing Practice (1982), states that nurses have a responsibility to engage in research so that knowledge in the field of mental health will be advanced. To help nurses achieve this aim, the ANA has enumerated the following process criteria:

1. Nurses should maintain inquisitiveness and open-mindedness in their practice of nursing.
2. They should apply the research findings of others to their own nursing practice.
3. They should participate in the development, implementation, and evaluation of research projects appropriate to their levels of education.
4. They should use responsible investigative standards whenever engaging in research.
5. They should ensure that the rights of human subjects are protected.
6. They should consult with and/or seek the supervision of experts whenever necessary.

Independent nursing practice

CURRENT STATUS

In the past few decades, mental health nursing has expanded both its clinical base and its range of clinical practice.* Recently, nurses have departed from the medical model and have developed a model that embraces the nursing process. Nurses

are now making nursing diagnoses, writing nursing orders, treating human responses to illness, and evaluating outcome effectiveness. Enough of this terminology has been legislated into nurse practice acts to enable some psychiatric nurses to expand their role from that of dependent practitioner to that of independent practitioner. Nurse-practitioners and clinical nurse specialists have thus become legally able to practice in an "expanded" or autonomous role. However, autonomy in practice should not be interpreted as an unsupervised or unregulated practice of nursing. Instead, nurses collaborate with other nurses and with other professionals in the giving and receiving of professional supervision.*

The expanded role of the nurse has provided an opportunity for many psychiatric nurses to become direct providers of mental health care. Along with this change in employee role a problem has arisen about payment for service. Although psychiatric nurses in private practice bill clients directly for services provided, these nurses have usually been unable to receive payment from clients' insurance companies or from such social programs as Medicare and Medicaid. This means that clients are not reimbursed for care provided by psychiatric nurses, although similar care provided by licensed social workers, psychologists, and psychiatrists will be reimbursed. In essence, clients are being financially penalized by third-party carriers for seeking mental health care from psychiatric nurses.

IMPLICATIONS FOR THE FUTURE

Third-party reimbursement for state-licensed nurse-practitioners and for certified psychiatric nurses is beginning to occur. In December, 1981, the U.S. Defense Department's Civilian Health and Medical Programs for Uniformed Services (CHAMPUS) approved the reimbursement of state-licensed nurse-practitioners and certified psychiatric nurses as CHAMPUS-authorized care providers ("Nurse Reimbursement Plan Approved for CHAMPUS," 1982).

---

*Refer to Chapter 2 for a history of psychiatric nursing.

*Refer to Chapter 9 for a discussion of professional supervision.

More recently, the Colorado Society for Clinical Specialists in Psychiatric Nursing (CSCSPN) successfully negotiated with Colorado Blue Cross/Blue Shield for third-party payment. Blue Cross/Blue Shield now holds that, as long as the supervision process set forth by the Colorado Insurance Statute (that psychotherapy done by psychiatric clinical nurse-specialists be supervised by a licensed physician or psychologist) is followed, claims will be paid. However, a letter from the clinical nurse-specialist's supervisor verifying the supervisory requirements must accompany every claim ("Third-Party Reimbursement," 1982).

Obviously, some progress is being made in recognizing nurse-practitioners and psychiatric clinical nurse-specialists as autonomous providers of mental health care. Yet much work still needs to be done to promote the autonomy and credibility of psychiatric nurses engaged in independent practice. As nurses become more politically active, as they establish networks of support, and as they advocate third-party payment for nurses, the autonomy and credibility of nurses engaged in independent practice will be advanced (Chaisson, 1982).

CHAPTER SUMMARY

Power, which is a dynamic of all interpersonal relationships, has many sources and forms, and it is the basis of many strategies. To have input into power systems that affect the direction of mental health care and professional nursing, nurses need to understand the interrelationship between power, politics, and planned change. Institutions, consumers, and nurses are major elements of the contemporary mental health delivery system. Within this system, issues related to quality of care, client rights, and allocation of resources often lead to power strategies and power struggles. Trends in mental health can indicate the issues around which future power struggles will revolve. Currently, some major mental health trends are consumerism, a questioning of the insanity defense, decreases in

funding for mental health research, and independent nursing practice.

SENSITIVITY-AWARENESS EXERCISES

The purposes of these exercises are to:

- Develop insight into the operation of power and politics in your own life
- Develop awareness of your own reactions to change
- Develop an understanding of how you can influence issues and trends in mental health

1. Think about a situation in which you have experienced planned change. The change may have occurred in your personal or professional life. Identify and describe:
   a. The factors that facilitated change
   b. The factors that impeded change
   c. The agent(s) of change
   d. The channels of communication among the people involved in the change situation
   e. Your reaction to the proposed change
2. Analyze and describe the following in regard to an institution (for instance, a health care agency, hospital, school) with which you are associated:
   a. The stated philosophy vs. the operational philosophy
   b. The regulation of behavior (expectations concerning acceptable and unacceptable behavior; negative and positive sanctions on behavior; achievement of upward mobility)
   c. The institutional variables (type of leadership, ideology, programs, resources)
   d. The type(s) of networks that exist between the institution and its social environment
   e. Instances in which you or others were victims of "institutional think"
3. Peruse your local newspaper for 1 month. Collect newspaper articles that relate to such issues or trends in mental health as consumerism, mental health research, the insanity defense, and independent nursing practice. On the basis of the articles you have collected, how would you describe the current state of each issue? What do you foresee happening with regard to each issue in the future? What emerging trends might influence the practice of psychiatric nursing on local, state, national, and international levels? What input can you have into future developments?

REFERENCES

American Nurses' Association Committee on Ethical, Legal, and Professional Standards
  1968 Code for Nurses with Interpretive Statements. Kansas City, Mo.: The Association.

American Nurses' Association Division on Psychiatric and Mental Health Nursing Practice
  1982 Standards of Psychiatric and Mental Health Nursing Practice. Kansas City, Mo.: The Association.

Annas, G., and J. Healey
  1974 "The patient's rights advocate." Vanderbilt Law Review 27:243-269.

Argyris, C.
  1972 The Applicability of Organizational Sociology. Cambridge: Cambridge University Press.

Ashley, J.A.
  1975 "Power, freedom and professional practice in nursing." Supervisor Nurse 1:12-29.

Babich, K.S.
  1981 "Useful research findings on violence: A summary." In Assessing Patient Violence in the Health Care Setting. K.S. Babich (ed.). Boulder, Colo.: Western Interstate Commission for Higher Education.

Barth, F.
  1959 Political Leadership Among Swat Pathans. London: Athlone Press.

Beigel, A.
  1977 "The politics of mental health funding: Two views." Hospital and Community Psychiatry 28(3):194-195.

Bennis, W., et al.
  1969 The Planning of Change. New York: Holt, Rinehart & Winston.

Blase, M.G. (ed.)
  1973 Institution-Building, A Source Book. Washington, D.C.: U.S. Government Printing Office (U.S. Dept. of State).

Borus, J.F.
  1976 "Neighborhood health centers as providers of primary mental health care." New England Journal of Medicine 295(3):140-145.

Borus, J.F., and G.L. Klerman
  1976 "Consumer-professional collaboration for evaluation in neighborhood mental health programs." Hospital and Community Psychiatry 27(6):401-404.

Brown, B.J., K. Gebbie, and J.F. Moore
  1978 "Affecting nursing goals in health care." Nursing Administration Quarterly 2(3):17-31.

Brown, B.S.
  1976 "The crisis in mental health research." Address presented at the 1976 Annual Meeting of the American Psychiatric Association.

Bumgardner, H.L., et al.
  1972 Institution Building: Basic Concepts and Implementation. Chapel Hill, N.C.: University of North Carolina (mimeographed).

Burgdorf, M.P.
  1979 "Legal rights of children: implications for nurses." Nursing Clinics of North America 14(3):405-416.

Burke, S.
  1979 "What the Washington professionals expect." American Journal of Nursing 79(10):1949.

Chaisson, M.G.
  1982 "Candidate's statement." The American Nurse 14(3): 20.

Clarke, A.R.
  1982 "Editorial comment." Perspectives in Psychiatric Care 20(2):64.

Connolly, P.M.
  1982 "Psychiatric and mental health nursing research." Pacesetter 7(3):3.

Creighton, H.
  1970 Law Every Nurse Should Know. Philadelphia: W.B. Saunders Co.

Curtin, L.L.
  1978a "Nursing ethics: theories and pragmatics." Nursing Forum 17(1):4-11.
  1978b "A proposed model for critical ethical analysis." Nursing Forum 17(1):12-17.

Daughterty, L.B.
  1978 "Assessing the attitudes of psychiatric aides toward patients' rights." Hospital and Community Psychiatry 29(4):225-229.

Donley, R.
  1979 "An inside view of the Washington health scene." American Journal of Nursing 79(10):1946-1949.

Downs, A.
  1967 Inside Bureaucracy. Boston: Little, Brown & Co.

Durkheim, E.
  1933 Division of Labor in Society. G. Simpson (trans.). New York: Macmillan, Inc.

Ennis, B.J., and L. Siegel
  1978 The Rights of Mental Patients: The Basic ACLU Guide to a Mental Patient's Rights. New York: Richard W. Baron Publishing Co., Inc.

Epstein, C.
  1974 Effective Interaction in Contemporary Nursing. Englewood Cliffs, N.J.: Prentice-Hall, Inc.

Gerrard, B.A., W.J. Boniface, and B.H. Love
  1980 Interpersonal Skills for Health Professionals. Reston, Va.: Reston Publishing Co., Inc.

Gonzalez, H.H.
  1976 "The consumer movement: the implications for psychiatric care." Perspectives in Psychiatric Care 14(4): 186-190.

Gordon, M.
  1969 "The clinical specialist as change agent." Nursing Outlook 17:37-39.

Grand Council of Nurses of the International Council of Nurses
  1953 International Code of Nursing Ethics. Sao Paulo, Brazil: International Council of Nurses.

Hallick, S.
1967 Psychiatry and the Dilemmas of Crime. New York: Harper & Row, Publishers, Inc.

Health Task Force of the Urban Coalition
1970 Rx. for Action. Washington, D.C.: U.S. Government Printing Office (The Urban Coalition).

Kohnke, M.F.
1982 Advocacy: Risk and Reality. St. Louis: The C.V. Mosby Co.

Landsberg, G., and R. Hammer
1978 "Involving community representatives in CMHC evaluation and research." Hospital and Community Psychiatry 29(4):245-247.

Leach, F.
1954 Political Systems of Highland Burma. Boston: Beacon Press.

Leininger, M.
1978 "Political nursing: essential for health service and education systems of tomorrow." Nursing Administration Quarterly 2(3):1-16.
1979 "Territoriality, power, and creative leadership in administrative nursing contexts." Nursing Dimensions: Power in Nursing 7(2):33-42.

Lewin, K.
1974 "Frontiers in group dynamics." Human Relations 15-41.

Lindman, F., and D. McIntyre
1961 The Mentally Disabled and The Law. Chicago: University of Chicago Press.

Lippitt, R., et al.
1958 The Dynamics of Planned Change. New York: Harcourt, Brace & World, Inc.

Maine, H.
1907 Ancient Law. London: John Murray.

Martin, N.H., and J.H. Sims
1956 "Thinking ahead: power tactics." Harvard Business Review 34:25-29.

McFarland, D.E., and N. Shiflett
1979 "The role of power in the nursing profession." Nursing Dimensions: Power in Nursing 7(2):1-14.

Miller, W., R.O. Dawson, and R.I. Parnas
1976 The Mental Health Process. New York: New York Foundation Press.

National Association for Mental Health
1974 "Citizens making a difference." Mental Health 58(4):16-17.

National Commission on Community Health Services
1966 "Health is a community affair." Cambridge, Mass.: Harvard University Press.

Nations, W.
1973 "Nurse lawyer is patient advocate." American Journal of Nursing 73:1039-1041.

"Nurse reimbursement plan approved for CHAMPUS."
1982 The American Nurse 14(2):19.

Offir, C.W.
1974 "Civil rights and the mentally ill: revolution in Bedlam." Psychology Today 8(5):60-62.

Peplau, H.E.
1953 "Themes in nursing situations." American Journal of Nursing 53:1221-1223.

Perrow, C.
1970 Organizational Analysis: A Sociological View. Belmont, Calif.: Wadsworth, Inc.

Psychiatric Nurses Association of Canada
1977 "Code of ethics." Canadian Journal of Psychiatric Nursing 18(6):8.

Rouslin, S.
1976 "Commentary on professional ethics." Perspectives in Psychiatric Care 14(1):12-13.

Ruiz, P., and M. Behrens
1973 "Community control in mental health: how far can it go?" Psychiatric Quarterly 47(3):317-324.

Sadoff, R.
1975 Forensic Psychiatry. Springfield, Ill.: Charles C Thomas, Publisher.

Scheflen, A.E., and A. Scheflen
1972 Body Language and Social Order. Englewood Cliffs, N.J.: Prentice-Hall, Inc.

Schell-King, M., and M.R. Finneran
1982 "The role of forensic psychiatry and the insanity defense." Perspectives in Psychiatric Care 20(2):55-64.

Scriven, M.
1967 "The methodology of evalution." In Perspectives on Curriculum Evaluation. AERA Monograph Series on Curriculum Evaluation, no. 1. Chicago: Rand McNally & Co.

Shapiro, M.
1974 "Legislating the control of behavior control: autonomy and coercive use of organic therapies." Southern California Law Review 47:237-356.

Shindul, J.A., and M.E. Synder
1981 "Legal restraints on restraint." American Journal of Nursing 81(2):393-394.

Steadman, H.J.
1982 "Insanity defense: some questions answered." This Month in Mental Health (September), p. 6.

Stone, A.A.
1975 "The right to treatment." American Journal of Psychiatry 132:1125-1134.
1979 "Informed consent: special problems for psychiatry." Hospital and Community Psychiatry 30(5):321-326.

Szasz, T.
1963 Law, Liberty and Psychiatry: An Inquiry Into the Social Uses of Mental Health Practices. New York: Macmillan, Inc.

"Third-party reimbursement"
1982 Pacesetter 7(3):5-6.

Torrey, E.F.
1973 Cited in "Tending the spirit." Wall Street Journal, March 26, pp. 1, 17.

Towery, O.B., and C. Windle
1978 "Quality assurance for community mental health centers: impact of P.L. 94-63." Hospital and Community Psychiatry 29(5): 316-319.

Ver Steeg, D.F.
1979 "The political process; or, the power and the glory." Nursing Dimension: Power in Nursing 7(2):20-27.

Votaw, D.
1979 "What do we believe about power?" Nursing Dimensions: Power in Nursing 7(2):50-63.

Warner, R.
1977 "Witchcraft and soul loss: implications for community psychiatry." Hospital and Community Psychiatry 28(9):686-690.

Willeg, S.H.
1970 The Nurse's Guide to the Law. New York: McGraw-Hill Book Co.

Zaleznik, A.
1979 Power and Politics in Organizational Life. Nursing Dimensions: Power in Nursing 7(2):64-74.

Zaltman, G., R. Duncan, and J. Holbek
1973 Innovations and Organizations. New York: John Wiley & Sons, Inc.

Zentner, J.L.
1973 "Organizational ideology: some functions and problems." International Review of History and Political Science 10(2):75-84.

Zimmer, M.J.
1974 "Quality assurance for outcomes of patient care." Nursing Clinics of North America 9(2):305-315.

ANNOTATED SUGGESTED READINGS

Donley, R.
1979 "An inside view of the Washington health scene." American Journal of Nursing 79(10):1946-1949.
The author discusses some of the insights gained into Washington politics as a result of her experience as a Robert Wood Johnson Health Policy Fellow. She suggests approaches for nurses who want to develop political power.

Gonzalez, H.H.
1976 "The consumer movement: the implications for psychiatric care." Perspectives in Psychiatric Care 14(4): 186-190.
Gonzalez discusses the historical development of the consumer movement in health care and then focuses on consumerism in mental health care. Implications are explored for utilizing consumers as active participants in mental health care: as mental health care providers, as doctors of the people, and as evaluators of treatment modalities. Issues and problems associated with consumerism in mental health are discussed.

Kohnke, M.F.
1982 Advocacy: Risk and Reality. St. Louis, The C.V. Mosby Co.
The author deals with the many aspects of advocacy. Among these aspects are the functions of advocacy, the importance of open-mindedness for advocacy, areas of proficiency that contribute to open-mindedness and the levels of advocacy (self advocacy, client advocacy, community advocacy).

McFarland, D.E., and N. Schiflett (eds.)
1979 Nursing Dimensions: Power in Nursing 7(2):1-86.
The entire issue is devoted to a discussion of the process of power and its implications for health care and nursing. Special emphasis is given to strategies for acquiring and exerting power; these strategies are compared to the usual nursing strategies in power situations. An annotated bibliography is included.

Ruiz, P., and M. Behrens
1973 "Community control in mental health: how far can it go?" Psychiatric Quarterly 47(3):317-324.
Ruiz and Behrens discuss the role of consumer representatives in developing knowledge about community mental health programs, learning how to effectively use power to achieve results, and determining what type of mental health services are most valuable for their community. The authors focus on Lincoln Community Mental Health Center in the Bronx, N.Y.

Schell-King, M., and M.R. Finneran
1982 "The role of forensic psychiatry and the insanity defense." Perspectives in Psychiatric Care 20(2):55-64.
The authors examine the relationship between the criminal justice and mental health systems within an historical framework. Several approaches to the problems of forensic psychiatry are explored: the traditional, the reform, and the rethinking. Special attention is given to the issues defining mental illness, the expert witness, and the insanity defense.

UNIT II

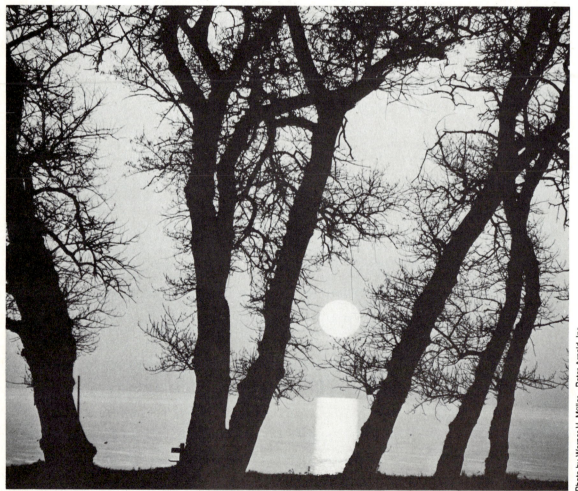

Concepts basic to understanding behavior and to nursing intervention

In this unit concepts that are vital to the understanding and practice of mental health nursing are presented. The first chapter in this unit discusses the sociocultural aspects of mental health nursing in a theoretical, as well as practical, sense. The cultural diversity of our society is examined, and discussions are included on how the nurse's cultural background may influence interactions with clients.

Chapter 5 looks at sociocultural factors that influence the composition, form, and dynamics of the family. Viewing the family as a social system, this chapter explores interrelatioships and interactions. The stages of human development are the focus of Chapter 6. The theoretical basis for nursing intervention for clients at all stages of the life cycle is provided. Chapter 7 presents the concepts of stress and adaptation. Discussions are centered on biological, psychological, and sociocultural factors and their relationship to stress and adaptation in mental health and mental illness.

Thoughts, emotions, needs, and ideas are communicated in various ways. Chapter 8 describes the process of communication and develops a theoretical basis for understanding communication in relation to culture and mental processes. The therapeutic use of communication skills and techniques is discussed in Chapter 9. Application of the nursing process to the establishment of a nurse-client relationship is the focal point of this chapter.

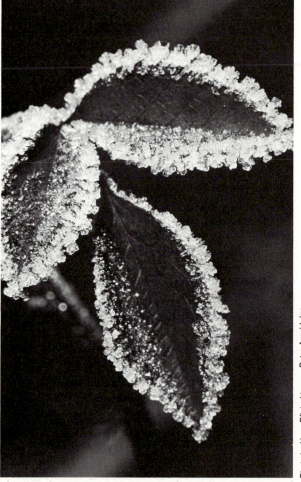

Photo by Hans Pfletschinger—Peter Arnold, Inc.

The sociocultural context of behavior

CHAPTER FOCUS

The population of the United States is composed of people from many different ethnic groups, each of which has its own culture. Through the process of enculturation, people learn the conceptual and behavioral systems of their culture. Enculturation is an essential mechanism for cultural continuity. When persons of differing ethnic backgrounds interact, some degree of another process, acculturation, usually occurs. Acculturation refers to the reciprocal retentions, losses, and adaptations that occur when members of two or more ethnic groups interact.

Because each culture codifies reality in its own way, members of different ethnic groups act upon different premises in behaving and evaluating behavior. When members of one ethnic group come into contact with the culturally coded orientations of another ethnic group, cognitive dissonance and culture shock may develop. Moving to a foreign country, moving to another neighborhood, or even entering a hospital may precipitate cognitive dissonance and culture shock, which engender stress and make people more vulnerable to mental illness.

Awareness of ethnic differences and their significance enables nurses to understand the cultural dimension of mental health and mental illness. In addition, a nurse's awareness of his or her own attitudes and the influence of ethnic heritage on them are essential to therapeutic nursing intervention. In order for nurses to engage in the therapeutic use of self, they must have a high degree of self-awareness and self-understanding. Attitude clarification helps them develop insight into many factors that influence their behavior.

THE UNITED STATES AS A MULTI-ETHNIC SOCIETY

The population of the United States is composed of many ethnic groups. An *ethnic group* is a collectivity of people organized around an assumption of common origin. The members of an ethnic group hold basically similar value and ideological systems and share systems of communication, social interaction, and world view. In addition, an ethnic group sees itself and is seen by others as a distinct category.

The characteristics that distinguish one ethnic group from another are not merely the sum of observable differences; they also include the characteristics that members of a group consider significant. Some characteristics may be emphasized by group members; others may be ignored or underplayed. Cultural traits that produce ethnic differences can be classified into two categories: (1) overt signs and signals, such as language, dress, and house-style, and (2) fundamental values establishing right from wrong and good from bad that serve as standards for judging behavior (Barth, 1960).

Novak (1973) describes several aspects of America's "New Ethnicity" movement: The movement acknowledges the United States as a multi-ethnic society, dispels the melting pot myth, and discourages cultural homogenization. Advantages of ethnic differences are emphasized, and ethnic consciousness raising is encouraged. Awareness of ethnic traditions and practice of ethnic customs are stressed. Involvement in the social and political needs of one's ethnic group is encouraged.

Despite the multi-ethnic nature of the United States, some social scientists believe there is a basic or mainstream American world view. Kluckhohn and Strodtbeck (1961) identify three aspects of any ethnic group's world view: people's relationship to other people, people's relationship to time, and people's relationship to the world about them. The British-American middle class is often referred to as mainstream America or as dominant American society. Central to the world view of this group are the following relationships:

1. Relationship to other people—individualistic and egalitarian
2. Relationship to time—extended future perspective and deferment of gratification
3. Relationship to the world—personal control, autonomy, goal-directed behavior, and self-determination (Schneider and Lysgaard, 1953; Kluckhohn and Strodtbeck, 1961; G. Spindler, 1977)

Dominquez (1975) holds that many minority ethnic group members consider assimilation into mainstream American society either impossible or undesirable. The Glazer-Moynihan study (1970) found that many people prefer to live in ethnic enclaves. An *ethnic enclave* is a geographic area in a city, town, or village that is populated by a minority ethnic group.

It has been suggested that it is the interaction of cultural heritage with immigration and post-immigration experiences that produces American ethnic group culture (Greeley and McReady, 1975). Greeley (1974) stresses that in the study of ethnicity it is important to differentiate between the concepts of ethnic identification, ethnic heritage, and ethnic culture.

Ethnic identification refers to where people place themselves on the "ethnic chart." For example, do people identify themselves as Hispanic-Americans? Afro-Americans? Sino-Americans? Some studies have indicated that the higher the educational, occupational, and income levels of immigrants, the more rapidly they identify themselves as Americans and become integrated into mainstream America (Rogg, 1974; James, 1977).

Ethnic heritage refers to the cultural history of people, and it may be perpetuated by ethnic schools, ethnic churches, and ethnic folk festivals. For example, *El Día de la Raza* (The Day of the Race), an Hispanic folk festival, is a time when various Hispanic ethnic groups come together to celebrate and to share with each other their distinctive folk dances, music, and foods.

Ethnic culture refers to attitudinal, value, and

behavioral patterns associated with an ethnic group. For example, North Americans and Latin Americans perceive time differently. In the United States, time is perceived as something fixed that can be divided into discrete segments. Time is valued for the pursuit of achievement and success. Promptness and adherence to schedules are highly valued, and efficiency is associated with doing one thing at a time. However, in Latin American societies, time is perceived as a relative and flexible phenomenon. Latin Americans tend not to adhere strictly to schedules, and they frequently function in a context where several things are going on simultaneously. These different orientations toward time can sometimes present problems in health care settings.

A mental health after-care clinic operated on an appointment basis. If clients were more than 15 minutes late for their appointments, they were not seen and had to reschedule their appointments. Clients who were habitually late for appointments were labeled "uncooperative," "unmotivated toward health," or "resistive to treatment."

Although the clinic's catchment area included a large Hispanic population, Hispanic clients were underrepresented on the clinic's roster. The nurse-anthropologist employed by the clinic was aware of the different conceptualizations of time held by North Americans and Latin Americans. She spoke with Hispanic clients who attended the clinic and with those who had been referred to the clinic but who did not attend. Both groups of clients cited the clinic staff's "rigidity" concerning promptness and appointment schedules as a reason why Hispanics did not attend the clinic.

The nurse-anthropologist discussed this situation with other staff members, and she explained to them the different orientations toward time held by Latin Americans and North Americans. The staff decided to develop a pilot program whereby on Monday, Wednesday, and Friday evenings clients could be seen without an appointment. The number of Hispanic clients attending the clinic increased measurably.

A fourth concept in the study of ethnicity is *ethnic interaction*. Ethnic interaction refers to the degree to which people's interpersonal relationships are based on ethnic affiliation. For example, Pasquali (1982) found that first-generation Long Island Cubans who had immigrated as adults were more likely to base friendships and marriage on shared ethnicity and that they were less likely to be integrated into American social networks than were first-generation Cubans who had immigrated as youths.

Equally important to the definition of an ethnic group is the way people outside an ethnic group perceive the ethnic group (Isajiw, 1974). For example, caucasian Americans may lump anyone who is oriental into the social interaction category of "Chinese," regardless of the person's ethnicity.

If such an ascribed category of social interaction is accepted both by the individuals who are being categorized and by others, then the category becomes established. If either party rejects the category, then alternatives may be proposed and compromises arrived at.

At a neighborhood health center, the Caucasian staff tended to view all black clients as having similar cultural backgrounds. However, the black clients rejected the category of "black American," and they educated the staff about the cultural differences among black people from the southern United States, from the Carribean, and from Africa.

Eventually, categories of social interaction become accepted by the media, the public, and by the minority group members themselves. When minority group members accept this "other definition" as Irish, Italian, or Chinese and stop thinking of themselves by their village or regional identities, immigrants have become ethnics (Horowitz, 1975).

Immigrants may accept the broad category of identity assigned by outsiders and identify themselves on a national rather than a regional or village level as a defense against the prejudice and hostility of society at large. Ethnic organizations may be formed and symbols may be created by immigrants who are unifying in national groups. Symbols may serve as representation of and stimulation for ethnic unity and ethnic consciousness (Sarna, 1978).

ENCULTURATION

Every ethnic group has its unique culture. *Enculturation* is the process of learning the conceptual and behavioral systems of one's culture. The goal of enculturation is to transform a person from a predominantly biogenic being (motivated by physiological states) into a predominantly sociogenic being (motivated by social values, sanctions, and constraints). To achieve this end, a culture must teach youngsters survival skills that provide for the biosocial continuity of society and standards and rules that govern behavior and the distribution of social and material assets (Honigmann, 1967). Through this process, members of an ethnic group learn how their ethnic group is distinguished from all others.

Basic group identity

Basic group identity, which evolves from membership in an ethnic group, results from shared social characteristics, such as world view, language, values, and beliefs. Isaacs (1975) points out that two concepts figure predominantly in the development of basic group identity: body and name.

The body is the most fundamental feature of basic group identity. Because exogamy (marriage outside the ethnic group) threatens the physical similarity of an ethnic group, many ethnic groups have taboos and constraints surrounding exogamy. Many ethnic groups have also created ways of physically distinguishing their members from all others (for example, through tatooing, scarifica-

tion, or molding the shape of head, nose, or lips).

Some people try to "pass" from their own ethnic group to an ethnic group of perceived higher status. Whether passing is achieved through intermarriage or other means, the degree of social mobility possible is closely associated with the degree of physical similarity to the ethnic group of higher status.

The name, or names, associated with an ethnic group carries much meaning. Names that ethnic groups give to themselves and others tell much about inter-ethnic relations. Both names and meaning may change over time (for example, "colored," "negro," "black").

Individual surnames may serve as badges of ethnic group identity and current ethnic orientation. For example, "Americanizing" a surname may indicate a desire to be assimilated into mainstream United States society.

Agents of enculturation

FAMILY

The earliest and generally most effective enculturating agent is the family.* The family experience is essential to the development of basic group identity. Ethnically specific (unique to an ethnic group) norms, values, role relationships, communication patterns, and world views are taught within the family context.

There are many different family forms, some of which are associated with specific ethnic groups. Two major types of family organization may be distinguished: extended and nuclear.

Extended families encompass three or more generations of kinsmen. The stem family of Japan (composed of eldest son, his wife and their children, and his parents) and the matrilocal family of the West Indies (composed of a woman, her daughters, and her daughters' children) are examples of extended families. The extended family has a potentially larger labor force and more options for the division of labor than does the nuclear

---

*See Chapter 5 for an in-depth discussion of the family.

family. The extended family also provides many adult members to share in child-rearing and with whom children can identify (Davenport, 1961; Scheflen and Scheflen, 1972).

In the United States, the nuclear family has long been regarded as the ''normal'' family form. This type of family, which consists of a man, a woman, and their children, emerged as an adaptation to the Industrial Revolution. As farms became mechanized and people began working in factories, large extended families were no longer an economic necessity (Scheflen and Scheflen, 1972).

At each stage of the life cycle, the two basic forms of family organization differ in their potential for meeting the needs of their members. The extended family provides members with security and dignity. Aging members have a place to live and usually hold positions of authority and respect. Children benefit from the presence of older family members, who help rear them and serve as role models. On the other hand, since respect and the exercise of family authority are usually the provinces of age, younger members of the family may live out much of their lives under the supervision of elders. In the extended family, security is often gained at the expense of personal growth and individualism.

The nuclear family usually encourages and facilitates the individual development of young members. However, nonfamily relationships and occupational demands tend to compete with and weaken family ties. Relationships with other relatives are often inadequate. Consequently, during periods of maturational or situational crisis, family members may not receive necessary support or security. For instance, during a divorce, parents may be distraught and unable to offer their children adequate emotional support. At the same time, the children may be physically and affectionally estranged from relatives who could serve as a support system. Aunts and uncles may live many miles away, and grandparents may be isolated from the family or may have little cross-generational contact. In the nuclear family opportunity for personal development is sometimes gained at

the expense of security (Scheflen and Scheflen, 1972).

Whether the ethnic family is extended or nuclear, it often gives its members conflicting messages: Succeed in mainstream America, but do not become part of it. Participate in society, but retain strong bonds with your ethnic group. At the same time, the ethnic family may try to protect children from discrimination by other ethnic groups. This protectiveness may deprive children of opportunities for full participation in mainstream American life and thereby prevent them from successfully competing in society (Gambino, 1974).

NEIGHBORHOOD

The concept of ethnicity centers around group identity. An ethnic group residing in an enclave feels a strong sense of belonging and community. According to Gans (1962), members of ethnic enclaves have a strong sense of ''neighborhood.'' Neighborhood constitutes a protective social milieu. It encompasses shops with familiar wares, social clubs, a church, often a school, and a supportive social network composed of reliable neighbors.

Neighborhood peer groups often form. Members may be bound together by age and sex, in addition to ethnicity. Because many residents of ethnic enclaves are born, live, and die in the enclave, the same peer group may be influential throughout a person's life. The neighborhood peer group provides support and a sense of belonging. It structures relationships within the neighborhood and with outside communities. It helps its members to cope with the conflict and tension that may be engendered when the values and customs of their ethnic group clash with those of mainstream America.

Within a neighborhood peer group, there is usually consensus about norms and role relationships. There is also pressure to conform. Studies such as those by Bott (1957), Gans (1962), and Young and Willmott (1957) have shown that when marriage is superimposed on peer networks, peer relationships tend to draw spouses into peer network activities and away from their conjugal relationship. Because neighborhood peer groups are often segregated by sex, spouses may receive emotional satisfaction and assistance from peer group members of the same sex. Women usually associate with childhood female friends and help each other with "women's work." Men usually associate with male childhood cronies and help each other with "men's work." The support that such peer relationships provide often reduces the need for emotional support and help from one's spouse and tends to weaken conjugal bonds.

The ethnic association is another type of neighborhood group that contributes to enculturation. In a multi-ethnic society like the United States, ethnic associations help reinforce ethnic identity and ethnic consciousness. Ethnic associations also help members cope with conflict and tension engendered by migration from one's homeland or contact with other ethnic groups. Associations such as the Landman Society (for Eastern European Jews) and the Sons of Italy establish new bonds of fellowship to replace those severed by migration and develop the rudiments of an ethnopolitical consciousness. Children of immigrants often have few, if any, memories of the homeland. Subsequent generations, born in the United States, not only may have few ties with their ethnic heritage but also may experience pressure to "Americanize." By reinforcing ethnic values, standards, and role relationships, ethnic associations serve as reference groups. They also provide mutual aid, promote the interests of the ethnic group, and facilitate the exchange of goods and services (Blau, 1964; Essien-Udom, 1964; Parenti, 1965; Eldersveld, 1966).

RELIGION

There is a historical association between ethnic groups and religious denominations. In addition to inculcating and reinforcing ethnic values, norms, and behavior, religious groups may act as political reference groups, militating for changes that will advance the ethnic group's aims. For example,

black religious sects in the southern United States spearheaded the move for desegregation and justice for Afro-Americans. Religious groups often try to advance ethnic goals by appealing to an abstract and idealistic moral order (Lenski, 1961; Manwaring, 1961; Stedman, 1964).

SCHOOL

When children reach school age, teachers join the ranks of significant others who are instrumental in enculturation. A teacher may be the first significant other with whom a child relates outside the family and the neighborhood. Especially to young children, teachers may represent the end product of the process of enculturation. Neighborhood schools in ethnic enclaves are sometimes staffed with teachers of similar ethnicity or with teachers who are knowledgeable about and supportive of the ethnic group's culture. However, when children of one ethnic group attend school with children of other ethnic minorities or with children from mainstream America, there may be little articulation between values taught at home and those taught at school (Dickerman, 1973).

Ethnic children may quickly realize that there are two value systems: one that reflects the values of their ethnic group and one that reflects the values of mainstream America. For example, Hsu (1970) points out that American values of equality before the law, of relying on lawyers to settle disputes on the basis of absolute concepts of legal right and wrong, and of personal growth and individual responsibility for becoming successful contrast sharply with Chinese values of deference to age, of a middleman or peacemaker settling disputes on the basis of situational or relative concepts of right and wrong, and of responsibility to one's extended family even at the expense of personal growth and individuation. Hsu also notes that while some Chinese-Americans may become anglicized, those who prefer to live in an enclave still hold much of the Chinese value system.

Ethnic children are usually not helped to view the two value systems as complementary. The school may try to socialize ethnic children into the culture of mainstream America by undermining and discouraging any manifestation of ethnicity. Behavior and customs taught and practiced at home may be derogated or forbidden in school.

Maria was a first-generation Italian-American. When she began kindergarten she was very outgoing and talkative. Her speech was accompanied by gesturing. The teacher was British-American and used little gesturing. The teacher frequently admonished Maria to "calm down" and "not to talk with your hands." Occasionally while Maria was talking the teacher would gently hold Maria's hands.

At the middle of the school year the teacher noticed that Maria had become very quiet. She spoke only when spoken to and then made only brief responses. The teacher consulted the school nurse.

The school nurse spent some time in the classroom observing Maria's behavior. The nurse, who was also Italian, noticed that Maria appeared very tense when speaking and that she used very little gesturing. The nurse shared this observation with the teacher. The teacher then disclosed that she had tried to help Maria learn to speak without gesturing. The nurse explained that this was an ethnic communication pattern and suggested that interference with it might be related to Maria's noncommunicative behavior. The nurse also referred the teacher to studies on ethnicity and communication.

The teacher decided she had been wrong to try to control Maria's gesturing and explained this to Maria. Maria gradually became more comfortable in the teacher's presence and more communicative.*

Thus criticism of ethnic children by teachers may be aimed at the core of the children's identity. Ethnic customs and values may be derogated or discouraged in the schoolroom, and ethnic literature, art, music, and heroes may be absent. This

---

*See Chapter 8 for a discussion of ethnicity and communication.

atmosphere may undermine ethnic identity and make it difficult for ethnic minority students to relate to the aims of formal education. Covello (1972) maintains that such students often find the experience of schooling an experience of cultural criticism.

In school, ethnic children become acquainted with ideas and behavior that are new and different and that may be held up as superior. The culture of mainstream America is attractive because it is the dominant, ''superior'' culture. The world of ethnic culture is attractive because it is familiar and secure. Thus conflict often occurs. Children may try to resolve this conflict through accommodation, which usually requires the maintenance of a dichotomy between public and private behavior. In public, ethnic children may reject ethnic behavior and try to use the behavior of mainstream America. In the private world of home and enclave, they may use ethnic behavior. For example, when they are at school, Chinese-American children may speak English and eat the ''American'' food that is served in the school cafeteria. When they are at home, the children may speak Chinese and eat such Chinese foods as rice, bean curd, snow peas, and water chestnuts. The degree of rejection of ethnic behavior depends largely on the ethnic composition of the school population (both students and teachers) and the ethnic homogeneity of the community. When a large percentage of the school population is composed of members of the child's ethnic group and when the child comes from an ethnically homogeneous nieghborhood, the probability of culture conflict is smaller than it is when school and neighborhood populations are ethnically heterogeneous (Covello, 1972; Gambino, 1974).

• • •

Ethnicity is inculcated through the process of enculturation. Family, neighborhood, church, and school serve as agents of enculturation. Kin, peers, clergymen, and teachers are profoundly influential in the transmission of norms, values, role relationships, communication patterns, and world view.

ACCULTURATION

During the process of enculturation members of an ethnic group learn the conceptual and behavioral systems of their culture. However, in a culturally plural society like the United States, members of different ethnic groups come into contact and interact with one another. The reciprocal retentions, losses, or adaptations of cultural patterns that result when members of two or more ethnic groups interact constitute the process referred to as acculturation (Barnett et al., 1954; Smith, 1973; L. Spindler, 1977).

The response of members of an ethnic group to inter-ethnic contact may be *assimilation* (becoming integrated with the dominant ethnic group), *separation* (developing, maintaining, or reinforcing ethnic enclaves), or *out-migration* (moving to another locale).

Peterson (1972) studied the reactions of Choctaw Indians to acculturative pressure. Out-migration was high in those Choctaw communities where job opportunities and social services (such as school and health facilities) were limited. Choctaws moved to Choctaw or Anglo communities that offered jobs and social services. Assimilation was high when job opportunities were available in Anglo communities and when Anglos were receptive to Choctaws (that is, when Anglos related to Choctaws as equals and offered them the prerogatives of Anglo status). Separation was high in those Choctaw communities that were large enough to provide necessary social services and where job opportunities were available in nearby communities.

Therefore, the degree of rigidity of ethnic group boundaries and the quality of inter-ethnic relationships influence the response of ethnic group members to acculturative pressures.

Ethnic boundaries

Every ethnic group has a unique culture. Ethnic groups function as systems and have the properties of systems. The properties of interacting ethnic groups influence the process of acculturation of ethnic group members.

Ethnic groups are bounded. Boundaries maintain the distinctiveness of an ethnic group. *Boundary maintenance mechanisms* are practices and types of behavior that exclude outsiders from the customs and values of a particular ethnic group. Such mechanisms protect the group from foreign influence and create a "we-they" orientation. Some examples of boundary maintenance mechanisms are ritual initiations, secret societies, fear of outsiders, social controls (such as gossip and rumor), racism, and ethnocentrism (Barnett et al., 1954; L. Spindler, 1977).

The degree to which an ethnic group uses boundary maintainance mechanisms largely determines how closed (resistant) or open (susceptible) the group is to acculturation pressures.

A community health nurse had recently been transferred from one district to another. The nurse had observed that the former district had been composed of third- and fourth-generation Americans of many ethnic backgrounds. Neighbors shared recipes for the preparation of ethnic foods. Teachers discussed the ethnic traditions of many countries. It was common for children and adults to have close friends with ethnic backgrounds different from theirs. Ethnicity did not seem to play a role in the selection of a physician.

The community health nurse's new district was different in many respects from the old one. The new district was composed largely of members of a single ethnic group. The residents were primarily immigrant of second-generation Americans. Local grocery stores sold traditional ethnic goods. While teachers in the school came from various ethnic backgrounds, the students were ethnically homogeneous. It was rare for children or adults to have friends from a different ethnic group. Ethnicity played a large role in the selection of a physician. People felt more comfortable with a physician who spoke their language and shared their customs. Residents were reserved in the presence of "outsiders" and seemed to mistrust them. The community health nurse was of an ethnic background dif-

ferent from that of the people in the district and initially had difficulty establishing rapport. Only after many months of attending local activities and events, shopping at local stores, talking with local merchants and residents, and otherwise demonstrating interest in and respect for their culture was the nurse accepted by the people in the district.

The residents of the first district described here exhibit open ethnic boundaries; there is much inter-ethnic exchange. The people in the second district exhibit closed ethnic boundaries. There is a very strong "we-they" orientation. Ethnocentrism and suspicion of outsiders operate to maintain ethnic boundaries, and acculturation is resisted.

Inter-ethnic relationships

In-group–out-group relationships among ethnic groups also influence the process of acculturation. Coser and Rosenberg (1957) point out that unique socio-politico-economic relationships may exist among the members of an ethnic group and differentiate that group from all other ethnic groups. This results in a "we" (in-group)–"they" (out-group) dichotomy. Relationships within a group are characterized by camaraderie, order, rules, and industry. Relationships between groups are characterized by hostility and conflict. Each ethnic group tends to view its own folkways as superior and right and those of other groups as inferior and wrong. Each ethnic group uses its culture as a standard for judging all other cultures (ethnocentrism).

A student nurse had been assigned to a pediatric unit to gain clinical experience. One client that the student cared for was a 4-year-old child who was recovering from meningitis. When the child was discharged from the hospital, the student decided to make a follow-up home visit. During the visit, the student observed the child eating a lunch of beans, rice, hearts of palm, and plantain. The student concluded that this meatless lunch was not very nutritious and that the family's eating habits were poor.

The family had recently emigrated from the Caribbean, where beans, rice, heart of palm, and plantain are traditional foods. The student nurse was unfamiliar with these foods and therefore viewed them as inferior. The student's judgment was influenced by ethnocentrism, a common in-group theme that contributes to in-group–out-group polarization.

Under certain acculturative conditions, an out-group may become a source of positive rather than negative reference. People may wish to belong to, feel loyalty toward, or emulate the behavior of an out-group and to reject the behavior of their own group. Emulation of out-group behavior tends to be in the direction of the technologically superior culture (Sherif and Sherif, 1953; Merton and Rossi, 1957; Hyman, 1960; L. Spindler, 1977).

Sherif and Sherif (1964) describe some conditions that influence the selection of a reference group:

1. The more unified an in-group is, the more likely that it will serve as a reference group for its members.
2. The more unified an in-group is, the more similar an out-group must be to it before in-group members will select the out-group as a reference group.
3. The more open an out-group is to new membership, the more likely that in-group members will select the out-group as a reference group.

Horowitz (1975) suggests that the more dominant and prestigious an ethnic group is, the more successful it will be in recruiting and in making itself appealing as a reference group.

Dohrenwend and Smith (1962) believe that the relative dominance of interacting ethnic groups can be determined by analyzing the following three conditions:

1. Which ethnic group(s) can recruit members of other ethnic groups into low-status positions (for example, slave, servant)?
2. Which ethnic group(s) can effectively exclude members of other ethnic groups from positions that confer status equal to or greater

than that enjoyed by members of the dominant group (for example, by segregating schools and neighborhoods)?

3. Which ethnic group(s) can assume high-status positions (such as teacher, physician, nurse, and social worker) in the activities of other ethnic groups?

The more completely these conditions are satisfied, the more complete is the establishment of a dominance-submission relationship between ethnic groups. This relationship may not be absolute. For instance, members of a minority ethnic group may be recruited into low-status positions in the economic activities of the larger society, but they may effectively exclude members of the larger society from the kinship and religious activities of the minority group.

When members of different ethnic groups interact, role relationships are established that usually reflect inter-ethnic status, power, values, and needs. These relationships provide culturally patterned ways for people of differing ethnic groups to interact (Barnett et al., 1954).

The Hsu family followed a very strong Chinese tradition when in their ethnic enclave. The family members spoke Chinese, wore traditional Chinese dress, ate Chinese foods, consulted a herbalist, and followed a Chinese value system. However, whenever they attended a family-practice clinic, they wore Western-style clothes, spoke English, and accepted prescriptions for Western medicines.

Inter-ethnic role relationships thus may produce private and public spheres of interaction, each with its appropriate behavior. By enclosing ethnic differences in a sphere of intra-ethnic articulation (private sphere), members of an ethnic group may maintain ethnic identity and still engage in a sphere of inter-ethnic articulation (public sphere).

The maintenance of dichotomous spheres of behavior is not the only option open to members of minority ethnic groups who wish to participate in mainstream America. Instead, they may try to "pass" and become assimilated into dominant mainstream society, or they may exaggerate their ethnic characteristics and use them to achieve status and desired socioeconomic rewards (Barth, 1960). Social scientists have been unable to determine the variables that influence the selection of an option or to speculate on the degree of success that any one option will provide minority group members who attempt to participate in mainstream society.

Indices of acculturation

The process of acculturation has two stages. In the first stage, cultural acculturation, members of a minority ethnic group accept and use the dominant ethnic group's language, customs, dress, and foods. Members of the minority group may be reluctant to alter their value system. Isolated ideas and values are altered more readily than those that are integral parts of the minority group's culture. In the second stage, structural acculturation, members of the minority ethnic group are incorporated into the dominant ethnic group's social networks (for example, play and peer groups, country clubs, and neighborhoods). This stage of acculturation necessitates acceptance by members of the dominant ethnic group and occurs more slowly than cultural acculturation (Barnett et al., 1954; Gordon, 1964).

In trying to measure degree of acculturation, anthropologists have considered the type and extent of inter-ethnic contact and the degree to which such contact results in identification with another ethnic group. Kelman (1961) hypothesizes that a change in ethnic identification occurs when people adopt types of behavior that are unique to another ethnic group. The new behavior enables them to establish a relationship with members of the other group and to define their self-image and roles according to the standards of the other group.

Chance (1965) and Shannon (1968) have developed criteria for determining degree of inter-ethnic contact:

1. Knowledge and use of the other culture's language.
2. Residential mobility
3. Occupational mobility
4. Access to mass media
5. National Guard or military service

Chance and Shannon have also developed the following indices for measuring identification with the culture of another ethnic group:

1. Preference for activities of another culture over those of one's own culture
2. Preference for foods of another culture when foods from both cultures are equally available
3. Preference for the clothing, hair styles, and cosmetic styles of another culture over one's own culture
4. Use of another culture's language
5. Acceptance of another culture's world view

Cultural assessment guide

Indices of acculturation can be used to develop a tool for assessing cultural orientation. Since people's cultural orientations and ethnic identities have strong influences on their values and behavior, nurses need to incorporate cultural assessment into overall assessment strategies. Information from the following areas should be included in such an assessment*:

1. Demographics. Client's name. Proper pronunciation of client's name. Client's age. If client is an immigrant, length of time in the United States and age at time of immigration. Place of current residence (for example, inter-ethnic neighborhood or ethnic enclave).
2. Family organization. Type of family. Generations represented. Members composing the family unit. Members vested with family authority. Members involved in child rearing. Sense of obligation to family members. Members residing in the same household or in different households. Interaction of family with society.
3. Sex-defined roles. Stereotyped male and female roles. Amount of independence permitted men and women. Degree of intimacy permitted between married men and women and degree of intimacy permitted between unmarried men and women.
4. Communication patterns. Languages spoken at home and outside home. Use of eye contact, touching, and gesturing. Interpersonal spacing. Use of humor. Use of proverbs.
5. Type of dress. Traditional ethnic dress or Western-style dress?
6. Type of food. Ethnic food or "American" food? Types of food preparation (for example, broiled, fried, baked; seasonings used). Food taboos. Use of food for health maintenance and/or treatment.
7. Relationship to people. Individualistic or group-oriented? Egalitarian or authoritative?
8. Relationship to time. Past-, present-, or future-oriented?
9. Relationship to the world. Personal control, goal-directed, or fatalistic?
10. Health care patterns. Definition of health and illness. Ideas concerning causes of illness (for example, germs, evil spirits, punishment for sins). Ideas concerning treatment of illness. Coping behaviors. Acculturative pressures. Minority status stressors. People consulted when ill (for example, family member, native healing specialist, physician, pharmacist) and order in which they are consulted.
11. Religious practices. Beliefs and rituals concerning birth, illness, and death. Nature of belief in a supernatural being or supernormal energy. Conceptualizations about the quality of life and the quality of death.

---

*Sources consulted in the preparation of this cultural assessment tool include Kluckhohn and Strodtbeck (1961), Spradley and Phillip (1972), and Mosley and Clift (1977).

CULTURE, COGNITION, AND CULTURE SHOCK

Codification of reality and behavior

Over a span of many years, people acquire and store information in their nervous systems. *Cognition* is the processing of information by the nervous system. This processing structures reality and gives meaning to human experience. Cognitive activity includes the focusing of attention, comprehension, problem solving, and information storage and retrieval (memory). When information acquired is consistent with other information being acquired or with information already stored, people experience a state of cognitive consistency or equilibrium (Jordon, 1953; Heider, 1958; Rodriguez, 1965; Estes, 1975).

One of the most important aspects of cognition is *coding,* which is the process of categorizing information. Information is sorted and then stored by means of various types of memory codes: iconic codes (visual images), echoic codes (auditory images), motor codes (motor skills), and symbolic codes (representative images) (Hunt and Lansman, 1975). Although culture influences all types of cognitive coding, symbolic codes are especially influenced by culture. For example, communication systems, one type of symbolic coding, vary from culture to culture. Even a sound such as hissing may communicate either approval (in Japan) or disapproval (in the United States).

All cultures provide a cultural code for perceiving, interpreting, and synthesizing reality. This culturally structured codification of reality is referred to as world view. *Culture* is an ordered system of shared and socially transmitted symbols and meanings that structures world view and guides behavior (Geertz, 1957). Members of an ethnic group, by virtue of their shared cultural background, usually have a common world view and similar values, ideologies, and standards of behavior. Although these thought and behavior patterns are similar among members of an ethnic group, they are not identical. Members of a group usually operate within the boundaries of established custom, but there may be a wide range of individual variation (Goodenough, 1961).

Because each culture codifies reality in its own way, members of dominant mainstream America may act upon premises for behaving and evaluating behavior that are different from those of members of minority ethnic groups. In the process of inter-ethnic contract and acculturation, change may occur in the culturally structured cognitive order of individual members of an ethnic group. Any such change involves learning new values, beliefs, and attitudes. Three conditions are necessary for such a change to occur:

1. Exposure. Adequate exposure to the cognitive system of another ethnic group must exist so that it may be learned.
2. Identification. Through the mechanism of emulation, another ethnic group must be used as a reference group and must provide motivation for change.
3. Access. Avenues of access to the valued resources of another ethnic group must be provided so that outsiders perceive that a change in their cognitive orientation will gain them desired rewards (Chance, 1965; Graves, 1967).

Individual members of an ethnic group, mindful of alternatives, make choices—usually between a traditional practice, value, or idea and a new one. Ogionwo (1969) analyzed how networks of information and influence are involved in the decision to adopt a new idea. He found that personal communication is more effective than mass media and that when mass media are used, broadcast media (radio and television) are more effective than print media (magazines and newspapers). Ogionwo also found that the flow of information is not simply from the source to the individual. Group interaction is also important. Family, friends, and social norms may all exert pressure on a person either to adopt or to resist a new idea.

A community mental health nurse identified a need for child care education for new parents. Counseling on a one-to-one basis proved unsuccessful. The nurse evaluated the program and realized that it had not considered the ethnic background of the clients.

The people in the community were immigrants and second-generation Hispanic Americans. In traditional Hispanic culture, child care is the sole responsibility of women. In addition, the extended family is central to Hispanic family life.

The nurse considered these cultural factors when revising the child care education program. The revised program was designed for the new mother and the female relatives in her extended family. This approach to child care education proved effective.

This vignette illustrates how important it is for nurses to recognize that informational flow is not simply from the nurse to the individual client. Group interaction is also important. The composition of the group and the influence of the group on the individual vary from culture to culture.

Cultural change and cognitive dissonance

When, through inter-ethnic contact and acculturation, change occurs in people's culturally structured cognitive orders, *cognitive dissonance* may develop. Cognitive dissonance is the state of disequilibrium and tension produced when two or more sets of information are at variance with one another (Festinger, 1957; Steiner, 1960; Kogan and Wallach, 1964).

When changes occur in value or ideological systems, people experience cognitive dissonance. They then try to resolve discrepancies in sets of information (such as conflicting value systems) and to reestablish cognitive consistency. People differ in their ability to tolerate cognitive dissonance and in their ways of resolving it and reestab-

lishing cognitive consistency (Festinger, 1957; Heider, 1958; Kretch et al., 1962).

People try to cope with the cognitive dissonance engendered by inter-ethnic contact and acculturative pressures by responding in one or more of the following ways:

1. Acknowledging only one set of information and denying the existence of sets of discrepant information
2. Reassessing the value of conflicting information so that one set of information assumes greater value than the others
3. Identifying differences between sets of discrepant information and trying to use one set to explain the others
4. Seeking new information that will be consistent with one set of information and not with the others
5. Tolerating the existence of sets of discrepant information (Festinger, 1957; McGuire, 1966; Wallace, 1970)

Steiner (1960) believes that persons who use a combination of coping responses are usually more successful in resolving cognitive dissonance than those who use only one response.

How or why people select particular responses for coping with cognitive dissonance has not been fully determined. Rokeach (1960) maintains that the more rigid and closed-minded people are, the more they will strive to maintain their existing belief systems. The more flexible and open-minded people are, the more receptive they will be to reconciling their existing belief systems with new or different information. The degree of people's open- or closed-mindedness is an indication of their readiness to change their belief systems. Berlyne (1960) suggests that open-minded people may even view cognitive dissonance as a challenge.

Close-minded people tend to reject or deny information that does not fit into their existing belief systems. They usually rely on the assessments of authority figures rather than on their own judgment. Closed-minded people also tend to consider fewer factors when making decisions. Open-minded people tend to respond in just the opposite way (Rokeach, 1960; Burke, 1966).

The potential impact of discrepant information on people's value and belief systems also influences the choice of coping responses. Degree of commitment to particular values and belief systems, degree of ethnocentrism, and degree of freedom to accept or reject discrepant information all influence the selection of coping responses (Zajonic and Burnstein, 1965; Abelson, 1968; Aronson, 1968; Kelman and Baron, 1968).

Cognitive dissonance and culture shock

Culture shock, which results from a drastic change in the cultural environment, is both precipitated by and a response to cognitive dissonance. Culture shock is engendered by unfamiliar cues of social interaction. When ethnic groups use dissimilar cues during interaction with each other, conflicts in communication and role relationships may result. Brink and Saunders (1976) have identified the following factors in social interaction as the ones that most frequently create cognitive dissonance and engender culture shock:

1. Different systems of communication
2. Unfamiliar physical environment
3. Isolation from family and friends
4. Foreign customs
5. Different or new role relationships

Any alteration in people's verbal or nonverbal systems of *communication* creates a barrier in the giving and receiving of behavioral cues. Even if people are familiar with the language of another ethnic group, they may have difficulty with nuances of meaning, styles of humor, and colloquialisms.

Alterations in the *physical environment* may also prove difficult. If people have recently immigrated to a country, utilities formerly taken for granted, such as electricity and telephone, may operate differently or be absent. House-styles,

clothes, shopping facilities, and food may also seem strange. It takes time and energy to learn to manipulate the mechanical environment. Fatigue and frustration may develop.

In addition, patterns of customary behavior and *role relationships* may be disrupted. People may have to become accustomed to new and different sex-linked roles, rules of etiquette, and status and kinship systems. Value and belief systems may also be challenged. Since people's ideological systems are usually implicit rather than explicit, they may not be aware of their own values and beliefs until they are questioned. They may realize only then that their standards and ideologies are different from those of their neighbors. These changes in life-style may create cognitive dissonance and result in culture shock.

Cognitive dissonance acts as a stressor and requires adaptive responses. The greater the number of changes required by the new cultural environment, the more difficult the cultural readjustment. Cultural readjustment is part of the process of acculturation. Having to unlearn old cognitive patterns may often prove more stressful than learning new cognitive patterns.

Oberg (1954) was one of the first to observe and describe the phases of adaptation to culture shock: excitement, disenchantment, and resolution. During the excitement phase, people begin to learn about their new country or neighborhood. They become acquainted with new customs, taste unfamiliar foods, sightsee, and begin to establish new work and social roles. As people begin to "settle in," they enter the disenchantment phase. Changes in life-style that earlier had seemed exciting now seem frustrating. Ethnocentrism surfaces as people tend to view the customs, values, and communications systems of other ethnic groups as inferior and infuriating. Feelings of inadequacy, loneliness, anger, and nostalgia predominate. If people remain in a new country or neighborhood and begin to learn the behavioral and communication systems of other ethnic groups, resolution of culture shock is under way. During this phase, new friendships are formed and feelings of inadequacy, isolation, and loneliness dissipate. With the termination of this phase, culture shock is successfully resolved.

However, responses to culture shock are not always adaptive. Spradley and Phillip (1972) have found that when people's usual coping responses prove ineffective and opportunity to learn new coping responses is unavailable, people may respond to culture shock with psychosis, depression, suicide, or homicide.

The following operational definition of culture shock describes the dynamic interrelationship between enculturation, cognitive dissonance, and culture shock:

1. People, through interaction with significant others, learn the skills necessary for participating in a particular ethnic group in a particular society.

2. When these people, through choice or force, interact with members of another ethnic group, the skills that were effective in their own culture may prove ineffective in varying degrees.

3. The people perceive the situation as stressful. Old role relationships, values, expectations, and types of behavior are either less effective or not effective. Culturally coded meanings for objects and events are not shared by members of the other ethnic group with whom they have to interact.

4. This drastic change in the cultural environment produces cognitive dissonance, which acts as a stressor and requires accommodation or readjustment of life-style and behavior. This situation is known as *culture shock*.

5. The people develop stress responses to the culture shock. During the process of cultural readjustment involved in resolving culture shock, they either (a) accommodate themselves to the other ethnic group by learning new behavioral, communication, and ideological systems and thus become acculturated or (b) are unable to learn the skills

required for cultural readjustment and become aggressive, depressed, or withdrawn. Mental illness may develop in the latter situation.

Culture shock and mental illness

Social scientists have found a relationship between culture shock and mental illness. Frost (1938) was among the first to study the incidence of mental illness in American immigrants. He found that the first 18 months in a new country is the period when they are most vulnerable. Dayton (1940) found that, for all age groups, the admission rate to psychiatric hospitals in the United States is significantly higher for foreign-born persons than for persons born in this country. More recently, Tyhurst (1955) corroborated the findings of Frost and Dayton by describing some of the maladaptive effects of migration. During the first 2 months in the host country, an immigrant usually experiences a general sense of well-being, with an associated increase in psychomotor activity. This hyperactivity serves to relieve tension. As the immigrant settles into the new country and encounters social difficulties engendered by unfamiliar language, customs, and values, culture conflict and emotional strain develop and gradually heighten. Flights into nostalgia often help an immigrant cope with the realities of culture shock. Approximately 6 months after having arrived in the new country, the immigrant may begin to evidence high anxiety, suspiciousness, depression, psychosomatic disorders, or any combination of these characteristics.

The incidence of psychiatric disorders in immigrants seems to be higher among women than among men. Several social scientists (for example, Murphy [1962]; Leighton et al. [1963]; Chesler [1972]) have observed that during periods of rapid sociocultural change, disjunctions often occur more acutely and more pervasively in the roles of women than in the roles of men. Such disjunctions contribute to greater role conflict among women than among men. For example, Pasquali (1982) found that among Cubans living on Long Island, the post-immigration role adjustment for women was tremendous. In Cuba, their role primarily had been one of supervisor of household help. After immigration, almost all of these women had to take jobs outside the home. In addition, their domestic role changed from supervising servants to doing housework and child care. These Cuban women suddenly had to juggle work roles with domestic roles, and this often contributed to over-burdening, role conflict, and role stress. Similar observations of role conflict and role stress have been made for Cuban women in other parts of the United States (Gil, 1968; Szapocznik and Kurtiness, 1980). Pasquali (1982) cautions that although Cuban men have not admitted to psychoneurotic or affective symptoms, it should not be concluded that they are not experiencing role conflict. It may be that the concept of *machismo* keeps Cuban men from admitting to feelings of stress and depression. Generally, when men cope maladaptively with stress, they develop what Chesler (1972) terms "male diseases." Such socially deviant behavior* as alcoholism, gambling, and aggressive acts have been termed male diseases by Chesler because they constitute an exaggerated stereotype of the male role.

The stress of culture shock is not limited to immigrants. Second- and even third-generation Americans may experience stress engendered by conflict between ethnic ideology and the ideology of mainstream America. Ethnic identity is formed early in life through interaction with family, peers, and significant others. Therefore, social networks are often composed of members of similar ethnic heritage. However, as Dickerman (1973) points out, to succeed in the United States and become assimilated into mainstream American society, members of minority ethnic groups must often deny much of their ethnic heritage. Ethnically ori-

ented customs, behaviors, beliefs, and values must often be unlearned and replaced by those of mainstream America. Such denial of ethnicity often requires people to disavow affiliation with family and other significant members of their ethnic groups. Dickerman maintains that disavowal of ethnic identity is demanded of all Americans who wish to participate in mainstream society but have not been born into it.

Spindler (1971), while studying the Menominee Indians of the United States, found a relationship between acculturative pressures and stress. He developed five categories that reflect degrees of social, economic, cultural, and psychological adaptation. Each category represents a different lifestyle:

1. Native oriented—continued and heavy identification with the traditional past; traditional values, customs, and social controls predominate
2. Peyote cult—synthesis of Christian and traditional behavior and beliefs
3. Transitional—some aspects of the traditional past and many of the values, attitudes, and practices of the Anglo-American lower class; goals of neither culture are meaningful
4. Lower-strata acculturated—cultural patterns and acquisitions of the Anglo-American working class; little social interaction with native-oriented Indians
5. Acculturated elite—cultural patterns and acquisitions of the Anglo-American middle and upper classes; almost no social interaction with native-oriented Indians

Spindler found that members of the transitional group exhibited free-floating anxiety. In an attempt to cope with their transitional stage of acculturation, many Menominee in this group withdrew from social interaction, consumed excessive amounts of alcohol, or both. Although members of the acculturated groups (lower strata and elite) also exhibited high anxiety, they tended to sublimate it into achievement of socially sanctioned mainstream American goals. In contrast, the native-oriented Menominee exhibited little anxiety, while

---

*Refer to Chapter 17 for a discussion of socially deviant behavior.

the members of the Peyote cult overtly expressed anxiety through Peyote rituals. Spindler's research thus indicates a relationship between culture shock and emotional stress. It also indicates that the way people try to cope with stress engendered by culture shock may be related to upward social mobility and degree of acculturation.

It should not be assumed that acculturation and social mobility *must* destroy ethnic ties. Gordon (1964) believes that while acculturation does occur during upward social mobility, detachment from one's ethnic group in either values or social relationships is not a necessary end result.

Culture shock and hospitalization

The transition from person to patient* may be marked by culture shock. In a total institution, such as a hospital, a significant number of persons are isolated from society, and their lives are organized according to the rules and regulations of a bureaucracy. People in total institutions fall into one of two categories: a large group of supervised inmates or a small group of supervisory staff. Social intercourse and mobility between the two groups are severely limited and usually formally prescribed. Through the bureaucratic management of blocks of people, total institutions try to provide for at least minimal gratification of human needs. A consequence of this enclosed, bureaucratically administered life is the molding of people's personalities and behavior. To change people into inmates (or patients), a total institution must use certain techniques, based on the principles of role loss and humiliation, that are built into its structure. These maneuvers are part of a "stripping process" that breaks down people's self-concepts and lifestyles so that they will more readily fit into the institutional mold (Goffman, 1961).

The stripping process may be facilitated in a number of ways. Such procedures as issuing hospi-

tal gowns, history taking, and confiscating personal belongings all succeed in undermining patients' self-images. Most people view wearing an open-in-the-back gown, even for a short time, as humiliating. Many people feel dehumanized when aides, technicians, nurses, and doctors do not know their names and have to check name tags to be certain they are talking with the right person. Being known by one's name is very important to one's self-image.

In addition, dependency is fostered by such common practices as being confined in bed, being served meals only at specified times, and having to ask for permission or assistance to get out of bed.

The abrupt transition from a familiar social system to an unfamiliar one is fundamental to the culture shock of hospitalization.* The following factors that are inherent in hospitalization may create cognitive dissonance and engender culture shock.

COMMUNICATION

A new language, "hospitalese," must be learned. People are asked if they have "voided." It is explained to patients that they will receive IMs, IVs, or ECT. Even previously familiar expressions may suddenly have different meanings. For example, instead of being an expletive, "S.O.B." stands for "short of breath." In addition, in psychiatric units nurses may or may not wear uniforms, and they may be addressed by their first or their last names. Such informal practices as nurses wearing street clothes and being called by their first names may facilitate nurse-patient communication. However, such informality may confuse some patients about the nurse's role and impede nurse-patient communication.

MECHANICAL ENVIRONMENT

People must become familiar with new mechanical devices and forms of transportation. In a general hospital, patients often must learn to use bedpans and call buttons and must allow themselves,

---

*The term "patient" is used here instead of "client," to denote a passive, acted-upon role.

*Brink and Saunders (1976) have also discussed this transition.

even when ambulatory, to be transported to various parts of the hospital in wheelchairs or on stretchers. Although patients in a psychiatric hospital usually encounter fewer mechanical devices, they may encounter physical restraints. They may also have to become accustomed to various types of surveillance systems, such as grating on windows, locked units, and suicide or escape precautions.

CUSTOMS

To fit into hospital routine, all patients must learn a new life-style. General hospital patients are expected to wear pajamas day and night. Patients in psychiatric hospitals often are not permitted to have access to such sharp objects as razors and mirrors. When to awaken, when to go to sleep, when to visit with family and friends, and when and what to eat are no longer matters of personal choice. While staff members may intrude into patient's domains—their rooms—patients are usually not permitted to enter the staff's domain—the nurse's station.

ISOLATION

Another characteristic of hospitals is the isolation of patients from their families and communities. Visiting hours are often brief (several hours twice a day) and may be scheduled at times when many people are at work. Children often are not allowed in hospital units. In some hospitals, patients do not have private telephones and may only have access to a telephone in the hall. Such a situation not only makes it difficult to place and receive calls but also violates a person's privacy. One's nearest human contact often is a hospital roommate. Roommates may or may not be compatible, and they may be from different social classes or ethnic groups. Thus a patient who views the mixing of socioeconomic and ethnic backgrounds as an invasion of privacy may be even further isolated from social interaction. Newspapers, television, or radio may become the major contacts with the outside world.

ROLE RELATIONSHIPS

Patients have to learn a new role, and it is a socially undesirable one. Our society values assertiveness and independence, but the role of patient is often characterized by dependence and subordination. Doctors, nurses, and aides often assume authority roles. Orders are passed from physicians and nurses to aides and finally to the patient. While staff members may both give and receive orders, the patient often can do only the latter. In addition, during the time that a person is assuming the role of patient, other role relationships—those of parent, spouse, employee, or student—may be temporarily interrupted. Occasionally, role reversals occur. For example, a self-supporting independent father may suddenly have to be cared for by his children.

• • •

An altered communication system, an unfamiliar mechanical environment, different customs, a sense of isolation, and new role relationships are inherent in the experience of hospitalization. These dramatic changes in life-style may create cognitive dissonance and result in culture shock.

During the first days of hospitalization, patients usually ask many questions and inquire into hospital routines. This period corresponds to Oberg's first phase of adaptation to culture shock (1954). In phase two, the disenchantment phase, patients become frustrated with hospitalization and respond with depression, anger, or withdrawal. When they learn the communication system and routines of the hospital, become friendly with staff and other patients, and demonstrate a sense of humor, they are beginning to resolve the culture shock of hospitalization. However, if patients stay in the hospital long enough to resolve culture shock completely, problems may develop. Unless they are in a long-term facility or a nursing home, such an adjustment is counterproductive. They feel ''at home''; they can function comfortably and easily within the framework of the hospital. They thus have become dependent and institutionalized. They are fearful of discharge and unwilling to face the resumption of life outside the hospital.

Culture, cognition, and the practice of nursing

NURSES AND CLIENTS AS MEMBERS OF ETHNIC GROUPS

Each person is born into a culture, and his or her enculturation includes assuming the cognitive system of that culture. It is important to remember that culture is persistent. Through the process of immigration, cultural patterns are transplanted from the country of origin to the new country, and then from the immigrant generation to succeeding generations. Even when a person from one ethnic group has extensive contact with people from other ethnic backgrounds, many of the thought and behavior patterns acquired during childhood persist.

Therefore, in the United States, both nurses and clients are usually influenced not only by the American cultural system but also by the cultural systems of their respective ethnic groups, of which British-Americans, Italian-Americans, German-Americans, Afro-Americans, and Sino-Americans are only a few. As a result of inter-ethnic marriage, some people have a mixture of ethnic heritages.

Ethnic heritage can be very influential.

James and Tony were nursing students. Although both young men had been born in the United States, their grandparents had been born in Europe. James was British-American, and Tony was Italian-American.

During a seminar discussion entitled "The Crying Client," James and Tony evidenced very different reactions. While both young men felt uncomfortable when people cried, James believed it was "unnatural and unmanly" for a man to cry. Tony did not see anything wrong with men crying.

James and Tony were influenced by different ethnic backgrounds. Each young man's ethnically

specific values, beliefs, and standards of behavior were reflected in his attitude about crying. James' British heritage sanctioned stoicism as a reaction to stress. Tony's Italian heritage sanctioned crying both for men and women as a response to stress.

An *attitude* is a verbal or nonverbal stance that reflects innermost convictions about what is good or bad, right or wrong, desirable or undesirable. People's attitudes, which are largely unconscious, are based on value systems that are influenced by their enculturation and on life experiences that are interpreted in terms of that enculturation. Nurses who regard their values, standards, beliefs, and perceptions of reality as absolutes may experience cognitive dissonance when they are confronted with other cultural systems.

After vacationing in the Caribbean, Jeanette decided to move there. Up to that time, she had lived in the northeastern United States. Initially, she was very happy with the move. She rented a house, did a good deal of sight-seeing, and went to the beach every day.

After a few months of becoming acquainted with her new environment, Jeanette began working as a nurse in a local hospital. The hospital was not air conditioned, and Jeanette found the heat oppressive. She could not understand how people could be expected to recuperate under such adverse conditions, and she became impatient with the staff, who thought that the heat was not an adversity. Jeanette also began to realize that her conception of time was different from that of the native population. While the natives viewed time as something flexible and relative and they did not strictly adhere to schedules, Jeanette highly valued adherence to schedules and punctuality. She became increasingly annoyed about "people's inability to be on time," and she began to view the native population as "irresponsible" and "unmotivated."

In addition, Jeanette was unable to reconcile folk healing practices with her belief in the efficacy of modern medicine. She felt that folk medicine was "ridiculous and dangerous."

Jeanette's interaction with a foreign culture resulted in cognitive dissonance and culture shock. The differences in value judgments between her and the native population served as stressors.

Opposing value judgments may also lead to value conflict. In the example of Jeanette, the following incompatible value judgments could constitute value conflict:

1. Jeanette's value judgments
   a. Absence of air conditioning during hot weather is an *unacceptable* situation for the recuperation of clients.
   b. Punctuality is *important*.
   c. Folk medicine is *bad*.
   d. Blending of modern medicine with folk medicine is *undesirable*.
2. Natives' value judgments
   a. Absence of air conditioning during hot weather is an *acceptable* situation for the recuperation of clients.
   b. Punctuality is *unimportant*.
   c. Folk medicine is *good*.
   d. Blending of modern medicine with folk medicine is *desirable*.

The differences between Jeanette's value judgments and those of the native population are what Meux (1980) terms the direct source of value conflict. Factors such as prejudice, concrete thinking, and stress, which may affect the perceptions and understanding of people about the degree of value judgment incompatibility operating in a particular situation, Meux considers direct sources of value conflict. People's value judgments are reflected in their attitudes about what is right or wrong, desirable or undesirable, important or unimportant.

ATTITUDE CLARIFICATION

The practice of nursing involves three levels of exploration: the factual level, the comprehension level, and the attitudinal level. For example, on the factual level a nurse may learn the definitions of defense mechanisms. On the comprehension level, he or she may consider the function of defense mechanisms and may differentiate between the adaptive and maladaptive use of defense mechanisms. On the attitudinal level, a nurse may explore questions such as the following: What do I consider healthy use of defense mechanisms? What do I consider unhealthy use of defense mechanisms? What defense mechanisms do I use? When do I use them? How often do I use them?

It is important that nurses become aware of their own attitudes. They need to understand how ethnic heritage influences attitudes—especially their attitudes about mental health and mental illness. Attitude clarification is one way that nurses may become more aware of their own attitudes. Because attitudes are often unconscious, a nurse may need to work with a colleague or supervisor who can provide objective information about behavior that reflects attitudes and who will assist in the clarification process. Attitude clarification can help nurses develop insight into some of the factors influencing their behavior.

The process of attitude clarification involves exploring alternatives and setting personal priorities. Using the work of Smith (1977) and Uustal (1977), we can identify the following six steps in this process:

1. An attitude should be the nurse's own attitude and not one that the nurse thinks is expected. For example, a nurse may believe that a person has a right to self-determination, even when suicide is a possibility. It is this attitude that needs to be acknowledged and explored, not an attitude that the nurse may believe is more acceptable to colleagues.
2. Alternative attitudes should be identified. If we again use the example of the permissibility of suicide, the following attitudes may be considered: nurses have a moral and/or professional obligation to prevent suicide; a person contemplating suicide is irrational and cannot be allowed to make such an important decision; suicide is sinful.
3. The consequences and significance of an attitude should be explored. What are the legal ramifications of ignoring a communication that indicates the possibility of suicide? What are the personal ramifications? What are the professional ramifications?

4. Personal priorities should be established. For example, does the nurse believe that being self-sufficient makes life worth living and that it is better to be dead than to be disabled, despondent, or dependent? Does the nurse believe that a person has a right to decide when to die?

5. An attitude should be affirmed. An attitude may be communicated to relatives, friends, or colleagues. For example, a nurse might say, "Mr. Jones is terminally ill. He is despondent. If I learned that he was saving pills to use to commit suicide, I would not try to stop him."

6. An attitude should be incorporated into a person's behavioral system. This is the point at which an attitude is acted upon. When the nurse who believes that a person has a right to decide when to die intentionally ignores clues to suicide, the nurse's attitude has been incorporated into his or her behavioral system.

Attitude clarification is an essential component of the practice of mental health nursing. In order for nurses to engage in the therapeutic use of self, they must have a high degree of self-awareness and self-understanding.* Attitude clarification helps nurses develop insight into many factors that influence their behavior. Raths, Harmon, and Simon (1966) have determined that people who are unclear about their own values and beliefs tend to be apathetic, inconsistent, irresponsible, and either compliant or nonconforming. Such behavior creates barriers to therapeutic communication. Attitude clarification helps nurses become more decisive, consistent, and reliable. These characteristics are fundamental to the formation of therapeutic relationships.

Very often nurses and their clients have different and somewhat conflicting attitudes. When these attitudes are radically different, frustration and misunderstandings may result. How often has a nurse tried to refer a client for psychotherapy, only to have the client hold tenaciously to the belief that "shrink therapy" is useless? How often has a nurse been taken aback at the stigma that is still attached to mental illness? The community health nurse who tries to help discharged psychiatric clients make places for themselves in the community is only too well aware of the prejudice that family, friends, neighbors, and employers still have about mental illness. How often has a nurse shaken his or her head in bewilderment over the number of people who spend a small fortune on over-the-counter drugs while condemning drug abuse?

Attitudes among health professionals frequently differ also. How often has a nurse shivered over incidents involving the too readily prescribed tranquilizer—especially in light of current research suggesting cross-addiction between tranquilizers and alcohol? How often has a nurse been astounded to hear colleagues refer disparagingly to persons with psychosomatic or psychoneurotic symptoms as malingerers and complainers? How often has a nurse encountered sexual bias?

Attitudes are deeply ingrained and are influenced by systems of cultural cognition and codification. Attitudes reflect beliefs, values, and standards of behavior. Attitudes are operative in all aspects of life. Thus it is unrealistic to think that nurses can be attitude free and totally objective. Through attitude clarification, however, they can become increasingly aware of their own behavior and less judgmental about others' behavior. Attitude clarification is essential to therapeutic nursing practice.

CHAPTER SUMMARY

The people of the United States come from various ethnic backgrounds. Each ethnic group has its own cultural system. Through the process of enculturation, people learn the conceptual and behavioral systems of their culture. When people from different ethnic backgrounds interact, some degree of acculturation usually occurs.

---

*See Chapter 9 for further discussion of the importance of self-awareness for therapeutic communication.

Because each culture codifies reality in its own way, members of different ethnic groups act upon different premises in behaving and evaluating behavior. Dissimilar culturally coded orientations often engender cognitive dissonance and culture shock. Moving to a foreign country, moving to another neighborhood, or even entering a hospital may precipitate cognitive dissonance and culture shock. Persons experiencing cognitive dissonance and culture shock are vulnerable to mental illness.

Awareness of ethnic differences and their significance enables nurses to understand the cultural dimension of mental health and mental illness. In addition, a nurse's awareness of his or her own attitudes and the influence of ethnic heritage on those attitudes is essential to therapeutic nursing intervention.

REFERENCES

Abelson, R.P.
1968 "Comment: Uncooperative personality variables." In Theories of Cognitive Consistency: A Sourcebook. R.P. Abelson et al. (eds.). Chicago: Rand McNally & Co., pp. 648-651.

Aronson, E.
1968 "Discussion: Commitments about commitment." In Theories of Cognitive Consistency: A Sourcebook. R.P. Abelson et al. (eds.). Chicago: Rand McNally & Co., pp. 464-466.

Barnett, H., et al.
1954 "Acculturation: An explanatory formulation." American Anthropologist 56:973-1002.

Barth, F.
1960 "Introduction." In Ethnic Groups and Boundaries. F. Barth (ed.). Boston: Little, Brown & Co.

Berlyne, D.E.
1960 Conflict, Arousal and Curiosity. New York: McGraw-Hill Book Co.

Blau, P.M.
1964 Exchange and Power in Social Life. New York: John Wiley & Sons, Inc.

Bott, Elizabeth
1957 Family and Social Network. London: Tavistock Publications Ltd.

Brink, P.J., and J.M. Saunders
1976 "Cultural shock: Theoretical and applied." In Transcultural Nursing: A Book of Readings. P.J. Brink (ed.). Englewood Cliffs, N.J.: Prentice-Hall, Inc., pp. 126-138.

Chance, N.A.
1965 "Acculturation, self-identification and personality adjustment." American Anthropologist 67:372-393.

Chesler, P.
1972 Women and Madness. New York: Doubleday & Co., Inc.

Coser, L.A., and B. Rosenberg
1957 Sociological Theory: A Book of Readings. New York: Macmillan, Inc.

Covello, L.
1972 The Social Background of the Italian-American School Child. Totowa, N.J.: Rowman & Littlefield.

Davenport, W.
1961 "The family system of Jamaica." In Working Papers in Caribbean Social Organization. S. Mintz and W. Davenport (eds.). Social and Economic Studies 10(4): 420-454.

Dayton, N.A.
1940 New Facts on Mental Disorders. Springfield, Ill.: Charles C Thomas, Publisher.

Dickerman, M.
1973 "Teaching cultural pluralism." In Teaching Ethnic Studies: Concepts and Strategies. J.A. Banks (ed.). Washington, D.C.: National Council for the Social Studies, pp. 5-25.

Dohrenwend, B., and R. Smith
1962 "Toward a theory of acculturation." Southwestern Journal of Anthropology 18:30-39.

Dominquez, V.R.
1975 From Neighbor to Stranger: The Dilemma of Caribbean Peoples in the United States. Antilles Research Program. New Haven, Conn.: Yale University Press.

Eldersveld, S.J.
1966 Political Parties: A Behavioral Analysis. Chicago: Rand McNally & Co.

Essien-Udom, E.U
1964 Black Nationalism, A Search for an Identity in America. New York: Dell Publishing Co., Inc.

Estes, W.K.
1975 "The state of the field: general problems and issues of theory and metatheory." In Handbook of Learning and Cognitive Processes. W.K. Estes (ed.). Hillsdale, N.J.: Lawrence Erlbaum Associates, Inc., pp. 1-24.

Festinger, L.
1957 A Theory of Cognitive Dissonance. Stanford, Calif.: Stanford University Press.

Frost, I.
1938 "Sickness and immigrant psychoses: Australian and German domestic servants the basis of study." Journal of Mental Science 84:801.

Gambino, R.
1974 Blood of My Blood: The Dilemma of Italian Americans. New York: Doubleday & Co., Inc.

Gans, H.
1962 The Urban Villagers. Glencoe, N.Y.: The Free Press.

Geertz, C.
1957 "Ritual and social change: a Javanese example." American Anthropologist 59:32-54.

Gil, R.M.
1968 The Assimilation and Problems of Adjustment to the American Culture of One Hundred Cuban Refugee Adolescents Attending Catholic and Public High Schools in Union City and West New York, New Jersey, 1959–1966. M.S.W. thesis, New York, Fordham University.

Glazer, N., and D.P. Moynihan
1970 Beyond the Melting Pot. Cambridge, Mass.: The MIT Press.

Goffman, E.
1961 Asylums: Essays on the Social Situation of Mental Patients and Other Inmates. New York: Doubleday & Co., Inc.

Goodenough, W.H.
1961 "Comment on cultural evaluation." Daedalus 90:521-528.

Gordon, M.
1964 Assimilation in American Life. New York: Oxford University Press, Inc.

Graves, T.D.
1967 "Psychological acculturation in a tri-ethnic community." Southwestern Journal of Anthropology 23:337-350.

Greeley, A.W.
1974 Ethnicity in the United States: A Preliminary Reconnaissance. New York: John Wiley & Sons, Inc.

Greeley, A.W., and W.C. McCready
1975 "The transmission of cultural heritages: the case of the Irish and the Italians." In Ethnicity—Theory and Experience. N. Glazer and D.P. Moynihan (eds.). Cambridge, Mass: Harvard University Press.

Heider, F.
1958 The Psychology of Interpersonal Relations. New York: John Wiley & Sons, Inc.

Honigmann, J.J.
1967 Personality in Culture. New York: Harper & Row, Publishers, Inc.

Horowitz, D.L.
1975 "Ethnic identity." In Ethnicity—Theory and Experience. N. Glazer and D.P. Moynihan (eds.). Cambridge, Mass.: Harvard University Press, pp. 111-140.

Hsu, F.L.K.
1970 Americans and Chinese: Reflections on two cultures and their people. Garden City, N.Y.: Doubleday Natural History Press.

Hunt, E., and M. Lansman
1975 "Cognitive theory applied to individual differences." In Handbook of Learning and Cognitive Processes. W.K. Estes (ed.). Hillsdale, N.J.: Lawrence Erlbaum Associates, Inc., pp. 81-110.

Hyman, H.H.
1960 "Reflections on reference groups." Public Opinion Quarterly 24:383-396.

Isaacs, H.R.
1975 Idols of the Tribe: Group Identity and Political Change. New York: Harper & Row, Publishers, Inc.

Isajiw, W.W.
1974 "Definitions of ethnicity." Ethnicity 1:111-124.

James, A.
1977 "Economic adaptations of a Cuban community." Annals of the New York Academy of Science 293: 194-205.

Jordon, N.
1953 "Behavioral forces that are a function of attitudes and of cognitive organization." Human Relations 6:273-287.

Kelman, H.
1961 "Processes of opinion change." In The Planning of Change. W.G. Bennis, K.D. Bennis, and R. Chin (eds.). New York: Holt, Rinehart & Winston.

Kelman, H., and R.M. Baron
1968 "Determinants of modes of resolving inconsistency dilemmas: a functional analysis." In Theories of Cognitive Consistency: A Sourcebook. R.P. Abelson et al. (eds.) Chicago: Rand McNally & Co., pp. 670-683.

Kluckhohn, F., and F. Strodtbeck
1961 Variations in Value Orientations. Evanston, Ill.: Row, Peterson & Co.

Kogan, N., and M.A. Wallach
1964 Risk Taking: A Study in Cognition and Personality. New York: Holt, Rinehart & Winston.

Kretch, D., et al.
1962 Individual in Society. New York: McGraw-Hill Book Co.

Kutsche, P.
1968 "The Anglo side of acculturation." In Spanish-Speaking People in the United States. J. Helm (ed.). Seattle: University of Washington Press, pp. 178-195.

Leighton, A.H., et al.
1963 Psychiatric Disorder Among the Yaruba. Ithaca, N.Y.: Cornell University Press.

Lenski, G.
1961 The Religious Factor. New York: Doubleday & Co., Inc.

Manwaring, D.R.
1961 Render Unto Caesar: The Flag Salute Controversy. Chicago: University of Chicago Press.

McGuire, W.J.
1966 "The current status of cognitive consistency theories." In Cognitive Consistency: Motivational Antecedents and Behavioral Consequents. S. Feldman (ed.). New York: Academic Press, Inc., pp. 2-46.

Merton, R.K., and A. Rossi
1957 "Contributions to the theory of reference group behavior." In Social Theory and Social Structure. R. Merton (ed.). Glencoe, N.Y.: The Free Press.

Meux, M.
1980 "Resolving interpersonal value conflicts." Advances in Nursing Science 2(4):41-69.

Mosley, H.J., and V.A. Clift
1977 "The evaluation of cultural dimensions in the curriculum." Cultural Dimensions in the Baccalaureate Nursing Curriculum. New York: National League for Nursing.

Murphy, J.M.
1962 "Cross-cultural studies of the prevalence of psychiatric disorders." World Mental Health 2:53-65.

Novak, M.
1973 The Rise of the Unmeltable Ethnics: Politics and Culture in the Seventies. New York: Macmillan Publishing Co., Inc.

Oberg, K.
1954 Culture Shock. Indianapolis: The Bobbs-Merrill Co., Inc.

Ogionwo, W.W.
1969 "The adoption of technological innovations in Nigeria: a study of factors associated with adoption of farm practices." Ph.D. thesis, University of Leeds. Cited in The Sociology of the Third World: Disparity and Involvement. J.E. Goldthorpe (ed.). New York: Cambridge University Press, pp. 220-224.

Parenti, M.J.
1965 "Black nationalism and the reconstruction of identity." In Personality and Social Life. R. Endelman (ed.). New York: Random House, Inc.

Pasquali, E.
1982 Assimilation and Acculturation of Cubans on Long Island. Ph.D. dissertation, State University of New York at Stony Brook.

Peterson, J.H.
1972 "Assimilation, separation, and out-migration in an American Indian Group." American Anthropologist 74:1286-1295.

Raths, L.E., M. Harmon, and S.B. Simon
1966 Values and Teaching. Columbus, Ohio: Charles E. Merrill Publishing Co.

Rodriguez, A.
1965 "One of the differential effects of some parameters of balance." Journal of Psychology 6:241-250.

Rogg, E.M.
1974 The assimilation of Cuban exiles: the role of community and class. New York: Aberdeen Press.

Rokeach, M.
1960 The Open and Closed Mind. New York: Basic Books, Inc., Publishers.

Sarna, J.
1978 "From immigrants to ethnics: toward a theory of 'ethnicization.'" Ethnicity 5:370-378.

Scheflen, A., and A. Scheflen
1972 Body Language and Social Order. Englewood Cliffs, N.J.: Prentice-Hall, Inc.

Schneider, L., and S. Lysgaard
1953 The deferred gratification pattern: a preliminary study. American Sociological Review 18:142-149.

Shannon, L.W.
1968 The study of migrants as members of social systems. In Spanish-Speaking People in the United States. J. Helm (ed.). Seattle: Univ. of Washington Press, pp. 34-64.

Sherif, M., and C.W. Sherif
1953 Groups in Harmony and Tension. New York: Harper & Row, Publishers, Inc.
1964 Reference Groups: Exploration into Conformity and Deviation of Adolescents. New York: Harper & Row, Publishers, Inc.

Smith, M.
1977 A Practical Guide to Value Clarification. La Jolla, Calif.: University Associates, Inc.

Smith, M.G.
1973 Afro-American research: a critique. In Work and Family Life: West Indian Perspectives. L. Comitas and D. Lowenthal (eds.). New York: Doubleday & Co., Inc., pp. 273-284.

Spindler, G.
1971 Dreamers Without Power: The Menomini Indians. New York: Holt, Rinehart & Winston.
1977 "Changes and continuity in American core cultural values: an anthropological perspective." In G. DiRenzo (ed.). Social Change and Social Character. Westport, Conn.: Greenwood Press, Inc.

Spindler, L.
1977 Culture Change and Modernization: Mini-Models and Case Studies. New York: Holt, Rinehart & Winston.

Spradley, J.P., and M. Phillip
1972 "Culture and stress: a quantitative analysis." American Anthropologist 4:518-529.

Stedman, M.
1964 Religion and Politics in America. New York: Harcourt, Brace & World, Inc.

Steiner, I.D.
1960 "Sex differences in the resolution of A-B-X conflicts." Journal of Personality 28:118-128.

Szapocznik, J., and W. Kurtiness
1980 "Acculturation, biculturalism and adjustment among Cuban Americans." In Acculturation: Theory, Models and Some New Findings. A.M. Padilla (ed.). Boulder, Colo.: Westview Press, Inc.

Tyhurst, L.
1955 "Psychosomatic and allied disorders." In Flight and Resettlement. H.B.M. Murphy (ed.). Paris: UNESCO.

Uustal, D.
1977 "The use of values clarification in nursing practice." The Journal of Continuing Education in Nursing 8:8-13.

Wallace, A.F.C.
1970 Culture and Personality. New York: Random House, Inc.

Young, M., and P. Willmott
1957 Family and Kinship in East London. London: Routledge & Keegan Paul, Ltd.

Zajonic, R., and E. Burnstein
1965 "The learning of balanced and unbalanced social structures." Journal of Personality 33:153-168.

ANNOTATED SUGGESTED READINGS

Barnett, H., et al.
1954 "Acculturation: an explanatory formulation." American Anthropologist 56:973-1002.
A classic exploration of acculturation, this article develops a theoretical framework that stresses the interaction between cultures in contact and factors that may facilitate or impede acculturation.

Brink, P.J., and J.M. Saunders
1976 "Cultural shock: theoretical and applied." In Transcultural Nursing: A Book of Readings. Englewood Cliffs, N.J.: Prentice-Hall, Inc., pp. 126-138.
This essay explores culture shock as a stress syndrome and the implications for nursing care. The authors discuss such categories as stressors, phases of culture shock, coping behavior, and hospitalization as culture shock.

Dunham, H.W.
1976 "Society, culture and mental disorder." Archives of General Psychiatry 33(2):147-156.
Dunham critically examines theories and hypotheses relating societal and cultural factors to the etiology or precipitation of specific emotional disorders. The author identifies many of the unresolved methodological difficulties involved in such research. The article concludes with a summary of definitive results that relate sociocultural factors to specific mental illnesses.

Marcos, L.R., and M. Alpert
1976 "Strategies and risks in psychotherapy with bilingual patients." American Journal of Psychiatry 133(11): 1275-1281.
The authors examine the effect of bilingualism on psychotherapy. If only one language is used in therapy, a large segment of a client's experience is excluded. If both languages are used in therapy, a client may change languages in an attempt to avoid emotionally laden material. The article concludes that monolingual psychotherapists need to assess the degree of language independence in bilingual clients.

Oberg, K.
1954 Culture Shock. Indianapolis: The Bobbs-Merrill Co., Inc.
In this classic discussion of culture shock, the author explores the nature and phases of culture shock and briefly suggests ways of coping with it.

FURTHER READINGS

Abernethy, V.
1976 "Cultural perspective on the impact of women's changing roles on psychiatry." American Journal of Psychiatry 133:657-666.

Broverman, I.K., et al.
1972 "Sex-role stereotypes." Journal of Social Issues 28:59-78.

Castaneda, C.
1971 A Separate Reality. New York: Simon & Schuster, Inc.

Chesler, P.
1973 "A word about mental health and women." Mental Health 57:5-7.

Fabrega, H.
1974 Disease and Social Behavior. Cambridge, Mass.: The MIT Press.

Favazza, A., and M. Oman
1972 Anthropological and Cross-Cultural Themes in Mental Health. Columbia, Mo.: University of Missouri Press.

Hill, R.
1971 The Strengths of Black Families. New York: Emerson Hall Publishers, Inc.

Jourard, S.
1964 The Transparent Self. New York: Van Nostrand Reinhold Co.

Paredes, J.A., and M.J. Hepburn
1976 "The split brain and the culture-and-cognition paradox." Current Anthropology 17:121-127.

Pasquali, E.
1974 "East meets West: a transcultural aspect of the nurse-patient relationship." Journal of Psychiatric Nursing and Mental Health Services 12:20-22.

Sapir, E.
1963 "Cultural anthropology and psychiatry." In Selected Writings of Edward Sapir in Language, Culture and Personality. D.G. Mandelbaum (ed.). Berkeley, Calif.: University of California Press.

Sizemore, B.A.
1973 "Shattering the melting pot myth." In Teaching Ethnic Studies: Concepts and Strategies. J.A. Banks (ed.). Washington, D.C.: National Council for the Social Studies, pp. 73-101.

Thomas, A., and S. Sillen
1968 Racism and Psychiatry. New York: Oxford University Press, Inc.

Tyler, S.A.
1969 Cognitive Anthropology. New York: Holt, Rinehart & Winston.

Wallace, A.F.C.
1970 Culture and Personality. New York: Random House, Inc.

Westermeyer, J.
1976 Anthropology and Mental Health. Chicago: Aldine Publishing Co.

White, E.H.
1974 Health and the black person: An annotated bibliography." American Journal of Nursing 10:1839-1841.

Wittkower, E.D., and R. Prince
1974 "A review of transcultural psychiatry." In American Handbook of Psychiatry (ed. 2), vol. 2. G. Caplan (ed.). S. Arieti (ed.-in-chief). New York: Basic Books, Inc., Publishers.

Zajonic, R.B.
1968 "Cognitive theories in social psychology." In The Handbook of Social Psychology. G. Lindzey and E. Aronson (eds.). Reading, Mass.: Addison-Wesley Publishing Co., Inc.

CHAPTER 5

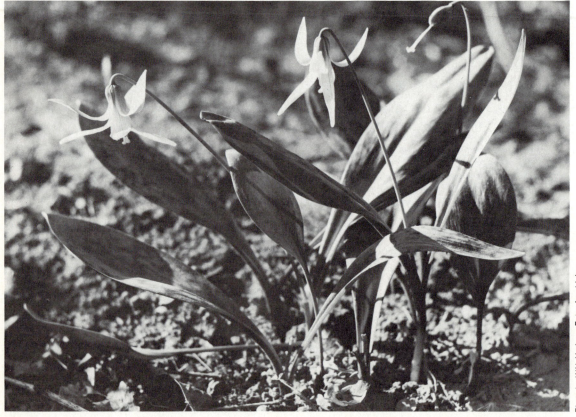

Photo by W.H. Hodge—Peter Arnold, Inc.

The family

CHAPTER FOCUS

Sociocultural factors have great influence on the composition, form, and dynamics of the family. The concept of ''family'' may vary depending on the stage of the developmental cycle that the family occupies and on the interactions, relationships, and organizational patterns among family members.

The family is a system and has the properties of any social system. There is an interrelationship between the family system and the context (physical, social, cultural, and emotional) in which it functions. This interrelationship is one of reciprocal influence.

THE NATURE OF THE FAMILY

The earliest and generally the most effective enculturating agent is the family.* Fundamental to any discussion of the family is a definition of the term ''family.'' Does it refer only to parent(s) and children? Does it include married children and their spouses? Does it encompass grandparents? Aunts and uncles? Cousins? Family friends or significant others?

Definition of the family

Any definition of the family must first shed the assumption that the nuclear family (parents and

*Refer to Chapter 4 for a discussion of the family as an agent of enculturation.

their children) is the basic or universal family form. Rather, when the family is viewed cross culturally, the fundamental relational components seem to be dyadic. Two dyadic relationships, because of their biological correlates, are essential to the formation of the nuclear family and to other family forms. These two relationships are the sexual dyad, which is the reproductive unit of society, and the maternal dyad, which is the temporal linkage between generations. The nuclear family is only one way of combining these two basic dyads. If other kin and other dyads are added to these two basic dyadic relationships, other family forms become recognizable (Adams, 1960). For example, if grandparents are added to the sexual and maternal dyads a three-generation extended family is formed.

An *extended family* encompasses at least three generations of kin. The stem family of Japan (composed of eldest son, his wife and children, and his parents) is an example of an extended family. The extended family has a potentially larger labor force and more options for the division of labor than either the nuclear family or the single-parent family. The extended family may be further characterized as follows:

1. Many adult members to share in child rearing and with whom children may identify
2. Provision of security to aged family members
3. Restricted opportunities for the personal growth of young adult family members because of the authority vested in elders
4. Extended kin support systems during situational and maturational crises (Scheflen and Scheflen, 1972)

In West Indian and Hispanic extended families the bond between mother and child may be very strong and it may be considered primary to all other relationships. Daughters often consider their mothers ''best friends'' and confide in them about problems and conflicts (Smith, 1956; Mintz and Price, 1976; Gilmore, 1980; Pasquali, 1982).

An 18-year-old unmarried Hispanic woman became pregnant. When she confided this to her mother, her mother offered to help her raise the child. During an antepartum examination, the nurse asked the young woman, who was accompanied by her mother, what plans she had made for the baby. When the young woman said her mother was going to help raise the baby, the nurse began to explain that there were other options available, such as placing the baby for adoption. The young woman's mother became very upset and interrupted the nurse by saying, "If you don't love your baby, who do you love? Not yourself. Not your mother. Nobody. Any man who comes to you is gonna say, 'If you don't love your children, you don't love me.' So the men will come and use you and say 'goodbye.'"

The nurse, who was not Hispanic, did not understand the primacy that many Hispanics give to the mother-child relationship. The nurse viewed the mother's behavior as "interfering, domineering, and rude." The nurse became defensive. The young woman rallied to her mother's aid and said to the nurse, "My mother is my best friend. She always has my best interest at heart." The counseling session ended abruptly.

Thus, the importance attached by some ethnic groups to the mother-child bond may not be understood by people with a different orientation to the family unit.

Another family form, at variance with the extended family, is the *nuclear family*. The nuclear family, long regarded by mainstream America as the ''normal'' family form, emerged as an adaptation to the Industrial Revolution. As farms became mechanized and people began working in factories and moving to cities, extended families were no longer an economic necessity. A nuclear family consists of a man, a woman, and their children. The nuclear family may be characterized as follows:

1. Many opportunities for the personal growth of children and young adults
2. Few adults who share in child rearing and with whom children can identify
3. Non-kin support systems during times of crisis
4. Inadequate extended family support systems during periods of situational or maturational crisis (Scheflen and Scheflen, 1972)

Another increasingly common family form is the *single-parent* family. Almost 7% of all American families are single-parent families, and most of these single-parent families (6.2%) are headed by women (Bureau of Labor Statistics, 1977). In the single-parent family, the sexual dyad that produced the children was temporary in nature either because it was not sanctioned by marriage or because the marriage was terminated by death or divorce. Sometimes the sexual dyad may be unrelated to the maternal or paternal dyad, as when a single woman or man adopts a child. The single-parent family, while offering many opportunities for the personal growth of children, may present some of the following difficulties:

1. The parent may look to the child for emotional support.
2. The child may manipulate separated parents, playing one against the other.
3. The child may become the pawn of separated parents.
4. The child may have to deal with evidences of the parent's sexuality (for example, affairs, live-ins).
5. The child may form positive relationships with parental lovers and then have to deal with feelings of loss when the lovers leave (Meagher, 1980; Critchley, 1981).

On the opposite end of the continuum from the single-parent family is the omnigenous (or "blended") family. The term *omnigenous family* refers to the family formed when parents divorce and remarry. Since many people divorce and remarry more than once, a complex kinship system of relatives and steprelatives may develop. An array of alliances and interpersonal relationships of differing meaning and intensity may also evolve. The strengths and weaknesses of an omnigenous family are not very different from those of the extended family (Tiger, 1978; Jordheim, 1980).

The basic forms of family organization differ in their potential for meeting the needs of their members. The extended family and the omnigenous family provide members with security. Children benefit from the collective presence of many adults, who help to rear them and who serve as role models. However, since age usually carries respect and the exercise of family authority, younger members may live out much of their lives under the supervision of elders. Therefore, in extended and omnigenous families, security is sometimes gained at the expense of personal growth. Nuclear and single-parent families usually encourage and facilitate the individual development of their young members. However, nonfamily relationships and occupational bonding tend to compete

with and weaken family ties. Relationships with extended kin are often inadequate. Consequently, during periods of maturational or situational crisis, family members may not receive necessary support or security. For instance, during a divorce, parents may be distraught and unable to offer their children adequate emotional support. At the same time, the children may be physically and affectionally estranged from relatives who could serve as a support system. Aunts and uncles might live many miles away and grandparents may be isolated in a nursing home. Therefore, in the nuclear or single-parent family, opportunity for personal development is sometimes gained at the expense of security.

Just as the definition of the family should not be restricted to the nuclear family but should be flexible enough to include kin that people regard as "family," the word "kin" does not refer only to people related by consanguinal or affinal bonds but also to fictive kin. *Fictive kin* are usually regarded as "just like family."

A Cuban client told a nurse: "This woman is not really my mother, but I call her Mamá Jolie. She and my mother were close friends all of their lives. They were always together, and this woman became like a mother to me. On Mother's Day, I always visit my mother and Mamá Jolie. Now that Mamá Jolie is ill and her children live in Cuba, I am the only daughter she has. I will help care for her when she leaves the hospital."

Fictive kinship is usually established through coparentage (godparentage) of a child or by longtime and close friendship with the entire family (Harris, 1956; Hutchinson, 1957; Miller, 1967; Pasquali, 1982). Fictive kinship binds people together in ties of affection and concern as well as in a sense of obligation, responsibility, and expectation concerning loyalty and exchanges of goods and services. Fictive kinship thus establishes a sense of relatedness among people unrelated by ties of consanguinity or affinity, and it helps people to adapt to their environmental conditions and changes (Stack, 1974; Gubrium and Buckholdt, 1982; Pasquali, 1982). For example, among the acquaintances of the elderly, there is often a sense of relatedness that enables them to establish confidant relationships and that serves as a support network or quasi-family. This quasi-family functions as a buffer against problems that the elderly may experience concerning aging and institutionalization (Lowenthal and Havens, 1968; Butler and Lewis, 1982).

In addition to discussing the various forms that the family may take and the members that it may encompass, when defining the family we also need to consider what stage of the domestic cycle the family occupies. Fortes (1958) has specified three phases in the domestic cycle: expansion, fission, and replacement. These stages are progressive and often overlap each other. Expansion begins with marriage and continues until completion of the natal family. It is physiologically limited by a woman's period of fertility, and it is structurally limited to the time when offspring are economically and jurally dependent on their parents. Davenport (1961) and Ashcraft (1966) argue that with some groups (for example, lower-class West Indian households), the period of expansion is extended beyond a woman's period of fertility. By absorbing children, such as grandchildren, the domestic group expands long after menopause has occurred. The next phase, fission, starts when the first child marries or leaves home and lasts until all children are married or leave home. This phase is sometimes called the "empty nest." However, because of economic problems, divorce, or other disruptive factors, adult children may return to the parental home after having left. This "refilled nest" often contributes to conflict in the family system and a need to renegotiate roles. Replacement begins when the first child establishes a family and continues as each succeeding child establishes a family. Replacement ends with the death of the ancestral parental pair. The children's families thereby take their place in society—a place vacated by the deceased parental pair. The domestic group thus goes full cycle.

Family versus household

Residents of a household may or may not be united by bonds of kinship. Also, members of a family may reside in different households. For example, after parents are divorced, children and their mother often live in one household while the children's father lives in another household.

Solien (1960) defines a household as a group of people bound together by common residence, economic cooperation, and the task of child rearing. A household is *not* concerned with the function of procreation. This is a function of the family. In those instances when family and household do not coincide, the household needs to be viewed as a separate but extremely influential adjunct or alternative to the family.

One type of household is a *commune*. Communal living is not new in the United States. The nineteenth century saw the rise of more than 200 communes. Many of these early Americans were participating in a life-style that violated the norm of monogamous family life. However, while a few communes, notably those of the Shakers, insisted on celibacy, most other religious communes have sanctioned monogamy. In secular communes, "free love" is often practiced. In both religious and secular communes, labor and money are usually shared among members (Jordheim, 1980).

Today communes are one way to collectively raise children. Commune participants share the bonding that sometimes becomes burdensome in nuclear and single-parent families. Bettleheim (1969) found that in communes, such as the Israeli kibbutz, children are bonded to their commune rather than to their parents.

Another type of household may be formed by cohabiting heterosexual couples. Macklin (1974) defines cohabitation as unmarried people sharing bed and board for a minimum of 4 nights a week and for at least 3 consecutive months. Cohabiting couples usually share household tasks and expenses. Often cohabitation is referred to as trial marriage, but Macklin found that the majority of cohabiting couples did not consider marriage a viable alternative to their present living arrangement. However, many cohabiting couples view themselves and their mates as being like spouses. They share bonds of affection and concern, and they have a sense of obligation, responsibility, and expectation concerning loyalty and exchange of goods and services. In these instances, cohabiting couples may be regarded as fictive kin rather than as unrelated people (Sedgwick, 1981).

Still another type of household may be formed by homosexuals. According to some social scientists (for example, Hoffman, 1968; Saghir and Robbins, 1973), lesbian dyads tend to be more stable than male homosexual dyads. In addition, many homosexual households include children. Often two gay partners live together with their children from a heterosexual relationship.

A homosexual orientation does not mean that people can not be dependabe, nurturing parents or that children raised by homosexual parents will become homosexual. The incidence of children living with their homosexual parent and their parent's partner seems to be greater among lesbian mothers than among gay fathers. Gay fathers seem to more frequently remain in their marriages while engaging in homosexual relationships than do lesbian mothers (Jordheim, 1980).

Thus, the definition of the family and the difference between the family and the household need to be considered when the nature of the family is examined. Social organization is flexible enough to permit different forms of the family to coexist in different parts of the world and even in different subsystems of the same society. Each of these different family forms may serve different functions and fill different needs of individuals and society. It is important for nurses working with families to include all the people that the client-family regards as family and to be aware of the cultural relativity of family form.

Functions of the family

A family system is more than a collection of actual or fictive kin. The concept of "family" includes interactions, relationships, and functional and organizational patterns that strive to effectively meet the needs of family members and the expectations of society. Family functions refer to what the family does; these functions include economic cooperation, procreation, child rearing (including socialization and enculturation), and the growth and development of family members. The family is further involved in information gathering, decision making, conflict resolution, and the promotion of acceptance, authenticity, trust, and cooperation among family members (Adams, 1960; Sedgwick, 1981). The emphasis given to family functions and the way that family functions are implemented will vary from culture to culture. The mental health status of individual family members is believed to reflect the level of family functioning.

It is important to view the *context* in which a family functions—in other words, the family's physical, social, cultural, and emotional environments. Context includes the nation, the state, and the neighborhood in which the family lives, the social institutions (for example, schools, churches, and organizations) with which it interacts, the social networks with which it relates, and the cultural, racial, and socioeconomic orientations of the family. The interaction between family and context is characterized by reciprocal influence: the context influences the family and the family influences the context. The degree of a family's involvement with or isolation from its context affects the family's ability to exert as much influence on its *total* environment as the environment exerts on the family. The environment may be especially influential in such areas of family functioning as exchange of ideas; incorporation of norms, expectations, and attitudes; effectiveness of support systems; and direction of goals (Sedgwick, 1981).

Five years ago, families A and B both moved from Korea to the United States. Family A moved into a Korean enclave. They share an apartment with already settled extended family members. All the adults in family A work at two jobs. They do not socialize with their neighbors. Because there are no adults at home when the children return from school, the children are told to stay in the apartment, to do their homework, and to complete household chores. They are not permitted to go out to play or to invite other children into the apartment. The members of family A have few friends in the neighborhood, have much difficulty speaking English, and have learned little about American norms and attitudes.

In contrast, Family B moved into an integrated Korean-American neighborhood. Although all the adults in family B work at two jobs, they have arranged their days off so that an adult is always home when the children return from school. The children in family B play with both Korean and American children, and the adults in family B have made friends with many of the parents of these children. The members of family B are conversant in English, and they have learned enough about American norms and attitudes to decide which are compatible with their life-style and which are not.

Thus, the effective functioning of the family is dependent on the relationship between the family and its context.

FAMILY PROCESS

Family theory

The models that family theorists use to study the operation of the family can be categorized as follows: (1) structural-functional analysis, (2) interactional analysis, (3) developmental analysis (Jones and Dimond, 1982).

The *structural-functional model* views the family as an open social system and explores the relationships between the family and other social institutions. For example, the contribution of status-role functions of family members to the maintenance of the family system may be examined. Individual family members are seen as reactive, rather than as action-initiating; they behave according to the demands or constraints of the family

system. In turn, the family system is viewed as a passive adaptor, rather than as a change-initiating agent, that functions to maintain the broader social system (Nye and Berardo, 1966; Sprey, 1969; Spindler, 1977; Adams, 1980).

In contrast to the structural-functional model, which looks at the functions of individual family members in family system maintenance, the *interactional model* focuses on the interacting personalities and interaction patterns of individual family members. The structural-functional model approaches the family as an open system and examines the relationships between the family and other social institutions, while the interactional model views the family as a self-contained unit. In the interactional model, the family system is analyzed by looking at the internal functioning of the family, such as its processes of communication, conflict resolution, and decision making (Hill and Hanson, 1960).

Like the two previous models, the *developmental model* focuses on individual family members. The family is viewed as an open social system. Within the context of the family, individual members are seen as holding dyadic positions (for example, wife-mother, daughter-sister). Norms prescribe acceptable role behavior, and changes in role behavior are studied over time. According to the developmental model, the needs and tasks of the family vary according to the phase of the developmental cycle it is in. The role behavior of family members fulfilling these needs and tasks is the focus of study. This analysis of family role behavior is conducted on three levels.

1. Alterations in the developmental tasks and role expectations of *children*
2. Alterations in the developmental tasks and role expectations of *parents*
3. Alterations in the developmental tasks of the *family unit* in response to cultural influences at various phases of the developmental cycle of the family (Jones and Dimond, 1982)

Each of the three family theory models focuses on the *health* of family systems. Nurses involved in primary prevention of family dysfunction need

Table 5-1. Comparison of family theory models

Family theory model	Boundaries of the family system	Unit of analysis	Focus of analysis
Structural-functional	Open	Individual family members	Relationships between the family and other social institutions
Interactional	Closed	Individual family members	Internal functioning of the family
Developmental	Open	Individual family members	Role behavior of family members over time

to be knowledgeable about family theory in order to accurately assess family dynamics and to promote optimal family functioning (Jones and Dimond, 1982). (See Table 5-1.)

Application of family theory to family process

The family is a dynamic system of interrelated parts that form a whole. As was previously pointed out, the family system includes members and their relationships with one another and with their physical, social, cultural, and emotional environments.

THE FAMILY SYSTEM

To understand the family as a system, one must have an understanding of general systems theory.

▶ Properties of systems

Central to all systems are the properties of *interrelatedness, flow of information,* and *feedback.* Any system, including a family system, must be able to interrelate with and incorporate a "full flow" of three categories of information in order to sustain effective functioning. These three categories are as follows:

1. External information—data concerning conditions outside the system, such as the nature of socioeconomic conditions (for example, an economic recession or political oppression) or the quality of support systems

2. Historical information—data of a historical nature that affects the system, such as a family rule that the present be interpreted in terms of the past or the interaction patterns of the families of orientation of one's parents

3. Internal information—data concerning conditions within the system, such as the existence of ambiguous or double-bind communication patterns among family members or the feeling of family members that they are trapped by the family (Buckley, 1967)

In turn, these three categories of information are used for feedback. Positive feedback facilitates change within a system, while negative feedback promotes system stability. For example:

1. Anticipated information: external information of an expected nature is fed back into the system and reinforces the system's stability or balance (an example of negative feedback).

2. Learning: new external information is fed back into the system and is used to alter the structure of the system (an example of positive feedback).

3. Self-awareness: new information about conditions within the system is fed back into the system and alters those conditions (an example of positive feedback).

Feedback thus has a regulatory function. It serves to monitor, reinforce, and correct the structure and conditions of the system. Because of feedback, change in any part of the family system affects the entire family. For example, when a family seeks counseling for one member (the identified client), positive feedback of two types, *learning* and *self-awareness,* is used not only to alter the behavior of the identified client but also to alter the structure and functioning of the family system.

Another property of any system, including a family system, is *homeostasis.* Homeostasis refers to the maintenance of equilibrium or to a steady state of balance. Many social scientists hold that because of the many forces of dysfunction and change that affect social systems, social systems are continuously in a state of flux and can only be in relative balance (Spindler, 1977). This state of flux and relative balance is referred to as *homeodynamics.*

Like other social systems, a family system continuously strives for homeostasis. Often the balance within a family system incorporates the pathological conditions of its members. According to Jackson (1957), when the behavior or condition of an identified client improves, it is not uncommon for another family member to experience an emotional or psychophysiological problem. This see-sawing of members evidencing dysfunction helps to maintain a family equilibrium.

When a family directs most of its energy into the maintenance of family equilibrium, there is little residual energy to channel into personal or family development. For example, in a family system that does not permit dissension, much energy is directed toward maintaining harmony among family members and hiding instances of family dissension from people outside the family.

The Anderson family almost always presented a united, harmonious appearance. The parents never disagreed with each other in front of the children, and they rarely disagreed in private. Neither the children nor the parents ever raised their voices to each other. If the children began to misbehave, a stern look from the mother would curtail the misbehavior. On the rare occasions that dissension in the family did occur, the Andersons pretended it did not exist.

One such instance of dissension happened

when Mrs. Anderson's brother, who had lived with the Andersons, died. Mr. Anderson had long resented the close relationship between Mrs. Anderson and her brother, a relationship that made Mr. Anderson feel "like an outsider in my own home." Thus, when Mrs. Anderson's brother died, Mr. Anderson did not attend the funeral. At the funeral, both Mrs. Anderson and the Anderson children acted as if nothing were amiss. Relatives noticed that Mr. Anderson was not at the funeral, and they wondered why, but no one, including Mrs. Anderson's sister, inquired for fear of "upsetting" Mrs. Anderson.

Obviously, the Anderson family used much energy to maintain an appearance of harmony and to mask dissension. Relatives facilitated and participated in this masking.

▶ Boundaries and boundary maintenance

Every system, including the family system, has boundaries. These boundaries may be distinct or ambiguous, flexible or rigid. In a social system, boundaries identify differences between social groups and maintain the distinctiveness of groups. Various forces may function as boundary-maintaining mechanisms (Spindler, 1977). Family secrets and family suspiciousness of people outside the family are examples of boundary maintenance mechanisms in a family system. The degree of boundary flexibility and boundary maintenance affects the way that a family system interacts with other social systems:

1. It defines who is entitled to family membership and who must remain outsiders
2. It determines the degree of differentiation permitted between family members and outsiders and the amount of emotional involvement that family members should invest in the family
3. It defines the frequency and types of extra-familial experiences available to family members and the criteria that should be used to evaluate extra-familial experiences (Hess and Handel, 1967)

The degree of openness (characterized by flexible boundaries and little boundary maintenance) or closedness (characterized by rigid boundaries and much boundary maintenance) also regulates the adaptability of the family system to its environment. Open family systems tend to be elastic in their interactions with other social systems and thus have a broad scope of adaptability. In contrast, closed family systems tend to be rigid in their interactions with the social environment and to ignore or misinterpret any input that comes from outside the family system. This interaction pattern severely restricts the family's scope of adaptability. Barnett et al. (1954) believe that the openness or closedness of social systems (of which the family is one) is related to the following factors: (1) multiple vs. single avenues of prestige and goal attainment, (2) well-defined vs. vague interpersonal relationships, (3) egalitarian vs. authoritarian social controls, (4) achieved vs. ascribed status, (5) situationally defined vs. prescribed activities, (6) alternative patterns vs. singularly specified patterns of behavior, and (7) the nature of self-corrective mechanisms.

Self-corrective mechanisms enable a social system to alter its functioning and to adapt internally. These adjustive mechanisms permit social systems, like the family, to counteract disruptive tendencies in society and to maintain equilibrium. Self-corrective mechanisms include such institutionalized measures of social control as force, enculturation techniques,* and socially sanctioned opportunities to relax restrictive rules (for example, socially approved occasions for role turnabout or for the display of competition between family members). Self-corrective mechanisms act to resolve conflict and to stabilize a social system.

---

*Refer to Chapter 4 for a discussion of enculturation.

The aforementioned Anderson family used most of its energy to maintain family equilibrium. The family interacted with the social environment predominantly as a unit. Family members had a few acquaintances but no friends, and the family rarely socialized with relatives. Mr. and Mrs. Anderson discouraged their children from having friends because "the behavior of other children is a bad influence. When they (our children) come home from playing with other children, we have to brainwash them into the right way to behave." Relatives were only permitted to talk to the Anderson children about activities and things, never about ideas, feelings, or relationships. Mr. and Mrs. Anderson feared that relatives might express opinions that were different from theirs and thereby influence the children in a direction other than the one set by the parents.

When the oldest Anderson daughter turned sixteen, she convinced her parents to let her have a party at home. She invited many of her classmates. Some of these classmates smuggled beer into the party and smoked cigarettes. Mr. and Mrs. Anderson were very upset by the behavior of these few teenagers. The Anderson parents used the incident to justify to themselves and to their daughter that to have friends would expose her to "bad influences."

Authoritarian parental controls, prescribed activities and behavior patterns, and such self-corrective mechanisms as the socialization of the Anderson children to view people outside the nuclear family as bad influences created within the Anderson family a rigid family structure that counteracted social influences inconsistent with the family's approach to life. Although equilibrium in the Anderson family was maintained through the use of self-corrective mechanisms, the types of self-corrective mechanisms that the family used restricted the family's ability to adapt to their social environment.

It should be noted that there are no completely open or completely closed family systems. Even the rigidly bound Anderson family interacted with outsiders when its members attended school, shopped for groceries, went to work, and so on.

▶ Family structure and role relationships

As with any social system, a family system operates according to rules and statuses. These rules and statuses usually, but not always, influence people to behave in a predictable fashion. It is on the basis of rules and statuses that roles are assigned (Spindler, 1977). For example, because parents usually have dominant status over young children, parents usually assume the roles of authority figures in the family. Family energy is directed toward helping members fulfill the roles that are essential for effective functioning of the family. Yet within any particular family, role assignments tend to be flexible and to change in order to reflect the stage of the developmental cycle that the family occupies (Fleck, 1972).

Factors such as illness or unemployment may interfere with family members' desire or ability to fulfill allocated roles. In such instances, role conflict and family disequilibrium may develop. Parental roles usually reflect the male-female division of labor in society (Fleck, 1972). Traditionally, in American society, husband-fathers have been instrumentalists (task oriented), while wife-mothers have been nurturers (Parsons, 1955). However, in contemporary American society, many men and women are renegotiating these traditional roles. During the period of renegotiation, role conflict and family disequilibrium may occur.

Role conflict may also be found in other areas of family life. Role reversal may occur, and this role reversal may produce role conflict. For example, aged and infirm parents, who are no longer physically or economically able to care for themselves, may have to rely on their children's assistance. In such situations, the roles of nurturer and provider, which are usually carried out by parents, are assumed by the children. Role reversal may also occur in times of social change, as when people immigrate to a new country.

When the Montaño family immigrated to the United States from Cuba, the family constellation consisted of Mr. and Mrs. Montaño, their 6-year-old son, their 5-year-old son, and Mrs. Montaño's parents. At the time of immigration, no one in the family spoke English. The adult Montaños had difficulty learning English. However, their sons, who at-

tended school with Americans, not only learned English but also learned many American customs. The children served as agents of acculturation and as translators for their parents and grandparents. At the age of seven, one son acted as a translator during such major family transactions as the purchase of a car and the signing of a business lease. Mrs. Montaño told a neighbor, "They (the children) know that we need them, not they need us."

Except for instances of role reversal, parents and other significant adults usually serve as role models for children.

▶ Power in the family

Power refers to the ability to act, to do, and to control others, while *authority* refers to the right to use power to command behavior, enforce rules, and make decisions (Leininger, 1979; McFarland and Shiflett, 1979; Votaw, 1979). In a family, authority is often based on the rank or position of members in the family hierarchy. For example, the mother and the father usually exercise absolute authority over young children, but, in the parents' absence, adolescent children may be "left in charge" of their younger siblings. Authority is thus delegated by the parents to the next in family rank.

At various stages of the developmental cycle of the domestic group, power in the family may need to be redistributed and diffused among family members in order to avoid a power struggle. For example, when children grow into adolescence, they usually want to assume some of the power held by their parents. Later in the developmental cycle, if adult children remain in or move back to the family home or if grandparents move in with the family, power and authority may again need to be redistributed. There may be times, however, when family members give ambiguous messages about the redistribution of power.

When their children were young, Mr. and Mrs. Johnson held all the power in the family and they exer-

cised it authoritatively. As their children approached adolescence, the parents encouraged their children to call them by their first names and to express opinions openly. Mr. and Mrs. Johnson told the children that they were the equals of adults and should not acquiesce in the opinions of adults simply because they were adults. Yet the Johnsons continued to unilaterally set curfews for their children and to have the final say about whom the children could date and when and where the children could go on dates.

When power is unambiguously redistributed, it provides opportunity for the personal growth of family members. Failure to redistribute power or the ambiguous redistribution of power may engender power struggles, limit the opportunities for personal growth of family members denied a share of family power, and otherwise act as a stressor in the family system. Unless the family finds another level on which to operate, family relationships may be endangered (Jackson, 1965).

Although power is a dynamic in all families, different orientations toward power may be evidenced by different families and even among different members of the same family. McClelland (1975) has categorized power orientations, ranking them from stage I to stage IV. Stage IV behavior is indicative of more social and emotional maturity than is stage I behavior. However, extremism in any stage may be pathological.

Stage I: "I am strengthened by others." Individuals rely on others for strength. If an association with a perceived powerful person is terminated, an individual may experience a loss of control and become hysterical or become dependent on food, drugs, or religion.

Stage II: "I can strengthen myself." Individuals gain a sense of power by exerting control over their bodies (for example, by becoming involved in exercise programs or self-awareness programs) or by amassing material possessions. Extremism in this stage may be exhibited through obsessive-compulsive behavior.

Stage III: "I can control others." Individuals obtain a sense of power by competing with, manipulating, or outsmarting others. The object is to dominate others. If carried to an extreme, people may engage in crime, personal violence, or smother love in order to gain control over others.

Stage IV: "I am influenced by others to carry out my obligations." An individual may subordinate his or her own desires and views to those of a higher authority. In the extreme, a person may be unable to differentiate between his or her personal desires and views and those of a higher authority. Such behavior is known as "messianism."

These categories of power orientation can be applied to power in the family. For example, the powerful person in stage I may be an authoritative parent on whom other family members totally depend. In stage IV, the higher authority on which decisions are based may be the "good of the family" or "the good of the children."

Sometimes a family member who nominally holds power is not the actual power holder. For example, the members of a family might say that the father is the authority figure, but a family therapist might observe that the mother is the family disciplinarian and decision maker. In this instance, the father *nominally* holds power but the mother *actually* holds power. In another family, the parents might consider themselves family authority figures when, in actuality, the children wield power by manipulating their parents.

CULTURAL INFLUENCES ON FAMILY PROCESS

The United States is a culturally plural society; it consists of people from various ethnic and religious groups. Culture influences the values, ideology, behavior, and life-style not only of immigrants but of second-, third-, and fourth-generation ethnic Americans as well (McGoldrick, 1982).

In the United States, the mass media, especially television, are extremely influential in the formation of people's impressions and attitudes about the world around them. Seal (1983), who has investigated the effects of television on children, believes that television is an important socializing agent, often rivaling parents and the school. An average child watches 4 to 6 hours of television a day. The effects of television are different for children than for adults. While most adults can differentiate between the play-acting world of television and the real world, children often cannot. Young children have difficulty distinguishing between the fantasy that is depicted in many children's programs and reality. As an example, Seal (1983) tells about a youngster who was asked if *Sesame Street*'s Big Bird is real. The child answered, "No, that's a costume. Under the costume is a real bird."

Adolescents also are influenced by television viewing. According to Seal (1983), they watch, almost exclusively, adult programs and believe that these programs depict reality. Two factors contribute to the credibility that adolescents give to television programs: (1) adolescents have limited life experience with which to compare the world depicted by television, and (2) television programing has the sanction of adults (the parents who allow and often encourage them to watch television and the adults who develop the shows) (Seal, 1983).

Through television viewing, children and adolescents learn to accept ethnic stereotypes. They incorporate into their self-systems stereotypes about the beliefs, customs, rituals, occupations, behaviors, and family forms of various ethnic groups. These ethnic stereotypes are usually disparaging, demeaning, and based on erroneous information (Seal, 1983). For example, the family ethics of Italian-Americans includes the importance of hard work, saving, self-sacrifice, and investing in real estate (including ownership of one's own home). Yet the stereotype often presented by the media is that Italian-American men are uneducated manual laborers who engage in domestic violence against their wives and children and that Italian-American women are uneducated domestic "slaves" to their families (Gambino, 1983).

Studies have shown that, in addition to stereotyping ethnic groups, television rarely presents positive images of them. Also, in the decade of 1971 to 1981, blacks and Hispanics experienced a decline in their representation in television programing, while the representation of white Anglo-Saxon types increased. This situation contributes to (1) a homogenization that ignores the diversity in values, attitudes, and beliefs of different ethnic groups in the United States; (2) a decrease in the exposure of the viewing public to the language patterns, dress, foods, family forms, and other behaviors of ethnics, and (3) a paucity of ethnic role models. As a result, the nuclear family is usually depicted on television as the "normal" family form, and ethnic family role models are missing, misrepresented, or disparaging (Miller, 1978; Seggar, Haffen, and Hannonen-Gladden, 1981; Seal, 1983; Gambino, 1983).

Because many health professionals, including nursing students and nurses, have incorporated ethnic stereotyping into their self-systems, it is important to become aware of these stereotypes and to understand the way in which culture influences family life, family behavior, and family process.

The way in which a person conceives of his or her environment (the person's system of cognition*) may be thought of as a map. People from different cultures have different cultural maps. This fact offers an explanation for differences in cultural behavior and for differences in conceptualizations of the family. The degree of agreement or disagreement between different cultural groups about the images, meaning, and priority given to the family is sometimes used as an index of the psychocultural distance between groups. For example, Szalay and Maday (1983) found that there is greater similarity, and thus less psychocultural distance, in the perceptions that black and white Americans have about the family than there is between whites and Hispanic-Americans or between blacks and Hispanic-Americans. Therefore, it

---

*See Chapter 4 for a discussion of culture and cognition.

should not be assumed that all minority groups have similar orientations toward the family. For example, black Americans include a broad network of relatives and friends-like-family in their definition of the family (Kennedy, 1980). Chinese-Americans extend their definition of the family to include ancestors and all their descendants, and these descendants may be very influential in child rearing (Hsu, 1970; McGoldrick, 1982).

A Chinese-American client explained to a community health nurse that when the American young couples in her neighborhood become ill, the grandparents often come to help out with the children. However, the grandparents are supposed to follow the rules of the house and not undermine the way in which the young couples have been raising their children. "With Chinese it is different. When grandparents visit, they can do anything they want with their grandchildren, even if it means going against the rules laid down by the parents. If Chinese parents should object to the overindulgence of the grandparents, they would be ridiculed, not sympathized with, by others. The same thing is true for the way that Chinese aunts and uncles care for their nephews and nieces."

Italian-Americans achieve identity as individuals through their roles, rights, and responsibilities in the family. The Italian-American family, therefore, provides its members not only with a sense of security but also with a sense of identity (Gambino, 1983).

In addition to ethnicity, social class may contribute to differences in family orientation. For example, families who occupy the middle socioeconomic stratum of American society tend to encourage self-expression and verbalization of differences among family members. However, families who occupy the lower socioeconomic stratum often have a ''nonintrospective orientation'' and they do not encourage verbalization of feelings. This is especially true for male family members

(Goode, 1964; Grey, 1969; Kohn, 1977).

Culture also influences the definition of life-cycle phases of individual family members. For instance, among Mexican-Americans, early and middle childhood usually encompasses a more protracted period of time than is customary among mainstream Americans. Mexican-American adolescence tends to cover a shorter period of time than does mainstream American adolescence. Moreover, among Mexican-Americans, middle age covers a larger block of time, permeating into what mainstream Americans define as old age.

Life-cycle rites of passage are also subject to cultural influence. For instance, among Cuban-Americans, a girl's fifteenth birthday signifies her social transition from girlhood to womanhood. The occasion is marked by a *fiesta de quince años* (fifteenth birthday party), at which the *quince años* girl is presented to that segment of society that constitutes the family's meaningful social relationships (James, 1977; Pasquali, 1982). Likewise, among Jewish-Americans, when a child turns thirteen, a bar (bas) mitzvah marks the social and religious transition from childhood to adulthood. Among Irish-Americans, death is seen as one of the most significant life-cycle transitions and they therefore stress wakes, while among Italian-Americans, marriage is an extremely important life cycle transition and they emphasize weddings (McGoldrick, 1982).

Cultural differences also influence the boundaries between families and the community. Hispanic-American families tend to have flexible boundaries. This boundary flexibility may be evidenced in child lending among Puerto Ricans (McGoldrick, 1982) or in preparing enough food so that unexpected guests may be invited to dinner among Cubans (Pasquali, 1982). For example, a Cuban woman told a nurse, ''The difference between Cubans and Americans is, if my child is in an American home at dinnertime, they send her home. If their child is in my house at dinnertime, I ask her to stay for dinner.'' In contrast to the flexible family boundaries of Hispanic-Americans, Italian-American and Greek-American families tend to have rigid boundaries. Although Italians may incorporate friends of long and close association into the family, the boundary between the family and "outsiders" is usually rigid. The rigid family boundaries among Greeks partially reflect Greek emphasis on the "blood line" and tend to discourage the adoption of children (McGoldrick, 1982).

All of the aforementioned differences in orientation toward the family demonstrate the significant role played by culture. Middlefort (1980) explains that it is not unusual for a subsystem in a family to assume dominance. When the cultural subsystem dominates family life, there may be a lack of individuation and an emphasis on one's relationship to and responsibility for the family. When the psychological subsystem dominates family life, the individual is stressed and the influence of the family on the individual is weakened. The individual's independence from the natal family may then be viewed as a goal and as an indication of emotional maturity. Middlefort believes that most psychotherapists view the psychological subsystem as the dominant subsystem in the family and ignore the cultural subsystem. Psychotherapists therefore espouse the importance of individuals achieving independence from the family hierarchy and especially from their parents. This apporach may not be appropriate for families in which the dominant family subsystem is the cultural.

GENOGRAMS

Construction of a genogram is one way for nurses to tap into the process of the family system over time. A genogram is an outgrowth of the genealogies that anthropologists have long used to learn about family relationships. Genograms depict family relationships over at least three successive generations.

Social scientists, such as Guerin and Pendagast (1976), have developed guidelines for the construction of genograms. These guidelines provide some consensus about the type of information that should be gathered and how this information

should be recorded. Male family members are represented by squares, famales by circles. Birth dates, death dates, marriage dates, separation and divorce dates, educational levels, occupations, and nature of relationships (for example, conflicts among members; with whom family alliances are formed) could be indicated alongside each symbol on the genogram. In addition, to present a more holistic picture, nurses might also indicate place of residence, ethnicity, major illnesses, religious affiliation (or absence of one), frequency and types of contact among family members (for example, visits, letters, telephone calls), fictive kin relationships, and immigration dates (where appropriate). This additional information can help nurses to begin to identify cultural orientations, extrafamilial relationships, and the physical and social distance that exists among family members. For example, family members may live in geographic proximity to each other but only infrequently interact with one another, or they may live at great geographic distance from one another but maintain frequent contact through visits, letters, and telephone calls. Possibly decisions are not made without the input of these geographically distant but socially close relatives. Fig. 5-1 shows a genogram that includes much of this information.

Genograms can be useful in two ways: (1) they can help clients gain better understanding of their own family systems, and (2) they can assist nurses to assess the dynamics of client-families and to identify family orientations and process patterns that have been perpetuated over generations.

CHAPTER SUMMARY

Family dynamics, family form, and who is defined as family are very much influenced by sociocultural factors. In addition to the various forms that a family may take and the members that it may encompass, nurses also need to consider what

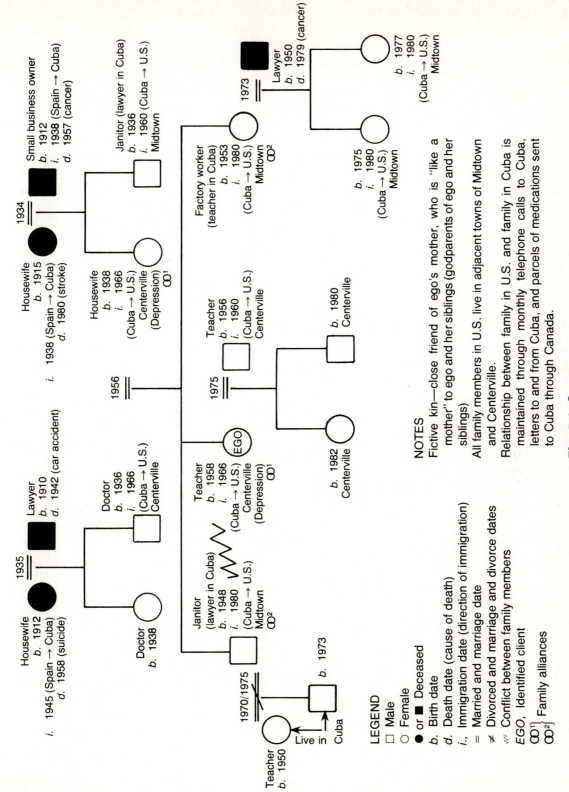

Fig. 5-1. Genogram.

NOTES

Fictive kin—close friend of ego's mother, who is "like a mother" to ego and her siblings (godparents of ego and her siblings)

All family members in U.S. live in adjacent towns of Midtown and Centerville.

Relationship between family in U.S. and family in Cuba is maintained through monthly telephone calls to Cuba, letters to and from Cuba, and parcels of medications sent to Cuba through Canada.

LEGEND

□ Male
○ Female
● or ■ Deceased
b. Birth date
d. Death date (cause of death)
i., Immigration date (direction of immigration)
= Married and marriage date
≠ Divorced and marriage and divorce dates
∿ Conflict between family members
EGO, Identified client
OO¹ ⎱
OO²⎰ Family alliances

stage of the developmental cycle a family is experiencing. The concept of ''family'' also includes the interactions, relationships, and organizational patterns among members that serve to effectively meet the needs of family members and the expectations of society.

The family is a dynamic system and has the properties of any social system. The effective functioning of the family system is dependent on the interrelationship between the family and its context (physical, emotional, cultural and social).

SENSITIVITY-AWARENESS EXERCISES

The purposes of these exercises are to:

- Develop awareness about the dynamics, strengths, and limitations of your own family system and the family systems of clients
- Develop awareness about family orientations and process patterns that have been perpetuated over generations in your own family and in client-families
- Develop awareness about the interrelationship between families and their context (physical, emotional, cultural, and social)

1. Construct a genogram of your family system. Be sure to include birth dates, death dates, marriage dates, separation and divorce dates, and immigration dates for family members. In addition, indicate educational levels, occupations, nature of relationships (for example, conflict among family members; alliances among family members), places of residence, ethnicity, major illnesses, religious affiliations (or nonaffiliation), frequency and types of contact among family members, and fictive kin relationships. On the basis of this genogram, how would you describe the dynamics in your family system? The physical and social distance among family members? The sociocultural orientation of family members? Next, construct a genogram for a client-family and answer the aforementioned questions.

2. Use one or more of the following techniques to describe your family's dynamics: reviewing the family photograph album, writing a family history, drawing a family picture, or role playing.

3. Using a tape recorder or taking notes, prepare a life history of a grandparent, great grandparent, or a sibling of such a family member (for example, a great aunt). This life history should contain the major people, relationships, and events in the person's life. You might start out by saying, ''Tell me about your life when you were a child.'' This question might lead you to ask, ''What was your life like when you were my age?'' or ''How was life the same (or different) then and now?'' A life history will help you to better understand the beliefs, conceptualizations, and perceptions of past events of this family member.

REFERENCES

Adams, B.
1980 The Family: A Sociological Interpretation. Chicago: Rand McNally & Co.

Adams, R.N.
1960 An Inquiry Into the Nature of the Family. The Bobbs-Merrill Reprint Series in the Social Sciences. New York: Thomas Y. Crowell Co.

Ashcraft, N.
1966 ''The domestic group in Mahogany, British Honduras.'' Social and Economic Studies 15:266-274.

Barnett, H., et al.
1954 ''Acculturation: An explanatory formulation.'' American Anthropologist 56:973-1002.

Bettleheim, B.
1969 The Children of the Dream. New York: The MacMillan Co.

Broderick, C.B.
1971 ''Beyond the five conceptual frameworks: a decade of development in family theory.'' Journal of Marriage and the Family 33:139-159.

Buckley, W.
1967 Sociology and Modern Systems Theory. Englewood Cliffs, N.J.: Prentice-Hall, Inc.

Bureau of Labor Statistics
1977 U.S. Department of Labor. Washington, D.C.: Government Printing Office.

Burr, W.R., et al.
1979 Contemporary Theories About the Family, 2 vols. New York: The Free Press.

Butler, R.N., and M.I. Lewis
1982 Aging and Mental Health: Positive Psychosocial and Biomedical Approaches (ed. 3). St. Louis: The C.V. Mosby Co.

Critchley, D.L.
1981 "The child as patient: assessing the effects of family stress and disruption on the mental health of the child." Perspectives in Psychiatric Care 5(5 and 6):144-155.

Davenport, W.
1961 "The family system of Jamaica." Social and Economic Studies 10:420-454.

Fleck, S.
1972 "An approach to family pathology." In Family Therapy: An Introduction to Theory and Technique. G.D. Erickson and T.P. Hogan (eds.). Monterey, Calif.: Brooks/Cole Publishing Co.

Fortes, M.
1958 "Introduction." In The Developmental Cycle in Domestic Groups. Jack Goody (ed.). London: The Syndics of the Cambridge University Press.

Gambino, R.
1983 Plenary Session Presentation at the National Conference on Ethnicity and the Media. Italian-Americans and the Media: Building a Positive Image. New York, April 9, 1983.

Gilmore, D.D.
1980 The People of the Plain: Class and Community in Lower Andalusia. New York: Columbia University Press.

Goode, W.J.
1964 The Family. Englewood Cliffs, N.J.: Prentice-Hall, Inc.

Grey, A.L.
1969 "Social class and the psychiatric patient." In Class and Personality in Society. A.L. Grey (ed.). New York: Atherton.

Gubrium, J.F., and D.R. Buckholdt
1982 Describing Care: Image and Practice in Rehabilitation. Cambridge, Mass.: Oelgeschlager, Gunn & Hain.

Guerin, P.J., and E.G. Pendagast
1976 "Evaluation of family system and genogram." In Family Therapy. P.J. Guerin (ed.). New York: Gardner Press.

Harris, M.
1956 Town and Country in Brazil. New York: Columbia University Press.

Hess, R.D., and G. Handel
1967 "The family as a psychosocial orientation." In The Psychosocial Interior of the Family. R.D. Hess and G. Handel (eds.). Chicago: Aldine Publishing Co.

Hill, R., and D. Hanson
1960 "The Identificaton of Conceptual Frameworks Utilized in Family Study." Marriage and Family Living 22:299-311.

Hoffman, M.
1968 The Gay World: Male Homosexuality and the Social Creation of Evil. New York: Basic Books, Inc., Publishers.

Hsu, F.L.K.
1970 Americans and Chinese: Reflections on Two Cultures and Their People. New York: Doubleday & Co., Inc.

Hutchinson, H.W.
1957 Village and Plantation Life in Northeastern Brazil. Seattle: University of Washington Press.

Jackson, D.D.
1957 "The question of family homeostasis." Psychiatric Quarterly Supplement 1:79-90.
1965 "Family rules: marital quid pro quo." In Family Therapy: An Introduction to Theory and Technique. G.D. Erickson and T.P. Hogan (eds.). Monterey, Calif.: Brooks/Cole Publishing Co.

James A.
1977 "Economic Adaptations of a Cuban Community." Annals of the New York Academy of Science 293:194-205.

Jones, S.L., and M. Dimond
1982 "Family theory and family therapy models: Comparative review with implications for nursing practice." Journal of Psychiatric Nursing and Mental Health Services 20(10):12-19.

Jordheim, A.E.
1980 "Alternate life-styles and the family." In Family-Centered Community Nursing: A Sociocultural Framework, vol. 2. A.M. Reinhardt and M.D. Quinn (eds.). St. Louis: The C.V. Mosby Co.

Kennedy, T.R.
1980 You Gotta Deal with It: Black Family Relations in a Southern Community. New York: Oxford University Press.

Kohn, M.I.
1977 Class and Conformity (ed. 2). Chicago: University of Chicago Press.

Leininger, M.
1979 "Territoriality, power and creative leadership in administrative nursing contexts." Nursing Dimensions: Power in Nursing 7(2):33-42.

Lowenthal, M.F., and C. Havens
1968 "Interaction and adaptation: Intimacy as a critical variable." American Sociological Review 33:20-31.

Macklin, E.D.
1974 "Cohabitation in college: going very steady; study at Cornell University." Psychology Today 8:53-59.

McClelland, D.
1975 Power: The Inner Experience. New York: Irvington Publishers, Inc.

McFarland, D.E., and N. Shiflett
1979 ''The role of power in the nursing profession.'' Nursing Dimensions: Power in Nursing 7(2):1-13.

McGoldrick, M.
1982 ''Ethnicity and family therapy.'' Family Therapy Networker 6:22-26.

Meagher, M.A.K.
1980 ''Separation, divorce, and subsequent coping problems of single-parent families.'' In Family-Centered Community Nursing: A Sociocultural Framework, vol. 2. A.M. Reinhardt and M.D. Quinn (eds.). St. Louis: The C.V. Mosby Co.

Middlefort, C.F.
1980 ''Ethnic and religious factors in family illnesses.'' Bulletin of the American Association of Social Psychiatry 1(3):16-21.

Miller, R.N. (ed.)
1978 Ethnic Images in American Film and Television. Philadelphia: Balch Institute.

Miller, S.
1967 ''Hacienda to plantation in Northern Peru: the process of proletarianization of a tenant farmer society.'' In Contemporary Change in Traditional Societies, vol. 3. J.H. Steward (ed.). Chicago: University of Chicago Press.

Mintz, S.W., and R. Price
1976 An Anthropological Approach to the Afro-American Past: A Caribbean Perspective. Philadelphia: Institute for the Study of Human Issues.

Nye, F.I., and F.M. Berardo
1966 Emerging Conceptual Frameworks in Family Analysis. New York: The MacMillan Co.

Parsons, T., and R.F. Bales
1955 Family, Socialization and Interaction Process. Glencoe, N.Y.: The Free Press.

Parsons, T.
1975 ''Some theoretical considerations on the nature and trends of change of ethnicity.'' In Ethnicity: Theory and Experience. N. Glazer and D.P. Moynihan (eds.). Cambridge, Mass.: Harvard University Press.

Pasquali, E.A.
1982 Assimilation and Acculturation of Cubans on Long Island. Ph.D. dissertation, State University of New York at Stony Brook.

Saghir, M.T., and E. Robins
1973 Male and Female Homosexuality: A Comprehensive Investigation. Baltimore: The Williams & Wilkins Co.

Scheflen, A.E., and A. Scheflen
1972 Body Language and Social Order. Englewood Cliffs, N.J.: Prentice-Hall, Inc.

Seal, C.
1983 ''Television entertainment.'' Paper presented at the National Conference on Ethnicity and the Media. Italian-Americans and the Media: Building a Positive Image. New York, April 9, 1983.

Sedgwick, R.
1981 Family Mental Health: Theory and Practice. St. Louis: The C.V. Mosby Co.

Seggar, J.F., J.K. Haffen, and H. Hannonen-Gladden
1981 ''Television's portrayals of minorities and women in drama and comedy drama, 1971-1981.'' Journal of Broadcasting 25:277-288.

Smith, R.T.
1956 ''The family in the Caribbean.'' In Caribbean Studies: A Symposium. V. Rubin (ed.). Seattle: University of Washington Press.

Solien, N.
1960 ''Household and family in the Caribbean.'' Social and Economic Studies 9:101-106.

Spindler, L.S.
1977 Culture Change and Modernization: Mini-Models and Case Studies. New York: Holt, Rinehart & Winston.

Sprey, J.
1969 ''The Family as a system in conflict.'' Journal of Marriage and the Family 31:699-706.

Stack, C.
1974 All Our Kin. New York: Harper & Row, Publishers, Inc.

Szalay, L.B., and B.C. Maday
1983 ''Implicit culture and psychocultural distance.'' American Anthropologist 85:110-118.

Tiger, L.
1978 ''Omnigamy: The new kinship system.'' Psychology Today 12:14.

Votaw, D.
1979 ''What do we believe about power?'' Nursing Dimensions: Power in Nursing 7(2):50-63.

ANNOTATED SUGGESTED READINGS

Jones, S.L., and M. Dimond

1982 ''Family theory and family therapy models: comparative review with implications for nursing practice.'' Journal of Psychiatric Nursing and Mental Health Services 20(10):12-19.

The authors compare and contrast theories of the family and theories of family therapy. Three theoretical approaches are discussed: the structural-functional, the interactional, and the developmental (or multigenerational). The importance of theories of the family and family therapy theories to family focused nursing are then explored.

Miller, J.

1981 ''Cultural and class values in family process.'' Journal of Marital and Family Therapy 7(4):467-473.

The author looks at some of the class- and culture-specific aspects of contemporary models of ''healthy'' family interaction. He urges that both sociodynamic and psychodynamic factors be recognized as operative in family systems.

FURTHER READINGS

Adams, B.

1980 The Family: A Sociological Interpretation. Chicago: Rand McNally & Co.

Epstein, N.

1978 ''The McMaster model of family functioning.'' Journal of Marriage and Family Counseling 4(4):19-31.

Levant, R.

1980 ''Sociological and clinical models of the family: an attempt to identify paradigms.'' The American Journal of Family Therapy 8:5-20.

CHAPTER 6

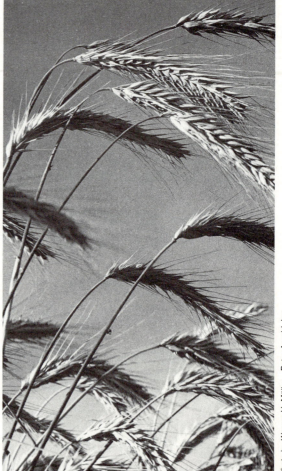

Photo by Werner H. Müller—Peter Arnold, Inc.

Human development

CHAPTER FOCUS

A nurse must understand that the process of human development is crucial to the accurate assessment of clients. There is a variety of perspectives on how and why a person develops in the manner he or she does. Cognitive, cultural, economic, physiological, and psychological factors are thought to influence the development of each personality in various ways, making it unique. In this chapter, an eclectic view of the operation of these factors will be presented. The role of culture and its impact on the socialization of a human being will be identified as one of the major factors in the process called ''development.''

Personality can be described as progressing along a chronological schema. The philosophies of human development of four major theorists—Freud, Sullivan, Erikson, and Piaget—will be discussed. Incorporated within this discussion will be the concept of vulnerability and its subsequent impact on healthy adaptation. Mental health and mental illness will be presented as reflecting a dynamic continuum on which types of human behavior can be placed. Such a continuum reflects the fact that health is a dynamic state, constantly interacting with external and internal forces.

Knowledge of the needs and tasks associated with a particular stage of development, and of the tools required to accomplish those tasks, is significant to nurses in making accurate assessments regarding recurrent behavior patterns and their implications. Data from such assessments can then be used to determine areas in which further learning is necessary in order for a client to develop appropriate skills to meet developmental tasks. A brief discussion of Maslow's hierarchy of needs will be presented, along with its implications for personality development. This portion of the chapter will present each developmental era—infancy, childhood, and so on—as an interrelationship of the many factors that influence the development of a person's unique personality. The concept of dying and death as the final phase of life will be discussed, and strategies of nursing assessment and intervention will be presented.

UNDERLYING DYNAMICS

Socialization and personality

The process of personality development is a complex one that is often misunderstood or misinterpreted because individuals who study personality do so according to their own inclinations. For example, a social-learning theorist might disagree strongly with a cultural anthropologist or a traditional psychoanalyst on the interpretation of a particular incident. Different strategies of intervention result. The question, however, is not which intervention is correct but rather which intervention is most effective in terms of client response and positive directional change. A therapist who refuses to see that an approach is, in fact, ineffective is not helping the client. Nurses therefore must be aware of the varying psychological, sociocultural, and biological factors present. They must have a basic understanding of each factor and its implications. Culture is the first of these variables that will be presented.

We assume that one function of a culture is to inculcate the young with prescribed conceptual, moral, ethical, and behavioral standards. The continuation of the society is thus ensured, and socialized beings are produced. Our focus as nurses, however, is the *individual* and his or her unique responses. We will be aware of shared personality characteristics, yet the critical emphasis will be on individuals and their socialization into roles within the culture as a whole.

A human being is not a closed system ruled or governed by a given nature; a human being is an open system. He or she creates and imposes order of an acquired nature. An individual exists within the framework of culture and society as a being whose needs, attitudes, values, and behavior are defined and made meaningful in the social and cultural milieu. A variety of social types, diversified in time and space, results. Individuals can be viewed as having a common structure of probabilities that can only be realized in a cultural context.

By first realizing that personality always comes into being in a cultural context, we can then consider how common cultural materials are utilized by individuals, rendering them unique beings. Although there are similarities in the composition of different personalities, individuals retain differences because of the unique ways they respond to and integrate various cultural patterns and traits. We can say that before their encounters with others, human beings are nothing substantial. They require the presence of others to stimulate the development of cognition, emotion, and, ultimately, sense of self.

Needs, as an aspect of personality, are noncognitive in origin. They can be divided into two categories: biological needs—such as thirst, hunger, and the need to eliminate—and needs acquired through interaction with society—such as the needs for affiliation and sense of self-worth. We need to bear in mind, however, that biological needs are themselves influenced by culture. For example, the need to eliminate is panhuman; however, each society has its own attitudes toward this need. What is considered modesty in one society might be considered inhibition in another. Nurses need to be aware that societal expectations are reflected in behavior clients use to meet needs.

Attitudes, as well as needs, reflect cultural orientation. Like needs, attitudes are major integrative forces in the development of personality; they give a sense of consistency to an individual's behavior. Attitudes are cognitive in origin: they are formed through interactions with the social environment. Attitudes serve to direct an individual's attention to his or her particular commitments and responsibilities. In a sense, they act as guidelines for the individual's present existence and help shape the future for the individual and for his or her progeny. An individual soon learns to attend to particular aspects of his or her environment on the basis of an attitudinal system. Ideas, social situations, and other people are grouped according to a person's "frame of reference," his or her own personal guidelines. Although overall cultural norms are reflected in an individual's tightly knit attitudinal system, they are integrated differently in each personality.

We have been placing various components of the individual into separate categories Thompson (1975) states that the construction of these parts into some semblance of a being within a cultural context requires an entity that acts as coordinator. That entity is the concept of self—a basic requirement for the sound psychological functioning of the human animal.

Self-concept is a major variable in the development of healthy patterns of behavior. A person's self-concept is the person's view of his or her own strengths and weaknesses; it is the person's perception of self based on reflected appraisals from the environment. Self-concept, then, is an accumulation of what others think of a person as well as the person's own exploratory activities that assist the person in understanding his or her world.

One of the most salient features of the self-concept is its ability to grow, to become more sophisticated in acquiring and applying knowledge and experience. In early infancy, the self-concept is virtually nonexistent. However, as infants begin to experience themselves as being different from their environment their motor activity increases. As children develop the tool of language, they become more capable of differentiating themselves from other objects and persons in the environment. Accomplishments bring positive reinforcement from significant persons, which serves to strengthen self-concept.

The mores of a culture are internalized and become such an integral part of a person that self-concept cannot be understood without cultural considerations. Internal needs and societal expectations are meshed to permit the individual as a social being to achieve a measure of consistency between the inner and outer selves.

The development of a positive self-concept allows an individual to experience a wide range of activities without feeling threatened. A perception of the world emerges that is unique to each person.

As positive experiences accumulate, an individual's self-concept is further enhanced. The individual who repeatedly encounters failure develops a poor self-concept, which is perpetuated through a phenomenon that amounts to a self-fulfilling prophecy. A person with a poor self-concept might continue to perceive his or her world in the most restricted sense unless the person can begin to perceive himself or herself as competent according to societal norms and values. A poor self-concept eventually results in maladaptive coping measures. One of our primary concerns as nurses is assisting such an individual to effect change that will potentiate a positive self-concept. This nursing function will be discussed further in this chapter, in the discussions of self-concept in relation to parent-child interactions and self-esteem.

It is evident that an individual can inherit biological characteristics, such as body size, weight, eye color, and hair color. However, the qualities that identify an individual as a human being are those which may not be genetically transmitted—thought patterns, emotions, and behavior responses, although some theorists indicate that certain types of behavior are in fact genetically transmitted. Those characteristics identified as congenital are passed on during the gestation period. However, our cultural heritage is acquired through our relationships with others. Even characteristics that seem to be predominantly biological can be related to cultural experience. For example, positive living conditions might be characteristic of a particular civilization because they are valued entities. The same factors might not be in evidence in another civilization, perhaps because they are not valued. A society might limit the availability of affection, physical warmth, and light. In such a case, an individual's physical growth as well as his or her emotional development might be retarded. Body size and weight might tend to be less than in a culture that placed a premium on factors that enhance these characteristics.

Locke and Rousseau were the first to oppose the view that the infant entered this world with a built-in set of responses—that he or she was a mini-adult who had already been programmed for eternity. Locke introduced the concept of the "tabula rasa"—that the newborn infant resembles a blank slate. The infant learns from the environment how, when and eventually why he or she should respond. Itard, in his famous work with the Wild Boy of Aveyron, expanded this concept. This young child of about eleven or twelve had the characteristic behavior of a wild animal, posturing himself on all fours, scratching and biting those who came near him. He had no awareness of social restrictions on behavior. He operated on an immediate-gratification principle. It was apparent that there was little instinctive basis for rules of socialization. The young boy had adapted to his environment as would any animal in similar circumstances. When the Wild Boy was found by Frenchmen in 1799, he was compared to persons living in a European cultural environment. By European standards he was a freak, a subhuman. Although this case is an extreme example, it serves to point out the individual differences that result from the socialization process.

It is of little importance to identify one specific factor—biological, psychological, social, cultural—as having more impact on development than another. Behavior and development have a multifactorial base.

However, recognizing the role of culture is particularly relevant in nursing. By recognizing the impact of culture on behavioral responses, the nurse makes available a broadened scope of assessment and intervention strategies. Let us consider some examples of what might have previously been identified as having a strictly biological base. The sensory nerve endings respond to heat and cold. However, this response can be culturally as well as biologically induced. A certain element of learned response develops as children are repeatedly warned not to touch something because it is hot. Parents are continually requiring children to put their coats on when the temperature falls to a certain point. Thus a child might not have been biologically triggered, yet he or she puts on a sweater. In addition, culturally determined dietary preferences affect nutrition, and culturally determined mating preferences affect genetic pools.

Biological factors can be subject to environmental modification. A child who has been locked in a closet for the first 2 years of life will probably be retarded in motor development. Culture provides a milieu in which an individual can exercise his various options. A person may be biologically ready for a higher-level task yet not have learned from his or her culture what the level means or how to reach it. The tools may be missing. We can look at a variety of situations in which a child may be identified as slow or backward based on the fact that he or she is biologically ready for a task but not performing it. For example, the sphincter of the bladder may be developed and functional, yet the child continues to wet his or her pants. Perhaps the child has not been socialized into a realization that this behavior is viewed negatively by the culture. A child's legs and arms may be coordinated sufficiently to propel him or her over to someone else; however, the question arises of what to do then. Is the answer to that question part of the process of socialization into a particular role by the culture? Socialization into roles continues into adulthood, and each individual may be socialized into a variety of roles. One of the prime examples of the socialization process is learning the roles of receiver of health care and health care provider.

In summary, we view the individual as emerging from a cultural context. A human being is born with the biological readiness to peform many functions; however, culture provides the basic materials for personality development, such as value systems, a knowledge base, and fundamental beliefs. Each individual then combines his or her biological and cultural equipment in a unique way to emerge as a personality different from all others. The culture in turn is molded by the individual in a sort of circular pattern. It is necessary to state at this point that, although individuals share personality traits, a true group personality never exists. As we pointed out in Chapter 4, we use the concept of "basic group identity" to refer to shared traits rather than to a single personality type that is characteristic of an entire culture.

Factors influencing personality development

It seems appropriate to the discussion of personality development that we provide an overview of some of the many "panphasic" factors, or factors that span all the developmental epochs. We suggest that these influences be called to mind as one assesses an individual in relationship to his or her developmental status. Too often human beings are simply categorized into eras, task groups, or age groups for diagnostic purposes without considering such factors as parent-child relationships, intelligence, self-concept, genetic transimission, age, sex, and child-rearing practices. We have identified three general categories for the purpose of discussion: psychological, biological, and sociocultural.

PSYCHOLOGICAL FACTORS

The parent-child relationship has been the center of attention during the past decade or so, particularly since the studies of Bowlby and Spitz. The primary concern of theorists has been the impact of the parent, initially the mother, on the early development of the child. Bowlby (1973) found that the infant develops a strong sense of attachment to the mothering figure and quite vigorously protests her (or his) leaving. The implication is that the persistent attitudes and styles of the parental figure are imprinted on the child at a very early age and that the resulting value system pervades the developmental span until some point in young adulthood, when the individual is able to strike out on his or her own.

▶ Family relationships

The nature of the family relationships that develop are crucial to each family member. It is within the family system that identification occurs, a major factor in personality development. We note that identification is particularly relevant to the oedipal phase but that it does, in fact, occur throughout the developmental cycle. Shifts in identification result from positive interpersonal relationships with others in the social system.

An infant who is isolated cannot develop into a mature, well-integrated individual. Indeed, physical growth itself must be facilitated by a system that nurtures, educates, and enculturates. The family unit is the chief molder of personality. It is a system that provides an atmosphere for the testing of unfamiliar techniques of adaptation. Within the family, one can become familiar with roles and institutions. There is a sense of stability and integration, a home base to which one may always return. The enculturating capacities of parents impinge upon children during whatever phase they may be in; they transcend all phases. Enculturation is a generational process. Each parent brings a value system and characteristics of personality into a mating relationship. Offspring are produced and the values and personality characteristics of the parents influence the development of those offspring.

It is important to note the deleterious influences that parents can have upon the personality development of children. The parent who feels little self-esteem and who has a poor image of himself or herself has difficulty responding to a child in a manner that promotes a positive self-concept in the child. For example, 7-year-old Jamie brings home his first homework assignment. After completing it, he asks his mother to check it for him. She repeatedly makes comments such as "Are you sure this is the way you were supposed to do it?" and "Did the teacher tell you this was alright?" These comments reflect the parent's inability to accept the child's actions as being correct and indicate the parent's dependence on an authority figure. She is uncomfortable with accepting the responsibility for her own actions, and this message is transmitted to her child. The child thus is led to question his own abilities, a situation that results in a distorted estimation of them.

The effect of parental influence may be quite positive during one phase of development and quite negative during another. A mother may develop a sound relationship with her infant, based on the comfort she experiences in being depended upon. However, if the mother is unable to relinquish this relationship, the child may suffer the consequences in later periods of personality development.

Self-concept evolves out of the parent-child interaction and functions as a mediator of development. Parents and children interact with one another; in this process a self-concept is continually evolving for each family member, as was discussed earlier. Each self-concept reflects the appraisals of significant others in the environment. Thus family life nurtures each child, providing strong affectional and relational bonds. As Satir (1975) points out in *Peoplemaking,* parents have the tremendous responsibility of facilitating the development of a positive self-concept and a sound sense of self-esteem.

It is necessary to identify the meaning of self-esteem as it relates to self-concept. An individual with a healthy self-concept is able to integrate the appraisals reflected from his or her environment and to accept his or her own strengths and weaknesses. Self-esteem grows out of this positive self-concept; individuals with high self-esteem feel they are worthwhile in spite of mistakes or defeats. They feel capable of achieving realistically determined goals and accept responsibility for their actions. They do not have to be right all the time; when they fail, they reassess their coping skills and develop another plan. They perceive failure not as total defeat but rather as an opportunity to develop an alternative plan of action.

Parents with high senses of self-esteem are able to provide an atmosphere in which children feel comfortable with their self-concepts and their emerging identities. There are no obligations attached to behavior and no conditions for reward. Unmet parental needs do not become a burden to the next generation. Each child is free to "be." Conditions within the family system are such that trust, a secure identity, and a sense of autonomy are valued. In appropriate situations, children are permitted to explore the decision-making process

and to experience independence. They are not forced to play out a symbiotic relationship to meet the needs of their parents.

Parents who are unsure of themselves or their own worth often unconsciously set up circumstances very much like ones they themselves experienced as children. Feelings of "bad me," guilt, and shame, which produce low self-esteem, are evoked in their own children just as they were evoked in themselves many years before. Unreasonable punishment and, ultimately, withdrawal of expression of love cause children of such parents to feel that their behavior must be unworthy if it has caused these responses from the persons they consider significant—their parents. They believe that they must truly be "bad." A pattern has been established that continues from generation to generation.

One needs to feel positive about one's self—aware of both limitations and strengths—before one can invest actively and positively in another human being. Such is the case in the parent-child relationship. If parents have experienced smooth developmental courses and if they are aware of their own needs, they will be more able to share a sound, nurturing relationship with their children.

▶ Self-concept

A positive self-concept, initiated in the toddler period and nurtured throughout the developmental span, enables an individual to meet each challenge as it comes and to deal with it appropriately. Problems are viewed not as insurmountable obstacles but as potential learning situations. It would be unrealistic to say that each possible impediment is viewed with gleeful delight. A person with a strong sense of self recognizes that he or she has a wide range of capabilities, yet also acknowledges his or her limitations. Such a person realizes that it is acceptable to work within the framework of those limitations. At each developmental level, the parameters of those limitations are altered. The individual with a healthy sense of self is able to adapt to those alterations.

Self-concept correlates with many factors, some

of which will be discussed at greater length later in this chapter. A person whose self-evaluations are negative tends to experience consistently high levels of anxiety, which in turn lead to less positive interactions with peers. An individual with a poor self-concept feels a sense of powerlessness to change his or her role, thus perpetuating a cycle of feeling victimized. This sense of inability to bring about change can be connected with the perception of an external locus of control—the feeling that one has no real opportunity to actively effect change, that it is in the hands of fate, so to speak. In contrast, a person with a positive self-concept has a sense of active participation in the environment and feels able to determine realistic life goals. These patterns serve to reinforce the notion that the self is the organizing factor in the personality.

Although each individual is unique, everyone is affected by interactions with his or her environment, and the process by which interactions affect a person is roughly the same for everyone. All aspects of human development interact, responding continuously to experiential and constitutional factors.

An individual's personality is a reflection of his or her input into the process of personality development. How one speaks to another person or how one puts thoughts into actions determines the response one receives from the environment. Environmental responses, in turn, determine behavior. Reciprocity exists in that the behavior of one individual has an impact on that of another, and vice versa. There is a continuous exchange of communication (both verbal and nonverbal) between persons (see Chapter 8). Future behavioral patterns are influenced by those interactions.

▶ Intelligence

One individual characteristic that is very relevant to personality development is intelligence. Intelligence is the aptitude or capacity for learning and includes problem-solving ability. Intelligence is biologically determined by virtue of the fact that a person inherits a nervous system. However, experiences provided by the environment may retard or facilitate the development of cognitive skills.

Differences in intelligence appear as early as infancy and gradually become more apparent during the childhood and adolescent years. The ability to reason through complex situations has many implications for personality development. Intelligence has a profound impact on many areas of development and behavior, such as talking, memory, understanding and applying new concepts, and creativity. It seems that children who learn rapidly and who can apply their knowledge develop a more positive self-concept—as a result of praise received from parents and teachers—than children who are poor achievers. They assume positions of leadership more frequently, recognize their limitations more readily, and are able to look at themselves and laugh when appropriate.

Intelligence was once considered completely hereditary. However, published studies have demonstrated that heredity is not the only factor. The effect of environment can no longer be negated. Children who were born to parents with low IQs who were then adopted by parents of average or high IQs have been shown to be able to reach the educational levels of their adoptive parents (McCandless and Evans, 1973)

Educational experiences play a definitive role in the development of intelligence, particularly during infancy and the preschool and adolescent periods. Thus parents need to provide an atmosphere that facilitates learning during these critical periods. Personality development will be enhanced, and a positive self-concept will be promoted.

▶ Loss

Object loss is discussed at length in the chapter on aggression against oneself (Chapter 18). However, it is relevant here to note the impact that loss has on personality development. Bowlby (1973) compares loss to separation from the mother figure. The manner in which loss is resolved, if in fact it is resolved, is crucial to the development of a positive sense of self and the ability to invest in trusting relationships. Although the interrelationship between positive self-concept and personality development has been emphasized several times in this book, we believe that it bears repetition. The sense of security one has in dealing with loss will be reflected in personality development over and over again. Since life is characterized by a series of losses, it is in this arena that nurses must focus to develop primary preventive strategies.

▶ Coping skills

The ability to cope with a variety of situations reflects an awareness of one's strengths and limitations and indicates a capacity to tap one's resources as necessary. Of great importance to personality development is the type of coping mechanism utilized as well as the degree and frequency to which it is called into play. For example, an individual may learn a coping skill such as the internalization of stress and its expression through a physiological route. This mechanism of reducing tension, learned in early interactions with significant persons in the environment, is then carried on throughout the life cycle. The nature of such early coping experiences and parental responses to them have a profound influence on future personality development. Coping skills that include an honest, open sharing of feelings provide the setting for the development of a sound sense of self. Coping skills that are rooted in, or fixated at, early levels of psychosexual development color the emerging personality. The terms ''oral personality'' and ''anal personality'' indicate levels of development in which individuals can be rooted. For example, the anal personality is characterized by a coping repertoire that includes retentive kinds of behavior with little sharing of feelings. An individual with this type of personality is stingy on a material level as well as an emotional level.

The nursing profession, by definition, had historically directed much of its effort toward secondary prevention. However, primary prevention efforts have awakened the awareness of parents on behalf of their children in order to facilitate the development of healthy coping skills during early childhood periods.

BIOLOGICAL FACTORS

The relationship of neurochemistry to the development of personality is a striking one. Two key hormones, androgen and estrogen, affect not only the biological sexual orientation but also the psychological assumption of sex roles. Aggression and maternalism are two types of behavior that are affected by these hormones. Androgen levels correlate positively with aggressive tendencies, and estrogen levels correlate positively with maternalistic tendencies. The neurochemical effect of hormones also has an impact on growth rates, weight, and bone ossification. Everyone grows at a different rate, a fact that is apparent if we look at a class of first-graders. There may be differences in height of as much as 8 inches. Size definitely affects the kinds of activities a child engages in and how he or she is perceived by peers. A boy who is considerably smaller than his classmates is often called a ''runt'' and may not be asked to participate in physical activities such as football or basketball. He may then assume a passive role among his peers. Because of a biological ''hand of fate,'' his personality development will have taken a particular course; the course might have been different if he had been larger. Thus a simple biological fact of life such as growth rate can have a wide-ranging effect on overall personality development. Again, the interrelatedness of biological and cultural factors is apparent.

The biological factors involved in personality development cannot be discussed without reference to the concept of maturation. Maturation is the process of developmental changes, a process that is controlled by genetic factors.

▶ Genetics

What is the significance of genetics to personality development? Various personal characteristics, such as physical appearance, motor activity, emotional reactivity, and energy level, are strongly related to genetic composition. Intellectual characteristics—and, to some degree, social characteristics—are shaped by heredity. As an individual matures, he or she experiences certain expected developmental changes. The timetable that controls these changes is laid down by genes yet may be vastly altered by environmental variables. Even under similar environmental conditions, it is quite possible that two male siblings will reach adolescence at very different times.

The task of nursing involves recognition of two basic facts: (1) each individual occupies his or her own given space on the developmental continuum, and (2) variables such as health care, stress, cultural expectations, and chronic illness affect an individual's rate of maturation irrespective of a genetic timetable. With these facts in mind, nurses can devise primary preventive strategies that promote optimum conditions for the development of each individual's unique personality.

▶ Age

Chronological age is probably one of the most common criteria used to categorize human development. Certain observable types of behavior have been identified for each particular age group. Within each age level, these common characteristics are studied in respect to frequency, variety, complexity, and organization. Mental age as well as chronological age need to be considered; individuals in the same chronological age group may have very different mental ages.

Obviously, there are significant limitations to the discussion of personality development in terms of chronological age. When age is considered alone, the very factors that we have just been discussing—genetic timetables and environmental influences—are negated. To say that a child is older is simply not sufficient to account for increased reading ability, for example. Many experiential factors need to be studied. Since environment plays such a great role in development, we need to identify what may be operating to influence reading ability.

Within an age level of children there is a wide range of variations. It is not appropriate, therefore, to say that a child of four will exhibit static characteristics. No child exactly fits the ''average'' mold. A nursing assessment must consider a range of developmental variations. Parents often believe that their child must exhibit characteristics X, Y, and Z by age 10, for example. They experience a sense of confusion, and panic frequently sets in, when the characteristics are not apparent. Both the child and the parents may then suffer severe consequences of the parents' misapprehensions. Prenatal and well-baby clinics provide excellent opportunities for nurses to discuss behavioral and biological expectations with parents. It is here that nurses can identify wide variations, thus preventing future difficulties in parent-child interaction as well as in the personality development of children.

When considering age as a factor in personality development, most studies have looked at children in ''average'' environments. This concept constricts one's view of development. More and more, researchers are identifying a variety of environments, both enriching and depriving ones, to broaden their perspectives on personality development. Again, just as biological and maturational factors cannot be put aside in the assessment of personality development, the role the environment plays cannot be ignored.

▶ Sexuality

Sexuality, including sex role behavior, attitudes, and values, is a powerful determinant of personality development. It influences the way persons are perceived, what types of occupations are available to them, and the way they view themselves.

Although sexuality is presented in this discussion of biological factors, it is important to note that psychological and sociocultural factors are equally relevant in the development of healthy sexual attitudes and behavior. Such attitudes and behavior in turn promote the growth of a healthy, adaptive personality. Concern for the development of a positive sense of sexuality has become an issue for the health professional. It is curious that this change has been such a long time coming, for few subjects touch each human being's life more powerfully. Until recent years the subject was considered taboo. Many educators, health professionals, and others felt that dissemination of information about sexuality would lead to an increase in promiscuity, homosexuality, and so-called sexual deviations, such as oral-genital sex and masturbation. As members of a rational, progressive society, we must realize that a person's interest in his or her developing sex drives and needs will not disappear magically if he or she is encouraged to ignore them. Sexuality is a component of a person's self-esteem and sense of identity. A person becomes aware of sexual differentiation prior to his or her knowledge of self as a member of other groups: the child is a boy or a girl before he or she is Irish, Catholic, or American (Hauck, 1970).

The issue of self-esteem is bound to how one feels about his or her body and the pleasure that is received from one's body. Self-esteem and sexuality are interwoven in the process of giving and receiving sexual pleasure. This process is connected to feeling comfortable within one's body. Cantor (1980) suggests that self-esteem implies an individual is worthy to live and enjoy life, including sexual experiences. Assaults to self in the form of physical illness, for example, can lead to loss of control over life and body, which in turn leads to decreased competence, self-esteem, and sexual confidence. Acknowledgment of the individual as a sexual being allows him or her to feel valued by others and affirms his or her sense of worth.

The terms "value" and "attitude" are important considerations in the area of sexuality. An individual may value a particular belief, object, or activity, which implies a consideration of its worth. Beliefs that are considered worthwhile guide actions or behavior. An attitude may be defined as a "feeling or emotion toward a fact or state" (Webster). Attitudes, like values, guide the manner in which individuals conduct themselves in the public dimension as well as in the private dimension. Sexuality is particularly influenced by one's attitudes and values. Wide differences exist even in Western culture as to what is considered "right" and "wrong." Definitions of "meaningful relationship," "love," and even "marriage" are often determined by individuals and may vary

from situation to situation. Confusion may arise when sexual roles and behavior seem no longer to be well-defined. Change, as always, produces feelings of anxiety and apprehension. However, increased sexual awareness should not be confused with open-ended permissiveness. For example, individuals during the adolescent years are seeking to test out their own emerging values and beliefs. Guidance in the form of direct, honest communication can facilitate the development of those values and beliefs. The pressure of peers and other external influences can confuse and overwhelm adolescents at a point in their lives when they are neither adults nor children. By acknowledging that identity incorporates one's sexual being, parents and significant other adults create an atmosphere in which discussions about relationships (one vs. several), intimacy, feelings, lovemaking (when to and when not to), childbearing, and alternative forms of sexual expression (such as homosexuality or bisexuality) can occur. Development of a sense of responsibility in regard to one's "right" to be sexual and to exercise choices in sexual expression comes out of respect for others as well as respect for self. An environment that encourages discussion of sexual issues and their ramifications can only reinforce that concept of respect. Affirmation of one's sexual being, which cannot be separated from one's physical, emotional, intellectual, sociocultural, and spiritual dimensions, enables one to strive for high-level wellness.

No single determinant can be said to account for sexual behavior. It results from the interaction of biological, psychological, and sociocultural factors.

Biological determinants of sexual behavior have historically been rooted in the concept of instinct. Sex, in one sense, is the innate drive to mate and to reproduce. Yet in lower animals there is no awareness that coitus leads to pregnancy—a fact that leads one to believe that humans as well as lower animals engage in sexual activity for pleasurable reasons. Sex appears to involve a psychological drive that is correlated with feelings of pleasure, which can be traced back to the "pleasure centers"

—the thalamus, the hypothalamus, and the mesencephalon. When these centers are electrically stimulated, animals experience pleasurable feelings of varying intensities.

One's sexuality is reflected in the complex interaction of the hypothalamus, the pituitary gland, and the gonads. This system is responsible for the stimulation and regulation of the hormones necessary for sexual development and activity. During intrauterine life the fetus seems to be under the direct influence of hormones, a situation that reflects a greater degree of genetic determination of sex roles and behaviors than is the case during the ensuing years of development. It appears that as an individual approaches adulthood, sexual roles and behaviors reflect the impact of cultural influences. Indirect data suggest that there is a prenatal influence, by fetal hormones, on the hypothalamus. This influence is exerted in a subtle manner throughout the life cycle. However, there needs to be an awareness of the interaction of these innate, biological factors and the environmental factors that facilitate the expression of those factors.

Thus it is inaccurate to view sexuality from the singular perspective of biological determination. Psychological factors may be considered expressions of underlying biological sexual instincts. For example, Freud believed that libido (sex drive) was the psychological representation of a biological sexual instinct. Psychological determinants may exist in the form of learned patterns of behavior. Motivation may be mediated through the brain yet have at its base such learned patterns. Sexual behavior, its expression and purpose, may be learned through psychological and sociocultural mechanisms.

Sexuality can be viewed as an interpersonal process in which one individual chooses to share with and relate to a significant other. The process involves the experiencing of interrelated emotional, psychological, and physiological changes that are pleasurable to each partner. Each person enables the other to realize his or her potential for sexual fulfillment while recognizing the partner's as well as his or her own strengths and limitations.

A person can experience sexual pleasure without a partner. The most common way of doing so is masturbation, or sexual arousal through either manual or mechanical stimulation of the sex organ —that is, the penis or the clitoris. Masturbation often has been described as "dirty" and considered inappropriate as a means of sexual satisfaction. The myth that masturbation leads to blindness and insanity has long been purported. It is no wonder, then, that masturbation has received little support as an alternative means of sexual stimulation. It is of particular importance that nurses recognize the fallacy of this interpretation of masturbation. They can help parents to see masturbation as a component of the normal growth and development process that occurs during the childhood period, a process that leads to a healthy sexual identity. A determination about the appropriateness of a child's use of masturbation as an adaptive measure may then follow. Masturbation may be a viable alternative for hospitalized clients as well as for persons who have no sexual partner. It is critical, however, that a nurse assess an individual's attitudes and feelings before suggesting masturbation. Achieving sexual satisfaction through this mechanism may be totally unacceptable to a client, and he or she may cut off communication with the nurse completely.

Gender identity. Sexual identity has traditionally been directly correlated with biological sex (maleness and femaleness), which may also be termed "core gender identity," and to its psychological attributes (masculinity and femininity), which may be referred to as "gender identity." However, recent changes in Western societal norms for men and women have led to a blurring of those characteristics traditionally identified as male and female. The sociocultural context of an individual provides the structure of values, attitudes, and beliefs from which one's sexuality is developed. Again, it is impossible—and inappropriate—to separate the biological dimension from the psychological dimension, or either of those dimensions from the sociocultural dimension.

Money and Erhardt (1972) proposed a model of psychosexual differentiation that reflects an integration of biological, psychological, and sociocultural dimensions. They believe that gender identity differentiation begins at conception and reaches its conclusion with the emergence of the adult. The sequence is initiated by the chromosomes. The undifferentiated gonads then transmit the message of gender identity through the hormonal secretions of their own cells. As a result of this process, genital dimorphism occurs—the external and internal sex organs develop to correspond to the chromosomal sex. At birth, the impact of social influences begins—sex is assigned by the use of names, the choice of colors (pink or blue), and the choice of toys (doll, football). The process of identifying oneself as male or female becomes part of social learning. As the child grows and develops, he or she receives reflected appraisals from the environment that serve to facilitate the development of self-concept and its component, body image. The child's understanding of gender identity becomes very concrete. He or she reaches puberty; accumulated learning shapes future behavior—sexual and otherwise. Sexual hormones secreted during this phase result in the development of erotic feelings. The culmination of this process of genital dimorphism, social learning, and secretion of pubertal hormones is what is termed adult gender identity. Money and Erhardt (1972) define gender identity as the "individuality of one as male or female as it is experienced in self-awareness and behavior—it is the private experience of gender role." They define "gender role" as "everything one says or does that indicates one is male or female—it is the public expression of gender identity."

In addition to incorporating the three dimensions mentioned previously, this model of psychosexual differentiation is related to the broader perspective of psychosocial development. An important task connected with identity formation is the development of a healthy, integrated sense of sexuality. Adolescence sees an upsurge in sexual activity; however, intimacy occurs only after an individual has achieved identity formation. As a person moves into adulthood, he or she shares in relationships—both in a physical sense and an emotional sense. Each person is an individual in his or her own right yet has the capacity to establish a continuing, sharing relationship—a relationship that can last until death. Thus, it is important to assess psychosexual differentiation *within* the framework of one's psychosocial development.

Sex-role stereotyping has been perpetuated throughout the years by both males and females. Neither group has been willing to risk being identified as "different." Sex roles are defined by characteristics representing masculinity and femininity. These categories emerge from the sociocultural framework inherent in each society. Traditionally, characteristics such as competitiveness, aggressiveness, and intelligence have been considered masculine in Western cultures. Female traits have included gentleness, warmth, and passivity, as well as tendencies toward being understanding and showing emotion.

Recently theorists in the field of human sexuality have suggested the concept of androgyny—the possession of human traits rather than those identified as either maculine or feminine. This concept, which involves a blurring of sex roles, can be viewed as a step toward positive mental health, because it does not require that a person be given a label based on whether a characteristic is appropriate. There is, however, concern that the concept of androgyny may increase the difficulty a child experiences in developing a sound sense of identity. It is important that children be clearly given the message that they are male or female to prevent ambiguity in core gender identity. They can then be encouraged to select from traits that are identified as "human" rather than "male" or "female." It is indeed important for nurses, counselors, sex educators, and other professionals to recognize that androgyny can be a threatening concept—an unknown. For example, a boy growing up in a tough neighborhood may feel extremely uncomfortable about assuming characteristics not acceptable to his group. He cannot be expected to assume traditionally feminine traits if he is going to be harassed by his peers. Thus the assimilation of human, rather than sex-linked, traits must occur over a period of time, because positive reinforcement from one's cultural group is a necessary ingredient in the process. It can be said, then, that the goal of mental health care is the introjection and expression of human traits.

Sex roles play a part in determining what is considered appropriate or inappropriate behavior. It is not possible to separate sex roles, sexual attitudes, and sexual behavior from one another. Each is interrelated with the others to produce a unique, complex, sexual human being. Likewise, one cannot separate biological, psychological, and sociocultural factors in the determination of gender identity. Each variable reinforces the others; one variable does not operate to the exclusion of the others. It is difficult to separate a biological imperative from one that is imposed by a culture.

Finally, the concept of sexual orientation is often confused with core gender identity or with gender identity. The term sexual orientation refers to sexual object choice. The orientation may be toward an inanimate object, as in fetishism. The orientation may also be heterosexual, homosexual, lesbian, bisexual, or ambisexual. Although societies often consider sexual orientations other than heterosexual to be deviant, any expression of sexual choice needs to be assessed in terms of its commitment to humanistic values. For example, an individual's sexual behavior must not harm or disadvantage another person. Each member of a relationship must freely consent to that relationship. Thus, heterosexual, homosexual, or lesbian relationships can be satisfying and enriching.

Sexuality and culture. Each society has a culture of sex. Sex is a part of embryonic life; its biological existence impacts upon consciousness as a force reflecting its instinctive nature. Yet enculturation provides the form and meaning necessary to define sexuality. Cultures vary from one society to the next as well as from generation to generation within one society.

Davenport (1977) suggests that the culture of sex is anchored in two directions. At one end, it is

linked to the potentialities and limitations of biological inheritance. On the other end, it is tied to the logic and internal consistency of the total culture. As one aspect of the total culture undergoes change, so must all the others. However, there are some inherent limitations because biological parameters cannot be exceeded. He further notes that *in order to understand one culture of sex, it is necessary to know how sexual performance is conceptually joined to the total culture.*

Traditions regarding intercourse, menstruation, contraception, and gender identity vary from culture to culture. For example, the pre–World War II Manus in Papua New Guinea considered intercourse between husband and wife as sinful and degrading. Women believed intercourse was something to be endured until a child was born. Intercourse outside the marriage was a crime that brought on supernatural punishments. Menstruation was such a well-kept secret that Manu men denied that women experienced monthly cycles.

The Polynesian cultures consider sexuality in a much different light. Infants and young children are encouraged in their expressions of sexuality, as are adolescents and young adults. In the latter group, members of both sexes are encouraged to masturbate and have premarital sex. The expression of sexuality is highly prized within the culture.

A culture that applies a negative connotation to sexuality is that of the Gusii of southwestern Kenya. The act of coitus itself implies hostility and antagonism. The man is expected to overcome the woman's resistance and, in fact, inflict pain and humiliation. Intercourse becomes a sort of ritualized rape, with some of the affective components as well. Women are expected to frustrate men by sexually taunting them. Overt expression of sexuality is punished from childhood throughout adolescence. Extramarital relationships bring on heavy punishment from the gods. An adulterous Gusii wife who continues to have intercourse with her husband may put him in mortal danger if he becomes ill or is injured in any way.

The Dobu, who constitute another Papua New

Guinea society, believe that women are sorceresses. Husbands are particularly vulnerable to sorcery during intercourse; therefore males must constantly decide between sexual gratification and the effects of sorcery.

Erotic codes vary from culture to culture as well. Acts such as the sharing or offering of food can be tinged with sexual meaning. In East Bay, a Melanesian society of the southwest Pacific, an act of sexual intimacy is the sharing of betel nuts and pepper between members of the opposite sex.

The use of language can be erotically stimulating as well. Davenport (1977) notes that Hawaiians clearly make sexual allusions through metaphor, pun, and multiple meanings. In addition, he identifies similarities between the Hawaiians and the Iban of Sarawak, whose issuances of compliments, scoldings, and expressions of respect and insult are couched in erotic terms.

The development of gender identity is also influenced by culture. Gilmore and Gilmore (1979) discuss male social impotence (lack of social power on the part of males) and gender identity conflict among men in the lower class in Spain. In the early life experience of males in this socioeconomic group, there is little or no contact with their fathers on a daily basis. Most time is spent in the "female" sphere, which is studiously avoided by the fathers, who spend much of their time in bars or taverns. Little socialization occurs between fathers and sons, even in adolescence. The dominant figure is female, in the form of mother, grandmother, or both. Power resides with the female, who is dispenser of all material goods as well as love and affection. Allowances are given by maternal figures, permission is granted to participate in activities by maternal figures, and maternal figures confer with teachers and other external authority figures. Further strengthening the female influence was the fact that, during the Franco period, working class women often were more able than men to maintain gainful employment, particularly in the service of wealthy and powerful employers. Therefore, the wife was often not only in control of the "private" sphere, or home life, but

was also superior economically in her position as wage earner. Thus, as Gilmore and Gilmore suggest, there has been an increasing degree of sex-role reversal and confusion as perceived by lower class males. Further evidence of the gender identity conflict has been noted by the authors during the festival *carnavale*. The upper class does not participate, considering it to be brutish and uncivilized. The lower class as a whole acts in ways that are normally unacceptable. Women drink and smoke, while men dress in female garb, often that of an old grandmother. It is the latter feature that is striking in relation to gender-role identity. It seems that this ritualized transvestism may be symbolic of the underlying gender identity conflict—the male's inability to control or satisfy the powerful maternal figure. Lower-class males then must compensate for a fragile male identification. The "macho" reputation is achieved in young adulthood by severing emotional and physical ties with the "female" sphere, thus producing the distant or absent father figure. The cycle is perpetuated as male children are brought into a world influenced predominantly by females.

Thus, as is shown by this example and the other examples of cultural variation cited in this chapter, sexual practices and attitudes cannot be viewed in isolation but must be seen in relationship to other aspects of the social system.

Sexuality and the nursing process.* With the advent of increased awareness of sexuality, including sex roles, attitudes, and behavior, it becomes imperative that nurses address the sexual health issues of their clients.

Woods (1979) in her book on human sexuality clearly defines the role of the nurse. She identifies seven major components of this role: facilitation of a milieu that fosters the client's sexuality as valid; provision of anticipatory guidance; validation of the normalcy of behaviors, thoughts, and feelings; education of clients; provision of intensive therapy when appropriate; counseling of clients; and consultation with schools, community groups, and

---

*See also chapter 9.

other health professionals. However, it has been noted in the literature that health professionals hesitate to initiate discussions of sexual health issues, while clients wait for permission to bring up the subject. Clients' questions about body image, resumption of activities of daily living, and alterations in function may reflect concern about sexual attractiveness or ability to engage in sexually pleasurable activities. A genuine listening attitude and use of specific skills in communicating honestly about sexual health can help clients and their partners to adapt actively and in a positive manner to their current life situations. The ability to listen, to be silent, to be patient, and to permit a client to discuss fears, anxiety, and depression affirms the client's sense of worth as a human being at a time when it is most vital.

In order to actualize these skills, a nurse needs to consider his or her basic knowledge level, attitudes, and comfort level as critical factors. In addition, the nurse must be keenly aware of self—individual value systems, fears, concerns, and vulnerabilities—when confronting the sexual health issues of others. Values clarification and desensitization through sexual attitude reassessment programs are often effective in helping health professionals to become more aware of their own belief systems and biases. They can then be more able to put aside their own needs when necessary in order to address those of their clients. It is only through the interactional process between client and nurse that sexual health issues are identified, goals set, and active problem-solving strategies implemented.

How do I assess my sexual beliefs and values? What issues are important for me to consider? Questions nurses might ask themselves include the following:

1. What do I consider "male" and "female" traits? Is there a dichotomy between the two?
2. What is "normal" sexual behavior to me? How do I feel about masturbation and oral-genital sex? What are variants of sexual behavior? How do I achieve sexual gratification?

3. How do I feel about alternative sexual lifestyles such as homosexuality, lesbianism, and transvestism?
4. How comfortable do I feel discussing sexual issues with a client? How comfortable do I feel discussing sexual issues with my partner?

According to Watts (1979) sexuality can be considered a psychophysiological system. Therefore, when conducting a sexual assessment, nurses should ask questions about sexual functioning at the same time that they ask questions relating to the reproductive and urinary systems. Detection of possible sexual dysfunctions (see Chapter 16) can be accomplished through a thorough sexual history.

Other areas that should be included in the sexual history and assessment are: developmental-level tasks; significant family interactions; sexual knowledge, attitudes, and values; current sexual activity; and satisfaction (or lack of it) in sexual relationships. As mentioned previously, the success of a sexual history depends to a large extent on how comfortable the nurse feels in dealing with the subject matter. It is imperative that nurses not neglect sexuality, since it is an integral component of the total individual. A healthy perception of one's own sexuality enhances the development of an adaptive personality.

The following can be used as guidelines for a sexual health assessment:

1. Utilize an honest, matter-of-fact approach that acknowledges the client as having sexual concerns and questions.
2. Maintain eye contact and sit comfortably close to the client.
3. Provide a sufficient amount of time for discussion—don't "run in and run out."
4. Utilize broad, general, open-ended questions to elicit information regarding sexual knowledge, perceptions of the impact of illness on sexuality, methods of sexual gratification, and attitudes relating to sexual issues.
5. Do not push the client into a discussion of sexuality. Leave the issue open for further

discussion at a later time. (Also, do not assume that because there are no questions, there are no concerns.)

6. Concerns about body image, activities of daily living, and return to pre-illness functioning can act as precipitants for discussion of sexual health issues. For example, statements that reflect general concern among all clients can be utilized: "Many people in your situation express concern about resumption of sexual activity."

7. Observation of the client during successive interactions provides information regarding comfort level (which issues are discussed and which are avoided), anxiety levels, unrealistic expectations of self or partner, guilt and shame, and level of psychosexual development.

8. Ask for clarification of unclear verbal and nonverbal communication: "When listening to you talk about your sexual preferences, I'm not sure what you are saying. Can you be more clear? I want to understand what this means for you."

9. Initiation of the discussion of sexual health issues acknowledges an individual as a sexual being and makes it possible for questions and concerns to emerge.

SOCIOCULTURAL FACTORS

Child-rearing practices, as a major component of the cultural context, had been relatively ignored by social scientists until the 1950s. Concepts such as Freud's Oedipus complex and the family romance were applied universally with little regard for cultural variations. This is not to say that these psychoanalytic constructs should be negated; instead their usefulness should be expanded. This can be accomplished most readily if they are linked to the cultural environment in which people and their symbols live. For example, Malinowski's (1927) study of the Trobriand Islanders, a society with a matrilineal and avunculocal psychological defense system, found that a male child developed a hatred of his mother's brother rather than his own father. Thus the Freudian concept has lim-

itations. The primary point to draw from this study is that although the family romance exists, it differs from culture to culture. Thus we could say that Freud's work, although substantially valid, is not necessarily completely valid for every culture.

Whiting and Child (1953) conducted a great deal of research in the area of cultural expectations, child-rearing practices, and individual development. They noted that excessive deprivation of affection during childhood could be correlated with pathological responses in later life and with related cultural beliefs.

As has been stated throughout this book, the impact of cultural context on personality development cannot be minimized. The interaction of biological, psychological, and cultural factors in the lifelong process called personality development cannot be ignored.

▶ Socioeconomic status

Socioeconomic status, social class, and social status are virtually synonymous. The educational level one's parents attained, the occupations they pursue, and the income they receive all contribute to one's social status. It is important to look at these functional correlates of an individual's particular class. What does being a part of an identifiable class mean? How do these correlates affect personality development?

Families of the middle class, whose members are often well-educated and have certain advantages, have often been compared with families of the lower class, whose members are often poorly educated and have few community resources. There is a marked difference in family stability between the two groups, with a concurrent effect on parent-child relationships. It is within the realm of these relationships that the effects of socioeconomic status on personality development can be noted. The middle class tends to raise children to be high achievers, to control their emotions, and to share thoughts and ideas with their parents. The environment is one in which cultural, physical, and intellectual opportunities are available and encouraged. Value is placed on the appreciation of music and art. Advantaged families may be more liberal than disadvantaged families in child-rearing practices, possibly because, as Zigler (1970) suggests, they have more time and the vocabulary to devote to democracy. Physical punishment is less likely to be used in advantaged families. In contrast, the frustrations of little money, time, and energy may cause the less advantaged family to release pent-up tension through excessive physical punishment or child abuse. Children from less advantaged families tend not to do well on standardized tests (possibly because of cultural variations) or to learn as quickly in school (perhaps because of a self-fulfilling prophecy on the part of teachers). Children from disadvantaged families also tend to feel less secure about their own self-concepts, a situation that has significant effects on personality development.

We do not mean to imply that a person from a lower-class family is always doomed to failure or that a person from a middle-class family always achieves his or her optimal level of being. The task of nurses is to recognize that the developmental rate can be seriously impeded by conditions of poverty. These conditions need not be restricted to less advantaged families as defined by socioeconomic criteria. As is seen more and more often, children from ''good'' families can experience difficulty in adjusting to life situations and can have poor self-concepts. A socioemotional poverty can exist in a setting in which material goods are provided but little else. Parents who are caught up in enhancing their own status may show little concern for the emotional needs of their children.

Such data can be useful in the area of primary prevention. By being aware that certain conditions promote positive personality development while others do not, parents can make efforts to provide situations in which learning and growth are facilitated.

▶ Religion

Religion is a factor that affects personality development in general and child-rearing practices, family stability, and self-concept in particular. Child-rearing practices may be heavily influenced by religious beliefs. For example, the Protestant ethic (''good, hard work will accomplish all'') may be transmitted to a child through a no-nonsense approach on the part of the parent. In such a family, the expression of feelings may be viewed as frivolous and unacceptable. In a family of another religious orientation, discipline may not be considered as important.

Knowledge, attitudes, and problem-solving methods may be influenced by religious affiliation. A child pursuing a parochial school education may develop attitudes and values somewhat different from those developed by a child in public school. Differences in motivational levels may be accounted for, in part, by differences in religious background. Even if religion does not play a particularly important role in a family's child-rearing practices, it still can have a profound influence on the development of moral and ethical standards.

▶ Education

Education, although the last factor to be discussed here, is one of the most influential in personality development. Differences in problem-solving capacity, initiative, creativity, and self-concept have been noted among children who have attended different schools. Our goal is not to trace these differences to their respective sources but rather to recognize their implications for the developing personality. Hoy and Applebury (1970) suggest that the most important aspects of the school experience are peer relationships and student-teacher relationships. Students generally see teachers as role models and agents for change. Unfortunately, however, some teachers are instrumental in giving students negative attitudes about themselves. If a teacher considers a student primarily in terms of the student's race, social class, or ethnicity rather than in humanistic terms, a self-defeating cycle can be produced.

It has been shown by various studies that schools are direct reflections of the communities in which they exist. Therefore, it is logical to assume that they meet the needs of their students. However, this is not always the case, particularly in school districts composed of large groups of minorities but administered primarily by members of the middle class (see Chapter 4 for further discussion). In order for individual development to be enhanced, the values of the school must be consonant with those of the community. Each group must be working toward the same end. For example, if a school supports the notion of a college education for all its students, but the community views its members as blue-collar workers with little need for a college education, the student is caught in the middle. In such a situation, the effectiveness of the school is impaired and the student is left with unmet needs and a feeling of frustration. Once the values and goals of community, teachers, and students are in consonance, the impact on personality development will be in a more positive, growth-promoting direction (McCandless and Evans, 1973).

• • •

Although a wide range of variables has been considered in terms of their impact on personality development, the most important concept is the interrelatedness of these factors. Biological factors are subject to environmental modification. A child raised in a vacuum, unable to learn from his or her environment, will be severely retarded in perceptual and motor development. Cognitive processes will also be affected. An individual's self-concept is greatly influenced by constitutional factors such as body height and weight. Genes determine the developmental timetable, but the timetable responds to environmental modifications.

Nurses are not as much concerned with determining the degree each component plays in the development of the individual personality as they are with recognizing that this interaction occurs and understanding its implications for the emerging personality.

Effect of early experiences on personality development

We have discussed in previous sections the impact of early life experiences on personality devel-

opment. Adaptive mechanisms in early life may be quite primitive, yet they act as prototypes for future reactions to stress.

Freudian theory has emphasized the fact that a "foundation for pathology" is laid in the early years. This concept may be taken a step further, away from strict psychoanalytic concepts, if we view early sociocultural or environmental experiences as being significant to the development of personality disturbances later in life. It can be said that, regardless of whether psychosexual development is maturational, the response of a child's caretaker and the environment in which the child exists at the time of each stage serve to influence personality development.

The energy that is invested in the tasks of each stage, the tension that arises in stressful circumstances, and the coping skills that emerge result in patterns that serve as models for future adjustment to the same circumstances. Freud (1916) states that as a consequence of each stage, a certain amount of libidinal energy is fixated at that stage, building certain defenses and expectations into the personality. Major psychopathology occurs when too much libido or energy is fixated at an early stage, because the coping patterns developed at those early stages are not applicable to problem-solving in adult life. In such an instance, the adult tends to use coping mechanisms that are not effective and that are not appropriate to his or her level of intelligence.

Probably the very first anxiety experience is that engendered by the birth process. The fetus moves quite rapidly from the warm, dark, quiet, and relatively safe environment of the womb into a bright, almost tumultuous environment. How does the infant respond to this barrage of stimuli? The adaptive mechanisms he or she develops become models for future adaptations.

The infant devises a number of methods of dealing with incoming stimuli. He or she selectively attends to stimuli, filtering out those he or she cannot or does not want to attend to. This cannot be done on a voluntary basis; however, the infant can focus on a specific activity that effectively blocks out other stimuli. He or she also becomes accustomed to a stimulus after it has been occurring for a long period of time. Anxiety then is no longer aroused.

What consequences do these experiences have in terms of personality development? Escalona and Leitch (1953) suggest that infants differ in responsiveness and in the speed at which they respond. It has been shown that there are infants who react more readily to stimuli—that is, startle more easily. A history of increased sensitivity to stimulation has been identified in children with pathology. Behavior patterns of the schizophrenic child may be maladaptive responses to this sensitivity. Such early mechanisms may serve to reduce anxiety initially, but they are ineffective in the long run.

Sleep is an effective method of reducing anxiety during infancy, and it is frequently utilized and reinforced. Can you recall instances when circumstances around you were overwhelming? It was quite comfortable to retreat to the bedroom, curl up in bed, and pull the covers over your head. Sleep relieves a person of the need to deal with anxiety. The development of this adaptive mechanism need not result purely from experiences during infancy. In adult life, one is told to "go to bed" or to "get some rest" in order to alleviate the anxiety of a tension-packed day. Sleep allows an individual the luxury of putting off dealing with a situation causing anxiety while realizing that it will be necessary to face the anxiety at some point. Sleep is but one mechanism of adaptation in the early phases of development.

Psychoanalytically oriented theorists believe that certain experiences may be perceived as being comforting because of their similarity to the birth process. A child, when anxious, may seek refuge in a warm, dark place—a place that is similar to the mother's womb. Although this view may stretch one's imagination, it is important to note that early experiences do set the stage for the use of certain adaptive mechanisms in later phases of life.

Factors such as self-concept, interactions with parents and significant others, socioeconomic background, and schooling experiences collec-

tively and individually affect the development of adaptive mechanisms in later life. For example, individuals who feel comfortable with their self-concepts are able to relate successfully to others. They are more likely to perceive themselves as integral parts of their surroundings and to provide themselves with sources of continuous information about those surroundings. Maladaptive mechanisms tend to occur when people perceive their environments as threatening. If, in the early phases of life, they encounter continuous negative reinforcement from parents and other significant people, they develop mechanisms to protect their already suffering self-concepts. Withdrawal from reality, submission, and psychophysiological responses are utilized to deal with tension. These patterns continue to develop throughout the early periods of life until they become entrenched in the adult personality.

Thus the early periods of life are fertile territory for the development of adaptive (or maladaptive) mechanisms. Nurses need to be cognizant of the many factors that affect personality development. As Freud first pointed out, we need to recognize the implications of early childhood experiences and response patterns in order to understand adult adaptive mechanisms.

THEORIES OF DEVELOPMENT

A wide range of published material is related to the development of personality. We will present the concepts proposed by four major theorists: Freud, Erikson, Sullivan, and Piaget. We believe that these theories present a broad base of knowledge from which students can develop their understanding of the dynamics of personality

Freud

Freud introduced the principle of epigenetics—the view that development follows a logical, sequential pattern. The critical tasks of each phase in the sequence must be completed in order to successfully move on to the next phase. If there is an interference in development at one of the stages, maladaptive behavior may result. However, since Freud's time it has been found that compensations are possible, to a certain degree. Deficiencies may be converted into strengths if they are recognized at an early stage.

In essence, Freud was arguing that sexual energy or libido is the prime motivator of human behavior. He viewed personality development in terms of libidinal investment, or cathexis, in the oral, anal, and phallic zones. He then correlated the process of physical maturation with the progression of the aforementioned zones.

Before Freud's view of psychosexual development is discussed further, his concept of the partitions of the mind—the id, the ego, and the superego—should be explained. The id represents the instinctual portion of the mind, controlled only by the blind strivings of Eros, the instinct of life, and Thanatos, the instinct of death. Thus the id is the origin of an individual's drives and motives. Normally, the actual forces of the id remain in the unconscious. Their effects are felt, however, as conscious perceptions of thoughts, desires, and feelings. The influence of the id is constantly and subtly felt by the ego, which is the rational, reality-based component. The ego results from interaction with the environment; this interaction forms a boundary for the mind. The ego is the portion of the psyche that others "see" first. It serves a decision-making function in that it determines what kinds and amounts of stimuli are allowed into the mind as well as what is permitted to leave. What we say and do, how we perceive situations—these functions are dictated by the ego. The ego acts as a mediator between the id and the superego, which is the conscience, the dictator of moral and ethical standards. The superego is a differentiation of the ego, as the ego is a differentiation of the id. Both differentiations are a result of the interaction of id and environment and concurrent cognitive development. However, the development of the superego results primarily from interactions with specific parts of the environment, such as parents.

At birth the infant is predominantly operating under the pleasure principle. He or she seeks immediate gratification for all needs and has little concern for the needs of others. He or she is all-encompassing, a concept that is supported by the orality or literally "eating alive" quality of the infant's responses to the mother. At the interfaces of the pleasure-driven id and reality there arise the beginnings of ego—the reality-oriented component of the mind. It is important to note that the thinking mechanisms associated with the initial, id-driven behavior can be connected to the dreams and fantasies of adults. This "primary process thinking" is frequently found in adaptive behavior of a regressive nature, such as in various types of psychosis. "Secondary process thinking" is related to reality situations.

Psychosexual development involves the concept of motivation. Freud believed that motivations remain constant throughout life but that the zones through which id gratification is sought vary. Much of motivation remains unconscious; however, in the course of the development of the ego, a person receives a limited insight into his motives. Knowledge that may not be conscious at the moment but that can be recalled at any time is said to exist in the "preconscious." Material that has never been permitted into conscious awareness, as well as repressed material, is said to exist in the "unconscious." The utilization of defense mechanisms to control anxiety points out the fact that individuals often do things for reasons they are unclear about or may even deny (see further discussion of defense mechanisms later in this chapter).

The oral stage of infancy encompasses approximately the first 15 months of life, in which children are unable to meet their most basic needs on their own. They depend upon others for that nurturance.

The channel of gratification is the mouth and lips, which are particularly sensitive. The stimulation of the mouth and lips sets off the sucking reflex. Libidinal energy is invested, or cathected, in the relevant channel of gratification, which in this psychosexual stage is the mouth. The gratifying objects are the mother's breast, a bottle, a pacifier, or the thumb. Energies of the infant are directed toward nursing, with the accompanying relationship to the parenting figure. The infant is unable to distinguish satisfying objects as being separate from his or her own body. They may, in fact, hold more attention than actual parts of the infant's own body. However, by approximately 9 months of age, the infant is able to discern the difference between self and the object of gratification.

Under favorable circumstances, the needs of an infant are met on a consistent basis. The way in which needs are met (or not met), particularly the responses of the parenting figure, have a great influence on an adult's ability to relate to another—to develop a sense of trust. If needs are met on a continuous basis by a warm, loving figure, a feeling of trust develops. We will discuss trust further when we consider the theories of Erikson.

It is interesting to note the paradox of infancy. It would seem that infants are totally helpless, dependent. However, their needs are met repeatedly without their actual recognition and identification of wanted objects. In a sense, then, there is an omnipotence inherent in the infant's personality. Parents of infants, who are often given to discussion of their problems, have frequently expressed the feeling that a mother's or a father's life revolves around the infant. Activities must be planned around the infant's feeding and sleeping schedule. A person cannot simply get in the car and go shopping; such an operation requires very careful consideration of the hours of wakefulness and the "irritable" periods. This feeling of not having one's own life sometimes reaches extreme proportions. In such circumstances a parent may use maladaptive forms of behavior to adjust.

Orality means more than just gratification through the mouth and lips. The infant actually "takes in" various kinds of stimuli in his or her environment, a process that lays the groundwork for future cognitive and emotional processes. Lest we focus primarily on feeding as the representation of the oral phase, we must be aware that the infant is particularly sensitive to tactile stimulation. This sensation is most highly developed in the oral, or infancy, period. The relationship to the mother's body is very important in this phase; it is an intrinsic component of orality.

Defense mechanisms to reduce tension develop in the phase of infancy or orality. Sublimation, introjection, projection, and denial act as initial tension-alleviating mechanisms in this period.

Sublimation is the directing of unacceptable libidinal energies into socially acceptable channels. These libidinal energies relate more specifically to sexual-aggressive drives or pleasure-seeking drives than to hunger, for example. Thumb-sucking provides physical pleasure; the infant is content with this mechanism, and it is more socially acceptable than sucking on the breast as a comfort measure. Gratification of the need is still achieved but in an indirect manner. The sublimation process also takes place in adults. A young woman on a weight-reduction diet collects thousands of recipes and thus sublimates her desire to eat. A man with intense hostile feelings becomes a lumberjack. The hostile energies are then channeled into vigorous wood chopping.

Introjection develops as a result of the infant's desire to be powerful, an attribute that the infant has ascribed to the parenting figures. The infant wants to incorporate this quality into his or her own personality. By doing so, the infant makes his or her self-esteem secure enough to last until a time when he or she is more able to accomplish tasks within the environment on his or her own. A healthy adult counterpart of this mechanism occurs as a result of the resolution of the grieving process. The bereaved person is able to incorporate qualities of the lost loved one, resulting in decreased separation anxiety and increased ability to invest in other relationships. However, introjection may be an unhealthy mechanism as well. For example, an individual may introject qualities of another person that will result in self-punishment (as when a person incorporates qualities of a punitive mother).

Coupled with introjection is the mechanism of *projection*. Projection involves the attributing of one's own unacceptable thoughts, wishes, fears, and actions to another person or object. In later life this mechanism is the basis for scapegoating. In infancy, mother and infant are perceived as one object by the infant, thereby facilitating the ascribing of feelings and wishes from self to the mothering figure. In later childhood, uncomfortable feelings are attributed to others. For example, a young child who is afraid of the dark might tell his mother that his teddy bear is afraid. In adult life, a person might place the blame for his or her failures on circumstances in the environment. The extreme form of projection is paranoia. Although projection is utilized to some degree by healthy individuals, it is a more pathological mode of adaptation than other defense mechanisms.

Denial develops somewhat later in the period of orality. This mechanism involves the rejection or disavowal of elements of reality that may be unpleasant or painful. The infant denies the presence of disturbing stimuli by closing his or her eyes. This is only a temporary adjustment technique, which eventually disintegrates when an individual is forced to confront reality. However, it is used quite regularly throughout life. The question for nurses thus becomes one of *when* to intervene and present reality without stripping the individual of this defense mechanism. Carter (1971) describes several examples of denial that may be seen in operation in the general population. Some people postpone diagnostic testing or, when confronted with results of tests, refuse to acknowledge that illness exists. Persons with chronic illnesses such as diabetes or cardiac problems sometimes ignore the disability and fail to take the prescribed medications or to follow the planned regimen. Each of these situations reflects a denial of painful information and an attempt to continue life on a "business as usual" level.

Since denial ranges along a continuum, it is important for nurses to determine whether denial is harmful or therapeutic in a given situation. Involved in this assessment is the nurse's understanding of his or her own feelings regarding the client and the illness. What are the nurse's own expectations of client behavior? Is the nurse fostering denial or preventing denial from following a natural course? Denial has many faces. Because of its complex nature, nurses must view its operation as multidimensional and must be aware that it has far-ranging implications. It is no longer sufficient to say that denial is healthy or unhealthy. A client's utilization of denial must be assessed carefully before its importance in the maintainance of a healthy, integrated ego can be understood.

It must be pointed out that defense mechanisms do not operate on a conscious level. Even in adulthood they operate below the awareness levels. The results of these mechanisms, however, are apparent.

The degree of libidinal energy invested during the oral phase is reflected in later activities such as gum chewing, nail biting, excessive eating and drinking, and smoking. All of these activities are said to satisfy oral needs. Problems that develop during the oral phase may prohibit the release of energy for utilization during later stages, thereby causing a fixation in that stage. In such a situation, the individual's physical development progresses according to schedule while psychosexual objectives remain the same as they were during that early period.

The toddler period is the stage in which the child begins to move throughout his or her environment, to exercise control, to be free to some degree. There is a shift of libidinal energy from the mouth as a channel of gratification to the anus. This area becomes highly sensitive and responds to stimulation. Baldwin (1967) suggests that the shift is not maturational but rather follows the attention that is directed toward the anus by the tiolet-training process. The focus of the anal period is toilet training. Here the child finds himself or herself in a bind. The child wants to please his or her parents by having a bowel movement in the right place at the right time, yet this intention impinges upon his or her developing sense of autonomy. The child also desires the immediate gratification of the pleasurable feeling of the act of defecating. The question becomes one of either delaying gratification in order to receive parental approval or risking disapproval for immediate pleasure. There is a sense of ambivalence, a combination of positive and negative feelings directed toward the same object or situation.

According to Freud, various features of the anal period are crucial to later development. The retention of feces and ''giving'' them to the parents increases the significance attached to possessions. The person fixated at the anal stage of development is often characterized as parsimonious and unable to tolerate ambiguity or confusion. The anal personality considers love objects as possessions and acts to control them rather than to permit them to act independently. This tendency may be reflected in the marital situation, with each partner ''belonging'' to the other.

The mechanism of sublimation is carried over into the anal phase, as are other mechanisms. Small children find pleasure in playing with feces, yet this is unacceptable to parents. Such activities as playing with mud, finger paints, sand, and modeling clay satisfy this instinctual drive in a socially acceptable fashion.

Reaction formation is the shift in feelings or attitudes from one point on a continuum to the extreme opposite point. The first utilization of this defense mechanism is the shift in attitude toward bowel and bladder function in order to avoid unacceptable impulses. For example, the desire to play with feces may be transformed into scrupulous cleanliness. Although the visible behavior is more socially acceptable, the original attitude is not erased. It is merely relegated to a lower level of consciousness. Another example, seen frequently in adult males, is concern about feelings of warmth and tenderness. Masculine characteristics of physical prowess are overdeveloped to replace unacceptable ''feminine'' traits.

Repression, one of the major defense mechanisms, arises during the anal phase in order to push unpleasant thoughts, feelings, and emotions out of conscious awareness. It is an attempt to prevent feelings of unpleasantness caused by the recollection of the desire to play with feces or of the sexual fantasies aroused by the parent during the phallic phase. Repression is the cornerstone of defense mechanisms, its major goal being to preserve ego boundaries.

Regression, the last of the primary defense mechanisms, is a return to an earlier stage of development, where modes of gratification were more satisfying and needs were met. The most important aspect of regression is that it happens *to* the ego; the ego is *acted upon* rather than doing the action. The child in the anal phase, feeling the pressure to conform to bowel and bladder training, may go back to the previous phase, in which he sought gratification primarily through the oral mode. Another example of regression in the toddler-age child is the seeking of attention from parents after the arrival of a new sister or brother, by soiling the diaper.

The phallic stage, or self-centered sexual stage, revolves around the concept of the Oedipus complex (or in the female, the Electra complex). There is a shift of libidinal energies from the anal region to the genitals. The male child directs his energies toward the mother, in direct competition with his father. He alternately loves and hates the father (ambivalence). The preschooler's ideas of sexual relations are often vague. The child sometimes places his hands all over the mother's body, particularly on the breasts. He imitates the way his father transmits affection to the mother. The mother tends to feel uncomfortable, particularly if she is unaware of her son's internal struggles at this time. The child, in any case, is not permitted to live out his fantasy. His feelings are condemned by both parents, yet those same feelings are accepted *between* the parents. The young boy fears the retaliation of his father in the form of castration. The subsequent aspect of this phase is the relinquishing of the sexual wishes because of fear of castration. Rather than be a rival of his father, the boy identifies with him. Hostility is repressed, as are sexual desires for the mother. In this way, the young boy begins to acquire masculine desires and values.

The Electra complex has not been as well defined as its male counterpart. Similar components exist: sexual desires are repressed, rivalry with the mother cannot be tolerated, so identification occurs, and acceptance of femininity results. The concept of castration anxiety is quite different for the female, since there is no penis. The resolution of this part of the complex lies in the fact that women can reproduce and men cannot.

The beginning of the resolution of the Oedipus complex occurs in the phallic stage, as does the beginning of the development of the superego. As we will see, this resolution is carried over into the latency period. To present a clear picture of the development of the superego, we will discuss the mechanisms of introjection and identification. The child takes on aspects of the personality of the parent of the same sex. This process, termed introjection, was discussed previously. As a result of this internal process, identification comes about. The child introjects the values, attitudes, and goals of his or her parents—a ready-made conscience—into his or her ego structure. Identification is the process whereby the child imitates the desired qualities of the significant other. This process concurs with the child's concrete cognitive level of development. Introjection serves as the basis of the superego, yet it can be carried to an extreme. In such a situation, an individual may replace his or her entire ego structure with the characteristics of the significant other, losing his or her own identity in the process. As a person matures, the superego becomes more readily based and less harsh and demanding. The development of the superego relieves the child's castration anxiety or penis envy.

Faulty resolution of the Oedipus complex has far-reaching effects on later personality development. It can be said that at the base of almost all neurotic difficulties lies an inadequate resolution of the Oedipus complex. The adult who is fixated at this phase of development is characterized by poor sexual identity and difficulty with authority figures.

The period corresponding to the grade school years is referred to as the latency period. As we noted, there is a tremendous flow of energy in the phallic stage. Then there is a quieting of that energy in the latency period, perhaps a "calm before the storm" type of effect. It is the valley between the two peak periods—the phallic and the genital

phases. A great deal of energy is devoted to intellectual pursuits. Sexual achievement and curiosity are replaced by a quest for knowledge and the motivation to achieve in school. Through sublimation, sexual drives are channeled into the socially accepted activity of the pursuit of education. The latency period is a time when culturally determined skills and values are acquired. The child moves out of the family system and is subjected to the values and attitudes of others. Throughout this period, the superego matures and becomes more organized, integrating the viewpoints of a variety of significant people in the environment.

The latency period, ranging from ages 6 to 12, is characterized by increasing sex-role development, which is facilitated by identification with the parent of the same sex. Testing of new sex roles can be seen in the development of sex-segregated gangs and cliques, which are quite common during this phase. Aggressive behavior, valued in males, takes the form of rebellion against authority. Reaction formation is in operation when the male child rejects not only sexuality but the whole opposite sex. This phenomenon can be noted in the attitude of boys toward girls in this age bracket. A 9-year-old boy would not be caught dead having a conversation with a girl! Adults fixated at this stage of development are often characterized by a lack of motivation and by an inability to appraise situations and solve problems creatively.

Freud did not actually include adolescence as a stage of personality development. It was his feeling that the personality is established by the beginning of adolescence. The genital stage differs from the phallic stage in that the genital stage is characterized by an overwhelming supply of sexual drives. But there is now a concern for others' feelings. The primary goal of this stage is the development of satisfactory relationships with persons of the opposite sex. The manner in which the Oedipus complex is resolved may have a definitive effect on an individual's choice of a partner. A girl often seeks out a boyfriend whose expectations in regard to her behavior are similar to her father's expectations about her mother. A man will often marry a girl who is quite similar to his own mother.

Table 6-1. Miscellaneous defense mechanisms

Defense mechanism	Definition	Example
Isolation	Ego allows actual facts of experience, either past or present, to remain in consciousness, but breaks the linkage between facts and the emotions that belong with them	Nursing student giving postmortem care walls off emotions usually elicited by dead human bodies
Displacement	Certain strivings or feelings are unconsciously transferred from one object, activity, or situation to another	Husband is mad at his boss, so he comes home and yells at his wife
Rationalization and intellectualization	Plausible reasons for one's behavior, feelings, and attitudes are constructed (rationalization)	Man cheats on his income tax but explains it away by telling himself, "Everyone does it"
	Anxiety is controlled through the transporting of conflict to the realm of secondary process thinking and talking (intellectualization)	
Undoing	A specific action is performed that is considered to be the opposite of a previously unacceptable wish or action; mechanism is related to the magical thinking of childhood	Ritual undoing of wrongs through penance

Table 6-2. Freudian stages

Developmental stage	Time period	Critical behaviors
Oral	Birth to 15 months	Mouth and lips are channel of gratification and means by which environment is explored
Anal	15 months to 3 years	Libidinal energy shifts to anal area; focus is on toilet-training and muscle control
Phallic (oedipal)	3 to 6 years	Libidinal energy shifts to genital area; introjection and identification initiate development of superego
Latency	6 to 12 years	Focus of energy is on intellectual development, maturation of superego continues; child moves out of family system (through school) and is subjected to others' values
Genital	12 years to early adulthood	Overwhelming supply of sexual drives; primary goal is developing satisfactory relationships with persons of the opposite sex

As a result of the Oedipus complex, the male identifies with the father. In the genital phase, repressed sexual feelings are allowed into consciousness, and acceptance of these feelings begins. It is at this point that libidinal energies are directed toward a relationship with the opposite sex.

Another major component of the adolescent phase is the development of a sense of self-worth. Inherent in this development is the defining of one's role in society. Up until this point, the adolescent had occupied a fairly secure role—he or she knew where he or she belonged, who his or her friends were. But during this phase of life he must move out of this comfortable niche and find his or her own place in society. This process can encompass a wide range of possibilities, such as further education, a vocation, and marriage. Finding one's place in society is, at best a difficult task.

An adult who is fixated at the genital phase of development is characterized by an inability to enter into an intimate relationship with another individual and by a tendency to "float" from one occupation or educational setting to another.

In addition to the defense mechanisms already presented, several others are commonly utilized. They are summarized in Table 6-1.

In summary, according to Freud two series of changes take place concurrently in the development of the personality. The first is the maturation of the ego, with the attending recognition of reality and development of defense mechanisms. The final product of this series is an interpersonally oriented being. Second, cognitive processes develop that permit an individual to assess and interpret his or her environment, to give meaning and rationality to what he or she perceives. This framework leads to the discussion of the view of development of another psychoanalyst—Erik Erikson.

Erikson

Erikson added a new dimension to Freud's psychosexual stages: psychosocial development. He viewed society as having a profound impact on the emerging personality. Erikson identified critical tasks for each phase of development. These graduated tasks must be met in order for a person to move successfully on to the next phase. Society assures the proper socialization of the child by providing him or her with opportunities for (1) role development, (2) attainment of independence, and (3) healthy expression of emotions. The accomplishment of these tasks occurs differently in each culture.

Development, according to Erikson, is a gradual process. The ultimate goal is an individual who not only feels comfortable with his or her own identity but also is sensitive to the needs of others in his or her environment: a *social* animal. Like Freud, Erikson believed that the success or lack of success of adaptation in one phase influences an individual's ability to master the critical tasks of the next period. It is not a question of a child selecting the tasks that he or she would like to master. Tasks occur on a continuum, each leading to the next, with an ever-increasing repertoire of coping abilities being made available on a regular basis.

A *sensory* phase lasts from birth to approximately 18 months. The most crucial task to be dealt with is the development of a sense of being able to rely on others, to establish a sense of trust. During this period infants are totally dependent upon others in their environment. As their needs are consistently met, they begin to attain a basic sense of trust. The significant relationships that occur during this phase set the tone for all future relationships. Infants who are able to trust others, to be confident that their needs will be met, are more likely to achieve a feeling of confidence in themselves. This feeling of trust in others and the increasing sense of self-confidence permit them to feel secure in the knowledge that their needs will be met should they find themselves in a helpless, dependent position in later life. Adults who have not experienced trusting relationships in early life will be more pessimistic in their expectations of others. Their relationships with others are frequently doomed to failure. Their lack of self-esteem is often projected onto others in the form of the attitude "He doesn't like me." This attitude elicits responses that reinforce it. The cycle then comes full circle. Individuals who do not have a

Table 6-3. Erikson's stages

Developmental stage	Time periods	Critical behaviors (tasks*)
Sensory	Birth to 18 months	Trust vs. mistrust; development of significant trusting relationships
Muscular	1 to 3 years	Autonomy vs. shame and doubt; child learns to function autonomously within the context of the environment
Locomotor	3 to 6 years	Initiative vs. guilt; increasing awareness of own identity and relationship to multiple other systems; increasing awareness of influence on others
Latency	6 to 12 years	Industry vs. inferiority; energies are directed toward creative activities and the pursuit of learning
Adolescent	12 to 20 years	Identity vs. role diffusion; transition from childhood to adulthood; achievement of integration of values, beliefs, attitudes acquired up to this point
Young adulthood	18 to 25 years	Intimacy vs. isolation; ability to extend self into intimate relationships with others
Adulthood	21 to 45 years	Generativity vs. stagnation; logical extension of young adulthood; relationships reflect successful achievement of intimacy and the ultimate goal of developing a family
Maturity	45 years to death	Ego integrity vs. despair; perception of life as a culmination of both positive and negative events; acceptance of one's own life as it is; ultimately a positive sense of self remains intact

*Term specifically used by Erikson.

basic sense of self are prevented from investing in open, two-way interactions with others.

The *muscular,* or toddler, phase approximates the period of ages 1 to 3 years. The critical task of this phase is the achievement of a sense of autonomy, as opposed to arousal of feelings of self-doubt. Lidz (1968) suggests that this cannot truly occur until the child achieves a sense of initiative, the critical task of the next developmental phase.

Perhaps the crucial concept here is the interrelationship of phases. Young children become independent of their parents as the parents provide opportunities to do so. They feel comfortable in seeking out new experiences in the environment because there has been the initial development of basic trust. They soon realize that they can take the initiative to explore their world, knowing full well that mother or father will be there if the need should arise. In this way children begin to feel independent, autonomous. They begin to be aware

of the effects their bodies have on the environment around them.

Parents greatly influence the degree to which children attempt to master their environment. When constant barriers, both physical and verbal, are placed in the path of the development of autonomy, there is little room for growth of initiative. Children feel they are ''bad'' for not conforming to rules and regulations. Parents who lack confidence in their own abilities often project their inadequacies onto their children. In such a case, the child does not feel capable of extending his or her horizons further into the environment. Again, a basic lack of trust in oneself prevents the development of a satisfying relationship.

The critical task of the next stage, the *locomotor* phase, is the achievement of a sense of initiative. During the period from ages 3 to 6 years, the developing child seeks to balance initiative and guilt. Erikson (1950) suggests the child achieves this balance by identifying with the parent of the same sex, thereby reducing the guilt produced by the rivalry between the child and that parent. As a result of this phase, the child develops a conscience that serves to regulate primary id impulses.

The locomotor phase is characterized by a greater organization of personality. The child gains an appreciation of his own sense of identity, his own place as a system in relation to many other systems. He becomes increasingly aware of his influence on others as well as of his limitations. In a later section, we will discuss the impact of the broadening range of cognitive processes on the child's personality organization and development.

The *latency* period, ages 6 to 12, is concerned with the task of industry versus inferiority. The child utilizes his or her energies in creative activities or in the pursuit of learning. The child seeks to become part of a group; a sense of belonging is crucial to this phase. The child begins to internalize the values and attitudes of those around him or her. There are new environments with which he or she now becomes familiar. The child finds a place for himself or herself among his or her peers. The child gains feelings of self-worth as a result of appraisals from other persons in the environment—adults, playmates, and schoolmates. Recognition that some people like him or her and value his or her word while others do not is critical to the development of a capability for a healthy self-evaluation. The quality of leadership is one that becomes apparent in this period. The child learns that he or she can lead; or the child sees himself or herself primarily as a follower. Or the child may see himself or herself as never being a part of the group and thus become habitually rebellious or alienated. In such a situation, the child often feels a sense of inferiority, which causes the child to act out in defiance against others—a protective shell made necessary by his or her lack of self-worth.

The *adolescent* phase, encompassing ages 12 to 20, is the transitional phase between childhood and adulthood. It is characterized by turmoil and change. There are individual variations in the rate of sexual maturation, as well as in the pace of emotional, intellectual, and social development.

The adolescent is expected to integrate all of his or her experiences up to that point into a coherent sense of self and to emerge as an adult.

The achievement of an integrated self requires the successful accomplishment of the tasks of previous phases. The child comes equipped with a basic sense of trust, an ability to make some decisions regarding his or her life, and an ability to relate to others individually and in groups. These factors enable the personality to gel into a workable, integrated whole.

During the transitional period the individual can prepare for independence, yet he or she is still under the protective umbrella of his or her parents. This situation may have a negative influence on successive development if parents do not permit children to exercise some of their options. If an adolescent remains in a children's world within the family but is confronted with adult expectations in the total society, a sense of role confusion results.

Erikson (1950) stresses the significance of the next phase—*young adulthood* or late adolescence, which lasts from ages 18 to 25. The crucial task of this phase is the achievement of intimacy as opposed to isolation. The young person must gain an ego identity that reflects an individual who is a human being in his or her own right. He or she is no longer considered someone's daughter or son. Once a firm sense of self has been established, the young adult is able to extend himself or herself into an intimate relationship with another individual. Interdependence—the sharing with another of all that one values without fear of loss of self—is the crux of this period. (It seems that an inability to achieve a true sense of intimacy in our current society is being reflected in a rising divorce rate, although the divorce rate is influenced by many other factors as well.)

The phase of *adulthood*, ages 21 to 45, is concerned with the task of generativity as opposed to stagnation. As young adults move through the life cycle, they begin to identify life goals, including occupational and marital choices. The period of adulthood thus is a logical extension of the period of young adulthood, during which the capacity for a sharing relationship develops. The adult's choices reflect the successful achievement of a sense of self-worth and belonging, and the transition from operating under parental values and attitudes to operating under one's own.

During this period, a dyad is often transformed into a triad with the addition of a child. The partners who feel comfortable with themselves and who have had their needs met are able to direct their love and energy into the development of a new human being. We have come full circle; the phases of development begin again—with another life.

The final phase of development according to Erikson, is *maturity,* in which the task is to accomplish ego integrity as opposed to despair. Individuals review their life experiences, considering those objectives they have successfully completed and those they have not. Persons who can accept their lives for what they have achieved undergo a renewed sense of ego integrity. Life has meaning for them, in both its positive and negative events. They do not despair for what might have been. The end of life is perceived as a culmination of their many experiences rather than as something to be feared. The older person has thought a good deal about death and has usually had many experiences with it. Death is a phase of development that one must pass through, with the ultimate goal being achievement of a positive sense of self in this final stage.

Sullivan

Harry Stack Sullivan believed that individuals need to be socialized in their environments. His theory was based on the premise that each individual seeks to avoid anxiety. Inherent in this theory is the view that coping mechanisms are developed in order to reduce anxiety. Sullivan differed from Freud and Erikson in that he viewed biological changes as the stimuli for emerging needs and growth trends.

As an individual grows, there are changes in his or her inherent ability to relate to objects and persons in the environment. Abilities and body parts are considered an individual's *tools*. The goal of each developmental phase is considered the *task*. For example, the task of the infancy stage is to receive fulfillment of needs from others in the environment. In order to accomplish this goal, the infant utilizes his or her mouth, the ability to cry. The mouth and the ability to cry are considered the tools. As the child moves through the stages of development, the tasks becomes more sophisticated, as do the tools. During late adolescence, the individual utilizes his or her genital organs and the

Table 6-4. Sullivan's stages

Developmental stage	Time period	Critical behaviors
Infancy	Birth to 18 months	Gratification of needs results in beginning level of trust
Childhood	18 months to 6 years	Learning to delay gratification in order to achieve longer-term rewards (i.e., parental approval)
Juvenile	6 to 9 years	Development of sense of belonging to one's peer group; "chum" relationships
Preadolescence	9 to 12 years	Primary relationships are with those of the same sex, switch of loyalty from family to peers
Early adolescence	12 to 14 years	Attempts to be independent while at the same time desiring dependence; primary goal is development of satisfactory relationships with members of opposite sex
Late adolescence	14 to 21 years	Achievement of an intimate love relationship without the fear of loss of self

process of experimentation (tools) to develop an intimate, loving relationship with another (task). Like Freud, Sullivan described the individual who successfully completed the tasks of each developmental phase as being interdependent, capable of forming a lasting relationship, and comfortable with his or her concept of self.

In order to facilitate the understanding of sullivanian theory, we will discuss some of its dynamic concepts. Reality orientation is referred to in terms of "mode." The prototaxic mode, occurring in infancy, is characterized by a lack of differentiation between self and the environment. Thus Sullivan's and Freud's concepts of self and its relationship to the environment are similar.

The parataxic mode is characterized by the breaking up of the undifferentiated whole. The resulting parts are illogical and disjointed and occur inconsistently. This mode is in operation primarily during childhood, but it also extends into the juvenile period. It is necessary for the child to separate the parts of the whole into discrete units so as to better understand their individuation and subsequent relatedness to the physical and social environment.

The ability to perceive whole, logical, coherent pictures as they occur in reality characterizes the syntaxic mode. The syntaxic mode is used as a means of understanding the environment and relating to others. In order to gain assurance that perceptions are real, adults seek consensual validation. They are then able to identify areas that need development as well as those that do not.

Sullivan refers to the organization of experiences that defend against anxiety as the "self-system." In order to make an accurate assessment of an individual's feelings of worth, it is important to understand the concepts of "good-me," "bad-me," and "not-me." The child, based on his or her interpersonal experiences, assumes one of the above postures. Behavior that is regarded as valued by the parents is then learned and incorporated by the child as good-me. Behavior that does not receive parental approval is identified as bad-me. The child perceives from verbal and non-

verbal cues that such behavior is not acceptable. For example, he or she may hear a parent talk about the unacceptability of tardiness. Behavior that generates large amounts of anxiety is denied and identified as not-me. A parallel can be drawn between the freudian mechanism of reaction formation and the concept of not-me. Each involves an unacceptable feeling being denied, the opposing feeling being verbalized, and anxiety being reduced for the moment. For example, a person who is experiencing feelings of hostility may say, "I love everyone as a brother." He or she may be saying, in effect, that the hostility is "not-me."

The focus of sullivanian strategies is to develop appropriate, healthy responses as components of the syntaxic mode. Reduction of anxiety caused by developmental deficits is also a primary goal. One of the purposes of the nurse-client interaction is to permit the client to identify these deficits and to correct them. (See Chapter 9 for discussion of nurse-client interaction.)

Sullivan identified six basic phases of development, which are similar to those of Freud and Erikson. In *infancy,* the period from birth to approximately 1½ years, the primary task is the development of basic sense of trust in others. The gratification of needs ensues as a result of the foundation of trust. The mouth, the ability to cry, the satisfaction response, empathic observation, autistic invention (see Chapter 21), exploration, and emergency responses such as rage and anxiety are the developmental tools—the means by which the child accomplishes the task.

As individuals move through the developmental phases, they increases their repertoire of coping mechanisms as each task becomes more complex. The focus of the *childhood* period, 1½ years to about 6 years, is learning to delay gratification in order to receive long-term reward—for example, parental approval. Through the use of mouth, anus, autistic invention, experimentation, manipulation, identification, and emergency responses such as anxiety, guilt, shame, doubt, and anger, children begin to develop a more realistic sense of their own influence on the environment, which leads to a greater sense of independence and self-worth.

The *juvenile* period, ages 6 to approximately 9, is characterized by the development of a sense of belonging within one's peer group. It is especially important for a child in this period to form satisfying relationships with children of his or her own age group. Sullivan refers to these as the "chum" relationships. Often the child will place his or her family second in order to meet the needs of his or her peers. The tools available to the child in this period include competition, compromise, cooperation, experimentation, manipulation, and exploration.

Following the juvenile period is *preadolescence,* which includes ages 9 to 12. During this time there is a marked switch of loyalty from family to peers. A friend of the same sex is the primary relationship. Exploration, manipulation, and experimentation, coupled with the capacity to love, consensual validation, and collaboration, are the primary tools of the period.

Early adolescence, ages 12 to 14, reflects the child's beginning attempts to be independent of parents and their set of values, attitudes, and beliefs. There is a sense of rebelliousness. It seems as though the child longs to be both independent and dependent at the same time, and anger arises from this seemingly impossible situation. The task at hand is learning to develop satisfactory relationships with members of the opposite sex. Another primary goal is the achievement of a sense of identity concurrently with a delineation of life goals. Lust, experimentation, exploration, manipulation, and anxiety are the tools most commonly utilized during this phase of development.

The last phase, *late adolescence,* encompasses ages 14 to approximately 21. The major task of this phase is similar to that of Erikson's late adolescent or young adulthood phase—achievement of an intimate, love relationship without the fear of loss of self. This is a culmination of the previous phases in that a sound sense of identity has developed, along with the ability to form trusting relationships with others. The appropriate tools of this period include genital organs, exploration, manipulation, and experimentation.

Sullivan believed that once an individual had completed the tasks of late adolescence, he or she would be capable of functioning interdependently in society. He thought it unnecessary to continue the discussion of personality development farther than this point, since the most crucial developmental tasks would already have been accomplished.

Piaget

Piaget describes personality development as a progression of cognitive processes. Initially the child is quite egocentric: he or she believes that all others in the environment share his or her feelings, thoughts, and beliefs. As the child matures, he or she becomes aware of others' viewpoints and develops an ability to integrate those concepts into his or her own framework.

Like the other theorists discussed, Piaget views development as a series of stages. When a stage has been completed successfully, the child moves on to a more complex one. For Piaget, mature, intelligent behavior is the ability to critically assess and problem-solve in virtually any situation. Thought processes progress from a concrete level to "formal operations," or abstract, logical thinking.

Four factors concurrently influence the development of cognition: biological maturation, experience with the physical world, social experience, and equilibration. Equilibration is the balancing and integrating of new experiences with those of the past as an individual progresses along the developmental course.

Two behavioral factors inherent in equilibration are *assimilation* and *accommodation*. Through the interaction of these two components, the child (and eventually, the adult) is able to reconcile and integrate any new behavior.

Assimilation is the ability to comprehend experiences. An individual is constantly being bombarded with new situations that require responses. What an individual learns as a result of new interactions with the environment needs to be incorporated into his or her already existing body of experiences. Thus new interactions are given meaning in terms of the experiences an individual has had up to that time. In other words, assimilation occurs.

When new concepts are introduced, a certain degree of upset or disequilibrium ensues, depending on the nature of the concept and its perceived effect. An individual directs his or her energies toward identifying and eliminating the cause of the disequilibrium. As the disequilibrium decreases, the perception of the event becomes more accurate. The process is termed accommodation. For example, the infant views the mothering figure as an extension of self. Through the process of development, the infant begins to differentiate self from environment. New experiences impinge upon the infant. The meanings of these experiences need to be integrated with the meanings of past experiences. The infant must change the manner in which he or she perceives the mothering figure in order to develop a differentiated self. Thus the process of differentiation occurs as a result of assimilation and accommodation, in that order.

In summary, assimilation is the mechanism whereby the comprehension of a new experience occurs, up to the point where previous experience left off. Therefore, assimilation frequently results in incorrect plugging in (because of lack of experience). Accommodation occurs to rectify the inaccurate plugging in. This leads to restoration of equilibrium at a higher level of functioning. A parallel can be drawn between disequilibrium and anxiety; the ultimate goals of an individual are the reduction of anxiety and the incorporation of experiences—and thus higher-level functioning—cognitive, emotional, psychological, and biological.

Piaget divides his cognitively based developmental schema into four periods. The first is the *sensorimotor* period, which lasts from birth to 2 years of age. This period is characterized by the infant's moving around in his or her environment. Meaning is attached to objects by way of manipulation. Young children begin to differentiate themselves from their environment through goal-directed behavior. One of the primary concepts children learn in this period is the permanence of objects, a concept that is basic to logical thought. Objects continue to exist, whether they are seen or not. Another concept that is basic to logical

Table 6-5. Piaget's stages of cognitive development

Developmental period	Time period	Critical behaviors
Sensorimotor	Birth to 2 years	Manipulation of environment through goal-directed behavior; child learns concepts of object permanence
Preoperational thought		Growing ability to utilize language as a tool; egocentrism,
Preoperational phase	2 to 4 years	or the belief that one's viewpoint is the only one, is a primary characteristic
Intuitive phase	4 to 7 years	Integration of concepts based on more than one dimension; increasing ability to comprehend rules and to recognize relationships
Concrete operations	7 to 11 years	Beginning use of logic and objectivity; reasoning is related to concrete or real events
Formal operations	11 to 15 years	Abstract thinking is reached during this period; emergence of self as well as recognition and validation of identity; development of relationships with others

thought is that objects retain their identity even though the context in which they appear changes. Children in this period learn that Grandma is the same person with her glasses off as she is with them on.

The second major period is that of *preoperational thought*. In order to describe the progression of cognition more clearly, Piaget divided this period into two phases—preoperational and intuitive.

The preoperational phase, ages 2 to 4 years, reflects the child's growing ability to use language as a tool to meet his or her needs. The seedlings of thought begin to appear as the child becomes more aware of the representation of objects by words. For example, a table is an object; we do not eat at the word "table" but at the actual object. The ability to make this distinction prepares the child for symbolic mental activity.

Children in this phase cannot categorize objects in more than one dimension—for example, an object cannot be both yellow and rectangular. They are capable of attending to only one primary characteristic at a time. They are also unable to classify a group of similar objects in terms of their multifactorial similarity.

Another general feature of thinking of the preoperational period is egocentrism. The child believes that his or her viewpoint is the only one—it is difficult for the child to understand thoughts, perceptions, and ideas as being different from his or her own. The child cannot understand why an event does not occur as he or she had thought it would. The child cannot allow for factors other than his or her own. When a parent admonishes the child, saying, "Don't do that—you wouldn't like it if someone did that to you," the child does not understand, because he or she is unable to place himself or herself in the position of another.

As children become older, they are able to conceive of groups or classes as having relationships. In the intuitive phase, ages 4 to 7, they comprehend basic rules and are able to integrate concepts based on more than one dimension. The number of objects in a group no longer changes as the context of presentation changes—another cornerstone of logical thought. For example, children are able to discern that one set of dots is equal in number to another set of dots even though the presentation is different (see illustration below). By the end of the preoperational period, children see that each block contains six dots.

In the period of *concrete operations,* ages 7 to 11, children begin to use logic and objectivity. Reasoning is related to concrete or real events—for example, all apples are fruit; then this apple is fruit. As a result of this phase, children can organize objects into hierarchies as well as reduce a whole into its component parts and combine it differently without causing a change in the whole.

The final step—abstract thinking—is reached during the period of *formal operations,* ages 11 to 15. By age 11, children are able to conceptualize a plan based on hypothetical events, consider more than one variable, and identify appropriate strategies of action. Potential relationships among objects can be visualized. As in the adolescent phases of Freud, Erickson, and Sullivan, there is emergence of self, recognition and validation of one's own identity, and then the development of relationships with others in the environment. The individual is able to reflect on himself or herself, review his or her experiences to that point, and evaluate their influence on self-appraisals.

Thus an individual's interaction with his or her environment is a fundamental premise of the piagetian philosophy of personality development. The child moves from simple cognitive processes, such as understanding object permanence, to formal, abstract thought processes.

MASLOW'S HIERARCHY OF NEEDS

The previous section dealt primarily with the phases of development a child must complete in order to reach maturity. Parallels among four theorists discussed were drawn when appropriate; the tasks or crises of corresponding phases often seemed to be similar. It is important to understand the implications of this statement: Nurses must not assess clients on the basis of only one developmental theory; they must correlate the relevant aspects of many theories.

Maslow (1954) views individuals from a perspective that is somewhat different from those of the four theorists discussed—but one that is equally important for health care providers to understand and apply. Maslow suggests that there is a priority or "hierarchy" of needs, that a person seeks to satisfy basic needs before moving on to complex ones.

The individual must be motivated to meet challenges, to satisfy needs. Motivation, a concept crucial to the understanding of human behavior, has been discussed in a variety of formats. It can be defined as the rationale or logical thought behind an individual's actions, plans, or ideas. A rationale operates on three levels—conscious, preconscious, and unconscious. Most of what motivates individuals operates on an unconscious level. This fact is of critical importance not only in a nurse's assessment of a client's behavioral responses but also in the nurse's understanding of his or her own reciprocal responses. Maslow proposed a list of five basic needs, each of which reflects a higher-level priority than the preceding one. The

needs are as follows: (1) physiological, (2) safety, (3) love and belonging, (4) self-esteem, and (5) self-actualization. What meaning do these needs hold for the development of nursing care strategies? Nurse and client could be operating on two different levels. Imagine, for example, that a community health nurse enters a woman's home to discuss her feelings about becoming a mother for the first time but that the woman does not seem interested. Observations of the surrounding environment reveal leaky ceilings, no food in the refrigerator, little furniture, tattered clothing. What are this woman's priorities of needs? Obviously, the nurse is concerned about a higher-level need (love and belonging) than the client. The client is concerned about physiological necessities and safety. Initially, lower-level needs must be satisfied. The client may then be more able to share her feelings about being a new mother. Nursing strategies must take into account the fact that lower-level needs must be satisfied to a greater extent than higher-level needs.

When the first three needs are, for the most part, satisfied, a person seeks out appraisals and assurance from significant others in the environment. He or she needs to feel a sense of self-respect and self-confidence. Individuals value the appreciation and recognition received from their peers; however, the last two of the five needs are rarely satisfied completely. Self-fulfillment needs and the recognition of one's potential for continued self-development tend to remain below the level of consciousness. These two needs thus tend to be unconscious motivators of behavior (Maslow, 1954). This fact should alert nurses to be critically aware of verbal and nonverbal behavior that may be motivated by a client's desire for self-respect, autonomy, and self-development.

Maslow's levels of need overlap, just as the phases of development of the various theorists overlap. Higher-level needs emerge before lower-level needs are totally satisfied. Most people tend to be partially satisfied in each area and partially unsatisfied.

CONTINUUM OF MENTAL HEALTH–MENTAL ILLNESS

We have noted that developmental "lags," fixations at early levels of development, or unsuccessful accomplishment of developmental tasks set the stage for mental illness. However, we must point out the fact that mental health, or mental illness, is not a static state. Behavior varies from minute to minute, day to day, month to month. Mental health can be likened to a series of peaks and valleys with plateaus interspersed periodically. Many factors interact, resulting in behavior. In addition, as we will note in succeeding chapters, culture influences the identification of mental illness. Sapir (1963) points out the role of culture as an etiological factor in mental illness—through child-rearing practices and stressful roles, for example—and as a symptom-molder, as in the case of syndromes peculiar to one culture. For example, in the United States, value is placed on rational, logical thought processes. Persons unable to behave in a rational manner are labeled "ill." The same behavior in another culture might be perceived as normal. Thus the criteria used to define and identify mental illness are linked to cultural heritage. It is necessary for nurses to appreciate the arbitrary, culture-bound bases of what is viewed as "normal." Oddities of behavior in another culture are easily identifiable as culture bound. However, the identification of psychiatric disorders within one's own society as being culture bound is not readily accepted.

Jahoda (1953) describes six characteristics developed in infancy and childhood that reflect positive mental health. The first of these indicators is a positive attitude toward oneself. A person who understands his or her strengths and accepts his or her limitations possesses a strong sense of identity and is relatively secure in his or her environment.

Appropriate growth and development, as well as achievement of self-actualizing ability, constitute the second positive indicator. Erikson's eight stages of man can be used to measure this particular criterion. The individual who is unable to successfully complete developmental tasks may become maladapted. Positive reinforcement of self-concept is of great importance in enabling an individual to achieve his or her maximum level of functioning.

The third indicator of positive mental health is the ability to integrate and synthesize life events in such a way as to maintain equilibrium and to reduce anxiety or make it tolerable. Each person develops a philosophy of life that reflects an assessment of the environment and his or her relatedness to, or isolation from, that environment.

Autonomy is the ability to make appropriate decisions and to be self-directed, with specific goals and objectives in mind. A parallel can be drawn between this fourth indicator of positive mental health and Erikson's second phase of development—autonomy versus shame and doubt. Can a person separate himself or herself from the environment and its social influences? Is he or she able to make decisions on his or her own and willing to accept the consequences of his or her actions, whatever they may be? Throughout the life span, vast amounts of energy are directed toward achievement of independence, which is an important indicator of mental health.

The fifth indicator of positive mental health is the ability to perceive reality without distortion. A person's perceptions of the "real" world as opposed to what is fantasized are influenced by cultural values and mores. Through consensual validation, a sullivanian concept, a person receives support from others in perceiving the environment validly. Similarly, we consider an individual to be mentally healthy if he or she is sensitive to another human being's wants and needs—that is, if the individual is empathic. One of the most significant indicators of mental disorder is the inability to grasp reality. However, this factor must be assessed in relationship to the predominant culture, as well as to family constellation and significant others.

The sixth indicator of positive mental health is

the ability to love others and to be loved. The ability to love others and be loved includes all aspects of interpersonal relationships, such as work and play. Environmental mastery is the crux of this criterion. The ability to adapt—to meet situations head-on, assess them appropriately, draw relevant conclusions, identify goals, and plan strategies—is a complex component of environmental mastery. The individual is no longer a slave of the environment; the individual is aware of his or her *impact* on other people, that he or she does

have input. Environmental mastery begins shortly after birth and continues through senescence. At each level, different tasks serve to increase an individual's ability to problem-solve in new and varied settings. Energy is directed toward mastering the tasks at hand. A paralyzed young adult devotes his or her energies toward mastering an environment that functions on the concept of mobility. A perceptually or visually impaired person seeks to master his or her environment. Each individual assesses his or her environment to discover what

Table 6-6. Overview of developmental stages

Stage of development	Play/social activities	Health promotion	Language/cognitive development
Infancy	Playing with self Understanding environment through movement Infant needs colorful, mobile, cuddly toys	Immunizations essential during this period Safety precautions relate to falls, burns, oral ingestion of foreign objects and poisons, drowning	Sensorimotor period—ability to recognize change and to adjust accordingly Vocalization begins about 4 months of age—relates to recognition of people and definition of needs; language in this phase is autistic; communication is goal-oriented by the end of the period

*According to Duvall (1971).

meaning it holds for him or her at the time. He or she then devotes energy toward the accomplishment of tasks that will reinforce environmental mastery.

Thus far in this chapter, some of the major aspects of personality development have been presented. Assessment of clients must be based on an overview of psychosexual, biological, cognitive, interpersonal, and social characteristics, as well as on other factors that combine to form an integrated, whole being. Table 6-6 illustrates such an

integration of the concepts we consider to be significant to the understanding of the unique personality of each client.

THE FINAL PHASE OF DEVELOPMENT—DEATH

Death—an unavoidable aspect of life yet probably one of the most difficult to accept—has achieved status as a legitimate health concern for

Text continued on p. 166.

Body image	Emotional development	Developmental tasks*
Diffuse feelings of hunger, pain, comfort, but no real body image; self not differentiated from environment; basis for positive perception of body image laid in early mother-child relationships By end of first year, internalization of sensory experiences into body image occurs Ego development and body image development occur simultaneously	Parent-child bonding crucial foundation for basic sense of trust and patterns of future relationships; essential that primary needs are gratified promptly	Achieve physiological equilibrium following birth Establish self as dependent person but separate from others Become aware of alive versus inanimate and familiar versus unfamiliar and develop rudimentary social interaction Develop feeling of and desire for affection and response from others Adjust somewhat to the expectations of others Manage the changing body; learn new motor skills; begin eye-hand coordination Learn to understand and control the world through exploration Develop beginning symbol system, preverbal communication Direct emotional expression to indicate needs and wishes

Continued.

Table 6-6. Overview of developmental stages—cont'd

Stage of development	Play/social activities	Health promotion	Language/cognitive development
Toddler	Play is primary mode through which child organizes world, releases tension, improves muscular coordination, and develops spaciotemporal perception Stage characterized by solitary or parallel activities	Primary concerns are respiratory infections and accidents; parents "childproof" the home by removing scatter rugs and sharp or breakable objects and putting poisons out of reach	Preoperational/parataxic period—learning through imitation; lack of understanding of cause and effect relationships Child communicates in an understandable manner yet may not use words with meaning Syncretic speech—one word represents a certain object; emotions, objects, actions are fused to have one meaning Speech is autistic, vocabulary enlarges
Preschool	Pre-gang stage; peers assume a new importance; child progresses from solitary play to cooperating with others in group; learns to follow rules, to compare self to others, and to be concerned about others; appraisals begin to come from persons other than parents—provides for reality testing and allows expression of emotion and creativity	Accident prevention—e.g., motor vehicles, burns, falling, drowning, child needs clear-cut safety rules explained consistently, simply; adult supervision is also warranted Immunization boosters Dental and medical check-ups important on a regular basis	Concept formation begins—child moves from lack of differentiation to awareness of objects as concrete and separate from the environment Inability to differentiate own feelings from external events—everything is important on an equal basis Language is used to get attention, to maintain interpersonal relationships, and to gather information Reading becomes significant factor in language development

Body image	Emotional development	Developmental tasks
Body image gradually evolves as a component of self-concept	Developmental task: autonomy versus shame and doubt—"Me do it!"	Settle into healthy routines
Child becomes more aware of his or her body as having physical and emotional components	Child relies greatly on parental responses and support; need for attention and approval acts as primary motivator for socialization process	Master good eating habits
Child not fully aware of the interaction of his or her body with the environment—i.e., the impact each has on the other	Toilet-training is major developmental accomplishment	Master the basics of toilet-training
Body products—e.g., feces—are not perceived as separate from self		Develop physical skills appropriate to stage of motor development
Self-concept develops from reflected appraisals of significant others; concept of "good-me" develops as a result of positive responses from others; critical period for development of positive self-concept		Become a family member
		Learn to communicate effectively with others
Ego boundaries become more differentiated, as do physical body boundaries; in part because of an increase in sexual awareness, an increase in motor coordination, more mature play experiences, and positive parental relationships	Child learns social roles and responsibilities and behaves more like adult counterparts	Settle into healthful daily routine of adequate eating, resting, and playing
Fear of mutilation is quite common in this period	Continuation of mastery of self and environment	Master skills of gross- and fine-motor coordination
	Developmental task—initiative versus guilt	Become a participating family member
	Child uses imagination and creativeness to greater degree	Conform to others' expectations
	Increasing awareness of feelings of love, hate, anger, tension—child learns modes of coping to reduce anxiety	Express emotions healthfully and for a wide variety of experiences
		Learn to communicate effectively with others
		Learn to use initiative tempered by a conscience
		Develop ability to handle potentially dangerous situations
		Lay foundations for understanding the meaning of life, self, the world, and ethical, religious, and philosophical ideas

Continued.

Table 6-6. Overview of developmental stages—cont'd

Stage of development	Play/social activities	Health promotion	Language/cognitive development
School age	Peer groups provide a broader circle of friends outside home environment Six- or seven-year old enjoys assuming roles —e.g., fireman, mailman, teacher, doctor, nurse Older school-age children enjoy table games of a simple nature, riding bikes, swimming Later in this period, creativity appears in the areas of music, art, dance, drama Predominant partner is "chum"—of same sex and age, actually is an extension of child's self; sharing of very special thoughts and feelings occurs	Illness occurs for first time as child enters school; upper respiratory infections are common Immunization boosters are important Safety precautions in relation to motor vehicle accidents and drownings	Stage of concrete operations—reasoning through real or imagined situations Child progresses to greater understanding of meanings and feelings Child uses language to establish relationships and to increase knowledge base Syntaxic communication is utilized—cause and effect relationships are beginning to be recognized Child learns to express feelings and thoughts in a way that is meaningful to others
Adolescence	Peer groups most important; status and recognition derived from the group; behavior defined by group members Sense of identity results from appraisals by others in the social setting	Mood swings quite common in this period Accidents involving motor vehicles of some sort are leading cause of death Obesity, excessive loss of weight (anorexia nervosa), acne, venereal disease, and pregnancy are current health issues	Period of greatest ability to acquire and use knowledge; adolescent is able to perform active problem-solving to reach realistic solutions; considers alternatives to problems; is highly imaginative—this can be a very creative time

Body image	Emotional development	Developmental tasks
School experience reinforces or weakens child's perceptions of body and self Fluidity of body image/self-concept, due to rapid physical, emotional, and social changes	Developmental task—industry versus inferiority Child progresses from self-centered to more other-directed behavior Child evidences concern for others—particularly "chum" in latter part of period More self-direction—continued imitation of adults Child still unaware of effects of self on others, yet becoming more tolerant of others' behavior	Decrease dependence on family and gain satisfaction from peers and adults Increase neuromuscular skills in order to participate in games and work with others Learn adult concepts, as well as concepts related to problem-solving Learn to communicate with others realistically Become active family member Give affection to, and receive affection from, family and friends without expecting immediate return Learn socially acceptable ways of handling and saving money Learn to deal with strong feelings Adjust to changing body image and come to terms with sex roles Discover healthy ways to become an acceptable person Develop positive attitude toward own and other social, racial, and economic groups
Body image and self-concept closely tied to identity formation; experiences of a positive nature enable development of positive body image; adolescent is sensitive to rapid change in physical characteristics; may be overly aware of a defect, resulting in undervaluation of self Body is the channel through which rejection or acceptance occurs	Developmental task—identity versus role diffusion completion of task rests on successful completion of previous tasks—leads to secure sense of self Values, attitudes, beliefs of parents are internalized Adolescent feels a sense of wholeness—recognizes uniqueness of self	Accept changing body size, shape, and function Learn a variety of physical skills Achieve a satisfying and socially acceptable sex role Find the self as a member of one or more peer groups; develop interpersonal skills Achieve independence from parents and other adults yet maintain interdependence Select a satisfying occupation in line with interests and abilities

Continued.

Table 6-6. Overview of developmental stages—cont'd

Stage of development	Play/social activities	Health promotion	Language/cognitive development
Adolescence —cont'd		Drug and alcohol abuse are, historically, very characteristic of period	
Young adulthood	Review of life options to decide what focus of life will be—e.g., marriage, work, family Person continues to have close circle of friends, usually based on similar interests, values, occupations Chooses social and recreational activities as pleasure-promoting as well as outlets for energy	Accidents—especially motor vehicle, industrial, drowning—are the leading cause of death	Full mental capacity has been attained, although knowledge may be increased in college or trade schools Person assumes more responsibility for own learning rather than expecting it to be handed to him or her Is able to make contributions to society of a social or intellectual nature
Middle age	Leisure time becomes a concern; as individual progresses toward retirement, assessment of leisure time is important; person needs to feel that it is acceptable to put aside time for leisure	Menopause—both male and female—occurs, with concurrent physiological changes Consideration of safety factors to prevent falls, burns Coronary artery disease is leading cause of death in men	Learning enhanced by individual's resource of life experiences Motivation to learn is greater—increasing numbers of individuals in this age bracket are continuing their education

Body image	Emotional development	Developmental tasks
		Prepare to settle into a close relationship with another individual based on love rather than infatuation
		Develop intellectual and work skills and sensitivity to others
		Develop workable philosophy of life, mature values, and worthy ideals
Body continues to be channel of connection to the world; disturbances of the body influence self-concept	Developmental task—intimacy versus isolation	Accept self and stabilize self-concept and body image
If body undergoes changes, person must explore those changes and incorporate them into existing picture	Inadequate resolution of identity crisis may lead to disturbances in sex role identity	Establish independence from parental home and financial aid
Body type and size influence personality development	Stress reactions, including physiological changes, may occur as a result of intolerable levels of anxiety	Become established in a vocation or profession that provides satisfaction and financial recompense
Illness causes changes in body image/self-concept that need to be integrated	Suicide is third leading cause of death	Learn to appraise and express love responsibly through more than sexual contacts
	Alcoholism and drug abuse are two other chronic problems	Establish an intimate bond with another
		Manage a residence
		Decide whether to have a family
		Find congenial social group
		Formulate a meaningful philosophy of life
		Become involved as a citizen in the community
Additional physical changes occur—graying hair, wrinkled skin, decreasing sensory functions	Developmental task—generativity versus stagnation	Rediscover and develop new satisfactions as a mate
Need to accept body changes as part and parcel of maturation process	Reassessment and evaluation of one's life are critical	Assist growing children to become more responsible
Need to recognize positive aspects of self, body, and other persons in age group	Acceptance of goals that were accomplished as well as those that were not	Create pleasant, comfortable home, appropriate to own values
	Enjoyment of watching children carry on traditional values and beliefs	Find pleasure in generativity and recognition in work
	Orientation toward needs and goals of others—willingness to extend self	Adjust to role reversal with aging parents
		Assume mature social and civic responsibilities

Continued.

Table 6-6. Overview of developmental stages—cont'd

Stage of development	Play/social activities	Health promotion	Language/cognitive development
Middle age —cont'd	Recognition of the era in which one was raised and subsequent values developed Relationship with spouse is especially important—provides security and stability in a period of much change	Other health problems include cancer, pulmonary disease, diabetes, depression, alcoholism	Ability to integrate cognitive function with experiential factors, resulting in more meaningful interpretation of life experiences
Older adulthood	Older individual often surrounds himself or herself with his or her few special friends; period characterized by great sense of loss—loss of close friends, loss of function/independence, and eventual loss of self Person is comfortable with daily routines and same people Needs to maintain contact with outside world in order to preserve reality orientation and to prevent loneliness Retirement affects number and type of relationships—person may feel cut off from meaningful people	Safety factors are of prime consideration; impaired sensory input hampers the accurate perception of environment; falls, burns, forgetfulness in regard to the taking of medications are examples of potentially dangerous situations Alterations in all major systems begin; regular physicals and early detection of illness help to reduce ensuing problems	Many factors affect learning: reduced motivation, sensory impairment, educational level, deliberate caution; capacity to learn continues—logical associations between words and events are easily recalled Apprehension in new learning situations Slowness in reaction time

several reasons. People are enjoying longer life spans, in many cases, because of the advances made by medical science. However, this fact can also create new stressors for families and clients around the issue of the quality of life. Many terminally ill clients are requesting that extraordinary life-support measures not be instituted, while their families and health care providers, especially nurses and physicians, are being caught in the throes of attempting to comply with these wishes. Clients, families, and health professionals are often unsure about how to support the wish to die with dignity. Is a client giving up hope too readily, or is he or she really ready to die?

Body image	Emotional development	Developmental tasks
		Develop and maintain active organization membership
		Accept and adjust to physical changes
		Make an art of friendship
		Use leisure time with satisfaction
		Continue to form a philosophy of life
Physical changes cause alterations in function and appearance and thus in body image; sensory deficits cause individual to believe that he or she is weak and less worthy; feels the loss of independence; perceives prostheses, hearing aids, glasses, etc. as being threats to wholeness	Developmental task—ego integrity versus despair; person defends his or her beliefs and life-style—because they hold meaning for the person; views life as worthwhile, productive rather than futile, and too short; individual who has had an intact ego throughout the life cycle is better equipped to deal with aging—feels completeness and satisfaction with his or her life; death then is not feared but accepted as part of life	Decide where and how to live out remaining years; find satisfactory home and living arrangements
		Continue a warm, supportive relationship with significant other
		Adjust living standards to a retirement income
		Maintain maximum level of health
		Maintain contact with children, grandchildren
		Maintain interest in people outside family
		Pursue new interests and maintain former activities
		Find meaning in life after retirement
		Work out significant philosophy of life
		Adjust to loss of loved one

Nurses as well as other health professionals frequently come into contact with persons who are dying, since most dying still occurs in the hospital, although there has been a concerted effort to facilitate the process of dying at home when it has been chosen by client and family. The nurse is frequently one of the individuals who is closest to the dying client. A holistic approach to care acknowledges that dying clients have a full range of human emotions, which can thrust them into the depths of depression or allow them, and those around them to experience a sense of peace. It seems also that the role of the nurse has assumed greater importance in a society where a reduction in the size of the nuclear family has left fewer family members available as support systems. In addition, a client's extended family may live far away, so that participation in the dying process may be limited to the client, the nurse, and one or two family members.

In Erikson's stages of development, the final stage is that of ego integrity versus despair. An individual can review life and accept what he has accomplished rather than despair over what could have been. Death can be viewed as a culmination of life's experiences, not something to be feared or denied.

The disengagement theory of Cummings and Henry (1961) states that an aging person and society participate in a mutual emotional, physical, and social withdrawal in preparation for the individual's death. However, the more recent literature, including that of Bernice Neugarten (1968), suggests that meaningful involvement in earlier developmental phases has a profound influence on activity level in later years. Contrary to the disengagement theory, physical, emotional, and social activity may constitute a vital force in an individual's life until death involuntarily causes disengagement. The latter theory provides a fundamental rationale for encouraging an individual to participate actively at whatever level he or she chooses in his or her final act of living—death. The dying process is a major life crisis; in order to participate in it, the individual must utilize his or her abilities to the maximum. Hine (1982) suggests that "people can experience their deaths as something they have to do rather than as something that is happening to them."

Stages of the dying process

Although each person who faces death experiences the situation uniquely, six stages are commonly associated with the process of dying. These stages, identified by Elizabeth Kübler-Ross as a result of her extensive work with the dying, were incorporated into her book *On Death and Dying* (1969).

The first stage is characterized by shock and denial. Many dying persons react with the statement, ''No, not me; it can't be true!'' Kübler-Ross says this reaction occurs whether a person is told at the outset of an illness or comes to his or her own conclusion at a later time. Denial is a healthy mechanism; at this point, it acts as a buffer. It also permits a person to collect himself or herself and to mobilize adaptive responses that are more effective on a long-term basis and that are most comfortable for him or her. The types of responses that the person develops depend upon previous experiences with loss situations, the time the person has to gradually prepare for death, and the manner in which the person received the information that he or she was going to die. Denial will be dropped when the individual feels that he or she will not be abandoned if he or she shares feelings.

Anger and rage are the responses associated with the second stage. ''Why me?'' That is the question the dying person most frequently asks of those around him or her. These feelings are often projected onto family and hospital staff at random, causing the arousal of many feelings in them that ultimately affect the responses of the client. At this point, the client feels that nothing is going well; the doctor is not helping him or her and the nurses do not care. The client directs anger at family members but at the same time desperately needs their support. He or she has difficulty sifting out and sharing emotions. Very often the client's anger takes the form of a desire to control his or her situation. Family and staff should allow the client to make some of the decisions regarding his or her own care.

After the period of anger, the dying person becomes less aggressive; in this third stage the client directs his or her energies toward bargaining for more time. This is an attempt at postponement, a delay for the accomplishment of some important task. Assume, for example, that a woman of 54 is dying of lung cancer. Her one wish is to see her daughter married. Once this wish has been realized, she sets another goal. Such a mechanism permits a client to cope with dying, but a piece at a time. These bargains are usually made with God and are kept secret. However, the message can be read between the lines. Bargaining enables the client to deal with dying a little at a time.

The fourth stage is depression. As the illness of the terminally ill client progresses, the client is no longer able to keep up a stoical appearance, and his or her rage is replaced by a great sense of loss. The client is going to lose everything—friends, family, all that holds meaning for him or her. Financial burdens may become heavier as a result of the loss of employment. Feelings of guilt and shame often accompany the depression.

Kübler-Ross calls the fifth stage ''preparatory depression.'' This type of depression helps to prepare the client for his or her future losses and thus eventually to give the client a sense of acceptance. It is important that a nurse recognize the client's need to express sorrow, to be sad. This is a quiet period with little need for words. A stroking touch is sufficient to let the client know that he or she is understood during this most difficult of times.

The final stage is acceptance. In this stage the client is neither depressed nor angry. He or she is able to admit being envious of the living, angry at those who do not have to die now. The struggle is over and the battle won. The dying person may prefer to be with one significant individual rather than to be surrounded with visitors. However, the client needs to know that he or she is not alone. This is the period of disengagement; it is especially important that family and friends understand the nature of this period.

Death is the final phase of growth (Kübler-Ross, 1975). It is essential that nurses accept the finiteness of their own and their clients' existences.

Although it is important to recognize the stages that the dying client passes through, they are simply a framework for understanding. Each person lives uniquely—and dies uniquely.

Sociocultural aspects of dying and death

Culture influences the kind of comfort measures and care that are given to a dying individual and the context in which the individual dies. For example, Mexican-Americans view the illness of one member of the family as a primary concern to the others. When possible, terminally ill people die at home among their family members and in familiar surroundings rather than in hospital settings (Gonzales, 1975).

Rural or elderly black Americans, Chinese-Americans, and native Americans may equate admission to a hospital for treatment with going there to die. Early diagnosis and treatment are resisted; an individual eventually enters the hospital on an emergency basis or in a terminally ill state, which reinforces the belief that hospitals are a place to die. Cultural orientation is reflected in the belief that individuals should not be alone at a time of trouble and one should be surrounded by family members at the time of death.

Hispanics often view illness and pain as a *castigo,* or punishment from God for their sins. Suffering can then be equated with penance, in which case comfort measures and pain medications are refused during the dying process in order to atone for sins (Baca, 1969).

Culture also influences individuals' attitudes about death as well as funeral practices and care of the body. Native Americans may view death to be the result of the violation of cultural taboos, while Haitians believe that voodoo can cause sudden deathy. Violent death such as suicide is often viewed as less acceptable than other forms of dying. For example, traditionally Roman Catholics who committed suicide were not permitted to be buried in consecrated ground. (For further discussion of suicide, see Chapter 18.)

Care of the body after death is determined by cultural beliefs. Muslim beliefs dictate that bodies must not be cremated nor be used as teaching cadavers. Organs cannot be donated, and an autopsy cannot be done. The Orthodox Jewish faith holds that the body should be buried in tact; thus cremation, embalming, and any cosmetic processes are not permitted. Some cultures view death as a part of life that needs to be prepared for. For example, Amish women sew the white burial garments for themselves and their family members. Instructions are left with friends and other relatives regarding the care of the body and the burial itself.

Spiritual aspects of dying and death

Spiritual and cultural aspects of dying cannot be easily separated. Often culture influences the spiritual beliefs that an individual considers most important. During the bargaining stage, clients may bargain with God or some other omnipotent being for more time in order to see or do "one last thing." Nurses need to consider spiritual beliefs or the lack thereof as they are working with dying clients and their families. For example, a client's spiritual background can help in preparing for death, through prayer, quiet meditation, or chanting or song. Family members may wish to have a quiet time each day with their loved one so they might pray together—saying the rosary or other appropriate prayers. Spiritual beliefs of clients and families can easily be overlooked when physical needs are present. Nurses need to be cognizant of clients' and families' desire for spiritual comfort through the visits of ministers, priests, or rabbis. Family members may wish to have their own clergy person, or they may feel comfortable with the hospital chaplain. It is necessary to assess spiritual beliefs on death as well as to recognize the importance of religious rituals for family and clients. It might be determined that the client or the family has no need or desire for consideration of spiritual beliefs. Nurses need to respect the right of clients to refuse spiritual counseling. Belief in a supreme being can take the form of spirituality rather than belief in God. Spiritual beliefs in whatever form deserve the respect of health care professionals as a component of a holistic nursing approach.

Paranormal experiences

Death is a physically degenerative process, yet there is evidence that suggests a radical alteration of consciousness and perception of reality that can-

not be perceived by the five physical senses, or "paranormal experiences." Hine (1982) hypothesizes that "it is possible that a gradual spiritualization of consciousness is what life is all about and that the altered states of consciousness observed at many deathbeds are simply the final and rapidly accelerating stages of the process." Grof and Halifax-Grof (1976) describe the knowledge gained from working with persons who have had near-death or paranormal experiences. These authors do not view deathbed hallucinations and visions as the delusions of an overmedicated client. They believe that the altered, higher state of consciousness is so overwhelming that it occurs outside the logical sequence of language as well as outside linear time and space. For example, often a client describes the experience of viewing all the events of his or her life as if they were occurring simultaneously—"my life flashing before my eyes." A client can also experience segments of his or her life juxtaposed but not in a chronological or rational manner. An example of this is a client's description of having been traveling with people who have long been dead. The experience is often confused by the fact that it seems real.

Clients report hearing health care professionals pronounce that they are dead yet having no sense of the loss of reality or the alteration of consciousness. A frequently described experience of clients who have undergone cardiac arrest is the feeling that they are watching the activities being performed as if they were outside of their bodies—a phenomenon known as autoscopic observation. Clients after near-death experiences describe following the body to the operating room, noting the details of the operation, and later being able to identify the staff members involved. During a client-support group for individuals with life-threatening arrhythmias, one woman stated that while undergoing cardioversion in the electrical studies laboratory, she perceived that she was watching everyone try to resuscitate her. She did not remember feelings of terror or panic but simply a warm, comforting sense that everything would be all right even if she died. Another client in the support group shared a similar experience during a cardioversion but remembers trying to shout down to himself, ''Wake up!''

Another near-death experience, similar to autoscopic observation, is transcendental observation, whereby the mind leaves the body and the environment and is transported to another place and time. For example, a client describes returning to the scene of an accident, after having been taken to the hospital, and observing the activities at the accident scene (Oakes, 1981).

Those who have had near-death experiences describe the mind being moved either through a tunnel or through darkness to a place of warmth, love, and brightness. The mind may be invited to enter the warm place or may be told not to enter because earthly activities have not been completed. The mind is then rapidly propelled backward and is reunited with the body, which is often accompanied by pain or discomfort. Negative apparitions in the form of hell-fire or monsters can occasionally occur.

Children and death

There is often a feeling of tragedy, of social injustice, when a young person is confronted with dying. Parents ask, ''Why the child? Why not me?'' Self-blame can be expressed in the form of statements such as ''I should have done more''— dooming the parents to eternally feeling themselves to be failures. The inability to respond honestly to the child forces the client to deal with his or her own grief alone. A child learns quickly that he or she is dying, whether it be from the whispers, the downcast eyes, or the sudden ending of discussion when he or she walks into a room (Waechter, 1971). Hollow cheerfulness and spoiling further isolate the child at a time when the child needs to be surrounded by the warm circle of his or her family. It is unfair to exclude the child from the anxieties and emotions of the rest of the family. Yet society would like to believe that children do not think of death, particularly their own. Epstein (1975) suggests that the strangeness of the hospital environment and the deliberate avoidance of the family *and* the hospital staff are responsible for the

child's hesitation to talk about his or her feelings. It is thought that children have no concept of death or lack the vocabulary to talk about it. Indeed they do lack the vocabulary if adults presuppose that the child ''doesn't understand.'' A child does, however, understand, but on his or her own level; adults must learn to deal with their own feelings and inhibitions in order to help the child to share feelings and fears.

What is a child's concept of death? Nagy (1948) identified three stages: until age 5, death is seen as reversible; from ages 5 to 9, death is personified; after age 9 or 10, death is seen as final and inevitable.

Children under the age of 5 view death as they would a separation; it is a temporary leaving that implies return at a later time. Death is associated with sadness and fears of separation. Fear of death can also be associated with expression of anger by parents, physical restraints during illness, and punishment for being bad. Children at this age do not recognize that when a person dies, all bodily functions cease and the individual is no longer able to be a part of the world as they know it.

Children from the ages of 5 to 9 are able to view death as a definitive separation from life. Death is frequently personalized in the form of a clown, an angel, or a bogeyman who takes people away in the night. Children in this age group often believe that they can avoid personal death by outrunning the ''death man'' or by locking him out. Parental admonitions of bad things happening can reinforce fears of death at this age.

Children over the age of 10 view death as inevitable and realize that they, too, will die one day. Death may be associated with being in a coffin and rotting. Parental views on reincarnation and an afterlife may be expressed by the child.

In general, children are surrounded by death— in the newspapers, on television, and in the movies. Nursery rhymes and fairy tales present death in both a realistic and a fantasy-like manner. The way a child copes with death is influenced by parental responses; experience with loss, violence, or illness in the family; teachings of significant adults; and the child's ability to integrate the experience. Feelings about death can be expressed through games or concern about sick pets. Honest, simple answers can dispel many of the myths and allay some of the anxieties children have regarding death.

The dying client

Caring for dying clients and their families should be based on the development of an approximated relationship, which Barton (1977) describes as a "need-discerning relationship that is more than just talking." A level of relatedness is promoted that facilitates both verbal and nonverbal communication. Needless prattle is unnecessary. The sincere listening of one individual to another or a simple touch may be all that is needed. There should be an appreciation by the nurse not only of the facts of clients situations but also of their wide range of experiences.

A relationship that is based on avoidance does not recognize or accept the concerns, needs, or perceptions of clients and their families. The nurse who focuses exclusively on seemingly relevant details, such as financial concerns, may avoid discussion of the client's personal experiences. Published studies indicate that nurses are quicker to respond to the physical needs of clients than to their emotional needs. In order to facilitate the expression of the client's feelings about the experience of dying, a nurse needs to understand the "metacommunication" that is being transmitted. "Metacommunication is a message about a message" (Satir, 1975). Metacommunication can also be described as the implicit content or the nonverbal interchange of an interaction. Understanding a client's metacommunication leads a nurse to a more accurate assessment and to more appropriate nursing responses. For example, a woman states during a physical examination, "I have a lump in my breast." This statement carries many implicit messages: "I have cancer." "Am I going to lose my breast?" "Will I die?" On the basis of unconscious personal priorities, the nurse responds to the client. However, communication may be cut off if the nurse does not

explore the implicit meaning of the client's message. The nurse's message also carries an implicit meaning. In order to clarify the metacommunication, the nurse might respond in this situation by saying, "It sounds as though you have some concerns—can you share them with me?" The client perceives her feelings as being legitimate and worthwhile. An open, direct relationship can then be developed.

Nurses often are overwhelmed by their own feelings while caring for dying clients. Barton (1977) describes a process of controlled distancing, "a therapeutic maneuver which permits the care-giver to maintain emotional integrity in the face of a continuous care process." It is sometimes critical that the nurse move back from the situation in order to more objectively understand what is occurring. This action allows the nurse to maintain a sense of control while at the same time maintaining sensitivity. A successful way of accomplishing controlled distancing is to become more aware of one's own identity and one's own feelings that dying arouses. Nurses need to share these feelings with their colleagues. A support system can readily be developed that fosters sharing, permits each nurse to feel comfortable with his or her feelings, and ultimately maximizes the relationship between nurse and client. Both nurse and client should be permitted to legitimately be persons.

Working with dying clients and their families also involves the assessment of physical needs, toward which, as mentioned previously, nurses generally direct most of their energies. Comfort measures, such as providing adequate pain management, positioning clients appropriately, and maintaining sufficient hydration, can be instituted by the nursing staff on the basis of assessment of the client and collaboration with the physician.

To maintain a position within his or her social context is a concern for the dying client. Once the diagnosis has been confirmed that an individual is terminally ill, the individual is labeled as "dying." What is the role of the dying person? Clients describe feelings of ambiguity, conflict, and incompatibility with others' wishes. Ambiguity is felt in the sense that the individual is living and wants to participate in that living. However, choices may be taken from him; a passive role can be thrust upon him, leaving him with little or no social identity other than as a dying person. He has gone from being Ed Jones, the father, the husband, the businessman, to Ed Jones, the individual who is dying. A feeling of being in limbo between life and death ensues. Health professionals may "expect," on a subconscious level, a client to die within a certain time frame. Frustration may even be expressed by staff members when this dying does not occur on schedule. The cause of this frustration may be that the staff members know no role for the dying person other than dying. The focus of care is *inappropriately* on the dying rather than on enabling the client to *live* while dying. From the latter frame of reference, the staff can encourage the client to participate actively in his or her care—to know when and how he or she can negotiate for himself or herself in the dying process. Maximizing the potential capabilities of the client and the family will reduce role strain. In this most unique and singular experience, the nurse can assist the client in experiencing his or her dying as a challenge, a final success, a fitting culmination to life.

Nursing intervention

THE DYING ADULT

A. Primary prevention
   1. Assist the client in developing mind, body, and spirit into an integral whole.
   2. Help the client to develop a holistic outlook on life, to view death as part of life and as an opportunity for spiritual growth.
B. Secondary prevention
   1. Assessment
      a. Assess stage(s) of dying process. Remember progression through stages is not lineal. Client may vacillate between stages or may experience two stages simultaneously.

b. Assess client's coping mechanisms and strengths—physical, emotional spiritual (such as beliefs in regard to death and religious rituals that are important), environmental (social and physical environment).
2. Implementation
   a. Assist client to work through denial and accept prognosis of death.
      (1) Accept client where he or she is. Don't push client to accept death.
      (2) Identify signs of denial:
         (a) Client attributes symptoms to a lesser medical condition.
         (b) Client goes from doctor to doctor looking for a better diagnosis.
         (c) Client participates in treatment because he *knows* it will cure him.
         (d) Client refuses treatment, believing symptoms will go away spontaneously.
         (e) Client knows the implications of illness, yet rejects belief that he or she will die.
         (f) Client complains that no one explains anything, yet things have been discussed several times.
      (3) Listen carefully to client's communication
         (a) Client may be pretending to be unaware of prognosis because client fears family, friends, and staff are not able to handle his or her expression of feelings and will abandon him.
         (b) Pick up cues. Client may give masked or covert cues that he or she wants to talk about death, testing nurse's readiness to handle communication about death.

(c) Respond to client's pace—e.g., client's request that you sit down *now* to talk may be a consequence of client's sixth sense that tomorrow he or she won't be able to talk.

b. Assist client to express anger and rage.

(1) Be alert to overt and covert (e.g., complaining and sarcasm) signs of anger.

(2) Ask client what he or she is angry about—often angry about energy and cheerfulness of staff and family, reflecting all that client is losing.

(3) Provide environment where client can acknowledge angry feelings—be receptive, not afraid of angry outbursts, not overly cheerful.

(4) Assist client to express anger appropriately—e.g., screaming, crying, talking, role playing, poetry, or artwork.

(5) Help client explore what client's death means to him or her—e.g., loss, anticipating pain, wanting to die.

(6) Involve client in planning and giving care.

(7) Be aware of own values regarding expression of anger, one's own difficulty in expressing anger can be placed on the client in the form of an expectation of particular behavior.

(8) Express anger that matches client's anger, affirming that expression of a feeling.

c. Assist client to work through bargaining.

(1) Allow client to verbalize about his or her wishes and expectations.

(2) Accept client's desire to gain more time rather than reject it as illogical or unreasonable.

d. Help client cope with depression.

(1) Help client to verbalize grief over impending losses (of friends, family, life).

(2) Allow client to express feelings of guilt (burden to family, not taking better care of self, etc.).

(3) Maintain nonjudgmental attitude regarding guilt.

(4) Assist client to make arrangements for significant others that will lessen guilt (e.g., social service referral, hospice care for help with bedside nursing, and supportive care).

(5) Unrealistic reassurance will block communication (e.g., "Don't cry, things will get better; don't worry, your family will take care of themselves").

e. Assist client with decathexis (preparatory depression stage).

(1) Allow client to go through decathexis—encourage client to see those individuals he or she would most like to. Help client to "let go" at his or her pace—be alert to cues of suicide.

(2) Explain to client, family, and staff that decathexis is normal and needs to be supported.

(3) Sit quietly with client; communicate via touch.

(4) Let client know you will stay with him and not abandon him or her in the death process.

f. Listen with respect to client's "deathbed hallucinations." Try to comprehend meaning of altered state of consciousness and support client. For example, if client says, "I'm trying to find my way" or "I can see death—I'm getting closer," nurse could reply, "You'll find your way." On one level this reply acknowledges client's struggle, on another level it supports his or her experience of getting actively involved in death process, and on yet another level it gives client permission to die.

g. Prepare family members for the physical and spiritual aspects of dying (e.g., cooling of body, breathing difficulties, coma, ''deathbed hallucinations''), mobilizing their coping mechanisms to better support client.

h. Assist client and family to decide on setting for death: home, hospital, hospice.
  (1) Consider the client and family as one unit of care.
  (2) Recognize need for physical, emotional, and spiritual support 24 hours a day, 7 days a week.
  (3) Utilize expertise of interdisciplinary team rather than shouldering total responsibility.
  (4) Utilize hospital chaplain or family spiritual advisor.
  (5) Respect right to refuse visits by clergy.

i. Assist client in the acceptance phase.
  (1) Respect client's wishes (regarding extraordinary means to preserve life, living will, etc.)
  (2) Provide an atmosphere where the client can contemplate his approaching death with peaceful expectation.
  (3) Assist family members in recognizing client's acceptance of death as a reality.

3. Evaluation
a. Evaluate effectiveness of nursing strategies to support client and family through phases of dying process.
b. Evaluate effectiveness of total care plan to enable client to transfer and utilize his or her energy to die in relative peace.

C. Tertiary prevention
  1. Be alert for prolonged and intractable use of denial or for the development of psychotic depression and suicidal ideation; if necessary, make referral to mental health clinical specialist or psychiatrist.
  2. Recognize bereavement needs of survivors and make appropriate recommendations (e.g., counseling, widowed persons groups, Parents without Partners).

THE DYING CHILD

A. Encourage communication through the use of comic strips.*
  1. Cut out several comic strips and remove the conversations, adding blank balloons for child's responses.
  2. Paste strips on plain pieces of paper.
  3. Be alert to overt expressions of concern for the child (i.e., activity, school work, social networks).
  4. Listen for *cues* indicating a readiness to discuss dying and death.

B. Encourage communication through playing with dolls. Encourage the child to manipulate a doll or family of dolls as he or she would like; the child can then act out his or her role, as well as others, in a world that seems less threatening than the real world.

C. Encourage communication through art, writing a short story or letter, and play.
  1. Each of these media also facilitates self-expression that is less likely to be hindered by defense mechanisms. Children may reveal their perceptions of relationships with family members, perceptions of support systems, awareness of their illness, and their knowledge regarding their treatment and progress.
  2. Encourage participation of family members in the child's expression of feelings and perceptions regarding his or her illness and death.
    a. Assist the family in the working through of the ''to tell or not to tell''

*Adapted from Epstein, 1975.

dilemma. Identify superficial advantages of not sharing information, while at the same time recognize disadvantages.

b. Help the family to recognize that the child has an awareness of what is going on at some level and needs simple, honest information.

c. Encourage support in the form of warmth, touching, affection, and presence.

PROBLEMS CONFRONTING NURSES WORKING WITH DYING CLIENTS

A. Inability of nurse to accept client's current stage of dying

1. Nurse encourages client to give up denial before he or she is ready, which increases denial and anxiety.

2. Nurse responds to client's anger with anger, avoidance, or punitive action.

3. Nurse doesn't accept decathexis and tries to reinvolve client in world.

4. Nurse doesn't respect client's philosophy regarding life and death, tries to force own values on client.

5. Nurse has not recognized own feelings about death, avoids dying clients.

6. Nurse has not resolved moral and ethical questions regarding euthanasia and allowing terminally ill client to discuss issues of ending life.

7. Nurse doesn't understand client's cultural and religious orientations toward death. This leads to misunderstanding and violation of client's and family's wishes regarding kind of care given, setting in which client dies, care of body after death, and funeral practices.

8. Nurse has not resolved own feelings about death, tries to avoid emotional pain of witnessing client in process of dying, tries to shield client from knowledge of own impending death or reinforces client's denial.

9. Nurse attempts to work through his or her own past experiences with the dying process—e.g., encouraging client and family to discuss dying before they are ready, because of own past experience with family members who allowed person to die without discussing feelings.

B. Inability of nurse to respond appropriately to near-death experiences

1. Nurse pushes or probes for account of near-death experiences—if client can't recollect, may fabricate an account; if client can recollect, pushing and probing may make client back off from giving account until he or she can find person whom he or she can trust and who will allow him or her to proceed at own pace.

2. Nurse views client's account as delusional, fanatical, or a scam, which blocks communication of near-death experiences and increases client's anxiety and fear of abandonment.

3. Nurse is very task-oriented and focuses on life-support systems to the neglect of personalized care, which increases client's anxiety and sense of depersonalization.

4. Nurse does not support client in recounting near-death experiences to family, which increases family's disbelief of client or leads to family reacting with emotional outburst; blocks communication of near-death experiences and increases client's anxiety and fear of abandonment.

CHAPTER SUMMARY

The process of personality development can be viewed from many perspectives. We have presented for discussion the many factors that influence this process.

There are numerous theories regarding the sequence of development. Our intention has been to present four major developmental theories, as well as to discuss Maslow's theory of the hierarchy of needs. It is essential that nurses assume an eclectic approach. The ultimate goal is to recognize each client as a unique human being. When a nurse keeps this fact in mind, a nursing assessment will reflect an accurate appraisal of all the elements that combine to form an integrated human being.

Dying and death have been presented as an integral component of human development, and strategies for providing holistic nursing care to dying clients—both children and adults—and to their families have been discussed.

SENSITIVITY-AWARENESS EXERCISES

1. Obituary exercise*
   a. Procedure
      (1) Write an obituary for your pet, for a significant other, for yourself.
      (2) For each obituary include the following:
          (a) Day, month, year of death
          (b) Age at which individual or animal died
          (c) Cause of death—lengthy illness, illness of short duration, accident
          (d) Scene of death—home, hospital, elsewhere
          (e) Type of service or arrangements for funeral—e.g., flowers, visiting hours, mass or other type of religious service
          (f) Accomplishments and/or merits of deceased
          (g) Who survives the deceased
   b. Purposes of exercise
      (1) Assists you in clarifying feelings about death and meaning of life and death; addresses the questions of how and when one would choose to die, which will ultimately affect perceptions of how others choose to die
      (2) Progression from a pet to a significant other to yourself enables you to gain some insight into the ability to confront the reality of death.
      (3) Facilitates discussion of the meaning of death

2. "Where do I stand" exercise* (for use with a group)
   a. Procedure
      (1) On a blackboard draw the following continuum:

My body will be disposed of in
an efficient manner and people
will not mention me when I am
dead.

I want everyone to grieve
for me every day of the rest of
their lives.

      (2) Go to the board and write in where you fit on the continuum.
   b. Purposes of exercise
      (1) Explores expectations an individual has of others in regard to his own death yet gives indirect clues as to how that individual would like to be treated should he learn he is dying
      (2) Decreases the possibility of confusing your own needs and desires regarding death with those of the client—believing you are doing what the client wants when in fact you are doing what you would like to have done yourself

3. "Confronting the conflict" exercise† (for use with small groups)
   a. Procedure
      (1) On a blackboard draw the following continuum:

It is ridiculous to suppose that
anyone might obtain satisfaction
from caring for a client who
dies shortly.

Great satisfaction can be
derived from treating a client
who dies shortly.

      (2) Mark the point at which you seem to fit.
      (3) Write a brief statement describing the level of satisfaction you believe would be derived

*Rationale adapted from Koestenbaum (1976).

*Adapted from Epstein, 1975.
†Adapted from Epstein, 1975.

from caring for a dying client. List specifics when possible.
b. Purposes of exercise
(1) Assists you in identifying conflicting feelings regarding your role in promoting health as well as in facilitating a good death
(2) Enables you to recognize some of the possible satisfactions involved in relating to a dying client

REFERENCES

Baca, J.E.
1969 "Some health beliefs of the Spanish-speaking." American Journal of Nursing 69:2172-2176.
Baldwin, A.L.
1967 Theories of Child Development. New York: John Wiley & Sons, Inc.
Barton, D.
1977 Dying and Death. Baltimore: The Williams & Wilkins Co.
Bowlby, J.
1973 Attachment and Loss: Separation, Anxiety, and Anger, vol. 1. New York: Basic Books, Inc., Publishers, pp. 101-120.
Cantor, P.
1980 "Self-esteem, sexuality and cancer-related stress." Frontiers of Therapy in Radiation Oncology 14:51-54.
Carter, F.M.
1971 Psychosocial Nursing (ed. 2). New York: Macmillan, Inc.
Cummings, E., and W. Henry
1961 Growing Old: The Process of Disengagement. New York: Basic Books, Inc., Publishers.
Davenport, W.
1977 "Sex in cross-cultural perspective." In Human Sexuality in Four Perspectives. F. Beach (ed.). Baltimore: Johns Hopkins University Press.
Duvall, E.
1971 Family Development (ed. 4). Philadelphia: J.B. Lippincott Co.
Epstein, C.
1975 Nursing the Dying Patient. Reston, Va.: Reston Publishing Co.
Erikson, E.
1950 Childhood and Society (ed. 2). New York: W.W. Norton & Co., Inc.
1968 Identity: Youth and Crisis. New York: W.W. Norton & Co., Inc.
Escalona, S., and M. Leitch
1953 "Early phases of personality development: a non-normative study of infant behavior." Monographs of the Society for Research in Child Development 17(1):33-49.

Flavell, J.
1963 Developmental Psychology of Jean Piaget. Princeton, N.J.: D. Van Nostrand Co.
Freud, S.
1916 A General Introduction to Psychoanalysis. New York: Liveright Publishing Corp.
Gilmore, M., and D. Gilmore
1979 "'Machismo': A psychodynamic approach (Spain)." Journal of Psychological Anthropology 2:281-299.
Gonzales, H.
1975 "Health care needs of the Mexican-American. In Ethnicity and Health Care. NLN Pub. No. 14-1625. New York: National League for Nursing.
Grof, S., and J. Halifax-Grof
1976 "Psychedelics and the experience of death. In Life After Death. A. Toynbee and A. Koestler (eds.). New York: McGraw-Hill Book Co.
Hauck, B.
1970 "Differences between the sexes at puberty." In Adolescence: Readings in Behavior and Development. E.D. Evans (ed.). Hinsdale, Ill.: Dryden Press.
Hine, V.H.
1982 "Holistic dying: the role of the nurse clinician." Topics in Clinical Nursing 3:45-54.
Hoy, W.K., and T. Applebury
1970 "Teacher-principal relationships in 'humanistic' and 'custodial' elementary schools." Journal of Experimental Education 2:161-170.
Jahoda, M.
1953 Current Concepts of Positive Mental Health. New York: Basic Books, Inc., Publishers.
Koestenbaum, P.
1976 Is There an Answer to Death? Englewood Cliffs, N.J.: Prentice-Hall, Inc.
Kübler-Ross, E.
1969 On Death and Dying. New York: Macmillan, Inc.
1975 Death: The Final Stage of Growth. Englewood Cliffs, N.J.: Prentice-Hall, Inc.
Lidz, T.
1968 The Person. New York: Basic Books, Inc., Publishers.
Malinowski, B.
1927 Sex and Repression in a Savage Society. New York: Harcourt Brace.
Maslow, A.H.
1954 Motivation and Personality. New York: Harper & Row, Publishers, Inc.
McCandless, B., and E. Evans
1973 Children and Youth: Psychosocial Development. New York: Dryden Press.
Money, J., and A. Erhardt
1972 Man and Woman, Boy and Girl. Baltimore: The Johns Hopkins University Press.

Nagy, M.

1948 ''The child's theories concerning death.'' Journal of Genetics and Psychology 73:3-27.

Neugarten, B.L.

1968 ''Adult personality: toward a psychology of the life cycle.'' In Middle Age and Aging: A Reader in Social Psychology. B.L. Neugarten (ed.). Chicago: University of Chicago Press.

Oakes, A.R.

1981 ''Near-death events and critical care nursing.'' Topics in Clinical Nursing 3:61-78.

Sapir, E.

1963 ''Cultural anthropology and psychiatry.'' In Selected Writings of Edward Sapir in Language, Culture, and Personality. Berkeley: University of California Press.

Satir, V.

1967 Conjoint Family Therapy. Palo Alto, Calif.: Science and Behavior Books.

1975 Peoplemaking. Palo Alto, Calif.: Science and Behavior Books.

Sheldon, W., S. Stevens, and W. Tucker

1940 The Varieties of Human Physique. New York: Harper and Brothers.

Stone, L.J., and J. Church

1968 Childhood and Adolescence: A Psychology of the Growing Person (ed. 2). New York: Random House, Inc.

Sullivan, H.S.

1953 The Collected Works of Harry Stack Sullivan. New York: W.W. Norton & Co., Inc.

Thompson, R.

1975 ''Culture and personality.'' In Psychology and Culture. Dubuque, Iowa: Wm. C. Brown Co., Publishers.

Waechter, E.H.

1971 ''Children's awareness of fatal illness. American Journal of Nursing 71:1168-1172.

Watts, R.

1979 ''Dimensions of sexual health.'' American Journal of Nursing, September, pp. 1568-1572.

Whiting, Child

1953 Child Training and Personality: A Cross-Cultural Study. New Haven, Conn.: Yale University Press.

Woods, N.F.

1984 Human Sexuality in Health and Illness (ed. 3). St. Louis: The C.V. Mosby Co.

Zigler, E.

1970 Social Class and the Socialization Process. Review of Education Research.

ANNOTATED SUGGESTED READINGS

Bartin, D.

1977 Dying and Death. Baltimore: The Williams and Wilkins Co.

Barton presents a multidimensional approach to the understanding of the process of dying. Spiritual, medical, and psychological issues are explored in depth. An outline that can be utilized by nurses as well as by other health professionals delineates the areas that need to be considered by persons who work with dying clients. Difficulties encountered by nurses, such as lack of adequate preparation to deal with dying clients, are identified and discussed.

Lidz, T.

1968 The Person. New York: Basic Books, Inc., Publishers.

This classical work presents an overview of the developmental cycle from birth to death. The discussion of each phase incorporates an assessment of biological, psychological, and cultural factors affecting growth and development. This excellent text provides a framework for a holistic understanding of the client as a person.

Watts, R.

1979 ''Dimensions of sexual health.'' American Journal of Nursing, September, pp. 1568-1572.

Watts presents sexuality as an integrated component of self that, like any other component, needs to be assessed. Brief synopses of sexual physiological responses and psychosexual development and gender identity, as well as a classification of disorders, are presented. The book explores sexuality concurrently with a review of the reproductive system of the female and the genitourinary system of the male.

FURTHER READINGS

Jourard, S.

1971 The Transparent Self. New York: Litton Educational Publishing, Inc.

Kastenbaum, R., and R. Aisenberg

1972 The Psychology of Death. New York: Springer Publishing Co., Inc.

Masters, W.H., and V.E. Johnson

1966 Human Sexual Response. Boston: Little, Brown & Co.

Michel, B., and E. Michel

1971 ''The nature and development of psychological sex differences.'' In Psychology and Educational Practice. G. Lesser (ed.). Glenview, Ill.: Scott, Foresman, & Co.

Rogers, C.

1961 On Becoming a Person. Boston: Houghton Mifflin Co.

CHAPTER 7

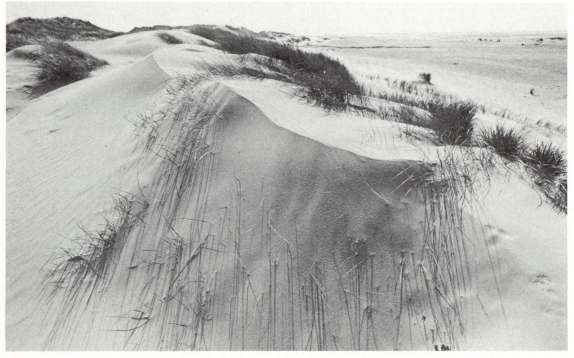

Photo by Klaus D. Francke—Peter Arnold, Inc.

Adaptation and stress

CHAPTER FOCUS

Adaptation, stress, anxiety—these are terms of significance for the health care team as well as for clients. The concepts these words represent will very often be the basis for clinical assessment and intervention.

A person's mental health fluctuates according to his or her ability to adapt to stress. Through the process of adaptation an individual meets needs that are dictated by internal and external factors. Adaptation may be equated with survival. The degree of ability to adapt inevitably influences the ability to survive. Adaptation may also be viewed as the changes an individual experiences as a reaction to stress. These changes act as a defense system by which a person attempts to deal with stress— whether by limiting its impact or by neutralizing its effects. Thus adaptation permits the whole person to continue to function in an effective manner. It promotes forward movement by reducing or alleviating the negative aspects of change. Adaptation can be viewed as a lifelong process that is neither permanent nor static; it involves constant change.

The nurse's role is unique. The nurse can be instrumental in helping a client to develop successful adaptive mechanisms in both the psychosocial realm and the physiological realm. Nurses are in a position to facilitate the efforts of the client to deal with obstacles that may interfere with the ability to respond appropriately and realistically to the demands of his or her environment, situation, or condition.

UNDERLYING DYNAMICS

Stress

What is stress? How does it differ from anxiety? What are the causes of stress? Are there different types of stressors? How does one adapt to stress? These are but a few of the areas that need to be discussed.

Selye (1956) describes stress as being nonspecific in nature and requiring a person to make some type of change. It is often perceived as negative and the source of all of life's miseries. Yet stress is a normal and useful response of the human system. In some cases stress is excessive and damaging, resulting in the need to avoid such situations.

The term "nonspecific" as used by Selye enables one to differentiate stimulus from response. The body's response is termed "stress," while those demands on the body that cause stress are termed "stressors." Every demand made on the body is specific, yet the body's response to stressors is nonspecific. For example, drugs exert specific actions on the body. Insulin reduces the blood glucose level, and diuretics increase the production of urine—each being a specific response. At the same time there is a common *nonspecific* response. Differing specific results occur, yet the nonspecific effects are similar. Both require adaptation even though the initiating stressors are different. It is unimportant whether stressors are positive or negative, pleasant or unpleasant; the nonspecific effect depends upon the adaptive demands made upon the body.

Mason (1975) suggests that stress is not so much a physiological concept as a behavioral one. He proposes that instead of a stressor eliciting a nonspecific hormonal response, it elicits a nonspecific behavioral response—that of emotional arousal. The significance of Mason's proposal lies in the idea that the individual must *perceive* the situation to be stressful in order for there to be a hormonal response to it.

Lazarus (1977) calls this perception "cognitive appraisal," which is important to the understanding of stress. Responses to stress can vary from situation to situation and from one time to another. The appraisal of the situation then determines the nature and intensity of the emotional response, but might also determine the coping mechanisms and their effectiveness.

Engel (1962) defines stress as any process, either in the external environment or within an individual, that demands a response from the individual. He views stress as an inducer of action rather than as an effect of that action. It is important to note that stress is not always a negative entity: pleasurable experiences such as marriage, delivery of a baby, or beginning a new job also produce stress. In fact, individuals are constantly under stress—even when they are asleep. Stress is inherent in the process of life—respiratory and cardiac activity and gastric secretion are but a few examples of physiological processes that may be considered stressors. It is not until stress becomes intensified and appears repeatedly that a person becomes aware of it.

Stress cannot be viewed as simply external in the social or physical environment or strictly within the individual as a psychological "weak spot." The stress response is an interactional process between personality and environment and is determined to a great extent by the individual's own perceptions.

The impact of the stressor also depends upon certain conditioning factors and the available coping mechanisms.

Conditioning factors

1. Physical aspects of environment (e.g., light, noise, crowding)
2. Previous experience with the stressor
3. General health status
   a. Nutritional status
   b. Exercise and leisure habits
   c. Amount of sleep
   d. Genetic endowment
4. Ego strength, self-esteem
5. Age
6. Developmental level

7. General attitude toward the world (evil and hostile vs. benevolent and hopeful—either can be adaptive or maladaptive)

Coping mechanisms

1. Denial
2. Withdrawal
3. Immersion in current system (e.g., work)
4. Crying
5. Laughing
6. Forced cheerfulness
7. Sleeping, dreaming
8. Attack
9. Compromise
10. Problem-solving activities

When examining the concept of stress, we need to consider several important facts. First, the person who is more emotionally mature is more capable of dealing with stress effectively, having a wider range of responses. Second, certain issues, such as the death of a significant person, will be stressful regardless of conditioning factors. Third, acute stress is less harmful than stress that continues chronically.

The key factor in understanding stress is understanding the perception of the event by the individual (which determines coping strategies and the impact on self-worth). Research and practice have indicated that health care professionals must direct their efforts toward prevention—helping clients to manage stress rather than become seeming victims of circumstance. In order to be effective, the nurse must be able to

1. understand the concept of stress.
2. recognize its signs and symptoms.
3. identify factors influencing perceptions of stressors and those altering effective coping with stress.
4. identify and implement strategies to reduce stress.
5. educate individuals about the management of stressors (e.g., nutritional and health counseling, use of relaxation techniques, biofeedback, methods of effecting change in lifestyle).

Adaptation to stress

Adaptation to stress occurs physiologically, psychologically, and culturally.

PHYSIOLOGICAL ADAPTATION

What occurs on the physiological level during a stress reaction? Stress stimulates the release of adrenocorticotropic hormone (ACTH) from the anterior lobe of the hypothalamus. Continued stimulation causes the production of cortical hormones. These hormones have various effects on the body, one of which is to act on the pituitary, when necessary, to reduce the production of ACTH. Stress acts first on the brain and then on the sympathetic nervous system to stimulate the production of norepinephrine and epinephrine. How is this hormone activity perceived by the individual? The body prepares itself for the stressor by increasing the heart

Table 7-1. Stress-related signs and symptoms

↑ Gluconeogenesis ⟶	Diabetes mellitus
↓ Gluconeogenesis ⟶	Hypoglycemia
↓ Excretion of intracellular potassium ⟶	Cardiac arrhythmias
↑ Vasoconstriction ⟶	Hypertension
↑ Anti-inflammatory response ⟶	Infectious diseases
↓ Immunity ⟶	Cancer
↑ Blood clotting ⟶	Coronary thrombosis
↑ Myocardial contractions ⟶	Altered cardiac demands
↑ CNS stimulation ⟶	Confusion, disorientation, thought disturbances

rate and respiratory activity; the pupils dilate to provide a wider range of vision; the skin may become cold and clammy and the person may become pale; "butterflies," muscle stiffness, weakness, increased perspiration, and chest pain often occur as well. Norepinephrine stimulates arteriolar vasoconstriction to increase blood pressure; the

Table 7-2. General adaptation syndrome

Alarm stage
    Stimulation of hypothalmus → stimulation of anterior pituitary → ↑ adrenocorticotropic hormone (ACTH)
    Catecholamine release → sympathetic nervous system activity → ↑ epinephrine and ↑ norepinephrine
    Posterior pituitary releases antidiuretic hormone (ADH)
    Sympathetic response:
        ↑ anti-inflammatory response
        ↑ respiration
        ↑ muscle tonus
        ↑ free fatty acids
        ↑ blood pressure
        ↑ cardiac rate
        Pupils dilate
        ↑ metabolism
    Parasympathetic response:
        Pupil dilation fixes
        ↓ cardiovascular output
        ↓ Muscle tonus
        Depletion of metabolic reserves
        Respiratory difficulty
Resistance stage
    Tissue anabolism
    ↑ antibody production
    ↑ hormonal secretion
    Hemodilution occurs
Stage of exhaustion
    Repeated GAS responses deplete body reserves, leading to increased risk of physical or emotional illness. Psychological exhaustion in the form of panic can result from prolonged anxieties and may incur psychotic episodes.

adrenal glands produce epinephrine, which stimulates the release of glucose by the liver; and peristaltic activity is slowed. Blood is diverted from the gastrointestinal tract to the cardiovascular system for the purpose of "fight or flight." The parasympathetic system may act simultaneously to produce diarrhea and excessive urination. (See Table 7-1).

Let us briefly look at Selye's (1956) general adaptation syndrome (GAS) as a correlate of the sympatho-adreno-medullary response to stress. Selye divides adaptation into three states or stages (see Table 7-2): Stage I is the initial "call to arms," which serves to alert the sympathetic nervous system. Stage II is the stage of resistance and prolonged abnormal physiological functioning in an attempt to deal with the stressors. Stage III is the final stage—exhaustion. Selye's emphasis on the pituitary-adrenal mechanism as a response to stress serves as a foundation for his concept of "diseases of adaptation." He sees stress—rather than inherent physiological defects—as responsible for the various disease states.

PSYCHOLOGICAL ADAPTATION

In order to effectively enable clients to cope with stressful situations, the nurse must understand the process of psychological adaptation. The three stages of adaptation that make up Selye's general adaptation syndrome can be correlated with a psychological model of adaptation. The alarm stage, which corresponds to a mild or +1 level of anxiety, alerts the system to stress. The client is able to perceive data. He or she can visualize connections. He or she can engage in problem-solving. However, the client may not be able to relieve the anxiety by his or her normal adaptive mechanisms. In such a case, anxiety increases and less adaptive types of behavior occur (for example, irritability, anger, withdrawal, denial, and silence). During the second phase, the resistance stage, characteristics of the moderate level of anxiety are apparent. Ego adaptive mechanisms may be called into action if anxiety continues to heighten. The mechanisms utilized are sublimation, rationalization, displacement, and compensation. Should these mechanisms fail, the client moves into the exhaustion stage, in which mechanisms of a more disintegrative nature are utilized for adaptive purposes. Unless the client changes his or her behavior, the client may become chronically ill and may even die. The exhaustion stage is correlated with a severe state of anxiety ($+3$ to $+4$); the client's attention is either focused on one particular detail or directed toward many scattered details. Adaptive mechanisms in this phase may include hallucinations, compulsive behavior, or severe psychophysiological illness.

Valiga and Frain (1979) have defined four levels of stress to assist nurses in their assessment of clients experiencing stress.

Level I—everyday living; use of energy to respond to habitual tasks

Level II—mild; new or less routine events (e.g., job interview); usual modes of coping alleviate stress

Level III—moderate; persistently stressful event; previous repertoire of coping strategies does not effect resolution; person expresses feelings of powerlessness, exhibits denial, depressive-elative mood swings, decreased social interaction, and decreased verbal communication; assistance from others to facilitate problem-solving is helpful

Level IV—severe; exhaustion phase of GAS; events are perceived as life-threatening; person exhibits extreme discomfort, purposelessness; if not controlled can lead to ulcers, asthma, psychosis; intervention focuses on development of intact resources of the individual (e.g., when physical reserves are currently unavailable, draw upon psychological strengths)

CULTURAL ADAPTATION

In order to live productively, individuals develop patterns of living and relationships with others that allow them to interact with the physical environment rather than be controlled by it. Cultural systems provide parameters for behavior and physiological functioning yet permit individual diversity. They allow individuals to adapt to various situations and problems and to be informed about the environment.

Adaptive changes often have been achieved through genetic, physiological, and constitutional means and have then been transmitted for generations through natural selection or conditioning by a culture.

Cultural adaptation in regard to mental health and mental illness may take place in a variety of ways. For example, modification of the environment may enable a client to adapt to a condition that interferes with optimum health.

Culture plays an important role in determining a client's definition of stress and how he or she responds to that stress. Alland (1970) views evolution of human behavior, or rather how one adapts, in light of Darwin's theory of biological evolution. Alland argues that there is an interrelationship between organic and social life that is significant to the understanding of adaptation.

Two types of cultural adaptation are significant. Inward-directed adaptation, including internal homeostasis or integration, results in continuous change and/or motion. Outward-directed adaptation is the result of encounters between a person and his or her environment. The total of these interactions results in the development of an effective self-regulatory system, one that is capable of functioning within a variety of environments.

The interaction between evolutionary concepts (the development of effective feedback or self-regulatory systems) and cultural concepts results in a change in the human system in the direction of a better environmental "fit." For example, organisms with higher developmental levels of homeostatic mechanisms will produce more offspring, leading to increased populations of these more highly adapted organisms. Eventually, less adaptable organisms will be overshadowed by organisms that more readily "fit" the environment.

It is important to note that both inward-directed adaptation and outward-directed adaptation have physiological, environmental, and cultural modes. Thus, cultural adaptation is as much a biological process as the inherent genetic process is.

How does this fact relate to the development of a "disease process"? Individuals are in a constant state of interaction with the environment. In the study of human stress, then, it is impossible to negate cultural and environmental factors, because they are interrelated with specific biological stressors. When the human organism adapts to reduce stress of biological origin, the organism also moves towards consonance with environment and culture.

Stress management

Stress management involves an active approach to determining the course of one's life. Stressors may be personal or individual; interpersonal, as within the context of a family, a nursing unit, or a classroom; or a complex interrelationship of both personal and group or professional. Assume, for example, that a nurse has not had much sleep prior to coming to work because she was up with her young baby during the night. She enters her unit to find that there have been several emergency admissions, two staff members have called in sick, and one client is near death. She experiences an overwhelming sense of lack of control and snaps out at a ward clerk who asks her where the operating room schedule is. In this situation, the nurse's lack of sleep and her possible concern over her young child's sleep habits increased her vulnerability when she was confronted with the scene in the unit. Initial problem-solving measures were not instituted. Stepping back and reviewing the events, possible stressors, and perceptions of the situation would enable the nurse to mobilize actions that would more effectively reduce stress.

The following techniques of stress management can be used by individuals who are encountering stressful situations:

1. Identify stressors you are experiencing ("self-monitoring"). Check your own feelings, and recognize symptoms of stress.

Ask yourself, "Is this stress work-related, home-related, or both? Am I anxious most of the time?"

2. Examine your behavior to determine what you are doing that might increase your stress level ("What triggers my stress? Unrealistic expectations of self? 'I must/should do . . .' rather than 'I would like to . . .'? Do I resist change?")

3. Examine coping strategies (avoidance, confrontation, etc.) and determine their effectiveness.

4. Identify what can be lived with and what cannot—set *priorities*. Is this a stressor that merits attention or one that takes care of itself?

5. Decide which stressors are within your control and which are not at this current stage. Identify what can realistically be changed and what cannot—don't waste energy on unrealistic goals.

6. Avoid use of overgeneralizations such as "I *always* make mistakes" or "Nothing will *ever* change."

7. Assume a positive frame of reference—i.e., "I can" rather than "I can't." Negative frames of reference use more energy and are less productive; reframe your thoughts from "This is terrible" to "What can I do, what are my choices?" Assume control rather than being the "victim"—manipulate the environment (e.g., change jobs, change activities or routine way of doing things, rearrange priorities, *make* choices and recognize consequences of actions). Controlling involves risk-taking—be a risk-taker! Utilize a problem-solving, action-oriented approach.

8. Use lists. When you can't cross something off in a reasonable period, reevaluate.

9. Use thought stopping. Monitor negative thoughts and actually instruct yourself to stop negativism.

10. Concentrate on "quick recovery." You can wallow in bad feelings for however long

you choose to, or you can return to rational thinking and decision making.

11. Use mental diversion. Prepare information as you need it (for a test, a presentation, etc.), and then focus on a favorite activity.

12. Take care of yourself. Focus on positive things that have been accomplished rather than on all negatives. Make appropriate use of leisure time and vacation days. Ensure appropriate nutrition: How do you eat? What do you eat? Ensure sufficient sleep: Are your sleep habits regular? Do you often feel fatigued? Get sufficient exercise. Make use of biofeedback, relaxation measures, guided imagery, transcendental meditation, or momentary relaxation (''quickie'') to reduce stress.

Biofeedback is the use of electrical, audiovisual, tactile, or other sensory modalities to assist in stress reduction. The above-mentioned measures are used to place, to some extent, normally involuntary functions of the nervous system under the voluntary control of the individual. Reduction of blood pressure and pulse rate, for example, can be effected through the use of biofeedback.

Guided imagery is an exercise involving calling to mind a scene that elicits a serene, peaceful mindset. For example, the individual imagines enjoying a sunny day at the beach, experiencing the smell of the salt water, feeling the ocean breeze and the warm sun, and running toes and fingers through the sand. This exercise is simple yet effective in promoting a quiet mental response that not only refreshes a person but also relaxes him or her.

Progressive relaxation is used to relieve muscular tension. The fundamental premise is that muscles cannot simultaneously be tense and relaxed. Individuals are asked to study and recognize within themselves the difference between tense and relaxed muscles. Thus, one can be more cognizant of the presence of muscle tension and can actively institute relaxation measures. Jacobsen (1978) describes a progressive muscle-relaxation program that helps individuals to sequentially tense and relax muscle groups, beginning with the neck and

head and moving through the extremities. This exercise program usually takes about 20 to 30 minutes and should be done two or three times weekly. It is a program that must be practiced if it is to work effectively. Individuals often feel uncomfortable initially doing the exercises, although their calming effects have been noted in the literature.

Group resolution of stressors may also be a method of stress management. It rests on the group's commitment to direct, open communication. Individuals must be assertive—both in the expression of anger and in the expression of affection—yet be respectful of others as human beings. There must also be a mutual willingness to resolve interpersonal issues, to reach shared goals, and to explore conflicts. When a group is unable to resolve a stressful situation, a consultant may be helpful in suggesting solutions.

Nurses are in a position in health care settings to assist clients to identify stressors, to implement strategies to reduce stress, and to evaluate their effectiveness. The nursing assessment of a client reveals psychological, physiological, and social history, as well as information relevant to the client's stress response: When does it occur? Is it rational? Is it a conditioned response to a specific stimulus? What demands are made on the client? What resources are available to the client? Planning and implementation of specific stress-reduction techniques will depend upon the data gathered as well as the client's preferences and usual coping strategies. Evaluation of the strategies can initially be done by the nurse, with the eventual goal being to have it done by the client.

In summary, the goals of stress management can be succinctly stated: to help individuals learn to be responsive to themselves, to alter their responses to stress, and to alter their environments in order to reduce stress.

Stress in the nursing profession

Stress has been identified as an integral component of societal structure. Each living organism experiences stress through the process of living; excessive stress can be harmful, yet at moderate levels stress acts as an initiator of action, a promoter of growth. Stress incorporates the physical characteristics of the environment as well as the sociocultural and psychological facets, all of which are part of the context of the nurse-client relationship. Thus, stress can arise from *within* the context of this multidimensional relationship. In addition, stress can be a product of the broader environment as well as a product of specific relationships within that environment—with clients' families, other health care professionals, and so on. In short, the stress that a person experiences as a result of being part of a helping profession must be addressed.

ENVIRONMENTAL STRESSORS

Very often the units in which nurses function are too small or their physical layouts are inappropriate. Long corridors, too little storage space, overcrowding resulting from the presence of equipment, and absence of windows are examples of possible stressors in the environment. Having a private space for nurses has been identified by one staff member of a very busy cardiac unit as being instrumental in reducing stress. In this particular situation there had been little space at the nurses' station, and the only other available area had been in the crowded locker room. It had been necessary to spend only several minutes in this windowless "closet" in order to understand why staff members did not utilize this area. Support from the head nurse as well as other administrators led to the construction of a space for nurses alone, indicating their importance in the hospital hierarchy.

Large intensive care units do not usually provide individual cubicles; clients and their nurses are separated by thin curtains. Although curtains can be drawn, there is very little sense of privacy. Every staff member is aware of what the others are doing. As one staff member of such a unit has noted, she doesn't have to ask for help; someone is always right there to offer. However, other staff members have expressed feelings of being in a "fish bowl"—a sentiment expressed by clients as

well. Some nurses from this same intensive care unit have expressed a preference for individual rooms, because then only those people who were involved in a client's care would be at the bedside.

Other physical factors in the environment can act as stressors. Noise levels in busy intensive care units were the first factor to be recognized as possibly contributing to stress. Turner, King, and Craddock (1975) found that the average minimum noise level exceeded 60 decibels. This level was noted during the early morning hours. Maximum levels, occurring between 1 PM and 7 PM, reached nearly 90 decibels. This is roughly the intensity of an automobile horn. According to these authors, daytime noise exceeding 50 decibels is perceived as annoying. Thus, it is not difficult to understand why clients complain about noise and feel as though they are getting no rest. Nurses may complain of headaches upon leaving a busy unit at the end of the day, possibly because of the increased noise level.

Light can also be a factor in contributing to a stressful environment. It is not a question of enough light but often the type of lighting, as well as glare, that becomes an issue. Often there are no windows to provide natural lighting, or windows face directly onto other buildings. A semidark, artificially lighted environment can lead to sensory deprivation and generalized feelings of lethargy and depression. For example, the gynecology-oncology unit of one large urban hospital is located on the ground floor of a building that is situated between several other buildings. Each window faces onto another building. It is impossible for staff or clients to determine what is happening in the outside world. This further isolates an already-isolated staff and client population. Nurses in this unit have expressed feelings of being "second class citizens," being in the "dungeon," and being the "death ward." They have identified their physical location as contributing to their lack of identity as a viable part of the hospital and ultimately to the development of stress in the unit.

Scheduling can also be a stressor. Much of the work force in the business world operates on a "9 to 5,'' Monday through Friday work week. Nurses, however, must provide 24-hour care to clients; someone must work during the evening and nighttime hours, seven days per week. New graduates must spend their allotted time on evenings and nights, while ''veterans'' may, in some institutions, work days permanently. Nurses may work 1 month of days then 1 to 2 months of evenings or nights. It is difficult to adapt to any one shift when shift rotation occurs frequently. The Stanford study (Steffen, 1980) concluded that staff members who do shift rotations (including nurses) exhibit greater incidences of digestive difficulties, disturbed sleep patterns, accidents, high anxiety levels, depression, and generalized dissatisfaction with life than do staff members who work regular hours.

Shift rotation not only affects the individual nurse but also has a profound impact on families and friends.

Several young nurses were discussing the demands of the nursing role with a psychiatric liaison clinical specialist. Many in the group spoke to the issue of being "out of synch" with the rest of the world. One young woman who was newly married voiced her concern for her marriage: "If I work days, I usually don't get off work exactly at 4:30—it's not due to disorganization but is usually due to a client being admitted right at change of shift, or a client's family having one last question. My husband is supportive but doesn't really understand why I can't leave when it's 4:30. In his world, what doesn't get done today will still be there tomorrow! When I work off-shifts, there may be two or three days when I don't even see him. I can understand how difficult it must be to have a family, be a wife, and pursue a career in nursing."

This is just one example of the impact shift rotation has on nurses and their significant others. Stress arises when men or women attempt to meet the demands of a schedule that may be changing monthly while concurrently attempting to maintain stable relationships with others.

A male nurse in a medical intensive care unit has described the stress he experienced having to work evenings and leave his pregnant wife alone. She taught school; he worked evenings and every other weekend. He had chosen to work evenings in order to continue his professional education during the day. After consultation with a psychiatric nurse liaison, he decided to change to a unit that required him to work only Monday through Friday, 9 AM to 5 PM. Although he was relinquishing a job he prized highly, he found it necessary to select a different type of position in order to decrease his own personal stress. As was noted in the Stanford study (Steffen, 1980), shift rotation can exact a physical as well as psychological toll from the staff.

NURSING AS A FEMALE PROFESSION

Various authors have noted that the nursing profession has emerged concurrently with the growth of the women's movement. Changes in roles and expectations have had a profound impact on the nurse as a professional being. The concept of the nurse as a career person is coming to the fore. Nursing is involved in the process of professionalization. More and more, individuals are entering nursing with a commitment to a career. The number of ''washing machine'' nurses, as Dr. Clifford Jordan notes, is decreasing somewhat. These individuals have moved in and out of nursing, often on the basis of personal economic need. Excellent nursing care has still been provided, yet a conflict has been created between nurses who have felt that their profession is a career and requires a commitment and those who view nursing as a job with little future orientation.

Although the number of male nurses is increasing, nursing is still predominantly a female profession. Change is occurring slowly; the problems noted by Lavinia Dock (1920) are very similar to those seen today. She pointed out that the status of nursing has depended in large part upon the status of women. In the past, women were not expected to make career commitments, nor were they rewarded for such commitments. Women were the nurturers and caretakers, assuming a passive, submissive role. Men were the breadwinners, the dominant force in the family. These same roles were often actualized in the hospital environment, with the doctor assuming the dominant role. Male physicians made decisions, wrote orders, and asked for charts and seats in the nursing station. Nurses followed orders, provided care, and were compassionate to their clients. Power and decision-making were ascribed to the male; independence was viewed as being unfeminine. Thus, today nurses still tend to experience difficulty in asserting themselves, in actively participating in decision making, and in effecting conflict resolution.

ISSUES CONFRONTING THE NURSING PROFESSION

Further powerlessness has resulted from the profession's inability to unite itself with common goals, expectations, and entry-level educational preparation. What other profession has three levels of entry into practice? Other conflicts exist in such areas as the right to collectively bargain, the issue of a job versus a career, the level of autonomy that is appropriate, and third-party payment. There is little consensus among nurses, and there is really no one professional organization that speaks to the needs of nurses as a whole. Grissom and Spengler (1976) suggest that women lack a basic trust for each other because of the inherent need to compete with one another for men.

Finally, the relatively low value placed on nursing's worth in our society is a source of stress. Although clients often express satisfaction with their care, monetary recompense indicates that society does not consider nursing a valuable service. The hospital bill reflects physicians' services and laboratory and other diagnostic tests, while nursing is considered under "bed and board." It has been noted that in some areas of the United States, nurses are paid less than garbage collectors, plumbers, tree trimmers, and supermarket clerks. This fact, coupled with the public's image of nurses as pro-

viders of technical services with little ability to use cognitive skills, acts as a source of stress. Ultimately, feelings of poor self-worth can lead to a devaluing of care and a disenchantment with the profession.

MEN IN NURSING

In a profession dominated by women, the male nurse is often viewed as unique or uncommon. Bush (1976) suggests that male nurses are suspected of being homosexual. Men who consider a career in nursing are frequently discouraged by parents and friends. During discussions of their career plans, they are often less able than other students to tell others about their occupational preference.

Male nurses experience stress in relation to role expectation. Traditional male attributes include assertiveness, self-control, and aggressiveness, yet the nursing role implies nurturance and warmth. How does the male nurse reduce the dissonance and act out his role? As the number of male nurses increases, perhaps the nursing profession will be able to deal more effectively with the issue of role expectation for both men and women.

It has been noted by Gulak (1981) that male nurses receive higher salaries than female nurses and that a larger proportion of them occupy administrative positions. However, male nurses sometimes feel that they are being "used" for their size or their strength rather than being considered nurses.

It seems that there are sources of stress for the male nurse in a female-dominated profession that arise out of being male with certain ascribed masculine characteristics. Female nurses, while accepting and valuing their male counterparts, can also resent their ability to generate higher incomes. In addition, women may fall back into the traditionally prescribed role of submissive responder and encourage male nurses to assume the initiative in decision-making and conflict resolution. In any case, stress for both male and female nurses may be the result of a lack of role integration in the profession as a whole.

SUPPORT GROUPS AS A STRESS-REDUCING TECHNIQUE

Support groups are a useful mechanism in reducing stress. A support group provides a place where members of a particular unit or floor can meet to share information about clients, to discuss ways of meeting the needs of particular clients, and to share feelings and frustrations concerning their work. In this type of group, a sense of acceptance exists and members receive comfort from sharing both positive and negative feedback without fear of repercussion. A feeling of ''I'm not in this alone'' allows individuals to explore various options without decreasing their senses of self-worth. Lewis and Levy (1982) suggest that meetings be used for catharsis, to help nurses to recognize and deal with their own feelings and limitations, and to identify strategies of intervention for clients (as well as for the solving of organizational conflicts).

Active support groups can be successful in mediating the effects of stress by encouraging a problem-solving approach to situations. Various issues can arise, depending upon the nature of the group; new graduates have different concerns from a group of management-level nurses. A support group does not provide therapy, nor should it be a ''bitch'' session. Gripes are a part of life; members need to express their feelings and then seek to resolve the issues.

Support systems are an essential component of the context of the nurse and his or her environment. Nurses must define their support resources—their peers, their administrators, and other health care professionals. Support must be drawn upon and returned in a mutual relationship. In this manner, the emotional well-being of nurses can be replenished by those who most understand.

Anxiety

Anxiety is a result of stress. Engel (1962) describes anxiety as the psychological response to great amounts of energy running unchanneled as a result of a stressful situation. As was previously stated, stress is the inducer, not the effect, of an action. Anxiety is often described as a feeling of apprehension, of impending doom. The behavior of a person who is experiencing anxiety can run the gamut from maintainance of a state of alertness to panic of such severity that the individual either becomes immobilized or attends to every minute cue in his or her environment. Anxiety is a subjective experience that results from a fear of an undetermined nature. Anxiety may have its roots in past experiences, or it may be produced by a threatened or perceived loss of inner control or by a threat to self-esteem. Feelings of isolation, helplessness, and insecurity are associated with anxiety.

Anxiety can be described as a motivating force; it activates an individual to make changes and to grow. Without mild to moderate levels of anxiety, an individual might remain in a static state with little energy to confront the daily issues of life. An individual who copes successfully with an anxiety-producing situation emerges feeling a greater sense of worth and competence. Successes only serve to reinforce a personal pride in one's problem-solving abilities. Anxiety at this level acts to promote a sense of well-being. This is not to say that in the process one does not feel uncomfortable, nervous, or threatened; however, the long-term result is a renewed confidence in oneself.

Freud used the term ''anxiety'' to refer to that anxiety which results from the trauma of the birth process itself. Then, throughout the developmental span, anxiety is generated by conflict between the id and the superego. The ego acts as referee between the two conflicting forces. Freud (1936) proposed that anxiety acts as a signal system, warning that a conflict may become overwhelming. He also believed that the object of anxiety is unconscious and related to earlier object loss. Freud differentiated fear from anxiety by arguing that fear has its origins in a threatening external event. It is an acute response whose precipitating factors are real and immediate, while anxiety has its origins in intrapsychic conflict. According to freudian theory, ego-defense mechanisms defend the ego against anxiety. These mechanisms operate outside the level of conscious awareness, acting to repress all material that is anxiety producing (see Chapter 6 for a discussion of defense mechanisms).

Sullivanian, or interpersonal, theory proposes that anxiety is a tension state that is transmitted through an empathic process from mother to infant, with the infant responding as though mother and self were one. In order for this process to occur, the ego must have some awareness of the environment. Sullivan (1953) believes that the infant fears disapproval from the mothering figure and that later experiences with significant others thus can generate feelings of anxiety if the individual perceives that his or her behavior will not receive approval. The lack of parental approval during childhood therefore affects adult interpersonal situations.

Peplau (1963) bases much of her theoretical framework on Sullivan's theory. She defines four levels of anxiety, which are summarized in Table 7-3.

General characteristics of anxiety, then can be identified as: (1) energy that cannot be directly observed, while its effects on behavior can be; (2) a subjective experience; (3) a physical, emotional, intellectual, sociocultural, and spiritual experience; (4) an emotion without a specific object; and (5) something interpersonally communicated.

Certain physiological and psychological changes occur as a result of anxiety. Physiological changes involve primarily the autonomic nervous system. Mild or moderate anxiety tends to increase physiological functioning, while severe levels slow down functioning and can ultimately result in death.

Table 7-3. Levels of anxiety*

Mild (+1)	Moderate (+2)	Severe (+3)	Panic (+4)
Person is alert; sees, hears, grasps more than he would ordinarily; goal-oriented learning is enhanced; recognizes anxiety May protect self by limiting close interpersonal relationships Uses coping mechanisms to relieve tension, such as nail biting, walking, crying, sleeping, eating, laughing, smoking, drinking Anxiety is controlled with little conscious effort	Perceptual field is narrowed, but person can attend to more if directed to do so (person makes use of selective inattention—i.e., directing attention to a primary focus with little attention to the periphery) Increased powers of concentration Problem-solving capacity still available	Perceptual field greatly reduced Person may become preoccupied with one detail or focus on many details simultaneously ("scattering") Selective inattention continues to be operative Physical and emotional discomfort increases: nausea, vomiting, dizziness	Attention is narrowed severely, or speed of scatter is sharply increased Feelings of awe, dread, terror are common; delusions and hallucination can appear Exhaustion and death occur if panic continues for prolonged period

*Data adapted from Peplau, H. 1963. "A working definition of anxiety." In Some Clinical Approaches to Psychiatric Nursing. S. Burd and M. Marshall (eds.). New York: Macmillan, Inc.; and Menninger, K. 1963. The Vital Balance. New York: Viking Press.

Physiological changes	Psychological changes
Tachycardia	Tension
Palpitations	Apprehension
Tremors	Indecisiveness
Muscle tension	Oversensitivity
Diarrhea	Tearfulness
Frequent urination	Agitation
Diaphoresis	Irritability
Dry mouth	Dread
Cold, clammy skin	Panic
Pallor	Powerlessness
Dilated pupils	Low self-worth
	Poor reality testing (delusions, hallucinations)

Clients express anxiety in a variety of ways, many times quite subtly. For example, a client may describe his or her admission to the hospital in terms of feeling ''shaky'' and ''nervous.'' Other client responses to anxiety-producing situations include: ''My heart is pounding,'' ''I have a lump in my throat,'' and ''My body felt cold and I was perspiring a lot.''

Mild levels of anxiety can help a person to cope with a stressor. For example, a student is preparing for an examination and notices details and logical connections she had not noticed previously. She describes herself as being ''on edge.'' This mild anxiety facilitates her use of problem-solving strategies, which enhance her learning.

However, a moderate level of anxiety may prevent a person from noticing connections between details:

Mr. A has been receiving an anticoagulant for approximately 1 year. He has been hospitalized for a pulmonary embolism and has been receiving appropriate treatment. In the discharge teaching phase, he pays close attention to the signs of bleeding but fails to hear instructions about restrictions on aspirin use and the necessity of having regular blood levels drawn. Mr. A frequently repeats questions and seems distracted.

Mr. A is able to recognize and respond to a limited amount of information. Some pieces of information assume great importance, to the exclusion of other significant information. This client's anxiety needs to be reduced to a mild level and then utilized in the problem-solving process.

Severe and panic levels of anxiety drastically impair functioning in all realms. Connections between details may no longer be apparent. Physical and emotional discomfort increase; feelings of dread, apprehension, and terror ensue. Thought processes are affected; loose associations, delusions, and hallucinations are called into operation to create a reality that is less threatening than the existing one. An individual may also exhibit dissociative responses, obsessive-compulsive behavior, conversion, or psychosomatic responses to severe levels of anxiety. At this point anxiety has gone beyond its service to the individual; the inability to cope appropriately with mounting levels of anxiety leads to the development of pathological behavior. Anxiety, then, can be viewed as the underlying dynamic of emotional illness. Symptoms of anxiety, as mentioned above, are attempts to control anxiety. The symptoms of anxiety also represent, at a symbolic level, an unresolved inner conflict.

Mild levels of anxiety are handled with little conscious thought or effort. Menninger (1963) has listed a number of coping mechanisms that are utilized to relieve the tension of day-to-day living:

Overeating
Drinking
Smoking
Self-discipline
Laughing, giggling
Crying
Cursing
Boasting
Sleep
Hobbies
Talking it out
Thinking things through
Physical exercise
Acting to alter
Fantasy formation and daydreaming
Dreaming
Use of religious faith
Symbolic substitutions (i.e., going on a shopping spree)

It is important to note that one must distinguish between the "normal" use of coping mechanisms in everyday living and the misuse of them. Coping mechanisms are only effective insofar as they permit individuals to live in a reality-based environment. (For further coping strategies, see the section on stress management, earlier in this chapter.)

Moderate, severe, and panic levels of anxiety require greater effort and energy to control the effects on self. These coping strategies can be divided into task-oriented and ego-oriented behaviors.

Task-oriented behaviors involve the use of one's cognitive abilities. Problem-solving activities are used to confront a situation and meet the needs presented. Assertive behavior is an essential component of problem-solving. Individuals are respected for their beliefs, and an outcome that is satisfactory for all those involved is the long-term goal. Compromise is not a win-lose situation but rather a strategy that implies gains on both sides. Task-oriented behaviors vary; in fact, they can be destructive when rights of others are violated in the process of meeting a need or solving a problem. In such a case, one individual's anxiety might be reduced at the expense of another's.

Ego-oriented behaviors are those mechanisms utilized by the ego to protect the self. Task-oriented behaviors may not be sufficient to resolve a situation. Ego-defense mechanisms then protect the individual from experiencing feelings of overwhelming inadequacy and the resulting loss of self-worth. These mechanisms are used with mild and moderate levels of anxiety. However, as the degree to which they are used and the frequency of use increase, distortion of reality may become apparent and interpersonal relationships may be disturbed. For the most part, these mechanisms are out of the realm of conscious control; therefore, monitoring of reactions becomes difficult. (For further discussion of ego-defense mechanisms, see Chapter 6.)

FEAR AND ANXIETY

The terms "anxiety" and "fear" are frequently used synonymously. Fear, however, is aroused by the presence of an actual threat, of a danger that is currently present. Fear and anxiety differ in that fear is relatively self-limiting. For example, a person might fear skiing down a mountain for the first time. He or she would perceive the situation as fearful, yet it is doubtful that the event would cause a prolonged feeling of loss of self-worth. The physiological symptoms aroused by a frightening situation are similar to those generated by mild to moderate levels of anxiety. The cognitive and emotional changes attributed to anxiety are not usually experienced by a person who is frightened.

CATEGORIES OF ANXIETY

Free-floating anxiety can be associated with panic-arousing feelings of terror and dread that cannot be connected with a particular causative factor. Individuals experiencing this type of anxiety have the sensation that it invades every inch of life, exerting its influence on every aspect of life. Relief behaviors include withdrawal, phobic responses, ritualism, and dissociative responses.

State anxiety is precipitated by an event or situation that is perceived by the individual as being outside of his or her realm of control. An example of a precipitant of state anxiety would be learning that a close female friend has been assaulted by a rapist. The situation can be identified as anxiety provoking; this is different from free-floating anxiety.

Some individuals experience, or are predisposed toward experiencing, high levels of anxiety simply as a result of their personalities. Often the underlying conflict that generates the anxiety has occurred early in development yet continues to recur. Such individuals—who are said to have habitual anxiety, or *trait anxiety,* are likely to respond to many situations by exhibiting behaviors indicative of moderate to severe anxiety.

An understanding of state and trait anxiety can be helpful in predicting and assessing a client's responses to stressful situations. Measuring tools such as the State-Trait Anxiety Inventory can be used to assist the nurse in establishing a relationship that will enable the client to successfully alleviate anxiety.

The freudian conception of anxiety—that it is

generated by instinctual drives approaching the ego, creating a sense of danger—is known as *signal anxiety*. If the id-based instinctual drives cannot be satisfied by the ego in an appropriate manner, the intrapsychic defense mechanisms are called into action by the ego.

A young woman in her thirties complained of nervousness, insomnia, palpitations, and gastrointestinal disturbances. She described her life as being quite miserable, her husband being the major source of that misery. Her description of her past experiences revealed that she had had a cool, rejecting mother and an alcoholic father whom she adored. Her husband, on the other hand, was a much more giving, loving person. At the time when her 8-year-old daughter began to develop a close relationship with her father, a reemergence of the woman's need for a relationship with her own father occurred. She experienced overwhelming feelings of anxiety as the original conflict reappeared, and she lashed out at her husband.

Separation anxiety is the anxiety that occurs when an individual is confronted with the impending or feared loss of a person who is considered significant. Children at various stages of development, such as the infant of 8 to 9 months, the toddler, and the school-age child, can experience this type of anxiety when facing separation from a parent or significant adult. "School phobia," a related condition, may be described as an anxiety response to being away from home for even short periods of time, rather than as an aversion to school per se.

In addition to being described in terms of levels (mild, moderate, and so on) and types (separation, signal, and so on), anxiety can be described in terms of duration. *Acute anxiety* has a sudden onset and may last from a few hours to a few weeks. Symptoms can be severe, such as rapid heart rate and pounding in the chest, increased respiratory rate, tachycardia, tremors of the extremities, nausea, diarrhea, and headache. Feelings of loss of control, apprehension, inadequacy, irritability, and decreased problem-solving ability occur as well. *Chronic anxiety* has no sudden onset but rather generates a constant, generalized feeling of apprehension or nervousness. Symptoms are much less pronounced than in acute anxiety yet may exert more impact on body systems because of their chronic nature. Chronically anxious individuals are *always* waiting for something to happen to them, always worrying about everything. Life is never fully enjoyed but is actually ruminated over. Chronic anxiety can be a combination of state, trait, and signal anxiety.

PRIMARY AND SECONDARY GAIN

The concepts of primary and secondary gain need to be discussed in relation to anxiety and relief behaviors. The primary gain resulting from phobic behavior, obsessive-compulsive responses, withdrawal reactions, and so forth is the reduction of anxiety, which is generated by internal sources as well as environmental forces. A secondary gain is an advantage an individual experiences as a result of the primary symptom or symptoms. For example, a mother of five children is hospitalized for hysterical paralysis. The symptoms prevent her from carrying on her responsibilities as wife and mother. Therefore, underlying dependency needs are met that otherwise might have been expressed in other, more destructive ways. Secondary gains include not only relief from responsibilities but also a mechanism by which to seek attention and a means by which to control others in the environment.

Although relief of anxiety is of great importance, secondary gains are often equally important. Secondary gains can interfere with the client's wish to recover and in some cases prevent recovery.

Although anxiety has a negative connotation, mild to moderate levels act in the service of the ego to promote learning. Without some level of anxiety, there would be no need for change. Anxiety acts as a motivating agent; it disrupts equilibrium sufficiently to promote the initiation of coping strategies or relief behaviors. Life would certainly be boring without some type of energizing force.

Therefore, anxiety and the adaptation that it brings forth serve as the foundation from which each person develops and preserves his or her sense of identity. The most healthy person is the one who has confronted anxiety-provoking situations and has actively taken steps to resolve them. Thus, repeated experiences with anxiety in limited amounts have growth-promoting potential. Anxiety serves to provide the energy necessary for adaptation.

Anxiety that is perceived as a threat can give rise to relief behaviors that protect or distance an individual from his or her anxiety. Intrapsychic defense mechanisms such as denial, projection, rationalization, and displacement can operate as part of a cluster of relief behaviors. These mechanisms can control anxiety for a limited period of time; however, at some point anxiety must be experienced as an energizing force that can be utilized as a growth-promoting force. When anxiety is continually avoided or denied, more severely dysfunctional behaviors occur, such as hallucinations, delusions, or other forms of psychotic behavior.

Stress, as an inducer of anxiety, may be seen as a precipitator of very individualistic responses on the part of clients, families, and nurses themselves. There continue to be unanswered questions: Why do some people respond in a psychophysiological manner while others respond in a phobic or compulsive manner? Why are some people able repeatedly to meet life's challenges with seemingly little difficulty while other people have great difficulty? In the next section, commonly encountered stressors and nursing intervention will be presented.

COMMONLY ENCOUNTERED STRESSORS

Threats to body image

As was discussed in Chapter 6, body image is an integral part of self-concept. Body image is reflective of the attitudes one holds about one's body.

Related to body image is sense of identity—one's perception of one's strengths and weaknesses and one's relationships to others.

Body image can be altered by the addition of artifacts or by a threat to body integrity. The disruption of body image can be caused by many situations, including weight loss or gain, surgical intervention, and pathophysiological and psychopathological conditions. Because certain areas of the body hold more meaning for an individual than others, threats to these areas may be considered more significant and require more action by the individual. Throughout the life cycle, varying dimensions of body image are developed and redeveloped. Feelings of self-worth may correlate with positive body image. An individual who has difficulty developing an integrated self-concept has a corresponding difficulty relating to others. It is only after the development of positive feelings about self that an individual seeks to invest in others.

Many factors contribute to the development of body image. The most pertinent factors include responses from others in the environment (such as parents and peers), one's own attitudes and emotions regarding the body, one's degree of independence and motivation, physical appearance, how well the body functions, and perception of body territoriality. Body image thus is multidimensional rather than unidimensional. Nursing assessment and intervention must include a survey of the various factors in an effort to develop a realistic appraisal and plan of action. Clients' feelings about particular aspects of body image depend on whether they perceive them as functional tools or as central personal attributes. For example, dentures may be accepted as a tool rather than as a central attribute, while hair may be viewed as essential to one's identity.

A sense of body space and self-concept emerges during the first year of life. As the child moves through the developmental stages, changes occur in the physical aspects of the body. During adolescence, the body is viewed as a social tool; however, as middle age and old age approach, the body becomes wrinkled, skin sags, and sensory functions decrease. As the actual physical appearance of the body changes, the feelings one has about oneself may also change. Therefore, it is important that nurses assess the impact that disturbances in body image have on an individual and his or her relationships with others.

Kolb (1959) groups body image disturbances into five categories: (1) neurological dysfunctions that affect sensorimotor status, such as paraplegia or hemiplegia; (2) metabolic dysfunction, such as thyroid disease or obesity; (3) dismemberment, such as loss of a limb; (4) personality dysfunctions, such as neuroses, psychoses, and psychophysiological diseases; and (5) dysfunctions related to progressive deformities, such as arthritis. Body image is a vulnerable entity. It may be distorted, as in a person experiencing pain, or diminished, as in a person with decreased sensory function. Although a client in pain often focuses attention on the area of pain, the whole self is consumed by the pain.

Threats to body image are sources of stress because body image is related to various areas of function. The choice of a life's work, sexual behavior, the ability to respond appropriately to stress, and relationships with others are related to the concept of self and body image.

Surgical removal of a body part (for example, amputation of a limb or removal of the gall bladder) or alteration of a body function (for example, colostomy or ileostomy) often constitutes a threat to body image. Gross changes in body size and shape may also serve as threats to one's self-concept. Changes result, for example, from the increases in weight caused by pregnancy or overeating and from excessive weight loss. Finally, pathological processes, such as coronary artery disease, cause changes in the functioning of critical body parts, such as the heart. Even though there may be no outward manifestation that the body is not functioning properly, one's self-concept is definitely altered.

Surgical removal of a body part such as a breast or a limb often causes the client to perceive himself or herself as no longer being whole. Breast cancer is on the rise in the United States, and its impact is being felt in all social classes. The changes in self-concept that result from a mastectomy depend upon the significance a woman places on the breasts and her perception of the seriousness of the threat posed by the loss of a breast. Various values are placed on the breast—it is a symbol of femininity for many, and it is often closely linked with sexual functioning. Loss of a breast may mean loss of a job, if performance in the job relies on use of the whole body, as in modeling. With the loss of a breast, a woman comes face to face with her feelings of self. She will depend on the reactions of significant others to help her assimilate the change in body image into the self-concept. The loss of a limb causes a similar disturbance in body image. The degree of the threat to self-concept that results from such a loss depends upon the value placed on the limb and the ability of the individual to successfully adapt to the loss.

A colostomy or an ileostomy often poses a threat to body image and self-concept. Defecation and urination traditionally have been considered private functions. Feces have often been considered dirty, both literally and figuratively, and odors and sounds related to bowel function have been considered taboo. Thus, to release feces into a small plastic bag that may leak or smell is often regarded as repulsive, and clients may display a tendency toward social isolation in order to protect their self-concepts. Very often they resist accepting the reality of body image change. However, the changes—the stoma, the odor, the plastic bag—need to be incorporated into a restructured body image.

Coronary artery disease is frequently described as a psychophysiological response to stress. Coronary artery disease therefore may be viewed both as a threat to body image and self-concept—a stressor—and as a *result* of maladaptation to stress. The heart is the "organ of choice" (refer to Chapter 16). It is important to recognize this dual position that coronary artery disease holds. The disease process is commonly interpreted in nursing assessments as being stress-induced; however, it is equally important to assess the impact that coronary artery disease has on body image and self-concept. (Coronary artery disease as a psychophysiological response to stress is discussed further in Chapter 16).

An increase in body weight is one of the prominent changes that occurs during pregnancy. Women often speak of feeling "like a balloon." A woman's body space enlarges, possibly restricting her movement through territory that had originally been familiar and accessible. Everyday functions such as bending down to tie shoes, driving a car, and turning around in a small space are no longer as easy to accomplish. The increased size may result in a disturbance in body image and a threat to self-concept, depending upon a woman's feelings toward the pregnancy.

Obesity and anorexia nervosa are considered psychophysiological responses to stress (see Chapters 15 to 17 for further discussion). However, as in the case of coronary artery disease, obesity and anorexia nervosa, which produces excessive weight loss, can be considered to be both stressors and stress responses. For example, obese persons may have body image disturbances that both result from overeating and contribute to overeating. This dual concept can be diagrammed as follows:

Stressor (increase or decrease in body size) → Possible disturbance in body image and altered self-concept

Stress response (overeating [obesity] or excessive weight loss [anorexia nervosa]) → Perpetuation of disturbance in body image and probably lowered self-concept

Thus it is critical that a nurse determine the impact of a client's body size on body image and self-concept. The physical changes that an individual experiences may result in increased anxiety levels and the utilization of pathological defense mechanisms.

Several commonly encountered stressors that may cause disturbance in body image and alteration of self-concept have been presented. In a nursing assessment, it is important to determine the client's perception of the meaning of a threat and its implications for his or her life-style. It is also important to note that age affects perception and adaptation to change in body image. For example, a young child might have fewer adjustment problems to a crippling illness than an adult. The client calls varying levels of defense mechanisms into action, depending on the seriousness of the threat. The goal of nurse and client is to recognize the implications of the alterations and to maximize the client's adaptive capacities.

Pain

Pain, which is associated with many disease processes, may be considered a stressor. Pain may also be considered a response to psychological stress, in either an adaptive or a maladaptive sense. Pain will be discussed in this section as a stressor —a personal, subjective experience that elicits various types of responses, depending on physiological, biological, and sociocultural factors. Pain may be defined as a stressor in that it causes anxiety levels to rise; the greater the pain, the higher the level of anxiety. Adaptation to pain may be retarded if the pain receptors are no longer functioning properly or if one's culture places restrictions on the expression of pain. In the latter instance, excessive denial of pain may be used to the detriment of a client's nursing care.

PAIN THEORIES

The gate control theory (Seigle, 1974) suggests that the small-diameter afferent fibers in the spinal cord transmit painful stimuli to the substantia gelatinosa. Impulses can be blocked at this point by the stimulation of the large-diameter afferent fibers or by the cerebral cortex mechanisms that control sensory discrimination, motivation, affect, and cognition. This process in turn "closes the spinal gate" and blocks transmission of pain impulses to the brain.

The gate control theory holds that in order to understand the client in pain, one must consider the following factors:

1. The person's memory

2. Past and present pain experiences
3. Present state of mind
4. Interpretation and response to pain
5. Conditions that increase anxiety (These conditions also increase pain.)

Nursing intervention based on the gate control theory focuses on altering sensory discrimination through the use of behavior modification, biofeedback, and distractions such as music, touching, and backrubs. Seigle (1974) suggests that acupuncture may stimulate the gating mechanism if the needles are inserted along specific meridians.

The specificity theory states that specific nerve cells respond to specific stimuli. These stimuli are always interpreted as pain. Some impulses are directed toward motor fibers of the reflex arc, which leads to an immediate response by the muscles. Other impulses cross to the opposite side of the spinal cord, where they ascend to the thalamus, which in turn leads to the perception of pain by the cerebral cortex and the interpretation of the location and intensity of pain.

The specificity theory explains the fact that tissue damage results in pain; however, it does not explain why the same damage occurring in different people or in different incidents can result in varying degrees of pain or perhaps no pain at all. In addition, this theory does not explain why pain is *not* alleviated by chordotomy, thalamotomy, or analgesics in some individuals, and it does not provide a rationale for the return of pain following surgical intervention (McCaffery, 1972).

The pattern theory suggests that a pattern of impulses is generated by the pain receptors, which consist of reverberating circuits formed by closed loops of nerve fibers in the spinal internuncial pools. The pattern serves as the basis of an internal code that supplies the message that there is pain.

The pattern theory explains why a normally nonpainful stimulus or the absence of painful stimuli following an injury produces a response that is perceived as painful. However, the theory does not explain the reasons why severing the spinal cord pathways does not alleviate pain in all circumstances (McCaffery, 1972).

FACTORS INFLUENCING THE PAIN RESPONSE

What influences the behavior of a person experiencing pain? Does each person respond according to a predetermined ''set''? Because cultural, physical, and psychological factors influence the pain response, it is important to recognize that a client may not fit into any specific category of responses. The following factors are presented as guidelines for nursing assessment and intervention.

The duration and intensity of pain will be reflected in client behavior. For example, the chronic pain involved in terminal cancer is best described as all-consuming. The focal point of behavior is relief of pain. Superficial pain, on the other hand, prepares the body for ''fight or flight.'' Additional factors that affect the perception of pain are sensory restriction and prolonged loss of sleep. Clients often experience more pain during the night than they do during the day, because the number of incoming stimuli decreases during the night, and their type and pattern change. The body responds to stimuli of lesser intensity during periods of quiet, such as nighttime; during the day the number and variety of stimuli bombarding the client are greater. The other factor, sleep deprivation, lowers the adaptive capacity of the client, thus intensifying the perception of pain. The client who has been undergoing a rigorous series of diagnostic tests, the preparations for which preclude normal sleep, may cry pitifully following the pinprick for a blood sample. This is not irrational behavior. It should be expected in light of our understanding of pain perception.

Traumatic life experiences can initiate or sustain pain, or increase its intensity. Past experiences with pain will also influence pain perception. Increased experience with pain will often lead to an increased perception that pain is threatening, which in turn leads to increased sensitivity to pain. Powerlessness regarding the cause of illness and the resulting pain reinforces an increased sensitivity to painful stimuli. Often the presence and attitudes of others influence pain perception. For example, a client who experiences annoyance from health care professionals regarding his or her expression of pain can have a more intense subjective experience with pain and a resulting fear of pain.

The client's perception of pain as a threat to life must be considered. As the perception of a threat to life, life-style, or body image increases, concurrent increases in anxiety, depression, pain intensity, and complaints about pain will occur. Subsequently, there will be an observable increase in the intensity of behavioral responses to pain.

Religious beliefs may have an impact on the meaning pain has for clients. Pain may be perceived as a punishment for not having followed God's teachings, or it may be accepted as part of God's plan—a component of life that is nonnegotiable but one that must be taken along with the good aspects of life. Clients who perceive pain as a punishment may pray for forgiveness, while those who perceive pain as a part of God's plan may pray for the ability to tolerate that pain.

The social acceptability of the body part involved influences clients' verbalization of pain. Pain experienced in the genitals or the rectum is frequently not expressed, because clients are embarrassed and do not know proper terminology to describe the location of the pain. In such a situation, a client will often select a health care professional on the basis of age, sex, occupational title (R.N., L.P.N., nursing assistant), and ethnic background to discuss pain perceptions with—someone who is as similar as possible to himself or herself. For example, an older man may experience difficulty discussing his hemorrhoids with a young female nurse who is close to the age of one of his granddaughters. He may feel much more comfortable sharing his pain perceptions with a male attendant.

Culture may dictate very detailed and specific responses to pain. Reactions to pain vary according to a person's age, sex, and occupation. Culture may also determine whether curative or palliative treatment is sought and whether the intensity and duration of pain are sufficient to merit reporting. Recognition of cultural influences allows a nurse to understand the significance of pain for each individual client as well as the overt response to that pain. Nurses thus can develop a wide range of approaches when intervening in the process of pain perception.

Since there are many ethnic groups within American society, nurses need to identify the influences that the culture has upon pain expectancy and pain acceptance. Zborowski (1969) has done extensive work in the field of pain perception and its cultural components. McCaffery (1972) supports Zborowski's belief that cultural background exerts more influence on behavioral response than the pain situation itself.

Each culture defines its own parameters of pain response, determines the necessity for pain relief, and dictates the type and duration of use of defense mechanisms employed to control increased levels of anxiety. For example, the "old Americans," typically third-generation Americans of white, Anglo-Saxon background, do not often verbalize pain. Their reflex response to pain is to withdraw rather than to cry out. These clients are frequently future-oriented and optimistic about treatment plans. They are often labeled "good" patients because they rarely ask for assistance. This type of behavior can be misleading to the nurse and can discourage the sharing of feelings regarding the pain experience.

Members of another group, Jewish Americans, may describe pain as being "terrific" or "unbearable." Tolerance or acceptance of pain is usually low. Outward expressions of the stress of a pain experience are considered acceptable. Crying and moaning elicit sympathetic responses from others and serve to draw others close to the client. Jewish-Americans are future-oriented yet pessimistic about their treatment plans. They may seek several medical opinions.

Latin Americans and Americans of a Mediterranean background respond in a manner similar to that of Jewish Americans. A low tolerance for pain exists, along with the need to verbalize one's inner response to a painful experience. There is, however, an orientation to the present; palliative relief is sought immediately.

Irish-Americans present another distinct response to the pain experience. The client is stoic, almost to the point of being unable to admit to experiencing pain. Withdrawal behavior is the means most frequently utilized to control overt responses. Pain is viewed as something one must face with the attitude of ''grin and bear it.'' This group is future oriented, and its members accept the validity of information provided by the health care team.

Black Americans also have parameters of pain response. There is a denial of the existence of pain until it reaches an emergency state. Clients describe pain in general terms, and there is a reluctance to seek pain relief.

Each cultural group has its own parameters of pain tolerance and response behavior. The goal of a nursing assessment is not to rigidly categorize each client's subjective pain experience on the basis of ethnic group. However, as Larkins (1977) points out, ''the experience of pain defies explanation in purely physiologic or biological terms; the sociocultural aspect of pain must be taken into account. The patient's cultural background influences not only attitudes towards pain but his response to it as well.''

An important consideration in the assessment of the expression of pain is the reward or gain that a client derives from that expression. For example, clients who verbally express pain may elicit a sympathetic response from family, staff, and friends. They are placed in a dependent, ''sick'' role that releases them from the responsibilities of the adult-parent-spouse role. Clients who need to receive such a reward for the expression of pain may be attempting to adapt to a situation that has become excessively stressful, such as the increased responsibility associated with a new job, marriage, or parenting. Psychogenic pain (for further discussion, refer to Chapter 16) is considered a psychological response used to control the anxiety caused by the arousal of previously unconscious conflicts. Pain, therefore, may be viewed from two perspectives—as a commonly occurring stressor and as a psychophysiological response to a stressful life situation.

Pain is a subjective personal experience. Pain responses are altered by physical and physiological factors as well as by cultural and psychological determinants. In order to decide upon and implement a plan of action, a nurse should consider the overt as well as covert expressions of pain and their implications. ''Bad'' clients are not necessarily the ones who are most vocal about their pain, nor are the ''good'' clients necessarily the ones who stoically keep their complaints to themselves. Observation of responses to the pain experience will promote the accurate assessment of the implications of that experience for each client.

Immobilization

Immobilization commonly causes stress that may affect all areas of function—physical, emotional, sociocultural, and cognitive. Prolonged immobilization has a profound impact on the psyche. Feelings of powerlessness occur. A reorganization of territory results. There may also be a redefining of self from young, strong, active, vigorous, and productive to weak, vulnerable, inactive, and nonproductive. There is a decreased physical ability and decreased energy level; full-time work is prohibited, yet there is little recreational ability available either. Clients perceive a sense of downward mobility, which in turn leads to a sense of loss of control and a decreased sense of self-worth.

In order to discuss the concept of immobilization as a stressor, we must consider the effect of immobilization on sensory status. When an individual is immobilized, there are multiple changes in the patterning and variation of incoming stimuli. One of the primary nursing actions is to identify each client's sensory status in order to maintain perceptual and responsive function. There is no clear-cut mechanism to determine at what point sensory overload or deprivation begins. But it is certain that there are gross changes in behavior when overload or deprivation occurs.

What occurs as a result of sensory overload or deprivation? The client experiences a decrease in the ability to solve problems. The ability to perform tasks requiring eye-hand coordination is decreased, as is perceptual alertness. Often there is disorientation to time, and the client feels as though his or her body parts were floating. Hallucinations and illusions are described vividly by clients who have spent extended periods of time in intensive- or coronary-care units, where restrictions regarding visitors, flowers, clocks, and reading materials are imposed. In these units, sensory overload may be experienced because of the constant humming of monitors or other types of machinery and the constant lighting, whether it be day or night. Clients rapidly lose orientation to time and place, since the familiar objects that act as cues are absent. Clients who are isolated in such units, as well as those who are restricted to their own homes or rooms, often experience a sense of overwhelming anxiety and depression.

Who fares well in these situations? Does everyone respond similarly, or are there persons who do not develop behavioral changes? The person who needs to be amused continuously—to be on the go or always engaged in some kind of activity—is the type of client who adapts poorly to sensory deprivation or overload. It has been found that, as in many other situations, clients who have developed successful adaptation mechanisms before their illnesses and whose egos are sound are better able to cope with the multiple effects of sensory deprivation or overload. This is not to say, however, that such clients rely solely upon their own resources for the development of adaptation mechanisms. Nursing intervention to prevent or reduce the effects of sensory deprivation or overload will be presented later in this chapter.

Immobilization and sensory deprivation or overload are stressors that are interwoven with one another. Each system of the body responds differently to prolonged periods of immobility. Often, immobilized clients must deal with many crises at once. For example, associated with immobilization are often changes in body image as well as in such normal bodily functions as breathing, urinating, and defecating. Concurrently, clients experience profound changes in emotional, social, and cognitive status. Nursing measures, therefore,

must be directed toward identifying these changes as stressors and mobilizing clients' resources in order to help them adapt to their new situations.

Loss

In recent research, loss and concurrent changes have been identified as predominant stressors; they have been shown to precipitate varying degrees of anxiety. Life changes correlate with major health disruptions. Individuals who experience many changes over a short period of time seem to be more susceptible to illness. Toffler (1970) believes that too much change in too short a period of time can cause adverse physical as well as emotional reactions. Although this statement is not necessarily true for all individuals, it is imperative that nurses recognize the correlation between change and illness.

Holmes and Rahe (1967) developed a "social readjustment rating scale" on which are ranked stressful life events of both a positive nature (such as marriage, pregnancy, and promotion) and a negative nature (such as death of a spouse, divorce, or illness). Each event is rated in "life change units" (LCUs); the number of LCUs ranges from 100 to 19. Holmes and Rahe's hypothesis was that the greater the number of LCUs, the greater the probability of a client experiencing a health crisis. Table 7-4 lists the various stressful events and their corresponding numbers of LCUs.

The scale ranks life events according to their "stress value"—that is, the amount of coping that is required to adapt to them. The stressors listed include those that are threats to physiological integrity as well as those that are threats to self-esteem. Clients perceive stressful events differently, depending on their past experiences and their current emotional and physical health. By observing clients' responses to stressors, nurses can formulate comprehensive nursing care plans.

Why do some people become ill as a result of stress while others are much more capable of adapting to stress with a minimal amount of health change? Are some people more vulnerable as a result of certain variables? Do some individuals

Table 7-4. Social readjustment rating scale

Rank	Life event	Mean value
1	Death of spouse	100
2	Divorce	73
3	Marital separation	65
4	Jail term	63
5	Death of close family member	63
6	Personal injury or illness	53
7	Marriage	50
8	Fired at work	47
9	Marital reconciliation	45
10	Retirement	45
11	Change in health of family member	44
12	Pregnancy	40
13	Sex difficulties	39
14	Gain of new family member	39
15	Business readjustment	39
16	Change in financial state	38
17	Death of close friend	37
18	Change to different line of work	36
19	Change in number of arguments with spouse	35
20	Mortgage over $10,000	31
21	Foreclosure of mortgage or loan	30
22	Change in responsibilities at work	29
23	Son or daughter leaving home	29
24	Trouble with in-laws	29
25	Outstanding personal achievement	28
26	Wife begin or stop work	26
27	Begin or end school	26
28	Change in living conditions	25
29	Revision of personal habits	24
30	Trouble with boss	23
31	Change in work hours or conditions	20
32	Change in residence	20
33	Change in schools	20
34	Change in recreation	19
35	Change in church activities	19

Reprinted with permission from Holmes, T., and R. Rahe. 1976. "The social readjustment rating scale." Journal of Psychosomatic Research 11:213-218. Copyright 1967, Pergamon Press, Ltd.

have better outside support systems, more optimistic outlooks on life, or better health habits? McNeil and Pesznecker (1977) sought to discover whether good health habits, strong support systems, and a positive outlook could act as forces in assisting people to adapt to increased change. They noted that although the above variables made slight differences in the likelihood that major illness would occur, change was still the most significant factor. There are many ways in which a nurse, particularly in a community setting, can intervene on the primary level to help persons experiencing stress. The goal is to help individuals become managers of their own life changes rather than simply to help them cope with the crises that occur as a result of those changes.

Loss, like change, cannot be avoided during a lifetime. As individuals move through the life cycle, they are continuously experiencing some degree of loss—the loss of instant gratification of all demands, the loss of total dependence through learning to crawl and to walk, the loss of control over the environment through illness, the loss of hearing and sight, the loss of close friends through separation or death, the loss of independence through the aging process, and, finally, the loss of their own lives. How well individuals adapt to new losses depends, to a great extent, on past experiences with loss. If they have been positive in nature, an individual can successfully assimilate new losses and changes. However, the more negative past experiences with loss have been, the greater the potential that a person will have difficulty in adapting to current losses.

This concept can be stated in another way: early modes of adaptation to loss are the foundation of future patterns. To cite an example, the infant who is being weaned from the breast may receive nonverbal messages that this is a traumatic experience, and the experience may therefore be a negative one. For a more positive picture, consider the situation of a school-age child who moves away from his best friend. He and his parents discuss his feelings as well as theirs. There are open lines of communication and a sense of honesty. There is an understanding of the meaning of the loss to all involved. The child develops healthy patterns of adaptation, which are supported by his parents. The course has been set for the continuation of these healthy mechanisms in the future.

NURSING INTERVENTION

In this section, anxiety and each stressor discussed in this chapter will be addressed in terms of levels of prevention and the nursing process.

ANXIETY

Primary prevention

Primary prevention is a critical concern for nursing. A person's ability to respond to anxiety depends on the person's ability to identify potential stressors in his or her life situation. Anxiety can stimulate a positive growth response. Continued anxiety, however, causes exhaustion and the eventual development of psychopathology or pathophysiology. The goal of primary prevention is to help people develop healthy patterns of coping with anxiety during the early years of life in order to prevent later maladaptive responses. The family becomes the unit of focus. Intervention with the family directs the family's attention toward (1) the development of a positive self-concept, including healthy feelings towards one's own body; (2) the facilitation of interaction with others in the environment; (3) the sharing of feelings in an open, honest, caring manner; (4) the utilization of the problem-solving process to resolve disagreements; and (5) the acceptance of each individual as a separate being with unique behavior. A healthy family environment provides an atmosphere in which members can communicate their needs and identify potential stressors without feeling ashamed or afraid of repercussions. Each member feels unique and important. To minimize the effects of stressors and resulting anxiety, family members support one another in their attempts to plan their lives. Children grow up feeling confident in their ability to cope and able to reach out for support from others when it is necessary.

Adult clients can be educated to recognize potential life stressors. Nurses and other members of the health care team can assist clients in managing their own environments through anticipatory planning—that is, by helping them to determine the number and types of stressors they can cope with comfortably. Education, role modeling, and supportive counseling with families and individuals are primary nursing measures for promoting effective coping patterns and healthy adaptation.

Secondary prevention

The nursing process provides the framework for secondary prevention.

ASSESSMENT

Nursing assessment of a client experiencing anxiety is based upon presenting behaviors, including the client's subjective description of feelings, previous experiences with similar anxiety-producing situations, effectiveness of coping strategies, and current support systems.

These questions will be helpful in the assessment process: Is the client's reaction to the stressor appropriate to the situation? If it is inappropriate, are cognitive functions impaired? What is the client's level of anxiety? Has the client repeatedly attempted the same coping strategy and failed? How does his or her behavior reinforce the anxiety? Are coping strategies effective or destructive? Is the anxiety acting in the service of learning and promoting growth? What is the effect of the client's family on his or her anxiety level? Are expectations of the family consistent with those of the client or in conflict? What function does symptomatic behavior (for example, psychosis) play in the family? What happens when symptomatic behavior decreases? What coping strategies are used by the family to resolve anxiety? What secondary gains can be attributed to symptomatic behavior? What sources of support, other than the family, are available to the client? Formulation of nursing diagnoses will be specific to the level of anxiety. Severe and panic levels of anxiety may result in distortion of thoughts, feelings, and behavior.

A complete nursing history is critical to the formulation of nursing diagnoses reflective of the issues facing the client. Anxiety affects cognitive ability, interpersonal relationships, physiological and psychological function, and sense of self-worth.

ANALYSIS OF DATA

Assessment of presenting symptoms, stimulus situations, maladaptive coping responses, and holistic health factors leads to an increased understanding of the client within the context of his or her current situation. After a thorough analysis of data, nursing diagnoses are formulated.

Those clients experiencing severe to panic levels of anxiety frequently need to be hospitalized. They are unable to care for themselves physically or participate in realistic decision making and activities of daily living. Nursing diagnoses reflect the need to reduce severe anxiety levels as rapidly as possible and to protect the client from self and others.

NURSING DIAGNOSIS

Alteration in activity (either immobilization or hyperactivity) related to a panic level of anxiety* engendered by underlying conflicts (for example, social role conflict, sex conflict) and a precipitating stressful life situation (behavior associated with DSM-III diagnosis 300.01—panic disorder)

PLANNING

The nurse may initially establish goals but, as therapy progresses, the client should enter into goal setting. Long-term goals for the client are as follows:

1. To work through the conflicts that are arousing anxiety
2. To learn to effectively cope with stressful life situations so that a panic level of anxiety is not generated

Short-term goals are as follows:

1. To learn to identify and describe feelings of anxiety
2. To identify and describe the precipitating stressful life situation and the associated feelings
3. To relate the precipitating stressful life situation to situations in the past that aroused similar feelings
4. To reevaluate the potency (in terms of stress) of the precipitating stressful life situation
5. To develop more effective coping behaviors
6. To avoid excessive use of secondary gain

---

*Refer to Chapters 7 and 13 for further discussion of intervention in anxiety.

IMPLEMENTATION

1. Be directive with the client—for example, "I am going to move you into a quieter space; I will stay with you until you're feeling more calm."
2. Listen with the intent to *hear*—use the "third ear."
3. Stay with the client while respecting his or her need for space.
4. Acknowledge overwhelming feelings of awe, apprehension, terror, or fear of "going crazy" as being *real* to the client.
5. Present a calm, honest approach that affirms your ability to provide control when the client is unable to do so.
6. Provide a protective environment, meeting physical needs until the client is able to do so:
   a. Proper diet, high protein
   b. Encourage fluids
   c. Small, frequent feedings
   d. Establish a routine of eating, sleeping, elimination
   e. Symptomatic relief of diarrhea and gastric hyperactivity
7. Reduce environmental stimuli by removing the client from situations that increase anxiety, such as a crowded day room.
8. Assist the client in identifying what stressor he or she feels comfortable dealing with.
9. Support present coping strategies rather than removing defenses prematurely. Current defenses *do* relieve anxiety even though they may be inappropriate. Criticism of defenses may lead to increased anxiety. For example, ritualistic behavior should not be interrupted initially.
10. Set limits on inappropriate coping strategies once anxiety has been reduced and a trusting relationship has been established.
11. Encourage participation in activities:
    a. Support the use of gross motor activities that require little concentration or problem-solving.
    b. Work individually with clients rather than involve them in group activities.
    c. Involve family members in activities.
12. Determine what types of comfort measures are preferred by the client—for example, warm milk, hot bath, soft music, favorite quilt or afghan.
13. Reduce the number of demands made on the client, since decision making is difficult. Allow choices in treatment, diet, and daily activities when appropriate.
14. *Cautiously* use tranquilizing medications; monitor for untoward effects.
15. Distinguish between anxiety and physical symptoms such as those of cardiac arrhythmias and myocardial infarctions.

It is critical that severe to panic levels of anxiety be addressed rapidly by the nurse. Once anxiety has been decreased to more manageable levels, nursing intervention is directed toward enabling clients to develop more effective ways of resolving stressful situations. This effort cannot be accomplished when clients are experiencing severe levels of anxiety.

• • •

Burd and Marshall (1963) suggest that the focus of secondary intervention with moderate levels of anxiety is threefold: recognition of anxiety, understanding its causes, and developing adaptive methods of coping with the stressors. Nursing diagnoses may relate to any situations that generate moderate levels of anxiety. One example will be given, as follows.

NURSING DIAGNOSIS

Moderate anxiety relating to impending cataract surgery

PLANNING

The nurse assists and guides the client in the establishment of goals. The long-term goals for a moderately anxious client involve the development of coping strategies that provide for the effective resolution of ongoing crises of daily living. The individual learns to maximize the growth-promoting aspects of mild levels of anxiety and to live within the parameters of that anxiety, since it is a facet of everyday existence. Short-term goals for the client include the following:

1. To learn to identify behavioral responses that are indicative of anxiety in a given situation
2. To participate in the scheduled set of activities each day for 2 weeks
3. To learn to identify potentially anxiety-producing situations
4. To learn to remove himself from situations that potentially will increase anxiety levels

IMPLEMENTATION

1. Help the client to recognize that he or she is anxious by acknowledging signs and symptoms you observe in him or her—for example, ''You look uneasy, upset, or concerned.''
2. Connect the observable behaviors with the feeling of being anxious—for example, ''After you spoke to your mother this morning, you paced for about twenty minutes and seemed to lose your concentration. How would you describe your feelings then?''
3. Refrain from giving false reassurances such as, ''Don't worry—you'll feel better later'' or a similar empty cliché.
4. Explore possible causative factors of anxiety: ''Can you tell me what was happening before you started to feel anxious?'' Direct intervention toward connecting the perceived stressor with possible underlying conflict.
5. Assist the client in identifying previous coping strategies and their effectiveness.
6. Support the client's use of effective coping strategies.
7. Identify maladaptive use of coping strategies; point out the client's responsibility for his or her behavior and support the client's ability to mobilize effective coping strategies. Provide comfort.
8. Assist the client in the appraisal of threatening situations—that is, within the context of past and current relationships.
9. Use the educative-supportive nature of the nurse-client relationship as the forum for the testing out of new behaviors and the provision of appropriate feedback.
10. Encourage the use of physical exercise, such as walking, jogging, and bicycling, to relieve anxiety.
11. Offer other methods of tension reduction as options—for example, progressive relaxation, yoga, meditation, biofeedback, or guided imagery.

The use of the problem-solving process is an integral component of nursing intervention to reduce moderate levels of anxiety. The use of an insight-oriented, educative approach helps the client to define anxiety and its causes and to utilize adaptive methods to resolve anxiety-producing situations. The nurse can then explore the motivational aspects of mild anxiety, that level of anxiety which acts to promote growth and prevent stagnation. As noted previously, a client who succeeds in reducing anxiety enhances his or her repertoire of coping strategies and increases his or her sense of worth as a human being.

BODY-IMAGE CHANGES
Primary prevention

The development of a positive self-image, including a positive attitude toward one's own body, is a critical focus of primary prevention. Positive feelings about one's body image permit open, direct, honest communication and the expression of feelings with others in one's environment. Feelings about one's own body emerge in the first year of life. There is a need to educate parents about the messages they convey to their children regarding body image. A positive sense develops as a result of positive appraisals from the environment, particularly from parents and significant others.

Secondary prevention

ASSESSMENT

Assessment reveals the meaning body image holds for the client and how his or her perception may change regarding self, depending upon the extent, duration, location, nature, and visibility of a body alteration. It is also important to note previous experience with successful coping strategies, availability of rehabilitation programs, availability of support networks, age of the client, degree of impact on life-style, and rapidity of onset of the change. The client's perception of body-image changes is a key factor in assessment. Since each individual is unique, this perception can vary from client to client.

ANALYSIS OF DATA

Assessment of presenting symptoms as well as coping strategies, changes in life-style, and perception of body-image changes leads the nurse to formulate a nursing diagnosis. The following diagnosis is intended to serve as a prototype for other changes in body image.

NURSING DIAGNOSIS

Diminished sense of self-worth secondary to surgical amputation of a limb

PLANNING

The nurse helps the client to establish goals. The long-term goal for the client is to integrate the body alteration into his or her body image and to emerge with a holistic sense of self-worth. Short-term goals for the client include the following:

1. To observe the stump 3 to 5 days postoperatively
2. To identify feelings regarding the stump at that time
3. To participate in dressing changes of the stump 5 to 7 days postoperatively
4. To identify feelings regarding the effect on his or her life-style

IMPLEMENTATION

1. Identify areas of concern to the client by listening and observing for nonverbal messages. Explore feelings and validate the client's statements in relation to his or her changed body image. Rather than probe directly into this emotionally charged area ask open-ended questions.
2. Emphasize the client's areas of strength—accentuate the positive! By mobilizing his or her own strengths, the client begins to regain a sense of worth and a more positive self-concept.
3. Encourage physical movement, since it enhances the client's ability to integrate body changes into a new body image. The client develops competence through mastering his or her own body again.
4. Facilitate the interaction of the client with others in his or her environment. Provide an atmosphere in which the client can gradually resume his or her previous social roles as well as develop new ones. It is imperative that nurses allow the client to progress at his or her own pace. It is often helpful for the client to discuss feelings with others who have experienced similar alterations. Nurses can act as resource persons by contacting support groups as is necessary.
5. Include the client in self-care activities that will increase the client's opportunities to become reacquainted with his or her body. Such activities as looking at a wound, participating in dressing changes, feeling the bandages or cast, and handling equipment (for example, colostomy bags, prostheses) are crucial in the restructuring of body image and self-concept.
6. Recognize that the client will take his or her cues from the nurse's reactions to his or her

changed body image. The client is acutely aware of responses from his or her environment, and the client assimilates those responses into his or her newly developing body image.

7. Facilitate the expression of unresolved feelings such as anger, fear, hopelessness, and dependence by providing open lines of communication at all times.

8. Include family and significant others in all aspects of the client's course of recovery. Encourage the sharing of feelings and concerns that they may have regarding the care of the client and his or her eventual resumption of previous roles (or assumption of new ones). As was previously noted, responses from significant others are crucial.

PAIN

Primary prevention

The focus of primary prevention is the development of healthy patterns of coping with stress in order to increase the client's ability to cope with pain and to decrease anxiety associated with the anticipation and the aftermath of pain. The client will then be better able to recognize and seek help for his or her pain.

Secondary prevention

The goal of secondary prevention is the assessment and relief of the client's experience with pain—recognizing the nature and meaning of pain.

ASSESSMENT

Assessment is directed toward eliciting the following information: nature, duration, and type of pain, what relief measures are useful, meaning and perception of this pain experience, previous experience with pain, cultural and spiritual influences on pain expression, congruence of verbal and nonverbal expression of pain.

ANALYSIS OF DATA

Following a thorough assessment of client perception and response to pain, nursing diagnoses can be formulated as they relate to specific situations.

NURSING DIAGNOSIS

Reduction in ability to cope with painful stimuli

PLANNING

The nurse helps the client to establish goals. The long-term goals for the client are to learn to cope with pain, which will reduce stress and decrease anxiety, and to develop healthy patterns of coping with anxiety (see nursing diagnosis of moderate anxiety, p. 202). Short-term goals for the client include the following:

1. To learn to identify the nature and duration of painful stimuli
2. To learn to verbalize painful experiences within the context of his or her society and culture
3. To develop more effective coping skills, which will reduce the effects of painful stimuli

IMPLEMENTATION

1. Recognize that the pain experience is real to the person who is describing it.
2. Explore the meaning of the pain experience with the client. Perhaps a desire for gain or reward is an important aspect of his or her behavior.
3. Remain with the client during the painful experience. Perceptions of pain increase during the night or at other times when the client is left alone to focus on the pain.
4. Reduce environmental stimuli of a noxious nature, such as excessive lighting and noise. Often a quiet, slightly darkened room serves to alleviate pain.
5. Provide periods of rest and relaxation. It has been noted that fatigue potentiates the pain experience.
6. Educate the client as to the various pain

relief measures that are available; this enables the client to maintain a sense of control over his or her pain. Pain relief measures include breathing exercises, relaxation techniques, and guided imagery.

7. Touch the client. Touching and other means of sensory input often reduce pain perception.

8. Observe verbal and nonverbal expressions of pain. Are they congruent with one another? For example, does the client describe excruciating pain while lying casually on the bed watching television? Does the client deny pain even though he maintains a rigid posture while in the supine position?

9. After careful observation of pain behavior, administer analgesics in a prudent manner. Document pain relief and attendant behavior.

10. Behavior modification and hypnosis are used successfully in the management of pain. Surgery such as chordotomy may be indicated in the case of intractable pain.

11. Assist the client to determine positions that reduce the pain.

IMMOBILIZATION

Primary prevention

The goals of primary prevention are to help the client adapt to immobilization and to enable the client to maintain a positive self-image in the face of prolonged immobilization.

Secondary prevention
ASSESSMENT

Assessment focuses on identification of physical, perceptual, and social deficits caused by immobility; the meaning of immobilization to the client; assessment of coping strategies; onset and duration of immobilization; previous experiences with immobilization; age at onset; and the availability of support systems.

ANALYSIS OF DATA

The assessment should provide an understanding of the presenting symptoms and their interrelationship with family dynamics, precipitating factors, and client coping strategies. Nursing diagnoses will reflect situation-appropriate changes in mobility.

NURSING DIAGNOSIS

Diminished mobility related to imposed bed rest

PLANNING

The nurse helps the client to establish goals. The long-term goals for the client are to adapt successfully to immobilization and to continue to feel a sense of self-worth in relation to family, occupation, and social relationships. Short-term goals for the client include the following:

1. To describe feelings associated with immobilization
2. To identify coping stretegies that assist him or her in resolving sensory overload or deprivation
3. To select options that will enable him or her to participate in activities of daily living

IMPLEMENTATION

1. Provide such physical activities as turning and moving of unaffected parts of the body within the confines dictated by the client's situation. Movement helps the client to determine his or her own body space, which may have been altered by the immobilization. Activity also serves to reduce the severity of the negative physiological effects of prolonged immobilization.

2. Identify individual effects of sensory overload or deprivation. For example, while one client may quietly accept all the medical procedures being done for him or her, another client may evidence hypersensitivity to the environment by being acutely aware of and involved in all the activities around him or her. This type of client needs to feel a sense of control over the environment. You can facilitate this control by providing

information and including the client in the care process.

3. Maintain sensory-perceptual stimulation by means of newspapers, television, radio, visitors, and so on.

4. Reduce environmental stimuli of a monotonous nature, including noise, lighting, and personnel impinging on the client's space.

5. Identify adaptation mechanisms, along with their efficiency levels, in the current situation and in past situations of a similar nature. What are similarities and differences? Accentuate ego strengths. How can they be developed in the client's best interests?

6. Describe the client's immediate environment, and explain the various sights, sounds, and smells. This enables the client to understand the patterns of what is going on around him or her.

7. Allow the client to resume activities at his or her own pace. Introduce changes in routine slowly and with brief explanations of rationale.

8. Structure the environment and activities so that the client is not expected to accomplish tasks that require in-depth problem-solving processes. Sensory overload or deprivation decreases his or her capacity to learn and to solve problems.

9. When you consider a roommate for an immobilized client, it is often wise to place the immobilized client with a person who is oriented toward and involved with his or her environment.

10. Provide an atmosphere of open communication whereby the client may verbalize concerns or fears relating to immobilization.

11. Point out inappropriate responses, such as prolonged hallucination, hostility, withdrawal, or belligerence, to the nursing team. Consultation with a psychiatric nurse-clinician or a physician may be necessary.

12. Include family members and significant others in the nursing care plan of the immobilized client. Assist them to recognize and understand the effects of prolonged immobilization (for example, sensory overload or deprivation). They may also be instrumental in enabling the client to resume his or her former social roles or to develop new ones.

13. The primary goal of nursing care is to recognize situations that may cause sensory overload or deprivation and the clients who are potentially at risk. Nurses should consider not only those clients who are physically immobilized but also those who have social, emotional, or cognitive impairments. Individuals in mental institutions or orphanages, the elderly, the blind, the deaf, and the mute—these are just a few of the target populations that are at high risk in regard to the effects of sensory overload or deprivation.

LOSS

Primary prevention

Primary prevention focuses on the early development of adaptive strategies to effect a healthy resolution of the crises of change and loss. Within the family setting, children can be encouraged to grieve openly and to share the positive and negative aspects of change and loss. It is imperative that individuals learn methods of coping in the early phases of life, since change and loss characterize every stage of the life cycle. Those who have learned effective strategies and have experienced successful resolution of the crises of loss and change will be less likely to experience major difficulties in later life.

Secondary prevention

ASSESSMENT

Assessment focuses on the client's strengths and the client's ability to make active choices regarding the course of his or her life. The client needs to prepare for change and constructively resolve issues of loss. The following are areas to consider in the assessment: previous life changes (within past year), effectiveness of coping strategies, presence of maturational crises, level of helplessness or hopelessness, level of ego strength, presence of support systems, previous experiences with loss, phase of grief, and perception of life following loss.

ANALYSIS OF DATA

The assessment should reflect the client's responses to loss, presenting symptoms, level of integration, and use of coping strategies as well as the impact of family and environmental dynamics. Nursing diagnoses will be formulated on the basis of individual situations. The following nursing diagnosis serves as a protocol for individuals experiencing loss.

NURSING DIAGNOSIS

Loss of current socioeconomic status in association with a change in job position

PLANNING

The nurse helps the client to establish goals. Long-term goals are as follows:

1. To resolve loss through an appropriate grieving mechanism
2. To integrate changes resulting from loss in order to move to a higher level of functioning

Short-term goals are as follows:

1. To verbalize anger, helplessness, and other feelings of loss
2. To identify and develop successful strategies for coping with loss
3. To mobilize available resources to assist in adapting to loss

IMPLEMENTATION

1. Encourage the verbal expression of feelings of anger, helplessness, fear, or hopelessness by maintaining open lines of communication.
2. Support the client yet allow the client his or her own time to grieve. Be there when the client feels the need to relate to another human being. (See Chapter 18 for further discussion of grief.)
3. Facilitate participation in activities of daily living. Support attempts to engage in such new behavior as managing the checkbook or putting on the storm doors.
4. Gradually encourage the client's reinvestment in new object relationships. Since this process often reemphasizes the sense of loss, it should be paced cautiously.
5. Identify ego strengths. Help the client to perceive himself or herself as a worthwhile human being who is capable of experiencing life to its fullest in spite of his or her loss.
6. Direct the client in anticipatory planning by preparing him or her for what changes and/or losses lie ahead. Persons who are most in need of such planning include expectant parents, couples contemplating marriage, adolescents who are experiencing maturational crises, clients in low-income housing projects, individuals whose spouses have chronic or terminal illnesses, couples that are separating or divorcing, clients who move frequently, clients who are about to experience menopause, and individuals who are about to retire. To focus on these groups before the onset of illness is a major nursing priority.
7. Assess the client's previous life changes in light of adaptive mechanisms used—their effectiveness or ineffectiveness in coping with the stress incurred as a result of the change or loss. What symptoms does the client have?
8. Educate the client—on either an individual or a group basis. The client learns through his or her relationships with group members and nursing staff how to become a manager of his or her own life. The client need not wait for a major health crisis to occur. Instead, the client's preparation for and understanding of change and loss enable him or her to develop successful adaptation mechanisms. Pressures of life will no longer seem insurmountable. Some changes may be delayed while the client is adapting to those of higher priority. The goal of intervention is

the recognition of changes and their impact on life-style.

9. Refer to community resources that may help the client adjust to changes in life-style.

EVALUATION

The client and, whenever feasible, the client's family and significant others (for example, house-mate, very close friend) should be included in estimating the client's progress toward attainment of goals. Any evaluation should encompass the following areas:

1. Estimation of the degree to which conflicts have been worked through
2. Estimation of the degree to which goals have been achieved and client functioning has improved (demonstrated by a decrease in maladaptive coping behavior and the learning of more effective coping behavior)
3. Identification of goals that need to be modified or revised
4. Referral of the client to support systems other than the nurse-client relationship
   a. People in the client's social network who are willing to serve as a support system
   b. Community agencies that help clients learn to live with stressors to which they may never completely adapt (e.g., ostomy clinics)
   c. Centers that specialize in helping clients to cope with specific stressors (e.g., pain clinics)

TERTIARY PREVENTION

The focus of tertiary prevention is on the assessment of maladaptive responses to anxiety, alterations in body image, lengthy immobility, painful stimuli, or situations that generate a sense of loss. Intervention at this level is directed toward helping the client to resolve maladaptive coping measures and to minimize further effects of these maladaptive measures.

CHAPTER SUMMARY

Each individual is in a continual state of flux, always responding to internal and external cues. Adaptation is the series of changes that occurs in response to stressors. The way an individual adapts to stress is influenced by cultural, physiological, and psychological factors. If a stressor is not perceived as very threatening, anxiety levels are mild. Mild anxiety can be utilized in the service of learning. As anxiety levels increase, however, problem-solving capacities become impaired and previously successful coping behavior becomes inadequate. If severe anxiety continues for a prolonged period, physical exhaustion and maladaptive patterns of behavior result. Recognition of anxiety levels and their implications for nursing intervention are critical to the process of healthy adaptation.

Several commonly encountered stressors that pose varying degrees of threat to self-concept have been presented. Key concepts in the understanding of these stressors include the perception of the event and the degree and type of coping mechanisms utilized. In some instances a change, such as an increase in body size, is both a stressor and the *result* of a stress response. Nurses need to keep in mind the difference between *stressor* and *stress response*.

Primary, secondary, and tertiary preventive measures in relation to stress, anxiety, and adaptation have been presented. Primary prevention directs its efforts toward identification and management of potential stressors. Secondary prevention involves the early detection of actual stressors and the implementation of nursing strategies to cope with them. Tertiary prevention deals with the assessment of maladaptive responses arising from prolonged periods of uncontrolled anxiety and intervention to keep these maladaptive responses from becoming permanent.

Evaluation of these three levels of intervention is an integral component of nursing practice. Nurses need to be aware of the implications of the stress response and the attendant anxiety levels—

both for themselves and for their clients. One goal of the nurse-client relationship is the identification of motivators of behavior. An understanding of anxiety and its effects on behavior enables nurse and client to explore present and future coping mechanisms. The nursing diagnosis and the subsequent nursing intervention should reflect this understanding. Nursing care of the person experiencing stress includes all areas of prevention—primary, secondary, and tertiary.

SENSITIVITY-AWARENESS EXERCISES

Stress-reduction measures

1. Progressive relaxation*
   a. Procedure
      (1) Lie very quietly in a comfortable position.
      (2) Loosen clothing.
      (3) Allow yourself to be relaxed; assume a mental posture that permits relaxation.
      (4) Follow a sequence beginning with the upper extremities and moving down through the trunk and lower extremities, tensing each group of muscles twice for 30 seconds and relaxing each group twice for 60 seconds. Produce tension in one group at a time. Do not tense muscles after they have become relaxed. (These instructions are often given on tape so that they may be followed more easily.)
      (5) Progressive relaxation should be practiced regularly, once a day each day. When it has been mastered, it can be used at any time as a self-regulatory measure. It does *not* work for everyone.
   b. Purpose: to help you note the difference between muscle tension and muscle relaxation. You will also be able to remember what it feels like to release the tension. Recall may then be used to effect muscle relaxation.
2. Breathing exercise†
   a. Procedure
      (1) Sit in a chair in a comfortable position, with loose clothing.

      (2) Control your breathing so that it is slow, deep, and regular.
      (3) Close your eyes and exhale slowly while pulling your abdomen in.
      (4) Inhale quickly through your nose, bringing in as much air as you can so as to fill the rib cage.
      (5) Draw in your abdomen and push the air out through your mouth.
      (6) Repeat steps 3 to 5 ten times.
      (7) Inhale slowly through your nose. Hold your breath for 10 seconds.
      (8) Exhale slowly through your mouth until your lungs are empty.
      (9) Repeat steps 7 and 8 five times.
   b. Purpose: to reduce stress by controlling your breathing. Tension and relaxation are mutually exclusive; therefore by focusing on relaxation you cannot be tense. This measure, as do the others, enables you to feel more in control of your situation, which also serves to reduce stress.
3. Guided imagery*
   a. Procedure
      (1) Find a quiet, comfortable place to sit.
      (2) Close your eyes and imagine a peaceful scene that has special meaning for you—a place where you have been or would like to go.
      (3) Visualize this scene in as much detail as you can. Imagine the smells, sounds, and "feels" of this place, such as the sun, the breeze, the scent of flowers, the trickling of a brook.
      (4) Experience the pleasure of this scene for a few minutes, and then slowly open your eyes.
   b. Purpose: to respond to symbolic stimuli, enabling you to feel as if you are *actually* experiencing the restful scene. You feel the effects of the imagery and stress is lessened.

Guide for developing your own stress profile†

Take a little time to reflect on the following questions as a guide to self-exploration.
1. How often do you feel tense, anxious, irritable?
2. How often do you eat, drink, or smoke to relieve tension?
3. Do you feel that you have more to do than you

---

*Adapted from Jacobsen (1978).
†Adapted from Ulene (1978).

*Adapted from Ulene (1978).
†From Sutterley, D.C. 1979. "Stress and health: a survey of self-regulation modalities." Topics in Clinical Nursing 1:1.

can accomplish each day? Do you always feel rushed?

4. Do you enjoy what you are doing? Are your daily tasks a source of pleasure and satisfaction?
5. Do you find time to relax regularly every day?
6. Do you have difficulty sleeping?
7. How would you rate your general state of health at present?
8. Do you consider your present weight to be a problem?
9. Do you eat a nutritious balanced diet (free from the excesses that can become ''stressors'')?
10. Do you exercise regularly?
11. Do you believe you are getting adequate exercise and do you enjoy it?
12. Do you believe you are physically fit? (Is your resting pulse rate above 80/min?)
13. Calculate your life change index; is it more than 300 for the year?
14. Do you try to recognize tension in yourself? (And how do others see you expressing your stress and tension?)

Ask yourself:
- What kind of tension you feel and under what circumstances.
- What were you thinking or feeling and how did you respond when under heavy stress?

Keep a log or diary to assist you in a self-examination to identify your own sources of stress (what bothers you).

Try to recognize your own manifestations of stress and tension (others may need to help you).

Stressors of altered body image, pain, and immobilization

1. Types of exercises
   a. Think about your body, its appearance and functioning. Identify one body part that you view as central to your body image. Next, imagine yourself with that body part multilated or dysfunctioning.
      (1) What feelings are evoked?
      (2) How do you think this change would affect your relationship with significant others? Your interaction with strangers?
      (3) What effect do you think it would have on your ability to establish a meaningful sexual relationship? At what point in the relationship would you disclose or discuss the alteration in your body?
      (4) What influences have your family, your society, and your religious and ethnic heritage had in the formation of your attitudes and feelings about this body part and your anticipated reaction to the alteration?
   b. Recall an incident in which you experienced pain that lasted a minimum of several hours. This pain may have been from something as common as a toothache or a severe headache or from something more complex (such as surgery, an accident, or an illness).
      (1) Describe the pain both verbally and pictorially (the picture may be abstract or concrete).
      (2) How old were you when you experienced this pain?
      (3) What were your feelings during your pain experience?
      (4) What occurrences or factors seemed to increase your perception of pain? Decrease your perception of pain?
      (5) What were your responses to your pain?
      (6) How long did your pain last?
      (7) What were your feelings and responses when your pain was over?
      (8) Ask family and friends to tell you their perceptions of your reactions during and after your pain experience.
      (9) How do your responses to pain compare with the responses of your family members to pain? With the responses of other members of your religious or ethnic group to pain?
   c. Spend an entire day in a wheelchair or immobilized in bed (this means you cannot ambulate and can only change position with assistance). Keep a diary of the day. (The entries in your diary may be written or may be made on a tape recorder. If you discontinue the exercise before the day ends, discuss why you made that decision.) Your diary entries should discuss the following:
      (1) How immobilization affects your physical, perceptual, and social functioning
      (2) How immobilization changes your life-style
      (3) Your feelings
      (4) The mechanisms you use to cope with immobilization
      (5) Assistance you receive from others
      (6) The reactions of others to your immobilization
      (7) Factors in the physical and social environ-

ment that facilitate or make more difficult your attempts to cope with immobilization

2. Purposes of the exercises:
   a. To facilitate the development of insight into factors that influence one's own perception of, interpretation of, and response to altered body image, pain, and immobilization
   b. To facilitate the development of sensitivity to clients who are experiencing altered body image, pain, or immobilization
   c. To increase understanding of the effect that one's family, ethnic heritage, religious affiliation, and society have on the perception of, interpretation of, and response to altered body image, pain, and immobilization

REFERENCES

Alland, A.
   1970 Adaptation in Cultural Evolution: An Approach to Medical Anthropology. New York: Columbia University Press.
Bush, P.
   1976 "The male nurse: A challenge to traditional role identities." Nursing Forum 4:390.
Burd, S. and M. Marshall (eds.)
   1963 Some Clinical Approaches to Psychiatric Nursing. New York: MacMillan, Inc.
Dock, L.
   1920 A Short of History of Nursing. New York: Putnam.
Engel, G.
   1962 Psychological Development in Health and Disease. Philadelphia: W.B. Saunders Co.
Freud, S.
   1936 A General Introduction to Psychoanalysis. New York: Pocket Books (1969).
Grissom, M., and C. Spengler
   1976 Woman Power and Health Care. Boston: Little, Brown & Co.
Gulak, R.
   1981 "Nurses salaries: Just beginning to catch up." RN 44:40.
Holmes, T.H., and R.U. Rahe
   1967 "The social readjustment scale." Journal of Psychosomatic Research 11:213-218.
Jacobsen, E.
   1978 You Must Relax (ed. 5). New York: McGraw-Hill Book Co.
Kolb, L.
   1959 "Disturbances of the body image." In American Handbook of Psychiatry, Vol. 1. S. Arieti (ed.). New York: Basic Books, Inc., Publishers.

Larkins, F.
   1977 "The influence of one patient's culture on pain response." Nursing Clinics of North America 12(4):156-162.
Lazarus, R.S.
   1977 "Cognitive and coping processes in emotion." In Stress and Coping: An Anthology. A. Monat and E. Lazarus (eds.). New York: Columbia University Press.
Lewis, A., and J.S. Levy
   1982 Psychiatric Liaison Nursing: The Theory and Clinical Practice. Reston, Va: Reston Publishing Co.
Mason, J.
   1975 "A historical view of the stress field." Journal of Human Stress 1:22.
McCaffery, M.
   1972 Nursing Management of the Patient with Pain. Philadelphia: J.B. Lippincott Co.
McNeil, J., and B. Pesznecker
   1977 "Keeping people well despite life change crises." Public Health Reports 92(4):343-348.
Menninger, K.
   1963 The Vital Balance. New York: The Viking Press.
Peplau, H.
   1962 "Interpersonal techniques: the crux of psychiatric nursing." American Journal of Nursing 62:53-54.
Peplau, H.
   1963 "A working definition of anxiety." In Some Clinical Approaches to Psychiatric Nursing. S. Burd and M. Marshall (eds.). New York: MacMillan, Inc.
Shilder, P.
   1950 The Image and Appearance of the Human Body. New York: International Universities Press, Inc.
Seigle, D.
   1974 "The gate control theory." American Journal of Nursing 74:498-502.
Selye, H.
   1956 The Stress of Life. New York: McGraw-Hill Book Co.
Steffen, S.M.
   1980 "Perceptions of stress: 1800 nurses tell their stories." In Living With Stress and Promoting Well-Being. K.E. Claus and J.T. Bailey (eds.). St. Louis: The C.V. Mosby Co.
Sullivan, H.S.
   1953 Interpersonal Theory of Psychiatry. New York: W.W. Norton & Co., Inc.
Sutterley, D.C.
   1979 "Stress and health: a survey of self-regulation modalities." Topics in Clinical Nursing 1:1.
Toffler, A.
   1970 Future Shock. New York: Random House, Inc.
Turner, A., C. King, and J. Craddock
   1975 "Measuring and reducing noise." Hospitals 49:85.

Ulene, A.
1978 Feeling Fine. New York: Ballantine Books.
Valiga, T., and M. Frain
1979 "The multiple dimensions of stress." Topics in Clinical Nursing 1:1.
Zborowski, M.
1969 People in Pain. San Francisco: Jossey-Bass, Inc., Publishers.

ANNOTATED SUGGESTED READINGS

Claus, K.E., and J.T. Bailey (eds.)
1980 Living With Stress and Promoting Well-Being: A Handbook for Nurses. St. Louis: The C.V. Mosby Co.
This timely compendium of articles serves to increase nurses' understanding of stress through a conceptual model of stress and its impact on individuals. Stress management techniques are presented for dealing with job-relocated stress. Measures to increase individuals' awareness of stressors are offered as well as strategies for coping effectively with the stressors of everyday living.

Jacobsen, S.F., and M. McGrath (eds.)
1983 Nurses Under Stress. New York: John Wiley & Sons, Inc.
This selection of articles examines the practice of nursing in its many environments. It considers nurses as individuals, members of organizations. A variety of stressors are identified and coping behaviors are explored thoroughly. This book comes at a time when nurses need most to learn to become more skillful in their own stress prevention and management.

Pasquali, E.
1975 "Personification: patient and nurse problems." Perspectives in Psychiatric Care 13:58-61.
The author discusses the problem of personification. She identifies the difficulties that occur when a client is unable to integrate an alteration in body image into his or her view of self. Appropriate nursing strategies are presented.

Peplau, H.
1963 "A working definition of anxiety." In Some Clinical Approaches to Psychiatric Nursing. S. Burd and M. Marshall (eds.). New York: Macmillan, Inc.
Peplau's classic discussion of anxiety presents the various levels of anxiety and their behavioral and physiological manifestations. This clear-cut and concise presentation serves as a framework for the understanding of anxiety and for the development of relevant nursing strategies.

Smith, M., and H. Selye
1979 "Reducing the negative effects of stress." American Journal of Nursing 79(10):1953-1957.
This article points out that nurses need (1) to have a sound understanding of the concept of stress, (2) to recognize the manifestations of stress, and (3) to apply strategies to reduce stress. Each individual responds differently to stressors, depending on past experiences, coping mechanisms, and perception of a stressful event. Consideration therefore must be given to all factors affecting the response to stress. The authors conclude that a holistic approach is necessary for the rehabilitation of clients. Education provides clients with the information to manage both potential and actual stresses.

FURTHER READINGS

Bell, J.
1977 "Stressful life events and coping methods in mental illness and wellness behaviors." Nursing Research 26: 136-141.
Breeden, S., and C. Kondo
1978 "Using biofeedback to reduce tension." American Journal of Nursing 75:2010-2012.
Garfield, C.A. (ed.)
1979 Stress and Survival: The Emotional Realities of Life-Threatening Illness. St. Louis: The C.V. Mosby Co.
Gruendeman, B.
1975 "The impact of surgery on body image." Nursing Clinics of North America 10:635.
Hurst, M., C.D. Jenkins, and R. Rose
1976 "The relation of psychological stress to onset of medical illness." Annual Review of Medicine 27:86-95.
Kerr, N.
1978 "Anxiety: theoretical considerations." Perspectives in Psychiatric Care 16:36-46.
Lambert, V., and C. Lambert
1979 The Impact of Physical Illness and Related Mental Health Concepts. Englewood Cliffs, N.J.: Prentice-Hall, Inc.
Maguire, P.
1975 "Emotional responses after mastectomy." In Contemporary Obstetrics and Gynecology. Boston: Little, Brown & Co., pp. 34-48.
Murphy, L., and A. Moriarity
1976 Vulnerability, Coping, and Growth. New Haven, Conn.: Yale University Press.
Selye, H.
1977 Stress without Distress. Toronto: McClelland & Stewart, Ltd.
Williams, C., and T. Holmes
1978 "Life change, human adaptation and onset of illness in clinical practice." In Psychosocial Nursing: Assessment and Intervention. D. Longo and R. Williams (eds.). New York: Appleton-Century-Crofts.

CHAPTER 8

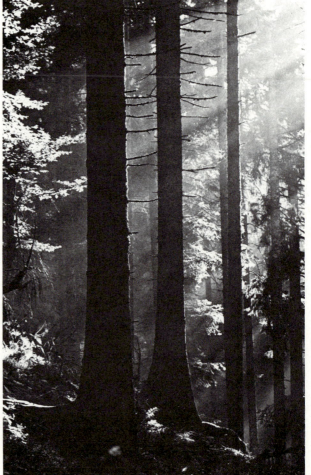

Photo by Werner H. Müller—Peter Arnold, Inc.

Basic concepts of communication

CHAPTER FOCUS

Communication is a process involving three levels of interaction: verbal, kinesic, and proxemic. Just as language varies from culture to culture, kinesic behavior and proxemic behavior are also culturally variable. When members of different cultures interact, dissimilar verbal, kinesic, and proxemic cues can contribute to misunderstandings and disruption of role relationships. Therapeutic communication involves more than learning a body of interviewing skills. It involves understanding the process of communication and the influence of culture on communication.

Ruesch and Bateson (1968) view communication as the social matrix of psychiatry. Until recently, health workers have focused primarily on verbal communication. Now they are beginning to recognize the importance of nonlinguistic communication—kinesics, the use of body parts in communication, and proxemics, the use of space in communication.

Silverstein (1977) states that meaning is communicated each time one member of a society interacts with another member. This is known as a *cultural event*. For instance, think of all the verbal and nonverbal ways that people communicate the message of dominance-submission.

The United States is a nation of immigrants. Its population is an ethnic mix. Even though most of its people speak English, they use ethnically patterned kinesic and proxemic behavior. Scheflen (1972) cautions that, even when people speak the same language, it cannot be assumed that there is shared meaning. Communication may be misunderstood; communication problems may arise. Knowledge of the process of communication and the influence of culture on communication may prevent the development of communication barriers and may help to establish therapeutic communication.

Communication is the act of imparting and exchanging ideas, information, and feelings with others. People communicate through both verbal and nonverbal expression. Verbal communication is spoken language; the words we use and the way we use them. Nonverbal communication embraces kinesics and proxemics: the way we move body parts and the way we use the space around us. The two modes of communication—verbal and nonverbal—are neither separate nor unrelated. Instead, they are different *levels* of communication that systematically interrelate to reinforce, supplement, or contradict one another. Dr. Albert Mehrabian (1969, 1972) has calculated that 7% of the total impact of a message comes from verbal expression, 38% from vocal expression, and 55% from facial expression. We can agree or disagree with Dr. Mehrabian's figures or argue that ''facial expression'' is too narrow a category and that all body movements need to be considered, but most of us will agree that verbal and nonverbal expressions interrelate in the act of communication.

VERBAL COMMUNICATION

''In the beginning was the word. . . .'' Verbal communication refers to spoken language, to the sounds (paralanguage) and words we use when we communicate. Language influences the way people perceive, interpret, and respond to the world around them. For instance, the grammatical forms of American Indian languages influence Indians' perception of relatedness. Many of these languages do not contain coersive or possessive words. The Wintu Indians of California cannot say ''I have a child'' or ''I took my child to the doctor.'' Wintu language does not permit such expression. Instead, the Wintu say, ''I live with the child or ''I went with the child to the doctor.'' Similarly, the Navaho Indians of Arizona and New Mexico guide rather than command their children to observe numerous Navaho taboos. Navaho parents do not speak of teaching children to obey or of punishing children. Instead, they explain that when a taboo is broken a specific unpleasant consequence follows. When a child violates a taboo, parents view it as a mistake that the child must rectify and not as a consequence of something that parents either did or did not do. As a result, neither parents nor children experience a sense of overwhelming guilt (Lee, 1959). Thus language plays an important role in

reinforcing the concepts of permissiveness and personal integrity that are central to the interpersonal relationships of many American Indians.

Any group of people can create arbitrary meanings for words and phrases. An ethnic group, an age group, a social class, or an occupational group may have its own vocabulary (Ervin-Tripp, 1977). For example, the abbreviation ''S.O.B.'' has a different meaning to nurses than to the general public. The shared meaning and understanding of language help to create and maintain a sense of identity, belonging, and exclusivity. In order to understand the way people communicate verbally, we must have some knowledge of the properties of spoken language.

Properties of spoken language

The basic components in the structure of language are phonemes, morphemes, and syntax. Phonemes and morphemes form the basic units of the expressive system (sound system) of language. A phoneme is a minimal unit of sound that distinguishes one utterance from another. For example, the /p/ sound in the word ''pet'' is a phoneme. In addition, there may be variants of a phoneme. For example, the aspirated /kʰ/ is a variant of the unaspirated /k/, as in /ski/ (s<u>k</u>y) versus /k^hē/ (key) (Gleason, 1961). Immigrants may have difficulty learning the phoneme variants of the language of the host country. This sometimes causes communication difficulties and stress.

A school nurse–teacher noticed that a 10-year-old Cuban girl who had immigrated three years before frequently came to the infirmary with complaints of headache and upset stomach. During a conference with the girl's teacher, the school nurse learned that although the girl was conversant in English, she had difficulty with phoneme variants. When she spoke in class, her classmates would laugh. The girl would then become embarrassed, quiet, and withdrawn. The school nurse recognized that the language problem was causing the girl stress and that it might undermine her self-concept. The school nurse therefore referred the girl to the school's speech therapist.

A morpheme is a *meaningful* sound that cannot be broken down into smaller meaningful sounds. Root words such as ''walk'' and ''trot'' and affixes such as ''ed,'' ''ing,'' and ''s'' are examples of morphemes. In addition, morphemes, like phonemes, can have variants. For instance, /z/ is a variant of the affix /s/, as in /ske̅z/ (skis) versus /räks/ (rocks). Phonemes and morphemes are related because every morpheme is composed of phonemes (Gleason, 1961).

Syntax, the third component in the structure of language, refers to structural cues and the arrangement of words into phrases and sentences. Syntax tells how a sentence should fit together (Bloomfield, 1933). In English, the usual order is subject—verb—object.

Types of structural cues include intonation, transition, and pitch. Taken together, pitch, intonation, and transition usually mark off phrases and sentences and tell us about their construction. For example, sentences that terminate with a rise in pitch are usually questions, whereas those that drop in pitch are usually declarative statements (Gleason, 1961).

Although spoken language changes, the rate of change is usually slow enough so that speakers of the same language are able to communicate. When linguistic variations cause communication difficulties between speakers of the same language, we say that the people speak different dialects (Bloomfield, 1933; Jesperson, 1967).

Although there is no definitive explanation for how sound change originates, we can consider how it spreads from person to person. Imitation of speech habits, both conscious and unconscious, is an important means of spreading phonemic change. People tend to imitate the sounds of foreign languages, of people of superior wealth and status, and of people in enviable positions. The spreading of phonemic change through imitation tends to be slow and it survives only when the pronunciation is easier, when the alteration is deemed superior, and when the sound change originates independently among many different individuals (Jesperson, 1967).

Culture and spoken language

Spoken language is culturally specific. The relationship between language and culture can be divided into the following two areas of exploration:

1. World view, which looks at whether culture is influenced by language or whether language influences culture
2. Sociolinguistics, which studies the relationship between language and the social context in which it occurs (Eastman, 1975)

WORLD VIEW

Some linguists believe that language structures thought and defines experience, thereby determining world view. Because members of a language community share a similar perception of the world, any given reality, whether physical or social, can be structured in various ways. Different languages utilize different structures. Therefore, there is no universal reality but many different realities. By understanding the meaning of a people's language, we learn about their thought processes, culture, and perception of reality (Whorf, 1956; Sapir, 1964; Lucy and Shweder, 1979).

Antilanguage is an example of language emerging from, creating, and reinforcing the social structure of society, in this case an ''antisociety'' (a society that runs counter to society-at-large). The role and function of antilanguage is to create an alternative reality that emphasizes certain ''anti'' aspects of society. Antilanguage words refer to the central activities of the counterculture and they express meanings and values that are not shared by the rest of established society. Antilanguage thus creates and maintains an alternative reality and an alternative social structure with its own system of values, sanctions, rewards and punishments (Halliday, 1976).

A nurse began working in an adolescent treatment program. Most of the youths in the program had been referred there because of drug abuse and juvenile delinquency. The nurse discovered that the youths had their own language, a language that he did not understand. For instance, there were many new words for police, drugs, and acts of vandalism. The nurse soon realized that this language served a dual purpose for the youths. It created and described the reality of their counterculture and, because it was not understood by members of "straight" society, it acted as a boundary-maintenance mechanism.

However, some anthropologists do not agree with the view that separate realities are generated by different language systems. These anthropologists argue that there is a universal reality and that different societies segment this reality differently. Language and the number of words in a language that refer to specific concepts permit the members of a language community to be more aware of and more articulate about certain aspects of their environment but do not create separate realities (Fishman, 1960; Berlin and Kay, 1969).

SOCIOLINGUISTICS

Some linguists seek to identify and describe the characteristics of and the interrelationships between language varieties, the functions of language, and the speakers. The basic unit of analysis is a speech community. A speech community is a social group that shares a similar understanding of the speech and rules of at least one dialect of the several dialects or languages that may be found within a particular locale (Fishman, 1968, 1971; Hymes, 1972).

Sociolinguists have found that people who speak a common language often use different rule systems. This sometimes leads to misinterpretation of communication. Two rules, the violation of which may cause misunderstandings, are the rules of alternation and co-occurrence (Ervin-Tripp, 1972). *Alternation rules* establish the alternatives available to a speaker, such as whether to address a person by title, first name, surname, or any combination of these options (Ervin-Tripp, 1972).

In one unit of a hospital, clients called student nurses by their first names and graduate nurses by their surnames. However, clients usually addressed the clinical nurse specialists by their titles and surnames (for example, Dr. Traube).

Ervin-Tripp points out that social categories such as kinship, sex, status, age, and type of interpersonal relationship influence the range of alternatives available to a speaker.

Rules of co-occurrence mandate the use of the same level of structure, be it lexical or syntactic (Ervin-Tripp, 1972). For example, the rule of co-occurrence is followed when a bilingual client uses Spanish syntax and pronunciation when speaking Spanish and English syntax and pronunciation when speaking English. Conversely, the rule is violated when a bilingual client uses the syntactic order of one language and the vocabulary of another language.

At times, different linguistic rule systems give rise to ethnic tensions. In a multiethnic society, stigma may be attached to linguistic rule systems that are different from those of the dominant language. Immigrants and other minority groups may then differentiate between public and private spheres of interaction. They may speak their native language in the private sphere and the dominant language in the public sphere (Eidheim, 1969; Gumperz and Hymes, 1972).

A community health nurse served a catchment area that had a sizeable Hispanic population. The English-speaking population resented the influx of Hispanics and openly voiced the belief that if Hispanics wanted to live in the United States, "they should at least learn to speak English." The community health nurse noticed that in the shops owned by English-speaking shop-keepers and in the neighborhood health station, where many of the nurses were bilingual, Hispanic clients spoke English. However, at home and at solely Hispanic social gatherings, Spanish was spoken.

Thus, spoken language is part of any communication system. It communicates needs, feelings, and intentions. The properties of verbal communication can be identified, described, and analyzed. In looking at the communication value of speech, we have seen the importance of understanding the interrelationship between language and the context in which it occurs. We will now explore another level of human communication: nonverbal communication.

NONVERBAL COMMUNICATION

Nonverbal communication is any type of communication other than verbal. We will focus on two areas of nonverbal communication: kinesics and proxemics. *Kinesics* refers to the way we use body parts when we communicate, and *proxemics* refers to the way we use space when we communicate. Observation will show that body movements and spatial arrangements *do* communicate significant information. We can think of kinesics as body language and of proxemics as space language.

Kinesics

Birdwhistle (1963, 1970), a pioneer in the field of kinesics, recognized certain similarities between spoken and written language and body language. His research was guided by two basic assumptions: that individuals are constantly maneuvering to accommodate the presence and activities of other individuals and that the system of kinesic movement is learned and ultimately analyzable. In order to understand the way people communicate kinesically, we must have some knowledge of the properties of kinesic behavior.

PROPERTIES OF KINESIC BEHAVIOR

Kinesic behavior is most often unconsciously performed. It is found both among primates and among other mammals. Socialization plays an important role in transmitting kinesic systems from generation to generation. Body movements are responsive to an individual's bio-psycho-cultural state and usually vary in form and meaning according to ethnic background, sex, age, and social class (Efron, 1942; Birdwhistle, 1970; Scheflen and Scheflen, 1972).

The point of origin, speed, and destination of a gesture, empathic assessment, a person's psycho-physiological state and cultural background, and the context in which a gesture is made are all involved in the way a person reads and responds to the body movements of another. For example, when a man with whom we are conversing raises his arm, we rapidly and unconsciously ask ourselves. "What is he doing? Is he friend or foe? What do I mean when I do that? What has happened in similar situations when someone has raised his arm like that? Who is he aiming at?'' The interpretation we arrive at and the way we respond will vary greatly—they depend on our answers to these questions. Certainly the raising of an arm by a stranger on the street has a different meaning from the same gesture performed by a friend at a cocktail party, an opponent in a sports arena, or a person receiving physiotherapy.

Body movements, then, are very important to our understanding of others and to being understood by others. Just as individuals have the physical capacity for producing thousands of sounds, but are limited by language to the use of only a very few, each individual, on the basis of culture, uses only a relatively small number of the many motions available for communication. Kinesic behavior can be classified according to function. Scheflen and Scheflen (1972) have distinguished and described three types of body movement that aid in communication: markers, reciprocals, and territorials.

Markers act as punctuation points and indicators:

During a group therapy session, it was observed that participants lowered their heads, eyebrows, and hands at the end of statements, but raised one or all of these body parts when they asked questions. Moreover, when one participant accused another of monopolizing the session, he pointed his head and right hand in the direction of the accused and said, "Harry doesn't give any of us a chance to get a word in edgewise."

Can there by any question that these group members were using their bodies to clarify or dramatize situations?

When people make one gesture as they say one word and another gesture as they speak the next word and so on, we say that they are using markers of speech. Gestures are also used to mark the beginnings and endings of sentences. For example, at the end of a sentence, people not only lower voice pitch, but also lower their hands and heads. On the other hand, when people ask a question, they raise their voices, heads, and eyebrows. When people have completed an idea, they usually signal this fact by shifting their eyes and heads and changing their posture. When they begin to express another idea, they again shift kinesically.

Whereas markers of speech involve only the speaker, markers of discourse involve both speaker and listener. People try to obtain speaking rights in one of several ways, depending on the situation. They may stand, as when making a formal presentation. They may remain seated, but lean forward and extend one or both hands into the space in front of them. They may lean back in their seats and either steeple their fingers or place the palms of their hands behind their heads. These latter types of posturing often indicate that the people about to speak have some status, and the posturings are usually differentiated by sex. Women tend to steeple, while men tend to place the palms of their hands behind their heads. Meanwhile, listeners are looking in the direction of the speaker, occasionally making eye contact with the speaker, and intermittently making such listening movements as nodding. In addition, if speaker and listeners are in rapport, they indicate this by posturing and moving in synchrony. Finally, when discourse is completed, a terminal marker signals the end of the encounter. Participants lower their eyes and engage in some parting ritual such as shaking hands, kissing, or palm brushing.

Reciprocals indicate affiliation between people. Reciprocals include bond-servicing behavior (behavior that reinforces interpersonal bonds, such as exchanging food and drink or giving affection and attention) and empathic behavior (such as looking sympathetic or exchanging winks and smiles).

Courtship behavior and quasicourtship behavior are also reciprocals. Courtship behavior is characterized by increased muscle tonus and preening. A message of intimacy is conveyed. Women protrude their breasts and display their wrists or palms. Men display their chests by straightening up, contracting abdominal muscles, and squaring their shoulders. Voices are kept low so that conversations will not be overheard. Quasicourtship behavior, on the other hand, contains qualifiers or metacommunication signaling that courting should not be taken seriously. Voices may be loud enough for conversations to be overheard. References may be made as to the inappropriateness of the situation for courting, or an incomplete postural-kinesic configuration may be given. For instance, participants may be facing each other, but their torsos may be turned toward other people or their eyes may dart around the room.

Quasicourtship behavior has a systems-maintenance function. In situations in which one participant either withdraws or is excluded, quasicourtship behavior calls back the errant participant and thereby maintains the interaction. Quasicourtship behavior thus facilitates rapport and sociability, necessary elements in group cohesion.

To avoid the misunderstanding of communication, nurses must be able to distinguish between courtship and quasicourtship behavior.

A student nurse observed a psychiatrist interacting with a 23-year-old female client in the sitting room of a large hospital. They were facing each other, with their bodies turned toward the staff in the nurses' station. The client frequently brushed hair away from her face, presenting the palm of her hand to the psychiatrist. The psychiatrist adjusted his tie several times. They were speaking loudly enough so that the student nurse could hear that they were discussing plans for the young woman's imminent discharge.

The student misinterpreted this quasicourtship behavior for courtship behavior and felt that the psychiatrist was encouraging his client's "seductive behavior." After talking the situation over with her instructor, the student was able to identify the behavioral qualifiers that signaled the message that courting should not be taken seriously (participants' torsos were turned away from each other and toward the rest of the staff, they were talking in a large sitting room and in the midst of other people, and they were speaking loudly enough so that their conversation could be easily overheard.)

Occasionally, individuals inadequately learn either the courtship behavior or the behavioral qualifiers. Since both sets of behavior are essential for quasicourtship, deviance or pathological behavior ensues when *either* set is performed in the absence of the other. Persons with schizophrenia often use courtship behavior without including behavioral qualifiers. Instead of quasicourting they court. We usually say that they are exhibiting inappropriately seductive behavior. Or an individual may be unable to deal with quasicourtship behavior and respond by "decourting"—withdrawing or criticizing. This type of behavior is often associated with such sexual dysfunctions as impotence and frigidity (Scheflen, 1965; Scheflen and Scheflen 1972).

Scheflen (1965) states that misinterpretation of quasicourtship behavior results, at the individual level, in a loss of courtship readiness and rapport and, at the social level, in a loss of group cohesion.

Other types of reciprocals, those of dominance and submission, indicate status. A dominant male may place his hands on his hips, scowl, or place the palms of his hands behind his neck. A dominant female may steeple her fingers. The person in the submissive position will usually "reciprocate" by lowering his or her head. It is important for a nurse who is working with a submissive client to avoid assuming a dominant role either verbally or kinesically. By being aware of reciprocals of dominance and submission, the nurse can be more attuned to patterns of dominance and submission in the nurse-client relationship.

Unlike reciprocals, *territorials* frame an interaction and define a territory. When people want to pass through or intrude on other people's territories, certain behavior patterns are displayed. The intruders will bow their heads, curl their shoulders inward so that their chests do not protrude, keep their arms at their sides and look downward. In addition, they may mumble a "pardon me."

A nurse noticed that whenever Mrs. Bowens walked past the library section of the sitting room, she looked downward and curled her shoulders inward. The nurse mistakenly assumed that Mrs. Bowen was intimidated by Mr. Jackson, who usually spent his free time in the library. After discussing the situation with another nurse, who was more knowledgeable about kinesics, the first nurse recognized that, since Mr. Jackson had staked out the library section as his territory, Mrs. Bowen was displaying normal behavior for passing through or intruding on another's territory.

We have seen how kinesic signals help interacting participants recognize what is happening. We will now explore the regulatory nature of kinesics.

REGULATORY NATURE OF KINESICS

Nonverbal behavior, especially kinesic behavior, serves to regulate the pace of a relationship and to monitor deviant behavior. Regulatory behavior occurs many times during an interaction. When deviance appears, a new pattern of behavior may emerge to monitor the deviant behavior; it will continue until the deviant behavior ceases.

A nurse-therapist had received a family's permission to videotape its family therapy session. After the session, the nurse studied the videotape and tried to identify group dynamics. She noticed that every time the husband-father leaned in to speak to her, he would lower his voice. This excluded the rest of the family from the interaction. The wife-mother and two daughters would then cross their legs and rub their noses. At the appearance of this behavior, the husband-father would lean back in his chair and raise his voice, so that the rest of the family could hear what he was saying. By interrupting any alliance with the nurse that excluded other family members, the wife-mother and the two daughters were monitoring the husband-father's behavior.

Thus we see how monitoring gestures and signals can occur synchronously among members of a group and can serve to check deviant behavior.

Whenever we try to interpret the meaning of kinesic behavior, we have to look beyond the individual or the group to the interrelationship between behavior and context. This is what is meant by a systems approach to understanding behavior.

Kinesic behavior is learned and passed on from generation to generation. Scheflen and Scheflen (1972) point out that the nuclear family or household is the first group to which a person belongs. It is here that most kinesic behavior is learned. Family or household members function interdependently to obtain food, affection, status, and self-esteem. Should a member deviate from culturally defined behavior, some of these ministrations can be withheld as a sanction. Therefore, at one and the same time, family interactions physically sustain a young child while servicing social bonds and teaching culturally approved values and behavior.

As individuals grow to maturity, they belong to other groups and expand their social networks. In each of these groups, they play specific roles. Should they deviate from expected role behavior, metacommunications occur that serve to discipline and reindoctrinate them or to keep them out of the mainstream of society. Bateson (1955) defines *metacommunication* as communication that tells how verbal communication should be interpreted.

A community health nurse was visiting with a woman who was the mother of a toddler and an infant. The nurse was discussing sibling rivalry with the mother. The toddler was sitting at the kitchen table eating cookies and drinking milk. As the toddler reached for a cookie, he knocked over the glass of milk. The mother jumped up and said sweetly, "Don't worry, Johnny—accidents will happen." However, from the frown on her face and her brusque behavior in cleaning off Johnny's wet clothes, both the community health nurse and Johnny were very aware that the mother was annoyed with Johnny's behavior.

The behavior that communicated the message of annoyance contradicted the verbal message; it indicated how the verbal message should be taken. This is the function of metacommunication. It can support or contradict verbal communication and thereby reinforce the values, behavior, and standards of society. Interactions continue in their customary manner, and unusual experience and information are kept to a minimum.

Taken together, metacommunication, marking, and territorial and reciprocal behavior serve to clarify ambiguous communication, signal deviance in an interaction, and bring about a return to conventional behavior. It is primarily through this regulatory function of kinesics that social order is maintained.

CULTURAL INFLUENCES ON KINESIC BEHAVIOR

Communication specialists like Birdwhistle (1952, 1970) and Scheflen and Scheflen (1972) believe that kinesic behavior is culturally variable. Ruesch and Kees (1969) agree with this view and have postulated that body movements are a function of their cultural context. Ruesch and Kees argue that climate, population density, mode of subsistence (for example, agricultural versus industrial economy), availability of raw materials, and historical heritage all influence the cultural specificity of body movements.

Some researchers have identified culturally specific body movements. For example, considerable time has been spent exploring the culturally specific form and meaning of eye movements. Ashcraft and Scheflen (1976) have found that while most British-Americans seek eye contact as a means of establishing affiliation and rapport, West Indians and Afro-Americans usually avoid direct eye contact, for such behavior invites the escalation of hostility. British-Americans often misinterpret the black American's avoidance of eye contact as being indicative or submissiveness or of having something to hide. Black Americans often misinterpret British-American eye contact as either a put-down or a confrontation. Hispanic women tend to hold eye contact slightly longer than women from other ethnic groups, and this behavior is often interpreted by non-Hispanic people as seductive.

Hall (1966) has found that even in the "British-American world" eye contact differs. The British tend to blink their eyes to show they are listening and understanding conversation, while Americans, who have conventions against staring, do not look directly into people's eyes. Instead, Americans indicate attentiveness by nodding and making listening noises. While an American's gaze wanders over the face and sometimes off the face, an Englishman's gaze is fixed on the eyes.

Needless to say, the cultural variability of the form and meaning of eye movements can result in many misunderstandings.

A young Hispanic nurse was assigned as primary nurse to an Irish-American male client. The client had been hospitalized for treatment of a myocardial infarct. The nurse spent much time listening to the man's fears, explaining his diet to him, and helping him to establish a prescribed exercise program. Because the young man was unaccustomed to women maintaining prolonged eye contact except when inviting or involved in intimate encounters, he interpreted the nurse's slightly prolonged eye holding as seductive behavior. He responded by inviting her out for a date. To the nurse, whose behavior was customary for someone from her Hispanic culture, the client's behavior was unwarranted. She could not see why this young man had acted as he had. In talking the situation over with a nurse-anthropologist, she was able to identify the kinesic behavior that had resulted in the misunderstanding. Once she understood the cultural dynamics of the situation, she was able to explain to the client that she was not trying to establish a social relationship and to point out why he might have thought that she was. The confusion was resolved, tension between them was lessened, and a more therapeutic relationship was established.

Misinterpretation of the culturally specific form and meaning of another's kinesic behavior can cause misunderstandings and produce barriers to communication. And without effective communication a therapeutic relationship cannot be established.

The cultural specificity of kinesic behavior is also revealed in the form and meaning of gestures. Scheflen and Scheflen (1972) have noted that British-Americans tend to gesticulate less frequently than persons from Mediterranean countries and Eastern European Jews. When British-Americans do gesticulate, they usually keep their forearms in fixed positions and move either or both hands from the wrist in a circle approximately 6 inches in diameter.

Effron (1942) found that, in a day-to-day communications, Italians tend to use their hands, faces, arms, and shoulders to emphasize and illustrate their words. Gestures can become so flamboyant that Italians need approximately an arm's length of lateral space in order to avoid striking things with their sweeping arms. Eastern European Jews tend to use motions to ''support'' words. Instead of the sweeping arm movement of Italians, which starts at the shoulder and involves the entire arm, they tend to hold the upper arm close to the body and use only the lower arm to gesture. Eastern European Jews usually stand within touching range as they converse. They are able to poke, pull, and push as they embellish, punctuate, and accent their conversations.

Scheflen and Scheflen (1972) observed that black Americans tend to gesticulate much like British-Americans but that working-class blacks often use more gestures than middle-class blacks. Black Americans generally gesticulate with the index finger and also display their palms more frequently than do British-Americans.

One might wonder of what import this knowledge of the cultural specificity of gestures is to nursing. We will look at two examples.

Ms. Galiano, a nursing instructor, was a second-generation Italian-American. After several years of teaching, she found herself becoming increasingly tense during clinical seminars. One day, she sat down and tried to identify the dynamics of the situation. Everything was similar to previous semesters with one exception: this semester her clinical group was sitting in a tight circle with barely 6 inches of space between the chairs. Ms. Galiano suddenly realized what was happening. Her clinical group was composed of British-American students and Eastern European Jewish students, none of whom needed lateral space for body movements. Ms. Galiano, however, used the gesticulatory behavior common to her ethnic group. In order to kinesically communicate, she needed lateral space. Without such space, her body language was being stifled. As a result, she was becoming tense. She explained the dynamics of the situation to the group. They spread open their circle and allowed Ms. Galiano the space she needed to gesticulate. The problem was solved. Both students and teacher had received a first-hand lesson in the role of kinesic behavior in the process of communication.

Ms. Thompson, a 60-year-old British-American, had been admitted to a psychiatric hospital. A student nurse established a one-to-one relationship with her. The student became concerned about Ms. Thompson's lack of body movement during their interactions. He told his instructor: "Either Ms. Thompson is scared to death of me or she's catatonic. She never moves." His instructor helped the student to look at the dynamics of the interaction. The student was of Eastern European Jewish extraction and used much gesturing and touching during conversation. Ms. Thompson was British-American and accustomed to little gesturing. Her behavior was neither rooted in fear nor pathological. It was completely normal for someone of her ethnic background.

Postures and gestures thus can have various causes and various meanings. Form and meaning are influenced by cultural context. Probably because culturally specific behavior is unconscious and not formally learned, it is one of the last types of behavior to be acculturated. As a result, when people of different ethnic backgrounds interact, misinterpretation of behavior may cause misunderstandings.

Body language, then, like speech, is very much a part of any communication system. Kinesic behavior communicates needs, feelings, and intentions that are universal, but the form and meaning of body movements are culturally specific. In looking at the communicational value of kinesic behavior, we have seen the importance of understanding the interrelationship between kinesic behavior and its context. We will now explore another level of human communication: proxemics.

Proxemics

The proxemic level of communication—the use of space—has only recently become an area for study. Hall (1966) was a pioneer in proxemic research. Scheflen and Ashcraft (1976) see space as neither thing-defined nor people-defined. They refer to bounded space as territory that is framed and used by people but that does not consist of people. Instead, it surrounds people or exists between them. It is defined by a relationship or pattern of behavior and movement. Therefore, a ''territory'' is more than just a space. It is a space that has been claimed by a person through body language and the claim has been acknowledged by others. People claim space either through the direction in which they orient their bodies or by the way they project their gazes or voices. Even though claims may be of a temporary nature, once a space has been claimed and the claim has been acknowledged, a territory has been established.

Mr. Jefferson was recovering from abdominal surgery. He spent a great deal of time in bed watching television. The television set was located on a shelf on the wall opposite his bed. Any time that a nurse came in to care for the person in the next bed, he or she had to walk through the space between Mr. Jefferson's bed and the television set. Each time that the nurse did this, if Mr. Jefferson was watching television, the nurse said, "Excuse me." By orienting his body and his gaze toward the television set, Mr. Jefferson had claimed this territory, and the behavior of the nurse acknowledged the claim.

Proxemics, as a legitimate area of research, grew out of studies of animal territoriality. Once it was recognized that animals organize space, it was a short step to the realization that human beings also organize space.

Animal behavioralists (Wynne-Edwards, 1962; Lorenz, 1966; McBride, 1964; Goodall, 1967) have observed that each animal species occupies a life-supporting ecological niche. Within each niche, groups mark off territorial boundaries that keep their members inside the territory and intruders out. Within their territorial boundaries, the members of the animal group are able to maintain visual, auditory, or olfactory communication. This communication can be maintained on a prolonged basis or only during the mating season, depending on the species.

Many animal behavioralists have studied distance regulation among animals. Hediger (1950, 1955, 1961) identified three types of distance: flight distance, personal distance, and social distance. Flight distance is the distance that a wild animal will tolerate between itself and an enemy before fleeing. Usually, the larger the animal the greater the distance it keeps between itself and a predator. For example, while an antelope has a flight distance of 500 yards, a lizard's flight distance is only 6 feet. Personal distance is the normal spacing maintained between animals of the same species. Dominant animals tend to have larger personal spaces than subordinate animals. Moreover, subordinate animals tend to yield personal space to dominant animals. Therefore, spacing often reflects social organization. Social distance, the third type of distance, is found only among social animals. It is the maximal distance that an animal will travel from the group before the animal begins to feel either psychologically threatened or physically and socially isolated (unable to maintain visual, auditory, or olfactory contact with the group). Social distance serves to contain a group of animals; it varies from species to species.

Christian (1960), Calhoun (1962), and Southwick (1964) have found that during prolonged overcrowding of animals, dominance hierarchies break down, territorial boundaries are violated, and a stress syndrome develops. The stress syndrome includes elevated eosinophil counts, adrenocortical hyperactivity, and enlarged adrenal glands. If left unchecked, the syndrome can result in the death of the animals.

PROPERTIES OF HUMAN SPACING

Now that we have looked at some studies of spacing in animal behavior, we will note some properties of human spacing. Scheflen and Ashcraft (1976) have been pioneers in the examination of the properties of space. By studying territories of orientation, these researchers have shown how we can better understand the ways in which human beings organize space.

Scheflen and Ashcraft use the term *point behaviors* to refer to the way in which body parts move within a space and orient themselves in some direction. For example, the gaze of an instructor's eyes may be directed toward a student in order to warn, reprimand, or focus attention upon the student. A nurse's head may be cocked so that it can be oriented toward a client. The small space that becomes the object and extension of point behavior is called a "spot."

Positional behaviors involve four body regions: head-neck, upper torso, pelvis-thighs, and lower legs–feet. These regions may be oriented in the same direction or in different directions. When saying a fast "hello" to classmates, a student may orient head, chest, and arms toward the class mates while orienting the lower part of the body in the direction in which he or she is walking. When a single body region or a cluster of body regions is pointed in a specific direction, it claims a space beyond that occupied by the body region. People usually avoid looking into or walking through this space. It is through such acknowledgment that a space is claimed and a territory established.

Besides being organized by identifying spatial orientations, space can also be organized by degree of affiliation. In Scheflen and Ashcraft's terminology, people who are affiliated ("with" one another) share *"with" space*. In "with" spaces, participants use body parts and regions to show that they are affiliated and that they share a similar spatial orientation. For example, a nurse and a client may, during the course of their interaction, assume congruent body positions or mirror-image stances ("book-ending") and thereby define a common focus of attention. In addition, people show they are affiliated by leaning toward each other, forming links through touching, and using arms and legs to demarcate spatial boundaries.

In *"non-with" spaces,* participants use body parts and regions to show that they have different spatial orientations and that they are unaffiliated with one another. For example, during a nurse-client interaction, the nurse and the client may assume stances that show that they are affiliated but may position their extremities to form a barrier between themselves and others. They are indicating that they are temporarily unaffiliated with the others.

So far we have looked at how body parts and regions define spatial orientation and organization. However, body parts and regions belong to and are part of the total body. When looking at the orientation of the total body in space, we are describing relationships. People may commit all or only part of their bodies to an interaction. We will now look at patterns of low commitment and patterns of high commitment.

While *low-commitment configurations* may result in the dissolution of a relationship, *high-commitment configurations* reinforce a relationship. Low-commitment configurations are characterized by the involvement of only one body part, the positioning of a body region so that a person is only partially oriented toward the focus, the maintenance of maximal interpersonal distance, the crossing of extremities, or the covering or immobilization of body regions so that body movements are minimal. High-commitment configurations are characterized by the involvement of several body regions, the positioning of body regions toward the focus of orientation, the maintenance of minimal interpersonal distance, the uncrossing of extremities, and the display of mutual point and positional behavior. In the following hypothetical situation, patterns of both high and low commitment affect an interaction.

Ms. Zender, a student nurse, was sitting outdoors with her client, Mr. Morrow. They were seated on chairs and facing each other. Each was leaning forward as they talked. After about 20 minutes, Ms. Zender gazed over at a softball game that was being played nearby. Within minutes, not only was she looking at the game but her head and upper torso were turned away from Mr. Morrow and toward the softball field. A silence fell between nurse and client. Five minutes later, Mr. Morrow said he had nothing more to say. He got up and left. Ms. Zender was frustrated and confused. She told her nursing instructor that the interaction had been going "so well and then suddenly Mr. Morrow got up and left." The instructor had been sitting outside and had observed the changing behavioral configurations. In the beginning of the interaction, both Ms. Zender and Mr. Morrow were engaged in high-commitment configurations. When Ms. Zender turned her gaze and her body toward the softball game, she changed her spatial orientation and assumed a low-commitment configuration. From that point on, the interaction deteriorated. Once the student became aware of her behavior, she stopped blaming Mr. Morrow for interrupting the interaction and recognized how her own spatial orientation had affected the interaction.

Spatial orientations and relations do not exist in isolation. They are formed by people who cluster together at a given time. Scheflen and Ashcraft (1976) use the term *formations* to refer to these clusters of people and the term *sites* to refer to the spaces these formations define and occupy.

One type of site, a solo site, is the space occupied when a person is alone or with very few other people. The size of a solo site is determined by such factors as ethnicity, age, affiliation, role, activity, social class, and sex. Scheflen and Ashcraft (1976) have found that a British-American or Afro-American man, when standing and conversing with acquaintances, usually occupies a site of approximately 1 square yard. Since persons from the Mediterranean area and from Eastern Europe are inclined to stand closer together, each person's site tends to be smaller than the site occupied by a British-American or a black American. Latin Americans stand even closer together than Mediterraneans. Since Cubans stand only about 18 inches apart when conversing, their sites tend to be even smaller than those of Mediterraneans or Eastern Europeans.

Another type of spacing, unaffiliated rows, is found when strangers sit side by side in a public area (for example, when strangers sit on a park bench). They may try to separate themselves from others by maintaining space around themselves, orienting themselves in different directions, or erecting barriers.

On the other hand, persons who know each other may show affiliation by huddling together and maintaining a distance from others, erecting barriers to separate themselves from others, and orienting themselves toward each other and away from the strangers present.

Obviously, it is important for nurses who work with clients of various ages, social classes, and ethnic backgrounds to recognize how these variables influence the way people occupy and use space and show affiliation.

A nurse was explaining hospital visiting regulations to a Cuban visitor. Both nurse and client were standing in a face-to-face formation. The nurse, who was British-American, suddenly began feeling very uncomfortable. She started moving around, side-stepping, and taking occasional steps backward. Every time she moved, the visitor would take a step toward her. Each person was doing a "distance dance." The British-American nurse was trying to maintain slightly more than an arm's length of space between herself and her client. The Cuban client was trying to maintain a much smaller (approximately half an arm's length) interpersonal space. Each was trying to establish and maintain the interpersonal distance that was common to his or her ethnic background, and each was confused by the distancing maneuvers of the other. Had the nurse been aware of what was occurring, she might have felt less uncomfortable and she might have been able to use her energy to interact more effectively with her client. Unfortunately, she did not have this awareness. Because she felt uneasy, she terminated the interaction prematurely.

Up to now, we have been focusing on relationships. Scheflen and Ashcraft (1976) have shown that another way to examine the properties of space is to look at the characteristics of fixed spaces and built spaces. Because it sets a focus of orientation, provides a place in which to interact, and defines what is going to happen, furniture establishes *fixed spaces*. For instance, wheeling a medicine cart into a hospital room, building a nurses' station in the center of a hospital unit, or placing a television set in the sitting room of a day hospital sets a focus and defines the type of activity that is going to occur.

Built spaces are bounded by such physical structures as curbs, walls, and fences. Areas may be marked off by lines or low barriers across which people can see and interact, or they may be marked off by walls through which participants cannot see one another. The latter type of built space obviously provides a greater degree of privacy.

The use of fixed and built spaces has many implications for nurses. Sommer (1969) observed that in a certain state psychiatric hospital all chairs were arranged in straight lines against walls. Although people sat side by side, rarely in the course of a day did they engage in more than two brief conversations. Sommer hypothesized that conversation was inhibited by the fact that clients had to turn their heads at a 90-degree angle in order to talk to persons sitting alongside. As a result, clients usually sat quietly, staring at the floor or ceiling. Sommer wondered why the chairs were arranged side by side and arrived at the following answers:

1. The arrangement made it easier to clean the room.

2. It was easier for nurses to supervise the unit.
3. The arrangement was a function of ''institutional sanctity.'' Since the furniture had always been arranged that way, it had become a fixed routine.

Rather than the environment being arranged to meet the needs of the people inhabiting it, the people had been arranged to fit the environment. Sommer received permission to rearrange the furniture. He began by placing chairs around square tables. He chose square tables because the boundaries of a square table can be determined and demarcated more easily than those of a round table. Shortly after the furniture was rearranged, client interactions increased in both number and duration.

We have seen how built and fixed spaces, point behavior, and positional behavior occur within some larger pattern of behavior. Types of behavior are hierarchically arranged and occur within a broad context that is both temporally and spatially defined. Now we will look at the way culture influences the meaning, ordering, and use of space.

CULTURE AND PROXEMICS

The organizational, social, and symbolic meaning and use of space have been explored by archeologists, social anthropologists, psychologists, geographers, and ethnographers.

Hall (1966) has looked at people's perception of space. He sees people as surrounded by expanding and contracting perceptual fields that at all times provide them with information. He believes that people interact in four spatial zones: intimate, personal, social, and public.

The *intimate zone* is the zone of physical contact. It is the area within 18 inches of the body. This is the zone of lovemaking and comforting. Sight is often blurred or distorted. The perception of odors, heat, and breath from another's body is heightened. The voice, if used, is kept to a whisper. Americans feel uncomfortable if forced into the intimate zones of strangers. For instance, when crowded onto an elevator, Americans respond by becoming immobile, holding their arms at their sides, fixing their eye on some spot, and tensing their bodies. Many nurses have experienced this same response when comforting clients with whom they have not established rapport, trust, and confidence.

The *personal zone* comprises the area 18 inches to 4 feet from the body. This area is sometimes visualized as a "bubble" that a person keeps between self and others. The bubble expands and contracts according to circumstances. At a small personal distance, one can hold and touch another person. At a great personal distance, one is just within reach when both parties extend their arms. Vision is not distorted, as it is in the intimate zone. In fact, a person is able to see the texture of the hair, the pores in the skin, and the three-dimensional qualities of objects. The breath and body heat of another person are imperceptible, and the voice level is moderate. During a nurse-client interaction, participants usually maintain personal distance.

Social distance is approximately 4 to 12 feet. At this distance people cannot touch one another. This is the distance at which most business is conducted; it is also the distance maintained by student and teacher during a classroom lecture.

Public distance, 12 to 25 feet or more, separates public figures from the public. It is used in formal situations. Fine details of the other person are lost, as is the three-dimensional quality of the body. This is the distance maintained between student and lecturer in a large lecture hall.

These zones of interaction are neither static nor absolute. They are related to the way people organize their senses, a process that is culturally determined. What is considered intimate distance in one society may be considered personal or public distance in another society.

Although there are areas of cultural similarity among societies of the Western world, there are also many areas of cultural difference. People who are unaware of these differences risk misunderstanding others and being misunderstood. Behavior that differs from that of the dominant culture is usually interpreted as rudeness, ineptness, or apathy. We will now explore some proxemic differences among cultures.

Scheflen and Scheflen (1972) have observed that when people place themselves in a vis-à-vis position for the purpose of communication, the amount of space between them depends on their ethnic background, their degree of intimacy, their previous relationship, the reason they assembled, and the amount of available physical space. Should the people interacting come from different ethnic backgrounds or have different ideas about the purpose and circumstances surrounding the interaction, they will have difficulty agreeing on the distance between them. They might do a "spatial dance" until they arrive at a spatial compromise. For example, Englishmen and British-Americans usually arrange themselves just beyond touching distance, and they touch very little while interacting. Latins and Eastern European Jews tend to position themselves within easy tactile range and to use varying degrees of touching during conversation. A nurse who has been culturally conditioned to use little touching while conversing may be made very uncomfortable by the small interpersonal distance and the use of touching by a client or a colleague, and vice versa.

What is regarded as intrusive behavior in one culture is not necessarily regarded as such in another culture. Ashcraft and Scheflen (1976) point out that while urban Americans and Englishmen try to avoid touching when in crowds and apologize if they do touch, this is not the case in all cultures. Frenchmen often collide with one another without apologizing, and Russians, who often slip on the ice, knocking one another down, usually get up without paying any attention to those they have knocked over. Moreover, Hall (1966) notes that while Germans become very upset by people who break into line ahead of them, Poles see nothing intrusive about crashing queues.

The definition of intrusive behavior* is also influenced by social class. Ashcraft and Scheflen

---

*Refer to Chapter 9 for a discussion of privacy and intrusive behavior.

(1976) have noted significant differences in the way members of the middle and lower classes define intrusiveness. Middle-class American family members usually lay claim to specific household chairs. There is mother's chair, and there is father's chair. Children are usually not permitted to sit in these chairs without parental permission or they must vacate them when the parent appears. On the other hand, in a lower-class home, where furniture may be at a premium, there are usually more family members than there are chairs. This shortage of chairs does not afford the luxury of ''owning'' a chair.

Status and previous claim to territory can also influence the definition of intrusiveness. For example, during staff report, nurses or students who are new to a unit might feel uncomfortable because they do not know where to sit. If the newcomers do not wait and see what the customary seating arrangements are, they may sit in another nurse's seat or in the seat ''reserved'' for the head nurse. Inadvertently, they have intruded on other people's spatial claims.

As we have seen, we all have a sense of territoriality that is operative in our daily lives. As we interact with others, we both acknowledge other people's claims to space and expect them to acknowledge our claims. Problems arise when the use of different spacing signals results in ambiguous or disputed claims. When this occurs, we do not realize that a claim has been made and therefore do not respect it.

DEVIANT PROXEMIC BEHAVIOR

We have discussed how the use of space can be misinterpreted by persons of differing backgrounds. However, some people exhibit behavior that is deviant even by the standards of their own ethnic, economic, or regional groups. Such people might touch persons with whom they do not have tactile rights, or they might fail to touch persons with whom they have such rights. They may orient their bodies away from persons with whom they are interacting, or they may stand at distances that are too close even for their own ethnic back-

grounds. Such deviant territorial behavior is called ''distance maneuvering.''

Ashcraft and Scheflen (1976) have advanced several possible explanations of deviant territorial behavior. One is decreased living space. Traditionally, less living space has been available to the poor and to city dwellers than to the wealthy and to suburbanites. Since 1900, the amount of living space has decreased for those living in the American Northeast, without an accompanying decrease in the number of persons in a household. Large apartments have been subdivided into small apartments. New, high-rise apartments have been built smaller than older apartments. Open spaces surrounding dwellings have given way to homes and industrial parks. The change that has taken place is obvious if one simply looks around and counts the number of vacant lots that exist now as compared to 10 to 20 years ago. How many people have the luxury of living on an acre or more of land? Space is indeed at a premium.

As population density has increased, we have developed behavior to try to ensure some modicum of privacy. Such territorial behavior includes not only actions that stake out private areas but also actions that show respect for privacy. Rooms in a house or an apartment are arranged so that a person goes from communal areas to increasingly private areas. The central hallway and the living room are open to guests, but access to the kitchen is usually only by permission. In fact, sometimes the kitchen is even off limits to certain family members. How often is a family member shooed away by a mother so that she may work in ''her'' kitchen? Bedrooms are very private areas. In fact, adolescents often mark this privacy with ''no trespassing'' and ''keep out'' signs. Rooms thereby become a means of ensuring some degree of privacy.

However, crowding can be defined only by looking at the context in which it occurs. For instance, Ashcraft and Scheflen (1976) have observed that children are better able to tolerate sleeping in a crowded bedroom if they can study and play in another room. Ashcraft and Scheflen have also found that crowding is culturally defined. While black Americans and British-Americans tend to disperse throughout the available space in a house, Puerto Ricans tend to cluster in one room. While Italian-Americans, British-Americans, black Americans, and Jewish Americans usually define being ''alone'' as being physically removed from *family members* (they go outside or into another room), Puerto Ricans usually define being alone as being physically separated from *strangers* but being among their families.

In light of such information, nurses need to recognize that the crowded and cramped living conditions of ghetto apartments have conceptually different meanings to people of different ethnic groups. If a nurse suggested to a harried Puerto Rican mother that she try to get some rest and privacy by relaxing in her bedroom away from the noise and activity of family members, the nurse would be imposing his or her concept of privacy on someone whose definition of privacy was very different. The Puerto Rican mother would probably view the idea as strange and unworkable. The nurse, unless aware of the ethnic variation in the definition of privacy, would not even realize that he or she was being ethnocentric. A misunderstanding might result as both nurse and client become frustrated in working toward their goal of decreasing the mother's sense of fatigue and harassment.

Patterns of proxemic communication vary. By looking at these patterns, nurses can discover cultural frames that influence the structure of a person's perception of the world. Since a person's perceptual structuring of the world influences his or her definitions and interpretations of the use and meaning of space, people of differing ethnic backgrounds often misinterpret the meaning of each other's proxemic behavior. Territorial intrusion occurs, and conflicts of varying intensity develop. When we study proxemic communication, we are studying how people of different cultures use their senses to screen perceptual data, admitting some information and filtering out other information. Culture therefore serves as a medium for proxemic communication.

RELATIONSHIPS AMONG LEVELS OF COMMUNICATION

We have heuristically examined all three levels of communication: verbal, kinesic, and proxemic. We will now consider how these levels are interrelated. For years, communication specialists have realized that the process of communication involves more than speech. Until recently, however, they have lacked the tools to study the nonverbal aspects of communication. They therefore have focused their attention on the aspect of communication that they have had the tools to study—the verbal aspect.

Scheflen and Scheflen (1972) explain that as language evolves and attempts are made to clarify and punctuate speech, specific body motions such as gestures, posturing, and spacing behavior begin to be used. Interactions thus come to involve the interpretation of kinesic and proxemic behavior, both as autonomous means of communication and as mechanisms integrated with speech.

The investigation of the relationships between various levels of communication probably owes its inception to the collaborative efforts of Traeger, Smith, Hall, and Birdwhistle. Fromm-Reichman later joined them. Research commenced on kinesics, proxemics, and metalinguistics. The process of communication was defined as including three coexisting levels: verbal, kinesic, and proxemic.

Out of this early research, interest was stimulated in communication as a system of interrelated levels. Birdwhistle (1972) recalls that ''circum-speech'' behavior was identified. Circum-speech includes such behavior characteristics of conversation as instrumentals, interactional behavior, markers, demonstratives, and stress kinesics. Instrumentals are such task-oriented movements as walking, smoking, eating, and knitting. People often carry on these activities while they are speaking. Interactional behavior is found in both verbal and nonverbal interactions. It includes shifts or movements of all or part of the body that increase, decrease, or maintain space between interacting individuals. Remember the ''spatial dance'' that people do when trying to adjust the distance between them? Markers are body movements that illustrate ambiguous words. For example, hand sweeps that indicate direction and accompany such phrases as ''here'' or ''there'' and head nods that clarify pronominal references are all markers. Demonstratives, like gestural mapping, are actions that accompany and illustrate speech. When people indicate with their hands that a toddler has grown ''this tall'' or that a melon is ''this big,'' they are using demonstratives. The term stress kinesics refers to movements of the hand, head, or eyebrow that serve to mark the flow of speech; these movements generally coincide with linguistic stress patterns. When students raise their eyebrows as well as the pitch of their voices to state in amazement, ''I received an 'A' on my nursing process paper,'' they are using a stress kineme.

Until recent years, we paid little attention to the interrelationship of linguistics, kinesics, and proxemics. Anthropologists, psychologists, and nurses focused almost all of their attention on verbal communication. What people said and how they said it were analyzed extensively. It was not until the 1950s that kinesic behavior became the object of study. Proxemic behavior was not studied until the late 1960s.

CHAPTER SUMMARY

People from different cultures not only speak different languages but also inhabit different sensory worlds. Selective screening of sensory data admits some information and filters out other information. An experience that is perceived through one set of culturally patterned sensory screens is quite different from the same experience perceived through another set. An encounter or interaction is one type of experience. When members of different cultural groups use dissimilar verbal, kinesic, or proxemic cues, assumptions, and orienta-

tions, misunderstandings can occur and role relationships can be disrupted. A sense of nonrelatedness to the members of the other cultural group can develop. Culturally influenced and acceptable behavior that is different from that of the dominant culture can be mistaken for deviant or pathological behavior.

REFERENCES

Ashcraft, N., and A. Scheflen
1976 People Space: The Making and Breaking of Human Boundaries. New York: Anchor Press.

Bateson, G.
1955 ''The message, 'This is play.' '' In Group Processes. B. Schaffner (ed.). Madison, N.J.: Madison Printing Co.

Berlin, B., and P. Kay
1969 Basic Color Terms: Their Universality and Evaluation. San Francisco: University of California Press.

Birdwhistle, R.
1952 Introduction to Kinesics. Louisville, Ky.: University of Louisville Press.
1963 Some Relationships Between American Kinesics and Spoken American English. Paper presented at the annual meeting of the American Association for the Advancement of Science.
1970 Kinesics and Context. Philadelphia: University of Pennsylvania Press.
1972 ''A kinesic-linguistic exercise: the cigarette scene.'' In Directions in Sociolinguistics: The Ethnography of Communication. J.J. Gumperz and D. Hymes (eds.). New York: Holt, Rinehart & Winston, pp. 381-404.

Bloomfield, L.
1933 Language. New York: Holt, Rinehart & Winston.

Calhoun, J.B.
1962 ''Population density and social pathology.'' Scientific American 206:139-146.

Christian, J.J.
1960 ''Factors in mass mortality of a herd of sika deer (Cervus Nippon).'' Chesapeake Science 1:79-95.

Eastman, C.M.
1975 Aspects of Language and Culture. San Francisco: Chandler and Sharp, Publishers, Inc.

Effron, D.
1942 Gesture and Environment. New York: King's Crown Press.

Eidheim, H.
1969 ''When ethnic identity is a social stigma.'' In Ethnic Groups and Boundaries. F. Barth (ed.). Boston: Little, Brown & Co.

Ervin-Tripp, S.M.
1977 "Language and thought." In Horizons of Anthropology, S. Tax and L.G. Freeman (eds.). Chicago: Aldine Publishing Co.

Fishman, J.A.
1960 "A systematization of the Whorfian hypothesis." Behavioral Science 5:323-339.
1968 Readings in the Sociology of Language. The Hague: Mouton.
1971 Sociolinguistics: A Brief Introduction. Boston: Newbury House Publishers.

Gesell, A., and G. Amatura
1946 The Embryology of Behavior. New York: Harper & Row, Publishers, Inc.

Gleason, H.A., Jr.
1961 An Introduction to Descriptive Linguistics. New York: Holt, Rinehart & Winston.

Goodall, J.
1967 The wild Chimpanzee. Washington, D.C.: National Geographic Society.

Gumperz, J.J., and D. Hymes
1972 Directions in Sociolinguistics: The Ethnography of Communication. New York: Holt, Rinehart & Winston.

Hall, E.T.
1966 The Hidden Dimension. Garden City, N.Y.: Doubleday & Co., Inc.

Halliday, M.A.K.
1976 "Anti-languages." American Anthropologist 78:570-584.

Hediger, H.
1950 Wild Animals in Captivity. London: Butterworth & Co.
1955 Studies of the Psychology and Behavior of Captive Animals in Zoos and Circuses. London: Butterworth & Co.
1961 "The evolution of territorial behavior." In Social Life of Early Man. S.L. Washington (ed.). New York: Viking Fund Publications in Anthropology, No. 31.

Hymes, D.
1972 "Models of the interaction of language and social life." In Directions in Sociolinguistics: The Ethnography of Communication. J.J. Gumperz and D. Hymes (eds.). New York: Holt, Rinehart & Winston.

Jespersen, O.
1967 "Causes of change." In Classics in Linguistics. D.E. Hayden, E.P. Alorth, and G. Tate (eds.). New York: Philosophical Library, Inc.

Lee, D.
1959 Freedom and Culture. Englewood Cliffs, N.J.: Prentice-Hall, Inc.

Lorenz, K.
1966 On Aggression. M. Wilson (trans.). New York: Harcourt, Brace & World, Inc.

Lucy, J.A., and R.A. Shweder
1979 "Whorf & his critics: linguistic and nonlinguistic influences on color memory." American Anthropologist 81:581-615.

McBride, G.
1964 A General Theory of Social Organization and Behavior. St. Lucia, Australia: University of Queensland Press.

Mehrabian, A.
1969 "Significance of posture and position in the communication of attitudes and status relationships." Psychological Bulletin 71(5):359-372.
1972 Nonverbal Communication. Chicago: Aldine-Atherton.

Ruesch, J., and G. Bateson
1968 Communication, The Matrix of Psychiatry. New York: W.W. Norton & Co., Inc.

Ruesch, J., and W. Kees
1969 Nonverbal Communication. Berkeley: University of California Press.

Sapir, E.
1964 "Conceptual categories in primitive languages." In Language in Culture and Society: A Reader in Linguistics and Anthropology. D. Hymes (ed.). New York: Harper & Row, Publishers, Inc.

Scheflen, A.E.
1965 "Quasi-courtship behavior in psychotherapy." Psychiatry: Journal For Study of Interpersonal Processes 28: 245-257.

Scheflen, A.E., and N. Ashcraft
1976 Human Territories: How We Behave in Space-Time. Englewood Cliffs, N.J.: Prentice-Hall, Inc.

Scheflen, A.E., and A. Scheflen
1972 Body Language and Social Order: Communication as Behavior Control. Englewood Cliffs, N.J.: Prentice-Hall, Inc.

Sommer, R.
1969 Personal Space. Englewood Cliffs, N.J.: Prentice-Hall, Inc.

Southwick, C.
1964 "An interesting subject for studies of socially induced stress responses." Science 43:55-56.

Traeger, G.L.
1964 "Paralanguage: a first approximation." In Language in Culture and Society: A Reader in Lingustic Anthropology. D. Hymes (ed.). New York: Harper & Row, Publishers, Inc.

Whorf, B. Lee
1956 "Language, thought and reality." In Selected Readings of Benjamin Lee Whorf. J.B. Carroll (ed.). New York: John Wiley and Sons, Inc.

Wynne-Edwards, J.C.
1962 Animal Dispersion in Relation to Social Behavior. New York: Hafner.

ANNOTATED SUGGESTED READINGS

Ruesch, J., and G. Bateson
　1968 Communication, The Social Matrix Of Psychiatry. New York: W.W. Norton & Co., Inc.
　　Ruesch and Bateson develop a theory of human communication that includes social context, networks (intrapersonal, interpersonal, group, and cultural), technical characteristics (coding and informational state), interaction, and self-correction. Communication is viewed as a system, and the interrelationship between communication, mental illness, and psychiatric intervention is discussed.

Sheflen, A.E., and A. Sheflen
　1972 Body Language and Social Order. Englewood Cliffs, N.J.: Prentice-Hall, Inc.
　　Scheflen and Scheflen examine kinesic behavior within the contexts of verbal communication, group processes, ethnicity, and social order. The book is divided into four sections: the fundamentals of kinesics, the regulatory nature of kinesics, communication in institutional and political control, and communication in the creation of deviance. Photographs are used to illustrate examples of kinesic behavior.

Scheflen, A.E., and N. Ashcraft
　1976 Human Territories: How We Behave in Space-Time. Englewood Cliffs, N.J.: Prentice-Hall, Inc.
　　The authors explore human territoriality within a context of space-time and show how territorial behavior is integrated into ever-enlarging contextual units. The book is divided into five parts: teritories of orientation, formations and sites, built territories, use of territorial forms, and territorial disturbance. A photographic format is used to illustrate the dimensions of human territoriality.

FURTHER READINGS

Boucher, M.L.
1971 "Personal space and chronicity in the mental hospital." Perspectives in Psychiatric Care 9:206-210.

Condon, W.W., and W.D. Osgood
1966 "Sound-film analyses of normal and pathological behavior patterns." Journal of Nervous and Mental Disorders 143:338-347.

Ekman, P., and W. Friesen
1972 "Constants across cultures in the face and emotion." Journal of Personality and Social Psychology 17:124-129.

Ekman, P., et al.
1969 "Pancultural elements in facial displays of emotion." Science 164:86-88.

Gerber, C.B., and D.F. Snyder
1970 "Language and thought." Perspectives in Psychiatric Care 8:230-237.

Newman, O.
1972 Defensible Space. New York: Macmillan, Inc.

Sarles, H.B.
1970 "Communication and ethology." In Anthropology and the Behavioral and Health Sciences. O. von Mering and L. Kasdan (eds.). Pittsburgh: University of Pittsburgh Press.

Scheflen, A.E.
1964 "The significance of posture in communication systems." Psychiatry 27:316-331.

CHAPTER 9

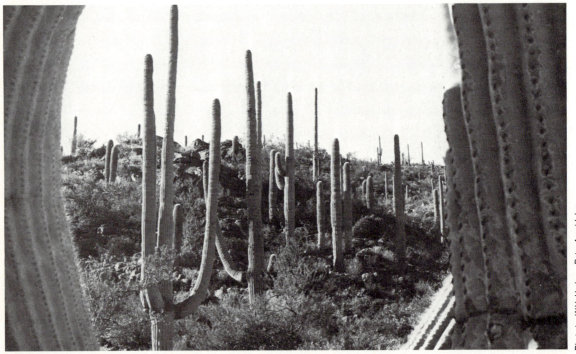

Photo by W.H. Hodge—Peter Arnold, Inc.

Therapeutic communication and the nursing process

CHAPTER FOCUS

The nursing process is the framework for nursing practice. Nurses and clients explore client experiences, nurses sustain clients in those experiences, and nurses communicate their assessments, plans, and evaluations to other health team members. The focus of therapeutic communication is the client's here-and-now experience. The task of the nurse is to sustain the client in that experience. The cultural backgrounds of nurses and clients influence their perceptions and interpretations of experiences, their responses to experiences, and their responses to communication cues. In addition, behavioral concepts relating to sexuality, privacy, humor, empathy, and touching figure prominently in the nurse-client relationship and in the ability of nurses to sustain clients.

THE NURSE-CLIENT RELATIONSHIP

Nurse and client as components of the relationship

Client and nurse bring the five dimensions of the self (biological, intellectual, psychological, sociocultural, and spiritual) to the therapeutic relationship. Together, client and nurse explore what the client is presently experiencing that is of import or concern to the client.

The elements of any experience are perception, interpretation, and response. The way people view

an event or a situation and the meaning it has for them affect the way in which they react. Many factors may influence one's perception, interpretation, and, ultimately, one's response to an event (Ujhely, 1968). These factors may be categorized as follows:

Biophysical factors

1. Organs or systems involved or affected by the event or situation
2. Degree of involvement: partial or total
3. Nature of onset: sudden or gradual; age at onset
4. Duration of involvement: short-term or long-term

Psychosocial factors

1. Past experience with similar events or situations

2. Values, attitudes,* and beliefs (influenced by religion, social class, ethnicity, and acculturation)
3. Present emotional state
4. Habitual ways of coping and problem-solving
5. Personality traits, such as rigidity, flexibility, introversion, extroversion
6. Situational factors, such as sick leave, insurance benefits, and supportive social networks

The influence that any given factor or combination of factors has on one's perception, interpretation, and response varies not only from situation to situation but also from person to person. Thus, a symptom such as occasional chest pain may be experienced differently by different people.

Client A, a 50-year-old Hispanic man, immigrated to the United States 10 years ago. He is married, and he has a 15-year-old son and a 10-year-old daughter. Although he understands English, client A speaks only Spanish at home. For the past 5 years, he has worked as a factory piece-worker. When he does not work, client A does not get paid. He has no health insurance.

Although client A knows that his father died in middle age, he does not know the cause of his father's death. When client A began experiencing chest pain, he initially ignored it. When the pain persisted, he consulted an espiritista (a Puerto Rican native healer) and he also prayed and did "good works." When client A finally decided to consult a physician, he sought a middle-aged, Hispanic doctor who spoke Spanish.

Client B is a 59-year-old second-generation Hispanic-American. He is married, and he has two married children. Although client B knows Spanish, he speaks English at home. For the past 10 years, he has been employed as a dairy manager in a supermarket. Client B belongs to a union whose benefits include 10 days of sick leave and health insurance.

At the age of 60, client B's father died from "heart trouble." When client B began experiencing

---

occasional chest pain, he was certain that he was developing the same type of heart trouble that had killed his father. Client B went to his family doctor, an American "who doesn't rush you in and out. Who spends time with you. Who asks about the family, and who isn't prejudiced against Spanish people."

Client C is a 37-year-old third-generation Hispanic-American. He is married, and he has a 10-year-old daughter and a 7-year-old son. Client C understands very little Spanish. English is the only language that he speaks. Client C is a junior executive with a bank. He has 30 days of sick leave, health insurance, and disability insurance that pays his salary if he is unable to work because of serious illness.

There is no history of heart disease in client C's family. Three weeks before his pre-promotion physical examination, he began experiencing occasional chest pain. Client C initially rationalized that the chest pain was "indigestion" and that it was caused by the anxiety he was experiencing about his upcoming promotion. He tried to relax by "unwinding with a few drinks at lunch and at home in the evening." When client C did seek medical attention, he went to "a young American doctor with up-to-date knowledge and the newest in office equipment."

These hypothetical situations illustrate the effects of biophysical and psychosocial factors on the perception and interpretation of an event and the response to it. In these vignettes, such factors as age at onset of chest pain, past experience with people who have experienced chest pain, coping patterns, type of employment, presence or absence of sick benefits, cultural background, and degree of acculturation influenced the frames of reference from which the three clients approached a similar event—occasional chest pain.

Likewise, when nurses and clients approach situations from different frames of reference, their perceptions, interpretations, and responses may differ. Nurses may identify certain client needs as priorities, but clients may not share this view. Also, nurses may have definite expectations about

---

*Refer to Chapter 4 for a discussion of values, beliefs, attitudes, and attitude clarification.

how clients experiencing a particular crisis should respond. If nurses are unaware of the factors that affect the experience, they may react with frustration and anger toward clients whose responses differ from their own.

A client, accompanied by his wife and two daughters, was brought into the emergency room. The client, a 47-year-old man, was having intermittent chest pain and he was experiencing severe anxiety. His family was crying and begging the physician and nurse to "do everything that can be done. Just don't let him die." The nurse felt that the client and his family were "overreacting." A diagnosis had not been made, and the nurse did not believe the client to be in immediate danger of dying. The nurse became annoyed and responded with impatience to both the client and his family.

The nurse was unaware that at the age of 47, both the client's brother and his father had died from heart attacks. To the client and his family, the client's intermittent chest pain was viewed as yet another family member suffering a heart attack that would probably result in death.

Had the nurse been aware of their frame of reference, the response of the client and his family may not have been viewed as an overreaction but as an appropriate response given the circumstances. Instead, because the nurse and the client and family had different frames of reference, the nurse responded with frustration and impatience and was unable to sustain the client and his family in their experience.

To cope with and profit from an experience, one must be able to learn from that experience. Learning is an active process that uses intellectual and perceptual capacities and acquired knowledge to explain events, to engage in problem solving, and to plan and implement change.

Both client and nurse bring intellect, perception, knowledge, and experience to the therapeutic process. Together, they explore the client's perception of events that the client regards as important or as matters of concern. Although occasionally comparisons may be made with past experience or reminiscing may occur, the *focus* is on the here and now—what the individual is presently experiencing. Clients can thus talk about events of concern or importance to them with assurance that only subject matter that they are psychologically able to tackle will be explored. Should the nurse introduce a topic, he or she might inadvertently select one that is traumatic to the client (Ujhely, 1968; Sayre, 1978). Nurses encourage clients to take the initiative in setting the focus by offering such broad opening questions as "What have you been thinking about?" or "What's been going on with you?"

Behavioral concepts and the nurse-client relationship

The *task* of nurses is to sustain clients in their experiences. Sustaining refers to all nursing interventions that are designed to help clients cope with and learn from their experiences (Ujhely, 1968). Attitudes and feelings about sexuality, privacy, humor, empathy, and touching figure prominently in the nurse-client relationship and in the ability of nurses to sustain clients.

SEXUALITY

Since people are sexual beings, the sexuality of nurses and clients may influence the nurse-client relationship in many ways. Feelings and beliefs about sexuality contribute to attitudes about sex. These sexual attitudes in turn may either promote or inhibit therapeutic communication and the ability of nurses to sustain clients in their experiences.

A holistic view of sexuality stresses the following concepts:

1. Human sexuality includes more than the act of intercourse. Sexuality integrates the physical, emotional, intellectual, sociocultural, and spiritual dimensions of human beings. The expression of sexuality enriches personality, communication, and love.
2. Authenticity and effective communication enrich human sexual functioning.

3. Human sexual behavior involves three aspects:
   a. Fantasy—mental images of engaging in sexual behavior alone or with others
   b. Emotion—subjective feelings and sensations that may be manifested by such observable signs as flushing, rapid pulse, and increased respiratory rate
   c. Behavior—sexual activity engaged in alone or with others
4. Sexuality is an integral part of the human condition. It continues throughout life and does not disappear as one ages.*
5. Human sexuality is influenced by a person's sociocultural background, especially by ethnicity, religion, and social class. For example, sociocultural factors may influence a person's conception of what is masculine behavior and what is feminine behavior. This conception often results in sex-role stereotypes. Sociocultural factors may also influence what a person views as appropriate sexual expression and appropriate sex objects.
6. At some point in most people's lives, they experience stress that is related to sexuality (Otto, 1978; Woods, 1979; Whipple and Gick, 1980).

The conceptions, feelings, and values that people have about human sexuality are often reflected in their attitudes about sex. Sexual attitudes include what people regard as "normal" and "abnormal" sexual behavior and how they feel about their own sexuality (Blondis and Jackson, 1982). The following sexual attitude self-assessment guide may help nurses identify some of their own attitudes about sex.

1. What type(s) of sexual activity do I consider "normal" or "abnormal" (for example, fellatio, cunnilingus, fantasy, masturbation)?
2. How frequently should people engage in sexual activity? If people engage in sex more frequently or less frequently than what I con-

sider satisfactory, do I regard them as undersexed or oversexed?
3. At what age is it acceptable for people to start engaging in sexual activity? (Which types of sexual activity?)
4. At what age is it no longer acceptable for people to engage in sexual activity? (Which types?)
5. With whom is it acceptable to engage in sex (for example, self, person of the same sex, person of the opposite sex)?
6. What is the primary purpose of sexual activity (for example, pleasure of self, pleasure of another person, procreation, maintenance of a relationship, establishment of a relationship)?
7. What is the appropriate context for sexual activity (for example, marriage, a meaningful relationship, a casual relationship)?

The feelings and attitudes that people have about sex usually vary over time and may be affected by motivational and situational factors (Blondis and Jackson, 1982).

Jennie Foster, a 65-year-old widow, met Tom Barrister, a 68-year-old widower. Jennie and Tom began going out. Their children were pleased that their parents had found companionship and encouraged the relationship. However, as the relationship between Jennie and Tom matured, their children found it "disgusting" and "embarrassing" to see Jennie and Tom hug and kiss each other. Jennie told a friend, "I would never mention this to my daughter, because she would think I was a dirty old woman, but I find Tom very seductive."

The children of Jennie and Tom felt that it was acceptable and desirable for their parents to share companionship. However, they apparently also felt that sexuality should disappear with age. It is not uncommon in our society for young adults to believe that elderly people should not experience any sexual feelings, let alone engage in sexual ac-

---
*Refer to Chapter 6 for further discussion of human sexuality throughout the life cycle.

tivity. This attitude about the sexuality of aged adults is reflected in the regulations of many nursing homes that prohibit heterosexual cohabitation among residents, including spouses.

An understanding of human sexuality and the development of self-awareness about and comfort with their own sexuality is necessary before nurses can help clients deal with sexual concerns. Nurses are primarily involved with activities of education, counseling, case finding, and referral. For example, when educating and counseling parents about human sexuality, nurses may assist them to foster in their children guilt-free attitudes about sex, thereby helping the children to incorporate their sexuality into their self-systems.

When counseling clients who have suffered disturbances of body image,* nurses may

1. explore client attitudes about their sexuality.
2. explore family relationships, support systems, and religious and ethnic heritages that have influenced client attitudes about sex.
3. explore how altered body image is affecting clients' senses of self as sexual beings as well as their sexual relationships and sexual functioning.

If sexual conflicts and sexual problems (for example, inorgasmia, impotence) are identified that are beyond the nurse's therapeutic expertise, referral should be made to sex therapists or to sex clinics.

When working with clients who are institutionalized for prolonged periods of time (for example, nursing home residents), nurses should try to ensure clients' privacy so that they can fulfill their sexual needs through either self-gratification or other means (this approach has also been suggested by Blondis and Jackson, 1982).

If nurses are uncomfortable with their own body images and sexuality and are unaware of their own attitudes about sex, barriers to therapeutic communication may develop. For example, some nurses may feel embarrassed when discussing sex and they may avoid opportunities for client education and counseling (Whipple and Gick, 1980).

---

*Refer to Chapter 7 for further discussion of body image.

A nurse in an oncology clinic was conducting an intake interview with a woman who 5 months before had had a mastectomy. The nurse was trying to determine how the woman was tolerating chemotherapy and how she was coping with her altered body image. Suddenly the woman began to cry as she told the nurse, "I dread having sex with my husband. The pressure of him leaning on my chest makes me feel like the left side of my chest is caving in, and when he penetrates me, I feel like I'm being torn apart. I even have some vaginal bleeding afterwards." The nurse became flustered and said, "You should discuss this with your gynecologist."

The nurse's comment blocked communication; the client no longer talked about her sexual concerns. The nurse's embarrassment prevented exploration of the client's feelings about herself as a sexual being after her mastectomy. The nurse's embarrassment also prevented client counseling concerning alternative coital positions that might avoid pressure on her chest and the importance of foreplay and nonhormonal vaginal lubricants in counteracting the drying effect of chemotherapy on the vaginal mucosa.

Sometimes the embarrassment that nurses may feel about sex may lead them to misinterpret or fail to understand client behavior.

Geoffrey White was scheduled to have an orchidectomy later in the week. He seemed unconcerned about the surgery and very jovial. He continuously joked about "hoping the doctor would sleep well the night before surgery and would have a steady hand." He also told many jokes about sex, and many of his comments to the nurses contained sexual innuendos. The nurses felt very uncomfortable with Mr. White. They tried to avoid going into his room. When they did have to interact with him, the nurses often were sarcastic or brusque with him.

The nurses' embarrassment about the client's sexual behavior interfered with their understanding of the meaning of his behavior. The nurses did not recognize that through sexual acting out the client was expressing concerns about his scheduled orchidectomy and about his sense of masculinity. Instead of trying to help the client explore his feelings and fears, the nurses' behavior conveyed rejection and disapproval of the client's sexuality.

This does not mean that nurses should not set limits on the sexual acting-out of clients. It is possible to recognize and intervene in the situation underlying sexual acting-out behavior while explaining to the client that it is inappropriate for him to try to place the nurse in the role of sexual partner (Blondis and Jackson, 1982). The nurse may also assess whether the client knows how to relate to a person of the opposite sex in a way other than on an overtly sexual level. If the nurse discovers that the client has difficulty in relating nonsexually with members of the opposite sex, this might be an area to work on during nurse-client interactions. By taking these approaches, the nurse is dealing with the client's sexual acting-out behavior in a therapeutic, nonjudgmental, and nonpunitive manner.

Nurses may be judgmental and punitive about sexual behavior that is different from their own. For example, they may view masturbation or homosexuality as "sinful" or sex-change operations as "unnatural," and they may convey these attitudes verbally and nonverbally to clients.

Judgmental attitudes and punitive behavior present barriers to therapeutic communication. To promote therapeutic communication and to sustain clients in their experiences, nurses need to feel comfortable with their own sexuality. Nurses also need to evaluate the sexual behavior of a client on the basis of its meaning for the client and its appropriateness to the nurse-client relationship. These principles should guide nurses in their interactions with clients, both males and females, heterosexuals and homosexuals.

PRIVACY

The way in which nurse and client define privacy and the types of privacy mechanisms they use may very much affect the nurse-client relationship. Privacy is a culturally specific concept. What is regarded as intrusive behavior by one ethnic group may not be regarded as intrusive behavior by another ethnic group.

A traditional American definition of privacy stresses individualism and the restriction of personal responsibility to the nuclear family (Altman, 1975). However, many first- and second-generation ethnic Americans (for example, Hispanic-Americans, Chinese-Americans, Italian-Americans) tend to be extended-family oriented; their sense of responsibility includes the extended family of real and/or fictive kin* (Goodman and Beman, 1968; Kutsche, 1968; Hsu 1970; Scheflen and Scheflen, 1972; Pasquali, 1982). This difference in orientation toward privacy may lead some ethnic clients to stereotype American health care practitioners as "cold" and "aloof."

A first-generation Cuban-American woman was very unhappy with the quality of antepartum and postpartum care that she had received when she had her first child. Physicians and nurses had taken health histories and had given health counseling to her and her husband but they had viewed her parents and mother-in-law as "outsiders" and had not included them in the family unit. This woman confided to a nurse-anthropologist that "the American doctors and nurses were so cold—they didn't care about me and my family. They were only concerned with me having my baby. In Cuba, your doctor knew the entire family and always asked how everyone was. He was like a member of the family."

Milgram (1970) has hypothesized about the relationship between the concepts of warmth/coldness and privacy. He suggests that city dwellers are often characterized as cold and aloof primarily because they have a restricted definition of personal responsibility to others, which underlies their in-

---

*Refer to Chapter 5 for a discussion of real and fictive kin.

terpersonal relationships and physical privacy-regulating behaviors.

The privacy-regulating mechanisms that people use are culturally influenced. Some ethnic groups tend to use many physical-barrier types of privacy mechanisms. Other ethnic groups tend to use many interpersonal-barrier types of privacy mechanisms. For example, Germans and middle-class Americans usually use physical barriers, such as closed doors, to convey the message that they want to be left alone (Hall, 1969). Physical barriers in general tend to convey the message that one wants to be left alone or that others should knock before entering one's domain (Kira, 1970; Altman, Nelson, and Lett, 1972).

Ethnic groups that infrequently use physical-barrier privacy mechanisms often use interpersonal types of privacy mechanisms. For example, Puerto Ricans tend to define privacy as being physically removed from strangers and public places but being with family members (Ashcraft and Scheflen, 1976). Many Cubans tend to have a concept of privacy that is similar to that of Puerto Ricans. Cubans may leave doors unlocked or ajar to provide ready entry to extended family members (real and fictive kin). This behavior should not be interpreted as meaning that Cubans do not value privacy. Instead, their concept of privacy is not individualistic but extends to the entire extended family. The time that Cubans spend with their extended family is time when interactions, situations, and experiences encountered during the day can be discussed, evaluated, and integrated (Pasquali, 1982). Similarly, the Chinese concept of privacy tends not to be individualistic but to extend to all members of the household. Within the home, space and possessions are not "owned" by any individual but are accessible to all household members. Even in houses with sufficient room, until they reach adolescence Chinese children may sleep in their parents' bedroom. Neither children nor parents feel that such a sleeping arrangement infringes on anyone's privacy. In sharp contrast to the few physical barrier types of privacy mechanisms within the Chinese home, high walls and many gates may demarcate and separate the people within the Chinese home from the world outside (Hsu, 1970).

Having time alone to evaluate one's interaction with the social environment is an important function of privacy. It is especially important when people are encountering situations that may be new or with which they have little experience. It provides an opportunity to validate perceptions, interpret experiences, and plan how to respond to new behavior and situations (Westin, 1970). This function of privacy is especially important for immigrants who are coping with the stress of culture shock and for clients who are coping with crises.

However, clients in crisis often are not afforded the privacy they need to evaluate interactions and situations. For instance, when people are admitted to hospitals, they usually must share rooms with strangers. In addition, personal privacy may be violated by a steady stream of health professionals (most of whom are also strangers) giving personal care and asking personal questions. History-taking often reveals information that usually is not told to strangers. These "normal" hospital practices may be regarded by clients as intrusions.

For those clients who habitually use physical barriers to guard their privacy, such staff practices as leaving hospital room doors open and not knocking before entering clients' rooms may be interpreted as invasions of privacy. Clients who have an extended-family orientation rather than an individualistic or nuclear-family orientation toward personal responsibility and privacy may view the practice in many special care units (for example, ICUs, CCUs) of restricting visitors to the nuclear family as evidence that health care providers are "cold" and "uncaring." Restriction of visitors also may deprive these clients of the support and feedback that they need from extended family members to evaluate and integrate their experiences with illness and hospitalization.

To help safeguard clients' privacy and thereby sustain them in their experiences, nurses need to be aware of how clients conceptualize privacy. Then they need to develop strategies that will enable clients to maintain as much privacy as possible.

Nurses might try some of the following strategies:

1. Whenever possible, give a client a choice about room assignment (for example, a private room or a semiprivate room; which of two semiprivate rooms) and roommates (for example, a roommate who smokes or one who does not smoke; a roommate who has many visitors or one who has few visitors).

2. Respect the physical privacy barriers that a client may erect. For example, if a client's door is closed, knock before entering. Unless contraindicated for safety reasons, allow a client who so wishes to keep the curtains drawn around the bed.

3. Obtain a client's permission before allowing students or other health team members to observe a procedure. Safeguard the client's privacy during the procedure through the use of screens or curtains and by draping the client.

4. Use interpersonal types of privacy-regulating mechanisms. For example, modulate your voice when discussing personal information with a client so that other people in the room will not overhear what is being said.

5. Try to schedule and coordinate client care so that a client will be allowed the time alone or with family that is needed to integrate experiences.

6. Recognize that unscheduled visits to a client's home may intrude on a client's privacy. Schedule home visits so that they are mutually convenient for nurse and client. This will enable the client to negotiate household routines and other visitors so that they will not conflict with the home visit.

While nurses have a responsibility for facilitating client privacy, they also have a responsibility for ensuring their own privacy. A first step in safeguarding their privacy is for nurses to become aware of how much privacy they require and what types of mechanisms they use to obtain privacy. Many nurses may need help to recognize that authenticity and humanism in relationships with clients and staff do not negate the right of nurses to personal privacy. Nurses do not have to answer probing questions from clients and staff about their personal lives (Blondis and Jackson, 1982). Most nurses also need time away from clients and the families of clients so that they can be alone or with colleagues. This time is necessary for them to integrate their experiences with clients and for them to express their emotions (for example, feelings about working with an angry client or about caring for a terminally ill client).

A recognition that, while all people have privacy needs, different people have different concepts of privacy and different ways of regulating privacy is essential to therapeutic communication and to the effective functioning of the nurse-client relationship.

HUMOR

Humor can decrease social distance by encouraging rapport, by decreasing anxiety, and by making the social structure of the health care setting seem more relaxed and flexible. However, humor can also be a means of expressing such feelings as aggression, hostility, and depression. It is, therefore, important that nurses understand the functions and purposes of humor so that they can use it to facilitate therapeutic communication and to sustain clients in their experiences.

Situations that produce humor vary from culture to culture, and there is no universal agreement on a definition of humor. However, humor is usually generated by the incongruous, the ludicrous, or the unexpected. In our culture, humor is characteristically described as follows:

1. It can be verbally or nonverbally communicated.

2. It is an indirect form of communication.

3. A continuum of laughter exists, ranging from laughing at to laughing with.

4. A sense of humor is a sign of mental health and maturity; it demonstrates an ability to laugh at one's *minor* misfortunes and to see oneself as one is seen by others (Lorenz, 1966; Robinson, 1970; Moody, 1978; DuBois, 1979).

The United States is a multi-ethnic society. It is

therefore important for nurses to understand that although humor is found cross culturally, both the style and the form of humor are culturally variable. For example, the style of British humor is usually viewed by Americans as understatement, while the style of American humor is usually viewed by the British as overstatement, exaggeration, or slapstick. Both the British and the Americans tend to view the style of Oriental humor as subtle and characterized by degrees of amusement.

The form that humor takes tends to reflect ties with other aspects of the culture. For example, one theme in traditional Hispanic culture is male dominance and female submissiveness. A man's good name is maintained through the reputations of the women to whom he is related (wife, sisters, daughters). Women are supposed to be virginal and faithful, and men are supposed to demonstrate their *machismo* through the consumption of alcohol, by engaging in premarital and extramarital sexual liasons, and by protecting the family (Murillo-Rhode, 1976; Gilmore and Gilmore, 1979; Pasquali, 1982). Hispanic humor often reflects this cultural theme. For example, ''loose women'' are frequently the object of jokes.

The purposes and functions of humor operate on both the individual and the societal levels. On the level of the individual, humor may

1. decrease anxiety, stress, and tension.
2. release angry, aggressive, or hostile feelings in a socially acceptable way.
3. deflect emotionally painful conflicts and situations. Repeated joking about a topic may indicate conflict concerning the topic; joking may be the way the person is trying to cope with feelings generated by conflict.
4. facilitate learning.
5. reflect self-acceptance, an adequate self-image, and sound mental health.
6. indicate underlying pathology. Inappropriate, aberrant, or uncontrollable laughter may be symptomatic of pseudobulbar palsy, amytrophic lateral sclerosis, or gelastic epilepsy. Inappropriate silliness is often found in people with Alzheimer's disease, Pick's disease,

and hebephrenic schizophrenia.

7. alleviate physical pain and stress, strengthen the immune system, and produce a sense of euphoria or physical well-being. It has been suggested that by stimulating the production of T-lymphocytes laughter strengthens the immune system and that by stimulating the endocrine system (especially the pituitary gland) to release endorphins,* laughter decreases pain and produces a sense of well-being (Moody, 1978; Cousins, 1979; DuBois, 1979; Abeles, 1982; Goldstein, 1982; Pasquali, 1980; Freud, 1961).

The following vignette illustrates how humor may operate on the level of the individual.

A nurse was trying to teach an adolescent boy with diabetes to give his own insulin injections. The boy was very angry about having diabetes, and he was resistant to the idea of daily insulin injections. The nurse began sharing with the client cartoons that dealt with people's feelings and attitudes about chronic illness and injections. The cartoons provided an avenue of release for the boy's angry feelings, and he was able to laugh at some of his fears about injections. He soon was finding cartoons that dealt with chronic illness and injections to share with the nurse. The humor that the nurse and client shared facilitated trust and decreased the client's anxiety. This relaxed atmosphere facilitated the young man's sharing of his concerns and learning about his diabetes.

On the societal level, humor serves to lessen intergroup conflict and to promote social solidarity:

1. Humor provides a means of expressing feelings and attitudes that might otherwise be difficult to express and permits these feelings and attitudes to be expressed in a socially acceptable manner.

---

*Laughter stimulates the manufacture of catecholamines (for example, epinephrine, norepinephrine, and dopamine). The catecholamines in turn stimulate the release of endorphins, which act as natural opiates.

2. Humor decreases social distance by functioning as a leveling mechanism. If people flaunt success, others may tease them or play down their successes.
3. Humor provides a means for individual feelings and concerns to be shared, thereby facilitating consensual validation and camaraderie.

Lorenz (1966) spoke to these societal functions of humor when he said, ''Barking dogs may occasionally bite but laughing men hardly ever shoot.''

The societal functions of humor may sometimes be institutionalized. For example, the anthropologist Radcliffe-Brown (1952) described one type of institutionalized humor, the joking relationship. A joking relationship refers to a relationship between two people where custom allows or, sometimes, prescribes the teasing or ridiculing of one or both participants in the relationship. When one person teases the other and the other person accepts the teasing good-naturedly and without retaliating, the joking relationship is said to be asymmetrical. This contrasts with a symmetrical joking relationship, in which each of the participants teases and ridicules the other.

When a man marries a woman, he forms relationships with her family. However, prior to the marriage, he had been considered and had considered himself an outsider to her family group. Although this situation may be modified, it is not totally changed by marriage. Similarly, although after marriage a woman usually maintains ties with her family, these ties are altered by her new and close relationship with her husband. Thus, marriage results in both attachment and separation, in both social conjunction and social disjunction. While social conjunction requires the avoidance of hostility, social disjunction involves divergence of interests and thus contains the seeds of conflict. The joking relationship permits the release of antagonisms that may be engendered by social disjunction, while the custom requiring that teasing be accepted good-naturedly avoids the eruption of serious conflict. Thus, the joking relationship serves both as a social release and as a social control.

Joking relationships are common in Africa, Asia, Oceania, and North America (Radcliffe-Brown, 1952). In the United States, mother-in-law jokes and nurse-doctor jokes are forms of asymmetrical joking relationships. For example, nurses may tease some doctors about the ''aseptic aura'' that doctors seem to think they have. The joking relationship permits the nurses to release their irritation about the physicians' poor aseptic techniques, while the custom that such bantering be accepted good-naturedly avoids serious conflict between the nurses and doctors involved in the joking relationship and allows them to continue working together.

Another type of institutionalized humor is the intercultural jest. Intercultural jesting serves to express aggression toward an outgroup or to express cultural conflict among acculturating groups. Intercultural jesting may have as its theme the pitting of folk medicine against medical science. For example, among Mexicans who reside along the Texas-Mexican border, the *curandero talla* (jest about a native healer) pits the *curandero* (native healer) against physicians. The following, paraphrased from Paredes (1968), illustrates the structure of the *curandero talla*:

A person becomes ill and consults several doctors who either cannot help him or who recommend painful and costly remedies. Then someone suggests that the patient consult a curandero. *The patient and family skeptically consult the* curandero. *The* curandero *scolds them for their skepticism and then asks, "What do the doctors say?" The family recounts the doctors' diagnosis and recommendations. The* curandero *listens indulgently and then orders a simple remedy such as goat turds. The patient experiences a full recovery and then confronts his physicians, who are astonished. The doctors are so curious about the cure that they visit the* curandero. *The* curandero *explains that he knew an herb would cure the patient but that he did not know which herb. Since goats eat all herbs, he prescribed goat turds knowing that the therapeutic herb would be present in the turd.*

Thus the *curandero talla* not only ridicules the hit-or-miss character of some folk remedies but also ridicules medical science. Paredes believes that these jests reflect the rejection that acculturating people may feel for their folk culture as well as the antagonism that they may feel toward American culture and what they perceive as uncaring American health care providers. Intercultural jesting thus helps to express the conflicts engendered by acculturation.

In Anglo-American society, jokes are also often made about modern medicine, especially about technology and medicine or about inept or callous health care givers. For example, comic strips abound with illustrations of nurses taking a client history while the client is bleeding to death, of interns administering intravenous fluids through the wrong orifice, and of people whose pacemakers need battery transplants or whose ''tiny timepieces'' all explode at the same time. These comic strips not only try to familiarize Americans with the new technology in health care but also reflect the feelings and fears that many Americans may be experiencing about health care (Pasquali, 1980).

Only when nurses understand the many purposes and functions that humor serves can they begin to understand the implications that humor has for the nurse-client relationship. Certainly a shared joke can strengthen the relationship if the humor occurs within an atmosphere of caring and respect. Also, because humor can serve as a release for emotion, can facilitate learning, and can alleviate physical pain and strengthen the immune system, nurses might creatively incorporate humor into their care plans.

A mental health nurse was giving grief counseling to a woman whose spouse had died 3 months earlier. In addition to helping the client work through her feelings of grief, the nurse was concerned about the woman's vulnerability to illness. Aware that the level of T-lymphocytes is lowered during grief reactions and of research suggesting that humor may stimulate T-lymphocyte production, the nurse

helped the client to select two television programs that made her laugh real "belly laughs" and encouraged the client to watch these programs daily.

However, if nurses want to use humor therapeutically, they need to consider the cultural backgrounds of their clients. What is suitable for joking in one culture may not be suitable in another culture. In addition, a joke may not be understood.

A cartoon that showed a dog dressed as a preppie and acting very "cool" was hung on a nursing school bulletin board. All the students thought it was "cute and funny." However, a first-generation Lebanese-American faculty member did not see the humor in the cartoon. Instead, he became upset because he interpreted the cartoon to mean that in the United States students are treated like dogs.

Clients may joke about situations that are emotionally painful to them or that are causing them conflict. Humor may be one way in which clients try to cope with feelings that are generated by conflicts.

A client who had hypertension and a family history of strokes was advised by her doctor to stop smoking and to lose 50 pounds. The client ignored the physician's advice. She joked, "I live to eat, not eat to live," and she teased friends and relatives who were dieting, saying that they were "trying to live forever." The client also told many jokes about people outliving their doctors.

The client's humor, explored in the context of her other behavior, suggested the presence of a problem. The client's compulsive smoking and eating, juxtaposed with her family history of cerebral vascular accidents, was engendering conflict. Her joking was one way that she attempted to cope with the anxiety generated by this conflict.

Institutionalized clients (for example, clients in hospitals or nursing homes), often engage in jocular griping among themselves about their low status in the health care hierarchy, about institutional routines, or about embarrassing and tension-producing procedures.

Three clients who shared a hospital room joked about "vampires [laboratory technicians] who come in several times a day to suck our blood [take blood samples]" and about the nurses who wake them at 5 AM to take vital signs and again at 11 PM to give them sleeping pills. The clients enjoyed cutting out and sharing comic strips that ridiculed hospital routines, and they frequently exclaimed, "We'll have to go home to get some rest."

By joking about their displeasure with hospital routine, individual complaints became shared and collective complaints. Not only does this facilitate consensual validation and camaraderie, but, in the process, people are able to step outside themselves and to laugh at the discomforts that they share with others (Pasquali, 1980).

Family and friends of clients may also use humor to handle their feelings about a loved one's serious illness, emotional instability, or imminent death. Humorous get-well cards are one vehicle for the expression of this humor, although many times these cards may seem unfeeling to seriously ill clients or to clients who are trying to cope with altered body image or impending death.

It is not enough for nurses to recognize that humor is serving a purpose for clients and for the families and friends of clients. Nurses need to listen for the messages (or themes) that underlie the humor. Once themes have been identified, nurses can use the nursing process to intervene.

Often nurses and other health team members can use humor to handle their own reactions to serious illness and to death. Sometimes the humor may be macabre. Macabre humor may be found among staff members in such high-stress situations as emergency rooms, operating rooms, and special care areas (for example, psychiatric units, oncology units, and cardiac care units). Although humor is one way of expressing their feelings, staff members need to learn to cope with feelings surrounding client care in more authentic ways. Nurses and other health team members also need to be very careful that clients and their relatives and friends do not overhear macabre humor and interpret it as callousness or lack of concern for clients.

An understanding of the functions and purposes of humor is important if nurses are to use humor to facilitate therapeutic communication and to sustain clients in their experiences.

EMPATHY

Empathy increases the ability of nurses to sustain clients in their experiences. Studies have shown that effective counselors are more empathetic with clients than are ineffective counselors (Fiedler, 1950; Heine, 1950).

Nurses may ask, ''What is empathy? What is the relationship between empathy and understanding?'' One way of viewing the relationship between empathy and understanding is to differentiate between ''understanding diagnostically'' and ''understanding therapeutically'' (empathizing) (Porter, 1949). Understanding diagnostically refers to a cluster of *intellectual* assessments of client behavior.

During an intake interview, a nurse noted that the client cried easily, was withdrawn, appeared disheveled, and complained of insomnia and appetite loss. The client's history revealed that his wife had died recently.

This level of understanding helps nurses to describe and analyze client behavior.

In contrast, understanding therapeutically, or empathizing, involves viewing a client's experience as the client perceives it and ''borrowing'' or tuning into the client's feelings (Gendlin, 1962; Bradley and Edinberg, 1982). Thus, empathy is the ability to use imagination and will to project oneself into the emotions and thoughts of another person without losing one's objectivity. The avoidance of subjective involvement and value judgments is an important component of empathy (Forsyth, 1980). Empathy facilitates an "I-thou" rather than an "I-it" relationship.

One way of projecting oneself into a client's phenomenological world is to develop an internal frame of reference (Rogers, 1942; Porter, 1950; Brammer and Shostrom, 1982). This means that the nurse tries to view a client's phenomenological world as the client perceives it. The nurse then tries to become, as Rogers describes it, the alter ego of the client's attitudes and feelings. When the nurse uses an internal frame of reference rather than an external frame of reference, he or she begins feeling *with* the client rather than feeling or thinking *about* the client.

A nurse was counseling a recently widowed woman. The client was very upset about her husband's death. The nurse assumed an internal frame of reference *and thought, "How does this woman view her husband's death? What does she see as the difficulties? How would she like to resolve those difficulties? How can I help her to clarify her thinking so that she can resolve the difficulties?"*

Compare the above situation with the following example:

A nurse was counseling a recently widowed woman. The client was very upset about her husband's death. The nurse assumed an external frame of reference *and thought, "What are the problems that I can identify? What solutions can I find for these problems? How can I help the client to recognize these problems and accept my solutions?*

Obviously, an internal frame of reference rather than an external frame of reference facilitates tuning into a client's phenomenological world and in-

creases a nurse's understanding of a client's experience.

Even though many therapists rate empathy as the most important quality of an "ideal" therapist, therapists sometimes fall short of this ideal (Raskin, 1974). Although there does not seem to be a connection between empathy and clinical understanding of client behavior, empathetic therapists seem better able to establish and maintain warm and accepting relationships with clients than do nonempathetic therapists (Fiedler and Senior, 1952; Fiedler, 1950; Luft, 1950). Empathy helps nurses to establish therapeutic communication with clients and to sustain clients in their experiences by

1. cutting through the deep sense of aloneness often experienced by clients.
2. increasing nurses' knowledge of client difficulties.
3. enabling nurses to give clients clues about how they (clients) may be feeling and how they (clients) are coming across to others (Blondis and Jackson, 1982; Bradley and Edinberg, 1982).

An empathetic response to a client not only gives the client a sense of being understood, but it also facilitates the client's self-exploration, thereby promoting client growth (Truax and Carkhuff, 1964; Bradley and Edinberg, 1982).

A nurse walked into a client's room and found her forlornly looking at a negligee that had been a gift from her husband. The client had recently had a mastectomy. The nurse placed a hand on the client's shoulder and said to her, "You look so sad." The client began to cry and told the nurse, "I wonder if I'll ever be able to wear this again?" The nurse sat down next to the client and answered, "Perhaps you would like to talk about your sadness." The client began to tell the nurse that she felt she had lost her femininity.

The nurse's ability to tune into the client's phenomenological world not only made the client feel that the nurse understood her concern but also gave the client feedback about how she was coming across to others. The nurse's sensitivity and accurate therapeutic understanding helped the client to express her thoughts and feelings, validate her experience, and minimize her sense of aloneness.

However, there may be obstacles to empathetic response. Language may be a barrier. Even when people speak the same language, different people may attach different meanings to the same words.* Therefore, nurses need to clarify with clients the meanings they attach to words and concepts. For example, a client may be referring to anger when talking about being "upset," while a nurse may associate anxiety with feeling upset.

Differences in life experience may also interfere with empathetic response. The discussion of experiential differences earlier in this chapter has implications for the development of empathy. When nurse and client are of different sexes, ages, or races or when they have different cultural or socioeconomic backgrounds, obstacles to empathy may be present. For example, a 22-year-old nurse who has never been seriously ill may have difficulty understanding the reaction to hospitalization of an 80-year-old, chronically ill client. Such experiential differences make it very important for nurses to focus consciously on the client's perception of the situation. This approach will help nurses to avoid making value judgments about a client's life-style or coping behaviors. Judgmental attitudes may lead nurses to reject or avoid a client and may contribute to closing nurses off from therapeutically understanding a client's experience.

Sometimes, similarities in life experience between client and nurse may lead to a nurse overidentifying with and sympathizing with a client. For example, a nurse may begin to feel sorry for or pity a client, or a nurse may become angry at the people with whom the client is angry. When this occurs, the nurse becomes very subjective and may be unable to help the client cope with the experience.

In direct contrast to the nurse who overidentifies

---

*Refer to Chapter 8 for a discussion of language and meaning.

and sympathizes with a client is the nurse who is reluctant to tune into a client's phenomenological world for fear of being exposed to the client's emotional pain. Should a nurse be afraid to "borrow" a client's emotional pain, then the nurse may wall himself or herself off from the client's experience.

Any of these obstacles may lead nurses to assume an external frame of reference, may block therapeutic understanding, and may produce an "I-it" relationship. Likewise, the ability of nurses to assume an internal frame of reference and tune into the phenomenological worlds of clients facilitates therapeutic communication.

TOUCHING

Touching is one way of communicating. By touching, people express such emotions as love, sympathy, hostility, and fear. Nurses often use touching to communicate care and empathy to clients. Holding a fearful client's hand or placing one's hand on the shoulder of a crying client may communicate more empathy or concern than any words might offer. Therefore, it is not surprising that many nursing activities incorporate touching. These activities range from such comfort measures as bathing clients and giving backrubs to such care-giving measures as changing dressings and irrigating ostomies.

Touching is also a means of exploring one's environment (Blondis and Jackson, 1982). Toddlers are always touching objects—furniture, toys, flowers, and so on. They are learning about the world they live in. As people mature, they continue to use touching to familiarize themselves with new environments. For example, clients who have only recently been admitted to a hospital unit may stroke, finger, or grasp bedcovers, arms of chairs, and magazines in an attempt to familiarize themselves with the objects in their environment and to become spatially oriented. Nurses need to become aware of the significance of touching and not to view it as random or meaningless movement.

Bradley and Edinberg (1982) point out that, for many nurses and clients, the high degree of touching that is customary in the nurse-client relationship can be at variance with the degree of touching that they have been conditioned to consider "normal" in social interaction. These nurses and clients may feel uncomfortable with the degree of touching involved in comfort- and care-giving nursing activities and with tactile communication of feelings. For example, some nurses and clients may interpret touching as aggressive or intrusive rather than as evidence of empathy and caring.* Generally, people who speak Latin-derived languages use more touching and are more comfortable with touching than are people who speak Anglo-Saxon–derived languages. On the cultural continuum of touching, Scandinavians tend to fall midway between Latins and Anglo-Saxons. However, even within the same cultural group, there may be a great deal of variation (Montagu, 1971).

Therefore, to avoid misinterpreting the use of touching, nurses need to be aware of both their own attitudes about touching and the attitudes of their clients. The following self-assessment guide might help nurses gain insight into their own attitudes about touching.

1. How much touching is customary among members of my family? My ethnic group?
2. In what context(s) do I and my family most use touching? Least use touching?
3. Among people of which age groups and/or which sex do I consider touching most acceptable? Least acceptable?
4. How do I feel when, during conversation, people touch me?
5. Does my reaction to being touched vary according to the part of my body being touched (for example, limb vs. trunk vs. genitals)?
6. Does my reaction to being touched vary according to the person doing the touching (for example, family member, lover, friend, professional care giver) and the sex of the person doing the touching?

---

*Clients who are suffering from some psychiatric disorders, such as schizophrenia, may have difficulty with ego boundaries. In such instances, touching should be used judiciously. Refer to Chapter 21 for further discussion.

7. How do I feel (or imagine I would feel) when I am the recipient of personal care (for example, a backrub, a bath, a dressing change, an ostomy irrigation)?

Communication themes

A communication theme is a recurrent idea or concept that underlies communication and ties it together. Peplau (1953, 1954) and Ujhely (1968) have pioneered in helping nurses listen for the meaning or messages being conveyed—the themes of communication. There are three types of communication themes: content theme, mood theme, and interaction theme.

The *content theme* is the idea that underlies or links together seemingly disparate topics of discussion. It is the "what" of communication.

Elvira Johnson, 31 years old, was hospitalized after an attempted suicide. She had been married for 3 years to Stuart Johnson, a successful insurance agent. Barbara, a student nurse began meeting biweekly with Mrs. Johnson to talk about her concerns. After 3 weeks, the student nurse became very disheartened and frustrated. She believed that Mrs. Johnson was using the time to socialize and that she was only talking about superficial topics. Barbara's verbatim notes showed that Mrs. Johnson frequently spoke as follows: "When I was younger, I had several girl friends. None of us were any beauties. We would go bowling or out for pizza. We had a lot of laughs. We didn't need boyfriends to have a good time."

"My husband is an insurance agent, and many of his clients are pretty young student nurses like you. They take out professional liability insurance." Then she would laugh and ask, "Do you think I can trust him with those students?"

"I had a beautiful wedding. Many friends were invited. My sister was my maid of honor, and my husband's best friend, Jeff, was his best man. They really are good friends—best buddies they call each other. I think if my husband had to choose between the two of us he would choose Jeff."

In discussing this interaction with her instructor, Barbara began to see that low self-esteem was a recurrent theme. Mrs. Johnson saw herself as an unattractive woman. She felt threatened by her husband's young clients and believed that her husband preferred his male friend to her. Mrs. Johnson had not been engaging in superficial conversation. The underlying message or theme in her interactions was that of low self-esteem. Once this theme was identified, nursing intervention could be planned.

The *mood theme* is the affect or emotion a person communicates. To identify the mood theme, one needs to listen for speech patterns and tone of voice. In addition, gestures, facial expressions, posture, and personal appearance should be observed. The mood theme reflects an individual's affect. Is the person angry? Hopeless? Apathetic? Any adjective describing a mood may be a possible mood theme. The mood theme is the ''how'' of communication.

Mrs. Barnes had recently been diagnosed as diabetic. A community health nurse was counseling her in diabetic care and helping her work through her feelings about being diabetic. The nurse noticed on each of her visits that Mrs. Barnes' 14-year-old son, Matthew, appeared listless. His face was expressionless. Regardless of what was happening or what he was speaking about, Matthew's face was expressionless and his voice was monotone.

The community health nurse identified Matthew's mood as apathetic. She recognized that this flatness of affect or apathy might be an indicator of deep emotional conflict. The nurse referred Matthew to a neighborhood counseling center.

By identifying the mood theme of apathy and recognizing its import, the community health nurse was able to make an appropriate referral.

The *interaction theme* is the idea or concept that best describes the dynamics between communicating participants. Are the partners in communication relating to one another in a pattern of domi-

nance-submission? Collaboration? Power struggle? Parallel play? If the interaction theme is reinforcing well-established patterns of pathology or if it is destructive of therapeutic communication, it may need to be identified so that the problem can be resolved.

After a 1-year stay in a psychiatric hospital, John Toomey was discharged to his home. Carlos Rodriquez, a psychiatric nurse, visited John on a weekly basis. Carlos' purpose was to help John readjust to living in the community. The focus of these visits was to assist John in finding employment, to teach him to shop for and prepare meals, and to help him to budget his money. Whenever John had to make a decision or initiate a plan of action he would ask Carlos "What do you think I should do?" Carlos would usually respond with his assessment of the best course of action. After several visits, Carlos realized that the interaction theme had become one of dominance-submission. He had taken the dominant role, and John had assumed the submissive role. Once Carlos had identified these dynamics, he pointed out to John the pattern their interactions had taken. Carlos explained that in the future he would help John explore alternatives and arrive at a decision but would not make the decision.

Had Carlos failed to identify the interaction theme, he might have continued to reinforce unhealthy patterns of communication and behavior.

These vignettes illustrate what is meant by content, mood, and interaction themes. Although these hypothetical examples have been drawn from nursing situations, any one or a combination of themes can be identified in any sequence of communication, be it social or therapeutic.

THE NURSING PROCESS

Identifying predominant communication themes and helping clients learn appropriate and effective coping behaviors require that nurse and client actively explore a client's experience within the framework of the nursing process.

Steps in the nursing process

The steps in the nursing process have been delineated in various ways by various authors. Basically, each way has been a form of the scientific method. Briefly outlined, the steps are as follows*:

1. Making an assessment—collecting data about a client†; aim: to gather information from the verbal and nonverbal communication of the client, the client's family and/or significant others
   a. Gather the following information systematically and continuously from one-to-one interactions, group therapy sessions, and recreational and unit activities:
      (1) The client's, the client's family's, and significant others' perceptions of the situation or problem
      (2) The client's intrapersonal, interpersonal, and sociocultural strengths and limitations
      (3) The client's verbal, kinesic, and proxemic behavior
      (4) The client's status: biological, intellectual, psychological, sociocultural, and spiritual
      (5) Factors that predisposed the client to the situation or problem
      (6) Factors that precipitated the situation or problem
      (7) The client's present environment (both social and physical)
      (8) The interaction of yourself and the staff with the client, the client's family, and significant others
   b. Verify the data.
      (1) Confirm observations and perceptions by obtaining consensual validation or additional information from the client, the client's family, significant others, and/or other sources (for example, records, psychological tests).
      (2) Communicate assessment information to other staff members, verbally and through charting. A particular form of charting may be done at the time of admission—the admission assessment. The following information is usually charted on admission:
         (a) The event that precipitated hospitalization
         (b) Prior psychiatric problems
         (c) Past school and childhood relationships; relationships with parents and siblings
         (d) Sexual and marital history
         (e) Relationships with children
         (f) Job; vocational and avocational history
         (g) Any special physical conditions
         (h) History of allergies
         (i) Medications taken recently or within the past 2 or 3 weeks (does the client have any medications with him or her *now?*)
         (j) Blood pressure, temperature, pulse and respiratory rates, weight and height
         (k) List of clothing and valuables
         (l) Phone number of family member or friend
2. Analyzing the data—making inferences based on the collected data*; aim: to understand the meaning of the client's behavior patterns
   a. Identify predominant themes and the interrelationship among these themes.
   b. Identify the interrelationship between themes, predisposing and precipitating factors, the client's overall health status,

---

*Adapted from National Council of State Boards of Nursing, Inc., 1980; LaMonica, 1979; Atkinson and Murphy, 1980; American Nurses' Association, 1982.

†Although the singular "client" is used throughout the discussion of the nursing process, it should not be interpreted as referring only to individuals. The term "client" also encompasses social units such as families and couples.

---

*This step of the nursing process may be facilitated through clinical supervision—either with the help of a teacher or supervisor or through "peer supervision," which implies a mutual exchange of ideas and suggestions among co-workers.

and the client's perception of the situation or crisis.

c. Formulate a nursing diagnosis that states both the behavioral problem (or impending problem) and its relationship to contributing factors (for example, depression related to the loss of a spouse; anxiety related to culture shock; grief related to post-mastectomy body image).

3. Planning client care—establishing goals and developing intervention
   a. Aim: to develop a plan of action for initiating change or for enabling the client to better cope with the existing situation
      (1) Determine whether the locus of decision making is predominantly with the nurse, predominantly with the client, or shared between nurse and client.*
      (2) On the basis of the locus of decision making, facilitate or encourage the participation of the client, the client's family, and/or significant others in setting goals and in establishing priorities among goals (several goals may be pursued simultaneously; highest priority goals relate to preventing a client from harming self or others).
      (3) Differentiate between long-term and short-term goals.
      (4) State projected outcomes (observable behavioral changes) of nursing actions.
   b. Aim: to design and modify a client care plan that is based on psychiatric nursing principles, the psychiatric literature, and the nurse's own experience with effective approaches to specific behavior problems
      (1) Anticipate client needs on the basis of the priority of goals.

      (2) Include the client, the client's family, and/or significant others in the development of intervention strategies.
      (3) Plan care that is congruent with the client's age, sex, locus of decision making, religion, and culture.
      (4) Identify nursing approaches that should be followed for specific behavioral problems.
   c. Aim: to cooperate with other health team members in the delivery of health care
      (1) Design a care plan that is consistent with the total therapeutic regimen.
      (2) Coordinate the client's treatment program (for example, unit, recreational, and occupational activities; group and one-to-one therapies).
      (3) Report and/or chart information that is pertinent to client care.

4. Implementing the care plan—instituting and completing nursing actions that are necessary for the achievement of established goals and the facilitation of growth-promoting behavior
   a. Aim: to counsel the client
      (1) Help the client to identify stressors and to develop effective means of stress management.
      (2) Facilitate the client's relationships with family, health team members, and/or significant others.
      (3) Inform the client about or ensure that the client is informed about mental health status, confidentiality, and, when applicable, retention status.*
      (4) Refer the client to appropriate community resources (for example, Alcoholics Anonymous, Alatot, Alateen, Alanon).
   b. Aim: to provide care that will facilitate the accomplishment of therapeutic goals
      (1) Establish a physical and social milieu

---

*Refer to Chapter 1 for a discussion of the locus of decision making.

*Refer to Chapter 3 for a discussion of retention status and confidentiality.

that ensures the client's safety.

    (2) Provide a physical and social milieu that promotes rapport, verbalization, the development of insight, and the trying out of more adaptive coping behaviors.

    (3) Provide care that compensates for gaps in the client's perception, interpretation, or response.

    (4) Encourage the client to participate in and follow the therapeutic regimen.

    (5) Modify care according to the client's needs or priorities.

    (6) Provide care that encourages self-actualization and emotional interdependence.

    (7) Supervise and coordinate the work of health team members for whom you are responsible.

    (8) Report and chart nursing actions and client responses to nursing actions.

5. Evaluating the care plan—determining the degree of goal achievement; aim: to include the client in estimating the client's progress toward the attainment of goals

    a. Estimate the degree to which goals have been achieved, crises have been resolved, and coping behaviors have become more effective.

    b. Identify goals that need to be modified or revised.

    c. Evaluate the effectiveness of nursing actions or approaches.

    d. Identify aspects of the milieu and/or nursing approaches that need to be modified or revised.

    e. Bridge the client to support systems other than the nurse-client relationship.

        (1) People in the social environment (for example, friends, relatives, clergy) who are willing to serve as support givers

        (2) Community agencies that offer help with problems that may arise in the future

The following vignette illustrates how the nursing process is used in mental health nursing.

Toby Jackson, a 69-year-old woman, was hospitalized for congestive heart failure. Because of her physical condition, for the past year her physical activity had been severely resricted. John, a student nurse, met biweekly with Mrs. Jackson. John had noticed that Mrs. Jackson took little interest in her physical appearance and rarely spoke with her roommate. Mrs. Jackson had told John, "When I was younger, I took care of my children and my home. I was widowed when I was 31, and I had to earn a living and support and raise those children all by myself. I was always busy. I took care of everyone. Now I can't even take care of myself. I'm no good to anyone." John replied, "It sounds like you define your value as a person by what you can do for yourself and others." Mrs. Jackson answered, "That's right. You have to keep busy and be useful. Otherwise, you're no good to anyone, even yourself."

John had gathered data about Mrs. Jackson's concerns and had validated his perception with the client. In supervision with his instructor, John looked at the meaning of the client's communication. He identified low self-esteem as one of Mrs. Jackson's predominant content themes, and he formulated the following nursing diagnosis: low self-esteem related to a decreased sense of productivity. This decreased sense of productivity was associated with the physical restrictions of congestive heart failure and hospitalization.

John determined that the locus of decision making could be shared between him and the client. John, in collaboration with Mrs. Jackson, established the following plan of care:

1. Long-range goals—assist Mrs. Jackson to

    a. accept both her strengths and her weaknesses.

    b. develop insight into sources of low self-esteem.

    c. develop feelings of adequacy and security.

2. Short-range goals—assist Mrs. Jackson to
   a. assess her level of self-esteem.
   b. recognize that low self-esteem is a predominant communication theme.
   c. recognize that feelings of low self-esteem are causing her discomfort and that new ways of coping should be explored.
   d. identify some positive qualities in herself.
   e. set realistic goals for herself.
   f. develop skills and talents that will build self-confidence.
   g. engage in activities that present a challenge but that can be readily completed and thus provide a sense of accomplishment.

The nursing principles on which the above client care plan was based are as follows:

1. Negative appraisals have contributed to Mrs. Jackson's feeling of low self-esteem. It is important to provide an environment that is nonjudgmental. The nurse should accept Mrs. Jackson's negative as well as positive attributes.
2. When an individual sets unrealistically high goals, the result will be failure. When failure consistently occurs, feelings of inadequacy are reinforced. The setting of challenging but realistic goals will help Mrs. Jackson to overcome some of her feelings of inadequacy.
3. Feelings of neglect tend to reinforce feelings of low self-esteem. It is important to approach Mrs. Jackson in a consistent, accepting manner and to make her realize that the nurse considers her a worthwhile person.

John's projected outcomes for his nursing intervention were that Mrs. Jackson would begin to take interest in her personal appearance (for example, attend to personal grooming, coordinate her clothes), that she would begin to converse with her roommate, and that she would communicate to others positive feelings about her self-worth. By the time the relationship between John and Mrs. Jackson was terminated, the client had begun to brush her hair each morning and to hold it in place with some brightly colored combs that her daughter had brought her. She also had begun to knit a sweater for her grandson. Mrs. Jackson and her roommate occasionally talked about her knitting. Mrs. Jackson told John, "If I can't help take care of my grandchildren, at least I can knit them some winter clothes. That will help my children with the clothing bills. That makes me feel good." Just prior to her discharge from the hospital, John referred Mrs. Jackson to a clinical nurse specialist in private practice who would work with Mrs. Jackson to accomplish more fully the established goals. In addition, John helped Mrs. Jackson to identify two people in her social environment, her clergyman and her oldest daughter, to whom she could express her concerns and on whom she could count for support.

The nursing process also involves the *charting of observations* of client behavior. In most mental health facilities, the nurse is not the only team member who charts observations. All team members are expected to record observations of clients with whom they work. The purposes of charting are as follows:

1. To facilitate the sharing of information among the entire staff
2. To provide information for planning and revising a treatment plan
3. To keep a record of changes in a client's behavior that may lead to a better understanding of client problems

Nurses should observe the following basic principles of charting:

1. Record accurately, using concise, simple language.
2. Be objective and nonjudgmental.
3. Give concrete examples. For instance, what was the *behavior* that suggested hostility? What *intervention* was taken? What *effects* did the intervention have?
4. Quote *exactly* what a client says. This is especially important in reporting delusions and hallucinations. Use quotation marks.
5. Sign, date, and record the time of each entry.
6. If a mistake is made, cross through it and initial.

Guide for assessment of mental health

The following guide has been designed to assist students to assess a client's mental health status, to establish goals and develop nursing strategies consistent with a client's perceptions and orientations about health and illness, and to communicate (verbally and through charting) information about a client's condition to other health team members.

1. Demographic data
   a. Name
   b. Address
   c. Age
   d. Sex
   e. Education
   f. Ethnicity (optional)*
   g. Religion (optional)*
   h. Living arrangements
   i. Marital status
2. Admission data
   a. Date and time of admission
   b. Manner of admission
      (1) Self
      (2) Relatives
      (3) Police
      (4) Other (describe)
   c. Form of retention (if hospitalized)
      (1) Informal retention
      (2) Voluntary retention
      (3) Involuntary retention
      (4) Emergency
      (5) Comments
   d. Reason for admission
   e. Client's primary complaint
   f. Client's premorbid personality
3. History of psychiatric problems
   a. Previous condition: date; problem
   b. Assistance sought: native healer; therapist; agency; clergyman; other (describe)
   c. Current levels of functioning and coping
4. Behavioral observations
   a. Thought patterns

      (1) Delusion*: grandeur; persecution; somatic; self-accusatory
      (2) Obsession
      (3) Ideas of reference
      (4) Phobia
      (5) Looseness of association
      (6) Flight of ideas
      (7) Fugue
      (8) Impaired judgment
      (9) Impaired insight
      (10) Impaired orientation to time, place, or person
      (11) Impaired memory
      (12) No observable thought disturbance
      (13) Comments
   b. Sensory processes
      (1) Hallucination*: olfactory; auditory; tactile; gustatory; visual
      (2) No observable sensory disturbance
      (3) Comments
   c. Speech patterns
      (1) Blocking
      (2) Word salad
      (3) Echolalia
      (4) Circumstantiality
      (5) Irrelevancy
      (6) Confabulation
      (7) Mutism
      (8) Neologism
      (9) Perseveration
      (10) Stuttering
      (11) No observable speech disturbance
      (12) Comments
   d. Affect
      (1) Elation
      (2) Depression
      (3) Ambivalence
      (4) Apathy
      (5) Anger and hostility
      (6) Anxiety
      (7) No observable disturbance of affect
      (8) Comments
   e. Motor activity

---

*Legislation protects people from being required to reveal ethnicity and religion.

---

*Quote *exactly* what the client says. Use quotation marks.

(1) Hyperactive
(2) Hypoactive
(3) Stereotypical: persistent; aimless; repetitive
(4) Perseveration
(5) Catalepsy: stupor; waxy flexibility
(6) Compulsion
(7) No observable disturbance in motor activity
(8) Comments
f. Level of consciousness
(1) Confusion
(2) Stupor
(3) Delirium
(4) Alert
(5) Comments
5. Physical appearance
a. Posture
(1) Sagging
(2) Rigid
(3) Curled into fetal position
(4) Bent
(5) No observable disturbance in posture
(6) Comments
b. Facies
(1) Drooping or sagging: deflected eyes; lusterless eyes; drooping eyelids; deep nasolabial folds
(2) Uplifted or retracted: smiling; retracted brow; wide open eyes; darting eyes
(3) Blank: staring into space; distant expression in eyes
(4) Mask-like or ironed-out
(5) Facial tic
(6) No observable disturbance in facies
(7) Comments
c. Mode of dress
(1) Overly neat
(2) Disheveled
(3) Bizarre
(4) Appropriate
(5) Comments
6. Physical status

a. Vital signs: pulse; temperature; respiration; blood pressure
b. Physical condition
(1) Medical problems: acute; chronic
(2) Physical aids (describe)
(3) Medications: date and time of last dose
(4) Allergies (describe)
(5) Physical signs and symptoms: skin rash; edema; sore throat (phenothiazine side effect?); unusual gait, fine hand tremor, or any extrapyramidal symptom
(6) Comments
c. Patterns of daily living
(1) Sleep patterns: restlessness; insomnia; narcoplexy; average number of hours of sleep
(2) Personal hygiene: kempt; unkempt
(3) Eating patterns: number of meals a day; compulsive eating; anorexia
(4) Drinking patterns: beverage; quantity consumed; frequency of consumption
(5) Sexual patterns: sexual orientation or preference; attitudes about sexuality; sexual activity
(6) Elimination patterns: constipation; diarrhea; urinary frequency; urinary retention
(7) Social patterns: recreation; work; intimacy; community involvement
(8) Comments
d. Level of self-care
(1) Personal hygiene
(2) Activities of daily living
(3) Comments
7. Cultural orientation
a. Place of residence: interethnic neighborhood; ethnic enclave
b. Family organization: nuclear; extended; members composing family unit; members vested with authority; members involved in child rearing; sense of obligation of family members to one another

c. Sex-defined roles: stereotyped male and female roles; amount of independence permitted men and women; degree of intimacy permitted between married men and women, unmarried men and women

d. Communication patterns: language spoken at home; language spoken outside home; use of touching and gesturing; interpersonal spacing

e. Type of dress: traditional ethnic dress; Western-style dress

f. Type of food: ethnic food; American food

g. Relationship to people: individualistic; group-oriented; egalitarian; authoritative

h. Relationship to time: past-oriented; present-oriented; future-oriented

i. Relationship to the world: personal control; goal directed; fatalistic

j. Health care patterns: ideas concerning causes of mental illness; ideas concerning treatment of mental illness; people consulted for treatment of mental illness (e.g., family member, native healer, mental health therapist, other [describe])

k. Comments

8. Effective social network
   a. Family
   b. Household members (if different from family)
   c. Friends
   d. Associates: employer; coworkers; neighbors; others
   e. Religious affiliates: clergyman; church elders; congregants
   f. Comments

9. Stressors
   a. Culture shock
      (1) Communication (foreign verbal, kinesic, and proxemic systems)
      (2) Mechanical environment (e.g., different types of food, housing, clothing, utilities)
      (3) Social isolation from family and friends

      (4) Foreign customs, standards, and/or values
      (5) Different or new role relationships
   b. Life changes
      (1) Affectional: marriage; birth; death; divorce; abandonment
      (2) Socioeconomic: promotion; demotion; unemployment; change of employment; change of residence; increased responsibilities
      (3) Biophysical: serious illness (acute or chronic); surgery; accident; loss of body part; sexual trauma (e.g., rape, incest)
   c. Other (describe)
   d. No significant stress
   e. Comments

10. Coping mechanisms
    a. Coping mechanisms used (describe)
    b. Effectiveness of coping mechanisms
    c. Client's perception of mechanisms that are effective in reducing stress
    d. Comments

11. Resources
    a. Personal: interests; leisure time activities; physical and mental abilities; educational achievement; other
    b. Social: interpersonal networks; economic support systems (e.g., health insurance, sick leave, union benefits); food, shelter, clothing; other
    c. Comments

12. Candidacy for active involvement in treatment program
    a. Developmental level
    b. Interactional ability
    c. Willingness to participate in treatment program
    d. Locus of decision making
    e. Client problems, plans, ideas, hopes, or complaints that may impact on the treatment plan or progress
    f. Areas of anticipated need for assistance from nursing staff
    g. Comments

Operation of the nursing process throughout the nurse-client relationship

The various steps of the nursing process tend to be associated with definite phases of the nurse-client relationship.

The nurse-client relationship is characterized by three phases: orientation, working, and termination. Initially a client may speak about many different areas but will not delve deeply into any one area. This is to be expected. During this stage, which is called the *orientation phase*, the nurse and the client are getting to know one another and the client is mapping out areas of concern. At this time, the nurse begins to collect data about the client. At some point, the client will begin to repeat areas and will assume a high commitment configuration and/or postures of affiliation. This should indicate to the nurse a readiness to discuss these areas in greater detail. This repetition also signals the beginning of the next step in the process of exploration: description and clarification. This step is also referred to as the *working phase* in a therapeutic relationship.

As a client observes and describes what he or she perceives of his or her experiences, the nurse assists the client in this description. The nurse encourages the client by saying, "Start at the beginning and tell me what happened" or "Tell me more about that." Occasionally the nurse might assist the person to clarify thoughts by seeking to clarify speech. We have all had the experience of being unable to put something into words until we have thought it out clearly in our heads. Therefore, when a client uses vague pronouns, speaking of "them," "they," "he," "she," or "it," the nurse needs to seek clarification. The nurse may ask, "Who is 'she'?" or "Who are you referring to when you speak about 'all of them'?"

Mr. Graff, a 62-year-old man, had been admitted to the hospital after slipping in the bathtub and fracturing his leg. Following surgery to reduce the frac-

ture, Mr. Graff was resting in his hospital bed. When his meal was served, he became very upset. He could not eat because he did not have his dentures. Repeatedly he ranted, "How do you expect me to eat when they took my teeth?" Nurses and aides hastily looked through his bedside stand and in his closet but found no dentures. Yet the hospital record indicated that he had been wearing dentures when he was admitted. The staff activity seemed only to further aggravate Mr. Graff. He continued to rant, "They took my teeth." Finally a nurse asked, "Mr. Graff, who took your teeth?" Mr. Graff answered, "My daughter and son-in-law took my teeth home with them. They were afraid they'd get lost or broken if left here. Now how am I going to eat?" Once the situation was clarified, a phone call was made to the daughter, and she brought Mr. Graff's dentures to him. The problem had been resolved.

Occasionally during the process of exploration, a nurse may have to provide information to compensate for some lack in a client's ability to perceive or to correct a client's tendency to subjectively and selectively perceive and interpret an experience. For example, a nurse might give concise instructions to a person experiencing moderate to severe anxiety or might try to help a client perceive an experience more objectively by expressing doubt as to the reality of a perception and asking, "Isn't that a bit unusual?" However, a nurse must be careful to word such an expression so that it does not threaten the client, increase the client's anxiety, and further distort the client's perception of reality.

Once a client has described and clarified an experience, he or she is ready to progress to the next step of exploration. It is at this point that the nurse and client *together* look at the data. They try to place events in sequence, to determine in what way the experience is similar to or different from other events, and to evaluate the impact of the experience on the individual. In helping a client explore an experience, a nurse might inquire, "What happened first?" or "In what way was this the same as (or different from) . . .?"

A 70-year-old woman, Mrs. Rich, had just completed the first week in a home for the aged. She appeared lonely and explained, "I feel so alone and afraid. I don't know anyone here. I have no one to talk to. I've never been in a place like this before. I've never even been in a hospital. I had all my children at home." A nurse inquired, "Was there ever a time in your life that you had some of these same feelings?"

Mrs. Rich thought a while and said, "Yes, when I was first married. My husband brought me to this small town where he had found work. I didn't know a soul, and all my family lived miles away. I felt so alone—I thought I'd never feel like I belonged. I'd go for long walks, and before long I'd begin to see some of the same faces. I'd sort of smile, and they'd smile, and before you'd know it we would be talking."

The nurse had assisted Mrs. Rich to find similarities between the present experience of loneliness and a past experience.

Once nurse and client have sifted through the data, putting events in sequence and establishing similarities to and differences from other experiences, the client is ready to draw conclusions and to formulate the meaning of the experience. The nurse assists the client in this process by facilitating summarization or by suggesting a tentative conclusion. The nurse might say, "Then what you are saying is . . ." or "What do you conclude from all this?" or "It sounds like what you're saying is . . . . Does that sound right to you?" In the case of Mrs. Rich, once she had made the comparison between her experience as a bride and her present experience in the nursing home, the nurse would be able to ask, "Might you be able to handle this new experience in a similar way?" Ideally, Mrs. Rich would state that it might be possible and would agree to give it some thought.

Now the client is ready to decide whether events should be allowed to progress as they have been or whether new behavior is needed to better cope with the experience. The nurse might inquire, "The

next time this happens, what might you do?" By asking a client to consider what behavior might be more appropriate in the future, the nurse encourages the client to formulate a plan of action. In the example of Mrs. Rich, once she had recognized similarities between her past and present experiences, the nurse would be able to help Mrs. Rich deal with the situation. Mrs. Rich might decide that since, in the past, taking long walks had helped to familiarize her with her new neighbors, she might start strolling around the nursing home and into scheduled activites.

"Perhaps," Mrs. Rich stated, "taking walks will help me get to know people." The nurse agreed that this plan was worth a try and suggested that they evaluate the results after a week. At the end of the week, Mrs. Rich proudly reported that she had made one "pretty nice friend" and that several other people were stopping and chatting with her.

Thus during the working phase, the nurse assesses and analyzes client data, helps the client plan a course of action, supports the client in trying out the plan, and assists the client in evaluating how effectively the plan has helped him or her cope with the situation. Should the evaluation show the new behavior to be ineffective, nurse and client need to identify the reasons why it does not work and to develop a new course of action.

The *termination phase* is the conclusion of the nurse-client relationship. It is often characterized by such relationship stalls as client avoidance of interactions (either missing sessions or leaving early) or client attempts to extend the relationship.

Because it was the end of the semester, Judith Johanson was terminating her relationship with both of her clients. Judith had told her clients at their very first meeting that their last interaction would be on May 7, and she had, in recent interviews, reminded them that their last interaction was imminent. Each client responded to termination differently. While for the past two sessions one client had made such excuses as being too tired or too busy to meet with the student nurse, the other client had told Judith, "You have helped me so much. I really appreciate it. Can I have your address so I can keep in touch with you?"

Judith discussed her clients' reactions to termination with her instructor. Judith decided to confront her first client with his behavior, and the client told Judith that he always had difficulty saying good-byes. Judith also explained to her second client that extending the relationship was not part of their original agreement and would change the relationship from a therapeutic to a social relationship.

In addition to the actual saying of good-bye between client and nurse, during the termination phase the nurse and the client summarize the problems that have been worked upon and discuss the degree of goal accomplishment. The nurse helps the client to assess the motivation and effort used in problem solving. This is also a time when the nurse might give feedback to a client about the client's strengths, therapeutic accomplishments, and areas to continue to work upon. The nurse might also share with the client something that the nurse has gained from their interactions. For example, a nurse might tell a client, "You have shown me that life experience is an important source of learning" or "You have helped me to better understand what it is like to experience such a life crisis." Time should also be set aside for the client to express feelings about the relationship—for example, what was helpful and not helpful, what areas were easier to talk about than other areas, feelings about termination. The nurse should discuss his or her feelings about termination with a colleague or supervisor. Finally, the nurse should help the client establish networks of support other than the nurse-client relationship (for example, significant others, rap groups, self-help groups) that may be of assistance in coping with problems that might arise in the future.

Thus, the termination phase focuses on the nursing process step of evaluation, and this phase ideally occurs over several weeks. When termination occurs prematurely because of the sudden discharge of a client from the health care setting, both the client and the nurse may have a sense of frustration and of unfinished business.

The operation of the nursing process throughout the nurse-client relationship can be summarized as follows:

Phase of the nurse-client relationship	Steps of the nursing process
Orientation	Assessment (begin to collect data)
Working	Assessment (continue to collect data, verify data)
	Analysis of data; planning of client care, implementation of the care plan, evaluation (begin to evaluate and revise care plan as needed)
Termination	Evaluation (continue to evaluate—goals attained, outcomes achieved, and effectiveness of nursing actions; bridge client to other support systems)

GUIDELINES FOR PROMOTING THERAPEUTIC COMMUNICATION

Using the nursing process and establishing and maintaining a therapeutic relationship require therapeutic communication. To therapeutically communicate with clients, it is necessary for nurses to understand psychiatric nursing principles, to use the supervisory process, to be knowledgeable about the "do's" of therapeutic communication, and to recognize barriers to therapeutic communication.

Principles of psychiatric nursing

Some of the important principles underlying psychiatric nursing intervention include:

1. Freud's dictum that *all behavior is meaning-*

ful and that most behavior, in the complex human organism, is designed to satisfy several needs. For example, an individual who strives to do a job well may be attempting to satisfy the following needs:

a. The need for approval
b. The need for security
c. The need for affection and companionship
d. The need for self-respect
e. The need for increased knowledge
f. The need to create and to express creativity

Several other needs could be added to the list. Pathological behavior also may represent attempts to satisfy needs. For example, a person who maintains a delusion of being persecuted by the FBI or the CIA may be satisfying the following needs:

a. The need to disown one's negative and aggressive thoughts and to project them onto the outside world
b. The need to feel important (as a result of being singled out)
c. The need to provide some reasons for the existence of a chaotic inner world and thus restore some measure of order to that world

2. Maslow's hierarchy of needs (Maslow, 1967). A person tries to meet the most pressing needs first and, in doing so, may not recognize other important (perhaps even life-supporting) needs. For example, a person who is in a manic state seeks immediate release of tension through physical exertion. Sometimes the need for rest and adequate food are completely ignored in deference to the need for physical release of energy. Individuals whose needs have been satisfactorily met in the past are generally able to tolerate delays in the satisfaction of present needs.

3. The humanistic-existential stance that *all human beings have potential for growth.* Many psychiatric clients have led chaotic lives in the past and are experiencing a multitude of severe problems in the present. A feeling of hopelessness about a situation can become contagious, affecting even the nurse, or it can take the form of a self-fulfilling prophecy. To be truly helpful, the nurse must appeal to, cultivate, and reinforce the client's "healthy part." This belief in an individual's potential for change and for growth is also the antidote for any other dissatisfaction that can arise out of the nurse's own hopelessness.

4. The use of "themes" as a way of collecting and organizing data about the needs, problems, and goals of a client

Matheney and Topalis (1965) have compiled a very useful and concise list of psychiatric nursing principles. The following discussion incorporates several of them, as well as some additional principles and some illustrations of important points.

In interaction with psychiatric clients, *consistency* is important. When there is intrapsychic turmoil, a consistent, fairly well-ordered outer world can be a calming influence that provides the client some security. A person who has the painfully low self-esteem that is so common with psychiatric clients may automatically blame himself or herself for inconsistency on the part of others. A "You're OK—I'm *not* OK" stance (Harris, 1969) is taken by such a client who tells himself, "I'm the sick one, so it must be *me* who made the mistake."

Acceptance as a worthwhile human being is what we are all looking for. Because of traumatic past experiences, the need of the psychiatric client for acceptance is extreme. However, acceptance of a client does not include automatic acceptance of all of the client's behavior. Self-destructive acts or aggressive acts that constitute a danger to other people are some obvious examples of behavior that cannot be accepted. *Limit setting* may be necessary in order to control some types of behavior, but the setting of limits can be done in a respectful, accepting manner that is therapeutic and not destructive of the client's self-esteem.

For example, when a nurse is involved in a one-to-one, confidential interaction with a client, and another resident of the unit keeps interrupting their conversation by asking to be included, some action is mandated. It would probably be most helpful if the nurse were firm in setting limits on such behavior, explaining to the interrupting person that the conversation is private. An appointment for a one-to-one conversation with the interrupter, or for a three-way casual conversation, could be made for the very near future. Such a response by the nurse recognizes the needs of both clients. It fosters self-respect and respect for others, and it helps promote the client's trust of the nurse.

When they first begin to work with psychiatric clients, nurses are often reluctant to employ any form of limit setting. This reluctance probably arises out of the fear that setting limits may hurt the client, whom they view as having suffered sufficiently already, and also out of the nurse's need to be accepted. *Therapeutic* limit setting, however, is not harmful, and it can be very beneficial for clients who are unable to exercise control over their own behavior. The validity of this statement has been demonstrated by the case of a young woman who, after having recovered from a period of confusion and florid psychosis, thanked her nurse for having set limits on some of her bizarre behavior.

In dealing with *unacceptable behavior,* nurses need to remember some important points. First, is the behavior truly unacceptable? The ability to express negative feelings verbally is a necessary part of living. Verbal expression of anger is more mature and socially acceptable than physical expression of anger. Therefore, the expression of negative feelings, although it can be threatening to the nurse, should be encouraged and supported. Nurses do, however, sometimes need to protect other clients—especially *vulnerable* clients—from verbal abuse.

When behavior is truly *unacceptable* or when *safety* requires that some amount of physical force be used, the least amount possible should be employed. An example of a situation that might prove very distressing to a nurse working with psychiatric clients would be the need for several staff members to restrain a client who simply must be given medication.

A small, frail-looking elderly woman who had a severe heart condition and who was also psychotic was expressing her psychosis with hyperactivity that was threatening her life. Sedation was absolutely necessary; the woman had only recently been admitted, and the behavior was a continuation and escalation of what had been happening at home. Since she refused all medication and exhibited a degree of strength that was extraordinary for her age and size, it was necessary for several staff members to restrain her while an injection was administered.

While it was not possible in this case, many such situations could be avoided through judicious use of medication *before* anxiety has escalated. A cooperative nurse-client relationship that facilitates good communication and close observation can alert staff and client to a build-up of anxiety or aggression that might be alleviated by appropriate use of sedative medication.

The legitimate goals of psychiatric nursing intervention allow for acceptance of individuals as they are and for the fostering of personal growth. Control of behavior, while sometimes necessary, is never completely benign, and it is certainly not one of the main goals.

In interacting and communicating with clients, *nurses use themselves as therapeutic tools.* But they should keep some important points in mind. Responding to clients' emotional or mental problems with an appeal to logic is usually not much help. If clients were able to be logical about their inner turmoil, they probably would not be in the hospital or clinic and under psychiatric care. Murray Bowen (1976), a noted family therapy theorist, points out that persons who are most vulnerable to emotional illness live in a feeling-dominated world in which it is often impossible to distinguish feeling from fact.

Sometimes clients deny or feel guilty about their real feelings. ''They aren't logical'' is a common remark. Allowing for the expression of feelings is probably the best course at such a time. For some clients, the ability to take a more logical stance toward their problems may be a longer-term goal. This is particularly true of acutely ill psychiatric clients.

Giving advice, like appealing to logic, usually is not helpful. If we could simply visit every psychiatric unit and hospital and advise clients of the best courses of action for their future, we could probably empty most of these facilities. Not only is giving advice a naive approach but also it does not allow for differing value systems. It would be better to remember that when people are troubled and looking for answers to their problems, they often have most of those answers inside their own heads. The way to help is to facilitate the process of getting to those answers. This is why *listening* can be such a valuable tool.

The nurse generally should avoid raising client *anxiety levels* unnecessarily. An increase in anxiety level will only exacerbate symptoms, because the symptoms of psychopathology are exaggerations of the normal defense mechanisms used to control anxiety. There are times, however, when some provocation of anxiety may be justified in order to facilitate growth. Encouraging a client to begin to participate in group therapy may be an example of such justified provocation. For clients who have had difficulty learning to relate to others at all and for clients who have never had a "group experience," the thought of participating in a group can be frightening. The nurse can help by *supporting* clients through the necessary stages. Clients can develop increased self-respect and optimism as a result of having accomplished a difficult task.

Support and reassurance, in the situation just described and indeed in any situation, must be given in a realistic manner and with authenticity if they are to be effective. Telling the truth is the best approach; sometimes the amount of information or detail may need to be modified, but for a nurse to lie to clients to protect their self-esteem is not a good idea. For example, a nurse who praises a client falsely or intentionally loses games in order to bolster a client's self-esteem is participating in self-defeating behavior. The client is likely to spot this dishonesty, and it may destroy any trust the client had in the nurse and result in a *decrease* in the client's self-esteem.

In using the nursing process in the psychiatric setting, the nurse often needs to analyze client behavior. The goal of this analysis is to try to understand what clients are attempting to communicate or what some of their needs may be. The analysis is done in the nurse's head, and the behavior should *not* be interpreted to clients. There are several reasons for this:

1. The nurse may indeed be right on target with interpretations that are made to clients, but clients may not be emotionally ready to accept the information or knowledge about their underlying motivations. Information of this kind can exacerbate psychotic or neurotic symptoms.
2. The nurse may be wrong in the interpretation; nurses are not mind readers.
3. Communications that even hint at mind reading are not helpful. Many psychiatric clients have habitually used unclear communication patterns, and verbalized interpretations of their behavior serve to reinforce these faulty communication patterns. In addition, some clients have delusions that other people can read their minds, and it is thus not therapeutic to reinforce these delusions through communications that might suggest mind reading.

Countertransference is a universal phenomenon in helping relationships. It can be a helpful tool in understanding clients, or it can be a significant nursing problem. Countertransference is experienced by the therapist; *transference* is experienced by the client. Both are intrapsychic concepts. Transference, as it occurs in the helping relationship, has been defined as "those feelings and attitudes that were originally experienced with regard to significant others in the past but are now displaced or projected upon the therapist" (Saretsky, 1978). Countertransference has been defined as

. . . the emotional process present in the therapist [that] . . . (1) is in relationship to the patient, (2) has a bearing on the therapeutic process, (3) involves unconscious feelings of the therapist, (4) has a component of conscious or unconscious anxiety, and (5) represents a blending of appropriate, defensive and fixated responses (Eisenbud, 1978)

A nurse must ensure that countertransference becomes an effective agent for, rather than an obstacle to, understanding and relating to a client. A nurse's acceptance and awareness of countertransference are the first steps in avoiding some of its pitfalls. To use the self as a therapeutic tool, one should know as much as possible about the tool. *Reasonable objectivity* is the ideal, but this does not mean cold underinvolvement (what was referred to years ago in nursing as "being professional"). Goldsborough (1969) points out that the therapeutic use of self is not effective unless a nurse is open to involvement and committed to going beyond the imparting of learned skills. Holmes and Werner (1968) see underinvolvement as being as damaging and as useless as overinvolvement. They cite three factors from which underinvolvement may arise: the need of the nurse for a facade, lack of knowledge of how to be effectively therapeutic, and apathy toward and dissatisfaction with one's work.

There is, therefore, an optimum level of involvement between nurses and clients in psychiatric settings. Maintaining that level is rather like walking a tightrope, with overinvolvement on one side and underinvolvement on the other. Perhaps a better way to describe the situation would be to refer to the "art" of psychiatric nursing—this branch of nursing is characterized by a dynamic state of relative equilibrium, as far as involvement with clients is concerned. How does the nurse reach this state of relative equilibrium? One thing that can help is the availability of an objective person with whom the nurse can discuss clinical work and problems—in other words, a person with whom the nurse can establish a supervisory relationship.

The supervisory process

Ideally, anyone involved in therapeutic relationships with psychiatric clients should also be involved in a supervisory relationship. Problems of countertransference, overinvolvement, manipulation, or mutual withdrawal between staff members and clients may all be dealt with through a supervisory process. In addition, increased self-awareness—a necessary and important goal for the nurse working in a psychiatric setting—can be promoted through the supervisory process. It is also helpful to have another source of ideas for modifying a care plan.

The supervisory process can be part of scheduled staff meetings or team conferences, or it can be the focus of separate meetings. Regardless of which format is used, meetings held on a regular basis, with sharing of clinical material and with peer supervision, can help to meet the goals of supervision. Where a fairly open and trusting atmosphere exists, interpersonal conflicts among staff members are appropriate topics for discussion. Otherwise, the effects of staff conflicts may be projected onto clients, and certain clients may even act out some of the conflicts.

Constructive supervision that involves the sharing of information can facilitate a dynamic, creative approach to carrying out the nursing process in a psychiatric setting.

"Do's" of therapeutic communication

It is not uncommon for students or for beginning practitioners to be fearful of "prying" or of "saying the wrong thing." All too often, principles and techniques of interacting abound with "don'ts." *Don't* pry! *Don't* ask questions merely to satisfy your own curiosity! *Don't* give personal information to clients! *Don't* push for too much too soon! Certainly, such don'ts are important to keep in mind, but a therapeutic relationship should not be based solely on them. There are also a great many "do's." During an interaction, it is just as important, if not more important, to be mindful of these positive guidelines. In fact, if nurses can focus on such positive parameters, they may find that they are better able to establish therapeutic relationships and more confident in establishing them. The following are some important "do's" of therapeutic communication:

1. *Do* select a quiet, private area in which to hold interactions. Imagine how it may feel to discuss personal feelings and problems within hearing range of others or in a place subject to frequent intrusion.

2. *Do* provide for comfortable seating arrangements. Standing is not conducive to in-depth interaction. People cannot stand for long in one place without becoming tired and restless. Also, sitting on a bed in a client's room is neither comfortable nor conducive to therapeutic interaction. The nurse should be seated in a chair. This enables the nurse to see the client without staring and without blocking the client's avenue of egress. It is often a good idea to sit down first and let the client arrange his or her chair so that he or she feels comfortable with the seating arrangement. Remember that staring may heighten anxiety. The client is already carrying around enough anxiety. The interview situation should not add to it.

3. *Do* provide an avenue of egress. An already anxious person frequently leaves an interview situation to get a cigarette or a drink of water. Whatever the reason given for a client's physical departure from the interview situation, leaving provides the client with an opportunity to gain both physical and emotional distance from what might be perceived as a stressful situation. Keep in mind that by providing an area of "escape" the nurse is also providing an area of reentry. If a client does not have to climb over people and furniture, he or she is much more likely to return to an interview.

4. *Do* be aware that behavior usually satisfies several needs at the same time. For example, bragging serves to build the braggart's self-esteem, but, by making others feel insecure, it may also serve to manipulate and control people. Eating is

another example of multipurposeful behavior. When people eat during a time of stress (for example, exam week) they may be meeting not only a physiological need but also a psychosocial need. Food symbolizes love and security. From infancy on, many people associate being fed with being cared for. Everyone has a special "security" food. For some, it may be chocolate; for others, warm milk. While eating such foods, people gain a sense of security and well-being.

5. *Do* keep in mind that when people are trying to satisfy a need that is of primary importance to them, they may either ignore or fail to recognize that other needs exist. Many community health nurses have encountered parents who must devote almost all of their time and energy to earning enough money to keep food on the table and a roof over their heads. As a result, these parents may give a lower priority than does the nurse to such preventive health measures as immunizations and annual physical examinations. This is an example of focusing on a felt primary need and ignoring other needs.

6. *Do* recognize that people should be accepted as they are. To accept people as they are means to recognize that they have strengths and weaknesses and positive and negative emotions. For instance, when clients are angry, allow them to express anger. Saying, "Calm down," "Be more rational," or "Put it all in the past and forget it" is not only fruitless but also ignores the reality and importance of their feelings.

7. *Do* allow people to proceed at their own pace. The less threatened people feel, the more quickly rapport can be established. People will also be better able to look at their experiences and to learn from them.

A student nurse had established a pattern of asking a client questions about her family. The student was "pushing" the client to talk about an area that was not of her own choosing. The client would tersely answer these questions and then fall silent.

The student soon became frustrated because the client would not "open up." One day the student developed laryngitis. Student and client agreed they would spend the allotted time sitting together. The student would listen to whatever the client wanted to talk about. Much to the student's amazement, the client began to talk about the difficulties she had experienced on her last weekend pass home!

Once the pressure to talk about traumatic material was lifted, the client was able to discuss areas that were meaningful to her.

8. *Do* observe client behavior. Are clients depressed? Elated? Apathetic? Do they appear alert? Confused? Hyperactive? Pay attention to physical appearance. Are clients appropriately dressed? Bizarrely dressed? Slovenly dressed? Do they hold themselves in a sagging posture? Do they move rigidly? What are their facial expressions? Physical appearance reflects how people feel about themselves. Nurses may learn much about their clients' emotional states by observing behavior and physical appearance.

9. *Do* remember that nonverbal behavior can only be understood in its context and that it may either reinforce or contradict the verbal statements or behaviors of either nurses or clients. Scheflen (1973) found that the following metabehaviors or metacommunications are frequently encountered in psychotherapeutic relationships:

a. Nose wiping. The back of one's index finger is run laterally between one's nostrils and upper lip. This behavior is often used when a person is lying or exaggerating or when a person is monitoring the deviant behavior of another person.

b. Mouth covering. One's hand is placed over one's mouth. This behavior characteristically occurs when a speaker is told to keep quiet or when a person says something that is prohibited or embarassing or that should not have been divulged.

c. Eye covering. The palm of the hand is used to cover the eyes. This behavior may be a monitoring behavior, or it may indicate that a person is trying to understand an idea or gain insight.

d. Eye pointing. The index finger is used to point to one's own eye. This behavior usually tells others to "pay attention."

e. Lint picking. The index finger and thumb are used to pick lint (real or imaginary) off one's clothes. This behavior often signifies that a person is saying something that would normally elicit censure from the lint picker but that, at the time, the lintpicker feels it would be inappropriate to censure the speaker.

f. Looking up. One looks up at the ceiling and then down at an individual. This behavior usually signifies that a person is going to say something that he or she considers significant.

g. Eyebrow raising, shoulder shrugging, deadpan facial expression. These behaviors characteristically are used to discredit unrealistic conceptions.

10. *Do* be consistent when interacting. Consistency facilitates the establishment of security, rapport, and trust in a relationship.

A nurse and a client decided that between 4 PM and 5 PM each day they would talk over the events of the day and assess how the client had dealt with them. One day, the client was particularly talkative and continued talking beyond the agreed-upon limit. The nurse reminded the client of their agreement and helped the client summarize and terminate their conversation.

Thus the nurse was consistent in maintaining the boundaries of their relationship. To talk an hour one day, half an hour the next day, and perhaps 2 hours another day would create an ambience of uncertainty. The client might begin wondering: "What is expected of me? How long will the nurse stay with me today? How much time do I have to discuss my problems?" As such feelings of uncertainty grow, it is very likely that the client will question the nurse's reliability. Certainly, if a particular need arose, a nurse and a client might agree to extend their time together. By doing so, they would be acknowledging that the situation warranted an exception to their usual arrangement. By maintaining the boundaries of the relationship, consistency and trust are reinforced rather than undermined.

11. *Do* try to keep client anxiety to a minimum. High anxiety decreases one's ability to perceive, and learning is less likely to occur. The nurse needs to help clients decrease their anxiety. Altering the environment may have a therapeutic effect. By controlling the noise level and avoiding overcrowding, the nurse can make the environment less stressful. For instance, in a crowded unit, it is important to provide a quiet area. It is not uncommon for very anxious individuals in a psychiatric unit to request some time in a seclusion room. The individuals recognize that by limiting external stimuli they may decrease their stress levels. A nurse's availability to anxious clients so they can verbalize their concerns may also help reduce anxiety. Finally, a nurse should remember that physical activity, such as gardening and participating in sports, serves to dissipate anxious energy and to help anxious individuals feel more comfortable.

12. *Do* explain routines and procedures in terms that people can understand. A nurse needs to assess the levels of anxiety and levels of understanding of clients, evaluate the influence of past experiences, and explain technical terminology. For example, when a nurse is establishing a therapeutic relationship, a client's past experiences with psychotherapy may have a great influence on the client's present experience. If a client has participated in a relationship in which a nurse pushed the discussion into an area that the client was not yet ready to explore, the client may be reluctant to enter into a new therapeutic relationship. In addition, if a nurse orients a client to the purpose of a therapeutic relationship by saying, "We are entering into a one-to-one relationship, and you can discuss your problems during these interviews,"

the client may hesitate to talk with the nurse for several reasons. The client may not understand what is meant by a "one-to-one relationship." The client may associate the word "interview" with probing questions. The client may be frightened by the focus on "problems." The client may feel that he or she does not have enough "problems" to fill up the "interview" time. When a nurse explains that during an interaction clients may discuss anything that is of interest or concern in their daily lives, the nurse is using vocabulary that is more understandable and less threatening.

13. *Do* offer clients realistic reassurance. To give false reassurance or to reassure clients before their situation has been explored blocks communication. For example, to reassure a crying person that everything will be "all right" before you know why the person is crying cuts off communication. To tell someone who has had mutilating surgery, "Things will look brighter once you get out of the hospital" is to deny that there will be difficult times ahead. By acknowledging that there will be some difficult times but that rehabilitation and psychotherapy will help with readjustment, a nurse offers realistic reassurance. The nurse thereby provides clients with opportunities to explore their concerns and also points out treatment modalities that will assist them in dealing with the stress caused by their situations.

14. *Do* remember that there is always potential for growth. There are no "hopeless," "hardcore" individuals. People who do not show progress or seem resistant to therapy may not yet be ready to change. Readiness to profit from therapy is not much different from readiness to learn how to walk or talk. People must see a need for change before change can take place. Also, it is possible that the staff may need additional knowledge of therapeutic tools to help clients work through difficulties. If client and nurse are ready and able to grasp an opportunity for therapy, there is potential for growth.

The process of therapeutic communication focuses on client experience. By helping clients to learn more appropriate and effective coping behavior, nurses encourage them to move beyond mere tolerance of a stressful situation to understanding and profiting from it.

Barriers to therapeutic communication

Up to now we have primarily concentrated on the unimpeded process of therapeutic communication. Therapeutic principles have functioned as guides to effective interaction. However, the process does not necessarily progress from stage to stage without some difficulties being encountered. Difficulties may arise out of characteristics of the client, the nurse, or both. We will describe some of the most frequently encountered barriers to the therapeutic process. It is important to note that these barriers are not restricted to the therapeutic process; they may be found in any situation in which two or more people interact.

EGOCENTRISM

Egocentrism is the attitude that one's own mode of living, values, and patterns of adaptation are superior to all others. This attitude is often accompanied by contempt for life-styles that differ from one's own. Egocentrism tends to manifest itself in superior, proselytizing, moralizing, rejecting, hostile, or aggressive behavior.

When a nurse and a client have different values, especially if one or both are unaware of how strongly they are influenced by these values, conflict may result.

A community health nurse had been visiting the Smith household to assist Mrs. Smith in the care of her 72-year-old mother-in-law. The mother-in-law had suffered a stroke that had left her aphasic and that had paralyzed her right side. After several weeks, Mrs. Smith confided to the nurse that she found it very time consuming and fatiguing to take care of her mother-in-law. Mrs. Smith said, "My primary responsibility is to my husband and children, and now I feel like I have no time or energy left for them." She feared that the strain was also

being reflected in her children. She pointed out that her 5-year-old son had begun bedwetting and that her 8-year-old daughter, complaining of stomach aches, had seen the school nurse three times in the past 2 weeks. Mrs. Smith said that she and her husband were considering placing her mother-in-law in a nursing home.

The nurse had strong feelings about the duty of children to care for their aged parents. In fact, he came from a family background that regarded it as disgraceful to place parents in a nursing home. He responded to Mrs. Smith, "Oh, that would be such a shame. I'm sure you'll be able to manage once you get a routine. After all, you have to remember that you're setting an example for your children. The way you treat your mother-in-law is probably the way your children will treat you when you're older."

The community health nurse inadvertently was imposing his values on the client.

Sometimes it is the client's values and attitudes that function as a barrier to therapeutic interaction.

Marcia Henderson, 22 years old, went to a neighborhood mental health center for counseling. Ms. Henderson complained of feeling "tired and sad." She added that she cried easily and had no appetite. During a subsequent session, Ms. Henderson asked the nurse, "What is your religion?" The nurse responded, "Catholic. Why do you ask?" Ms. Henderson replied, "Oh, no reason, I'm just nosey I guess." At the following session, Ms. Henderson requested another nurse, explaining, "I'm living with a man whom I have no intentions of marrying. I can't talk about this to someone who's Catholic. I don't want any moralizing at my expense."

The client's values and attitudes led her to assume that the nurse would pass judgment on her. The client erected a barrier to the therapeutic process and terminated the relationship.

Thus problems may arise when a nurse and a client have different value systems. Conflict is especially apt to result when participants are unaware of the influence their values exert on them. Even the most self-aware people have values that operate outside their full awareness. Only as nurse and client become more aware of the values that influence their thoughts and feelings can they begin to free themselves from subjectivity and to accept that another person's value system can be adaptive. (See Chapters 4 and 6 for discussion of attitudes.) Egocentrism then ceases to exist as a barrier to effective communication, and nurse and client can begin to set mutually agreed-upon goals.

DENIAL

Denial is the unconscious evasion or negation of objective reality. Denial functions to reduce anxiety, to stabilize and define relationships, and to retain or regain a sense of autonomy.

When either nurse or client uses denial, a barrier to the therapeutic process is erected. Eventually, the nondenying participant becomes bored, frustrated, or angry with the other's systematic avoidance of certain topics and may respond either by ignoring the pattern of denial or by confronting the use of denial. Ignoring the pattern of denial serves to reinforce its use. Confronting denial too early or too severely almost certainly will threaten the denying individual, provoke anger in the individual, and cause the individual to try to cope with reality by further reliance on denial. The therapeutic process then becomes characterized by anxiety.

A student nurse, Marty Hendricks, was working with Julie, a verbally and physically abusive adolescent girl. Without any observable warning, Julie would suddenly lash out at people. Recently she had severely scratched her psychiatrist's face.

During supervisory conferences, Marty consistently assured his instructor that he felt comfortable in Julie's presence, that he trusted Julie, and that he did not think Julie would strike out at him. The more his instructor questioned him about his feelings, the more adamantly he asserted that he was unafraid. The instructor believed that Marty was denying reality and decided to stop challenging his description of his feelings and instead to be in-

creasingly supportive of him during this experience. As Marty began to feel more comfortable with his instructor and less threatened by possible recriminations from her, he began to talk about how he felt "uneasy" with Julie.

Thus, challenging people's use of denial can cause them to feel threatened and to rely increasingly on denial as a way to cope with reality. When attempts are made to alleviate the anxiety underlying denial, the need to use denial usually decreases.

RESISTANCE

Resistance is conscious or unconscious reluctance to bring repressed ideas, thoughts, desires, or memories into awareness. By preventing the entry of such threatening material into consciousness, resistance functions to maintain an individual's security or self-esteem.

Therapeutic intervention involves helping clients explore experiences that are of concern to them. If clients try to avoid material that threatens their self systems, attempts to help them verbalize feelings, evaluate patterns of behavior, or examine interpersonal relationships may be met by resistance. Should a nurse fail to recognize clients' use of resistance and try to force them to talk about painful areas from which they feel a need to retreat, the nurse may only succeed in increasing their anxiety.

Peter Mulally had been experiencing auditory hallucinations. The nurse assigned to work with Peter noticed that whenever she questioned him about the content of these hallucinations, he would change the subject. The nurse became very impatient with his behavior and began pressuring him to talk about the hallucinations, explaining, "I can't help you unless I know what's troubling you." Peter began rocking back and forth in his chair. Instead of changing the subject, he got up and walked away.

Resistive behavior, then, can escalate when a nurse does not recognize that resistance is being used to avoid extremely anxiety-producing material. Had the nurse allowed the client to retreat from the areas that were painful to him, the client's anxiety might have decreased rather than increased. At the same time, the nurse would have contributed to an atmosphere of trust. The client might eventually have felt free to explore threatening material without fearing loss of security or self-esteem.

The use of resistance is not restricted to clients. Sometimes nurses use resistance.

Joan Bellows, a student nurse, was consistently absent the last day of each clinical experience. During her community mental health experience, her instructor pointed this pattern out to her. Joan responded, "I'm coming down with a cold and don't want to talk about it right now." The instructor said, "Maybe you'll feel like discussing it some other time."

As the day for terminating with her client approached, Joan's instructor again pointed out her habit of being absent on the last day of each clinical experience. Joan explained, "One time I was sick. Another time I had car trouble—and the last time the alarm clock didn't ring and I overslept." The instructor replied, "Sometimes good-byes are difficult to say."

The next time Joan and her instructor discussed Joan's plans for termination with her client, Joan began to cry. She explained that she never could say good-bye to anyone and would do anything to avoid good-byes. She was ready to talk about an area that until then had been too painful to explore.

Given an accepting relationship, individuals can be helped to deal with previously resisted material. By gradually calling attention to their resistive behavior and slowly and nonjudgmentally exploring or pointing out possible reasons for the behavior, a nurse can facilitate the resolution of resistance. Individuals can then begin to deal with the threatening material. It is important to remember that since resistance is a mechanism used to maintain secur-

ity and self-esteem, attempts should not be made to pointedly confront people using resistance or to argue them out of resistance.

• • •

Characteristics of the client, of the nurse, or of both may set up barriers to the therapeutic process. Egocentrism, denial, and resistance are three frequently encountered barriers. However, they need not be insurmountable. If they are recognized and understood, steps can be taken toward resolution of the difficulties and reestablishment of the therapeutic process.

Listening is essential for effective communication. Listening requires moving beyond the words used in order to hear the meaning or messages (themes) being conveyed. In the process of therapeutic communication the focus is on the client's experience as the client perceives it. Client and nurse become actively involved in moving beyond mere tolerance of the experience and toward an increased understanding of the situation and a plan for developing appropriate and effective coping behavior. During this exploration, some barriers to therapeutic communication may arise. Once these barriers have been understood, they can be surmounted and therapeutic communication can be reestablished.

CHAPTER SUMMARY

Therapeutic communication involves more than learning a group of interviewing skills. It involves understanding the process of communication and the role that nurse and client play in establishing and maintaining therapeutic communication. The focus of therapeutic communication is the client's here-and-now experience. The task of the nurse is to sustain the client in that experience. The nurse and the client actively explore the client's experiences within the framework of the nursing process. The cultural backgrounds of nurse and client affect their perceptions and interpretations of experiences, their responses to experiences, and their responses to communication cues.

Many factors may influence therapeutic communication and the ability of nurses to sustain clients in their experiences. Chief among these factors are behavioral concepts relating to sexuality, privacy, humor, empathy, and touching. With this knowledge, barriers to effective communication may be avoided and therapeutic communication may be promoted.

SENSITIVITY-AWARENESS EXERCISES

The purposes of these exercises are to:

- Develop insight into some of your own customs and communication behaviors
- Develop awareness of the customs and communication behaviors of others
- Develop sensitivity to differences in customs and communication behaviors that may contribute to culture shock in immigrants and culture conflict in ethnic Americans
- Develop awareness of the impact of culture on the nurse-client relationship

1. Look at the kinesic and proxemic patterns used by you and your family in the following situations:
   a. At the dinner table
   b. Standing and conversing
   c. Sitting and conversing
   Especially note interpersonal distances maintained, how territorial boundaries are established and acknowledged, and the degree to which gestures and touching are used.
2. When conversing with your family or friends, alter your usual kinesic and proxemic patterns in the following ways: use more gesturing and touching; use less gesturing and touching; increase your interpersonal space by 6 inches; decrease your interpersonal space by 6 inches.
   a. How did you feel with each of the above alterations in your usual nonverbal communication pattern?
   b. How did the people with whom you were conversing react? (For example, they tried to reestablish spatial distance; they withdrew when you tried to touch them; they moved further away to give you more room to gesture.)
   c. Ask the people with whom you were interacting how they felt.
   d. What cultural factors might have influenced the reactions and feelings of the people with whom you were interacting?
3. Role play that you are visiting a foreign country. You become ill and you go to a hospital. You are not familiar with the language or customs of the country. Try to make your symptoms or discomfiture known to the "health practitioners" without using verbal language. Remember that your life may depend on your ability to make yourself understood. At the end of 5 minutes, look at:
   a. Your feelings during the experience
   b. The behavior you demonstrated
   c. The behavior and reactions of the "health practitioner." Ask the "health practitioner" what his or her feelings were.
   Now reverse roles and reenact the exercise. How do reactions compare with the first enactment?
4. Examine a relationship that you have established with a client. Look at the effects that attitudes about sexuality, privacy, humor, empathy, and touching have on the relationship.
5. Analyze and describe how your cultural background (for example, ethnicity, religion) influences or may influence your perception, interpretation, and response in such health-related experiences as physical illness, emotional illness, and hospitalization. How might your perception, interpretation, and response affect your ability to sustain clients having similar experiences?

REFERENCES

Abeles, J.H.
   1982 "Letters." The Sciences 22:3.
Altman, I.
   1975 The Environment and Social Behavior: Privacy, Personal Space, Territory, Crowding. Monterey: Brooks/Cole Publishing Co.
Altman, I., P.A. Nelson, and E.E. Lett
   1972 The Ecology of Home Environments. Catalog of Selected Documents in Psychology 2:65.
American Nurses Association Division on Psychiatric and Mental Health Nursing Practice
   1982 Standards of Psychiatric and Mental Health Nursing Practice. Kansas City: ANA Publications.

Ashcraft, N., and A.E. Sheflen
1976 People Space: The Making and Breaking of Human Boundaries. Garden City, N.Y.: Anchor Press/ Doubleday.

Atkinson, L., and M.E. Murphy
1980 Understanding the Nursing Process. New York: MacMillan, Inc.

Blondis, M.N., and B.E. Jackson
1982 Nonverbal Communication with Patients: Back to the Human Touch. New York: John Wiley & Sons, Inc.

Bowen, M.
1976 "Theory in the practice of psychotherapy." In Family Therapy. P.J. Guerin (ed.). New York: Gardner Press, Inc.

Bradley, J.C., and M.A. Edinberg
1982 Communication in Nursing. New York: Appleton-Century-Crofts.

Brammer, L.M., and E.L. Shostrom
1982 Therapeutic Psychology: Fundamentals of Counseling and Psychotherapy. Englewood Cliffs, N.J.: Prentice-Hall, Inc.

Cousins, N.
1979 Anatomy of an Illness as Perceived by the Patient: Reflections on Healing and Regeneration. New York: W.W. Norton & Co., Inc.

DuBois, R.
1979 "Introduction." In Anatomy of an Illness as Perceived by the Patient: Reflections on Healing and Regeneration. N. Cousins. New York: W.W. Norton & Co., Inc.

Eisenbud, R.
1978 "Countertransference." In Psychoanalytic Psychotherapy. G. Goldman and D. Milman (eds.). Reading, Mass.: Addison-Wesley Publishing Co., Inc.

Fiedler, F.E.
1950 "The concept of an ideal therapeutic relationship." Journal of Consulting Psychology 14:339-345.

Fiedler, F.E., and K. Senior
1952 "An exploratory study of unconscious feeling reactions in fifteen patient-therapist pairs." Journal of Abnormal Social Psychology 47:446-453.

Forsyth, G.
1980 "Analysis of the concept of empathy: illustration of one approach." Advances in Nursing Science 2:33-42.

Freud, S.
1961 "Jokes and their relation to the unconscious." In The Complete Psychological Works of Sigmund Freud (orig. 1928). J. Strachey (ed.). London: Hogarth Press.

Gendlin, E.
1962 Experiencing and the Creation of Meaning. New York: The Free Press.

Gilmore, M.M., and D.D. Gilmore
1979 "'Machismo': A psychodynamic approach (Spain)." Journal of Psychological Anthropology 2:281-299.

Goldsborough, J.
1969 "Involvement." American Journal of Nursing 69:65-68.

Goldstein, J.H.
1982 "A laugh a day—Can mirth keep disease at bay?" The Sciences 22:21-25.

Goodman, M.E., and A. Beman
1968 "Child's eye-views of life in an urban barrio." In Spanish-Speaking People in the United States. J. Helm (ed.). Seattle: University of Washington Press.

Hall, E.T.
1959 The Silent Language. New York: Fawcett World Library.
1969 The Hidden Dimension. Garden City, N.Y.: Doubleday & Co., Inc.

Harris, T.
1969 I'm OK—You're OK. New York: Grossman Publishers.

Heine, R.W.
1950 An Investigation of the Relationship Between Change in Personality from Psychotherapy as Reported by Patients and the Factors Seen by Patients as Producing Change. Ph.D. dissertation, University of Chicago.

Holmes, M., and J. Werner
1968 Psychiatric Nursing in a Therapeutic Community. New York: MacMillan, Inc.

Hsu, F.L.K.
1970 Americans and Chinese: Reflections on Two Cultures and Their People. Garden City: Doubleday Natural History Press.

Kira, A.
1970 "The bathroom." In Environmental Psychology: Man and His Physical Setting. W.H. Ittelson and L. Rivlin (eds.). New York: Holt, Rinehart & Winston.

Kutsche, P.
1968 "The Anglo side of acculturation." In Spanish-Speaking People in the United States. J. Helm (ed.). Seattle: University of Washington Press.

LaMonica, E.L.
1979 The Nursing Process. Reading, Mass.: Addison-Wesley Publishing Co., Inc.

Lorenz, K.
1966 On Aggression. M.K. Wilson (trans.). New York: Harcourt, Brace & World, Inc., p. 294.

Luft, J.
1950 "Implicit Hypotheses and clinical predictions." Journal of Abnormal Social Psychology 45:756-759.

Maslow, A.H.
1967 "A theory of metamotivation: the biological roots of the value of life." Journal of Humanistic Psychology 7:93-127.

Matheney, R., and M. Topalis
1965 Psychiatric Nursing (ed. 4). St. Louis: The C.V. Mosby Co.

Milgram, S.
1970 "The experience of living in cities." Science 167: 1461-1468.

Montagu, A.
1971 Touching: The Human Significance of the Skin. New York: Harper & Row, Publishers, Inc.

Moody, R.A., Jr.
1978 Laugh After Laugh: The Healing Power of Humor. Jacksonville, Fla.: Headwaters Press.

Murillo-Rhode, I.
1976 "Family life among mainland Puerto Ricans in New York City slums." Perspectives in Psychiatric Care 14: 174-179.

National Council of State Boards of Nursing, Inc.
1980 National Council Licensure Examination for Registered Nurses. Chicago: The Council.

Otto, H.
1978 The New Sex Education. Chicago: Follett Publishing Co.

Paredes, A.
1968 "Folk medicine and the intercultural jest." In Spanish-Speaking People in the United States. J. Helm (ed.). Seattle: University of Washington Press.

Pasquali, E.A.
1980 "Comic strips in the classroom." In Teaching Tomorrow's Nurse: A Nurse Educator Reader. S.K. Mirin (ed.). Wakefield, Mass.: Nursing Resources, Inc.
1982 Assimilation and Acculturation of Cubans on Long Island. Ph.D. dissertation, State University of New York at Stony Brook.

Peplau, H.
1953 "Themes in nursing situations." American Journal of Nursing 53:1221.
1954 "Utilizing themes in nursing situations." American Journal of Nursing 54:325.

Porter, E.H., Jr.
1949 "Understanding diagnostically and understanding therapeutically." In Trends in Personnel Work. F.C. Wil-liamson (ed.). Minneapolis: University of Minnesota Press.
1950 An Introduction to Therapeutic Counseling. Boston: Houghton Mifflin Co.

Radcliffe-Brown, A.R.
1952 Structure and Function in Primitive Society. New York: The Free Press.

Raskin, N.
1974 Studies on Psychotherapeutic Orientation. AAP Psychotherapy Research Monograph. Orlando, Fla: American Academy of Psychotherapy.

Robinson, V.M.
1970 "Humor in nursing." In Behavioral Concepts and Nursing Intervention. C.E. Carlson (ed.). Philadelphia: J.B. Lippincott Co.

Rogers, C.R.
1942 Counseling and Psychotherapy. Boston: Houghton Mifflin Co.

Saretsky, L.
1978 "Transference." In Psychoanalytic Psychotherapy. G. Goldman and D. Milman (eds.). Reading, Mass.: Addison-Wesley Publishing Co., Inc.

Sayre, J.
1978 "Common errors in communication made by students in psychiatric nursing." Perspectives in Psychiatric Care 4:175-183.

Scheflen, A.E.
1973 Communicational Structure: Analysis of a Psychotherapy Transaction. Bloomington: Indiana University Press.

Scheflen, A.E., and A. Scheflen
1972 Body Language and Social Order. Englewood Cliffs, N.J.: Prentice-Hall, Inc.

Truax, C.B., and R.R. Carkhuff
1964 "The old and the new: theory and research in counseling and psychotherapy." Personality and Guidance Journal 42:860-866.

Ujhely, G.
1968 Determinants of the Nurse-Patient Relationship. New York: Springer Publishing Co., Inc.

Westin, A.
1970 Privacy and Freedom. New York: Atheneum.

Whipple, B., and R. Gick
1980 "A holistic view of sexuality-education for the health professional." Topics in Clinical Nursing 1:91-98.

Woods, N.F.
1984 Human Sexuality in Health and Illnes (ed. 3). St. Louis: The C.V. Mosby Co.

ANNOTATED SUGGESTED READINGS

Blondis, M.N., and B.E. Jackson

1982 Nonverbal Communication with Patients: Back to the Human Touch. New York: John Wiley & Sons, Inc.

The authors discuss the role that nonverbal communication plays in nurse-client interaction. Special attention is given to the interpretation of nonverbal cues and to the use of nonverbal techniques for more effective nurse-client interaction. Included in the book are such topics as pediatrics and parenting, sexual behaviors, geriatrics, death and dying, crisis intervention, and the nursing process.

Bradley, J.C., and M.A. Edinberg

1982 Communication in Nursing. New York: Appleton-Century-Crofts.

This book takes both an experiential and a theoretical approach to nurse-client interaction. Vignettes and verbatim excerpts of conversations illustrate topics dealt with, such as interviewing techniques, communication stalls, and empathy. Situations and suggestions that facilitate experiential learning are included.

Sayre, J.

1978 "Common errors in communication made by students in psychiatric nursing." Perspectives in Psychiatric Care 4:175-183.

Sayre discusses errors in communications that are frequently made by students and that impede therapeutic intervention. The author takes a chronological approach, identifying communication errors that may occur in the orientation, working, and termination stages of a relationship. Verbatim transcripts of student-client interaction exemplify the communication errors being discussed.

Scheflen, A.E.

1973 Communicational Structure: Analysis of a Psychotherapy Transaction. Bloomington: Indiana University Press.

Scheflen explains that the interpersonal processes of therapeutic relationships can be analyzed using a behavioral systems approach, with emphasis on nonverbal behavior. Diagrams of communicative positions and verbatim transcripts of a filmed psychotherapy session illustrate the points Dr. Scheflen makes in this context analysis.

FURTHER READINGS

Boucher, M.L.
  1971 "Personal space and chronicity in the mental hospital."
      Perspectives in Psychiatric Care 9:206-210.
Carlson, C.E. (ed.)
  1970 Behavioral Concepts and Nursing Intervention. Phila-
      delphia: J.B. Lippincott Co.
Gerber, C.B., and D.F. Snyder
  1970 "Language and thought." Perspectives in Psychiatric
      Care 8:230-237.

Greiner, D. (ed.)
  1979 Topics in Clinical Nursing. Communication (entire is-
      sue) 1:1-112.
Haveliwala, Y.A., A.E. Scheflen, and N. Ashcraft
  1979 Common Sense in Therapy. New York: Brunner/
      Mazel, Inc.
Sarles, H.B.
  1970 "Communication and ethology." In Anthropology and
      the Behavioral and Health Sciences. O. von Mering and
      L. Kasdan (eds.). Pittsburgh: University of Pittsburgh
      Press.
Scheflen, A.E.
  1963 "Communication and regulation in psychotherapy."
      Psychiatry 26:126-136.

UNIT III

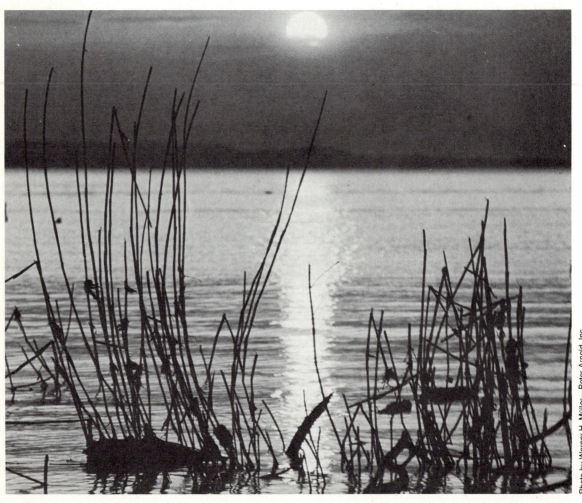

Therapeutic settings and modalities

This unit focuses on types of therapeutic settings and modalities. Chapter 10 introduces the concept of the therapeutic milieu and discusses the interrelated and sometimes overlapping roles and functions of the members of the mental health team. The role of the nurse is explored, and, in keeping with the holistic health approach of this book, the client is viewed as an integral part of the mental health team.

Chapters 11, 12, and 13 focus upon nursing functions in relation to group therapy, family therapy, and crisis intervention. In Chapter 14, community mental health services are presented as a system of interacting health and welfare subsystems. These subsystems are oriented toward a defined community, or catchment area. It is emphasized that community mental health services not only should address the psychosocial needs of the community served but also should consider the sociocultural background of its residents. The history and the current status of the community mental health movement are explored. In addition, the organization of community mental health services is discussed in terms of primary, secondary, and tertiary prevention, and the roles and functions of community mental health nurses are described.

CHAPTER 10

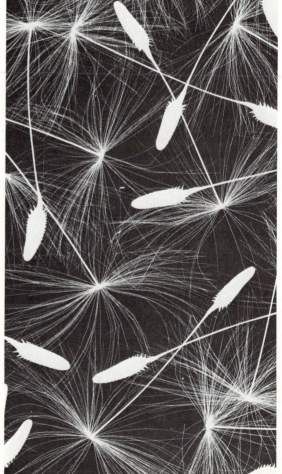

Photo by Werner H. Müller—Peter Arnold, Inc.

The therapeutic milieu

CHAPTER FOCUS

In addition to individual-relationship therapy, the nurse who works in a psychiatric setting is usually involved in important elements of milieu therapy. According to Fann and Goshen (1977), milieu therapy is "a therapeutic approach to hospital psychiatry in which the entire hospital environment is designed to facilitate rehabilitation. This includes occupational therapy, recreational therapy, team approach, work assignments and education of all who work in the hospital and participate in the care of patients." Although Fann and Goshen specify a hospital setting, milieu therapy can also be provided in various outpatient settings.

While professional nurses carry the greatest responsibility for maintaining a therapeutic milieu, they work cooperatively with other members of the interdisciplinary health team. In working as collaborative members of interdisciplinary teams, nurses find that their functions and responsibilities overlap or even duplicate those of other team members. Because of the nature of nursing education and clinical nursing experience, nurses bring some unique attributes and abilities to team participation. Health teaching from a holistic point of view is a prime example. In psychiatric settings the natural tendency is to focus on psychosocial problems. But a human being is also a biological organism. The nurse, with knowledge of physiology, psychology, sociology, nutrition, pharmacology, and health in general, can be the catalyst that helps the team members to approach the client as a whole person. In addition, nurses are the only professional members of the team who are always present in the milieu—24 hours a day, 7 days a week. Indeed, maintenance of the therapeutic milieu is the responsibility of the nurse. Thus the nurse can be instrumental in managing the milieu in a way that facilitates a consistent progression in the psychosocial growth of the client.

The mental health team within a therapeutic milieu differs from the traditional hierarchical or authoritarian structure found in many health facilities, in which decisions are made at the top and passed down through lines of authority. In the mental health team concept, authority and accountability are shared by team members, although the responsibilities that define professional practice are retained by the specific professionals. The client is considered to be an important, participating member of the team; the "community meeting" or "staff-client meeting" is one vehicle for accomplishing this in a therapeutic milieu. The mental health team and these concepts are briefly discussed in this chapter.

Treatment modalities that may be integral parts of milieu therapy include art, music, poetry, movement therapy, and psychodrama. These sometimes adjunctive therapies will be discussed in this chapter. Individual, family, and group therapy—also crucial elements of a milieu—are discussed in subsequent chapters.

HISTORY AND DESCRIPTION

"Milieu" is the French word for "middle" or "middle place"; in English we use it to mean "environment."

Milieu therapy implies use of the *whole environment* as a therapeutic agent—hence Maxwell Jones' term "the therapeutic community."

A useful definition of milieu therapy is "scientific manipulation of the environment aimed at providing changes in the personality of the patient" (Cumming and Cumming, 1962).

The concept of therapeutic community, or milieu, therapy is a spin-off of Maxwell Jones' work (1953) in Britain. Jones, a Scottish psychiatrist who has also done a great deal of work in America, developed a treatment modality that uses the environment—its physical facilities, various therapies, and interpersonal relationships—to foster a healthy personality. A therapeutic community is a protective setting. It provides relationships that will help its residents learn more effective and more socially acceptable means of coping. The therapeutic community becomes a microcosm of society. The individual is made to look at how he interacts and functions in this small and specially structured segment of society. Individuals who are acting out their inner conflicts are confronted by the entire community with their hostility, alien-

ation, manipulation, insensitivity, lack of responsibility, and poor judgment.

UNDERLYING ASSUMPTIONS

Maxwell Jones outlined what he saw as five basic principles of a therapeutic community:
1. Responsibility for treatment belongs not only to physician and staff but also to the residents.
2. Social distance between staff and residents is reduced; this may permit free discussion of the behavior of staff members as well as the behavior of residents.
3. A democratic atmosphere is cultivated.
4. Open communication in the form of shared feelings and information is strongly encouraged.
5. Deviant behavior is controlled and social learning takes place through the mechanism of resident-staff meetings (Erikson, 1982).

Skinner (1979) has further delineated the underlying assumptions of a therapeutic community:
1. Staff members focus on residents' assets in order to encourage growth.
2. Each interpersonal interaction is seen as an

opportunity to improve communication skills.

3. Participation in unit government provides (a) a vehicle for helping clients to meet their needs for autonomy and (b) a structure for meeting the needs of the group as a whole.
4. Individuals are responsible for their own actions.
5. Peer pressure is the medium through which the community itself develops and which enforces community behavioral norms.
6. Inappropriate behaviors are examined and dealt with as they occur.
7. Group discussion and the use of temporary seclusion (this only when the rights of others are in jeopardy) are techniques that are favored over punishment and restriction.

A therapeutic community is characterized by a team approach. Residents are part of the team and share in the responsibility and the process of decision making. They are included in the planning and implementation of treatment approaches and in the evaluation and reevaluation of their effectiveness. All aspects of the therapeutic community are seen as presenting opportunities for residents to examine their behavior and, when indicated, to grow in the direction of more socially acceptable behavior. There are three phases to treatment in a therapeutic community:

1. Adjustment to the setting
2. Observation, examination, and discussion (often confrontation) of adaptive and maladaptive responses (socially acceptable and unacceptable behavior)
3. Development of new, socially acceptable patterns of coping and communicating

Residents are included in all phases of treatment (both planning and implementation). Many different types of therapy may be used to facilitate change in behavior: encounter therapy, sociodrama, recreational and work activities, educational therapy, and community government.

Community government is an outstanding characteristic of a therapeutic community. Jones (1953) and Cumming and Cumming (1962) view community government as a primary means of implementing the goals of milieu therapy. Meetings are used to inculcate the social standards, values, and behavior that may never have been internalized by acting-out individuals. Community government provides opportunities to explore behavior, try out new roles, make decisions, and engage in problem solving. In the process, group identification is fostered.

Late one afternoon, Jean was admitted to a therapeutic community that worked with drug abusers. After a brief orientation to the house in which the community members lived, Jean was introduced to the residents and staff. Then she was shown to the room that she would share with two other girls. Jean settled in, had dinner, and then attended a group "sing." Residents played guitars, sang, and generally had fun. After the sing, Jean was told to help others clean up. She was directed, rather than asked, to take some responsibility for the evening's recreation. After helping with the clean-up she went to bed.

At 6 o'clock the following morning, a bell rang. The residents got up and busied themselves with washing, dressing, and straightening their rooms. During orientation Jean had been told that unless her section of the room passed morning inspection, she would not be able to join others at breakfast. Jean was hungry, so she quickly tidied up her dresser and made her bed. Then she went down to breakfast.

After breakfast, everyone attended a community government meeting. The "president" presided. He led a discussion of jobs that needed to be done in the house, activities that had to be planned, and problems that had arisen. Then he read a list of names of people who had been repeatedly ignoring rules. Each person was permitted to speak in his own defense. However, if he attempted to rationalize or manipulate he was "blown away." This means that in front of the entire group one of the several staff members who had formerly been addicts would verbally attack the offender's behavior. Then the community would decide how to handle the situation. It is important to emphasize that the person's behavior, not the person himself, was at-

tacked. Next, the president read the names of those residents whose behavior had improved and who were eligible for privileges. The entire group, including the person under consideration, decided whether privileges had been earned. Then work assignments were made. The community's house was run entirely by the staff and the residents. Community members were assigned to groups for cooking, doing laundry, shopping, and housekeeping. Jean was assigned to the housekeeping group.

Thus the residents are fully involved in every aspect of life in a therapeutic community. From the very first, Jean was included in the routine and incorporated into the process of community socialization.

According to one writer (Abroms, 1969) the goals of milieu therapy are the same as those of any other form of psychiatric care: to *set limits* on symptomatic behavior and to foster the learning of some basic *psychosocial skills*.

Psychosocial skills

Abroms has organized the teaching of psychosocial skills into four broad categories: orientation, self-assertion, occupational activities, and recreational activities.

Orientation can be as basic as the adjustment to time, place, and person that is necessary for a confused person. It can be as general or as extensive as the fostering of an understanding of the workings of an institution's social system, which would be appropriate to a tertiary-care, transitional-service setting.

Self-assertion implies the learning or relearning of direct, self-regulated ways of expressing feelings or attitudes—for example, learning to "talk it out" in the encounter groups of a therapeutic milieu for drug abusers. The adoption of such socially accepted behavior is evidence of growth from a stage in which chemical substances were used to avoid the pain of interpersonal relationships.

Occupational activities can include the learning

of basic skills for managing one's life, such as the ability to adhere to a schedule. These activities may also include formal occupational or vocational counseling, training, and placement.

Recreational activities are important to help clients develop the ability to engage in various leisure pursuits, to enjoy them, and to cooperate with others in enjoying them. The development of such ability helps to increase a client's self-confidence and self-esteem.

Setting limits

In discussing the types of behavior that necessitate the setting of limits, Abroms describes "five Ds" of pathology and lists them in order of decreasing severity:

1. *Destructiveness*—suicide, homicide, and other forms of behavior that harm persons or property
2. *Disorganization*—for example, the autistic and bizarre behavior and thinking of an acutely psychotic person
3. *Deviancy*—for example, acting-out behavior, illegal activities, and rule breaking
4. *Dysphoria*—for example, depression, hypochondriasis, schizoid detachment, elation, obsessions, and phobias
5. *Dependency*—avoiding responsibility for one's own feelings, thoughts, and actions

---

PHYSICAL STRUCTURE OF A THERAPEUTIC MILIEU

Structure and physical surroundings are important in enhancing therapy—ideal hospitals and units are set up in such a way as to provide a homelike, attractively decorated setting for the clients. Nursing stations are open and accessible and are not "cages" where staff members can retreat and withdraw from clients. The use of street clothes instead of uniforms by staff members has been part of the effort to minimize interpersonal barriers between staff and clients. The present-day architecture of psychiatric settings has the same purpose. Furniture is arranged to promote increased socialization among clients and between clients and staff. Fortunately, the large, barren day room with chairs rigidly placed against the wall has, for the most part, disappeared. Safety is considered without the obvious accoutrements of an old-style "asylum." For example, instead of barred windows, the newer facilities use a special break-proof glass in a tamper-proof window. Rooms are designed with the goal of maximum utility. Pleasant day rooms convert from sitting rooms to dining rooms to recreation rooms to group therapy rooms. Often the clients' bedrooms are designed to look more like comfortable and attractive motel rooms than hospital "sick rooms." Children's psychiatric facilities are designed in family-type arrangements—units are set up to resemble a home living situation as closely as possible, with a central living room, a kitchen, several bedrooms, and an outside yard.

PROGRAM OF A THERAPEUTIC MILIEU

Several important elements may be, and usually are, integral parts of the program of a therapeutic milieu:

1. Some form of *self-government*. Self-government can be accomplished in the form of structured meetings such as client-staff meetings, large community meetings, and clients' business meetings. An expectation in many facilities is that patients or residents will have some input into all of the unit activities. Some units expect clients to participate in team decisions about their fellow residents, around such issues as weekend passes, discharges, and changes in status while in the hospital. Meetings may provide a healthy, open forum for the discussion of everyday living problems in the unit. For example, at a meeting in one facility, the staff members' habit of not knocking before entering clients' rooms during the daytime hours was brought up by some of the annoyed clients. Feelings were expressed, ideas were exchanged, and clients and staff were able to work through a potentially milieu-destructive situation in a growth-enhancing manner. Usually community meetings are held on a once-a-week basis, and, because all members of the community should have an opportunity to participate, they tend to run longer than other group meetings (1½ to 2 hours). Six techniques for running a constructive therapeutic community meeting, as outlined by Russakoff and Oldham (1982), follow.

a. *Roll call* or *attendance* is taken. The unexplained absence of a staff member or a client may provoke fantasies of danger unless it is explained. New members of the community may be introduced at this time. Embarrassing questions about "why they are here" are avoided so that new residents can adjust comfortably to the milieu.

b. *An agenda* is created openly, within the meeting; this prevents the development of a potentially disorganizing "secret agenda." Too many or too few items on the agenda can lead to a discussion as to possible meanings (for example, excessive silence may indicate the clients' reluctance to talk about an earlier, upsetting event). "Emergency" issues can be given high priority in the agenda.

c. *Information gathering* is an important process. There should be no reliance on secrecy; relevant information should be presented openly. Interpretation of issues is avoided before the information-gathering process has been adequately addressed. Reality issues are clarified *before* proceeding to fantasy; this is particularly important when there are psychotic clients in the community, in which case it is best to maintain a concrete focus in the discussion. Information is best solicited from the entire community rather than singling out specific clients (for example, "What do members of the community understand about this?"). This helps maintain the focus as a *community* meeting.

d. An issue is brought to a conclusion before

another topic is introduced. This helps the more disorganized clients to follow the proceedings.

e. *Separation experiences* are addressed. For example, clients who are being admitted or discharged are noted. This is especially important for psychotic clients, for whom issues of separation are of primary concern.

f. *A supportive beginning and a supportive ending* to each meeting are necessary. Disruptive endings defeat the efforts of some disorganized clients to involve themselves in this important socializing event. Disruptive endings also may affect the behavior of clients after the meeting, while ending with a fairly benign issue helps clients to maintain social attitudes.

2. *Graded responsibility*. Treatment plans often reflect the principle of allowing the client to proceed at his own pace. Graded responsibility is a system that can demonstrate to the client his own progress in a very real way as he passes through "levels," "groups," or other structures for conveying status. This system also allows a reduction in responsibility for the client who needs a situation in which he can temporarily regress. For example, he may need a "quiet room" in which he can be isolated whenever he feels the need for fewer stimuli. A quiet room, if it is to be a therapeutic experience, must be used by staff and clients in a way that is protective of self-esteem and that does not imply any sort of punishment by the staff. (However, it should not provide clients with a means of avoiding responsibility.) Some units have "open charting" systems wherein clients may read their own charts at any time—the belief is that this practice fosters trust in the staff and the expectation of responsibility for oneself.*

3. Programs that provide *sufficient stimulation and activity*. To prevent unnecessary, nonthera-

peutic regression, most units or hospitals use recreational and occupational therapy situations and activities to maintain the clients' link between hospital and community.

4. *Individualization of treatment*. Overall rules and regulations are necessary to run any sort of community. However, since the needs of clients vary, their treatment must be individualized.

5. An *optimistic philosophy*. The philosophy of one therapeutic milieu may differ somewhat from that of another milieu, depending on the client population each serves. The needs of acutely psychotic or confused clients differ from the needs of acting-out, sociopathic individuals. Certainly, the needs of adolescents differ from those of a geriatric population. Maxwell Jones did his original work with sociopathic individuals, but the basic principles can apply to several settings. One part of any milieu's philosophy, however, remains crucial: there needs to be *an air of optimism about the prognosis for mental disorders*. This is necessary for clients *and* staff.

6. An *adequate communication system for staff*. It is to be hoped that optimum communication will help resolve conflicts among personnel and prevent any harmful projection of staff problems onto the clients. Staff members need to feel secure in their positions, and they need to obtain job satisfaction. A staff member who feels good about himself and about his job is a much more effective therapeutic agent than one who does not have these feelings. Adequate communication among staff members regarding the problems, progress, and daily activities of clients is likewise important. The *confidentiality* principle that operates within a therapeutic milieu is *not* one of confidentiality between client and single therapist, although the client must be assured that no personal information will leave the unit. Client–single therapist confidentiality is not compatible with the fact that each staff member must be an actively involved member of the therapeutic team. Complete and full communication among staff members is crucial to a program's success. Since observation of clients' behavior is an important and valuable part of milieu therapy, the

---

*However, clients in psychiatric facilities may not be automatically entitled to access to their records. For example, in New York state, it is the law that, in addition to consent by the client, consent by the Commissioner of Mental Health is required before a facility can allow access.

results of observation need to be shared with all staff members for maximum benefit to the client. Such information can be used effectively to modify treatment plans, and it can also help dilute possible distortions resulting from negative countertransference situations (see Chapter 9 for discussion of transference and countertransference). Some important ways of communicating among staff members include report meetings, weekly case conferences, and charting of observations.

SPECIAL THERAPIES WITHIN THE MILIEU

In addition to the more conventional forms of individual and group therapy, other types of therapy are used in a therapeutic milieu. Among these special types of therapy are poetry therapy; psychodrama; art therapy; graffiti therapy; dance, exercise, and yoga groups; music therapy; and videotape therapy. A brief description of each of these modalities follows.

Poetry therapy

Poetry is a useful tool for reaching many psychiatric clients. Poetry therapy can be handled in more than one way. A single poem may be chosen ahead of time by the leader for the group members to react to in a personal way. The leader may choose a poem that he or she thinks is particularly meaningful to many of the patients in the group, that addresses the problems, feelings, and lifestyle of the group members. It is hoped that the feelings the poetry evokes will be communicated and discussed by the group members. Many of Robert Frost's and Walt Whitman's poems seem ideally suited to such a purpose, but the choice is as wide as the therapist's experience with poetry. Another way of proceeding is for the leader to present several poems, representing different themes, to the group and have each member choose the one that is most meaningful to him and discuss it in a personal way. Still another method is

to have the members write their own poetry—an activity that can have the added benefit of increasing an individual's self-esteem through creativity.

Whichever method is used, the poetry serves to stimulate self-understanding (perhaps even catharsis), self-expression, and interpersonal interaction and to increase self-esteem. According to Arthur Lerner (1973), the important qualities of an effective poetry therapist are an acquaintance with a wide variety of poems, a genuine concern for people, an authentic love of poetry, and sensitivity and openness to the possible meanings of poems.

Psychodrama

Psychodrama, a form of group therapy that was originally developed by the late Dr. Jacob Moreno, is becoming widely used in short-term psychiatric units and in such places as alcoholism rehabilitation centers. Various institutes and continuing education courses train professionals in psychodramatic techniques, which focus on dramatizing an individual's conflicts, problems, and past and present relationships. A therapist directs the scene, and other clients or staff members play key roles or act as ''alter egos'' (roughly, persons who provide uninhibited versions of what the client is saying). There are opportunities for insight development through such methods as role reversals and for catharsis through such activities as conversations with a dead parent. The therapist keeps the action rolling as a stage director does, steps in to protect when necessary, interprets at times, and intentionally reduces group anxiety at the end through the use of a low-key ''sharing session.'' Warm-up techniques and gimmicks are used at the beginning of the session to promote group and individual interaction. Psychodrama is a powerful tool and should not be used in psychiatric settings except under the supervision of a trained person.

Art therapy

Art therapy is useful in three ways:
1. It can be used as a tool for stimulating self-

expression in a client (particularly clients who have difficulty expressing their feelings —for example, regressed schizophrenics or children before they can express feelings or conflicts verbally).

2. It can be used as a diagnostic tool from which modifications in a treatment plan can be made.

3. It can provide opportunities for increasing self-esteem and for promoting sublimation and personal growth.

Deep, analytical interpretation of a person's conflicts can be made on the basis of the art he produces. Interpretation, of course, should only be done by persons who have extensive knowledge of psychoanalysis and art therapy and diagnosis. However, using art therapy to stimulate expression, provide recreation and sublimation, increase interpersonal interaction, and enhance self-esteem is an appropriate method for nurses who work with psychiatric clients. Various materials may be used —water colors, oil paints, crayons, modeling clay, felt-tipped pens. Felt-tipped pens are particularly useful—they are easy to store and use, inexpensive, and colorful. Sometimes a group leader will offer a theme to the group and ask the members to draw their responses to it (for example, ''What do you look forward to?'' ''What was your happiest time?'' ''What makes you sad?''). Group members usually need a good deal of encouragement and support—an invariable complaint is ''I simply cannot draw at all!'' They need to be reassured that artistic ability is not a requirement; it often helps if the leader is willing to participate in the project as a member of the group. Each drawing is viewed by the group, and discussion follows. Any interpretation of a drawing is best given by the person who produced it. Another way of using art therapy is to have the group participate in the production of a large mural or collage. Such an activity promotes cooperation and interaction among members.

A specialized form of cooperative art therapy is *graffitti therapy,* which is a way of stimulating clients' expressions of self and communication with others. Participants are provided with a large piece of brown paper or a blackboard, and they are given pencils, crayons, chalk, or other writing instruments with which to scribble messages and comments. Clients are free to write whatever they choose (as long as it is socially acceptable to the community) and to remain anonymous. Themes or topics may be suggested, and staff *and* clients are encouraged to participate.

Movement therapy

Several forms of movement therapy are used in psychiatric settings; dance, exercise, and yoga are examples. Movement therapy provides several benefits. It can increase physical well-being and self-esteem and reduce anxiety. Exercise and dance can be particularly helpful to those depressed clients who tend to immobilize themselves in despair. Such group activities can also encourage interpersonal interaction—and, to put it simply, they can be fun. Rhythmic dance movements to music have been found to be especially beneficial for psychotic children—such movements help them to improve body coordination (Gunning and Holmes, 1973). Many nurses working in psychiatric settings who have had training in dance, yoga, or calisthenics—or who simply have an interest in these arts—are participating in movement therapy groups.

Music therapy

Music therapy has a long history in psychiatric care. The ancient Greeks believed that music could be a healing agent for persons in disturbed emotional states. In the seventeenth century, music was a specific part of the treatment of madness.

The goals of music therapy include increased self-esteem through pride in achievement, increased interpersonal relating, improved abilities to communicate and problem-solve, and an increased attention span. Music therapists are trained in psychology, sociology, anthropology, and education. They have a background in music, and they are required to complete a 6-month clinical internship. Some elements inherent in music are thought to have specific curative effects (Parriot, 1969). For example, a consistent rhythm is seen as having a calming effect, a regular but interrupted rhythm is thought to hold a person's attention and to create suspense, and an uneven or irregular rhythm is said to produce surprise and humor. In addition, music can encourage reminiscence, which is considered therapeutically valuable for geriatric clients. A "sing-along" featuring favorite tunes from the past is one possibility. While nurses may not be trained music therapists, many of them can certainly use their musical talents—or encourage clients to use theirs—to make use of the therapeutic value of music.

Videotape therapy

Some clinicians, units, and hospitals are using videotape equipment as a therapeutic modality. For instance, the technique of videotaping family therapy and group therapy sessions and having the participants view the tapes immediately afterward has been used to increase awareness of self and of communications patterns. The technique has also been used to help staff members to increase their own self-awareness. *Informed consent* is a very necessary requirement in the use of videotaping equipment.

• • •

While nurses are not art therapists, occupational therapists, or recreational therapists, their interest in—and recognition of the therapeutic value of—various activities can encourage clients to participate in them. Nurses may also encourage their clients in these various activities by participating along with them. Because nurses are often able to spend longer periods of time with clients than activity therapists can, nurses may be more knowledgeable about individual interests and talents and thus may be able to suggest activities to the therapists. Nurses then can observe and report on the effects of these forms of therapy. In addition,

nurses can plan and participate in activities that promote interpersonal communication, sharing, decision-making ability, and cooperation. Unlike activity therapists, nurses do not use activity groups for diagnosis and interpretation of clients' behavior. Instead, they use these groups to promote socialization—the learning of communication skills and social values.

Group therapy and activity therapy are important parts of the treatment of emotionally ill persons. Such therapy results in personal insight, the learning of socially acceptable behavior, and the development of positive group identification, all of which facilitate an individual's integration into social groups and the learning of social values and constraints.

THE ROLE OF THE NURSE

Standards of Psychiatric–Mental Health Nursing Practice, developed by the Division on Psychiatric–Mental Health Nursing Practice of the American Nurses' Association (1982), clearly states the nurse's responsibility for a therapeutic milieu: "The nurse provides, structures and maintains a therapeutic environment in collaboration with the client and other health care providers."

Milieu therapy and the primary nursing model

The use of primary nursing as the model for nursing care delivery is gaining in popularity throughout the United States. The model's popularity is, for the most part, well earned. This trend is bringing back the personal, involved, and professional aspects of nursing care in a variety of settings. It has been particularly effective in medical-surgical units of general hospitals. Psychiatric units probably are among the last of the holdouts against assimilation of the model into nursing practice.

The most obvious reason for the difficulties encountered in applying primary nursing in psychiatric units is a basic antagonism between the principles of milieu therapy and those of primary nursing. For example, milieu therapy necessitates a close, cooperative team effort in which *all* staff members work together to facilitate the growth and autonomy of the client. This effort makes possible flexible, fluctuating roles among workers. Primary nursing, however, is defined as "individualized, total patient care by the same care giver from the time of admission to discharge" (Smith, 1977). In the primary nursing model, assignment of staff members to clients is sometimes done in an *arbitrary* manner. The staff of a therapeutic milieu, though, ideally includes persons of a variety of ages, ethnic groups, and professional disciplines and of both sexes. Such a staffing pattern is specified so that a client's relationship with the staff can vary according to his changing needs and abilities. The goal is to help the client increase his ability to relate to others by having him interact with several different people. Arbitrary assignment of staff members to clients can defeat this purpose. In addition, arbitrary assignment may fail to adequately address the problems of countertransference in workers who should not be expected to work equally well in an intensive relationship with all clients.

Primary nursing also implies an *exclusive* staff-client assignment. This exclusivity can be a problem within the therapeutic milieu because it may lead to excessive dependency on one staff member. Abroms (1969) has described excessive dependency as one of the "five Ds" that milieu therapy aims to decrease. Exclusive assignment of a client to one worker may erode staff responsibility for *all* clients. Such assignment may be interpreted by the client as meaning that he *must* wait for his staff member to be on duty before he seeks counseling.

Another problem with an unmodified primary nursing model superimposed on a therapeutic milieu is the word "primary" itself. In one unit where such a model was introduced, the term "primary therapist" was objected to by the admitting psychiatrist, who had been the clients' therapist for many years and who continued to view himself in that role. The term was changed to "primary nursing therapist," which created another problem, since other members of the interdisciplinary team (such as social workers and occupational and recreational therapists) legitimately objected to the designation. Perhaps a better choice would be "primary milieu therapist."

Primary nursing, as it is performed in traditional medical-surgical settings, does not take into account the special needs and problems involved in the treatment of certain types of clients, such as one who is in the middle of an escalating and exhausting *manic* episode (see Chapter 18). The behavior of such a client is too demanding, too taxing of the coping abilities of any *one* staff member for a prolonged period of time. For the sake of both client and worker, the care of such a client needs to be shared. Caring for a chronically schizophrenic client is another example of a situation that can require the involvement of more than one staff member. Such involvement would help prevent a client's devastating reaction to the inevitable interruptions in a therapeutic relationship, such as a staff member's sickness, vacation, or termination of employment.

Primary nursing, as practiced in medical-surgical units, has had as one of its legitimate and laudable goals the assignment of personnel to clients on the basis of nursing care problems and the educational background of staff members. In many psychiatric units, the interdisciplinary team includes both staff members whose educational preparation is equivalent to that of a baccalaureate nurse and staff members who have more complex educational and experiential backgrounds than the baccalaureate nurse.

Finally, some of the traditional nursing functions that require a *professional* nurse as a primary giver of care (such as the administration of medication and the administration and supervision of treatments) are, because of the nature of the disabilities of clients in psychiatric units, of secondary importance. Medication routines are fairly simple—intravenous infusions and complex monitoring procedures and machines are not usually used.

These are some of the problems inherent in attempts to transfer without modification the primary nursing model to the psychiatric unit. However, there *are* benefits that primary nursing could provide for the psychiatric client who is hospitalized. For instance, the continuity of care from emergency room admission to discharge from the facility would certainly be enhanced. There might also be a built-in mechanism for avoiding the "woodwork client" phenomenon—the not-so-interesting client becoming lost in the shuffle. The phenomenon of the "problem client," whose taxing behavior elicits avoidance from staff, is another situation that might be prevented through primary nursing. Certainly, it has been reported that primary nursing can lead to increased job satisfaction. Psychiatric nursing, with its long tradition of therapy involving one-to-one relationships, seems expecially compatible with a primary nursing philosophy. Because the benefits may be as numerous as the problems in adapting the primary nursing model to milieu therapy, what is needed is a creative blending of the goals of primary nursing with the requirements for an effective and therapeutic milieu. *Primary care* that is flexible in its administration and not arbitrary in its assignment could be one aspect of the total milieu that enhances the effectiveness of treatment.

Liaison nursing: reaching out from the therapeutic milieu

Liaison nursing has become an important part of the health care system. Clinical specialists in psychiatric nursing provide consultation services for their nursing colleages in medical-surgical, parent-child, and geriatric settings. They also provide these services to other professionals, such as physicians and social workers. Another aspect of liaison nursing is the giving of care directly to clients in settings outside of the psychiatric unit. For example, the anxious client awaiting life-threatening surgery, the severely depressed victim of a stroke, or the family of a dying person may all be included

in the case load of a psychiatric nurse involved in liaison nursing.

The liaison nurse may be called in to conduct group sessions for staff members who are working in high-stress environments such as terminal care units, intensive care units, or pediatric patient units. The goal of these sessions is to help staff members to discuss and express their feelings about the difficult and painful aspects of their work and to provide group support for individuals who are experiencing stress.

Thus, the functions of the psychiatric nursing clinical specialist who performs liaison work may include consultation; client assessment; teaching of staff, clients, and their families; and direct intervention with clients. In a hospital, a good deal of this intervention with clients may be in the form of crisis intervention.

THE MENTAL HEALTH TEAM

People are treated for mental illness in a variety of settings—for example, community mental health clinics, day-care centers, psychiatric hospitals, and psychiatric units of general hospitals. These facilities become part of the social network or support system of an individual, and they are social systems in and of themselves. Some people (for example, workers and "outpatients") spend part of the day within such a system, while others ("inpatients") spend all of their time there. Each of these systems is rather like a self-contained society; subcultures may evolve with their own customs, rules, and mores (Goffman, 1961). Goffman and the Cummings (1962) are among many social scientists who have studied the psychiatric facility as a social system.

In most psychiatric facilities the formulation of treatment plans for clients is the responsbility of several different health care workers. The way this group of individuals works together as a team can be crucial to the success of a treatment plan. A relationship based on mutual respect and equality not only facilitates the team's functioning but also promotes the well-being of the client.

In a therapeutic milieu or community a certain amount of blurring of the distinctions between the roles of the various team members is considered appropriate. This role blurring may include the designation of an interdisciplinary team leader. While some agencies follow the medical model, in which a psychiatrist serves as team leader, other agencies allow any member of the helping professions to fill the role. Role blurring is based on the belief that the best person to help an individual is one who has developed a meaningful relationship with him or her. This belief does not negate the fact that each of the disciplines brings something unique to the team and to the overall care plan for a client. The nurse, as a cooperating member of the team, needs to have an understanding of the roles and functions of the other persons who make up the team.*

The most crucial member of the team is the client. It is important for nurses or any health professional to remember that no amount of treatment can be successful if the client is not engaged as a responsible partner in a therapeutic alliance. In the last analysis, it is the client who will, in one way or another, decide the outcome of therapy. Today, in many enlightened treatment centers, this fact is acknowledged through efforts to include the client in the process of making decisions about treatment or about goals for the future. Unfortunately, however, this philosophy is not always carried through; too often the client's views are considered *after* the ideas of other team members.

Most units and facilities allow clients some form of self-government within the overall treatment plan. The amount of self-government varies considerably. In some units clients participate only in once-a-week "client-staff" or "community" meetings that deal with here-and-now situations affecting staff and clients. In other units clients are expected to be responsible for many day-to-day decisions. Such decisions may involve the plan-

ning of recreational events and outings, the granting of weekend passes, and changes in the status of individual clients. In such units, clients also may be involved in decisions about discharge. In some alcoholic rehabilitation units, before clients are readmitted to the community, they must meet with the entire treatment staff to discuss what the clients see as their problems and their goals, as well as their potential degree of commitment to their treatment plans. Some facilities have "open charting" —clients are allowed to read their own charts at any time. All of these policies are based on the belief that encouraging an individual to be responsible for himself or herself and to assume responsibility for his or her peers will facilitate recovery and growth.

Inspired in part by the "radical therapists" (see Chapter 21), consumer advocacy* is beginning within the ranks of the mentally ill—or, more accurately, among recovered, or formerly mentally ill, persons. Advocacy takes energy, and someone in the midst of trying to cope with severe mental illness has little strength to spare. A significant portion of this advocacy is also carried out by relatives of clients, and they have been successful in making some major changes in large state-run facilities. Their efforts have caused federal and state funds for certain mental health institutions to be withheld until services and facilities were improved.

Clients have won some important court cases concerning their rights to freedom and to adequate and appropriate treatment while under psychiatric care. In addition to the right to treatment, other rights are being promoted by advocacy groups, including the following:

1. The right to the least restrictive form of housing
2. The right to education (particularly in the cases of mentally handicapped and emotionally ill children)

---

*For a detailed description of the roles of the various team members, see Chapter 1.

*Advocacy and the community as a client are discussed in Chapter 15; the nurse's role as a client advocate is discussed in Chapter 3.

3. Employment rights, including restrictions on the use of institutionalized persons to perform labor without receiving *at least* the minimum wage as well as protection against discrimination in employment in the community
4. The right to live in the community without being subject to discriminatory zoning ordinances
5. The right to refuse treatment (Trotter, 1975)

The roles and functions of each member of the health team will vary according to the needs of the population being served and the organization of the particular agency.

Certain professional responsibilities, however, may not be divided among the members of the mental health team. The physician, for example, always retains professional responsibility for such functions as prescribing medications. The nurse shares with the physician the responsibility for the administration of drugs and the evaluation of their effectiveness and side effects.

But many aspects of psychiatric treatment can be provided by all professionals and by some paraprofessionals. Individual and group therapy and maintaining a therapeutic milieu are some examples. It is in these areas, in which there is an overlapping of professional roles and responsibilities, that the professional expertise and experience of particular team members determine who is responsible for intervention. For example, a nurse with training and experience in crisis intervention or psychodrama would be the team leader when these therapeutic modalities are employed. Or a member of the team who is of the same ethnic group as a client may be more effective than other team members when ethnicity is an important consideration in therapy. Evaluation of client behavior and of the effectiveness of treatment plans are additional areas in which team leadership may shift from one team member to another.

In addition to the crucial ingredients of personal identity and integrity, the effective interdisciplinary team member has the ability to

1. accept the perspectives of others.
2. trust the knowledge and expertise of members of other disciplines.
3. function in an interdependent manner.
4. form new attitudes, values, and perceptions when necessary.
5. negotiate roles with other members of the team.
6. tolerate a constant review and challenge of ideas.
7. take risks.
8. accept a ''team'' philosophy of health care.
9. be problem and patient oriented rather than status or profession oriented. (Given and Simmons, 1977)

CHAPTER SUMMARY

Because of the nature of nursing education and nurses' clinical experience, milieu therapy is probably the area in which the responsibility of the nurse is most evident. The nurse brings a background in science and the humanities, as well as an understanding of psychiatric nursing principles, to the mental health team.

Milieu therapy usually includes some form of self-government for clients, such as community or client-staff meetings. Therapeutic limit-setting and graded responsibility are also important elements of the milieu.

Milieu therapy for clients who are experiencing emotional or mental problems often includes art, poetry, music, movement therapy, and psychodrama. Nurses who work in psychiatric settings are involved in varying degrees in these treatment modalities.

Ideally, members of the mental health team work together to engage the client in cooperative, goal-oriented involvement in his own treatment. Team members share in the evaluation of clients and in planning, implementing, and evaluating treatment programs. Team leadership may shift or rotate among team members, depending upon which member has the greatest expertise in a given situation or the most information about a given client.

Within the milieu, efforts are directed toward fostering responsibility for self and others and toward facilitating growth.

REFERENCES

Abroms, G.
1969 "Defining milieu therapy." Archives of General Psychiatry 21:553-560.
American Nurses' Association Division on Psychiatric–Mental Health Nursing Practice
1982 Standards of Psychiatric–Mental Health Nursing Practice. Kansas City, Mo.: ANA Publications, pp. 11-13.
Cumming, J., and E. Cumming
1962 Ego and Milieu. New York: Atherton Press, p. 5.
Erickson, R.
1982 "Viewing the therapeutic community through Adlerian spectacles." Journal of Group Psychotherapy 32:201-216.
Fann, W., and C. Goshen
1977 The Language of Mental Health, ed. 2, St. Louis: The C.V. Mosby Co., p. 87.
Goffman, E.
1961 Asylums: Essays on the Social Situation of Mental Patients and Other Inmates. Garden City, N.Y.: Anchor Books.
Given, B., and S. Simmons
1977 "The interdisciplinary health-care team: fact or fiction?" Nursing Forum 16(2):165-184.
Gunning, S., and T. Holmes
1973 "Dance therapy with psychotic children." Archives of General Psychiatry 28:707-714.
Jones, M.
1953 The Therapeutic Community: A Treatment Method in Psychiatry. New York: Basic Books, Inc., Publishers.
Lerner, A.
1973 "Poetry therapy." American Journal of Nursing 73(8):1336-1338.
Parriot, S.
1969 "Music as therapy." American Journal of Nursing 69(8):1723-1726.
Russakoff, L., and J. Oldham
1982 "The structure and technique of community meetings: the short-term unit." Psychiatry 45:38-44.
Skinner, K.
1979 "The therapeutic milieu: making it work." Journal of Psychiatric Nursing-Mental Health Services 17(8):38-44.
Smith, C.
1977 "Primary nursing care—a substantive nursing care delivery system." Nursing Administration Quarterly 1(2):1.
Trotter, R.J.
1975 "Open sesame: the Constitution and mental institutions." Science News, vol. 108, July 12, 1975, p. 31.

ANNOTATED SUGGESTED READINGS

Baker, B.
1982 "The use of music with autistic children." Journal of Psychosocial Nursing and Mental Health Services 20(4):31-34.
The author describes four phases of intervention into isolation patterns of autistic children through the use of music therapy: Phase I (breaking the shell), Phase II (shifting awareness), Phase III (building competence), Phase IV (building relationship with others). The interventions to break patterns of isolation include repetition; continuity in the environment; use of musical and rhythm instruments; imitative games; and bridging trust between the child and significant others.
Benfer, B.
1981 "Defining the role and function of the psychiatric nurse as a member of the team." Perspectives in Psychiatric Care 18(4):166-177.
Benfer presents a clearly organized delineation of the variables that affect the functioning of the interdisciplinary mental health team, with particular attention being paid to the functioning of the psychiatric nurse. Phases of group development in relation to interdisciplinary teams are reviewed, and the topic of "organizational politics" is briefly discussed.

Carser, D.

1981 "Primary nursing in the milieu." Journal of Psychiatric Nursing and Mental Health Services 19(2):35-41.

Definitions of primary nursing and of milieu therapy are included as well as a brief historical overview of the concepts. The relationship between the two concepts is examined, with some discussion of potential problems and solutions.

Devine, B.

1981 "Therapeutic milieu/milieu therapy: an overview." Journal of Psychiatric Nursing and Mental Health Services 19(3):20-24.

A historical and current overview of milieu therapy and its application to particular patient populations. A review of some research findings on therapeutic communities is provided, and some issues in milieu therapy are touched upon.

Islam, A., and D. Turner

1982 "The therapeutic community: a critical reappraisal." Hospital and Community Psychiatry 33(8):651-653.

A critical assessment of the concept of the "therapeutic community." As a "protest movement" the authors believe that the therapeutic community has achieved some degree of success. However, they suggest that its therapeutic value should be reassessed in light of recent research and presently changing social conditions.

Lipkin, G., and R. Cohen

1973 Effective Approaches to Patients. New York: Springer Publishing Co., Inc.

This manual describes problem behavior, discusses the underlying dynamics of the behavior, and suggests helpful approaches. The work is a practical, concise, and informative guide to working with clients with emotional problems.

Puskar, K.

1981 "Structure for the hospitalized adolescent." Journal of Psychiatric Nursing and Mental Health Services 19(7):13-16.

This article notes the various types of structure available to the hospitalized adolescent. The "six c's" of structure for the adolescent are reviewed: consistency, communication, clear rules, clear consequences, clear roles, and consultation-education for the staff. Strengths and weaknesses of an approach based on the six c's are briefly discussed.

FURTHER READINGS

Byrne, A., et al.

1972 "Graffiti therapy." Perspectives in Psychiatric Care 9(1):34-36.

Challela, M.

1979 "The interdisciplinary team: a role definition in nursing." Image (Sigma Theta Tau) 11(1):9-15.

Ciske, K.

1979 "Accountability—the essence of primary nursing." American Journal of Nursing 79(5):890-894.

Fink, P., et al.

1973 "Art therapy: a diagnostic and therapeutic tool." International Journal of Psychiatry 11(1):104-125.

Fitzgerald, R., and I. Long

1973 "Seclusion in the management of severely disturbed manic and depressed patients." Perspectives in Psychiatric Care 11(2):59-64.

Hyde, N.

1970 "Play therapy: the troubled child's self-encounter." American Journal of Nursing 71(7):1366-1370.

Leone, D., and R. Zahourek

1974 "'Aloneness' in a therapeutic community." Perspectives in Psychiatric Care 12(2):60-63.

Lewis, A., and J. Levy

1983 Psychiatric Liaison Nursing: The Theory and Clinical Practice. New York: Prentice-Hall, Inc.

Lyon, G.

1970 "Limit setting as a therapeutic tool." Journal of Psychiatric Nursing and Mental Health Services 8(6):17-21.

North, M.

1972 Personality Assessment Through Movement. Boston: Plays, Inc.

Pesso, A.

1969 Movement in Psychotherapy. New York: New York University Press.

Romoff, V., and I. Kane

1982 "Primary nursing in psychiatry: an effective and functional model." Perspectives in Psychiatric Care 20(2):73-78.

CHAPTER 11

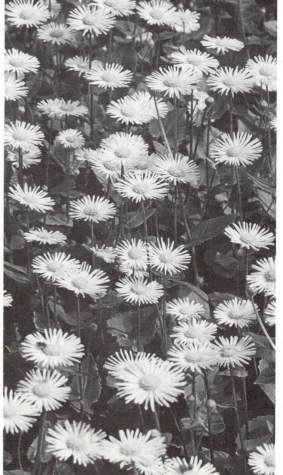

Photo by Werner H. Müller—Peter Arnold, Inc.

296

Group therapy

CHAPTER FOCUS

Group therapy is a treatment modality that is well established in psychiatric inpatient units, in outpatient clinics, and in community mental health centers. It originally received the impetus for its growth from economic factors during World War II (more people could be treated at one time), but it soon became apparent that group therapy provided important therapeutic benefits that were different from and in addition to those of individual psychotherapy.

In accordance with their various levels of educational preparation, professional nurses working in psychiatric settings have assumed the roles of group leader, group therapist, and co-therapist. The role of group therapist is the responsibility of the master's-degree clinical specialist in psychiatric nursing.

This chapter focuses on the curative factors inherent in group therapy, some guidelines for intervening as an effective group leader, and some important phenomena that occur in therapy groups. A knowledge of group dynamics can aid the nurse in working with colleagues and as a team member in any setting. A guide for the assessment of group process is included, and the use of the nursing process within a group situation is outlined.

Cartwright and Zander (1967) have defined groups in general. They describe a group as being made up of members who
1. engage in frequent interactions.
2. define themselves as members of the group.
3. are defined by others as belonging to the group.
4. share norms with other group members.
5. participate in a system of interlocking roles.
6. identify with one another through role models or ideals held in common.
7. find rewards within the group.
8. pursue interdependent goals.
9. have a sense of group unity.

10. tend to act in a unitary way toward the environment.

Therapy groups are a specific type of group. They differ from social groups (such as clubs, fraternal organizations, and lodges) in that they are specifically aimed at changing the maladaptive coping behavior of their members. A definition of group therapy has been provided by Kaplan and Sadock (1972). They describe it as a type of treatment involving two or more clients participating together in the presence of one or more therapists, who facilitate both emotional and rational or cognitive interaction to effect changes in the maladaptive behavior of the group members.

Group therapy came into existence at the turn of the century when a Boston physician, Dr. Joseph H. Pratt, used it to enhance the medical treatment of tuberculosis patients by attempting to deal with their emotional problems. During and immediately after World War II, when there was a shortage of psychiatric personnel, group therapy was seen as an economical form of psychotherapy. Eventually, a body of theory developed surrounding group treatment, and it became quite evident that in addition to its economic advantages group therapy had other important advantages over individual therapy. These advantages include provision of a protective environment for trying out new patterns of behavior, opportunities for learning new patterns of behavior, and the availability of a role model for interpersonal relating (the leader or leaders and other group members). There is also the opportunity for multiple transference situations *(see Chapter 9)* within the group, which can lead to the development of greater insight.

CURATIVE FACTORS IN GROUP THERAPY

One authority (Yalom, 1975) has delineated the curative factors that group treatment can offer:

1. *The instillation of hope.* Seeing the progress of others in the group, a group member feels hopeful about receiving similar help.
2. *Universality.* When a group member sees that others in the world share similar feelings or have similar problems, anxiety is decreased.
3. *Imparting of information.* Interpersonal relating, developmental tasks and stages, medications and other somatic treatments, and the structure of the setting are only a few areas in which information may be shared.
4. *Altruism.* The opportunity to support and to help increase self-awareness in another group member gives the helping individual increased self-esteem. It also encourages a preoccupied individual to become less self-focused.
5. *Corrective recapitulation of the primary family group.* Multiple transference opportunities are available in group treatment to help develop insight into one's background and its effects on present relationships. (The individual displaces and projects feelings and attitudes onto the therapist *and* onto other group members.)
6. *Imitative behavior.* The group leader, a recovering group member, or a group member who has already mastered a particular psychosocial skill or developmental task can be a valuable role model.
7. *Interpersonal learning.* The group offers many and varied opportunities for relating to other people on a here-and-now basis.

TYPES OF GROUPS

There are several ways of using group therapy and many ways of describing groups.

Play therapy groups are specifically used for therapy with children, because children have limited verbal abilities. Conflicts and problems are acted out in play, and interpersonal learning takes place.

Psychoanalytically oriented group therapy is an ''uncovering'' type of therapy aimed at helping group members delineate and understand their intrapsychic and interpersonal conflicts and problems. The group and the leader may follow any one of the various theoretical schools of psycho-analysis, such as Freudian, Sullivanian, or Jungian. This type of group therapy is most often done in an outpatient setting, with clients who are neurotic rather than psychotic and who are functioning on an adequate level of adjustment.

Repressive-inspirational group therapy provides the framework for such self-help groups as Alcoholics Anonymous and Overeaters Anonymous. Repressive-inspirational groups try to alter socially unacceptable behavior while developing and emphasizing socially acceptable qualities. These groups, which consist exclusively of acting-out (socially deviant)* or formerly acting-out individuals, usually meet in a community setting.

Michelle had been overweight for as long as she could remember. Even in kindergarten she had been taunted by other children, who gave her the nickname "fatty." She had been on and off diets all of her life. She would lose 50 or 60 pounds and then regain them. Now that Michelle was the mother of two children, she was afraid that her children would follow her poor eating habits and develop weight problems. She joined Overeaters Anonymous. With the support of the group members, all of whom either had been or were presently overweight, she was able to acknowledge her problem—that she ate when she was unhappy and that eating was a means not only of satisfying hunger but also of feeling secure. Michelle and another member of Overeaters Anonymous were teamed as "buddies." When one of them experienced an uncontrollable craving for food, she called her buddy and "talked it out." If necessary, the other person came to the house and stayed with her buddy until the craving for food passed. In this way, food binges were avoided.

It is obvious that a fundamental idea behind repressive-inspirational therapy is that with the help of persons who have experienced the same problem, acting-out individuals can face up to their socially

---

*Refer to Chapter 17 for further discussion of acting-out or socially deviant behavior.

unacceptable behavior, vow not to repeat it, and help others who are struggling with the problem.

Although nurses may not be directly involved in repressive-inspirational groups, they do play important roles as facilitators and resource persons. In hospitals, self-help groups such as Alcoholics Anonymous and Narcotics Anonymous frequently hold meetings for people who are potential members. Nurses who have established some degree of rapport with acting-out individuals can be influential in encouraging them to attend a meeting of the appropriate group. When nurses provide members with adequate time, privacy, and space for meetings, they give people the message "This is important therapy." In the community, community health nurses, occupational health nurses, and school nurse–teachers serve as important sources of information. In their role as case finders, these nurses come in contact with many people who may be in need of but unaware of existing self-help groups. It is often through the encouragement and support of such nurses that acting-out individuals make their initial contacts with these groups.

Encounter groups, or T-groups (the "T" stands for "training in human relations"), originated with Kurt Lewin in 1946. Lewin had been asked by the Connecticut Interracial Commission to help resolve some of the state's interracial problems. He and his colleagues assembled some of Connecticut's black and white leaders in an attempt to help them resolve their differences. Lewin appointed four observers to record the group process. After each session, these recorders discussed the group's dynamics with the group's leaders. Group members insisted on being present at these "postmortems." Lewin found that the conferees learned more from these feedback sessions than from the group meetings themselves. This was the inception of encounter group therapy.

Encounter groups focus on the here and now—on what group members experience as they meet. Members are urged to be completely candid and to shed their facades of adequacy, competence, and self-sufficiency. These groups are peer-oriented rather than leader (authority)-oriented. Members are encouraged to tell one another how they come across to others (that is, to provide feedback). Brutal verbal attacks often develop. Encounter group therapy seems to crack the shell of maladaptive communication patterns used by acting-out individuals. They then can begin to develop insight and to change their behavior. An encounter group thus functions as a microcosm of society.

Yablonsky (1965) describes an encounter group session at Synanon, the original therapeutic community for drug addicts in the United States. The meeting becomes an emotional battlefield. Complete candor is the order of the day. Maladaptive defenses and socially unacceptable behavior of members are repeatedly attacked. The encounters are designed to help acting-out persons see themselves as society sees them. They are forced to see both their strengths and their weaknesses.

Although nurses do not usually participate in encounter sessions, it is important for them to understand the therapeutic function of what might appear to be destructive group techniques.

A student nurse was trying to establish a therapeutic relationship with Jamie, who had been using alcohol since elementary school and drugs since he began high school. Jamie, aged 16, was now part of a therapeutic drug community. One of the treatment modalities used by this community was encounter group therapy. After a session in which the group had "attacked" Jamie's behavior and attitudes, Jamie complained to the student nurse. The student, who was not acquainted with encounter therapy, sympathized with Jamie and told him that it sounded as though he was being scapegoated. She explained, "They are probably ganging up on you so that no one will focus on them."

When the student recounted this episode to her instructor, the instructor explained the therapeutic rationale underlying the group's approach. After that, the student was able to support Jamie through the experience by helping him listen to what the group was saying. She also helped him realize that although his socially unacceptable behavior was under attack, he as a person was not being rejected.

As members of health teams, nurses need to be involved in developing and implementing therapeutic goals. It is also the function of nurses to sustain acting-out individuals during their experiences with encounter therapy. Moreover, because nurses work closely with families, it is important for nurses to understand the therapeutic rationale underlying encounter group therapy so that they can explain it to family members. Otherwise, the families of acting-out individuals could become alarmed at what might appear to be a brutally destructive or punitive group process.

The approaches of all health team members must be coordinated in order to ensure that the therapeutic goals of encounter group therapy are implemented and that socially acceptable behavior is promoted.

*Activity group therapy** is task oriented. A variety of recreational and occupational forms of therapy is used for the purpose of assessing and developing social and leisure skills. Activity groups are found in both hospital and community settings. The goals of activity group therapy are as follows:

1. To encourage communication
2. To facilitate the expression of feelings
3. To provide opportunity for decision making
4. To increase a person's concentration span
5. To teach a person how to cooperate, share, and compete

Activity group therapy is especially well suited for acting-out individuals. Such persons are action oriented—they try to cope with inner conflicts by doing and not by talking. Activities necessitating gross physical movements therefore provide socially acceptable outlets for the hostility and aggressiveness that underlie most acting-out behavior. Woodworking, sports, and arts and crafts are only a few of the activities that are suitable for acting-out individuals.

---

*See Chapter 10 for a discussion of various types of activity group therapy.

A group of student nurses brought construction paper and paints to a unit for newly admitted acting-out individuals. One young man had been admitted after he had taken LSD and experienced a "bad trip." He would not talk about the experience. Midway through a session in which the clients were using the art supplies, the young man sat down at the table. He picked up a piece of green construction paper and, using the colors yellow, purple, orange, red, and black, drew a demonic face. One student asked, "Who is that?" the young man answered, "That's how I felt—just like a devil." He was beginning to admit his experience and to assimilate it into his self system.

Activity therapy thus can facilitate communication and the expression of emotion. In addition, when people set up the equipment for an activity, share materials and tools, and put everything away afterward, they are engaged in interaction, interplay, and interdependency.

Few formal demands are made on activity group members. In this relatively nonthreatening atmosphere, they can "do" to things rather than to people. This is an important phase in the treatment of acting-out behavior. It serves the dual purpose of redirecting and sublimating aggression and hostility. New, socially acceptable behavior can supplant the older, socially unacceptable behavior.

Multifamily therapy groups and *couples groups* are composed of more than one family unit. These groups help members to work with the problems of intrafamily communication and relationships. Individuals and families help one another in a supportive, learning atmosphere. For example, the multifamily therapy group is commonly used to help the families of clients who are hospitalized with schizophrenia to be supportive factors in the clients' recovery.

In *groups for persons with special problems*—for example, colostomy groups, laryngectomy groups, and mastectomy groups—feelings are expressed and support and suggestions are offered in a way that helps members adjust to and accept their changed body images and decreased ability to function. Members are encouraged to function at their maximum potential levels. These groups can be "self-help" groups, or they can have varying degrees of professional leadership or involvement.

Other groups found in community and hospital settings include *sensory awareness groups, transactional analysis groups* (based on the theory of Eric Berne [1967]), and *problem-solving* or *brainstorming groups,* which are found in business and used by the staff members of health care facilities.

Therapy groups may be short-term, open-ended groups—the type most often formed in the psychiatric units of general hospitals—or they may be of the closed, long-term type found in community outpatient settings. "Open-ended" simply means that as one group member is discharged and leaves the group, another member may be added. The composition of the group is flexible and always changing. A closed group begins with a certain composition, and if someone leaves the group, no additional member is added. And while a closed group may be long term, there is often a specific time at which it is to disband.

PHASES OF A GROUP

As in individual treatment, there are phases to the life and natural history of a group. Most ongoing groups will proceed from the *orientation phase* through the *working phase* toward *termination.* Testing of the therapist and the group norms tends to occur in the early, orientation stage, which is generally characterized by only superficial discussion of the group's area of concern. The emerging group responsibility, cooperative therapist-client efforts, and identification with the leader occur in the working phase. Group cohesiveness then becomes evident. As in individual treatment, the termination phase requires that the leader prepare the group well ahead of the group's ending. A summary of the group's history and progress and the formulation of any future plans for individuals are appropriate during this phase.

Baruch Levine (1979) has delineated four phases in a group's development according to the directionality of relationships among the group members and the therapist: the parallel phase, the inclusion phase, the mutuality phase, and the termination phase (see Figs. 11-1 to 11-3). A change in the direction of relationships represents the evolution from one phase to another. Levine has also outlined the three recurring crisis themes in the life of a therapy group: authority, intimacy, and separation.

The parallel phase is the phase in which all relationships tend to be directed toward the group leader or therapist. The name is derived from the concept of "parallel play" in childhood social development. The amount of time spent in this phase depends on the level of psychosocial development of the individual members. For instance, an outpatient group of clients with neurotic problems may move rapidly to the next stage, whereas a group of clients who are chronically suffering from schizophrenia may spend the entire existence of the group in the parallel phase. This phase corresponds to the *orientation phase* described above.

During the inclusion phase there is a decrease in the centrality of the therapist in group relationships, and member-to-member relationships tend to increase. Members are beginning to share a more equal distribution of power within the group. For example, a group of adolescents becomes capable of and involved in some degree of self-government within the group. This inclusion phase occurs in the first half (roughly) of the *working phase* described earlier.

In the mutuality phase, relationships extend from most or all members to most or all members and the therapist. Everyone feels accepted and included, and there is a sharing of power. Initial empathy is developing and being facilitated. While members feel emotionally linked to one another, they also feel free to express themselves. Less work is expended on the group as a system and more on accomplishing the therapeutic task. The mutuality phase occurs in the latter half of the *working phase*.

The termination phase is mostly a phenomenon of closed groups but can also be associated with members leaving an open-ended group. The direction of relationships changes as members disengage from other members and the therapist and move toward outside relationships. Ideally, therapeutic goals have been reached. The nature of this phase may reflect the degree to which the crises of authority, intimacy, and separation have been resolved.

These crises are interrelated with all other forces operating in the group. Crises can occur at any phase, but some are usually associated with specific phases. *Authority crises* usually arise at the onset of a group's existense, and they are challenges to the power of the therapist. The resolving of the first authority crisis usually marks the transition from the parallel phase to the inclusion phase. Authority crises can recur at any time during the life of the group.

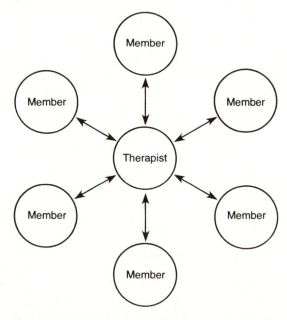

Fig. 11-1. Lines of relationship in the parallel phase (extreme situation). (From Levine, B. Group Psychotherapy: Practice and Development. © 1979. Reprinted by permission of Prentice-Hall, Inc., Englewood Cliffs, N.J.)

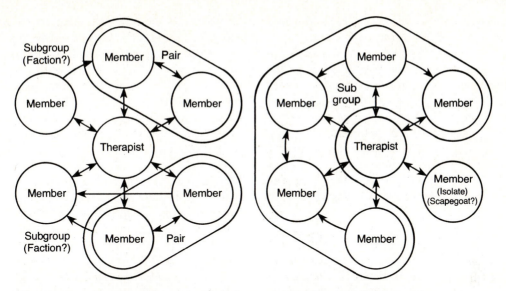

Fig. 11-2. Two of the many possible patterns of relationship during the inclusion phase. (From Levine, B. Group Psychotherapy: Practice and Development. © 1979. Reprinted by permission of Prentice-Hall, Inc., Englewood Cliffs, N.J.)

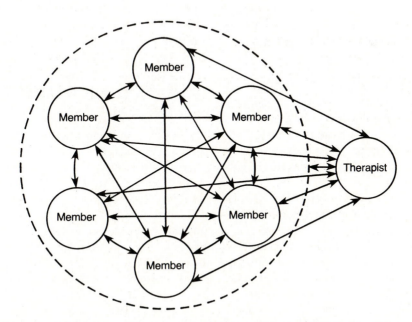

Fig. 11-3. Lines of relationship in the mutuality phase. (From Levine, B. Group Psychotherapy: Practice and Development. © 1979. Reprinted by permission of Prentice-Hall, Inc., Englewood Cliffs, N.J.)

Intimacy crises occur as intimacy develops among group members. Although these crises tend to recur throughout the group's existence, often the first resolution of an intimacy crisis occurs at the beginning of the mutuality phase. Pseudo-intimacy may be appropriate in adolescent groups, where peer conformity pressures are phase-appropriate, but pseudo-intimacy in adult groups may signify a premature forcing of intimacy on the group by the therapist. This could be detrimental to individual members, who might believe that the other group members actually experienced a degree of intimacy that they only simulated and are actually incapable of at this time.

Separation crises occur during various phases; they are often brought on by absences of members or therapist or by fears of members or therapist. These crises are not resolved if members continue to deny and repress their feelings about separation. Members of an effective therapy group tend to develop effective ways of resolving separation crises throughout the evolution of the group.

COMPOSITION OF A GROUP AND FREQUENCY AND DURATION OF MEETINGS

The size of a group and the frequency and duration of meetings can, of course, vary greatly. As a general rule, however, an ongoing therapy group meets once a week, its optimal size is eight to ten members, and a session lasts an hour to an hour and a half.

A group may be *homogeneous*—that is, composed of people who share characteristics such as age, sex, diagnosis, or particular problem—or it may be *heterogeneous*. There are advantages to each situation, and which is chosen generally depends upon the goals of the group.

Clients whose special needs tend to be best met within a homogeneous structure include adolescents, acute psychotics, alcoholics, isolated elderly persons, and seriously handicapped persons

(Fried, 1972). In contrast, middle-aged parents and young adults who are having difficulty bridging the generation gap in their own families may be able to improve communication and increase empathy through experiences in groups that are heterogeneous in terms of age. Heterogeneity and homogeneity of groups are concepts that can be related to the holistic health status of the client and any of the five dimensions of self (biological, intellectual, psychological, sociocultural, and spiritual). For example, homogeneity in regard to physical status can be an important consideration in the composition of a group of postmastectomy clients, while heterogeneity in regard to sociocultural background can provide a cross-fertilization that stimulates personal growth in group members.

Scheidlinger (1982) points out that in addition to heterogeneity and homogeneity, the concept of *balancing* is an important one. He cites as examples of unbalanced groups those comprising one man and several women, those comprising one withdrawn, socially constricted individual in a group of impulsive personalities, and those comprising members who are all withdrawn and constricted.

PHENOMENA OCCURRING IN GROUPS

Various communication problems are encountered in groups. One such problem is *monopolizing*. Group meetings have definite time limitations, and a person who monopolizes the conversation uses it up and deprives the other group members. This can lead to a sense of injustice in the group members and anger toward a group leader who fails to intervene (Sampson and Marthas, 1981). The evident signs of the monopolizer are:

1. Incessant, compulsive talking
2. Inability to listen
3. Interrupting others
4. Finishing others' thoughts and sentences
5. A tangential, confusing style of talking

6. A ''dream quality'' to what is being said
7. Restlessness and inattentiveness among the other group members
8. Symptoms of frustration and anger in other group members, especially against the leader

Ways of intervening with the monopolizer include:

1. Verbally reflecting the behavior
2. Interpreting the underlying meaning of the behavior (for example, relating it to anxiety)
3. Reflecting the group feelings about it
4. Confrontation of the group in regard to their reasons for allowing the monopolizing (Sampson and Marthas, 1981)

Intellectualizing tends to occur in a client who has difficulty dealing with feelings. Intellectualizing all group topics is a way of defending against internal conflicts and the emotional reactions that may be attached to them. Talking in the abstract and generalizing about everything are signs of intellectualizing. An atmosphere that encourages expression and exploration of feelings and direct confrontation of the group member's tendency to intellectualize are ways of intervening.

Using a *semantic argument* is one way for a member to attempt to control the situation (including control of others). Laborious discussions about exactly what is meant and philosophizing in general are ways of avoiding real issues, internal conflicts, and painful feelings. It is best to confront the individual and bring the topic back to the individual's feelings (for example, ''But how does all of that apply to you and your feelings?'' ''In what way do you find these things affecting your life personally?'')

Circumstantiality is a tendency to digress into numerous and unnecessary details and inappropriate thoughts before getting to the main idea. The effects of circumstantiality are similar to those of monopolizing—and, indeed, circumstantiality can result in monopolizing. Often the individual who communicates this way in group does so in other areas of life and is unaware of the devastating effects on interpersonal relations. Gentle but direct and consistent confrontation is usually helpful.

Tangentiality is a disturbed communication pattern in which the group member is unable to express ideas directly. Instead, the individual goes off on ''side trips'' with other, loosely related ideas. The main idea is not expressed. This way of communicating can be very confusing to the other group members. For this reason and because the individual is often unaware of the detrimental effects on interpersonal relating, there needs to be direct, consistent confrontation when tangentiality occurs in a group session.

Another type of problem in groups is *scapegoating,* which is the ''tendency of human groups to project onto others such emotions as fear, aggression, and guilt—emotions they must negate in themselves . . .'' (Scheidlinger, 1982). Scapegoating may be carried out against a group member who is present at a meeting, or it may be directed toward an individual who is not present. The leader must protect the scapegoated individual, point out what the group is doing, and use the phenomenon as a means of increasing the self-awareness of individual group members.

Transference can be directed toward the leader or toward other members of the group. Within any one group there may be transference reactions based on past or present relationships with mother, father, siblings, husband, wife, children, or boss. If one person's transference reaction is based on two or more relationships, the phenomenon is called *multiple transference.*

Relationships among group members can take several forms. For example, there may be pairing, subgrouping, or polarization. Such developments can be destructive if they interfere with honest and constructive confrontation or if they result in scapegoating or infighting. *Pseudomutuality* within a group can also interfere with honest relating and communicating. Sometimes *sadomasochistic* relationships will erupt between group members. Such relationships are often reflections of the way members relate outside of the group, and they can be used as learning opportunities. Some group members may display their tendencies to *withdraw* and *isolate* themselves or to *conform* as a pattern of relating.

Catharsis, an outpouring of emotional tension through verbalization or display of feelings, can occur in any group session. It can be a tension-reducing and growth-enhancing phenomenon. A cathartic release of pent-up emotions has been known to be a crucial turning point in a group member's life. In addition, an individual's strong expression of emotions has effects on the other group members; it is a vital part of the group process. It may be instrumental in producing group cohesiveness (Yalom, 1975).

Group members often assume various *roles* within the group. These roles serve various functions for the group, and they also may serve an unconscious, intrapsychic function for the individual assuming the role. Examples of some roles include *the peacemaker, the group catalyst, the leader, the protector, the attacker, the interpreter,* and *the assistant therapist.* The group member who assumes the role of assistant therapist or that of group catalyst can be very helpful to a leader. Often this individual is insightful and able to confront constructively and appropriately. However, this behavior may also be an attempt to avoid looking at one's own personal problems and to avoid being exposed to the group process.

A group leader should be aware of *seating arrangements.* Where an individual sits in relation to the leader may be an important clue to his or her personality. Members who always sit next to the leader may be indicating a need to associate with the leader for some reason—perhaps for protection. Habitually sitting directly opposite the leader may indicate a desire to engage in direct communication or confrontation with the leader. That ''pairing'' has occurred between two group members may be demonstrated by their choice of seats. The need to withdraw or isolate oneself or the feeling of being threatened by the group may result in placing one's seat at a point *outside* the group circle. While all group members are expected to sit within the circle, an exception to the rule may need

to be made for a threatened and timid schizophrenic client (Berne, 1966, p. 56).

It is sometimes helpful for co-therapists to sit opposite one another to maximize nonverbal communication between them and to enlarge their view of the nonverbal communication of other group members.

APPROACHES TO GROUP THERAPY

Group treatment may be based on any of the many schools of psychotherapy (Freudian, Sullivanian, transactional analysis, gestalt, Jungian, and so on), or it may be based on an eclectic viewpoint. Leadership style varies: it may be directive or nondirective, authoritarian or democratic, or laissez-faire.

As a general rule and for most group therapy situations, it is best for a leader to start out in a somewhat authoritarian role (authoritarian only in the sense that the leader gives the group its basic ground rules and perhaps states some goals for the group sessions). As the members begin to express trust and confidence in the leader, the leader gradually relinquishes this moderately authoritarian role by fostering interaction among the group members. The goal of the leader is to become a ''facilitator,'' a ''referee,'' a ''consultant,'' or a ''clarifier,'' or to assume any combination of these roles.

Carl Rogers is the originator of ''client-centered'' psychotherapy. He views the therapeutic process as allowing the client to grow through increased understanding of self. The therapist uses a nondirective technique of consistently reflecting the client's feelings. Rogers also applies this philosophy to group therapy; he sees the leader as a facilitator of the group's own potential for self-discovery and growth. Rogers (1971) has described several characteristics of an effective group leader.

1. The leader is a *facilitator* rather than a *direc-*

tor of the therapeutic process; he or she works toward becoming a participant and toward being able to move comfortably back and forth between the stances of leader and participant.

2. The leader is responsive to *meaning* and *feelings,* which are more important than the details of *what* happened to the group member. However, it may be necessary to explore these details before getting to the meaning.

3. The effective leader accepts the group where it is *now.* This implies an acceptance of the individual group member and the member's degree of participation. The group may not accept a particular member's degree of participation, but the leader must. Silence is acceptable if it is not unexpressed pain.

4. Sympathetic understanding of the individual member's intellectualizations and generalizations and the ability to select the self-referent meanings of these and respond to them are crucial.

5. The facilitating leader operates in terms of his or her own feelings but with a degree of caution. A leader who is *too* expressive *too* early in the group's evolution may be unaware of his or her feelings, and may be doing a kind of "acting-out" by expressing feelings without adequate thought.

6. The leader should confront appropriately and provide constructive feedback without attacking a group member's defenses. The group leader should use his or her *own* feelings responsibly and therapeutically in confronting group members and providing them with feedback.

7. An effective leader is able to use self-disclosure in a manner that is tempered by professional conscience and that serves a therapeutic purpose.

8. An effective leader avoids excessive planning and group "gimmicks." Gimmicks are used only as a last resort, because they rarely work.

9. A leader who is successful at being therapeutic tends to avoid interpretive comments, which only serve to make group members self-conscious. Commenting on group process* can be helpful sometimes but should not be overdone.

The following are some techniques that are effective in group therapy.

1. Provide a safe, comfortable atmosphere. Generally, when people feel secure, they are able to participate more easily in self-disclosure. Putting group members "on the spot" and attempting to force self-disclosure are the actions of an inexperienced and misinformed group leader. An exception to this is the highly confrontational format used by groups of clients who abuse drugs or alcohol.

2. As a general rule, focus on the "here and now." While some discussion of past events can be helpful, a client's obsession with them may be his or her way of avoiding current problems in living. Berne (1967) has described this game played in group therapy situations as "archeology."

3. Use any transference situations, as they become evident, as learning and insight-development opportunities. Point out the *differences* between the transference object and the group member's significant other. The increasing ability to be aware of one's own distortions is a sign of improving mental health.

4. Whenever necessary, protect individual members from verbal abuse or from scapegoating. This is an *important* role of the leader, and it also enables the leader to act as a model for constructive communication and interpersonal relating.

*Group *process* refers to everything that happens within a group—who talks to whom, who "pairs" with whom, who sits where, the tone of the group, who acts as "assistant therapist," the "norms" of the group, the degree of group cohesiveness, and so on. Group *content* simply refers to *what* is discussed.

5. Whenever appropriate, point out any change a group member has made. For example, one group member in an inpatient unit was not able to tolerate sitting with her group for an entire session. But with encouragement she gradually became able to stay for the entire session and then even began to participate. Another group member, who was prone to using a good deal of circumstantiality, was able, after participation in the group, to control this behavior effectively. In both of these situations, positive reinforcement provided ego support and encouraged future growth.

6. Handle *monopolizing, circumstantiality, hallucination,* or *disclosure of delusional material* in a manner that protects the self-esteem of the individual but that also sets limits on the behavior in order to protect the other group members. Other group members may feel threatened by psychotic behavior because they do not know how to respond to it, because they are afraid that they, too, may come to such a point, or both. Disclosure of delusional material is particularly threatening to other group members. Quite often, the delusional beliefs have *not* been totally accepted by the individual and thus are somewhat open to therapeutic intervention. Since there is usually this doubt on the part of the delusional client, it often helps to connect the beliefs to real feelings—of fear, anxiety, anger, and so on. For example, a leader might say, "Sometimes when we get frightened or feel insecure, we become suspicious of other people." The next step is to avoid dwelling on or exploring the delusional material in the group session. These steps on the part of the leader can help decrease the anxiety within the group, which is partially the result of members not knowing how to respond to their fellow group member.

7. Develop the ability to intuitively recognize when a group member (particularly a new member) is "fragile." Chances are that the member is indeed in a precarious mental and emotional state and should be approached in a gentle, supportive, and nonthreatening manner.

8. Use silence effectively, to encourage self-responsibility within the group. Silence should not be allowed to continue when it is nonproductive or when it becomes too threatening to the group members. A good rule of thumb is that usually the most anxious person in the group will break the silence—sometimes it is the leader.

9. Laughter and a moderate amount of joking can act as a safety valve and at times can contribute to group cohesiveness.

10. The "assistant therapist" in the group can be a useful phenomenon. A group member may assume this role, and is often extremely insightful in providing valuable feedback and suggestions. The group leader should be able to use this help without allowing the assistant to completely avoid group attention or to avoid dealing with personal problems.

11. Role playing and role reversals can sometimes be useful in short, modified versions. They may help a member develop insight into the ways he or she relates to others.

12. The promotion of interaction among group members is one of the main goals. Some techniques include:
    a. Reflecting or rewording comments of individual group members
    b. Asking for group reaction to one member's statement
    c. Asking for individual reactions to a member's statement
    d. Pointing out any shared feelings within the group
    e. Amplifying an individual situation to include either some or all of the group members
    f. Summarizing at various points within the session and at the end (Smith, 1970)

13. Encourage the cohesiveness of the group. Group cohesiveness includes all of the factors, both evident and subtle, that interplay to encourage individuals to remain in the group. The following factors may enhance group cohesiveness:
    a. The ability of the members to be *interdependent*
    b. A uniformity of standards among group members concerning behavior, communication, goals, and so on
    c. A mutually supportive attitude
    d. An attitude of responsibility toward one another
    e. An atmosphere that is protective and that enhances security and self-esteem

    The following factors may contribute to group dissolution:
    a. Frequent absenteeism of members or leader
    b. Loss of a leader
    c. Addition of new members without adequate preparation
    d. Canceled meetings
    e. Structural changes—time, day, size of group
    f. Subgrouping, pairing, or polarization

THE NURSING PROCESS IN GROUP THERAPY

An understanding of the phases of group development, the crises that occur in the life of a group, the various phenomena that can occur in groups, and some ways of intervening in groups can help the nurse to apply the nursing process to group therapy. This section will deal with assessing, analyzing, planning care, implementing the plan, and evaluating the effectiveness of the plan.

1. Making an assessment; aim: to gather information from verbal and nonverbal communication of the group and of the individuals within the group
   a. Gather the following information about group dynamics systematically and continuously from group therapy sessions:
   (1) Individual clients' perceptions of their situations or problems (content themes)
   (2) Predominant themes of the group as a whole (content *and* process themes)
   (3) Kinesic and proxemic behavior of individuals within the group (process themes)
   (4) The predominant theme of the present group environment (for example, hostility, parallel play, resistance, cooperation)
   (5) Biological, intellectual, psychological, sociocultural, and spiritual similarities and differences among group members (holistic health status)
   (6) Factors predisposing individuals within the group to their particular situations or problems
   (7) Factors precipitating particular situations or problems within the group
   (8) Strengths of individuals within the group
   (9) The directionality of relationships: leader to members, members to leader, among members
   (10) The particular phase of group development (for example, orientation, working, termination *or* parallel, inclusion, mutuality, termination)
   (11) Various types of phenomena occurring within the group process (for example, pairing, scapegoating, monopolization)
   (12) Current crises of group development (for example, authority, intimacy, separation)
   (13) The degree of power held by the leader as opposed to the members. This changes in accordance with the phase of the group's development

and/or the influence of group crises

(14) The interrelationships among group phenomena, roles, behavior, interpersonal relationships, content themes, phases, and crises

b. Verify the data.

(1) Confirm observations and perceptions by obtaining consensual validation from individuals within the group, through group consensus, and/or through other sources (records, psychological tests, pre-group and post-group meetings with others, such as co-leaders and staff members)

(2) Communicate assessment information to the other staff members verbally, in post-group sessions, in written group reports, and through charting on individual clients' records. Group session reports are written assessments of the therapy session that usually include:

(a) Identification of predominant group themes

(b) Identification and description of individual "content" themes

(c) Identification and description of individual verbal and nonverbal "process" themes

2. Analyzing the data; aims: to understand the nature of individuals' situations or problems and to understand the structure and developmental phase of the group and current themes and crises

a. Formulate nursing diagnoses that state the predominant themes of individuals and their relationships to contributing factors (for example, low self-esteem and unexpressed anger related to an impending divorce and the earlier loss of mother—precipitated in current group session through absences of regular group leader)

b. Formulate a nursing diagnosis that states the predominant social environment of

the group and its relationship to contributing factors (for example, group resistance and hostility related to absence of regular leader during vacation time)

3. Planning client care

a. Aim: to develop goals (individual and group) and a plan of action for initiating changes in individuals that will enable them to better cope with their existing situations and/or problems

(1) Depending on your assessment of the distribution of power within the group (centrality of leader vs. greater degree of "shared" power within the group) and/or group crises, help and encourage the group and individuals to set goals and establish priorities among goals (for example, need to discuss feelings around impending discharge of one member vs. need to plan for social event next week).

(2) Differentiate between long-term goals and short-term goals.

(3) State projected outcomes to the group.

b. Aim: to identify and modify group goals, taking into consideration individual capabilities, strengths, and weaknesses and the group status. Modifications should be based on group theory, group therapy principles, psychiatric literature, and the group leader's own experience with effective approaches to group interaction and development.

(1) Anticipate group and/or individual needs based on the priority of goals.

(2) Include all members of the group in the development of group interaction.

(3) Plan and work toward goals that are appropriate for the group members in terms of age, sex, locus of decision making, and intellectual, sociocultural, biological, psychological, and spiritual status.

(4) Identify group therapy interaction techniques that are helpful for specific group phenomena.

c. Aim: to cooperate with other health team members in the delivery of health care

  (1) Provide a group atmosphere that is consistent with the total therapeutic environment.

  (2) Allow for flexibility to meet the varied needs of individuals within the group.

  (3) Report and/or chart information that is pertinent to client care and to smooth functioning of the therapeutic milieu.

4. Implementing the care plan; aim: to facilitate group interaction and movement toward established group and individual goals

  a. Promote the individual's and the group's experience and use of the curative factors in group therapy (for example, universality, instillation of hope).

  b. Facilitate interaction among group members through knowledge and use of some of the techniques of group psychotherapy.

  c. Follow guidelines for effective leadership in group therapy.

5. Evaluating the care plan

  a. Aim: to include the client in estimating the client's progress toward attainment of goals

  (1) Toward the end of session, summarize and ask for summarizing input from the group regarding themes and phenomena of that particular group session.

  (2) For ongoing groups, schedule periodic individual sessions for group members to evaluate individual progress.

  b. Aim: to evaluate the effectiveness of the current care plan in group therapy

  (1) Periodically evaluate the development and changes in the group in regard to crises.

(2) Participate in pre-group and post-group sessions with other staff members and with co-therapists.

PRE-GROUP AND POST-GROUP STAFF MEETINGS

To facilitate an effective use of the nursing process in a group therapy session, it is helpful for staff members to meet, share information, and plan possible strategies for intervention. The pre-group meeting is generally in the form of a report that is given by staff members to the group leader or leaders. Each group member's history and present status are reviewed, and any potential problems of interaction between group members and/or between group members and the staff are discussed. Any known group trends or crises can also be addressed at this time.

Post-group sessions are useful in helping the staff to evaluate the whole group process. Staff members can share and discuss their observations and interpretations about the group and the individual members, and some problem solving may be done at this time. The post-group session also provides an opportunity for "peer supervision" and learning. Feedback about staff members' participation is available while it is still fresh in the minds of the participants.

The following guide has been developed to aid nurses both in making an assessment and in establishing goals for group therapy.

GUIDE FOR ASSESSMENT OF GROUP PROCESS

1. Description of group
  a. Type of group (e.g., activity, encounter, remotivation, psychodrama)
  b. Theoretical framework
  c. Goals of group
  d. Size of group

e. Composition of group
  (1) Age of members
  (2) Sex of members
  (3) Ethnic backgrounds of members (optional)*
  (4) Physical health status of members
  (5) Behavior exhibited by members
  (6) Educational levels of members
  (7) Communicational levels of members (e.g., verbal; mute; speak a foreign language)
  (8) Reality testing levels of members
  (9) Other (describe)
2. Physical setup of group (describe)
  a. Furniture (e.g., table and chairs or chairs only)
  b. Ventilation (Smoking vs. nonsmoking may be a group issue.)
  c. Distractions (noise from other areas; privacy)
3. Characteristics of group
  a. Group phase or stage (orientation, working, termination *or* parallel, inclusive, mutuality, termination)
  b. Level of cohesiveness
  c. Level of anxiety
  d. Level of conflict
  e. Level of resistance
  f. Crisis theme (authority, intimacy, separation)
  g. Other (describe)

4. Patterns of group interaction
  a. Communication patterns
    (1) Silence
    (2) Semantic argument
    (3) Intellectualization
    (4) Monopolization
    (5) Scapegoating
    (6) Other (describe)
  b. Behavior patterns
    (1) Physical activity
    (2) Withdrawal
    (3) Detachment
    (4) Cooperation
    (5) Competition
    (6) Other (describe)
  c. Social patterns
    (1) Group norms
    (2) Group rules
    (3) Roles (e.g., peacemaker, assistant therapist, leader, protector, attacker, interpreter)
    (4) Alliances among members (subgroups)
    (5) Conflict between alliances
    (6) Other (describe)
5. Patterns of leadership
  a. Approach of leader(s)
    (1) Laissez-faire
    (2) Democratic
    (3) Power struggle
    (4) Authoritarian
    (5) Other (describe)
  b. Competence of leader(s)
    (1) Provides relaxed, nonjudgmental atmosphere
    (2) Protects group members from disruptive communication patterns (scapegoating)

---

*Legislation protects people from being required to reveal ethnic background.

(3) Accepts all feelings, attitudes, and ideas as valid themes for group discussion

(4) Responds to verbal and nonverbal communication

(5) Facilitates communication and problem solving by:
  (a) Encouraging group members to clarify and describe feelings, attitudes, and ideas
  (b) Summarizing as needed

(6) Facilitates group cohesiveness by:
  (a) Asking for feedback and validation
  (b) Giving responsibility to the group
  (c) Encouraging the group to make decisions
  (d) Permitting the group to review and revise goals as indicated
  (e) Developing leadership among group members

(7) Other (describe)

CHAPTER SUMMARY

Group therapy is a valuable treatment modality. Nurses who work in psychiatric settings are involved, according to their educational preparation, as group leaders, group therapists, and co-therapists.

Some of the therapeutic benefits of group therapy may be similar to those of individual treatment, while other benefits are unique to group therapy. The curative factors of group therapy have been delineated, and the important characteristics that facilitate effective group leadership have been outlined.

It is possible to recognize a group's phase of development, current ''crises'' facing the group, and the emergence of various phenomena within the group. Effective use of the nursing process within a group situation is based on knowledge and sensitive understanding of these dimensions of the group process.

REFERENCES

Berne, E.
   1966 Principles of Group Treatment. New York: Oxford
      University Press, Inc.
   1967 Games People Play: The Psychology of Human Rela-
      tionships. New York: Grove Press, Inc.
Cartwright, D., and A. Zander
   1967 Group Dynamics: Research and Theory (ed. 3). New
      York: Harper & Row, Publishers, Inc.
Fried, E.
   1972 "Basic concepts in group psychotherapy." In The Evo-
      lution of Group Therapy. H. Kaplan and B. Sadock
      (eds.). New York: E.P. Dutton & Co., Inc., pp. 27-50.
Kaplan, H., and B. Sadock (eds.)
   1972 The Origins of Group Psychoanalysis. New York: E.P.
      Dutton & Co., Inc.
Levine, B.
   1979 Group Psychotherapy: Practice and Development. En-
      glewood Cliffs, N.J.: Prentice-Hall, Inc.
Rogers, C.
   1971 "Carl Rogers describes his way of facilitating encoun-
      ter groups." American Journal of Nursing 7(2):275-
      279.
Sampson, E., and M. Marthas
   1981 Group Process for the Health Professions (ed. 2). New
      York: John Wiley & Sons, Inc.
Scheidlinger, S.
   1982 Focus on Group Psychotherapy: Clinical Essays. New
      York: International Universities Press, Inc., p. 119.
Smith, A.J.
   1970 "A manual for the training of psychiatric nursing per-
      sonnel in group psychotherapy." Perspectives in Psy-
      chiatric Care 8(3):106.

Yablonsky, L.
   1965 Tunnel Back Synanon. New York: MacMillan, Inc.
Yalom, I.
   1975 The Theory and Practice of Group Psychotherapy (ed.
      2). New York: Basic Books, Inc., Publishers.

ANNOTATED SUGGESTED READINGS

Dublin, R.
   1981 "Concurrent group and family treatment for young
      adults." Social Casework 62(10):614-621.
      This article discusses some of the benefits of concurrent
      group and family treatment for young adults with seri-
      ous emotional problems. Case material on individual
      clients is presented, as well as the interrelationships
      with family dynamics and family treatment. Family
      treatment is seen as a natural outcome of the increased
      self-awareness and self-esteem that is inherent in in-
      volvement in group process.

Ernst, C., S. Vanderzyl, and R. Salinger
   1981 "Preparation of psychiatric inpatients for group ther-
      apy." Journal of Psychiatric Nursing and Mental Health
      Services 19(7):29-33.
      This article reports and discusses a study of the effec-
      tiveness of formally structuring the preparation of group
      participants in an inpatient setting. In this method cli-
      ents and therapist discuss purpose, goals, plans, and
      the roles of members and leader. Any preexisting atti-
      tudes toward therapy and therapy groups are also ex-
      plored. Instructional aids in the form of a film and writ-
      ten material are used. A review of the literature sup-
      porting a planned program of preparation for potential
      group members is included in this article.

Mackey, R.

1980 "Developmental process in growth-oriented groups."
Social Work 25(1):26-29.

The author examines how the changes that take place in individuals within a group occur. Several definitions of the term "group process" are discussed, and studies of group process by well-known group theorists are reviewed. A five-stage model of group development (Garland, Jones, and Kolodny) is presented. This includes (1) preaffiliation, (2) power and control, (3) intimacy, (4) differentiation, and (5) separation.

Marcovitz, R., and J. Smith

1983 "Patients' perceptions of curative factors in short-term group psychotherapy." International Journal of Group Psychotherapy 33(1):21-39.

A study of the mechanisms of change as perceived by clients in inpatient group psychotherapy is presented. The Yalom (1975) Curative Factor Q-Sort was used to determine the most helpful mechanisms of change (as perceived by clients). The author concluded that (1) a here-and-now orientation is best, (2) the teaching of concepts and the clear delineation of goals are important, (3) clients benefit from being encouraged toward self-responsibility and responsibility toward others, (4) sufficient time for expression of feelings is crucial, (5) it is important to foster an attitude of acceptance and respect in regard to differences within the group, and (6) praising risk-takers may encourage others to do the same.

Rogers, C.

1971 "Carl Rogers describes his way of facilitating encounter groups." American Journal of Nursing 71(2):275-279.

This excellent article describes Carl Rogers' philosophy of working therapeutically with groups. It is particularly helpful for nurses leading or participating in group therapy sessions in the psychiatric units of general hospitals. Appropriate, therapeutic use of self and self-disclosure is discussed.

Yalom, I.D.

1983 Inpatient Group Therapy. New York: Basic Books, Inc., Publishers.

Short-term psychiatric inpatient group therapy is an art unto itself. This excellent primer for clinicians who work with inpatient groups includes appropriate goals, common problems (e.g., rapid turnover of group members), and specific goals and techniques for different levels of functioning.

CHAPTER 12

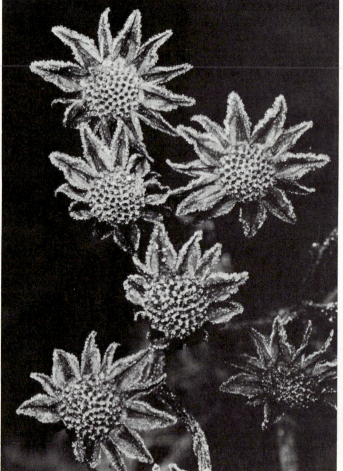

Photo by Hans Pfletschinger—Peter Arnold, Inc.

Family dysfunction and family therapy

CHAPTER FOCUS

The family is a system and has the properties of any social system. As the family system operates within its context, it may become vulnerable to stressors that affect family structure and family function. Alterations in family membership, sociocultural strains, maturational events, and disordered family relationships may stress the family system into dysfunction.

Nurses need to be aware of the models of family theory and family therapy that can be used in treating dysfunctional families. Among these models are the structural model, the interactional model, and the developmental (multigenerational) model. Nurses should also recognize that cultural presuppositions may be inherent in some aspects of these family models. Therefore, as nurses engage in primary, secondary, or tertiary prevention of family dysfunction, they should be aware that their assessments, interpretations, and goals may be value laden.

Throughout the United States, there is a growing tendency to view the family, rather than the individual, as the client of choice for the delivery of health care. Nurses, whether they are general-duty nurses, mental health nurses, occupational health nurses, or community health nurses, are becoming increasingly involved with the mental health needs of families. To effectively work with families, nurses need to become knowledgeable about family dysfunction and family therapy.

DYSFUNCTION WITHIN THE FAMILY SYSTEM

Stressors on the family system

As the family system interacts with other social systems, it may become vulnerable to any number of stressors that may impair its structure and function. Chief among these stressors are:

1. Changes in family membership—loss of a family member through divorce, separation,

death, chronic illness, or hospitalization or addition of a family member through birth, adoption, or incorporation (for example, grandparents move into the household)

2. Sociocultural strains—environmental pressures such as inadequate support systems, community disorganization, discrimination, inadequate housing, culture shock, overcrowding, and economic difficulties

3. Maturational events—transitions between developmental stages, such as marriage, entrance of a child into school, and retirement

4. Disordered family relationships—imbalance in the internal structure of the family, caused by such factors as double-bind communication, parental overburdening, overbonding to the family, and psychosomatogenesis.

Thus the family as a system is vulnerable to stress from its environment. The degree of stress that may be engendered depends on the nature of the stressor and the family's perception, interpretation, and response to the stressor. The following discussion focuses on the ways in which some of these stressors contribute to family dysfunction.

CHANGE IN FAMILY MEMBERSHIP

Vulnerability factors associated with a change in family membership include the ages of family members at the time of the change,* the emotional make-up of family members, and the nature of relationships among family members (especially between parents and children.)

The addition or loss of a family member may force a reorganization of the family system and may engender stress in the family system. This stress may threaten the emotional, social, and interpersonal security of individual family members, and it may influence their ability to accomplish developmental tasks.

During the infancy period, the infant's primary relationship is with the care giver (who is usually the mother). Loss of this relationship not only can result in a decrease in the quality and quantity of

———————
*Refer to Chapter 6 for a discussion of human development.

the infant's nurturing, but also can contribute to later difficulties with attachment or object permanence (Critchley, 1981).

However, it is during the preschool period that children are most vulnerable to the emotional, social, and interpersonal insecurities associated with change in family membership. For example, the birth of a sibling may engender jealousy in a preschool child. The hospitalization of a parent or parental divorce may cause a preschool child to experience separation anxiety and fear of abandonment. In addition to these reactions, a preschool child may respond to the loss of a parental relationship with repression and denial. The inability of the still present parent to authentically express feelings in front of the child may reinforce the child's denial and repression. Preschool children may also become regressed, withdrawn, hyperactive, and anorexic, and they may have temper tantrums, gastrointestinal upsets, and sleep disturbances. These responses are usually transient; there is no cause for alarm unless they become permanent. Since this is the stage in which children normally lay the foundation for satisfactory object relations, parental depression, overprotectiveness, or anxiety (parental responses to change in family membership) may interfere with the ability of preschool children to form object relationships (Irvine, 1965; Critchley, 1981).

It is during the school-age stage that children face the developmental tasks of industry and autonomy. At this time children become very involved with friends and with school activities. The involvement of children with the family is usually minimal. Change in family membership reinvolves children with the family, and this reinvolvement may interfere with childhood achievement of industry and autonomy.

If a change in family membership is due to the death of a family member, children may experience guilt feelings about having been unkind to or having wished for the demise of the family member. If a child dies, parents may idealize the dead child and they may create an unrealistic model for surviving children to follow. School-age children may respond to the stress of change in family membership with guilt, withdrawal, sadness, hostility, anxiety, and/or poor school grades. The persistence or intensification of any of these reactions, or the development of somatization, socially deviant behavior (lying, stealing), or depression, may signal the onset of a psychopathological condition* (Glaser and Strauss, 1964; Irvine, 1965; Markusen and Fulton, 1971; Critchley, 1981).

Young school-age children usually have difficulty using such coping behaviors as fantasy, denial, and structured activities to deal with the emotions engendered by a change in family membership. If the change was produced by divorce, a child may develop problems associated with strong and conflicting loyalties to both parents. For example, the loss† through divorce of a relationship with Father may be experienced by a child as rejection, loss of security, and paternal deprivation. The child may respond to this situation by blaming and becoming angry with his or her mother. At this age, resignation to parental divorce usually occurs within 1 year. Young school-age children achieve this resignation by increasing their psychological distance from both parents, thus coping with the turmoil engendered by conflicting parental loyalties (Kelly and Wallerstein, 1977).

Because older school-age children are better able to use coping behaviors of fantasy, denial, and structured activities and are better able to understand the situations surrounding changes in family membership, they are usually better able to cope with family membership changes than are younger school-age children. However, the increased ability of older school-age children to cope with family membership changes does not mean that difficulties do not arise. For example, an older school-age child may feel shame about parental divorce. He or she may evidence such symptoms as headaches and stomaches, as well as depression, poor self-esteem, school problems, and anger

toward the parent he or she perceives as causing the divorce. Age-appropriate tasks of identity formation and the development of mutuality and reciprocal support in interpersonal relationships may be undermined. If the parents use the parent-child relationship to decrease their own loneliness and insecurity, the child may become overburdened with adult responsibilities. This overburdening may interfere with the child's ability to form peer relationships. Such difficulty in relating to peers may lead some older school-age children to precociously engage in sexual experimentation in an attempt to form close interpersonal relationships (Wallerstein and Kelly, 1976; Kalter, 1977; Critchley, 1981).

When adolescents experience a change in family membership, they may try to cope by distancing themselves from the family. Adolescence is the developmental stage when children try to achieve independence from their families through a high degree of participation in school, work, and social events, and if a change in family membership occurs at this time, involvement in these activities may intensify more than is usual. Danger may be signaled when adolescents use excessive sexual activity or socially deviant behavior as a means of accomplishing family distancing (Glasser and Strauss, 1964; Markusen and Fulton, 1971; Sorosky, 1977; Berg-Cross, 1977; Critchley, 1981).

Sometimes late adolescents and young adults (aged 18 to 25 years) become overly concerned about family financial problems that result from change in family membership or concerned about the effect of family membership changes on younger siblings. Other times, they assume a disproportionate responsibility for household tasks or they become confidants to their parents. Any of these situations may produce overburdening. By interfering with the ability of late adolescents and young adults to establish their own identities, to enter into intimate relationships, with other people, and to become interdependent, this overburdening may hinder their ability to accomplish the developmental task of this life stage—intimacy vs.

---

*See Chapter 15 for a discussion of psychopathology in children.

†Refer to Chapter 18 for further discussion of loss and grief.

isolation (Erikson, 1950; Critchley, 1981).

Family membership changes also affect adults and their ability to accomplish developmental tasks. The tasks of the adult stage of life is generativity as opposed to stagnation. This is the period of life when the capacity to enter into a sharing relationship develops. A dyadic relationship may be formed, and the relationship may be extended by the addition of children. The birth of a child, especially of a first child, may arouse feelings in the parents of anxiety, inadequacy, and disenchantment with the parenting role (LeMasters, 1965). The death of a child may transform a family triad back into a dyad. If a spouse is lost, the sexual dyad itself is disrupted. Loss of family members may lead adults to question their life goals and to feel that they have not been successful in life. Critchley (1981) has found that after a divorce, the adults involved may feel anxious, depressed, angry, helpless, or insecure and that they may try to cope with their loneliness and insecurity by using one of their children as a confidant. When parents lose a child, they may respond to the child's death by engaging in self-blame. They may feel that they should have been able to prevent the child's death, and they may view the child's death as evidence of their failure to successfully perform their parenting roles (Glaser and Strauss, 1964; Markusen and Fulton, 1971).

The final phase of development, according to Erikson (1950), is ego integrity as opposed to despair. Older adults who are faced with family dismemberment may experience many of the same reactions as do young and middle-aged adults. However, for some older adults, in reviewing their lives, the loss of a family relationship may become a cause for despair.

Mr. and Mrs. Rockford were in their sixties. When their son, who had been married for 10 years, announced that he was getting a divorce, the Rockfords were shocked. After the divorce, their daughter-in-law obtained custody of the children and she moved out of the state. Mr. and Mrs. Rock-ford had been very close to their grandchildren, and they were accustomed to seeing them on a weekly basis. They knew that they would now only see their grandchildren infrequently and that they would not be part of their grandchildren's growing up. They despaired over what might have been.

Mrs. Fulicetti, who was 70 years old, lived with her daughter, her son-in-law, and their children. When Mrs. Fulicetti's son-in-law died, she felt sad and she despaired. At the funeral and in the days afterward, Mrs. Fulicetti frequently said, "I'm an old lady. God should have taken me. I've lived my life. My son-in-law had his life ahead of him and a family that needed him."

Yet some older adults respond to family dismemberment with sadness and anxiety but without despair. They have had much experience with the establishment, maintenance, and termination of relationships. They are able to look at the loss of a family member within the perspective of a life that has contained both positive and negative happenings, and they do not despair over what might have been.

SOCIOCULTURAL STRAINS

In families that are characterized by overcrowding, scarcity of resources (food, fuel, money, clothing), or instability (for example, inadequate support systems, interrupted interpersonal relationships, or lack of routine in daily living), parental overburdening may develop. Minuchin (1967) refers to these families as disorganized or disadvantages families. In such families, parents may only have sufficient time and energy to fulfill their children's need for physical nurturing. Children's psychosocial needs may not be recognized. Parents may view discipline only as a means of controlling children and not as a way of teaching and guiding children in socially acceptable behavior. Thus, although undesirable behavior may be punished, desirable behavior may go unacknowledged and unrewarded. As a result, the children from these family systems may experience the following problems:

1. An inability to recollect events so that they can be drawn upon for guidance in similar life situations
2. An inability to recognize subtle variations in interpersonal behavior. The behavior of others is either interpreted as aggressive or not understood at all.
3. An inability to respond to situations with moderation. The children are either passive or aggressive, intensely involved or totally uninvolved (Minuchin, 1967).

Sociocultural stress is also experienced by many ethnic families.* Ethnic families often try to become acculturated to American society while at the same time attempting to preserve ethnic traditions, customs, and behaviors. Ethnic parents may give their offspring a self-contradictory message: become successful in American society, but maintain strong ties with your ethnic group. If ethnic parents have experienced discrimination, they may become overly protective in their attempts to protect their children from discrimination. In addition, ethnic children, who in school are exposed to American life-styles, often become acculturated more rapidly than their parents. The children may then assume the tasks of acculturating their parents. This role reversal may produce overburdening in the children, a situation that may not only produce tension in intrafamilial relationships but may also deprive the children of opportunities to successfully compete in American society and to develop the social skills necessary to relate to people outside the ethnic group. In some instances, the children may respond to these stressors with alienation from American society. This alienation may be expressed in one or both of the following ways: (1) developing an antisocial attitude and trying to gain upward mobility in American society through socially deviant behavior† or (2) banding together in an ethnic peer group gang, or cult (Scheflen and Scheflen, 1972; Gambino, 1974).

Sociocultural stress may be further experienced

when ethnic persons marry outside their ethnic groups. The ethnic identities of the inter-ethnic couple may weaken. For example, an ethnic language may not be spoken at home and ethnic foods may not be prepared. For the offspring of inter-ethnic marriages, ethnic identity may become more optional than ascriptive. Children may opt to identify more with the ethnic heritage of one parent than with the heritage of the other parent, or they may ignore the ethnic heritage of one parent (Parsons, 1975). The parent whose ethnic heritage is not chosen may feel slighted or resentful.

In addition, differing concepts of male-female relationships may cause tension in inter-ethnic marriages. For example, while Mediterranean and Latin American male-female relationships are often strongly influenced by a tradition that includes a double standard and male domination of women, American male-female relationships are usually more egalitarian (Colecchia, 1978; Gilmore and Gilmore, 1979; Pasquali, 1982). Therefore, during the early years of marriage, inter-ethnic couples may have to make many adjustments concerning sex-defined role expectations and behaviors.

Different definitions and concepts of "family" may also create tension in inter-ethnic marriages. For instance, the extended family is a central force in the lives of many people of Asian, Hispanic, and Mediterranean descent (Hsu, 1970; Scheflen and Scheflen, 1972). Should such a person marry someone with a nuclear family orientation, the spouse may become resentful, impatient, or jealous of the degree of involvement with extended family members.

*Refer to Chapter 4 for further discussion of ethnicity.
†Refer to Chapter 17 for a discussion of social deviance.

A Hispanic man who had married a British-American woman complained: "My grandparents, aunts, uncles, and cousins have always been a very important part of my life. When we first came to the United States from Cuba, we all lived together. Even when we all had enough money to get our own places to live, we lived near each other. We still have a close-knit family. I feel secure knowing that no matter how bad things get, I have any number of people who will help me and who care about me. With my wife, it's a very different situation. Her idea of a family is her mother and father and her sister and brother. She has aunts and uncles and cousins, but she's not as close to them as I am to my relaitves. My wife always thinks my family is taking advantage of me. She doesn't understand how it is with us—how we all feel responsible for each other."

Thus, because of different conceptualizations of male-female relationships and of the family, tension and conflict may be engendered when people with different ethnic backgrounds marry. This tension and conflict may be compounded if offspring opt to identify more with the ethnicity of one parent than with the ethnicity of the other parent.

MATURATIONAL EVENTS

Events that mark the transitions between developmental stages can produce stress and tension in the family system. Marriage, parenthood, the entry of a child into kindergarten, and retirement are only a few of the maturational events that may force a reorganization of the family system. There may need to be a reassignment of family roles, a reordering of status positions, a reassessment of values, a re-channeling of communication, and a restructuring of ways to fulfill the needs and expectations of family members (LeMasters, 1965; Williams, 1974). The tension and disorganization that accompany these changes lead to maturational crises. Maturational crises* are predictable developmental events that occur at transition points in the life cycle (Williams, 1974).

A classic study by Klein and Ross (1965) of children's entry into kindergarten illustrates how a maturational event can generate stress within the family system. Klein and Ross found that the entry of a child into kindergarten was marked by tension within the family and by altered patterns of behavior. The way in which tension was expressed

varied from family to family and even differed among members of the same family. The following reactions were observed in children: (1) physical complaints such as anorexia, fatigue, and nausea; (2) increased use of or regression to such behaviors as bedwetting and thumb sucking; (3) hyperirritability, expressed in fighting with siblings or other children, talking back to parents, and uncooperativeness; (4) increased reliance on their mothers; and (5) such miscellaneous signs of stress as appearing "worried" or "keyed up," not wanting to attend school, and being either very talkative or very quiet.

Klein and Ross noted that parents usually experienced a sense of loss when their children entered kindergarten. Kindergarten entry also led to parental concern about value conflicts between the school and the family in the following three areas: (1) individuality vs. group conformity; (2) control of aggression vs. assertiveness and self-defense; and (3) learning to relate to the opposite sex vs. premature heterosexual interest.

Discomfit with shifts in parental roles was also evidenced. Many parents became annoyed when their children looked to the teacher as an authority figure and role model. Parents frequently experienced feelings of inadequacy about their ability to motivate and discipline their children as compared to the teacher's ability.

Klein and Ross also observed that at the same time that family members were reacting to the entry of a child into kindergarten, they began to display such growth behaviors as increased independence from the family, assumption of responsibility for oneself, and development of interests and activities outside of the family milieu.

Thus, the entry of a child into school, just like other maturational events, may engage families in role shifts, value reassessments, and other changes that alter family equilibrium, generate tension, and force a reorganization of the family system.

DISORDERED FAMILY RELATIONSHIPS

The way in which children are socialized within the family helps to mold their subsequent behavior

---

*Refer to Chapters 7 and 13 for a discussion of maturational crises.

as adults. Children learn from adult family members patterns of communication, means of coping with conflict, and ways to tolerate stress and alleviate anxiety (Albee, 1970; Lee, 1970; Satir, 1972).

Lucy grew up in a family that focused on health and illness to an extreme degree. When Lucy's father came home from work each evening, he would feel her forehead to see if she had a fever. This ritual of "feeling" Lucy's forehead replaced the kiss that is a common form of parent-child greeting in other families. In addition, whenever there was conflict between Lucy's parents, the conflict would be put aside when one parent complained of a severe headache. Lucy cannot ever remember her parents sitting down and trying to resolve a conflict. As Lucy grew into early adolescence, she began experiencing severe "migraines." These headaches were usually triggered by parental dissension. Extensive neurological examinations could uncover no physiological basis for Lucy's headaches.

The intrafamilial coping patterns of Lucy's family have been described by Minuchin et al. (1978) as being characteristic of a psychosomatogenic family.* In the psychosomatogenic family, children learn from adults that not only is psychophysiological dysfunction a concern common to all family members but also that it is a way to deal with conflict in the family. Instead of engaging in problem solving that would lead to conflict resolution, the family avoids the conflict by focusing on psychophysiological symptoms.

When intrafamilial behavior patterns deviate consistently and markedly from society's standards, family dysfunction may be engendered and family members may encounter difficulties interacting with their social environment (Fleck, 1972). The primary reasons for intrafamilial behavior patterns that deviate significantly from social norms

are parental overburdening and family overbonding.

Parental overburdening may be found most often in nuclear and single-parent families. Because these families are often both emotionally and geographically distant from extended family members, there may be too few adult family members to effectively care for children and to provide adults with whom children can identify. The total burden of child rearing then falls on the parents.

Searles (1965) and Scheflen and Scheflen (1972) see in parental overburdening the seeds of family dysfunction. Family members who remain in these families without avenues of mobility may develop overbonding to and overdependency on the family. There are three patterns that overbonding and overdependence may take (1): Clinging, overdependent children, who are afraid to be separated from the family, often develop phobias, hypochondriasis, or psychophysiological dysfunctions. (2) Children who are so strongly bonded to the parent of the opposite sex that they develop sexual attachment to that parent may become frozen in their emotional growth. They are often referred to as having unresolved Oedipus complexes. (3) Family members of any age who are overbonded to the family may become alcoholics or drug abusers. They may use alcohol or drugs to become assertive and confident enough to break away from the family, function independently, and relate to outsiders. However, they inevitably experience failure, lose confidence, and return to the family. Alcohol or drug abuse may at this point make them so helpless that the family takes them back and protects them.

Overbonded persons are often the identified clients in family systems. However, in all instances of overbonded, overdependent clients, we find that this is not solely the problem of the identified clients. Other family members are also locked into this overbonded relationship. In addition, these heavily bonded people tend to be vulnerable to double-bind situations,* in which they are confronted with paradoxical alternatives that

---

*See Chapter 16 for further discussion of the psychosomatogenic family and coping through psychophysiological responses.

*See Chapters 8 and 21 for further discussion of double-bind situations.

can be neither resolved nor avoided. Bateson and others (1956) believe this is the basis for schizophrenia.

Satir (1967) and Lidz et al. (1958) point out that disordered family relationships that generate identified clients are disappointing and destructive to all members of the family because:

1. The behavior of the identified client shatters the hopes of family members, especially of parents, to impress the community with the family's ideals.
2. The angry and rebellious behavior of the identified client can destroy parental expectations that their child will like them.
3. The socially deviant behavior of the identified client can be devastating to parents who look to their child to fulfill their own ambitions.
4. The behavior of the identified client may emphasize marital conflicts and divide the family, putting children in the position of having conflicting attachments and loyalties.
5. The identified client not only internalizes parental marital conflicts but continues to act out the family drama with other men and women long after the parents have died.
6. The identified client's labeling by the family as sick, bad, or different contributes to the development of low self-esteem in the client.
7. The identified client (and often other family members) is inadequately prepared to cope with life outside the family system. Family, especially parental, perceptions, interpretations, and responses to the environment tend to be incongruent with what members of other families experience. Since facts have to be consistently modified to meet emotionally determined needs, the family provides training in irrationality.

Violence within the family

Although categories of stressors have been discussed individually, they often interrelate to produce family dysfunction. To illustrate this interrelationship of stressors, we will look at violence within the family.* Domestic violence is a symptom of family dysfunction. In the United States, domestic violence has increasingly come to the attention of nurses and other health professionals.

Because domestic violence is rarely reported, it is difficult to determine its exact incidence. For example, Harris (1979) estimates that only 10% of wife abuse is ever reported to the police and that half of the women who experience abuse do not mention it to anyone, including other family members. Contrary to popular belief, family violence is not restricted to any social class, religion, race, ethnic group, or educational level. Societal attitudes that the family is sacred, that family matters should be kept private, and that the family should not be interfered with have contributed to society's tolerance of family violence (Lichtenstein, 1981).

Violence within the family refers to physical behavior that results in the infliction of physical harm by one family member onto another family member (Scott, 1974; Brown, 1981). Domestic violence may be divided into two categories:

1. Nonbattering behavior: one family member shoves, slaps, or throws objects at another family member.
2. Battering behavior: one family member kicks, bites, punches, uses an object to batter, or uses (or threatens to use) a gun or knife on another family member (Harris, 1979).

Although child abuse† and wife battering are the most commonly reported types of family violence, any member of the family may be a victim. In fact, because of the social stigma attached to a man being beaten by a woman, many husbands hesitate to tell anyone that they are being abused. The following statements of male clients speak to this reticence.

---

*See Chapter 17 for an in-depth discussion of violence, its theoretical framework, and nursing management.
†See Chapter 15 for a discussion of child abuse.

"My wife used to tie me up while I was sleeping and then beat the hell out of me. For years, I didn't tell

anyone because I was afraid they would think I was not a real man."

"About 6 months after we were married, my wife started to beat me. It's been going on now for 2 years. I really love her, but I can't go on like this. I'm too ashamed to tell people about it. I would go to a support group where there are other men who are experiencing the same thing, only I don't know of any such groups."

The factors most frequently identified as contributing to violence within the family are multiple. They include:

1. Family disorganization: Parental over-burdening or loss (through death, separation, divorce, or hospitalization) of significant others who served as role models for children or support systems for other family members may contribute to the breakdown of the family system. Such a breakdown may result in the loss of social controls that families usually impose on their members and may lead to:
   a. Inadequate development of social controls. The expectations and examples set by parents and other significant role models are especially influential on a child's ability to develop internal controls over behavior. If a child fails to internalize the expectations and controls over behavior that are sanctioned by society, he or she may use violent behavior as an adult.
   b. Learning of violent behavior. A child who grows up in a context of domestic violence is apt to learn that violent behavior is an effective way to solve problems. Children who observe violence in their own families or who are victims of physical abuse are apt to become child or spouse abusers as adults.
2. Sociocultural strains: environmental pressure such as inadequate support systems, community disorganization, poverty, overcrowd-

ing, and rapid social change may generate frustration and aggression, which may lead to:
   a. Anomie and alienation. There may be an absence of, or a failure to identify with, clear and shared standards of behavior and values. In addition, there may be a deterioration of the social roles around which people can organize their lives and order their social relationships. If children become estranged from socially approved purposes and goals, they may not incorporate the sanctions and constraints of society, and they may resort to domestic violence as adults.
   b. Incorporation of exaggerated stereotypes. Societal sex-role stereotyping of men as aggressive and independent and women as submissive and dependent may produce situations in which less powerful and secure men have to ''prove'' themselves by taking what more powerful and secure men either already have or can readily obtain. This social environment contributes to the use of violence by men against women and children as a means of attaining power in the family (Detre et al., 1975; Ashcraft and Scheflen, 1976; Halleck, 1978; Finley, 1981; Lichtenstein, 1981; Brown, 1981).

Such a multi-stressor approach speaks to the complexity of violence within the family and to the multigenerational transmission of patterns of family violence. Studies have shown that people who are child or spouse abusers have usually themselves been victims of child abuse (Smith and Hanson, 1975). Also, women who have been victims of child abuse are three times more likely to be abused by their husbands than are women who have not experienced childhood domestic violence (Harris, 1979).

Although violence within the family usually refers to physical abuse, a pattern of verbal abuse among family members, in the form of threats and derrogation, is also symptomatic of a dysfunctional family system. This is an area of family behavior that nurses need to be attuned to and in which more research needs to be done.

Vulnerability of families to dysfunction

To summarize the discussion of family dysfunction, it may be helpful to borrow the concept of "balancing factors" from Aguilera and Messick (1978). The interrelationship between such balancing factors as the way a family perceives a stressor (which is influenced by the stage of the domestic cycle occupied by the family, the cultural heritage of the family, and the ages of family members), the adaptability of the family social system, and the nature of family patterns of relating and communicating can either throw a family system into disequilibrium and dysfunction or contribute to a family system's maintenance of equilibrium and sound functioning. These opposing processes are diagramed in Fig. 12-1.

Although an entire family may experience a stressor or a series of multiple stressors, many factors may determine why one family member develops severe impairment of functioning while others do not. Chief among these factors are the

ages and developmental levels of family members; parental preference for one sex; parental reactions to fretful, colicky behavior in infants; nonresponsiveness of an infant; a high level of anxiety between spouses; a low degree of emotional involvement between spouses; and the holistic health status of family members. In addition, the following *pathological patterns of relating* may increase a family member's vulnerability to dysfunction:

1. *Scapegoating.* The process of consciously or unconsciously singling out one child to be the carrier of family problems has been termed scapegoating by family theorists. Possible explanations for a child's acceptance of this role include the fear of annihilation of the family system if he or she does not accept the role and the desire to defend against unconscious incestuous feelings.

2. *Emotional divorce.* Emotional divorce occurs when emotional investment between the spouses has been withdrawn. They may be "staying together for the children" or for any number of other reasons, but there is little real involvement with one another.

3. *Pseudomutuality.* Pseudomutuality includes the actions, conscious and unconscious, that

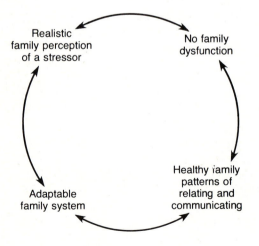

Fig. 12-1. Interrelationship of family balancing factors.

represent an attempt by family members to make the family system appear smooth-running and conflict-free to the outside world. This pattern of relating involves the creation of a facade; in reality, there is much overt and covert conflict and confusing communication.

4. *Coalition across generational boundaries.* Sometimes a parent tends to enter into or even initiate conspiracies and alliances with a child. Such a conspiracy, which is usually against the other parent, undermines the marital relationship and instills guilt and fear in the child, who has a self-perception of betraying one parent and being too close to the other. For example, assume that a child has asked his father for money to buy an ice cream cone from a street vendor. The father replies, ''No, it's 15 minutes before your supper!'' The child then asks his mother, who has overheard the exchange. She might respond in one of the following ways:
   a. ''No, your father is right; it's too close to supper!''
   b. ''Ok, here's the money, but let's not tell your father!''
   c. ''I don't agree with your father, and I will tell him so—here's the money.''
Response 1 is probably the healthiest; response 3 indicates a certain amount of marital discord—disagreement over child rearing. However, it is a healthier response than response 2, since the conflict is out in the open and the child is not engaged by the parent in a conspiracy against the other.

Pathological patterns of family communication may also contribute to a family member's vulnerability to dysfunction. The following are pathological ways of communicating with a family:

1. *Vagueness.* Vague ways of communicating, with a tendency to use universal pronouns (''they'') and loose associations, lead to ambiguity and to confusion on the part of the listener.
2. *Tangentiality.* Tangentiality means never really answering a question or responding to a statement in a direct way. This ''going off on tangents'' confuses a listener, who is not sure whether a question has been answered or, if it has been answered, what the response was.
3. *Double-bind communications.* A double-bind communication* involves the giving of two conflicting messages at the same time. One message may be verbal and the other nonverbal—for example, saying something affectionate to a child when body language says the opposite. Or both messages may be verbal: ''Son, your mother and I want you to be an independent person who makes his own decisions, so we have decided that you must go to a school out of town.'' A person who receives such a message is usually not aware that it contains two conflicting messages, but the conflict serves to immobilize and confuse the person. ''Damned if you do and damned if you don't'' messages are also double-bind messages—for example, a mother asking her adolescent schizophrenic son, ''If your father and I were drowning and you could only save one of us, which one would it be?''
4. *Family myths.* Some families engage in a perpetual denial of reality. For example, a father who is an alcoholic tyrant may have a wife who denies this fact to the world and to herself and insists that her children participate in the myth that the father is a sober and loving person. Any attempts by a child to state the real facts or to discuss feelings about them are met with strong denial and guilt-producing accusations.
5. *Mystification.* Mystification is a habitual communication process that might include any or all of the patterns described above. The following are some key characteristics of this process:
   a. Children being mystified do not realize that the family uses faulty communica-

---

*Refer to Chapter 21 for a discussion of double-bind communication and schizophrenia.

tion patterns and thus blame themselves for their confusion.

b. Children unconsciously sense that to question these patterns would threaten the equilibrium of the family system and their security.

c. The family continually uses these ways of communicating.

FAMILY THERAPY

Family systems theory and family therapy began in the mid-1950s (Bowen, 1978). In the United States, individuals and groups initially worked independently in the area of family treatment. They eventually began to communicate with each other, and a body of theoretical knowledge evolved. Today, family therapy is an effective tool for alleviating emotional problems. Graduate psychiatric nursing programs include family systems theory and clinical courses in family therapy as parts of their curricula. Psychiatric nursing clinical specialists are often actively involved as family therapists; many have increased their understanding and knowledge through participation in workshops and enrollment in family therapy institutions throughout the country.

Family therapists

In conducting family therapy, the goals of the therapist are to clarify and improve *family communication patterns* and *family relationship patterns*. The family itself is viewed as the client. It is thought that through reinforcement of healthy, clear boundaries between individuals, family members will be able to relate to one another in a meaningful way—in a way that protects healthy individual autonomy. There will not be the threat of loss of self through engulfment *or* the need to defend against this threatened loss through destructive distancing maneuvers. When necessary, the family therapist protects family members who are potential scapegoats and acts as a role model for more

mature functioning in the family environment. The therapist *clarifies* and *educates* and thus *facilitates* healthier functioning within the family system. In working with a family, a therapist usually wants to know something of the family history of both the husband and the wife. This information is helpful in assisting the family members to connect their past experiences to the present situation and to gain insight into their tendencies to use certain patterns of communicating and relating.

On the basis of how therapists work with families, Beels and Ferber (1973) have identified two types of family therapists: (1) *conductors,* who use their own dynamic personalities to give direction to the family, and (2) *reactors,* who let the family take the lead and then follow in that direction. Regardless of the approach that a therapist uses, the therapist's *use of self* is an important aspect of family therapy. Not only do therapists need to work through the relationships in their own families of origin and procreation, but they also need to work through their own ethnic identities. This helps therapists to resist being "triggered" by problematic relationships and ethnic characteristics found in their own backgrounds. In addition, when therapists learn about the orientation of the cultural groups from which they draw clients, they are less likely to be ethnocentric about values, attitudes, and behaviors that are different from their own (McGoldrick, 1982).

Models of family therapy

The approach devised by Jones and Dimond (1982), which was used to discuss models of family theory in Chapter 5, will be used to discuss models of family therapy.

STRUCTURAL MODEL

The family is viewed as an open system whose impetus for change arises from two sources: (1) biopsychosocial alterations in family members, and (2) interactions with other social systems. To fulfill family functions, the family group may differentiate into subsystems on the basis of age, sex, interest, or abilities (subsystems can consist of one or more family members). For example, in a given family the following subsystems may exist to carry out specific family functions: (1) the spousal subsystem, to fulfill conjugal functions; (2) the parental subsystem, to fulfill parenting functions; and (3) the sibling subsystem, to facilitate peer socialization. In addition, family members follow scripts or ''transactional patterns'' that regulate their lives and their relationships. These scripts are reinforced by systems of constraints. General rules that order family organization are known as *generic constraints*. For instance, in most families, parents have more authority in family matters than do children. The ways in which generic constraints are modified by a family are referred to as *idiosyncratic constraints*. For example, how parents specifically carry out their authority in the family and how parental authority differs from the authority of children may vary from family to family.

Minuchin (1974) and his followers are structural therapists. They view the demands for change that constantly face the family as potentials for family dysfunction. When faced with demands for change, individual family members, family subsystems, and the family as a whole may respond either with growth behaviors or with maladaptive behaviors. Maladaptive behaviors are dysfunctional transactional patterns for organizing family life and family relationships. The *goal* of therapy is to help the family learn new, alternative scripts or transactional patterns.

Parents came to a nurse–family therapist with complaints about their 8-year-old daughter destroying books. The mother was a university professor, and she spent much time reading and preparing lesson plans. The father was a law student, and he spent many hours studying. The nurse–family therapist found that the parents were not spending enough time with their daughter. The child tore up books when she was left to her own devices because her parents were busy reading or studying.

The nurse–family therapist assigned the parents the task of setting time aside each day for the purpose of teaching their daughter about the proper use of books. They might read aloud to one another, go to the library together, or, by following instructions in a book, create something (such as baking cookies or constructing a kite).

The activity of teaching their daughter about the appropriate use of books became an avenue for the parents to learn to spend time with their daughter. Thus, a new script was developed for family relationships.

INTERACTIONAL MODEL

The family is viewed as a communication system composed of interlocking subsystems (the individual family members). The process of family interaction, including rules that regulate relationships, is the focus of analysis. Family dysfunction occurs when the rules that govern family interaction become vague and ambiguous. This leads to confusion about what family members can expect from one another. Jackson (1965), Satir (1967), Haley (1962), and their followers are interactional therapists. The *goal* of therapy is to help the family clarify the rules that govern family relationships.

The Browns sought help for their 7-year-old son Peter. Peter's behavior at school had become disruptive. He teased his classmates, talked in class, and "resisted settling down to work."

After talking with Peter and his parents, a nurse-therapist determined that Peter's disruptive behavior was an attempt to unite his parents. Peter had learned that when his parents focused their attention on his disruptive behavior, they would stop arguing. The nurse-therapist therefore helped the Browns to focus on their marital relationship—not on Peter's behavior or on their parenting behavior. Central to the discord in their marital relationship was ambiguity in their communication of expectations. For example, Mrs. Brown "expected" that, since she had recently taken a job outside the home, her husband would help with the house-

work. Mr. Brown "assumed" that, if his wife wanted his help, she would ask for it. Neither person had ever clearly communicated what was wanted or expected from the other.

The nurse-therapist helped the Browns to see that each of them operated as if the other person were a mindreader. Messages were not clearly stated, and, because they did not communicate the expectations and wishes of the sender, the messages were incomplete. The nurse-therapist then helped the Browns to learn to communicate more clearly and completely with one another. Once the Browns learned to deal with their communication problems, their son Peter no longer needed to use disruptive school behavior to try to unite his parents.

The activity of clarifying rules for family interaction and of communicating expectations clearly to one another became an avenue for dealing with family dysfunction.

DEVELOPMENTAL MODEL

Because Bowen's (1971) multigenerational model focuses on reciprocal role relationships *over time* and thus takes a longitudinal approach to family therapy, Jones and Dimond consider it a quasi-developmental model. Bowen views the family as an emotional system. Change in one family member leads to change in other family members in a predictable, chain-reaction pattern. By using the following set of interrelated concepts, family dysfunction may be explained. If there is a high degree of *differentiation of self* among family members, family members are able to cope with changes and stress without becoming emotionally ill. Well-differentiated family members are characterized by authenticity in interpersonal relationships and by an ability to distinguish between thoughts and feelings. They are able to have "I" positions (ideas, plans, beliefs, and goals) that are their own and not their family's. They therefore can participate in the family system without being an "emotional domino" in the system (Friedman, 1971). People who have low levels of differentiation of self become fused with those with whom they have intimate relationships. Much of their energy is devoted to

finding affection and approval. Decisions tend to be based on feelings and cues from the family rather than on independent, objective thinking. People who have low degrees of differentiation of self tend to have high degrees of unresolved emotional attachment to their parents or to experience *emotional cutoff* (emotionally withdrawing from or denying the importance of one's parents, thereby creating an emotional disconnectedness between parents and child). In addition, the *sibling position profiles* (personality characteristics for each sibling position) of people with poor self-differentiation often are more typical of sibling positions other than their own. For example, an oldest child may exhibit the profile usually associated with a youngest child.

Generally, a person takes as a spouse someone with a similar degree of differentiation. The *nuclear family emotional system* refers to patterns of interaction and emotional functioning among parents and children in the nuclear family. These patterns are often "replicas" of what has happened in one's family of origin. Within the nuclear family, relationships are composed of interlocking *triangles,* the fundamental building blocks of the family. A triangle can be composed of a dyad that holds inside, comfortable positions and a third person, issue, or organization that holds an outside position. When relationships in the triangle become tense, the "outsider" may be brought into a closer position, or a family member holding an inside position in the triangle may try to avoid stress and obtain comfort by moving into the outside position. The classic family triangle is the mother-father-child triangle, and the tensions in this triangle, as in any triangle, are usually in flux (see Fig. 12-2).

Within the nuclear family, spouses may try to control ego fusion in any of the following ways: through overt conflict between spouses; through functional impairment of one of the spouses (for example, through alcoholism, physical illness, obesity, schizophrenia); or through functional impairment of one or more "triangulated" children (for example, through socially deviant behavior, physical illness, schizophrenia). This last method

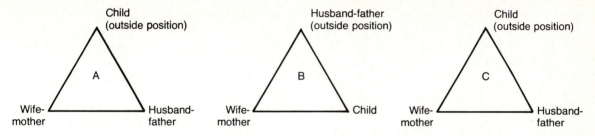

Fig. 12-2. Dynamic tensions of triangulation. Triangle A illustrates the family triangle with the spouse-parents holding inside positions and the child in the outside position. As tension increases between the spouse-parents, the child moves into an inside, "confidant" relationship with the mother, and the father escapes from the marital tension to the outside position in the triangle (triangle B). Later, when the child engages in behavior that is unacceptable to both parents, the wife-mother and husband-father realign themselves and the child again holds the outside position in the triangle (triangle C).

of controlling ego fusion among family members is referred to as the *family projection process*. When it is carried out over generations, it becomes the *multigenerational transmission process;* patterns of interacting and coping (for example, priorities, goals, attitudes) and unresolved issues can be passed down from generation to generation and can cause stress in the family members on whom they are projected. Illness thus is viewed as the transmission of insufficient differentiation across generational lines. The *goal* of therapy is to help family members attain a higher level of differentiation.

Larry was the identified client in the family. During several interviews with the family, the nurse-therapist learned that Larry's parents and grandparents had always valued education. In addition, it was customary in the family for parents to decide what careers their children would pursue.

Larry's father, his two uncles, and his grandfather were lawyers. When they went to law school, they had attended local universities and had lived at home. Larry's father said this was because they were a close-knit family.

Larry's parents had brought Larry up with the expectation that he would attend college. Larry wanted to be a veterinarian, but his parents did not want him to go out of town to veterinary school. Instead, they decided he would attend a local uni-

versity that had a law school. Larry would become a lawyer like his father.

Although Larry was unhappy with his parents' decision, he fulfilled his parents' expectations. Years later, Larry told a therapist, "I still wonder how my life would have been if I could have become a veterinarian like I wanted. But I also wanted to please my parents. If I had said 'No,' all hell would have broken loose. My parents would have thrown me out of the house and probably disowned me. Then what would have become of me?"

Larry had taken on the expectations and wishes of his parents. This was a behavior pattern that had been occurring in the family for generations, and it was a consequence of a low degree of differentiation. The therapist's goal would be to help Larry and his family attain higher levels of self-differentiation so that the lack of differentiation that had been transmitted over generations to Larry would not be projected onto Larry's children.

Cultural influences and family therapy

FAMILY DYNAMICS

The point was made in Chapter 5 that family organization and family dynamics vary according to cultural context. Although many family therapists are becoming increasingly aware of cultural variability, family theory and family therapy models are often culture bound and predicated on the family model of a "normal" middle-class, white, urban nuclear family (Haveliwala, Scheflen, and Ashcroft, 1979; Miller, 1981).

The assessments and goals of many family therapists tend to reflect this ethnocentrism. For example, self-direction, self-disclosure among family members, trusting in others, and independence are viewed by such therapists as Satir, Jackson, Haley, and Bowen as goals for any "healthy," well-functioning family system regardless of its cultural orientation. Yet self-direction and self-disclosure are characteristics that tend to be found in and valued by mainstream middle-class and upper-class families. These families usually have a sense, born out by experience, that their opinions, decisions, and actions can influence their fate. However, family therapists need to recognize that not all family systems encourage self-direction and self-expression and that this does not necessarily make them dysfunctional family systems. Some ethnic groups, such as the Chinese, do not encourage open expression of feeling among family members (Hsu, 1970). Also, many families in the lower stratum of American society often have a "non-introspective orientation" (Kohn, 1977; Miller, 1981).

Similarly, family styles of relating to others may also be culturally influenced. Banfield's study (1958) of southern Italian families revealed that an attitude of suspicion toward those who are not family and the maximization of material, short-range goals at the expense of people outside the family were acceptable patterns of family behavior. Spiegel (1959, p. 169) found that among Irish-American families dependency training is an important aspect of socialization. It is reinforced "through the mutual care and aid offered by the extended family, religious, and community networks."

It is therefore important for family therapists to be aware of the cultural variability of family organization and family dynamics so that their as-sessments, interpretations, and goals will not be value laden. A report by the Committee on the Family of the Group for the Advancement of Psychotherapy (1970) cautions therapists to be mindful of the cultural context of families when assessing family functioning.

FAMILY HEALING SPECIALISTS

All societies have healing specialists. In contemporary American society, psychiatric clinical nurse specialists, psychiatric social workers, psychologists, and psychiatrists can be trained as family therapists. In other cultures, such a role might be assumed by native healers, including *curanderos* (Central Americans), root doctors or *hoodoo* men (Afro-Americans), shamans (native Americans and Eskimos), and *babalawos* (Cubans and Yorubas).

The difference between family therapists and native healers is not as great as it may appear at first glance. Drawing on the study of Torrey (1977), we can look at some of the similarities between family therapists and native healers.

▶ Identifying and labeling the problem

A family therapist may speak of family fusion or of a closed family system as a source of family distress. A native healer may identify violation of a taboo or spirit possession as the source of family distress. In either case, identifying the problem conveys to the client-family that someone understands and cares. The very act of labeling the problem implies that it can be treated. Moreover, underlying the process of labeling is the assumption that, since the family therapist or native healer can identify and place the problem within a framework that the family can understand, he or she must share the client-family's world view. When world view is not shared between the therapist or native healer and the client-family, treatment is usually ineffective.

The parents of a Mexican-American girl were told by an Anglo-American family therapist that their daughter's depression and listlessness were related to their dysfunctional marital relationship. Therefore, the parents should become involved in marital therapy. They knew that their daughter was suffering from susto *(magical fright). They consulted a* curandero, *who performed the necessary* limpia *(spirit-cleansing ritual).*

An Anglo-American family would have found referral to a *curandero* as irrelevant as this Mexican-American family found the family therapist's approach.

▶ Personal qualities of the specialist

Among family therapists, empathy, authenticity, and nonpossessive warmth are important to the therapeutic process. Few studies have been done on the personal qualities of native healers; however, because people from different cultural groups conceptualize health and illness differently, the personal qualities of healers probably also vary. As was mentioned before, though, the ability of family therapists and native healers to share (or at least to understand) the world view of their client-families is a quality that is important to both.

▶ Expectations of client-families

Client-families usually have expectations in regard to the treatment they seek. In the vignette about the Mexican-American family, the family's expectation was that a *limpia* ritual would be performed to treat the daughter. Family therapists and native healers contribute to the expectations of client-families. For example, both family therapists and native healers are specialists in their societies, and some portion of client-family expectation is based on this expertise. In Western society, family therapists are accorded the status of professionals. Native healers are revered and sometimes feared because of their unique knowledge and power, a power that followers often believe is mystical or occult.

In addition, both family therapists and native healers have completed training programs, and

they may be "certified." Family therapists either have finished graduate programs that focus on family therapy or have taken courses in family theory and have had supervised clinical practice. Native healers, such as *babalawos,** have had a long preparatory period. This period is devoted to obtaining knowledge about herbs, learning rituals and divining procedures, and acquiring self-knowledge and self-control (González-Wippler, 1975). Some native healers may even have to pass a test at the end of their training period that "certifies" them as practitioners. For example, at the end of their training, Tenino Indian shamans are evaluated by already practicing shamans for the personal characteristics and fitness that are required for their exercise of power (Murdock, 1965).

▶ Techniques of therapy

Both family therapists and native healers try to ease family tension and resolve family conflicts. Family therapists may use such techniques as sculpting (constructing a live family portrait that depicts family alliances and conflicts), scripting (developing new family transaction patterns), and other creative arts (reviewing family photograph albums, writing family histories, drawing family pictures, constructing genograms, or role playing). Such techniques have been developed by Sedgwick (1976, 1978) and others to help families learn about, and to assist therapists in assessing, family dynamics, strengths, and weaknesses.

Native healers may use such techniques as rituals, spells, and divining. An example of the use of special techniques by native healers is the *curandero's* ritual treatment of *susto*.

---

*Babalawos are the high priests of Santería. The cult of Santería is a syncretization of Catholic and Yoruba beliefs, rites, and traditions.

Maria Sanchez appeared apathetic, listless, depressed, and withdrawn. She had no appetite and she ate little food. When she slept, she was restless and she had nightmares. The Sanchez family be-

lieved that Maria's *tonalli (soul) had been claimed by an evil spirit and that she was suffering from* susto *(magical fright). They brought Maria to a* curandero *who would perform the culturally prescribed* limpia *ritual.*

The purpose of the limpia *was to reclaim Maria's soul. Maria and her extended family members participated in the* limpia. *Spirit forms were cut from bark paper. These bark paper forms were used both to absorb evil spirits and to protect the participants at the* limpia *from evil spirits. A chicken was sacrificed. After the* limpia, *Maria's behavior improved and she once again became a functioning member of her family.*

The ritual techniques of a *curandero* accomplish the same ends as the techniques of the family therapist. A *curandero* acknowledges that a person is suffering from *susto* (also known as *espanto,* a culture-bound syndrome found among Central Americans). *Susto* is related to stress engendered by a self-perceived failure to fulfill sex-role expectations. Once a person is identified as suffering from *susto,* he or she is relieved of normal sex-role expectations and is made the focus of extended family attention. Although the *susto* sufferer is the identified client, *susto* indicates that there is a schism in the extended family. The culturally prescribed *limpia* ritual is a process for resolving the schism (all family members participate) and reincorporating the *susto* sufferer into the extended family (O'Nell and Selby, 1968). Thus, like the techniques of family therapists, the techniques that native healers use may serve to ease family tension and to resolve family conflicts.

• • •

It is important that nurses recognize that family dysfunction must be understood and treated within its cultural context. Family therapists and native healers share many similarities. Native healers should not be viewed as charlatans. In fact, the World Health Organization has recommended that Third World nations revive and expand their tradi-

tional health care systems (Returning to Traditional Healers, 1979). It has also been suggested that native healers and psychotherapists coexist and, whenever possible, work together so that the problems of families may be understood and treated within their cultural contexts (Horn, 1973).

NURSING INTERVENTION

PRIMARY PREVENTION

The focus of primary prevention is on the promotion and maintenance of healthy patterns of family interaction and functioning—on what family members say, on what they do, and on how they interact with one another in various situations. Nurses engaged in family-centered nursing function as teachers. They educate families, both family units and individual family members, about the following:

1. Potential sources of family stress
2. Effective coping patterns for dealing with stress
3. Life-style changes that may decrease family vulnerability to stress
4. Revision of family roles to accomodate maturational and situational changes in life-style
5. Family strengths that may support family functioning
6. Family weaknesses that may jeapardize family functioning (Jones and Dimond, 1982)

To engage in primary prevention activities with families, nurses need to understand the theories* that explain family functioning. Structural theory will help nurses understand the basic functions of a family. Interactional theory will help nurses identify dynamics of interaction among family members. Developmental theory will aid nurses in rec-

---

*Refer to Chapter 5 for a discussion of family theory.

ognizing family needs and tasks over time.

In addition to understanding family theory, nurses should be knowledgeable about stressors and their potential impact on family functioning. Nurses can then assist families in anticipating, preparing for, and ameliorating the effects of stressors on the functioning of the family.* For example, parent-child nurses and community health nurses may help parents anticipate the effect that the birth of a baby or the incorporation of a grandparent into the household may have on their marital relationship and on the needs, tasks, and interactions of other members. Strengths on which the family may rely and weaknesses from which the family needs protection may also be identified.

When a family has experienced a stressor, the nurse's role in primary prevention is to ameliorate the impact of the event so that it does not precipitate family dysfunction. For example, if the mother of a family has a mastectomy, the nurse may refer her to Reach to Recovery or to other mastectomy support groups. If a family member dies, the nurse may refer other family members to such grief support groups as widows and widowers groups (for bereaved mates) and The Compassionate Friends (for bereaved parents). Referrals to such self-help groups assist family members in coping with family stressors. Families are thereby helped to maintain equilibrium and to avoid dysfunction.

Moreover, knowledge about the influences of culture on family form and family dynamics is vital if nurses are to promote culturally acceptable patterns of family functioning. Should the cultural context not be considered, nurses might mistake culturally acceptable family functioning for family dysfunction.

---

*See Chapter 13 for a discussion of the nurse's role in anticipatory guidance and crisis intervention.

Nurses in the labor and delivery suite of a hospital whose catchment area included Chinese and Japanese enclaves observed that American and Asian fathers-to-be behaved very differently. Most of the American men either coached their wives through labor and delivery or waited in the solarium until their wives had delivered. In contrast, most of the Asian men brought their wives to the hospital and then returned home to wait the birth of their children. The nurses thought the Asian parents-to-be were "emotionally divorced," and they began to regard the Asian families as dysfunctional.

Only after conferring with a nurse-anthropologist were these nurses able to understand that in the Chinese and Japanese cultures, women have traditionally assisted women during childbirth. Men traditionally have been uninvolved. The reasons for this sex-role behavior include: (1) Chinese and Japanese men and women usually do not openly express emotion in public; (2) traditionally, Chinese and Japanese men view childbirth as women's work; (3) Chinese and Japanese women usually would be embarrassed to have their husbands present during the functioning of the female body.

Instead of promoting the culturally approved patterns of family functioning, the nurses had viewed the noninvolvement of Asian fathers-to-be and the absence of the expression of emotion between Asian spouses as evidence of emotional divorce. The nurses had identified family dysfunction where there was none. Their lack of knowledge about the cultural context of client-families had led them to inaccurately assess family functioning.

Understanding of family theory, family stressors, and cultural influences on the family system are therefore essential if nurses are going to promote and maintain healthy patterns of family interaction and functioning.

In addition, because overcrowding, poverty, and scarcity of resources may act as sociocultural stressors on the family system, nurses need to be aware of changes in local and national social programs. Nurses, as informed citizens and as client advocates, need to militate for social change. When budgets are streamlined, money for social services is usually cut. Yet this type of economizing often contributes to family stress. Promoting social changes that prevent socioeconomic stress or improve living conditions for families is an essential component of primary prevention of family dysfunction.

SECONDARY PREVENTION

The focus of secondary prevention is on intervention into family dysfunction and restoration of functional patterns of family behavior. Knowledge about principles of family therapy helps nurses understand the dynamics that contribute to family dysfunction. The symptoms of individuals are seen as developing from and feeding back into relational struggles and conflicts within the family system. The goal of nursing care is to help family members to function more effectively in their role relationships and interactions (Jones and Dimond, 1982). The nursing process provides the framework for intervention with client-families.

1. Assessment; aim: to gather information from verbal and nonverbal communication of family members
   a. Gather information systematically and continuously from interactions with individual family members and with the family as a unit. This information should include:
      (1) The family's perceptions of the stressor, situation, or problem
      (2) The family's interaction patterns, role relationships, and sociocultural strengths and limitations
      (3) The family's verbal, kinesic, and proxemic behavior
      (4) The holistic health status of individual family members: biological, intellectual, psychological, sociocultural, and spiritual
      (5) Factors that precipitate the situation or problem
      (6) The family's present environment (physical, social, cultural, and emotional environment)
      (7) The interaction of the nurse with individual family members and with the family as a unit
   b. Verify the data.
      (1) Confirm observations and perceptions by obtaining consensual validation or additional information from individual family members, the family as a unit, and/or other sources (for example, family photograph album, family Bible, genogram).
      (2) Chart family assessment information.
2. Analysis of the data; aim: to understand the nature of the family's dysfunction
   a. Identify family dynamics, family role relationships, and family stressors.
   b. Identify the interrelationship between family dynamics, family role relationships, predisposing and precipitating factors, the holistic health status of family members, and the family's perception of the stressor, situation, or problem.
   c. Formulate a nursing diagnosis that states both the family's dysfunction and the contributing factors (for example, disorganized role relationships related to the hospitalization of the husband-father; parental overburdening related to inadequate support systems; parent-child role reversal related to culture shock).
3. Planning client care
   a. Aim: to develop a plan of action for initiating change in a family or for enabling a family to better cope with the existing situation
      (1) Refer the family to a family therapist. Nurses who work with families in community or institutional settings but who are not family therapists should not attempt to provide family therapy. After assessing a family, analyzing the data, and making a nursing diagnosis concerning family dysfunction, these nurses should refer the family for counseling.
      (2) Nurses who are family therapists should:

(a) Determine whether the locus of decision making is predominantly with the family or is shared between nurse and family

(b) In accordance with the locus of decision making, assist or support the family in setting goals (for example, clarify the rules governing family relationships; decrease fusion among family members) and in establishing priorities among goals

(c) Differentiate between long- and short-term goals

(d) State projected outcomes (for example, wife-mother and husband-father will renegotiate roles; parents will develop adequate support systems)

b. Aim: to design and modify a care plan that is consistent with the family's beliefs and orientations and that is based on principles of family theory and family therapy, psychiatric literature, and the nurse-therapist's own experience with effective approaches to specific types of family dysfunction

(1) Anticipate the needs of the client-family on the basis of its priority of goals and the life stages of family members.

(2) Include all family members in the development of intervention strategies. It is important that all persons who are defined as family members be included (for example, extended kin, like-family).

(3) Plan strategies that are congruent with the life stages of family members, the life cycle of the domestic group, and the cultural orientation of the family.

(4) Identify family therapy approaches that should be followed for specific types of family dysfunction (for example, teach the family new or alternative scripts for family relationships; help the family clarify the rules that govern family interaction).

4. Implement the counseling plan; aim: to counsel the family

a. Help the family to identify stressors and to develop effective coping strategies.

b. Facilitate the development of trust among family members.

c. Facilitate self-expression among family members if this is consistent with their cultural orientation.

d. Provide information to, or clarify misconceptions of, family members. For example, a child may feel that she is responsible for her alcoholic father's incestuous behavior, while the wife-mother may feel that she is the cause of her husband's alcoholism. These misconceptions should be clarified. Information about protective services and state laws concerning incest and child protection should be given.

e. Refer the family or individual family members to appropriate community resources (legal services, social services, support groups).

f. Support the family members in their decision making.

5. Evaluate the counseling plan; aim: to include the family members in estimating the family's progress toward attainment of goals

a. Estimate the degree to which goals have been achieved, crises have been resolved, and family functioning has improved.

b. Identify goals that need to be modified or revised.

c. Evaluate the effectiveness of family therapy approaches.

d. Identify aspects of family therapy approaches that need to be modified or revised.

e. Bridge the family to support systems other than the family therapy relationship.

(1) People in the social environment (friends, extended family members, native healers, clergy) who are willing to serve as support systems for the family

(2) Community agencies that offer help with problems that the family may encounter in the future (for example, agencies that offer services to families experiencing maturational or situational crises)

The following family process assessment guide has a threefold purpose: it has been designed to assist nurses in assessing a family's functioning, in establishing goals, and in developing nursing strategies consistent with the family's cultural orientation.

1. Demographic data*
   a. Names of family members
   b. Ages of members
   c. Sexes of members
   d. Relationship between members: affinal; consanguinal
   e. Educational levels of members
   f. Occupations of members
   g. Ethnicity (optional)†
   h. Religion (optional)†
   I. Other (describe)

2. Family organization*
   a. Type of family: nuclear; extended; blended; single-parent
   b. Type of system: open; closed; boundary-maintaining mechanisms (describe); norms; rules
   c. Members involved in child rearing
   d. Members vested with authority
   e. Sense of obligation among family members
   f. Family roles: peacemaker; protector; attacker; provider; interpreter; rescuer; other
   g. Sex-defined roles: stereotyped male-female relationships; amount of independence permitted men and women
   h. Other (describe)

3. Family world view
   a. Relationship to people: individualistic; group oriented; egalitarian; authoritarian
   b. Relationship to time: past oriented; present oriented; future oriented
   c. Relationship to the world: personal control; goal directed; fatalistic
   d. Other (describe)

4. Family spiritual orientation
   a. Ideology
      (1) Nature of belief in a supernatural being or supernormal energy
      (2) Nature of belief in communion between a supernatural being or supernormal energy and people alive or dead
      (3) Conceptualizations about the quality of life and the quality of death
      (4) Nature of belief in life after death
   b. Inner life
      (1) Frequency and type of inner-life activity (meditation, yoga, prayer)
      (2) Interrelationship between family members' spiritual life and the other parts of their life (for example, family meditates when under stress; family prays when in trouble)
   c. Other (describe)

5. Family perceptions and definitions
   a. Family
   b. Privacy
   c. Intimacy
   d. Health (mental and physical)
   e. Illness (mental and physical)
   f. Presenting family problem (for example, which family members identify a problem; clarification of discrepant views of the problem)
   g. Other (describe)

---

*When time for assessment is limited these factors should be assessed first. Other factors can be assessed as the nurse is working with the family.

†Legislation protects people from being required to reveal ethnicity and religion.

6. Family health care patterns
   a. Ideas concerning causes of illness (mental and physical)
   b. Ideas concerning teatment of illness (mental and physical)
   c. People consulted in times of crisis or for treatment of mental and physical illnesses (family member; native healer; mental health therapist; clergyman; pharmacist; physician; other)
   d. Other (describe)
7. Family living arrangements
   a. Type of residence: multifamily dwelling; single-family dwelling; one-room dwelling; other
   b. Environment of residence: urban; suburban; rural; inter-ethnic neighborhood; ethnic enclave
   c. Time in residence: length of time in present residence; length of time in previous residences
   d. Family members living in another household (describe relationship)
   e. Persons other than family members living in the household (describe living arrangements)
   f. Sleeping arrangements: number of rooms serving as bedrooms (differentiate between rooms functioning solely as bedrooms and those that have other functions); family members sharing bedrooms; family members not sharing bedrooms
   g. Eating arrangements: family members eat together; eat alone; eat in shifts
   h. Privacy arrangements: rooms or sections of rooms reserved for specific family members; furniture (for example, chairs) reserved for specific family members
   i. Other (describe)
8. Family interaction patterns*

---

*When time for assessment is limited these factors should be assessed first. Other factors can be assessed as the nurse is working with the family.

a. Communication patterns
   (1) Verbal
       (a) Language spoken at home
       (b) Language spoken outside home
   (2) Kinesic
       (a) Touching
       (b) Gesturing
   (3) Proxemic
       (a) Interpersonal spacing
       (b) Fixed and/or built space
   (4) Themes
       (a) Double-bind messages
       (b) Manipulation
       (c) Scapegoating
       (d) Intellectualization
       (e) Blame placing
       (f) Validation
       (g) Other (describe)
b. Behavior patterns
   (1) Physical acting out
   (2) Isolation
   (3) Differentiation
   (4) Cooperation
   (5) Competition
   (6) Overdependence
   (7) Other (describe)
c. Social patterns
   (1) Alliances
       (a) Among family members
       (b) Between family members and members of social network
       (c) Conflict between alliances
       (d) Resolution of conflict between alliances
   (2) Dissemination of information
       (a) Sources of information
       (b) Pattern of communicating information
   (3) Social interaction
       (a) Social network: relatives; friends; employers; coworkers; neighbors; clergy; other (describe)
       (b) Community involvement: school; church; labor union;

neighborhood; other (describe)
(c) Patterns of recreation
(d) Patterns of intimacy
(4) Other (describe)
9. Family role relationships*
a. Authority
(1) Nominal authority figure(s)
(2) Actual authority figure(s)
(3) Patterns of authority
(4) Implementation of authority: direct; delegated
b. Decison making
(1) Nominal decision-making figure(s)
(2) Actual decision-making figure(s)
(3) Patterns of decision making
(4) Implementation of decisions
c. Regulatory
(1) Peacemaker figure(s)
(2) Protector figure(s)
(3) Interpreter figure(s)
(4) Attacker figure(s)
(5) Domineering figure(s)
(6) Submissive figure(s)
d. Other (describe)
10. Family stressors*
a. Changes in family membership: loss of a member through divorce, separation, death, or hospitalization or addition of a member through birth, adoption, or incorporation (for example, grandparents move into the household)
b. Sociocultural strains: environmental pressures such as inadequate support systems, community disorganization, discrimination, inadequate housing, culture shock, and poverty
c. Maturational events: transitions between developmental stages, such as marriage, entrance of a child into school, and retirement
d. Disordered family relationships: imbal-

ance in the internal structure of the family; related to such factors as double-bind communication, parental overburdening, overbonding to the family, and psychosomatogenesis
e. Other (describe)
f. No significant stress
11. Family coping mechanisms*
a. Coping mechanisms used (indicate whether mechanisms are used only by specific family members)
b. Effectiveness of coping mechanisms
c. Family's perception of mechanisms that are effective in reducing stress
d. Other (describe)
12. Family resources*
a. Familial: interests; leisure time activities; physical and mental abilities; other
b. Socioeconomic: interpersonal support systems; economic support systems (health insurance, sick leave, union benefits); food, shelter, clothing; other

TERTIARY PREVENTION

Families may have to continue to exist in environments that contributed to the development of family dysfunction. After the termination of family therapy, ongoing support in the form of *rehabilitative* services may be needed. Tertiary prevention programs are available in the following areas:
1. Educational training. Depending on the ages, interests, and abilities of family members, continued education, including college and vocational training (or retraining), may be indicated. Education increases self-esteem and prepares family members to be as financially self-reliant as their potential permits. This may help to reduce the impact of

*When time for assessment is limited these factors should be assessed first. Other factors can be assessed as the nurse is working with the family.

*When time for assessment is limited these factors should be assessed first. Other factors can be assessed as the nurse is working with the family.

chronic sociocultural stressors on family functioning and to limit the degree of family dysfunction.

2. Self-help groups. Some self-help groups function to limit the degree of dysfunction in already dysfunctional families. Such groups are composed of people who have learned or who are learning to cope with chronic stressors and with family dysfunction. For example, after divorce (a type of family dysfunction), Parents Without Partners helps single parents to cope with the social and emotional demands of parenting and to avoid parental overburdening, thereby preventing the development of further family dysfunction. Spouse support groups and Parents Anonymous offer help to abusive family members. Support groups are also available for the victims of family abuse and for families with mentally ill members.

3. Voluntary rehabilitation groups. The purpose of voluntary rehabilitation groups is similar to that of self-help groups. What differentiates them from self-help groups is that their members may not have experienced the same stressors that the client families have experienced. The Salvation Army and the St. Vincent de Paul Society are examples of voluntary rehabilitation groups. Emergency aid in the form of financial assistance, housing, and food is usually available. In addition, counseling, assistance in finding employment and housing, work projects, and leisure time activities may be offered. Family abuse shelters may be operated by religious, quasi-religious, or secular groups. Such shelters not only offer temporary assistance for battered family members, but often also bridge family members to agencies that provide economic assistance, legal services, support groups and assertiveness training programs. Thus, voluntary rehabilitation groups help to reduce the impact of chronic life-style stressors on family functioning and to limit the degree of family dysfunction.

CHAPTER SUMMARY

Throughout the United States, there is a growing tendency to view the family rather than the individual as the client of choice for the delivery of health care. To effectively work with families, nurses need to become knowledgeable about family organization and family process.

The family is a system and has the properties of any social system. As the family interacts with other social systems in its context, it may become vulnerable to stressors that affect family structure and function. Chief among these stressors are changes in family membership, sociocultural strains, maturational events, and disordered family relationships. Combinations of these stressors may interrelate as they influence family functioning.

Several models of family therapy may be used with dysfunctional families. These models are the structural model, the interactional model, and the developmental or multigenerational model. However, nurses should be aware that cultural presuppositions may be inherent in some aspects of these models. It is important for nurses to be mindful of the culture-bound aspects of family therapy models so that their assessments, interpretations, and goals will not be value laden. Whenever possible, family therapists and native healers not only should coexist but also should collaborate to ensure that family dysfunction will be understood and treated within its sociocultural context.

Nurses who work with families may engage in activities of primary, secondary, and/or tertiary prevention of family dysfunction. Primary prevention focuses on the promotion and maintenance of healthy patterns of family interaction and functioning. The focus of secondary prevention is intervention into family dysfunction and restoration of functional patterns of family behavior. The nursing process provides the framework for intervention with client-families. Tertiary prevention focuses on limiting the degree of family dysfunction and providing rehabilitative services.

SENSITIVITY-AWARENESS EXERCISES

The purposes of these exercises are to:
- Develop awareness about the vulnerability of your own family and of client-families to stress
- Develop awareness about the interrelationship between families and their context (physical, emotional, cultural, and social)
- Develop awareness about your own feelings and attitudes when working with dysfunctional families

1. Using the family process assessment guide in this chapter, assess the dynamics, strengths, limitations, stressors, coping patterns, health care patterns, and sociocultural orientations (toward family, privacy, intimacy, health, illness, and spirituality) of your own family. On the basis of this assessment, discuss your evaluation of your family's functioning. What level(s) of prevention (primary, secondary, and/or tertiary) are indicated? Repeat this exercise, this time assessing a client-family.
2. Look at the nature of stressors that have impaired or that are presently impairing the structure and functioning of your own family system. How did your family cope with each stress situation? How did the stress affect the ability of individual family members, including yourself, to accomplish their developmental tasks? How did the responses of each family member to the stress situation affect the responses of other family members?
3. Use one or more of the following techniques to describe the conflicts and alliances in your family system: sculpting (constructing a live family portrait), drawing a family picture, role playing.
4. Use the following self-assessment tool to become more aware of your own feelings and attitudes about working with dysfunctional families:
   a. What personal needs of my own do I try to meet when I work with dysfunctional families?
   b. When I work with dysfunctional families, to what extent do I feel helpless? Frustrated? Angry? Pity? Overwhelmed?
   c. How do my feelings vary according to the stressors the family is encountering? According to the family's coping patterns?
   d. To what extent do I try to cope with my feelings by avoiding the client-family? Blaming the client-family? Pushing the client-family to make a decision or to implement a decision?
   e. To what extent do I focus on the problems and limitations of the client-family?
   f. To what extent do I focus on the strengths and resources of the client-family?

REFERENCES

Aguilera, D.C., and J.M. Messick
1981 Crisis Intervention: Theory and Methodology (ed. 4). St. Louis: The C.V. Mosby Co.

Albee, G.W.
1970 "Short, unhappy life of clinical psychology." Psychology Today 4:42-43.

Ashcraft, N., and A. Scheflen
1976 People Space: The Making and Breaking of Human Boundaries. New York: Anchor Press.

Banfield, E.G.
1958 The Moral Bases of a Backward Society. Glencoe, N.Y.: The Free Press.

Bateson, G., et al.
1956 "Toward a theory of schizophrenia." Behavioral Science 1:251-264.

Beels, C., and A. Ferber
1973 "What family therapists do." In The Book of Family Therapy. A. Ferber, M. Mendelsohn, and A. Napier (eds.). Boston: Houghton Mifflin Co.

Berg-Cross, G.
1977 "The effects of divorce: a research review with a developmental perspective." Journal of Clinical Child Psychiatry 6:15-20.

Bowen, M.
1971 "The use of family theory in clinical practice." In Changing Families: A Family Therapy Reader. J. Haley (ed.). New York: Grune & Stratton.
1978 Family Therapy in Clinical Practice. New York: Jason Aronson, Inc.

Brown, L.
1981 "Theoretical frameworks for understanding violent behavior." In Assessing Patient Violence in the Health Care Setting. K.S. Babich (ed.). Boulder, Colo.: Western Interstate Commission for Higher Education.

Colecchia, F.
1978 "Women, ethnicity and mental health: the Italian woman, impressions and observations." In The Italian Immigrant Woman in North America. B.B. Caroli, R.F. Harney, and L.F. Tomasi (eds.). Toronto: The Multicultural History Society of Ontario.

Committee on the Family of the Group for the Advancement of Psychotherapy
1970 Treatment of Families in Conflict. New York: Jason Aronson, Inc.

Critchley, D.L.
1981 "The child as patient: assessing the effects of family stress and disruption on the mental health of the child." Perspectives in Psychiatric Care 11(5 and 6):144-155.

Detre, T., D. Kupfer, and S. Taub
1975 "The nosology of violence." In Neural Bases of Violence and Aggression. W. Fields and W. Sweet (eds.). St. Louis: Warren H. Green.

Erikson, E.
1950 Childhood and Society (ed. 2). New York: W.W. Norton & Co., Inc.

Finley, B.
1981 "See Evil—Play Evil." Gray Matter Newsletter, fall, p. 4.

Fleck, S.
1972 "An approach to family pathology." In Family Therapy: An Introduction to Theory and Technique. G.D. Erickson and T.P. Hogan (eds.). Monterey: Brooks/Cole Publishing Co.

Friedman, E.H.
1971 "The birthday party: an experiment in obtaining in one's own extended family." Family Process 10(3): 345-359.

Gambino, R.
1974 Blood of My Blood: The Dilemma of Italian Americans. New York: Doubleday & Co., Inc.

Gilmore, M.M., and D.D. Gilmore
1979 "'Machismo': A psychodynamic approach (Spain)." Journal of Psychological Anthropology 2:281-299.

Glaser, B.G., and A.L. Strauss
1964 "The social loss of dying patients." American Journal of Nursing 64:119-121.

González-Wippler, M.
1975 Santería. Garden City, N.Y.: Anchor Press.

Haley, J.
1962 "Whither family therapy?" Family Process 1:69-100.

Halleck, S.
1978 "Psychodynamic aspects of violence." In Violence and Responsibility: The Individual, the Family and Society. R. Sadoff (ed.). Jamaica, N.Y.: SP Medical & Scientific Books.

Harris, L.
1979 A Survey of Spousal Violence Against Women in Kentucky. Kentucky Commission on Women, study no. 792701.

Haveliwala, Y.A., A.E. Scheflen, and N. Ashcraft
1979 Common Sense in Therapy—A Handbook for the Mental Health Worker. New York: Brunner/Mazel.

Horn, Patrice
1973 "Newsline." Psychology Today 3:17

Hsu, F.L.K.
1970 Americans and Chinese: Reflections on Two Cultures and Their People. New York: Doubleday & Co., Inc.

Irvine, E.E.
1965 "Children at risk." In Crisis Intervention: Selected Readings. H. Parad (ed.). New York: Family Service Association of America.

Jackson, D.D.
1965 "Family rules: marital quid pro quo." In Family Therapy: An Introduction to Theory and Technique. G.D. Erickson and T.P. Hogan (eds.). Monterey: Brooks/Cole Publishing Co.

Jones, S.L., and M. Dimond
1982 "Family theory and family therapy models: comparative review with implications for nursing practice." Journal of Psychiatric Nursing and Mental Health Services 20(10):12-19.

Kalter, N.
1977 "Children of divorce in an outpatient population." American Journal of Orthopsychiatry 47(1):40-51.

Kelly, J., and J.S. Wallerstein
1977 "Brief interventions with children in divorcing families." American Journal of Orthopsychiatry 47(1):23-29.

Klein, D.C., and A.R. Ross
1965 "Kindergarten entry: a study of role transition." In Crisis Intervention: Selected Readings. H. Parad (ed.). New York: Family Service Association of America.

Kohn, M.I.
1977 Class and Conformity (ed.2). Chicago: University of Chicago Press.

Lee, P.R.
1970 Utilization of Allied Health Manpower—Future Prospects. Paper presented at a meeting of the American Academy of Pediatrics, San Francisco, October 20-22, 1970.

LeMasters, E.E.
1965 "Parenthood as crisis." In Crisis Intervention: Selected Readings. H. Parad (ed.). New York: Family Service Association of America.

Lichtenstein, V.R.
1981 "The battered woman: guideline for effective nursing intervention." Issues in Mental Health Nursing 3:237-250.

Lidz, T., A. Cornelison, S. Fleck, and D. Terry
1958 "The intrafamilial environment of the schizophrenic patient. IV. Parental personalities and family interaction." American Journal of Orthopsychiatry 28:764-776.

Markusen, E., and R. Fulton
1971 "Childhood bereavement and behavior disorders: a critical review." Omega 2:107-117.

McGoldrick, M.
1982 "Ethnicity and family therapy." Family Therapy Networker 6:22-26.

Miller, J.
1981 "Cultural and class values in family process." Journal of Marital and Family Therapy 7(4):467-473.

Minuchin, S.
1967 Families of the Slums. New York: Basic Books, Inc., Publishers.
1974 Families and Family Therapy. Cambridge: Harvard University Press.
Minuchin, S., B. Rosman, and L. Baker
1978 Psychosomatic Families. Cambridge: Harvard University Press.
Murdock, G.P.
1965 "Tenino shamanism." Ethnology 4:165-171.
O'Nell, C., and H. Selby
1968 "Sex differences in the incidence of susto in two azpotec pueblos: an analysis of the relationship between sex role expectations and folk illnesses." Ethnology 1:95-105.
Parsons, T.
1975 "Some theoretical considerations on the nature and trends of change of ethnicity." In Ethnicity: Theory and Experience. N. Glazer and D.P. Moynihan (eds.). Cambridge, Mass.: Harvard University Press.
Pasquali, E.A.
1982 Assimilation and Acculturation of Cubans on Long Island. Ph.D. dissertation, State University of New York at Stony Brook.
"Returning to traditional healers to improve third world medicine"
1979 Newsday, May 7, part II, p. 7.

Satir, V.
1967 Conjoint Family Therapy. Palo Alto, Calif.: Science and Behavior Books, Inc.
1972 "Family systems and approaches to family therapy." In Family Therapy: An Introduction to Theory and Technique. G.D. Erickson and T.P. Hogan (eds.). Monterey: Brooks/Cole Publishing Co.
Scheflen, A.E., and A. Scheflen
1972 Body Language and Social Order. Englewood Cliffs, N.J.: Prentice-Hall, Inc.
Scott, P.B.
1974 "Battered wives." British Journal of Psychiatry 125: 433-441.
Searles, H.F.
1965 Collected Papers on Schizophrenia and Related Subjects. New York: International Universities Press.
Sedgwick, R.
1976 "Family mental health: a sociopsychological approach." In Current Perspectives in Psychiatric Nursing: Issues and Trends, vol. 1. C.R. Kneisl and H.S. Wilson (eds.). St. Louis: The C.V. Mosby Co.
1978 "Photostudy as a diagnostic tool in working with families." In Current Perspectives in Psychiatric Nursing: Issues and Trends, vol. 2. C.R. Kneisl and H.S. Wilson (eds.). St. Louis: The C.V. Mosby Co.
Smith, S.M., and R. Hanson
1975 "Interpersonal relationships and child-rearing practices in 214 parents of battered children." British Journal of Psychiatry 127:513-525.

Sorosky, A.

1977 "The psychological effects of divorce on adolescents." Adolescence 12:123-136.

Spiegel, J.

1959 "Some cultural aspects of transference and counter-transference." In Individual and Family Dynamics. J.H. Masserman (ed.). New York: Grune & Stratton.

Torrey, E.F.

1977 "What Western psychotherapists can learn from witch-doctors." American Journal of Orthopsychiatry 42(1): 69-76.

Wallerstein, J.S., and J. Kelly

1976 "The effects of parental divorce: experiences of the child in later latency." American Journal of Orthopsychiatry 26(2):256-269.

Williams, F.

1974 "Intervention in maturational crisis." In Nursing of Families in Crisis. J.C. Hall and B.R. Weaver (eds.). Philadelphia: J.B. Lippincott Co.

ANNOTATED SUGGESTED READINGS

Erickson, G.D., and T.P. Hogan (eds.)

1972 Family Therapy: An Introduction to Theory and Technique. Belmont, Calif.: Wadsworth Publishing Co., Inc.

This book is a collection of readings about family therapy. Chapters deal with the historical perspectives of family therapy, models of theory and practice, various family therapy techniques, and recent developments in family therapy. Bowlby, Bell, Ackerman, Jackson, Haley, Scheflen, and Satir are among the many contributors to this book.

Jones, S.L., and M. Dimond

1982 "Family theory and family therapy models: comparative review with implications for nursing practice." Journal of Psychiatric Nursing and Mental Health Services 20(10):12-19.

The authors compare and contrast theories of the family and theories of family therapy. Three theoretical approaches are discussed: structural-functional, interactional, and developmental (or multigenerational). The importance of theories of the family and family therapy to family-focused nursing is then explored.

McGoldrick, M.

1982 "Ethnicity and family therapy." Family Therapy Networker 6:22-26.

The author discusses the importance of family therapists recognizing the effects of cultural differences on family process and family therapy assumptions. She further explores the need for family therapists to understand their own ethnic identities so that they will not be "triggered" by the ethnic characteristics of their client-families.

FURTHER READINGS

Foley, V.

1974 An Introduction to Family Therapy. New York: Grune & Stratton.

Resnikoff, R.O.

1981 "Teaching family therapy: ten key questions for understanding the family as patient." Journal of Marital and Family Therapy 7(2):135-142.

Smoyak, S. (ed.)

1975 The Psychiatric Nurse as a Family Therapist. New York: John Wiley & Sons, Inc.

CHAPTER 13

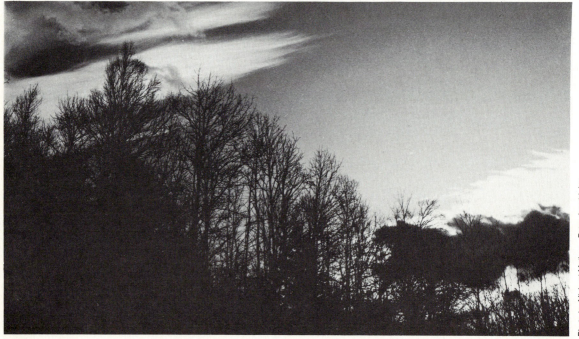

Photo by Michael Mather—Peter Arnold, Inc.

346

Crisis intervention

CHAPTER FOCUS

Crisis can be viewed as an integral component of everyday life situations. Crisis may be growth promoting and has the capacity to enhance one's self-esteem through the use of effective problem solving. A crisis may be situational, maturational, or social. One type of crisis may be compounded by another at any given time. Response to crisis depends on many factors: perception of the precipitating event and its impact on the future; available support systems; repertoire of effective coping strategies; personal vulnerabilities and emotional support.

Crisis theory provides a conceptual framework from which to provide active intervention. The methodology of crisis intervention follows a sequence of steps similar to the nursing process. Assessment of the presenting issues is made through data collection, and a plan is determined. Strategies are implemented, and evaluation is an ongoing process. Ego defenses are supported while more adaptive strategies are explored.

Nurses function as part of the interdisciplinary team in the use of crisis intervention as a therapeutic modality. Nurses may employ crisis techniques in their work with high-risk groups such as clients with chronic diseases, new parents, and bereaved persons. Crisis intervention techniques are not restricted to outpatient settings. They are effective in all units of general hospitals as well as in community settings. Nurses may also use crisis intervention in dealing with intragroup staff issues and client management issues.

CRISIS THEORY AND INTERVENTION

History

The philosophical base of crisis theory can be found in the works of Freud and others in the psychoanalytic movement. Freud noted that individuals' current behaviors are influenced by their genetic past. Early life experiences have a profound effect on later development. He also noted that individuals who were able to identify and mobilize coping strategies to resolve their conflicts were more likely to experience satisfaction in their lives. The psychoanalytic model, with its individualized approach, was helpful in assisting clients in their adaptation to stressful situations. The process of analysis was very costly, lengthy, and available to only a limited number of individuals.

The early 1940s saw the emergence of preventive psychiatry with its focus on maintenance of mental health and the prevention of mental illness. It was at this time that therapists in the field began to use certain psychoanalytic techniques such as catharsis and emphatic listening to facilitate individuals' healthy resolution of stressful experiences.

One of the leaders in the development of crisis theory was Eric Lindemann. His comprehensive study (1944) of bereavement following the Coconut Grove fire in Boston in 1943 laid the groundwork for our current understanding of the grieving process. He determined that there was a well-defined sequence of responses that bereaved individuals experienced following that catastrophic event. His observations revealed both physiological and psychological symptomatology. Lindemann's study further revealed that morbid grief reactions might also occur under certain circumstances. The morbid grief response represents a distortion of the acute grief response. He suggested that the most frequent distortion was that of a delayed reaction, which occurs, for example, sometime after the individual is confronted with a significant loss and at a time when he or she is facing other, more significant tasks. Lindemann (1944) presents the example of a young girl who lost her parents and her boyfriend in the fire and was seriously burned herself. During the course of her hospitalization she showed no signs of distress until approximately the tenth week, when she began experiencing tightness in her chest, feelings of emptiness, and a preoccupation with her deceased parents. Individuals may also attempt to hurry their way through the grieving process or to deny their grief by becoming engrossed in other activities or disposing of possessions of the deceased individuals. Lack of acknowledgement of the sense of loss and the accompanying feelings serves only to distort the grief response and delay reinvolvement with others.

Lindemann's observations defined a sequence of responses to loss that can be applied to any situation where individuals experience loss—whether it be loss of self-worth, of independence, of function, of status, or of a significant person or love object. Individuals throughout the life cycle experience loss at many different points. The significance of Lindemann's work lies in the fact that the knowledge of these stages can enable nursing and other helping professions to facilitate individuals' adaptation to potentially stressful events. Crisis intervention, as Lindemann envisioned it, would provide brief, active, collaborative therapy to mobilize clients' own resources within their own communities. The Wellesley Project was set up by Lindemann and Caplan as a community-wide program designed to provide crisis intervention services.

Concurrently, during World War II soldiers who were experiencing stress-induced reactions were treated immediately at the front rather than being sent back home. These men were able to return to combat and did not need further treatment in an inpatient setting. Glass (1957) substantiated these findings in his observations of troops in the Korean War.

Gerald Caplan (1964) developed a theory of individuals in crisis, and defined crisis intervention as a modality of treatment. His major emphasis was on the role that the community and its members play in the prevention of mental illness and maintenance of mental health. Caplan presented the concept of primary, secondary, and tertiary levels of prevention as essential factors in community mental health practice. Primary prevention may be viewed as a two-pronged focus involving social and interpersonal action. Social action directs its attention to social and political groups to generate necessary community reform. Large social issues, such as poverty, inadequate housing, poor educational services, and fragmented or nonexistent health services, are the target of social action intervention. Interpersonal action focuses on individuals and assists them in using effective problem-solving strategies.

Primary preventive techniques include educating individuals and providing consultation and crisis intervention. Education about stressors—physiological, environmental, emotional—assists individuals to modify their lives to reduce or eliminate the effects of those stressors. This concept applies to communities, families, and individuals. For example, recent warnings about dioxin helped public health officials to alert affected communities and to institute screening measures to prevent possible physiological effects in the future. Consultation and crisis intervention can be used with clients and families in the general hospital setting to facilitate their adaptation to the crisis of illness with its concurrent role changes and alterations in body image and independence levels. Individuals are encouraged to identify their own stressors (see the Holmes and Rahe scale in Chapter 4) and pursue strategies to reduce their vulnerability. As individuals' coping strategies increase, their sense of vulnerability decreases. Being aware of potential stressors increases a feeling of control and allows individuals to be managers of their own lives. Other examples of primary preventive strategies include parenting classes for new parents, couples groups for those considering marriage, support groups for women in their middle years, and groups for divorced individuals. Counseling in the

form of individual support may also be provided for the above-mentioned groups, as well as for those who are retiring and for those individuals and families who are transferred frequently by employers. Situations that present *potential* crises can be identified and worked through to prevent increased vulnerability. Success, however, depends mainly on the individuals' ability to be responsive by modifying their situations, on their previous coping skills and levels of success, and on their support systems.

Secondary prevention includes actions designed to reduce the number of existing cases by early diagnosis and treatment. In this level, the goal is to provide services that prevent lengthy periods of disability. The assumption can be made that either primary preventive services were unavailable or that the affected individual was unable to benefit from these services. From a nursing perspective, it is important that individuals be assessed accurately and be referred to appropriate resources immediately. Short-term therapy as opposed to prolonged hospitalization focuses on the return of individuals to their communities. Crisis intervention may be viewed as part of secondary prevention in that its goal is the healthy resolution of crisis and the return to at least a precrisis level of functioning.

Tertiary prevention involves techniques to reduce the long-term effects of mental disability. Rehabilitation programs are a way to assist individuals to return to their previous occupations and social roles or to enable them to learn new skills. Crisis intervention is an integral component of tertiary prevention—individuals are assisted in developing new methods of coping with stress and reaching their maximum rehabilitative states.

The evolution of community psychiatry and crisis theory was further influenced by the Report of the Joint Commission on Mental Health and Mental Illness (1961). The book *Action for Mental Health* documented the need for short-term crisis-oriented services based in the community. It noted a dearth of services, long waiting lists, and inappropriate, expensive therapies. The report further stated that 42% of people in crisis went to their clergymen or their family physicians rather than seeking mental health professionals. Large numbers of people were not receiving services when or where they needed them. The entire mechanism of providing psychiatric services needed revision. Through federal funding in 1963 and 1965, community mental health centers were developed to provide the comprehensive services necessary to meet the needs of large communities within their own community environments. Paraprofessionals or ''indigenous workers'' were identified as valuable resource persons who could be of great support in crisis situations. Crisis intervention techniques as a short-term problem-solving modality were found to be the appropriate method of treatment. Inpatient and outpatient crisis programs have demonstrated their effectiveness in meeting the needs of the masses and have reduced the need for long-term hospitalization. Crisis intervention as a valid modality of treatment has earned its place in community psychiatry.

Lastly, the Suicide Prevention Movement, begun in the late 1950s, was spearheaded by the efforts of Norman Farberow and Edwin Schneidman at the Los Angeles Suicide Prevention Center. Their work added to the development of crisis intervention techniques as appropriate strategies for meeting the needs of suicidal clients. As a result of their efforts, the suicide prevention movement grew, as did the number of centers providing crisis intervention services.

Definition of crisis

A crisis is a situation that cannot be readily resolved by an individual's normal repertoire of coping strategies. Anxiety increases, the individual becomes more immobilized, and a sense of disequilibrium results. Crises are time limited in the sense that either positive or negative outcomes result within a four- to six-week period. Crises are perceived as threatening and arise from precipitating events usually related to loss (or the *threat* of loss), illness, a change in status, new responsibil-

ities at work, or birth of a child. The event may have occurred recently or within the last few weeks or months, and the individual may not connect the event to the actual crisis situation. It is important to note that crisis is defined by the individual—not all stressful situations are crises. If an individual views a situation as being overwhelmingly stressful, the individual may be unable to resolve the situation and a crisis results. A state of crisis has growth-promoting potential. It may act as a catalyst to jar old habits and evoke new responses. Crisis has the potential to strengthen an individual's adaptive capacity and sense of self-worth. Crisis intervention as a short-term modality focuses on the resolution of the immediate issue through the mobilization of social, environmental, and intrapersonal resources. All individuals experience crisis throughout life. Reaching out for help in a time of crisis and effecting resolution serves to promote an overall sense of control and well-being. It is through this process that individuals emerge at an even higher level of functioning than in the pre-crisis state.

Phases of crisis

Caplan (1964) has described four phases of crisis.

PHASE I

A perceived threat acts as a precipitating event that generates increased anxiety. Normal coping strategies are called into action. If these measures are ineffective, the individual moves into the second phase.

PHASE II

The ineffectiveness of the phase I coping mechanisms leads to further disorganization. The individual experiences a sense of vulnerability and lack of control. Immobilization may occur, or the individual may attempt to cope with the situation in a random fashion. If the anxiety continues and there is no resolution, the individual enters phase III. Here the individual is most amenable to the helping process.

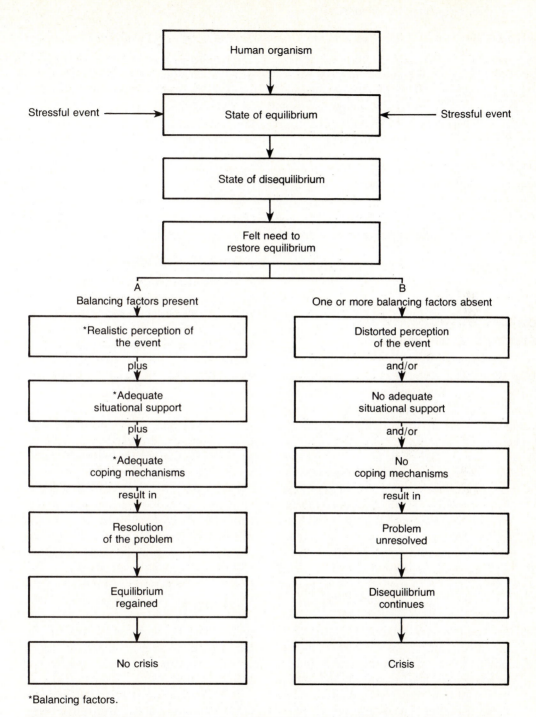

*Balancing factors.

Fig. 13-1. Paradigm: the effect of balancing factors in a stressful event. (From Aguilera, D.C., and Messick, J.M.: Crisis intervention: theory and methodology, ed. 4, St. Louis, 1982, The C.V. Mosby Co.)

PHASE III

A redefinition of the crisis is attempted in this phase with the hope that familiar coping measures will be successful. New problem-solving measures may also effect a resolution. Feelings are dealt with and decisions are made. The individual may return to a precrisis level of functioning.

PHASE IV

The fourth phase is characterized by severe psychological disorganization. Responses similar to those found in severe to panic levels of anxiety occur. Profound cognitive, emotional, and physiological changes are noted in this phase. At this point in time, more extensive treatment may be necessary if negative outcomes are apparent.

Factors influencing the perception of crisis

As noted above, a crisis is defined by the individual. Aguilera and Messick (1982) have developed a paradigm that explores several balancing factors that can affect the manner in which a crisis is resolved (see Fig. 13-1). A healthy resolution is dependent upon the following three factors:

1. Realistic appraisal of the precipitating event. Recognition of the cause-and-effect relationship between the event and feelings of anxiety is necessary for effective problem-solving to occur. Distortions in perception impair problem-solving, thus increasing already high levels of stress.
2. Availability of support systems. It is critical to mobilize existing support systems in order to prevent feelings of isolation and vulnerability.
3. Availability of coping measures. Over a lifetime, a person develops a repertoire of successful coping strategies that enable him or her to identify and resolve stressful situations. Although these coping strategies may not be successful immediately in new stress-producing situations, the person recognizes that they have succeeded in the past and will do so again.

Types of crises

Initially crisis had been defined as either maturational or situational. Chamberlin (1980) suggested a third category, "unanticipated social crisis," which includes catastrophic events involving multiple simultaneous losses. A person may experience more than one crisis at a time. Often a maturational crisis is compounded by a situational crisis. An adolescent who is struggling with his or her changing body image is confronted with the diagnosis of leukemia. The stressors of both crises may be so overwhelming that the individual may find it necessary to seek help.

MATURATIONAL CRISES

Maturational crises can be defined as the predictable processes of growth and development that evolve over a period of time. The ultimate goal of these processes is maturity. Erikson (1963) describes the developmental sequence of the eight stages of man—each of which is characterized by a major task that is resolved on a continuum. The transition points—or those junctures where individuals move into successive stages—often generate disequilibrium. Individuals are required to make cognitive and behavioral changes and to integrate those physical changes which accompany development. The extent to which individuals experience success in the mastery of these tasks depends on previous successes, availability of support systems, influence of role models, and acceptability of the new role by others. Williams (1971) suggests that success in previous transition periods lays the foundation for successes in stages that follow. Unresolved issues cause susceptibility to crisis and influence the ability to cope with the disequilibrium that can accompany transition points. In fact, unresolved dependency issues, for example, may be found as an underlying factor in individuals experiencing depression and gastrointestinal disorders.

Gender identity confusion may result in an unclear concept of oneself as a sexual being. A person may then have difficulty in establishing intimate relationships with members of the same sex or with members of the opposite sex. Conflict with authority figures may begin in adolescence and later have a profound impact in the young adulthood phase in the form of abusive or acting-out behavior. Any form of conflict, whether it be around the issue of values, sexuality, or dependency, generates anxiety and has the potential for creating a crisis for the individual involved (Baldwin, 1978). Appropriate intervention depends on the determination of the presence of unresolved issues so that further disequilibrium and personality disorganization can be prevented.

Role models who act as mentors function as available support systems as well as examples of the appropriate manner in which to behave as one moves along in the maturational process. Support systems are a crucial factor in responding successfully to the stress associated with transition points. (Each phase requires new, more sophisticated modes of responding that often generate much anxiety.) Individuals need a safe, trusting environment where new roles can be tried out without fear of repercussion or embarrassment.

The transitional periods or events that are most commonly identified as having increased crisis potential are adolescence, marriage, parenthood, midlife, and retirement. This is not to say, however, that crises cannot occur at other transition periods. The following is a case study of a maturational crisis—a crisis of parenthood:

Marian J., a 34-year-old white, single woman presented at the mental health clinic two months after the birth of her daughter, Rebecca. Marian stated that she felt depressed most of the time. She described sleeping difficulties, poor appetite, lack of energy, increasing frustration with the baby, and feelings of hopelessness and helplessness. Marian had previously been employed as a fashion designer for a large dress firm in New York City. She was college educated, came from an upper-middle-class Catholic family, and had no siblings. Her parents were currently living in a retirement community in Florida. Further exploration of Marian's situation revealed that she had planned the pregnancy, had no desire to marry the father, and planned to return to work when the infant was six months old. Day care facilities were provided by her place of employment. Marian stated tearfully that she had not realized taking care of a baby would require so much time and attention. She felt frustrated when the baby did not adhere to any schedule and seemed to cry a great deal. When asked about support systems, Marian said that her friends and co-workers were supportive of her decision to have the child; however, she felt out of the mainstream of activities. As Marian described it, she "could no longer just pick up and go." Although she had been aware that there would be changes in her routine after the birth of the baby, she clearly had been unaware of the extent of the impact of the arrival of the child. Marian also stated that her parents were of little support; her father could not understand her decision and refused to talk to her, while her mother expressed a desire to offer assistance. However, her mother felt caught between her father and Marian and therefore decided to remain in Florida "to keep peace."

Assessment of Marian's crisis situation revealed difficulty in adjustment to the new role of parent (including unrealistic expectations of self); loss of previous status as an employed person; lack of available support systems; and lack of a role model as possible precipitants of the crisis. Biochemical changes related to the pregnancy also merited exploration as a basis for her responses. Intervention was directed toward assisting Marian in redefining expectations of herself as a parent; mobilizing appropriate support systems, such as new-mothers groups; reconnecting Marian with selected friends by encouraging her to spend some time each day just for herself; and exploring the possibility of communicating with her mother and father in Florida.

SITUATIONAL CRISES

A situational crisis is one that is precipitated by an *unanticipated* stressful event that creates disequilibrium by threatening one's sense of biological, social, or psychological integrity (Aguilera and Messick, 1982). The severity of the crisis is, however, determined by the individual's own perception of the situation and the impact of the balancing factors previously discussed. A situational crisis poses the threat of loss—whether it be loss of health, loss of a loved one, or loss of job status through either a promotion or a demotion. Role change occurs that influences not only the individual but family and significant others as well. It is interesting to note that an individual's perception of crisis may change from moment to moment or from situation to situation. Each stressful event has the potential to create a crisis; the impact of the stressor depends on the effectiveness of coping strategies, previous experience with the stressor, availability of support systems, and flexibility of individuals in their current situation. Examples of events that can precipitate situational crises are prematurity, status and role changes, death of a loved one, physical or mental illness, divorce, change in geographic location, and poor performance in school.

Caplan (1964) suggests that a critical factor in the definition of a situational crisis lies in the concept of hazardous event. Because of its unpredictable nature, the presence of a hazard enhances the possibility of individual, family, or group disorganization. Situational crises have the potential to promote positive growth and change or to create multiple disruptions. The following is a case study of a situational crisis—a crisis of physical illness:

Mr. W., a 58-year-old white, single male, was admitted to the local general hospital with dizziness, syncopal episodes, shortness of breath, and feelings of pressure in his chest. After several days in the CCU, he was transferred 60 miles by ambulance to a large urban teaching hospital for further diagnostic studies. His preliminary diagnosis was ventricular tachycardia, a lethal arrhythmia initiated by an electrical deficit in the heart. During his first two days in the unit, he was quiet and remained in his room most of the time. After he had completed the first set of diagnostic studies, Mr. W. seemed more agitated. He frequently paced the hallways

and snapped at the nurses. Concurrently his physicians told him that he would need further studies (which were quite painful and frightening). He was also told that the medications used thus far to control the arrhythmia had not been successful. One evening he was sitting on the edge of the bed crying when the nurse entered to give him his medications. He snapped, "Why should I take these—they aren't helping anyway" and threw them to the floor. Exploration with Mr. W. of his current state revealed the following data: his insurance was running out in ten days; he lived alone and bills were going unpaid; his current job status was uncertain because he was no longer going to be able to work with heavy machinery (he was too young to retire, yet too old to find other employment); he feared he would be unable to receive Social Security disability payments. Mr. W. described his brother and sister-in-law as support systems. When asked whether they would be interested in learning cardiopulmonary resuscitation, Mr. W. stated that he didn't want them to "assume that kind of responsibility."

As in a maturational crisis, there is a ripple effect. Physical illness, in Mr. W.'s case, threatened to precipitate other crises: loss of function, retirement, and possibly loss of life. Assessment focused primarily on the precipitating event and the client's perceptions of the impact of the event on life-style in general. Intervention was directed toward resolving the individual stresses resulting from the onset of the life-threatening physical illness.

SOCIAL CRISES

A relatively recent addition to the discussion of crisis is the concept of ''social crisis.'' Chamberlin (1980) describes social crises as accidental, uncommon, and unanticipated crises that result in multiple losses and radical environmental changes. Social crises include natural disasters which impact on large numbers of people—floods, earthquakes, major fires. Violence and large-scale tragedies resulting from man's actions are also considered social crises—for example, group hostage-taking and riots, nuclear accidents, mass killings (as in the Tate-LaBianca murders), contamination of large areas by toxic wastes, wars, rape, and persecution of large groups of people because of ethnicity or race. This type of crisis is unlike maturational and situational crises because it does not occur in the lives of all people.

Because of the severity of the effects of social crises, coping strategies may not be effective. Individuals confronted with social crises usually do not have previous experiences from which to draw. Support systems may be unavailable because they may also be involved in similar situations. Mental health professionals are called on to act quickly and provide services to large numbers of people and in some cases whole communities.

Effects of a social crisis may occur months after the event, being manifested in high levels of psychological stress on both individual and community levels. Evidence of the importance of identifying and intervening in social crises is found in the American Psychiatric Association's delineation of criteria for posttraumatic stress disorder*:

A. Existence of a recognizable stressor that would evoke significant symptoms of distress in almost everyone
B. Reexperiencing of the trauma as evidenced by at least one of the following:
    1. Recurrent and intrusive recollections of the event
    2. Recurrent dreams of the event
    3. Sudden acting or feeling as if the traumatic event were occurring, because of an association with an environmental or ideational stimulus
C. Numbing of responsiveness to or reduced involvement with the external world, beginning some time after the trauma, as shown by at least one of the following:
    1. Markedly diminished interest in one or more significant activities

2. Feeling of detachment or estrangement from others
3. Constricted affect
D. At least two of the following symptoms that were not present before the trauma:
    1. Hyperalertness or exaggerated startle response
    2. Sleep disturbance
    3. Guilt about surviving when others have not or about behavior required for survival
    4. Memory impairment or trouble concentrating
    5. Avoidance of activities that arouse recollection of the traumatic event
    6. Intensification of symptoms by exposure to events that symbolize or resemble the traumatic event

Typology of crisis

Burgess and Baldwin (1981) have described crisis situations as "critical points of attention in health care delivery." Secondary prevention can be practiced as a part of crisis intervention through the detection of emotional illness and the referral of clients to appropriate agencies. Burgess and Baldwin stress the importance of establishing structure in crisis intervention, placing emphasis on the development of contracts with clients that facilitate crisis resolution. These authors also place emphasis on the working through of maladaptive responses, and the support for those responses, and on the development of strategies that are more effective. Burgess and Baldwin suggest that a "typology of crisis" seeks to understand and present interventions for client populations that have previously been neglected in the literature and in practice.

Assessment of a crisis is focused on identifying its effects on individuals, the community, the state, the nation, and perhaps the world. Intervention occurs in two phases: the first phase deals with the immediate effects, while the second phase is more concerned with the posttraumatic issues, as noted in the diagnostic criteria for posttraumatic stress disorder.

Baldwin (1978) originally developed the following classification system, which is based on sever-

---

*From American Psychiatric Association. 1980. Diagnostic and Statistical Manual of Mental Disorders (ed. 3). Washington, D.C.: APA.

ity of crisis. As one moves from class 1 to class 6, the crisis becomes more severe, and the locus of the stressor moves from external to internal.

CLASS 1—DISPOSITIONAL CRISIS

Butcher and Mandel (1976) define a dispositional crisis as a problematic situation that presents a sense of immediacy. The clinician's role may be to provide information, make a referral to an appropriate agency or discipline, or provide administrative leverage. Examples of dispositional crises include: meeting the parenting needs of one's children; experiencing stress resulting from the behavior of a substance abuser in the family; and being unable to study properly because of a roommate's lack of concern for study hours.

Strategies for intervention involve clarification of the issues and providing the necessary services and support.

CLASS 2—CRISES OF ANTICIPATED LIFE TRANSITIONS

There are normal life crises that are anticipated to some degree by clients and over which they may or may not have control. In some cases clients request help prior to the actual onset of the transition, while in other cases clients seek help during or following the transition. Examples of such transitions include going away from home for the first time, midlife career changes (going back to work or school or changing jobs), retirement, and separation and divorce.

The emphasis in strategies of intervention is on assisting clients in developing an understanding of the changes that will occur or are occurring and exploring what those changes mean. Effects on current life-style and family systems are assessed, and more adaptive coping strategies are developed. Group approaches have been useful in providing support to these client populations.

CLASS 3—CRISES RESULTING FROM SUDDEN TRAUMATIC STRESS

Crises of this nature are precipitated by powerful external stressors that are unexpected and over which the client has little control. Clients feel overwhelmed, and coping strategies are immobilized. Examples are sudden death of a spouse, family member, or significant other; rape; natural disasters such as floods; and war combat stress.

Providing or mobilizing support following the impact of the stressor is the initial goal of intervention. Clients are encouraged to acknowledge both positive and negative emotions resulting from a situation that has not been encountered previously. Clients are assisted in exploring other methods of coping that will be effective in meeting the changes that result from the stressor.

CLASS 4—MATURATIONAL/ DEVELOPMENTAL CRISES

These crises result not from an external source of stress but rather from one that is more internal and that is based on the psychodynamics of the individual client. These crises result from ineffective attempts to resolve interpersonal situations that are related to more deep-rooted developmental issues such as dependency, power, value conflicts, intimacy, and sexual identity. Attempts to attain emotional maturity are unsuccessful and repeated patterns of relational difficulties are often noted. Examples of crises reflecting power, intimacy, and sexual identity issues in particular are child abuse and incest.

Strategies of intervention focus on assisting the client to identify and understand the nature of the developmental issue that is the underlying precipitant. Clients are encouraged to respond to the manifest problem while concurrently developing coping strategies to resolve the developmental conflict.

CLASS 5—CRISES RESULTING FROM PSYCHOPATHOLOGY

Preexisting psychopathology may act to precipitate a crisis or may be instrumental in impairing or complicating crisis resolution. Such a crisis is precipitated by unresolved internal issues that are triggered by events within a relational context. Individuals in this class present with multiple problems that impact on several areas of functioning. Crises of this nature are frequently seen in borderline personalities, severe neuroses, characterological disorders, and nonorganic psychoses.

Intervention is directed toward resolving the presenting issue by developing problem-solving skills and manipulating the environment to effect changes in behavior. Stabilization of function to its maximal level is the primary goal. Referral to appropriate long-term therapy is made once the immediate crisis has been resolved.

CLASS 6—PSYCHIATRIC EMERGENCIES

In these crises, overall functioning is impaired and clients are no longer responsible for their actions. Crises of this type include acute psychoses, drug or alcohol intoxication, and impulse-control problems such as suicidal or homicidal behavior and uncontrollable anger and aggression.

Intervention with this type of crisis may be difficult in that the client can only provide limited information while service must often be instituted immediately. The goals are to work quickly and effectively to assess the medical and psychological condition; to assess the precipitant; and to provide intervention as rapidly as possible, particularly in life-threatening situations.

• • •

The importance of Baldwin's "typology of crisis" lies in the fact that it enables mental health professionals to understand more thoroughly the nature of a particular crisis. Strategies of intervention can therefore be made more appropriate to the crisis situation, and they can be more effective in resolving the particular issues of the situation.

CRISIS THERAPY AS A MODEL OF NURSING INTERVENTION

Individuals are most amenable to the helping efforts of health professionals and are most likely to make attempts to change ineffective coping strategies during times of crisis. Previously used coping methods may have maintained some form of equilibrium; therefore, change and growth would have been limited. However, a person does not initially consider a crisis situation to be growth promoting. The overwhelming emotional shock waves resulting from a crisis frequently distort perceptions and prevent action. Nursing intervention by skilled clinicians enables a client to emerge from a crisis with effective coping skills, a better understanding of self within the context of his or her environment and relationships, and a sense of competence regarding the ability to resolve issues.

Crisis intervention is used in a variety of settings in group and individual approaches. Because of its early association with community psychiatry, crisis intervention was frequently thought to be a useful modality only in community mental health centers. However, it has become apparent that crisis intervention is useful in many settings. Crisis intervention techniques may be successfully used by clinical specialists in liaison positions in general hospital settings. Nurses may work with families of clients who are in intensive care settings, assisting them in their adjustment to their loved ones' life-threatening situations. Clients and families are helped to adapt to body image changes and loss of independence and function and to come to grips with the potential or actual loss of life. Particular populations at risk, such as cardiac clients, clients undergoing dialysis, transplant clients, clients with cancer, and clients who have other chronic illnesses that affect life-style, support systems, and sense of self, potentially can benefit from group experiences as a means of resolving crises. Age is no barrier to crisis; crises occur in childhood, in young and middle adulthood, in geriatric and obstetrical populations. Emergency rooms are frequently the scene of potential and actual crisis situations for individuals and families. Each unit in the general hospital setting presents the potential for the use of individual and group crisis intervention strategies.

The community also has the potential for crisis intervention. Nurses function in community health centers, providing direct physical and psychological care for their clients. Nurses can use crisis intervention in industrial health settings, as well as in school and camp environments.

Crisis intervention techniques are frequently employed by mental health nurse–clinical specialists in their work with nursing staff members to resolve client management problems and intragroup staff issues. In such a situation, the clinician not only assists the staff in processing and resolving client and staff issues but also acts as a role model in the use of crisis intervention techniques.

Burgess and Baldwin (1981) suggest that mental health professionals who use crisis intervention techniques must develop skills at the following levels:

1. *Conceptual*—provides a framework for understanding client problems and for problem-resolution (that is, the behavioral model)
2. *Clinical*—Gestalt model techniques for effecting change; they evolve from the conceptual framework
3. *Communication*—effective skills create a nonthreatening atmosphere where clients can explore the impact of crisis on their lives.

Crisis intervention can then assume its place as a valid form of therapy, with a conceptual framework and a rationale evolving from that framework. The myth that crisis intervention is a holding action—a "one-shot" type of therapy that is practiced by paraprofessionals who have no specialized skills—can be dispelled (Burgess and Baldwin, 1981).

PHASES OF CRISIS INTERVENTION

The phases of crisis intervention as a therapeutic tool parallel the steps of the nursing process.

Assessment

Accurate assessment is a key factor in the appropriate use of crisis intervention techniques. Data are collected regarding the presenting problem and precipitating event. An exploration of the precipitating event is necessary in order to facilitate the development of effective coping strategies. Burgess and Baldwin (1981) present the following model for assessment:

1. Assessment of the precipitating event
   a. Time and place. It is often difficult for client and therapist to define the event within the client's recent past. Usually the event is clarified through the process of resolution.
   b. Interpersonal dimensions. Crisis is related to the context of the client's relationships, whether they be those of the past or the present.
   c. Affective reactions. Emotional responses to crisis are expected and should be explored and *affirmed*. Clients have the *right* to experience emotional disequilibrium. The nature of the responses must be accurately and quickly determined to protect clients from their own impulses (suicidal, homocidal, or other aggressive acting-out behaviors). Feelings commonly experienced are: +3 and/or +4 anxiety, fear, embarrassment, anger, guilt (see Chapter 4).
   d. Client's request for help. A request for help may be directly or indirectly conveyed and may be adaptive or maladaptive in nature. Requests for help enable the therapist to understand in some measure how the client has problem-solved in previous situations. The clients may wish support, therapy, an authority figure, or nothing (Lazare et al., 1972). Lazare further suggests that response to the request is critical in that a lack of response may lead to progressive deterioration of client behavior.
2. Assessment of psychodynamic issues. Assessment involves the exploration of the crisis precipitant within the context of current experiences. However, it is the role of the

therapist to identify past traumatic experiences that may be analogous to current ones and to identify any events that may cause anticipatory fear of reexperiencing an old trauma. An event occurring in the present environment may recall similar affect and behavior from past traumatic experiences. For example, a Vietnam veteran might experience a crisis response when confronting a situation in his present life that triggered feelings of inadequacy and helplessness similar to those experienced during his tour of duty in Vietnam.

3. Assessment of present coping strategies. When individuals experience a crisis, coping strategies that are a part of their normal repertoire are no longer effective. Assessment of these strategies offers information regarding the crisis and the client's understanding of the need for the use of particular coping strategies within the context of various relationships.

   a. Maladaptive coping responses. What would happen if the client were to modify behaviors and resolve the presenting problem? The assessment must evaluate the gains experienced through the use of maladaptive responses: security may be maintained at the cost of healthy equilibrium, and uncomfortable feelings such as anger, guilt, loss, and shame may not need to be confronted. Exploration of the need for maladaptive coping strategies leads to a more in-depth understanding of the crisis itself.

   b. Definition of alternative strategies. Once clients understand their use of maladaptive coping strategies, they are able to conceptualize and define more effective coping strategies. Nurses can present possible alternatives that can be tested by clients as a means of educating clients in relation to their own levels of emotional maturity.

4. Assessment of pre-crisis functioning

   a. Client's usual repertoire of coping strategies. Exploration of coping strategies employed prior to the onset of the crisis will reveal the range of responses called on in various situations. It may be determined that the client has a limited scope of coping measures when confronted with a situation that produces feelings of inadequacy or helplessness but that coping strategies used to resolve anger are quite effective. The process of exploration allows the client to gain insight into usual responses to situations that require adaptation and change.

   b. Emotional style and communication skills. Assessment of emotional style reveals a client's capability to respond fully to events in his or her life. For example, does the client experience emotions such as anger or affection, or does he or she keep them in check so as not to lose control? Clients may not even be aware of feelings they are experiencing until the feelings are pointed out to them. The more open clients are to the expression of their emotions, the more able they will be to recognize the cause-and-effect relationships between emotions and particular events.

   c. Social support system. A person exists within the context of many relationships; in fact, a person cannot exist without some type of relatedness to others. Assessment of support systems indicates the number and depth of relationships. A client may have many superficial relationships but no one to actually count on. Through an exploration of relationships, the nurse may note the circumstances in which relationships are initiated and how much energy is expended by the client in maintaining the relationship. Solitary time is important to most individuals; it must be determined whether the client spends time alone because the client wants to or because no one wants to spend time with him or her. Often individuals in the client's community may be called upon to provide support, such as the corner grocer, the postman, or a clergyman, or the client may be invited to join a group of similar individuals as part of a support system.

d. Personal vulnerabilities. All individuals feel vulnerable at some time in life; however, vulnerability is not characteristic of life in general. Vulnerable areas are often at the base of crisis experiences where coping strategies have not been developed. An assessment of these areas may reveal issues that were in part responsible for the onset of the crisis itself.

e. Self-report of personality. It is important to listen and *hear* clients' descriptions of themselves. How balanced are their lists of strengths and weaknesses? Do they describe themselves as basically good, or do they constantly put themselves down? Adjectives used to describe self are also important. Perceptions of self prior to the crisis can be compared to current perceptions. The client's sense of self and personal strengths can be used in crisis resolution.

5. Related areas of assessment. The following areas, when present, are integral parts of a comprehensive psychosocial assessment: suicidal behavior, substance use and abuse, recent medical history, and recent psychiatric history.

Following an accurate assessment of the presenting problem, a nursing diagnosis may reflect problematic issues within varying contexts of the client's life. The American Psychiatric Association has defined the criteria for posttraumatic stress disorder, which is a diagnostic category presenting symptoms and behaviors characteristic of a traumatic event of any nature. This category may be used as a corollary for the determination of a nursing diagnosis (see diagnostic criteria for posttraumatic stress disorder, p. 355).

Planning

Following data collection and analysis, client and nurse must collaborate on defining goals and interventions to resolve the identified issues. The locus of decision making in the crisis intervention process is shared for the most part. The assessment plan is primarily nurse-directed. However, in the planning and implementation phases, the relationship assumes a more collaborative nature; in fact, a well-skilled clinician will facilitate the client's development of adaptive strategies rather than solve the problems himself or herself. Through the assessment process the nurse gains a clearer understanding of how to maximize client strengths and provide appropriate client support.

Implementation

The third phase is implementation of the plan designed by client and nurse. In this phase the nurse maintains a goal-directed focus in order to facilitate the client's resolution of the presenting issue within a limited time frame (six to eight sessions).

During the intervention phase the nurse uses already developed communication skills to help the client understand the impact of the crisis and resolve presenting issues. The nurse encourages the open expression of feelings by affirming the client's right to experience those feelings. The nurse may also protect the client from harmful impulses resulting from an overwhelming sense of helplessness and depression. Clarification of issues facilitates client perception of cause-and-effect relationships, and an understanding of the emotional affect generated by the crisis develops. Because of the client's feelings of vulnerability, efforts by the nurse are directed toward ego support and acknowledgment of effective coping strategies. Mobilization of support systems is initiated, and the client is encouraged to employ those resources appropriately.

Jacobsen et al. (1968) suggest that crisis intervention may occur at a generic level or at an individual level. The *generic* approach assumes that there are generalized patterns of behavior in any crisis. The working through of grief is an example of a defined sequence of responses to loss. This pattern of response is not only applicable to loss through death but also to loss of function, loss of role status, or loss of independence. Intervention at the generic level focuses on facilitating the client's movement through the prescribed phases to reach resolution. Individual psychodynamics are not emphasized. *General support* is provided, giving clients a sense that they are not alone and that problem resolution can be effected. *Environmental manipulation* seeks to alter the current situation that may be potentiating the effects of the crisis. For example, assume that a young doctoral student has been feeling overwhelmed by her studies and her full-time job. With support from a nurse, the student seeks to reduce her stress by temporarily reducing her job to part-time status during the semester in which she has the heaviest course load. Feelings of helplessness are alleviated, and she is able to resolve the crisis successfully. *Anticipatory guidance* assists clients in responding to the crises of life that most individuals experience, such as death of a loved one, birth of a child, and the transition from one developmental phase to the next. Nurses can present parameters of expected cognitions, emotions, and actions based on what is known to be the experience of the majority of individuals in similar situations. A sense of control is re-established when clients feel that what they are experiencing is similar to the experiences of others. The universal statement ''Many times clients have expressed . . .'' indicates to the client that these feelings and perceptions are shared and understood. This does not deny, however, the uniqueness of the individual. Further exploration of feelings can be pursued. Through anticipatory guidance, clients can be prepared to cope with anticipated events and transition periods and reduce the potential of another crisis response in the future.

The *individual approach* differs from the generic in that there is an emphasis on individual psychodynamics as they exist within the context of relationships. The individual approach focuses on specific needs of a client and on the resolution of a situation peculiar to that client. This approach can be effective in situational and maturational crises. It is often employed when the generic approach has not effected crisis resolution. The individual approach reflects an understanding of unresolved emotional issues of the past, such as dependency and value conflicts, and their connection with the occurrence of behaviors in the past. The intent, however, is not to restructure the personality. Crises that involve impulsive, acting-out behavior, such as aggression directed toward self or others, need to be addressed by an individual approach rather than the generic, to protect clients from themselves and to protect others from the impulsive behavior.

Evaluation

Evaluation, the fourth and final step in crisis intervention, involves a review of the effectiveness of the strategies. Has crisis resolution occurred? Have goals been met, and has positive behavioral change been effected? Have adaptive coping strategies been developed and used? What have clients learned about themselves, their responses, and their potential for healthy adaptation in the future? The evaluation phase acts as a period of summation, during which clients can review events of crisis situations, their responses, and the ways in which they were able to resolve the issues. Other areas that need further exploration are identified, and measures to meet those needs are discussed. Nurse and client share the decision making in this phase and determine whether referral to another agency or health professional is appropriate.

CLINICAL CASE STUDY

The following case study will illustrate the four phases of crisis intervention.

Jack H., a 36-year-old white male, presented at the local mental health center complaining of feeling depressed and highly anxious. Symptoms included insomnia, loss of appetite, inability to concentrate, and tearfulness. He described the onset as occurring two weeks earlier when he was told of the date of his divorce hearing. His children were in the custody of his wife, and he was unable to see them regularly. His job was in jeopardy because of his inability to concentrate. The family had lived in the current home for only six months; therefore, available support systems for Jack were limited. His parents were divorced, lived several hundred miles away, and were unaware of his current difficulties. Jack described his marriage as "having its ups and downs," but he never expected his wife to file for divorce. He still loved her but she was unwilling to seek counseling, stating he would never change. Jack commented that he had "always been a failure and that this was just another example." He admitted that the marriage was not as good as it could be but felt that divorce was the ultimate sign of failure.

Assessment

Analysis of data reflected the following nursing diagnoses: ambivalence, loss of self-worth, and guilt feelings, all secondary to failure of marriage.

Planning

Goals were developed to assist Jack in reorganizing and resolving feelings of guilt and ambivalence. Jack's usual method of coping was to involve himself with his work. Because of his inability to concentrate, this method of coping was ineffective, which served to increase his anxiety lev-

els. His environmental supports were limited. He had spent his time either at work or with his family. He identified a person he could talk to but did not like to "bother him." Jack stated he was willing to work on his feelings. He demonstrated an active desire to resolve his issues.

Intervention was directed toward:
1. Long-term goal: return to pre-crisis level of functioning or higher
2. Short-term goals:
   a. Develop an intellectual understanding of the cause-and-effect relationship between the event and the emotions
   b. Implement new coping strategies such as developing supportive relationships at work and in his condominium complex
   c. Actively participate in the divorce proceedings and child custody action
   d. Take a two-week leave of absence from work

Implementation

Nursing intervention included the use of a generic approach based on the response to loss while at the same time considering the psychodynamics of Jack's own parents' divorce and its current effect on his life.

Support provided by the nurse enabled the client to explore feelings and new measures of coping in a nonjudgemental, unbiased, empathic environment. Jack's level of anxiety was reduced and his feelings of worthlessness were challenged as he and the nurse identified his strengths. Reduction of anxiety made more energy available to actively participate in the divorce proceedings rather than be a passive recipient of the event's effects. Jack came to recognize that both he and his wife had responsibility for the failure of the marriage; it was not his alone. He also began to recognize the feelings that he had experienced during his parents' divorce and the effects of those feelings on his current behavior.

By the completion of the sixth session, Jack was experiencing less anxiety and had a clearer perception of his role in the marriage and impending divorce. He was able to make decisions regarding his job, the custody of his children, and his future relationships with his wife and other women. Jack's support systems were still somewhat limited. He made plans to join an exercise club in his condominium complex.

Evaluation

As a result of Jack's more active involvement in directing the events of his life, he felt an increased sense of competence, self-worth, and control. His inability to concentrate, lack of appetite, and insomnia were decreasing, as was his anxiety level. Those coping measures that had been effective prior to the crisis were so once again. He had also developed new coping strategies that added to his repertoire for future use. Jack and the nurse reviewed the experience and the manner in which Jack had successfully used problem-solving techniques. The defined goals had been achieved.

CHAPTER SUMMARY

A crisis can be defined as a situation that cannot readily be resolved by an individual's normal or available repertoire of coping strategies. Events that precipitate crises may be anticipated, as in the case of the transition from one developmental phase to another. Situations of an external nature that threaten one's sense of biological, psychological, or social integrity may also precipitate crises.

Crisis theory provides a conceptual framework for active intervention. Contracts are time-limited to six to eight sessions in which presenting issues are explored, interventive strategies are implemented, and clients learn to modify behavior as necessary. Further referral is made if it is appropriate. Crisis intervention is no longer considered to be a ''band-aid'' approach or ''one-shot'' therapy. It is a valid modality of treatment practiced by clinicians who are skilled in the use of crisis strategies.

The methodology of crisis intervention involves a sequence of steps similar to those of the nursing process. An assessment of the presenting issue is made through data collection and analysis. A plan is determined through a collaborative effort with the client. Strategies of action to enhance coping measures are implemented. Finally, the effectiveness of the plan is reviewed, and a determination is made in regard to further action. Steps are followed sequentially and may be returned to as appropriate.

Nursing intervention is based on sound therapeutic communication skills. Ego defenses are supported while more adaptive strategies are explored. Manipulation of the environment alters stressful situations so that individuals are able to explore more effective resolutions.

Crisis intervention can be used in many settings and formats. Group crisis intervention reaches larger numbers of individuals. Examples include parenting groups, groups of at-risk clients such as those with cardiac disease, and families of clients in intensive care settings. Crisis techniques can be used in all general hospital units, as well as in community settings, including schools and industries. Nurses may also employ crisis strategies in dealing with intragroup issues concerning a nursing staff and in dealing with client management issues.

REFERENCES

Aguilera, D.C., and J. Messick
1982 Crisis Intervention: Theory and Methodology, ed. 4. St. Louis: The C.V. Mosby Co.

Baldwin, B.
1978 "A paradigm for the classification of emotional crises: indications for crisis intervention." American Journal of Psychiatry 4:538.

Burgess, A., and B. Baldwin
1981 Crisis Intervention Theory and Practice: A Clinical Handbook. Englewood Cliffs, N.J.: Prentice-Hall, Inc.

Butcher, J.M., and G. Mandel
1976 "Crisis intervention." In Clinical Methods in Psychology. I. We (ed.). New York: John Wiley & Sons, Inc.

Caplan, G.
1964 Principles of Preventive Psychiatry. New York: Basic Books, Inc.

Chamberlin, B.C.
1980 "The psychological aftermath of disasters." Journal of Clinical Psychology. 41:238-243.

Erikson, E.
1963 Childhood and Society. New York: W.W. Norton & Co., Inc.

Glass, A.T.
1957 "Observations upon the epidemiology of mental illness in troops during warfare." In Symposium on Preventive and Social Psychiatry. National Research Council (ed.). Washington, D.C.: Walter Reed Army Institute.

Jacobsen, G., N. Strickler, and W. Morely
1968 "Generic and individual approaches to crisis intervention." American Journal of Public Health 47:339.

Joint Commission on Mental Health and Mental Illness
1961 Action for Mental Health. New York: Basic Books, Inc.

Lazare, A.F., F. Cohen, A. Jacobsen, and E. Williams
1972 "The walk in patient as a customer: a key dimension in evaluation and treatment." American Journal of Orthopsychiatry 23:872.

Lindemann, E.
1944 "Symptomatology and management of acute grief." American Journal of Psychiatry 32:141.

Williams, F.
1971 "Intervention in maturational crises." Perspectives in Psychiatric Care 17:240.

ANNOTATED SUGGESTED READINGS

Baldwin, B.
1978 "A paradigm for the classification of emotional crises: implications for crisis intervention." American Journal of Orthopsychiatry 48(3):538.
This article presents an integrated crisis theory based on the author's development of six classes of crisis. Formats of intervention are well defined for each class. The comprehensive and pragmatic nature of this work serves to fill the gap left by other crisis theories.

Burgess, A., and B. Baldwin
1981 Crisis Intervention Theory and Practice: A Clinical Handbook. Englewood Cliffs, N.J.: Prentice-Hall, Inc.
This text presents a conceptual framework for crisis intervention as well as Baldwin's typology of crisis and strategies of intervention. It also explores in depth various types of crises that have not been discussed elsewhere, such as incest, women returning to work, and Vietnam War combat stress.

Lindemann, E.
1944 "Symptomatology and management of acute grief." American Journal of Psychiatry 101:141.
This article, which evolved from the author's study of the survivors of the Coconut Grove fire in Boston, describes the grieving process. The article played an important role in the emergence of crisis intervention as a valid method to cope with the grief response.

FURTHER READINGS

Dixon, S.
1979 Working With People in Crisis: Theory and Practice. St. Louis: The C.V. Mosby Co.

Donovan, J.M., M.J. Bennet, and C. McElroy
1979 "The crisis 'group'—an outcome study." American Journal of Psychiatry 13:906.

Goldstein, D.
1978 "Crisis intervention: a brief therapy model." Nursing Clinics of North America 13(4):657.

Harrison, D.
1981 "Nurses and disasters." Journal of Psychosocial Nursing 19(2):34.

Hoff, L.A.
1978 People in Crisis: Understanding and Helping. Menlo Park, Calif.: Addison-Wesley Publishing Co.

Lancaster, J., and D. Berkovsky
1978 "An ecological framework for crisis intervention." Journal of Psychiatric Nursing 16:17.

Puryear, D.
1979 Helping People in Crisis. San Francisco: Jossey-Bass, Inc.

Sheehy, G.
1976 Predictable Crises of Adult Life. New York: E. P. Dutton & Co., Inc.

CHAPTER 14

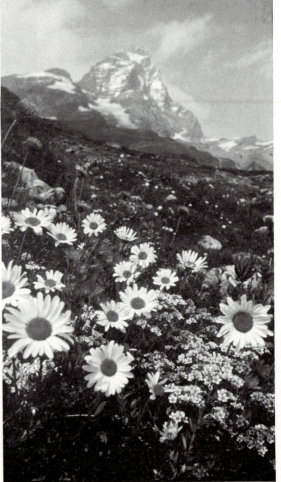

Photo by H. Grhscher—Peter Arnold, Inc.

Community mental health

CHAPTER FOCUS

Mental health care has been undergoing an evolutionary, some even say a revolutionary, process for more than a quarter of a century. The community mental health movement has been an important part of this process since its implementation on a nationwide basis in the 1960s.

The Comprehensive Mental Health Centers Act, passed by the United States Congress in 1963, along with subsequent legislation, has changed the mental health care delivery system. The 1963 legislation was unique in that it increased the involvement of the federal government in mental health care. Prior to the passage of the community mental health legislation, major responsibility for mental health care was a function of state and local governments and the private sector. The federal government had been involved only in funding research, education, and a few other aspects of mental health care and in providing health services to special groups such as the armed forces and veterans. The legislation established national guidelines for mental health services and provided some funding in the form of grants for construction and staffing of mental health centers. The guidelines were broad enough to allow programs to meet local and regional mental health needs.

Community mental health care involves a complex, multifaceted approach to meeting one of the nation's major health problems. Concepts of community mental health place emphasis upon reducing the incidence of mental disorders through locally available and comprehensive services for prevention, early treatment, and rehabilitation. As a means of achieving these objectives and of bringing mental health care into the mainstream of modern health practices, an integrated system of health, social welfare, and other human services was conceived.

Implementation of the goals of the community mental health movement is an evolving process in which communities; governmental, health, and social agencies;

professional practitioners; and consumers develop collaborative, cooperative programs to promote mental health. Because of variations in population density and the multiplicity of ethnic and sociocultural groups in the United States, the mental health needs and the organization of mental health services to meet those needs vary considerably from one community to another. Certain concepts, however, are characteristic of all community mental health programs. Among these concepts are the following:

1. Emphasis on preventive psychiatry and the availability of comprehensive services for the prevention, treatment, and rehabilitation of mental disorders
2. Provision of mental health services in a setting in which there is the least possible disruption of social and kinship support systems and the least possible interference with personal and civil liberties
3. Responsiveness to consumer needs through community involvement in the planning and evaluation of programs to meet mental health needs
4. Provision of mental health services by interdisciplinary mental health teams

The community mental health movement has had a major impact upon the treatment of persons with psychiatric disorders. There has also been an influence upon the roles and functions of health professionals involved in providing health services. As a basis for understanding current mental health practices, this chapter will focus on major aspects of community mental health. The present status of community mental health care and some of the factors that have influenced the realization of the goals of the movement will be discussed.

CONCEPTS UNDERLYING COMMUNITY MENTAL HEALTH CARE

The community mental health movement embraces a broad-spectrum approach to meeting mental health needs. Theoretical concepts place emphasis on the interrelationship of biological, psychological, intellectual, spiritual, and sociocultural forces inherent in a *holistic view* of the individual interacting with the environment (see Chapter 1). Developments in psychopharmacology and biochemical research and advancements in the knowledge of the effects on mental health of such sociocultural stressors as poverty, racism, and unemployment have emphasized the importance of a holistic approach to mental health promotion (Greenblat 1977).

The community mental health concept uses *systems theory,** taking an *ecosystem approach* to the organization of services to meet the mental health needs of communities. A human ecosystem is the environment, physical and social, of which the individual is a part and with which he or she interacts. The unit of analysis of human ecosystems is usually the family or the community (Wilkinson and O'Connor, 1977). An ecosystem approach to community mental health is based on the following assumptions:

1. Alteration in the number of admissions to a local community mental health agency will not only affect the operation of other local mental health agencies but also the resources, economy, and composition of the community (for example, there will be a

---

*Refer to Chapters 1 and 5 for discussions of systems theory.

change in the number of people employed and the amount of income earned).

2. There is a relationship between the environment and behavior. For example, overcrowding, inadequate housing, urban renewal, and migration influence behavior.

3. There is a relationship between human behavior and such elements of the immediate social environment as the family, school, and place of employment.

4. Social structure and the physical environment interrelate and influence the well-being of community members (both individuals and families) and communities.

5. Community mental health professionals will have an inadequate data base if they assess only one aspect of the ecosystem. This may lead to ineffective intervention (Kelly, 1966; Rapaport, 1977).

Therefore, from an ecosystem perspective, mental illness occurs when communities are unable to obtain adequate resources or to equitably distribute resources to their members. The origin of psychopathology is not located solely in the individual but within the entire ecosystem, of which the individual is one interdependent part (O'Connor, 1977).

Community mental health nurses facilitate the effective functioning of human ecosystems by engaging in primary (anticipatory), secondary (corrective), or tertiary (rehabilitative) preventive intervention.* Because human behavior is both affected by and affects the family and the community, all three levels of intervention may be engaged in serially or simultaneously (Lancaster, 1980). For example, secondary and tertiary activities may be aimed at treating and rehabilitating both the perpetrators and victims of violence (a symptom of system dysfunction), while primary activities may be aimed at preventing a recurrence of the overcrowding, inadequate housing, and parental overburdening that may contribute to future dysfunction in the ecosystem. In addition to an ecosystem

approach, any of the following conceptual models may be used in community psychiatry.

The *medical model,* as its name implies, involves the organization of mental health services in much the same way that services in an acute care hospital are organized. The major focus is upon the individual and the individual's symptoms and pathology. Treatment is oriented toward the amelioration of symptoms through brief psychotherapy and somatic and activity therapies. The medical model is often found in inpatient psychiatric units of general hospitals. These units provide short-term hospitalization for community residents who are in crisis, as a part of the community mental health system. Such units usually have outpatient clinics, which provide additional and longer-range services.

The *public health model* embraces many of the aspects of the public health movement that were so effective in eliminating communicable diseases. An approach based on this model is concerned with decreasing or eliminating mental disorders from the population or community, in addition to providing treatment and rehabilitation services. A community is a geographically defined area with a population of 75,000 to 200,000 people. A community, for purposes of community mental health, is also known as a catchment area. Preventive efforts in a catchment area include case finding, consultation, and education of community groups. In addition, community members participate in planning, implementing, and evaluating programs to meet mental health needs. Mental health workers functioning in the public health framework may have an eclectic view of the nature of mental disorders. Such a view makes use of several theoretical constructs as a basis for understanding and intervening in psychopathology. For example, the concepts of personality development of Freud, Erickson, and Sullivan may be used in consultation and education programs with parents and school systems as a means of primary prevention. Or vulnerability to stress may be understood in terms of psychodynamic theory. This may be combined with a view of the interaction between individuals

---

*Levels of preventive intervention will be discussed in more depth later in this chapter.

and the sources of stress in their environment, such as poverty—a view that is inherent in systems theory. Mental health workers then might join with community groups in social and political action to reduce the level of stress in the environment.

Within a catchment area there may be many ethnic and sociocultural groups, each of which may consider itself a community (Hume, 1974) and within which mental health needs and beliefs and practices related to health and illness may vary considerably. Thus the involvement of the members of such communities in mental health programs is important.

The *social model,* which traces its origins to Adolph Meyer but which has more recently been expanded by many social scientists, focuses upon the way in which the individual functions in society. Schulberg (1969) points out that, when this model is used, mental disorders are no longer perceived as primarily intrapsychic processes but are viewed as reflections of disequilibrium between the individual and the environment. He terms this model the ''problems in living'' model. Factors such as poverty and segregation often inhibit or prevent a person from assuming socially expected roles and functions. The behavioral responses to such deprivations and frustrations are often viewed as being normal within the social context rather than as symptoms of pathology. Mental health workers in community agencies that function according to the social model attempt to become cognizant of the problems, attitudes, and broad aspects of the environment as they apply to a particular population and not simply to the individual. Ideally, the resources and strengths of the community are mobilized in helping individuals and families to cope with crises and problems of daily living. Mental health workers may also join with community groups to improve the social milieu through social and political action.

The *holistic health model** focuses on the biological, psychological, intellectual, sociocultural,

---

*Refer to Chapter 1 for an in-depth discussion of holistic health concepts.

and spiritual dimensions of clients. Since the 1970s, holistic health concepts have been incorporated into some community mental health centers. In other instances, community holistic health centers have been established. In keeping with the holistic health philosophy of client-as-partner, the client's personal health inventory (which includes current health status and life stressors), personal goals, sociocultural orientations, and spiritual beliefs are reviewed. The health team and the client then agree on courses of action, which may include appropriate referrals. Holistic health centers may offer a range of services that include nutritional counseling, herbal treatments, accupuncture, reflexology, instruction in meditation and stress management, spiritual development, and such self-healing therapies as visual imagery. Because the emphasis of holistic health is on progress toward wellness, education and social support are aimed at health promotion and illness prevention. Lancaster (1980) points out that community mental health nurses who have master's degrees are prepared both as psychotherapists and as nurses. Because they have integrated the mind-body aspects of the person, they are excellent candidates for functioning within the holistic health model.

FACTORS INFLUENCING THE COMMUNITY MENTAL HEALTH MOVEMENT
Scope of the mental health problem

World War II, which brought universal conscription of young men for military service in the United States, focused national attention on the extent of the nation's mental health problems. Levenson (1974) notes that ''approximately 40% of the 5,000,000 men rejected for military service for medical reasons, during this time, were rejected because of some neuro-psychiatric defect.'' Levenson further notes that such disturbances were responsible for the greatest number of medical discharges from the armed services during the war.

Levenson (1974) also notes that in 1945 there were approximately 450,000 people in state psychiatric institutions in the United States and that the number had increased to 550,000 ten years later. The impact on the state budgets, which had to be increased to provide essential services, and on capital spending, to expand the institutions to meet the mental health needs of the steadily increasing institutional populations, was profound. In many states, the cost of mental health services became a major budgetary expense—and therefore a sociopolitical concern that served to focus attention upon the mental health problem.

The ever-rising costs of services gave impetus to the use of newer therapeutic modalities, particularly chemotherapy, and focused the attention of the federal government upon the nation's mental health needs.

Legislative action

In 1955 the United States Congress passed the Mental Health Studies Act, which directed that a Joint Commission on Mental Health and Mental Illness be appointed to study "the needs and resources of the mentally ill in the United States and to make recommendations for a National Mental Health program" (Joint Commission on Mental Health and Mental Illness, 1961). The Joint Commission, appointed by the National Institute for Mental Health, was an interdisciplinary group drawn from 28 national organizations concerned with mental health. The American Nurses' Association and the National League for Nursing were among the professional organizations supporting the study.

In 1961 the Joint Commission issued its final report in the form of a book entitled *Action for Mental Health: A Program for Meeting the National Emergency*. The report included the following recommendations:

1. To promote publicly supported research and the development of research centers. The report noted that education and scientific knowledge should be regarded as national resources.
2. To achieve better use of present knowledge and experience. The report recommended that "psychiatry and the mental health professions should adopt and practice a liberal philosophy of what constitutes and who can do treatment. . . ." The report noted that certain examinations and treatments should be done by physicians and that psychoanalysis and related forms of insight therapy must be conducted by persons with special training. It recommended, however, that nonmedical mental health workers "with aptitude, sound training, practical experience and demonstrated competence should be permitted to do short-term psychotherapy."
3. To increase the number of mental health professionals. The report recommended federal support of education in the mental health professions. The report also recommended that the mental health professions conduct national recruitment drives and training programs for all categories of mental health workers and that professional leaders become actively engaged in supporting constructive legislation for general and professional education.
4. To increase federal funding for mental health care and improvement in mental health services
5. To improve services provided to people with emotional disturbances. Among the recommendations were increases in the number of community mental health clinics and of psychiatric units in general hospitals; provision of counseling services in the community as secondary prevention measures; improvement in facilities for the chronically ill as tertiary prevention measures; and dissemination of information aimed at increasing public understanding and attitudes about mental illness.

President Kennedy's interest in mental health gave further impetus to the community mental health movement. In 1963 he spoke to the crisis in mental health. Congress responded by passing the Community Mental Health Centers Act, which allocated monies for mental health care and developed guidelines for mental health services.

The Community Mental Health Centers Act incorporated many of the recommendations of the Joint Commission. The basic principles of the act included the following:

1. Providing services for mental health care that are readily available to community residents
2. Providing comprehensive services to meet the varying needs of community residents
3. Providing services appropriate to the individual's problems

The original intent of the act was to establish 2,000 community mental health centers, in locations throughout the nation, to serve populations of from 75,000 to 200,000 people (Levenson, 1974). Although many mental health centers were built or organized as a result of the act, the original goal of 2,000 was not achieved.

A major effect of the Mental Health Studies Act and subsequent legislation on nursing and other, nonmedical health professions was a resolution of the problem of who was qualified to do short-term psychotherapy. The practice of short-term psychotherapy by qualified nurses, social workers, and other professionals became accepted.

Many additional legislative actions have been taken, and the legal procedures for the protection of clients' civil rights appear to be firmly established. Although the changes that have resulted are not usually referred to as one of the revolutions in psychiatry, they have indeed revolutionized many aspects of mental health care. The Department of Health, Education, and Welfare established the following guidelines for Medicaid reimbursement for institutions providing mental health care:

1. Deprivation of liberty and failure to provide treatment violate the fundamental principles of due process of law.
2. Individual treatment plans should be developed, medical orders filed and periodically reviewed, and a Citizen's Commission ap-

pointed to monitor the enforcement of client rights* (Stone, 1975).

The various states revised their mental health laws to protect clients' civil rights. For example, the New York State Mental Hygiene Law, revised in 1973, set stringent controls on involuntary admission to state hospitals and established the clients' rights to appeal and to review by the courts. This law also established a Mental Health Information Service, under the jurisdiction of a state court, through which lawyers are provided to represent clients and protect their rights. Other states have similar laws.

Although the right-to-treatment issue has not been completely resolved, that clients have a right to treatment has become fairly well-established policy and has been reaffirmed in the goals set forth by the President's Commission on Mental Health.

Report of the President's Commission on Mental Health

Shortly after taking office, President Carter established a Commission on Mental Health. The Commission, a 20-member interdisciplinary group whose honorary chairperson was the President's wife, Rosalynn, submitted its report to the President in April, 1978. The Committee members were selected from among the leaders of national organizations concerned with mental health care, among them the American Nurses' Association and the National League for Nursing. Serving on the Commission was Martha L. Mitchell, Chairperson of the American Nurses' Association Division of Psychiatric Nursing Practice. Three additional registered nurses served on task panels.

The Commission identified several mental health needs. Among them were prevention of mental illness, removal of financial barriers to mental health care, better distribution of mental health care providers, and improvement of services

---

*Refer to Chapter 3 for a discussion of due process of law and client rights.

to persons most in need, including children, adolescents, the elderly, minorities, and people with chronic mental health problems.

The following were among the major recommendations of the Commission:

1. A mental health service system through which services could be provided in the least restrictive settings so that the maximum possible independence of clients could be maintained (The report noted that community-based services should be the keystone of the mental health system.)

2. Improved services for the underserved groups already mentioned, through a new federal grant program

3. Continued phasing out of large state hospitals and upgrading of services in those that remain (Also recommended was community planning of services for formerly hospitalized clients.)

4. Protection of the civil rights of persons needing mental health care

5. Stipulation that clinical services be rendered only by, or under the direct supervision of, a psychiatrist or a psychologist, social worker, or nurse with an earned master's or doctoral degree

6. Coordination of mental health services and integration of a mental health system into other human service systems; inclusion of a mental health component in health systems agencies' plans

7. Recognition and strengthening of natural social support networks in mental health services and development of linkages between social support systems and mental health service systems as a means of improving mental health care

8. Giving more attention to prevention, with a strong emphasis on primary prevention of mental disorders

9. Expansion of the knowledge base through research and rebuilding of the nation's mental health research capacity

10. Improving public knowledge and understanding of mental health problems

11. Changing present laws governing third-party payment for mental health care to include additional health care providers and to give clients a broader choice of providers (Report to the President of the President's Commission on Mental Health, 1978)

Legislation that allowed the implementation of these recommendations to begin was passed by Congress and signed by the President in 1980.

CHARACTERISTICS OF COMMUNITY MENTAL HEALTH SERVICES

Concepts of preventive psychiatry

The purposes of primary prevention services are to identify potential health problems and to plan and implement preventive programs. Primary prevention services involve a cooperative effort between mental health professionals and institutions and organizations in the community. Although the individual health professional may practice mental health prevention as a part of the provision of professional services in any area in which he or she may function, preventive programs on a community-wide basis are a cooperative endeavor among health care and social welfare systems, educational institutions, courts and penal institutions, police precincts, industrial organizations, and health and safety organizations. Additional community resources may include the news media, social and religious groups, and individual residents. For example, an emergency room nurse who becomes aware of a drug abuse problem in a local high school population might institute a collaborative relationship with community agencies to provide preventive measures such as health education and to refer students and families to mental health facilities. Developing a program for prevention of drug abuse in this particular population would involve a variety of additional steps. Working with other professional persons, such as school nurses, teachers, and school officials, could be an initial step in the assessment of the extent of the potential danger. Health and welfare institutions could be sources of information about the availability of facilities for early treatment. Planning educational and other programs for prevention of drug abuse would involve collaboration among law enforcement agencies, community groups such as the Parent-Teacher Association, religious organizations, local news media, and mental health consultants.

Secondary prevention, the objectives of which are early identification and effective treatment of mental disorders, also necessitates a cooperative effort between community agencies and residents and mental health practitioners. Clients with mental health problems may come to the attention of, or seek assistance from, a community mental health center, a general hospital, private practitioners, or various health services. Or clients may seek assistance from family, friends, religious leaders, or other members of the community who are not health professionals. In some situations, people in need may not seek assistance from anyone. A community health nurse visiting a home may be the first health professional to identify depression in an elderly man living alone and to recognize that he is in need of treatment. Or a parent-child nurse providing services in a well-baby clinic may identify an emotional disturbance in a new mother. School nurses and teachers, nurses in medical-surgical units or other units of general hospitals, operators of "hot line" telephone services for drug and alcohol abusers and persons contemplating suicide, and persons working in abortion clinics and emergency rooms all may be involved in secondary prevention of mental disorders.

Tertiary prevention is oriented toward providing treatment and rehabilitative services, in the least restrictive setting possible, to persons with chronic psychiatric disorders and to persons who are developmentally disabled. Many clients who have been hospitalized for long periods of time suffer from the effects of institutionalization, or the "so-

cial breakdown syndrome." Rehabilitation of such clients often requires therapeutic measures designed to remotivate and resocialize them. In addition, the provision of basic subsistence needs and sheltered living facilities is often essential to any therapeutic endeavor.

Gerald Caplan (1964) noted several principles that are important in the rehabilitation of the psychiatric client. Among them is that rehabilitative treatment should be instituted as soon as a psychiatric problem has been recognized and a diagnosis has been made. According to Caplan, the major goals of rehabilitation are to maintain or reestablish social network systems and to counteract or reverse the social breakdown syndrome.

The term "social breakdown syndrome" was introduced in 1962 by the American Public Health Association's Committee on Mental Health (Greenberg, 1974). This syndrome begins when individuals who are experiencing psychiatric symptoms become unable to meet the behavioral expectations of their culture and develop feelings of isolation and estrangement. Such feelings are intensified by being labeled mentally ill and being admitted to a mental hospital. Long-term hospitalization then tends to foster helplessness, isolation, dependence, compliance, and identification with fellow clients. The social isolation and the loss of minimum social skills are major components of chronic mental disability. Beard et al. (1978) note that the debilitating effects of long-term hospitalization are reflected in apathy, inactivity, excessive dependence, and profound deficiences in the skills of daily living.

The community mental health movement and current treatments for major psychiatric disorders are oriented toward preventing or reversing the social breakdown syndrome. Brief hospitalization for treatment of acute psychotic states, in a therapeutic milieu, with follow-up care in outpatient departments of mental health centers in the community is used to achieve this goal.

The support systems that compose the social network include family, neighborhood, and religious and other groups through which individuals receive the physical, emotional, and psychological support that is essential to their well-being. Social contact, a sense of belonging and participation, and opportunities for achievement and mastery in interaction with group members also foster a sense of well-being (Caplan, 1974).

Although the family is often the most important part of a social network, a major psychiatric disorder may cause a breakdown in a person's relationship with the family. A family member who is regarded as mentally ill may be stereotyped and thus become alienated from the family. Nurses may ameliorate or prevent such stereotyping and alienation of psychiatric clients by working with family members as part of the treatment and rehabilitation process and by facilitating communication between clients and their families and other social network systems. Treatment in community settings, with minimal restrictions on clients' freedom and maximum opportunity for the maintenance of social contacts, is another important measure.

For some clients with chronic disabilities or for clients who have experienced long-term isolation from their social support systems, efforts to develop new social networks may be necessary. Ethnic and religious groups and community mental health services may provide such networks. For example, Alcoholics Anonymous often serves as a major social support system for persons with disorders related to alcoholism.

Essential services

The Community Mental Health Centers Act of 1963 established guidelines for mental health care and defined five essential services that a health center must provide to be eligible to receive federal funds. The five essential services were (1) around-the-clock inpatient care, (2) outpatient clinic services, (3) facilities for partial hospitalization (for example, day or night hospitals), (4) walk-in facilities for emergency services, and (5) community consultation and education services for prevention of mental illness and promotion of mental health.

The 1963 legislation listed additional services that could be provided but that were not mandatory: diagnostic services, rehabilitation services, research, and evaluation and training of mental health workers.

A subsequent law, the Mental Health Centers Act of 1975, required that all of these services be provided. In addition, this legislation required services for special groups—particularly children, the aged, ethnic minorities, and persons with special problems such as drug or alcohol addiction—and recommended coordination of health and human services systems to meet mental health needs.

The 1975 legislation had less of an impact on mental health care than the earlier legislation, in part because federal funding to implement the legislation was not provided and in part because of the evolving nature of community mental health. Some of the recommendations of the 1978 report of the President's Commission on Mental Health were similar to the stipulations of the 1975 Mental Health Centers Act.

Organization of services

The manner in which community mental health services are organized and the programs that are developed to provide comprehensive services may vary from one community to another. Many factors can influence the way in which community mental health programs are implemented. Variations in geographic distribution of population, population density, and mental health needs necessitate variations in the organization of mental health services. Socioeconomic factors and the availability of already existing mental health and human services systems may also affect the ways in which programs are planned to meet mental health needs. Many patterns of organization have developed (Macht, 1978). In some communities, services are organized under the auspices of a single agency, often with a single center serving as the hub of a mental health program. In other communities, several agencies develop a collaborative arrangement or system to promote community mental health. Such a system is referred to as a multiple-agency system.

The ideal toward which the community mental health movement strives is a system characterized by a collaborative endeavor of all agencies and personnel providing human services. Macht (1978) points out that to promote such collaboration, 26 states have established human services or human resources departments.

In a single-agency system, primary, secondary, and tertiary services are organized under one center, although some services are frequently provided in satellite clinics or other facilities in the community. In a multiple-agency system, services are divided among several agencies. For example, a voluntary hospital might provide in-hospital emergency and diagnostic services. Follow-up clinics and transitional services might be provided by non-profit organizations, branches of state, local, or federal government, or the private sector. Outreach programs and services to meet the needs of special groups such as children or the elderly might be offered through a variety of resources in the community. Each type of agency would collaborate in the training of mental health professionals and the planning of primary prevention programs.

Many large state hospitals have decentralized their operations by making their various units relatively autonomous and assigning each one to a particular community or catchment area. In addition to providing in-hospital treatment for persons with acute and chronic disorders, such units may function as community mental health centers that can provide further treatment, follow-up services, and health supervision in a community. Follow-up and satellite clinics are often staffed by members of an in-hospital mental health team. Such clinics offer clients some level of continuity of care and often provide special services such as the following:

1. Day and night treatment centers and follow-up clinics
2. Occupational and recreational training and rehabilitation programs
3. Transitional services such as halfway houses, foster homes, and supervised hostel arrangements
4. Vocational counseling centers and sheltered workshops
5. Emergency services, such as crisis intervention, and other brief forms of therapy to provide support to clients in their homes in crisis situations

Rehabilitation programs for clients whose chronic disabilities lead to institutionalization and the social breakdown syndrome may need to include special or long-range therapeutic measures and mental health services to prepare them for discharge from the hospital and to enable them to function in the community. Such measures may include a variety of therapies and activities designed to promote social, cognitive, and daily living skills.

Special living arrangements may be necessary for some clients. Halfway houses, for example, serve as transitional living facilities between the hospital and independent living in the community. For clients who have chronic disabilities or health problems that necessitate a continuing form of supervision, foster homes, adult homes, health-related facilities, or nursing homes may be used.

CURRENT STATUS OF COMMUNITY MENTAL HEALTH

During the past two decades there has been remarkable progress in the implementation of the community mental health concept. This progress is reflected in major changes in services for the treatment of persons with psychiatric disorders and developmental disabilities.

Stickney (1974) has aptly described the characteristics of public mental institutions, which were the major resource for mental health care for about a century prior to the mental health movement. He notes that such institutions "became progressively more overcrowded, underfunded, understaffed and stagnant.'' Others have described such institutions as warehouses for people.

Long-term hospitalization in institutions has largely given way to brief hospitalization in times of crisis and the development of treatment and prevention services in local communities throughout the country. State hospital populations have declined, despite a relatively stable number of admissions or, in some institutions, even a slight increase in admissions. For many persons with chronic disabilities, forms of supervised housing in the community have replaced the institution as a home. This pattern has become increasingly prevalent as the constitutional rights of persons with mental health problems have been affirmed by the courts.

There has been an increase in the number of mental health professionals, a phenomenon that has been made possible by government funding of professional education. Government funding has been important in improving the quality of care. For example, many nurses have earned graduate degrees in psychiatric nursing through government-funded educational programs. These nurses' contributions to nursing literature and research and to the quality of care provided in the agencies in which they are employed attest to the value of government funding of higher education. Unfortunately, the level of such funding has declined in recent years.

Progress has also been made in primary prevention, including public education about mental disorders and promotion of collaborative efforts between health and social service systems for the improvement of mental health care.

Despite the progress that has been made, many problems and difficulties lie ahead. Borus (1978) refers to the community mental health movement as being ''in a state of developmental crisis.'' As in any developmental crisis, he points out, there exist both the opportunity for growth and development and the danger of regression to a less healthy state.

Much criticism has been leveled against the community mental health movement in recent years by health professionals and the public at large. Community mental health has been accused by many authors of moving too far too fast, of failing to live up to early expectations and promises, and of moving people out of the back wards into the back alleys. That problems would be encountered and criticisms would arise as a result of a change in health care of the magnitude of that brought about by the community mental health movement was to be expected. Challenges to longstanding beliefs, attitudes, and practices and to areas of vested interest were threatening to many people.

In many communities, for example, there has been public resistance to the presence of mental health treatment and rehabilitation facilities. This problem has been exacerbated in some areas because of the large numbers of people with chronic disorders who have been housed or ''dumped'' in some communities. The problem, to some extent, reflects a lack of funding by state, local, and federal governments, which could have made possible the wider distribution of the mental health facilities necessary to provide care and treatment for persons with chronic disorders.

The maldistribution of health professionals is another major concern, particularly since the persons most in need of mental health services often reside in poor neighborhoods or in rural areas, where few health professionals practice and where the services that are available are often provided by local residents or self-help groups with inadequate preparation. Borus (1978) points to the ''lack of adequate and stable rewards'' as one of the causes of the maldistribution of health professionals.

Although there is general acceptance among health professionals of the concept of community mental health, there are differences of opinion concerning the scope and function of community programs. Schulberg (1969) points out that one school of thought holds that the focus of treatment and rehabilitation efforts should be on persons who seek help. This group is critical of the broader concepts of primary prevention, maintaining that too little is known about primary prevention at the present time. To other mental health professionals, a holistic orientation toward the treatment of mental health problems and a public health approach in developing programs for the total population of a community involve primary prevention and outreach programs in addition to treatment and rehabilitation services. The latter view has prevailed in many areas. But implementation of programs based on this view has been a slow and evolving process. Christmas (1979) points out that there are problems in developing the cooperative, collaborative effort essential to the concept of a system of human services to meet mental health needs. But, as she also observes, change, although slow in coming, eventually does occur. There is a need at all levels of government for legislation and funding to provide improved prevention, treatment, and rehabilitation facilities, professional education, and support of research.

There is also a need for continuing education of the public about modern concepts of mental health to overcome long-held myths and negative attitudes about psychiatric disorders and to gain public support for mental health maintenance programs and treatment and rehabilitation services. Although the community mental health movement has made progress in educating the public, much remains to be done, particulary seeking assistance from members of the communications media and from local, state, and federal legislators, all of whom are in a position to benefit the movement.

Deinstitutionalization

In the past 20 years, state mental hospitals have experienced a decline of 66% in the number of residents. The total of all client populations has decreased from approximately 559,000 to 191,000 people (Bachrach, 1979). The practice of discharging chronically mentally ill clients into the community is known as deinstitutionalization. According to the Report of the Task Panel on Deinstitutionalization, Rehabilitation, and Long-Term Care (1978), planning for deinstitutionalization is often

inadequate. The desire to shift the cost of care for chronically mentally ill clients from the state to the federal government often results in discharging clients into the community without ascertaining whether community service facilities exist. There is usually little assessment of client needs and level of functioning and little consideration of whether hospital or community is the best treatment setting for a particular client. Clients are frequently discharged from a state institution into a hostile community. The lack of aftercare and support services to facilitate the transition from a highly structured hospital setting to a less structured community setting may have a devastating effect on a client.

ORGANIZATIONAL STRESSORS

Factors inherent in providing care to chronically mentally ill clients in the community may produce organizational stress and ineffective and inefficient delivery of care. Stern and Minkoff (1979) identify six organizational stressors:

1. Goal of community mental health. The goal of the community mental health movement —to reintegrate clients into the community —is not compatible with the needs of most deinstitutionalized clients. Many chronically mentally ill clients do not have access to social networks, community support, or aftercare services necessary for reintegration into the community. Nurses and other mental health professionals who are strongly committed to the community mental health movement may experience stress when reintegration into the community cannot be effectively implemented for deinstitutionalized clients. Mental health professionals may try to deal with this conflict by engaging in blame placing (blaming clients or the community) and rejecting deinstitutionalized clients.

2. Ideal of community mental health. Many nurses and other mental health professionals hold that community mental health centers should serve the entire community. Treating deinstitutionalized clients is time consuming.

If community mental health professionals work with deinstitutionalized clients, they have less time to serve the rest of the community. This dilemma may cause conflict and stress. Many nurses and other mental health professionals resolve the conflict by concentrating on primary and secondary prevention to the exclusion of tertiary prevention. This approach results in the abandonment of deinstitutionalized clients.

3. Threat to professional esteem. Among nurses and other mental health professionals, status and professional recognition tend to be associated with the care of acutely ill, rather than chronically ill, clients. Acutely ill clients may be viewed as more challenging and more satisfying to work with than chronically ill clients. In addition, the education of most mental health professionals does not provide the special skills needed to work with chronically mentally ill clients. These factors tend to threaten professional esteem.

4. Threat to professional ability. There is a dearth of research dealing with chronic mental illness. Those treatment strategies that are available are often ineffective with deinstitutionalized clients. Craig and Hyatt (1978) found that when nurses work with deinstitutionalized clients, they may experience frustration, helplessness, and hopelessness. For this reason, nurses and other mental health professionals often try to avoid treating deinstitutionalized clients and may delegate this responsibility to nonprofessionals.

5. Reality of chronicity. Chronic mental illness is rarely cured. Many nurses and other mental health professionals judge their effectiveness by their ability to cure clients. To satisfy their need for client progress, many mental health professionals may pressure deinstitutionalized clients to alter their behavior, may establish short-term goals that deal only with dysfunction, and may ignore long-term goals that would deal with problems related to chronicity. A power struggle between client and therapist may develop over control or the definition of the therapeutic relationship (Craig and Hyatt, 1978).

6. Reality of deinstitutionalization. The discharge of chronically mentally ill clients into the community may present many problems. Communities may be hostile and resistant. Families may feel overwhelmed. Clients may feel isolated and insecure in their new community surroundings and may wish for the security associated with hospital routine. Aftercare facilities for deinstitutionalized clients may be inadequate.

According to Scheper-Hughes (1982), because the cost of many programs for deinstitutionalized clients are financed by Medicaid monies, the focus of these programs is usually on medical and psychiatric treatment and sheltered-workshop types of employment. Yet what is most often needed by deinstitutionalized clients are such supportive services as adequate housing, provision of nutritious food, and a place to "hang out." Deinstitutionalized clients who spend their days in libraries, public parks, diners, and donut shops are usually viewed either with suspicion or as public nuisances (Evans, 1978).

The need for a nonstressful place to "hang out" has been supported by several large-scale outcome studies of aftercare facilities for deinstitutionalized schizophrenic clients. Those aftercare facilities that offer intensive psychiatric and social work services have poorer results in areas of symptom relief, relapse rates, and development of social skills than those centers that offer many hours of recreational therapy, socializing, and occupational therapy. Intensive insight-oriented and milieu therapies can be overwhelming and anxiety producing for "fragile" schizophrenic clients (May, 1976; Linn et al., 1979).

The need for a place to spend free time and the desire to socialize with people like oneself are common human needs and are found among many deinstitutionalized clients. The despair and isolation experienced by deinstitutionalized clients who have been "dumped" into a community without any support systems contribute to a high suicide rate among deinstitutionalized clients (Scheper-Hughes, 1982). Studies have shown that some deinstitutionalized clients who live in single room occupancy hotels, rooming houses, or apartments with other deinstitutionalized clients have been able to establish and maintain social support systems among themselves (Sokolovsky et al., 1978; Scheper-Hughes, 1981). It is vitally important that community mental health workers facilitate the formation and maintenance of such client support systems.

IMPLICATIONS FOR THE FUTURE

The gestalt of the community mental health movement may need to be altered to include the hospital as an integral part of the community. The hospital and the community mental health agency will need to cooperate with and complement each other. The hospital may need to introduce creative approaches to chronicity and to increase the type and number of services for chronically mentally ill clients. To prevent duplication of services, hospitals and community mental health agencies may need to cooperate in planning programs aimed at problems associated with chronicity. This approach necessitates a recognition of such unique service needs of chronically mentally ill individuals as resocialization, housing, vocational rehabilitation, and employment opportunities.

The goal of reintegrating all mentally ill clients into the community may need to be reexamined. Long-term institutionalization may be indicated for people who are so severely chronically ill that the structure and nursing care available in hospitals are necessary. For people who are mildly or moderately chronically ill, reintegration into the community may be a viable alternative to institutionalization. However, it will be necessary to provide adequate aftercare and supportive services and to involve communities in planning and delivering services. In addition, to obtain continuous information about the needs of chronically mentally ill individuals, outreach programs for deinstitutionalized clients

may need to be developed (Schulberg, 1977; Stein and Test, 1978; Bachrach, 1979).

The education of nurses and other mental health professionals may also need to be reexamined. Clinical specialization and in-service education programs for the care of chronically mentally ill individuals will need to be encouraged. Development of skills that are effective in the treatment of chronically mentally ill clients may lessen the threat to professional esteem that many nurses and other mental health professionals often experience and may help to keep professionals involved in the care of chronically mentally ill clients (Stern and Minkoff, 1979).

Impact of decreased funding

The Community Mental Health Centers Act of 1963 allocated monies, using a "seed money" concept, for community mental health centers. The concept of seed money was based on the belief that community mental health centers should gradually become less dependent on National Institute of Mental Health (NIMH) funding. Federal regulations for non-poverty areas stipulated the following funding formula to finance community mental health centers' operational costs: 80% NIMH funding during the first year of a center's operation; 65% funding during the second year; 40% during the third and fourth years; 35% during the fifth and sixth years; and 25% during the seventh and eighth years. In some instances, NIMH funding was continued through the twelfth year of a community mental health center's operation. Poverty areas received 90% NIMH funding for the first two years of operation, and then the funding was gradually decreased to 30% in the eighth year. NIMH money was to be "matched" by gradually increasing amounts of nonfederal monies. Thus, community mental health centers would progressively become financially independent of Federal grant money and would find other sources of revenue (Weiner et al., 1979).

It was assumed that Medicare, Medicaid, and

other third-party payments would largely replace NIMH funding. Client fees for direct services and local grant monies would presumably augment third-party reimbursements. In actuality, Medicare and Medicaid have refused to reimburse community mental health centers (Weiner et al., 1979). In addition to the lack of Medicare and Medicaid reimbursements, state and local governments have experienced budget cutbacks and have not been ready sources of grant monies (Weiner et al., 1979).

Therefore, although most community mental health centers in their eighth year of operation have been able to find sufficient funding to supplement their dwindling NIMH seed money and have not had to compromise their services, those community mental health centers in their tenth or twelfth years of operation have been experiencing a financial crunch and they have responded by altering their service priorities. The pattern that is emerging is that centers usually increase such readily reimbursable and traditional services as inpatient care and emergency care but sacrifice such less profitable and nontraditional services as partial hospitalization, home visiting, education, and consultation (Naierman et al., 1978; Weiner et al., 1979; Woy et al., 1981). If Federal and state funding continues to be cut, the balanced mix of essential services that these community mental health centers provide will be jeopardized (Woy et al., 1981).

In 1981, the Omnibus Budget Reconciliaton Act incorporated the mental health services support programs formerly administered by NIMH into an alcohol, drug abuse, and mental health (ADM) services block grant. Because states have the option of transferring grant monies between alcohol, drug abuse, and mental health categories, it is likely that 47% of the monies will be spent on mental health care. It is anticipated that the funds appropriated for community mental health services will decrease at least 25% to 34% and possibly more if states withhold Federal block grant money to cover administrative costs. In addition, if Congress accepts President Reagan's New Federalism, it is possible that ADM block grants may not be renewed and that ADM block grants will be an intermediate stage in the eventual phasing out of Federal support for ADM services (Pardes, 1982a, b; Beigel, 1982).

The impact of decreased funding for community mental health centers is already being felt. Community mental health centers are serving fewer acutely seriously ill and chronically ill clients and more of the "worried well," who require shorter periods of treatment. In addition, there has been a decrease in the number of professional community mental health center staff members and an increase in the number of paraprofessional staff members. This change in staffing pattern probably reflects an attempt on the part of administrators to retain as many staff positions as possible, in the face of shrinking budgets, by employing fewer professionally prepared people (Beigel, 1982; Winslow, 1982).

IMPLICATIONS FOR THE FUTURE

Whether the community mental health movement can survive during a period of economic uncertainty is a question that is frequently raised and one that is important both for the public at large and for mental health professionals. Federal budget reductions have already been made in the area of community mental health, and it is unlikely that state and local governments will be able to supplant these funds. Therefore, community mental health centers may decide to turn to private insurance as a means of recouping these monies. However, such third-party reimbursement may necessitate a change in community mental health services from long-term treatment programs (which are not covered by private insurance) for seriously and chronically ill clients to short- and medium-term treatment programs (which are covered by private insurance) for less seriously ill clients. An emphasis on providing services that are reimbursable by private insurance may concomitantly de-emphasize partial hospitalization, consultation, and education

—services that are not covered by private insurance. However, if community mental health centers, in marketing their services to the private sector, seek direct service revenues and service contracts, as well as private insurance reimbursement, then partial hospitalization, consultation, and education services may continue to be part of the comprehensive services offered by community mental health centers (Beigel, 1982; Winslow, 1982).

Several factors favor the continuation and possibly the expansion of the community mental health movement, even during a period of economic uncertainty. One factor is economic. Providing services through which to treat people with psychiatric disorders and disabilities in the community is less costly—in both human and economic terms—than maintaining large inpatient populations in public hospitals. Although it is necessary in times of fiscal restraint to establish priorities in relation to mental health programs, economic considerations favor the community mental health approach. Prevention of disorders is also far less costly in human and economic terms than secondary and tertiary programs.

Another factor that augers well for community mental health programs is the court actions that have upheld the constitutional rights of persons with psychiatric problems. Our legal system is based on precedents established by decisions of the courts. The many lawsuits adjudicated in state courts across the nation and in the United States Supreme Court during the past two decades have established precedents and upheld clients' constitutional rights concerning mental health care, including the right to such care in the least restrictive setting.

The strong commitment to the community mental health movement that has been demonstrated by many mental health professionals and many consumers of health care holds promise for the development of the movement in the future. Participation in social, political, and community action to promote mental health programs and facilities is an important function of nurses and members of the other health professions.

CULTURE AND COMMUNITY MENTAL HEALTH

Cultural background of the community

For health care givers to effectively meet the mental health needs of a given community, they must understand the cultural background of that community. The cultural background of community residents affects their conceptualization of and response to mental health and mental illness. Zola (1966) has identified a "fit" between sociocultural background, value orientations, and coping behaviors. This "fit" may be seen in the way members of different ethnic communities (or different ethnic groups within a particular community) handle anxiety. For example, Italians, who tend to be vocal and demonstrative in times of joy, may deal with their anxiety through open expression of it. This coping behavior not only helps Italians to dissipate their anxiety but also helps them in their interaction with other Italians. The dramatic expression of anxiety helps Italians become simpatico with influential or supportive people and protects them from the envy of others. The Irish, on the other hand, tend to view life as somber, full of suffering, and something to be endured with silence. Irish-Americans thus are apt to handle anxiety-producing events with denial, to ignore discomfort, and to show little emotional affect, and they may endure anxiety-producing events for a longer period of time and with more stoicism than Italians. Italians may be more expressive in verbalizing their anxiety and seeking help than are the Irish. Community mental health nurses whose cultural backgrounds are different from the background of the members of the community that they serve may view the responses of expressive clients as excessive and undignified, or they may overlook the mental health needs of stoic clients. Nurses and other community mental health professionals may become angry with clients who need the services of the community mental health center but who are reluctant to seek help.

A community may comprise various minority groups, which display different and distinct orientations and responses to health and illness. Flaskerud (1982), however, has identified a cluster of characteristics that many minority groups share. Among these characteristics are:

1. A victim orientation. Some minority groups are the victims of institutionalized racism or discrimination, or they may experience the stigma in American society that is attached to illegal alien status or poverty. Many minority groups are segregated in ghettos or on reservations.

2. Communication problems.* A language barrier (both verbal and nonverbal) may exist between minority group members and members of mainstream America. Differences in cultural orientation and life-style may result in differences in perception, interpretation, and response to events and situations.

3. Definition of the family.† Members of many minority group cultures have an extended kin family orientation that encompasses many households and several generations. There usually is a sense of responsibility for one's extended family and an inclusion of extended kin in problem solving. This orientation is different from that of mainstream Americans, who tend to view the nuclear family as "normal" and who engage in problem solving on a nuclear family level or on an individual level.

4. Respect for the elderly. In various minority groups, elderly family members may be looked to for advice, and their advice is usually followed. Elderly family members may also be the authority figures in the family. This is different from the situation in many mainstream American families, which tend to be egalitarian or to devalue elderly family members.

5. Fatalistic orientation. Many minority groups tend to be fatalistic and to believe that their existence and health are at the mercy of the environment and/or God. They may feel that they have little personal control over their fate except to remain in harmony with the environment and/or God. On the other hand, mainstream Americans usually believe that they can control what happens to them—that they are "masters of their fate."

6. Holistic orientation toward health and illness. Many minority groups view health and illness as complex physical, psychological, and spiritual conditions. When they become ill, this holistic orientation is usually reflected in a mixture of somatic, spiritual, and emotional complaints. This is especially true for Hispanic and Asian-Americans (Padilla et al., 1975; Smith Kline Corporation, 1978a). Native healers, rather than traditional community mental health professionals, can relate to this admixture of complaints, conceptualize health and illness in the same way as do minority group clients, and involve extended family members in the therapeutic plan (Woods, 1977; Weaver and Sklar, 1980).

Utilization of community mental health services

Among the various cultural groups in American society, there are differences in attitudes toward accepting mental health care and using community mental health centers. Community residents who are members of the lower socioeconomic class or who are members of minority racial or ethnic groups may be apprehensive or suspicious of a community mental health staff that is predominantly white and middle class. These minority group community members may associate community mental health centers with other mainstream American–controlled institutions, such as the police and the courts, that they have found repressive (Warner, 1977). Also, the previously

---

*Refer to Chapter 8 for a discussion of culture and communication.
†Refer to Chapter 5 for a discussion of culturally influenced family forms.

discussed cluster of shared differences between many minorities and mainstream Americans may further contribute to a sense of alienation of minority group residents from community mental health centers. Sue (1977) reports that 50% of ethnic Americans fail to return for a second session at a community mental health center. This is despite the fact that Black Americans and Native Americans are proportionately overrepresented on community mental health center intake roles. (Asian-Americans and Hispanic-Americans are proportionately underrepresented.)

Even within the same cultural group, attitudinal differences based on sex may exist. In many cultures it is more acceptable for women than for men to express emotional distress and to seek help for their problems. This is a major factor in explaining why, throughout the United States, women not only use community mental health facilities more often than do men but also seek help earlier in the course of their problems than do men (Kerson, 1981).

In addition, a lack of knowledge about the services offered by the community mental health center and the fees it charges may contribute to underuse of the facility. The existence of a sliding scale, based on income, is often unknown to community residents.

Implications for nursing

To better meet the mental health needs of minority group community residents, community mental health nurses need to be knowledgeable about the cultural backgrounds of clients and potential clients and to adapt approaches to their clients' cultural orientations. The following adaptations of approach may increase the use and effectiveness of community mental health center services:

1. Community mental health nurses should collaborate with other community mental health workers and with community leaders in designing comprehensive services that address the problems of poverty, housing, unemployment, discrimination, and social and medical problems.

2. Community mental health nurses should act as client advocates for clients who are using the community mental health center or other agencies.

3. Community mental health nurses should be sure that health center services are readily available to *all* community residents. This may mean locating the center in an ethnic area, lobbying for adequate public transportation, and making home visits to clients who are homebound or who do not have babysitters. It may also mean the scheduling of ample evening and weekend hours and walk-in appointments so that financially needy clients will not have to take off from work to attend the community mental health center (Sue, 1977; Warner, 1977).

4. Community mental health nurses should use family therapy and should encourage other professional team members to use such therapy and, when culturally appropriate, to include extended kin in the family grouping.

5. Community mental health nurses should take a holistic approach to client problems. They should also use crisis-oriented therapy that focuses on clients' presenting problems and that offers concrete goals and results (Flaskerud, 1982).

6. Community mental health nurses, whenever possible, should converse with ethnic clients in their native languages. Otherwise, nurses should urge that indigenous workers be hired to act as translators and culture brokers between community mental health professionals and clients (Lorion, 1974; Sue, 1977; Weaver and Sklar, 1980).

7. Community mental health nurses should facilitate the incorporation of native healers into community mental health centers. Native healing may be used in conjunction with traditional Western therapies, or a system of mutual referrals may be set up between native healers and community mental health workers (Padilla et al., 1975; Campbell and Chang, 1973; Warner, 1977).

8. Community mental health nurses should assess the levels of acculturation of clients.* Nurses should also be aware that, because children often acculturate more rapidly than their parents, intergenerational problems may develop (Pasquali, 1982).

9. Community mental health nurses should work with clergy and pastoral counselors to help clients with the spiritual components of their problems (Padilla et al., 1975; White, 1977).

10. Community mental health nurses and other community mental health professionals should include community leaders and community residents in planning and evaluating community mental health center services. In addition, community members should be encouraged to use the physical facilities of their local community mental health center for community meetings and activities (Campbell and Chang, 1973; Padilla et al., 1975; Ho, 1976; Windle et al., 1979).

11. Community mental health nurses should use culturally acceptable interactional approaches in order to establish rapport with ethnic clients. For example, nurses should be supportive rather than confrontive with Hispanic-American clients (Padilla et al., 1975), set a leisurely pace and ask about physical health with Asian-American clients (Smith Kline Corporation, 1978a), and use self-deprecating humor with Native American clients (Edwards and Edwards, 1980). Nurses should also remember that maintaining eye contact with Asian-American, Black American, Native American, and Hispanic American clients is usually considered rude behavior or an indication of hostility (Scheflen and Scheflen, 1972; Smith Kline Corporation, 1978a, b; Edwards and Edwards, 1980).

Such a culturally comprehensive approach to the delivery of community mental health services to American minority groups has been used in a community mental health center serving a Filipino-American population (Yee and Lee, 1977):

The purpose of the project was primary prevention of disorders that might arise from culture conflict. The community mental health workers viewed the resolution of culture conflict as the "process of achieving balance between opposing cultures." To help the target population, Filipino-American adolescents, mobilize the strengths and resources of their Filipino culture and use these strengths and resources as psychological and supportive mechanisms when interacting with American society, the community mental health workers established the following project goals. Filipino-American adolescents would:

1. *Develop self-awareness and a positive self-image*
2. *Develop value clarification skills (with both Filipino and Western values) so that balance, not blending, between the two cultures might occur*
3. *Develop communication skills that would facilitate interaction with family and peers*
4. *Develop such cultural social support systems as family, church, and peers*

To implement these goals, the community mental health workers collaborated with local high school administrators and teachers. The mental health project was integrated into the school's already existing Filipino bilingual-bicultural course. The community mental health workers functioned as "guest speakers on communication and culture." During ten weekly sessions of fifty minutes each, the following topics were covered: basic communication skills, self-identity, generational values, and self and society. Didactic teaching was limited to ten-minute lectures. Active student participation in the sessions was encouraged with such techniques as role playing, small group discussion, game playing, and role modeling. For example, two Filipino role models, a woman, Maria Clara, and a man, Jose Rizal, personified all that is considered ideal for Filipino women and men. Presentation of such role models facilitated discussion of personality traits that are highly valued by Filipinos

---

*Refer to Chapter 4 for a discussion of acculturation and its assessment.

but that may be at odds with Western values.

Such exercises promoted self-exploration, fostered pride in Filipino heritage, facilitated acceptance of intergenerational and intercultural value differences, and helped Filipino-American adolescents to clarify their place in American society. As a final exercise, adolescents were asked to identify with one of three sociogram sculptures: (1) Anglo life-style, (2) Filipino life-style, (3) Filipino-American life-style. Because in Filipino culture direct statements about one's feelings and attitudes are considered impolite, the focus of self-exploration was always on the students' social and family roles rather than on their "gut reactions."

The community mental health workers included evaluation of the project's effectiveness as an ongoing aspect of the project. After each session, the mental health workers and the teacher and then the mental health workers alone would analyze aspects of the session that had gone well, aspects that had gone poorly, and aspects that could have been handled differently. At the end of the ten weekly sessions, eight high school students were hired and trained to ask open-ended evaluation questions of the student participants. Primarily, the mental health workers wanted to know what the student participants found most helpful and least helpful about the sessions and to elicit suggestions for making the program more valuable. Students, rather than project workers, conducted these evaluations, because the mental health workers recognized that the Asian standard for good manners might influence student participants to answer politely and affirmatively any questions asked by "ousiders" and adults.

At all times, the community mental health workers collaborated with and kept community groups and leaders informed about the project's purpose and progress. Community role models that shared a common cultural background with the students were incorporated into the program. Both English and Tagalog, the national language of the Philippines, were spoken during the sessions.

Such a multifaceted approach, which operates within the cultural parameters of the target population and which demonstrates respect for the community and its strengths, is necessary for an effective community mental health program.

Community mental health nurses, because of their educational and experiential backgrounds, are especially well suited to work with minority group clients. Flaskerud (1982) points out that with their public health background, nurses are comfortable with home visits and with family counseling. In addition, generalist and holistic health perspectives help nurses to understand the view of many minority groups that health and illness are complex physical, psychological, and spiritual conditions. Moreover, their educational background enables nurses to understand and intervene in both health and illness. Each of these attributes emphasizes the capacity of community mental health nurses to understand and to work with the subtle but important relationship between community mental health and culture.

COMMUNITY MENTAL HEALTH NURSING

A community approach to mental health may require an adjustment in the tasks of mental health nurses. Community mental health nurses need to focus on activities in primary mental health care for the community in general and for subcultures within the community. This means that nurses should participate in programs that promote or reinforce the strengths and effective coping behaviors of members of a particular community. Community mental health nurses also should identify high-risk populations and provide services that reduce stress and deal with other psychosocial factors before healthy emotional functioning is disrupted.

Levels of practice

Community mental health nurses engage in a variety of levels of practice that involve assessing, planning, implementing, and evaluating mental health services for communities of people. Nurses function in organizational, advisory, advocacy, direct service, and consultative positions in community mental health agencies. The American Nurses' Association Division on Psychiatric and Mental Health Nursing Practice (1982) has identified *process criteria* (criteria focusing on nursing activities) and *outcome criteria* (criteria focusing on observable or measurable end results) for the practice of community mental health nursing. Process criteria specify that:

1. Nurses use their knowledge of systems theory and community and group dynamics in the analysis of community systems.
2. Nurses are cognizant of the influence of sociopolitical issues on community mental health problems.
3. Nurses encourage the participation of community members in the assessment and development of programs to address the mental health needs of the community.
4. Nurses are activists in articulating community health needs to such appropriate individuals and groups as legislators and regional and state planning boards.
5. Nurses engage in didactic and experiential teaching programs that meet the community's mental health needs.
6. Nurses serve as consultants in designing and implementing community mental health programs.
7. Nurses explain available mental health programs to members of the community.
8. Nurses collaborate with health team professionals and with community members in developing, implementing, and evaluating mental health programs.
9. Nurses identify populations at risk in the community and delineate areas of scarcity in community services.
10. Nurses assess the strengths and coping behaviors of individuals, families, and the community in order to promote, maintain, and improve their levels of mental health.
11. Nurses are knowledgeable about, refer cli-

ents to, and facilitate the use of appropriate community resources.
12. Nurses collaborate with inter-agency personnel to facilitate continuity of care for consumers of agency services.

Outcome criteria specify that:

1. The activities of nurses in primary, secondary, and tertiary mental health care are documented.
2. Mental health services that address the needs of the community are provided.
3. Nurses assume leadership roles in voluntary and governmental community health groups.

Qualities of community mental health nurses

Whether nurses in community mental health agencies are functioning as staff nurses prepared at the baccalaureate degree level or as clinical specialists prepared at the master's or doctoral degree level, they need to have a sound understanding of the unique contributions of nurses to the community mental health team. They also need high degrees of assertiveness and flexibility. Without these qualities, community mental health nurses may find that they are losing their identities in the role blurring that is common among community mental health professionals or that they are jeopardizing their effectiveness by being nonassertive in interdisciplinary altercations and exploration of roles. Topf and Byers (1972), in their review of community mental health literature, found a high degree of role fusion or job co-occurrence among psychiatrists, psychologists, social workers, and nurses. These members of the multidisciplinary community mental health team all engage in individual, group, and family therapy; supervision, education, and consultation; program development and evaluation; administration; research; and aftercare. However, home visiting and liaison activities are usually viewed as a contribution of nurses only.

Community mental health nurses also need to be clinically competent, knowledgeable about change theory, community organization, and the politics of institutions, and innovative, so that they can define their roles, demonstrate to colleagues the contributions nurses can make to community mental health programs, develop their own case loads, and engage in community outreach and consumer advocacy programs (Ujhely, 1972; Clark, 1978).* In addition, community mental health nurses often are responsible for training community paraprofessionals or indigenous community workers. During these training sessions, nurses sometimes find that they must reexamine their own perceptions, value systems, purposes, and functions (Richards, 1972).

Thus, community mental health nurses need to be knowledgeable, assertive, flexible, and innovative in order to achieve their goals and to maximize their effectiveness in planning and delivering mental health care to communities.

Community assessment

To effectively function as community mental health nurses, nurses need to be aware of the strengths, deficits, and needs of the community they are serving. Lancaster (1980) has identified three types of information that nurses need to know about the community:

1. Community attitudes. The attitudes of health professionals, special interest groups (for example, neighborhood associations or parents of emotionally disturbed children), and community residents toward mental health needs and services should be elicited. This process necessitates ongoing dialogue between consumers, other health care providers in the community, and community mental health nurses.
2. Community strengths and limitations. The availability of trained mental health workers, such as psychiatric nurses, social workers, and psychologists, and of nonpsychiatric

health professionals, such as community health nurses, physicians, clergymen, and teachers, should be determined. In addition, such physical resources as already functioning mental health clinics, halfway houses, hospitals, and nursing homes should be identified and their accessability to and use by the community evaluated. Finally, any overlapping of services or fragmentation of services that are already available to the community should be identified.
3. Target population. The geographic catchment area should be delineated. The size of the population in need of mental health services (currently and potentially needy clients) should also be determined, and then this population should be segmented according to specific characteristics (for example, ethnicity, social class, religious beliefs). Finally, the needs, problems, attitudes, and perceptions of the target population, as well as their desire for change and the direction in which they want that change to occur, should be determined.

The following community assessment guide* has been designed to help nurses assess communities and to identify areas for community intervention:

1. Physical description of the community: Geographic parameters of the community; territorial distribution patterns (zones of business and residence; shopping, cultural, recreational, and health facilities; areas of overpopulation and underpopulation; multiple-family dwellings and single-family dwellings; inter-ethnic neighborhoods or ethnic enclaves)
2. Target population: Age, sex, and types of family and/or household groupings; ethnic composition of the community (ethnic groups represented; degree of acculturation and assimilation; degree of interaction among ethnic groups); socioeconomic levels

---

*Refer to Chapter 10 for further discussion of the role of the nurse and the mental health team.

*Sources consulted in the preparation of this assessment guide include Leighton (1959), Clark (1978), Lancaster (1980), and Robinson (1978).

of the population (income levels represented; proportion of population in each income level; occupational groups represented; educational levels represented); spiritual orientations of the population (beliefs and rituals concerning birth, illness, and death; nature of belief in a supernatural being and/or supernormal energy; conceptualization about the quality of life and quality of death); health status of the population (support systems; strengths; prevalence of physical and mental disorders; acculturative pressures; minority status stressors)

3. Community resources: Existence of schools, health facilities, shopping areas, recreational facilities, self-help or support groups, and neighborhood action groups; availability of these resources (accessible by public transportation or by walking; open on week-ends and in the evening); degree of satisfaction of community residents with community resources (perceived fit between community needs and services; overlap of services; fragmentation of services; cultural barriers or facilitators to use of community resources such as personnel who speak the language of minority group consumers)

4. Community attitudes about deviance: Attitudes about mental illness (fear mentally ill people; include mentally ill relatives and friends in their social networks); attitudes about social deviance* (reject people who have a history of social deviance; try to emulate social deviants); attitudes about treatment facilities for deviants (feelings about locating treatment facilities within the community; prevailing view that deviants should be treated/should be punished)

5. Community functioning: Decision-making patterns (decisions are based on adequate/inadequate information; are made by default; are arrived at by community consensus); communication patterns (patterns reflect ste-

reotyping of or distance maneuvers between groups; nature of formal and informal communication channels; efficiency or fragmentation of communication patterns); leadership patterns (identifiable community leaders; leadership shifts according to the situation at hand; leadership is concentrated among a few groups; leadership is distributed throughout the community; degree of trust between community leaders and community residents); power patterns (location of power in the community; perception of how power is used)

6. Community integration: Incidence of "broken" homes (for example, dysfunctional families); incidence of violent, criminal, or delinquent behavior; adequacy and use of recreational facilities; adequacy of associations (degree to which people group around such common interests as religion, work, or recreation; cohesiveness of existing groups); presence of isolation factors (poor transportation systems; absence of telephones; poor interpersonal relationships)

7. Community attitudes toward change: Perception of change (views about how customs, life-styles, and institutions will be affected by change; past experiences with change); forces facilitating or inhibiting change (relationship between change agents and the community; degree of awareness of need for change; degree of anticipated personal suffering or personal benefit from change; degree of involvement of community residents in planning for change; previous degree of openness of the community to change)

8. Community health care patterns: Prevalent definition(s) associated with specific community groups of health and illness; ideas concerning causes of illness (for example, evil spirits; punishment for sins; stress); ideas concerning treatment of illness; people consulted when ill (family member; native healing specialist; physician; pharmacist) and the order in which they are consulted

*Refer to Chapter 17 for a discussion of social deviance.

A comprehensive community assessment will provide community mental health nurses with the information necessary for identifying community mental health problems and for planning community mental health services that will address those problems. Lancaster (1980) lists five essential aspects of effective community mental health planning: (1) awareness that uncoordinated inter-agency planning tends to produce fragmented services or duplication of services; (2) recognition of the importance of involving the community in or obtaining community support for plans; (3) ability to define the range of essential services that will be provided to the community; (4) collaboration between mental health professionals and community residents; and (5) awareness of the importance of a systems approach to planning.

CHAPTER SUMMARY

The community mental health concept embraces an interacting system of health, welfare, and social services oriented toward meeting the mental health needs of a community. Programs are organized to provide mental health services for populations in geographically defined communities termed catchment areas. Each catchment area may have a population of from 75,000 to 200,000 people. Programs to meet community needs are, ideally, developed through a cooperative effort between health and social agencies, community organizations, and residents of the community served.

Although many factors influenced the development of the community mental health movement, the Community Mental Health Centers Act, passed by Congress in 1963, was a major factor in the implementation of mental health programs on a national basis. The act provided some federal funding for mental health care and established principles and guidelines to meet comprehensive mental health needs of residents in their local communities. Subsequent legislative actions further

defined mental health care and upheld the constitutional rights of persons who have psychiatric disorders.

Although it continues to be an evolving process, the community mental health movement has significantly changed the treatment of mentally retarded persons and persons with psychiatric disorders. Before the community mental health movement, mental health care had usually been available only in public hospitals, where long-term hospitalization was often a major form of treatment.

The community mental health concept uses a public health approach to meeting mental health needs. This approach involves primary, secondary, and tertiary prevention. Primary prevention seeks to reduce the incidence of psychiatric disorders, secondary prevention seeks to reduce the disability rate through early and effective intervention, and tertiary prevention seeks to prevent or reduce the severity or duration of long-term disability.

The characteristics of agencies providing mental health services and the ways in which mental health teams function vary from one agency to another and according to the philosophies and professional orientations of health team members. The mental health services offered also vary according to the priorities established by a particular community.

SENSITIVITY-AWARENESS EXERCISES

The purposes of the following exercises are to:
- Develop awareness about your own attitudes and the attitudes of others toward mental health care and community mental health facilities
- Develop knowledge about the functioning and use of a local community mental health center
- Develop insight into the strengths, deficits, and needs of your community and/or your client's community
- Develop an ecosystem perspective to community mental health

1. Using the community assessment guide in this chapter, assess your community and/or your client's com-

munity. From the data obtained from your assessment, identify and describe:
   a. Community attitudes about community mental mental health needs and services
   b. Community strengths and limitations (physical, cultural, technological, and social)
   c. Size and composition of the target population. Be sure to include the ethnic and socioeconomic characteristics of the target population, as well as health status and attitudes and perceptions about mental health and mental health care.
   d. Implications for primary, secondary and tertiary intervention
2. Using the community assessment guide in this chapter, assess the functioning and integration of your community and/or your client's community. Identify and describe:
   a. Decision-making patterns
   b. Communication patterns
   c. Leadership patterns
   d. Power patterns
   e. Incidence of "broken" homes
   f. Incidence of violent, criminal, and/or delinquent behavior
   g. Adequacy and use of recreational facilities
   h. Adequacy of associations
   i. Isolation factors
3. Interview neighbors, health professionals, other professionals (for example, teachers, clergy) and small business owners. What are their attitudes about mental illness? About social deviance? About types of treatment and aftercare services that should be offered? About the location of treatment and/or aftercare facilities in their own community?
4. Visit a community mental health center and assess the following:
   a. Availability to clients (for example, intake procedures, hours open, length of waiting list, accessibility by public transportation or walking, fee scale)
   b. Staff-client interaction (for example, degree of rapport between staff and clients, incorporation of native healers or indigenous workers into the health team, use of client's native language)
   c. Treatment services (for example "fit" between clients' cultural orientations and therapeutic modalities, use of traditional versus nontraditional treatment modalities, types of essential and recommended services)

REFERENCES

American Nurses' Association Division on Psychiatric and Mental Health Nursing
   1982 Standards of Psychiatric and Mental Health Nursing Practice. Kansas City: American Nurses' Association.
Bachrach, L.L.
   1979 "Planning mental health services for chronic patients." Hospital and Community Psychiatry 30(6):387-393.
Beard, M.T., C.T. Enelon, and J.G. Owens
   1978 "Activity therapy as a reconstructive plan on the social competence of chronic hospitalized patients." Journal of Psychiatric Nursing and Mental Health Services 16(2):33-41.
Biegel, A.
   1982 "Community mental health centers: a look ahead." Hospital and Community Psychiatry 33(9):741-745.
Borus, J.F.
   1978 "Issues critical to the survival of community mental health." American Journal of Psychiatry 135(9):1029-1035.
Campbell, T., and B. Chang
   1973 "Health care of the Chinese in America." Nursing Outlook 21(4):245-249.
Caplan, G.
   1964 Principles of Preventive Psychiatry. New York: Basic Books, Inc.
   1974 Supportive Systems and Community Mental Health: Lectures on Concept Development. New York: Behavioral Publications.
Christmas, J.J.
   1979 "The many faces of psychiatry—innovation, initiative or inertia." Journal of Psychiatric Treatment and Evaluation 1(1):11-15.
Clark, C.C.
   1978 Mental Health Aspects of Community Health Nursing. New York: McGraw-Hill Book Co.
Craig, A.E., and B.A. Hyatt
   1978 "Chronicity in mental illness: a theory on the role of change." Perspectives in Psychiatric Care 16(3):139-144.
Edwards, E.D., and M.E. Edwards
   1980 "American Indians: working with individuals and groups." Social Casework 61(8):498-506.
Evans, D.M.
   1978 "Alienation, mental illness and the partitioning of space." Antipode 10(1):13-23.
Flaskerud, J.H.
   1982 "Community mental health nursing: its unique role in the delivery of services to ethnic minorities." Perspectives in Psychiatric Care 20(1):37-43.
Greenberg, E.M.
   1974 "The social breakdown syndrome and its prevention." In American Handbook of Psychiatry (ed. 2), vol. 2. G. Caplan (ed.). S. Arieti (ed.-in-chief). New York: Basic Books, Inc., Publishers.

Greenblat, M.
1977 "Introduction to psychiatry and the third revolution." Psychiatric Annals 7(10):7-9.

Ho, M.K.
1976 "Social work with Asian Americans." Social Casework 57(3):195-201.

Hume, P.B.
1974 "Principles of community mental health practice." In American Handbook of Psychiatry (ed. 2), vol. 2. G. Caplan (ed.). S. Arieti (ed.-in-chief). New York: Basic Books, Inc.

Joint Commission on Mental Health and Mental Illness
1961 Action for Mental Health: A Program for Meeting the National Emergency. New York: Basic Books, Inc.

Kelly, J.G.
1966 "Ecological constraints on mental health services." American Psychologist 21:535-539.

Kerson, T.S.
1981 "The impact of ethnicity on community mental health." Journal of Nursing Education 20(3):32-38.

Lancaster, J.
1980 Community Mental Health Nursing: An Ecological Perspective. St. Louis: The C.V. Mosby Co.

Leighton, A.H.
1959 My Name Is Legion. New York: Basic Books, Inc.

Levenson, A.I.
1974 "A review of the Federal community mental health centers programs." In American Handbook of Psychiatry (ed. 2), vol. 2. G. Caplan (ed.). S. Arieti (ed.-in-chief). New York: Basic Books, Inc.

Linn, M.W., E.M. Caffey, C.J. Klett, G.E. Hogarty, and H.R. Lamb
1979 "Day treatment and psychotropic drugs in the aftercare of schizophrenic clients." Archives of General Psychiatry 36:1055-1066.

Lorion, R.P.
1974 "Patient and therapist variables in the treatment of low income patients." Psychological Bulletin 81(6):344-354.

Macht, L.B.
1978 "Community psychiatry." In Harvard Guide to Modern Psychiatry. A.M. Nicholi, Jr. (ed.). Cambridge: Belknap Press of Harvard University Press.

May, P.R.A.
1976 "When, what and why? Psychopharmacotherapy and other treatments in schizophrenia." Comprehensive Psychiatry 17(6):683-693.

Naierman, N., B. Haskins, and G. Robinson
1978 Community Mental Health Centers—A Decade Later. Cambridge: ABT Associates.

O'Connor, W.
1977 "Ecosystems theory and clinical mental health." Psychiatric Annals 7:63-77.

Padilla, A.M., R.A. Ruiz, and R. Alvarez
1975 "Community mental health services for the Spanish-speaking surnamed population." American Psychologist 30(9):892-904.

Pardes, H.
1982a "Q & A." Hospital and Community Psychiatry 33(5): 345.
1982b "NIMN report." Hospital and Community Psychiatry 33(7):525-526.

Pasquali, E.A.
1982 Assimilation and Acculturation of Cubans on Long Island. Ph.D. dissertation, State University of New York at Stony Brook.

Rapaport, J.
1977 Community Psychology: Values, Research and Action. New York: Holt, Rinehart & Winston, Inc.

Report of the Task Panel on Deinstitutionalization, Rehabilitation, and Long-Term Care
1978 Task Panel Reports Submitted to the President's Commission on Mental Health, vol. 2. Washington, D.C.: U.S. Government Printing Office.

Report to the President of the President's Commission on Mental Health
1978 Washington, D.C.: U.S. Government Printing Office.

Richards, H.
1972 "Implications for nursing in the training of paraprofessional workers in the community mental health setting." In The Nurse in Community Mental Health. E.P. Lewis and M.H. Browning (eds.). New York: The American Journal of Nursing Co.

Robinson, K.M.
1978 "Working with a community action group." Journal of Psychiatric Nursing and Mental Health Services 16(8): 38-42.

Scheflen, A.E., and A. Scheflen
1972 Body Language and Social Order: Communication as Behavioral Control. Englewood Cliffs, N.J.: Prentice-Hall, Inc.

Scheper-Hughes, N.
1981 "Dilemmas in deinstitutionalization." Journal of Operational Psychiatry 12(2):90-99.
1982 "A proposal for the aftercare of chronic psychiatric patients." Medical Anthropology Quarterly 14(2):3-15.

Schulberg, H.C.
1969 "Community mental health: Fact or fiction?" Canada's Mental Health Supplement, No. 63. Ottawa: Department of National Health and Welfare.
1977 "Community mental health and human services." Community Mental Health Review 2(6):1-9.

Smith Kline Corporation
1978a Cultural Issues in Contemporary Psychiatry: The Asian Pacific American. Continuing Education Services (audiotape).
1978b Cultural Issues in Contemporary Psychiatry: The Hispanic American. Continuing Education Services (audiotape).

Sokolovsky, J., C. Cohen, D. Berger, and J. Geiger
1978 "Personal networks of ex-mental patients in a Manhattan SRO hotel." Human Organization 37(1):5-15.

Stein, L.I., and M.A. Test
1978 "An alternative to mental hospital treatment." In Alternatives to Mental Hospital Treatment. L.I. Stein and M.A. Test (eds.). New York: Plenum Publishing Corp.

Stern, R., and K. Minkoff
1979 "Paradoxes in programming for chronic patients in a community clinic." Hospital and Community Psychiatry 30(9):613-617.

Stickney, S.
1974 "Wyatt vs. Stickney: the right to treatment." Psychiatric Annals 4(8):32-45.

Stone, A.
1975 "The right to treatment." American Journal of Psychiatry 132(11):1125-1134.

Sue, S.
1977 "Community mental health services to minority groups." American Psychologist 32:616-624.

Topf, M., and R.G. Byers
1972 "Role fusion on the community mental health multidisciplinary team." In The Nurse in Community Mental Health. E.P. Lewis and M.H. Browning (eds.). New York: The American Journal of Nursing Co.

Ujhely, G.B.
1972 "The nurse in community psychiatry." In The Nurse in Community Mental Health. E.P. Lewis and M.H. Browning (eds.). New York: The American Journal of Nursing Co.

Warner, R.
1977 "Witchcraft and soul loss: implications for community psychiatry." Hospital and Community Psychiatry 28(9):686-690.

Weaver, C., and D. Sklar
1980 "Diagnostic dilemmas and cultural diversity in emergency rooms." Western Journal of Medicine 133(4): 356-366.

Weiner, R.S., J.R. Woy, S.S. Sharfstein, and R.D. Bass
1979 "Community mental health centers and the 'seed money' concept: effects of terminating federal funds." Community Mental Journal 15(2):129-138.

White, E.H.
1977 "Giving health care to minority patients." Nursing Clinics of North America 12(1):27-40.

Wilkinson, C.B., and W. O'Connor
1977 "Introduction and overview." Psychiatric Annals 7:10-15.

Windle, C., J. Neal, and H.K. Zinn
1979 "Stimulating equity of services to nonwhites in community mental health centers." Community Mental Health Journal 15(2):155-168.

Winslow, W.W.
1982 "Changing trends in CHMCs: keys to survival in the eighties." Hospital and Community Psychiatry 33(4): 273-277.

Woods, C.M.
1977 "Alternative curing strategies in a changing medical situation." Medical Anthropology 1(3):26-54.

Woy, J.R., D.B. Wasserman, and R. Weiner-Pomerantz
1981 "Community mental health centers: movement away from the model?" Community Mental Health Journal 17(4):265-276.

Yee, T.T., and R.H. Lee
1977 "Based on cultural strengths, a school primary prevention program for Asian-American youth." Community Mental Health Journal 13(3):239-248.

Zola, K.
1966 "Culture and symptoms—an analysis of patients' presenting complaints. American Sociological Review 31: 615-630.

ANNOTATED SUGGESTED READINGS

Falskerud, J.H.
1982 "Community mental health nursing: its unique role in the delivery of services to ethnic minorities." Perspectives in Psychiatric Care 20(1):37-43.
This article, while not overlooking diversity among ethnic groups, identifies some of the shared characteristics of ethnic groups. These shared characteristics distinguish ethnic group members from the mainstream American therapists who often predominantly staff community mental health centers. From this perspective, the author draws implications for culture-based intervention and identifies the unique qualities that nurses bring to community mental health.

Lancaster, J.
1980 Community Mental Health Nursing: An Ecological Perspective. St. Louis: The C.V. Mosby Co.
This recent work provides a good theoretical background in community mental health. A holistic view of the individual interacting dynamically with his or her environment is the approach used by the author. The book also provides a preventive approach to meeting mental health needs. There is some discussion of particular mental health problems, as well as the problems of various age groups, persons who abuse drugs or other substances, and other persons at risk.

Robinson, K.M.
1978 "Working with a community action group." Journal of Psychiatric Nursing and Mental Health Services 16(8): 38.
This article provides a theoretical framework and a process for assessing the functioning of a community action group. Using systems theory and group dynamics, the author provides a step-by-step description of a community action group and the role of professional nurses serving in a consultant capacity to the group. The steps and principles outlined can be used for assessing and promoting positive change in any group.

UNIT IV

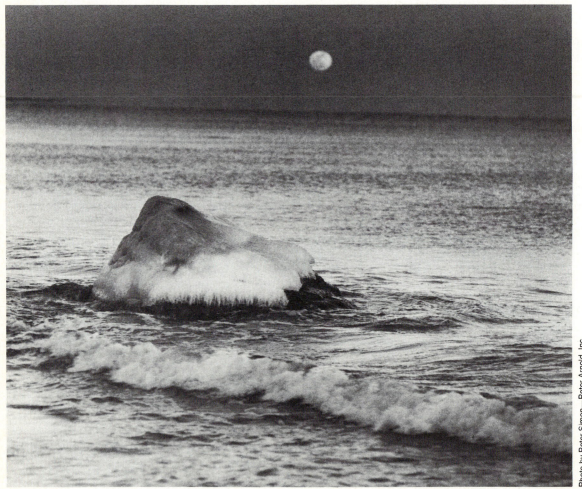

Client behavior and
the nursing practice

The fourth section of this book focuses on major psychogenic and psychiatric conditions of children, adolescents, and adults. Although each chapter looks at the development and/or implications of particular disorders throughout the life cycle, Chapter 15 explores in depth and within a family context selected disorders that are specific to children and adolescents.

Within a holistic health framework, patterns of coping with stress are discussed. Various types of maladaptive behavior are viewed as ways of coping with stress. The DSM-III categories associated with specific maladaptive behavior patterns are given.

The patterns of coping with stress that are discussed in these chapters range across the mental health continuum. The earlier chapters deal with conditions that involve relatively little interference with psychosocial adaptation, and the later chapters deal with conditions in which there may be great interference with psychosocial adaptation.

Each chapter provides a theoretical foundation for understanding client experiences and for using the nursing process. Treatment modalities are discussed in relation to particular mental health problems. In addition, each problem is explored in terms of primary, secondary, and tertiary prevention.

CHAPTER 15

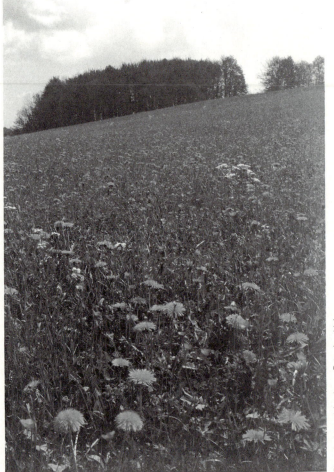

Photo by Löwenlahnwiese—Peter Arnold, Inc.

Coping with the conflicts and stressors of childhood and adolescence

CHAPTER FOCUS

The Report of the Joint Commission on Mental Health of Children (1969) identified several factors that act as precipitants for the development of emotional disorders; these factors include faulty life experiences, relational difficulties between parent and child; adjustment reactions to school and social experiences; internalized conflicts; and adjustment difficulties related to physical handicaps and severe ego dysfunction. More than 80% of emotionally disturbed children fall into the first two categories—life experiences and relational difficulties. Nurses in school health, community health, family practice, and camp settings, in addition to nurses in well-child clinics, should be able to identify these potential factors and intervene at a primary level. Nurses can act as educators and as support and resource systems for the family within which a child exists. Thus, the focal point of nursing assessment and intervention is twofold: assisting the child to modify unhealthy behaviors and enabling the family to develop more effective means of communication and more effective parenting skills.

This chapter begins with descriptions of selected disorders of childhood and adolescence; primary characteristics of each are discussed to provide guidelines for nursing assessment. Specific underlying etiologies are also discussed. Emphasis is placed on a holistic approach to the understanding of childhood and adolescent disorders and subsequent interventions. The authors stress the importance of an assessment that reflects a multifactorial approach to the development of these disorders.

Modalities of treatment reflect a varied approach as well. Individual therapy, milieu therapy, groups for both parents and children, and family therapy are explored in depth. Somatic therapy, including psychopharmacology and electroconvulsive therapy, is presented as it relates specifically to children and adolescents.

The final section of the chapter covers the nursing process. Primary prevention focuses on screening for risk—identifying children and families who may be in potential difficulty as a result of poor environmental factors, a lack of knowledge regarding parenting, or a lack of appropriate problem-solving skills. Secondary prevention is explored in light of the increased emphasis on case finding and early diagnosis. Specific diagnoses are presented relative to the disorders of childhood and adolescence discussed in the earlier section. Family diagnoses are also discussed. Long- and short-term goals and nursing strategies are specifically delineated for each diagnosis. General outcome criteria are included at the conclusion of the discussion of secondary prevention. Tertiary prevention involves the use of therapeutic measures directed toward ensuring the optimum level of functioning in cases where there is chronic dysfunction. Residential placement is included in the discussion of tertiary prevention.

The purpose of this chapter is to give nurses a greater understanding of emotional disorders of childhood and adolescence, as well as of specific interventive techniques. The emphasis on a holistic approach provides guidelines that facilitate nurses' comprehensive assessment and intervention with children and adolescents and with their families.

HISTORICAL PERSPECTIVES

In 1972, Fagin cited the findings of the Report of the Joint Commission on the Mental Health of Children (1969) that 1,400,000 persons under the age of 18 needed professional psychiatric help. At that time a third were receiving some form of assistance from mental health facilities, while 3% were being treated in residential living centers. In 1978, the President's Commission on Mental Health supported the findings noted by Fagin. The Joint Commission further delineated the problems that seemed to act as precipitants for the development of emotional disorders. These are:

1. Faulty life experiences and training
2. Surface conflicts between children and parents, such as relational difficulties among siblings and adjustment difficulties in the areas of school, social relations, and sexuality
3. Internalized conflicts of a deeper nature that lead to neurotic responses
4. Adjustment difficulties related to physical disorders and handicaps
5. Adjustment difficulties related to severe mental disorders such as psychotic behaviors and mental retardation.

The Joint Commission noted that approximately 80% of the children who need treatment fall into the first two problem areas. These children are able to live within the context of their families and the larger environment. Treatment, when appropriate, can be provided for both child and family on an outpatient basis. Often school nurses, community health nurses, or family nurse practitioners are able to identify troublesome areas and provide education, support, or referral to mental health professionals when it is necessary. Tertiary care is most appropriate for the remaining 20% of the identified population. In some instances, as with severe psychosis, institutionalization and close supervision are necessary.

Since a child exists within the context of his or

her family, the provision of services has been influenced by the family system. Children, particularly young children, are not often encouraged to seek out mental health services, nor are they often able to seek out such services. Parental attitudes toward mental health professionals and their practice are often negative. Yet parental expectations, previous experiences within parents' own families of origin, and parents' lack of clear communication patterns serve as the basis for the development of emotional and mental disorders. It is important to identify high-risk families, to connect members of these families with appropriate resources, and to assist parents in becoming more effective.

One difficulty in the provision of services relates to family members' lack of awareness of their own problems. Often parents themselves do not realize that they have questions regarding parenting. For example, parents may not be aware that consistency is important in a relationship with a child. It must be emphasized also that children under the age of three do not often come to the attention of those who provide mental health services. It becomes critical for nurses in well-baby clinics and other health facilities, such as health maintenance organizations (HMOs) and hospital emergency rooms, to be able to assess accurately the developmental status and emotional response of a child, as well as the parent-child interaction. If undetected, emotional difficulties may establish maladaptive patterns of behavior, leading in turn to future adjustment difficulties. It was noted by the Joint Commission that in childhood the foundations in all areas of development, including physical, social, emotional, and intellectual, are laid for the ensuing years. Negative experiences learned in the parents' families of origin can be played out in the current family system, leaving open the possibility of generating similar maladaptive methods of coping. Supportive-educative services are not uniformly offered to parents and families; it is only when children begin to display inappropriate behaviors that resources are made available.

Other factors that impact on provision of services include socioeconomic background, cultural and religious values, and attitudes toward mental health services (see Chapter 14 for further discussion of attitudes toward mental health services). Socioeconomic status has a profound influence on families' abilities to use mental health services. There are too few programs in which fees are based on a sliding scale or in which reduced fees available for parents in lower economic brackets. Often it is this population that is most in need of services, yet services are too costly or federally sponsored programs such as Medicaid do not cover psychiatric expenses.

Cultural and religious values not only may influence familial child-rearing practices but also may dictate certain norms, values, and expectations that may conflict with societal norms and expectations. Mental health services and the providers of services may be viewed with apprehension. The family may draw together to protect a child who is experiencing difficulty rather than expose the family to the scrutiny and intervention of outsiders. Cultural and religious values do have a significant influence on children, yet one needs to remember that each child is unique and needs an environment in which expectations of behavior and communication are clear.

ROLE OF THE NURSE

Statistics indicate that a large number of children and youth are in need of some level of psychosocial intervention. Nurses, as the largest group of health care providers, potentially possess assessment skills and the ability to design and implement relevant plans of care for this population. Furthermore, nurses have limitless opportunities for contact with children and families. However, Fagin (1972) states that few nursing students are exposed to child psychiatric concepts in their undergraduate curricula. Some mental health concepts relating to childhood and adolescence may be incorporated into the pediatrics component, yet insufficient attention is directed toward this area because of the large amount of biophysiological information currently taught relative to health care of children. Therefore it can be said that nurses currently complete their undergraduate studies with little or no knowledge of child and adolescent psychiatric problems and interventions. With the current focus of nursing assessment and intervention directed toward the concept of family, it would seem logical to discuss issues of the child and adolescent within the context of the family system.

Intervention with children who are experiencing difficulty coping with life situations or with those who display psychotic behaviors can be an emotionally upsetting experience for nurses. Feelings of vulnerability are aroused in the nurse. A sense of overwhelming inadequacy to deal with the child and the other members of the family may also be felt by the nurse when confronted with the extensive patterns of behavior and the wide variety of developmental tasks to be accomplished throughout childhood and adolescence. These factors often seem incomprehensible to health practitioners, as well as to families who are moving through those phases.

The primary role of the nurse is to understand the child within the context of the family. Before they can accomplish this, nurses must be aware of their own values and beliefs regarding family: their roles within their own families, expectations of behavior, how feelings are expressed, what the lines of communication are. Nurses may perceive other families as behaving inappropriately in terms of the nurses' own values and experiences within their own family systems. A family that is already experiencing distress can detect feelings of ambivalence or a blaming attitude on the part of a nurse, which immediately places a barrier between nurse and family. The family then takes a defensive position that does not allow open communication to occur. The child's maladaptive behavior may then escalate as he or she responds to the increased anxiety level within the family system. Nurses should be aware that feelings of guilt and failure in the parental dyad can be quickly reinforced by nurses' thoughtless comments.

Nurses may become easily frustrated with parents who do not promptly change their patterns of child-rearing when it has been demonstrated that these behaviors may be less effective than others. It is difficult to change lifelong patterns—even more so when disequilibrium in the family is already occurring. Individuals tend to revert back to old behavior patterns or become immobilized in the face of escalating anxiety. Even though parents may understand intellectually the need for more open communication or for changing a maladaptive manner of responding, it is much more difficult to operationalize those changes and to become emotionally committed to them. Parents bring their own experiences from childhood, which influence their behaviors as parents as well as their expectations of their children. In some situations parents do not communicate their expectations to one another, creating an ambiguous situation for the child.

Nurses need to feel comfortable with their own feelings and with their expectations in regard to roles in the family system. After accomplishing these objectives, a nurse can create an atmosphere within which the members of a family can discuss alternative coping strategies and can explore their feelings and gain support from one another and from the nurse, thus emerging as a more healthy unit in a holistic sense.

It must be noted that adults are prepared for the jobs or careers they intend to pursue; however, they undergo little or no preparation for their most critical task—parenting the next generation. With that thought in mind, nurses should believe that parents are most likely doing the best they know how, based on their own experiences and their current physical, social, economic, emotional, educational, and religious resources. It is part of nursing to support the parental role when appropriate—to be empathic and to set realistic goals for the family as a whole unit and for the child who is demonstrating maladaptive methods of coping.

DISORDERS OF CHILDHOOD

It is important to note here that disorders should be assessed in relationship to the prescribed developmental tasks as stated by Piaget and Erikson (see Chapter 6). Nurses need to be cognizant of children's senses of self and their relationships to others, their perceptions of body image, and their ability to perform age-appropriate intellectual functions. Various tools can be used to assess these areas; they will be discussed later in this chapter, in the section on the nursing process. There are many disorders of childhood; several have been selected and will be discussed in depth.

Lewis (1979) notes that differential diagnosis in children is often difficult. Certain traits may be classified into a "syndrome," which implies a specific etiology, a specific treatment, and a specific prognosis. For example, short attention span and hyperactivity have been associated with minimal brain damage, yet there is no proof that this single diagnosis represents a factual assessment and an appropriate basis for intervention in regard to these two identifiable behaviors. DSM-III sought to correct this "clustering" of behaviors into one category by identifying specific disorders: attention deficit; conduct disorder; anxiety disorders; reactive attachment disorder; eating disorders; disorders with physical manifestations; developmental disorders; and pervasive developmental disorders.

Attention deficits

Attention deficit disorders may be seen either with or without hyperactivity. The term is more descriptive than qualitative in nature. Lewis (1979) suggests that short attention span may be due to fatiguability, which may result from the amount of time it takes the child to process information or from the amount of information impacting upon the child's perceptual system at any given time. He also states that this type of behavior may be worse at the end of the day, perhaps resulting from anxiety. Further signs of attention deficit disorders include clumsiness, confusion of right and left and front and back, lack of symmetry of five finger-hand movements, and intellectual and memory faults. Children who are hyperactive are described as restless, impulsive, and quarrelsome. Their be-

havior often distracts others in the same environment and makes it impossible for themselves or others to maintain task orientation and to complete objectives. The inability to complete assignments or follow directions may lead a child to cope in a maladaptive manner by withdrawing, being negativistic, playing the class clown, or denying any difficulty exists. It is important for nurses to recognize that whatever the behavior, children are labeled in a negative or derisive manner, which then acts as a feedback mechanism to generate further socially unacceptable behavior.

Conduct disorders

Children who have assaultive tendencies, who start fights for no apparent reason, who are cruel to animals and others, and who are malicious with intent are categorized as having unsocialized aggressive reactions. Kalb (1979) suggests that these children experience little or no guilt when committing these deeds, suggesting that a healthy superego development has not taken place. Often parents are rejecting in nature and do not provide the continuous, consistent relationship necessary for a child to develop a strong identity and intimate relationships with others later in life.

Socialized aggressive children are those children who participate in a group or groups for the purpose of engaging in antisocial behavior such as stealing, truancy, and staying out late at night. In this situation, children are substituting support from their peer groups for unavailable or inadequate support from their parents. The conduct disturbance sometimes serves to enhance feelings of self-worth and to provide courage and a sense of independence in the face of anxiety-provoking situations. In other cases, the aggressive disorder may bring punishment that assuages those guilt feelings that may have arisen.

Conduct disorders may be further manifested by sexually promiscuous behavior, lying, fire setting, or cheating. Regardless of the behavior, nurses must seek out the reasons underlying that behavior—whether it be for attention and gratification, to control anxiety, or to bolster self-esteem.

Reactive attachment and withdrawal

Shyness, withdrawal, inability to relate socially to peers, and oversensitivity characterize children who are experiencing disorders in social relatedness. These children often demonstrate excessive worrying and submissive behaviors. Within the family system, activity is not tolerated well and is often punished. Because these children do not form intimate relationships with peers, they engage in daydreaming to provide the support they are not receiving from significant others. If withdrawal continues, it is likely that impairment of reality will increase. Affective impoverishment becomes more apparent as the child seeks to create a world that is less punitive.

Reactive disorders bear discussion because they occur frequently—individuals cannot progress from infancy through adolescence without some level of stress occurring as a result of life events. Individuals who do not experience stress and are not confronted with the need to change in order to progress in their development might be considered a poor risk for adjustment in future life situations. Through confrontations with situations that require individuals to adopt alternative behaviors, they learn that change can be effected and that they can be in control of their lives. They may also learn that in failing, learning can occur. However, as Kessler (1979) points out, there is a fine line between normal adaptive responses and pathology. There is a complex interrelationship among the nature and impact of the stressor, current and past experiences with stressors, the level of support from significant others, and the current emotional and physical health of the child. Particularly with younger children, it becomes difficult to predict how a child will adapt to stressful situations. It is important to note here that infants and preschool children are more vulnerable to the impact of stressors for those reasons noted above. Children at this age have limited coping strategies; at the same time, however, they may be more flexible in their coping if they have the appropriate support systems. The critical factor in reactive dis-

orders is the identification and amelioration of traumatic stressors. This will reduce the risk of lasting alterations in the child's personality.

Reactive responses may be subtle in nature; therefore, assessment must be directed toward identifying changes in behavior—for example, increased withdrawal, night terrors, bedwetting, eating problems, and hyperactivity—as well as identifying the stressor causing those changes. Intervention requires parental involvement and the willingness to consider the behavioral response of the child within the context of the family rather than as a singular event solely involving the child. Parents who are able to consider their own reactions and expectations and their influence on their children are more able to respond clearly and consistently to their children's needs. When there is little role confusion and ambiguity between parent and child and when needs of parents are not confused with needs of the children, there is decreased risk of development of maladaptive coping responses.

School phobia may be considered as a form of separation anxiety in children (Coolidge, 1970). Evidence of school phobia has been noted as early as nursery school age; however, the highest incidence is in the kindergarten to grade three category. Coolidge suggests that this disorder is seen primarily in upwardly mobile families, in which great emphasis is placed on education and achievement. An examination of the family dynamics reveals individuals who are ambivalent or unclear about their parenting roles. Parents may feel a strong sense of protectiveness toward their child while resenting the dependent relationship that has developed. The parents' fear of separation and uncertainty is transferred to the child. The phobia results after a traumatic event that the child interprets as a threat to his or her own life as well as to the lives of the parents, such as the loss of a grandparent or the extended business trip of a parent.

Assessment reveals anxiety in massive proportions that leads to somatic symptoms such as nausea, vomiting, headaches, and, on occasion, fevers. Once the child is permitted to remain at home, symptoms subside and there is a return to normal activity. Differentiation between normal refusal to go to school and school phobia is essential. Critical factors in the assessment process include previous episodes of school refusal, current traumatic events as precipitating factors, and the parents' ability to clearly define their role and to manage the episode as part of normal growth and development.

Depressive responses

Depressive disorders in childhood are not identified as a separate category in DSM-III, and such a category has not been included in previous diagnostic manuals. Cytryn and McKnew (1979) suggest that this omission perpetuates the myth that children do not experience depressive reactions when in fact they do. Accurate diagnosis of childhood depression is made difficult by the widely divergent symptoms found in this category. Clinical symptoms are age related and are often quite different from the clinical picture of depressed adults. Cytryn and McKnew (1979) state that the depressive process manifests itself in three ways:

1. Fantasy. Depressive themes are demonstrated in dreams or spontaneous play or are elicited through projective testing. Fantasy is present in almost all children who are diagnosed as experiencing a depressive reaction.
2. Verbal expression. Depression is evident through talk of hopelessness, suicide, and being worthless, unloved, and unattractive.
3. Mood and behavior. Observable signs include psychomotor retardation, sadness, crying, anorexia, and sleep disturbances. Masked depression evidences itself in hyperactivity, aggressiveness, school failure, delinquency, and psychosomatic symptoms.

This last category is characterized by the least stability on the part of the child. The authors note that the first line of defense is the development of depressive fantasy, which enables the child to project or deny through fantasy life. Acute depressive reactions are marked by verbal expression of depression, whereas mood and behavior changes are most frequently noted in chronic depressive reactions. At this last level, the preceding defenses against depression have failed, thus permitting mood and behavior changes to surface.

It is important to note that in childhood there are several factors that enhance the ability to defend against depression. During infancy, the maturational process, which promotes a sense of hope and fulfillment and the ability to substitute love objects (since object constancy has not yet been attained), serves to counteract the depressive process. During preschool and latency, the still-rich fantasy life, immature reality testing, and ability to substitute love objects allows for the containment of depressive symptoms at the fantasy level. As the child moves into adolescence and young adulthood, depressive symptoms are expressed through verbal means, and mood and behavior changes are noted. More mature reality testing and verbalization of feelings counteract the use of fantasy life and other more primitive defenses used in earlier life. Thus, the frequency of overt depression in adult life is greater than in earlier stages of life. (Even in adult life, overt depression does not occur in situations where denial and other primitive mechanisms are in operation.)

As in other childhood disorders, family dynamics are of crucial importance. Cytryn and McKnew (1979) state that families of depressed children present a varied clinical picture. Several themes are apparent: frequent separations; sudden loss of significant love object; rejection and denigration; loss of involvement; lack of awareness of childhood distress symptoms; and parental depression. Early detection requires an assessment of the family—its nodal events and parental attitudes—as well as an understanding of the child within the context of other relationships, particularly those involving school and peers.

Pervasive developmental disorders

It was maintained in the literature prior to 1979 and in DSM-II that children with severe impairment of relatedness and behavioral aberrations fall into the category of childhood psychosis. The term "psychosis" currently is not used diagnostically in the assessment of children. The term "pervasive developmental disorders" has been determined to incorporate previous psychopathology, namely, infantile autism, childhood schizophrenia, and symbiotic psychosis. Thus, the classic works of Bender and Kanner refer to infantile autism and childhood psychosis. Although the terminology has now been altered to more accurately reflect the disorders, these classic works and others will be reviewed as primary sources on etiology and behavioral characteristics.

Disorders first diagnosed in infancy or childhood reflect alterations in thinking, affect, speech, and perceptions. These children display an inability to relate to others, clinging behavior with the parenting figure, body image distortion, and difficulty with speech or no speech at all. There may also be poor development of locomotor, fine motor, and visual-motor skills, which results in erratic and peculiar patterns of functioning (Fish and Ritvo, 1979). It is important to note that the degree of personality disorganization varies from time to time within the same child, as well as among children having the same disturbance. This variability increases the difficulty of accurate assessment. However, the following key characteristics have been identified.

INFANTILE AUTISM

Infantile autism is characterized by profound disturbances of speech, perception, and neurological functioning in children under the age of 30 months. Kanner (1955) noted that few cases of autism are seen. In fact, less than 1% of the children he evaluated for autism were actually autistic. Autistic children, as a group, seem to reflect altered behavior patterns from birth. Chess et al. (1970) identified the "difficult temperamental type"—those children who exhibited less adaptability to change, irregular feeding and sleeping patterns, and less desire to interact with others in the environment—as being more likely to develop behavior problems as they progressed through childhood. Thus, although it is difficult to diagnose autism in the first year of life, it seems that autistic children demonstrate erratic behavior that begins early in the developmental process.

▶ Speech, language, and thought disturbances

Autistic children exhibit all levels of speech retardation. Some remain mute, whereas others may speak only in the present tense even when referring to past occurrences. Fish and Ritvo (1979) state that a critical characteristic is the coexistence of jargon and unintelligible speech with mature speech. As the percentage of unintelligible speech increases, the prognosis for these children worsens. Comprehension of speech may vary: some children are oblivious to meaning, whereas others may be unable to understand subtle or abstract meanings.

Kanner (1955) suggests that rigid echolalic speech can be identified in children whose speech has progressed beyond jargon and simple words. Literal repetition of statements and questions indicates that there is no change in the use of pronouns nor in the inflection of voice.

Formal thought disturbance is reflected in conceptualization and logic of thought. There may be a lack of connectedness between sentences, distorted grammar, pronoun reversal, and sudden irrelevancies. Kanner (1955) further notes that words can be condensed or distorted to create neologisms. These children have been observed to create worlds characterized by endless illogical connections and juxtapositions that hold little if any meaning for themselves and those around them.

▶ Perceptual and motor disturbances

Many children demonstrate unpredictable and disorganized responses to environmental stimuli. Inappropriately exaggerated responses to insignificant stimuli, with inattention or shortened attention to new or obvious stimuli, have been noted. These children do not use visual cues to learn about their environment but rather manipulate their environment through their mobility. Those objects in the environment that move can be readily discerned. Autistic children have difficulty separating an object figure from its background, creating the need to move objects while inspecting them. During assessment, lack of response to voices or loud noises is often seen. Kanner (1955) states that autistic children do not adapt to a wide variety of activities or use of different objects. There is attention to specific details of objects without regard for the object as a whole. There is little creative or imaginative play as is found in age-appropriate children. Brightly colored toys and objects attract the attention of autistic children.

Motor development is characterized by simple, repetitive movements such as hand flapping, finger twiddling, rocking, and whirling. Infants are fascinated by movement of any kind, yet autistic infants demonstrate this interest to excess. This need for motion is carried further into forms of self-stimulation such as banging of the head and rocking.

▶ Affect and mood

Kanner (1955) observed that the ''blank expression'' of autistic children reflects the indifference of these children to those around them. Temper tantrums and outbursts of tears, rage, and other aggressive responses are initiated when the child's routine or need for ''sameness'' is interrupted. Bender (1947) describes excessive anxiety that tends to be precipitated by change in the environment or disruption of normal activities. The flat affect may be incongruent with thought processes, and it does not necessarily correlate with changes in the environment; in fact, it may occur in the absence of stimuli. Although anxiety is common in many childhood disorders, the illogical eruptions demonstrated by autistic children are a distinguishing feature.

▶ Social relatedness

Autistic children are often viewed as aloof and distant. The avoidance of eye contact has been noted as early as six months. Kanner (1955) differentiates this inability to relate to others from withdrawal from relationships in that the latter requires a previously existing relationship. Autistic children are unable to relate to others from the very beginning of life. Although clinging and symbiotic behavior may also be observed, there is little if any emotional attachment to other persons. Less severely autistic children may interact periodically but are unable to sustain a lasting relationship. These children infrequently initiate social relationships and are often observed as being isolated and preoccupied.

CHILDHOOD-ONSET PERVASIVE DEVELOPMENTAL DISORDERS

Disturbances in thought, affect, social relatedness, and behavior emerge in children between ages thirty months and twelve years. Children in this category may have experienced a relatively symptom-free relationship within the family system. Precipitating factors of a severe nature such as loss of a parent through death or separation, repeated separating, sexual abuse, or violence often initiate high levels of anxiety, resulting in ego fragmentation. It is important to note that no one factor leads to the onset of symptoms. There is a complex interrelationship of factors that must be considered during the assessment process.

Children who develop symptoms after the first three years of life seem to have a more favorable prognosis than children diagnosed as autistic in the infancy period. Areas similar to those in infantile autism are affected: thought processes, behavior, affect, and relatedness. Those areas are assessed in relation to continuing age-appropriate characteristics. Thus, characteristics noted in the infantile autism group will be observed in varying degrees in this group. The following behaviors are characteristic of childhood-onset developmental disorders.

▶ Speech, language, and thought disturbances

Speech may have developed appropriately up to the point of diagnosis. Elective mutism may be present, as well as impairment of nonverbal communication. Cognitive function is impaired, including insight and judgment. Bizarre fantasies and preoccupation with unusual thoughts may also be observed. Echolalic repetition characterizes speech; distorted syntax and fragmented speech patterns result. Although delusions and hallucinations occur in later years, they are not apparent in childhood disorders. Looseness of association and lack of logical connections also characterize this group of children.

▶ Perceptual and motor disturbances

Extreme hypoactivity or hyperactivity may occur, as well as ritualistic movements such as rocking, turning, and whirling. Perception of body boundaries is also impaired. Bender (1947) noted that drawings of the human body are often distorted, with an emphasis on peripheral details such as hair, extremities, and fingers. There is also a distortion in the perception of the relationship of one's own body to other objects in the environment.

▶ Affect and mood

As in the infantile autism group, these children display inappropriate affect with mood swings that range from rage to passivity and apathy. Their responses to dangerous situations do not approximate the normal response. As noted previously, illogical anxiety that has no apparent relationship to external events is also exhibited by these children.

▶ Social relatedness

A striking characteristic is the lack of attachment to and hence the withdrawal from peers and peer groups. There is a social distance that is maintained throughout relationships. A lack of response to the feelings of others as human beings and little sense of cooperative interaction can be observed. These children experience much anxiety when changes occur in their environment, and they lack flexibility in adaptation to new persons or events in their surrounding territory. Distorted perception of body boundaries is reflected in these children's inappropriate touching of others and taking of objects belonging to others as if they were their own.

• • •

The Report of the Joint Commission (1969) states that less than 10% of children with psychiatric disorders are severely impaired; when impairment is severe, the treatment may be long-term and costly. Many times residential treatment centers are the most effective and appropriate sources of therapy. However, there remains a profound impact on the families of these children. Supportive interventions must also be provided for the family as a whole to assist family members in coping with the hospitalized child and with their own feelings and behaviors.

CHILD ABUSE

Child abuse as defined by Feigelson-Chase (1975, p. 1) is the "deliberate and willful injury of a child by a caretaker—hitting, beating up with a belt, cord or other implement, slamming against a wall, burning with cigarettes, scalding with hot water, locking in a dungeon, hog-tying, torturing, even killing." Child neglect refers to parental lack of care in the provision of necessities such as food, clothing, and shelter. The definitions of abuse and neglect do vary from state to state.

Child abuse in the form of infanticide and abandonment has its beginnings early in history. Infanticide as a sacred ritual was depicted in the Bible. Abraham was asked by God to sacrifice his first-born son, Isaac, as a sign of piety. Feigelson-Chase notes that the sacrifice of first-born sons in ancient Palestine was quite common. Perhaps the most well-known cases of infanticide were those ordered by Pharaoh in the Old Testament and Herod's slaughter of the innocents from which Jesus was saved. Infanticide was often practiced to satisfy the perceived demands of religious beliefs or superstition; however, population control was also a primary reason. It was not uncommon in the Alaskan, Chinese, Scandinavian, Polynesian, African, and Australian aborigine cultures to kill children. Sumner (cited in Feigelson-Chase) notes that in Tahiti members of the higher social class were not required to kill their children, while members of the lower caste were permitted only one or two children; the rest were killed.

In many instances throughout Europe in the 1700s, infanticide was the only alternative for unmarried pregnant women. If pregnancy were discovered they would be excommunicated from the Church and forced into isolation. On the other hand, the penalty for infanticide was often death. Sacking—putting the guilty mother in a sack and throwing her in a river—was a terrible death. Frederick the Great substituted decapitation as punishment, based on his belief that it was more humane. As late as 1890, infanticide was still practiced in Europe, primarily among people in the lower class. Mothers—often assisted by lovers or husbands—murdered their children to hide their shame or to relieve themselves of the responsibility of raising the children.

The Japanese practiced infanticide for centuries. Feigelson-Chase notes that the custom of *mabiki* or "thinning out" was practiced by Japanese farmers who killed their second and third sons. Girls were spared because they could be sold as servants or sent to be geishas. The rate of infanticide in Japan experienced peaks and valleys based primarily on the need of society for increased industrial and military growth.

Thus, child abuse is not new to us; its existence has been documented throughout our history. And child abuse cannot be viewed solely within the context of the family; rather, it must be viewed within the larger context of society, as an instrument of social control. Wherever poverty and all of its ramifications can be found, there is the likelihood of child abuse.

Epidemiology

Dr. C.H. Kempe first used the term "battered child syndrome" in the literature in 1962. He described the physical abuse experienced by infants and preschoolers who were defenseless and unable to communicate what was happening to them. Cur-

rently, the Centers for Disease Control (CDC) reports that the incidence of child abuse in the United States is on the increase. Estimates reveal that hundreds of thousands of children die from abuse or neglect, which cannot be substantiated in all cases. Further reports from the CDC indicate that 20% of the cases involve children who have been abused before and that 22% involve multiple trauma.

Abuse tends to be more common among families in the lower socioeconomic bracket; however, it does occur in middle- and upper-income families. In the higher-income cases, parents may be ambivalent about their parenting roles and unable to accept and cope with the attendant responsibility (Gladston, 1979). Reporting of these cases is more unlikely.

Until recently sexual abuse and incest have been considered taboo subjects. Dr. Ann Burgess has brought the issue of child molestation to the public's attention. She noted in her presentation in 1981 at the second annual Psychiatric Mental Health Symposium that statistics showed that sexual abuse of children was on the rise. Frequently the abuser is an acquaintance of the family and many times holds a respected position in the community. She further noted that men who molest young boys are often involved with the boys in Boy Scouts, Little League, church groups, or other group activities. In one instance, in November 1983, two pediatricians in New York City were accused of child molestation in their practice.

Incest as a form of sexual abuse has recently achieved nationwide attention through a television presentation. The January 1984 airing of *Something About Amelia* portrayed the plight of a father who had sexual relations with his daughter and the impact on the family. The role of the psychiatrist in the treatment of sexual abuse victims has received national attention as well. In January 1984 in the state of California, a psychiatrist was required to reveal the name of an incest victim's abuser, who was then brought to court. This legal development will have a profound impact on the success of treatment of incestuous families.

Characteristics of victims of abuse

Physical signs of abuse are quite apparent to the observer. Fresh bruises and welts as well as old scars can be seen. A history of old fractures of the skull and long bones such as those of the legs and arms are also seen. Gladston (1979) states that these children may be well-fed and well-dressed and their injuries attended to appropriately; however, the etiology of the injuries is not often recognized. Parents will bring the abused child to various clinics—never using one consistently—thus making it more difficult for health professionals to draw a clear picture from the data. Parents frequently reflect concern about their child's status as well as ambivalence about their role as parents. The child's body becomes a battleground for the simultaneous feelings of love and hate experienced by the abusing parent. Specific marks on the body such as human bite marks, bruising of the genitalia, excoriation and/or bruising at the wrists and ankles, hand or thumb imprints on face and neck, black eyes, and missing teeth are key assessment factors. Children who experience neglect and abuse may be inappropriately dressed (for example, no socks and shoes in winter), malnourished, and physically disheveled and unclean.

Patterns of behavior

Abused children have little sense of self—deriving what they can from parents who have never developed their own senses of self-worth. This poor sense of self is projected downward to the child, and the cycle goes on. These children have few peer contacts, often remaining socially isolated because parents are not happy with any of their friends. They may tend to be very close to parents, yet withdrawn. There is a suspiciousness on the part of these children when they are in contact with other adults, particularly when questions are asked about the injuries. The child's intense attachment to parents often confuses diagnosis because there seems to be a deep concern for one another. Other major characteristics include inordinate amount of time spent at school with little desire to go home, delinquency and other socially aggressive behavior, teenage pregnancy, depressed mood, assuming a parental role in the family system with concurrent age-inappropriate behaviors, wearing clothing that hides scars and bruises, avoiding direct eye contact, and not answering questions until checking with parents. When an abused child is hospitalized for his or her injuries, it may be noted that there is frequently little protest when parents leave and affect is flat. The child may be fearful of other adult contact in the hospital setting while desiring hugging and cuddling. Although the behaviors described reflect both ends of the behavioral spectrum, it is important to consider that this variation may in fact be due to the ambivalence in the parental relationship—the desire to cling and the fear of further physical and emotional abuse. The development of a trusting relationship is a critical element of nursing intervention and a difficult one at best. In summary, Gladston (1979, p. 589) states that "child abuse is an act that reflects the human capacity to entertain two intense and mutually contradictory emotions simultaneously." He further suggests that child abuse lies on the spectrum of human violence somewhere between homicide and suicide.

ADOLESCENT MENTAL HEALTH

Adolescence has been described as one of the major developmental periods. Erikson views adolescence as a period of great physical and emotional change, the goal being a beginning sense of identity—a separation from parents as the primary support system. Self is the focus of development in adolescence. Peer groups guide identity in such areas as dress, activities, academic excellence, and college selection. It has also been called a period of "turmoil" and "adjustment." Adolescents themselves find this time one of ambivalence—the exhilaration of the adult life ahead mingled with the desire to run back to the "nest" and be taken care of. It is maintaining this delicate balance within the family system that contributes to the successful mastery of this period.

Physical changes are apparent in this period. Early in adolescence, secondary sex characteristics emerge with the attendant biological changes. Penis size increases, and breasts develop; the female begins to display the rounded figure; and pubic hair appears in both sexes. Menses may begin as early as age eleven. Voice changes in the male occur. As adolescence progresses, hormonal and growth activity lead to further changes. Males begin to lose their gawkiness; muscle mass increases to fill out the body. Females experience an increase in estrogen as the body prepares for ovulation and pregnancy becomes a possibility. Females experience continued growth and fullness in the breasts and hips. A primary physical change throughout adolescence is the occurrence of acne. Endocrine activity experiences an upsurge in this period, leading to increased production of the sebaceous glands. Adolescents find these varied physical changes difficult to adjust to, and their adjustment is compounded by the emotional swings common to this period.

Emotional changes are wide and varied. Adolescents are noted for their heightened sensitivity to events around them, as well as to their own bodies. Initially, adolescents are uncomfortable discussing the changes they are experiencing.

Elizabeth had just begun her menses. Her mother noticed some pink-tinged tissues in the bathroom. When she openly brought the issue to Elizabeth's attention, Elizabeth promptly turned red and began to deny the occurrence. The mother continued to gently acknowledge the naturalness of this phenomenon and provided support until Elizabeth seemed to be less threatened by the situation.

Often adolescents feel a lack of control over their own bodies and over external events, as is demonstrated by this vignette.

Abrupt changes in mood, impulsive behavior, fluctuations between responsibleness and "flakiness," dress styles, and overt rebellion against parental values are often at the core of adolescent-parent struggles. As noted earlier, beginning at early adolescence peer groups become the major shaping forces, which is frequently frightening to parents. Adolescents' need to control often drives parents and adolescents into struggles that result in benefits to no one. Jay Haley (1980) noted in his book *Leaving Home* that some struggle must occur in order for the adolescent to separate and develop as an individual; however, the essence of the struggle is critical. Those "minor" struggles, over issues such as curfews and styles of clothing and hair, have less serious consequences than those that involve major value conflicts. Haley's point, which is a valid one, is that separation cannot occur unless there is some force that activates the separation.

Critical to the parent-adolescent relationship is the maintenance of a delicate balance of control. Although adolescents struggle for independence, parental limit-setting and expectations are necessary, particularly in early adolescence. Those parents who want to be "friends" to their children promote further role confusion at a time when the adolescent needs clarity. The major focus of parenting is on the provision of support and guidance as the adolescent moves toward independence. To actualize this support, parents must have a clear definition of their own roles and expectations, must be able to tolerate the mood swings and other behaviors that are a part of the emerging individual, and, lastly, must be able to separate out their own goals, desires, *and* unresolved conflicts.

Adolescent depression and suicide

Depression in adolescents may be expressed through apathetic behavior: they show decreasing interest in self, peers, school, and activities, and social isolation becomes an increasingly prominent facet of life-style. This behavior pattern may be confused, however, with the moodiness, social isolation, and depression that are so characteristic of the healthy adolescent. As Jones (1980) noted, when this behavior does not occur, parents begin to wonder whether the adolescent is emotionally healthy. The key factor is the adolescent's acting upon his or her morbid wishes and fantasies.

Dr. Susan Blumenthal (*New York Times,* August 7, 1983) stated that "teenage suicide has become a devastating public health problem." She continued by pointing out that more than 5,600 men and women under the age of 25 committed suicide in 1981. It has been noted also that increasing numbers of younger children (ages 8 to 12) are considering and in some instances actually carrying out suicide. Many suicides go unreported because they are considered accidents; self-destructive behavior may emerge in the form of high-risk activities such as driving fast, parachuting, hang gliding, or doing something on a dare. Adolescents tend to operate on impulse; if they are unable to control impulses and to activate appropriate problem-solving mechanisms in times of high stress, they may inadvertently kill themselves. Precipitating factors may include failure in school, pregnancy, and perceived loss of significant relationships. Stress levels become intolerable, and the ability to problem-solve decreases. The suicide attempt often becomes a method of communication—a means of expressing ambivalence toward assuming an adult role or a measure to reduce the overwhelming feeling of anxiety that threatens to engulf the adolescent.

Evans (1982) provides insight into the concept of suicide among youth. In his article, he suggests that suicide is a growing problem in the United States, which seems to stem from several factors: lack of or termination of a significant relationship (for example, parent, girlfriend, boyfriend); loss of options to effect change in one's life; social change; and family alienation.

Hart and Keidel (1979) specify candidates for suicide as adolescents who do not show the characteristic signs of turmoil and who have certain risk factors such as family history of suicide, previous suicide attempts, depression, substance abuse, and social isolation. However, this theory does not consider the large number of adolescents who, during the process of adolescence, are subjected to these risk factors and do not commit suicide.

Cline (1978) suggests that there are particular personality factors inherent in the suicidal adolescent. The psychoanalytic approach presents the suicidal adolescent as angry about parental "rejection" as he or she attempts to separate. This sense of anger toward the love object is internalized, thus leading to destruction of self.

Teicher and Jacobs (1966) support a theory that considers a suicide attempt in the context of an adolescent's total life events rather than as a rash event or a singular episode. Suicide is considered a final alternative in the problem-solving process; it is used when other courses of action have failed. These authors suggest a sequence of events that reflects family problems in childhood: inordinate struggle with the family for independence; loss of a meaningful relationship; and, finally, perceived loss of all social attachments. The solution is suicide.

Durkheim (1951) in his treatise on "anomie" suggested that suicide resulted from social alienation, or a sense of social insecurity. McAnarney (1979) builds upon Durkheim's theory; however, he contends that suicidal behavior emerges from the powerlessness and normlessness of the family rather than of society as a whole.

In summary, the etiology of adolescent suicide is varied. It is a complex interrelationship of factors: internal constitution and temperament; ability to communicate needs; existence of meaningful relationships; availability of support systems; parental stability and support; and the ability to problem-solve and use effective coping strategies. Suicide may be the adolescent's one remaining means of revenge, the final cry for help, or the only perceived method to manipulate the environment.

Substance abuse

The use of drugs and alcohol among adolescents reflects society's trend toward pills and alcohol as a measure of tension relief. Countless ads on television and in magazines and newspapers tell us how we can relax with a Bud or invite a special friend over to enjoy a Harvey's Bristol Cream. Pills are touted as relieving menstrual cramps and tension headaches. Medicine chests often resemble mini-pharmacies. Thus, adolescents are growing up in a society where drugs are used to relieve tension and to create a sense of well-being. Peer pressure and the desire to achieve a sense of relatedness are often the basis for substance abuse. The "high" experienced by adolescents creates the illusion that they can share intimate relationships with others. However, when the "high" is gone, the isolation returns—and the cycle begins again. A combination of drugs and alcohol can be dangerous, even resulting in death. Although adolescents may recognize the dangers of substance abuse, the desire to be like their peers and the belief that "nothing will happen to me" create an unnecessarily risky situation.

As adolescent drug users become increasingly part of the drug subculture, their energies are directed solely toward the acquisition of drugs. Some may sell to other adolescents to support their own habits; others may steal or engage in various forms of criminal activity. Hospitalization may be viewed as a means to avoid imprisonment. Treatment is not likely to be taken seriously, and such clients are often resistant to intervention. Manipulation is a characteristic behavior that is used to create disorganization among the members of the hospital staff, and it also serves to keep the client in control. (For further discussion of substance abuse, see Chapter 17.)

Eating disorders

Anorexia nervosa, which was initially recognized in the latter part of the nineteenth century, has gained increasing attention over the last three decades. Its symptoms can range from minimal manifestations to starvation and even death. Although anorexia will be discussed in greater depth in Chapters 16 and 19, it is important to note here because the primary age of onset is between 15 and 25 years. Anorectics are usually female and come from middle- and upper-class families where excellence is the expectation. The anorectic displays a perfectionistic, achievement-oriented attitude. Sanger and Cassino (1984) note that the idea of becoming fat disgusts the anorectic and she perceives herself as being fat even when emaciation becomes life threatening. Bruch (1970) notes that in families of anorectics there is little differentiation of boundaries; thus the anorectic feels she has little control, even over her own body. To exert control and assume independence, she chooses not to eat. The family system supports this pattern of somatization rather than direct expression of feelings. Therefore the anorectic strives for perfection and seemingly acquiesces to parental control. A polite exterior is maintained by the family while rigidity is the primary characteristic of the internal family function. Bruch (1970) maintains that the only object of control that the adolescent female has is her own body. She further notes that mothers of anorectics have often given up their own careers—and perhaps control over their own lives— to become submissive housewives. These mothers' ambivalence, anger, and lack of control are then projected onto their daughters. Also, perhaps a sense of frustrated hopes and ambition is projected onto the daughter in the hope that the daughter will achieve and succeed where the mother has not.

The clinical picture may present depression and anxiety. There may be a withdrawal from activities and friends, which may be viewed as "normal" for an adolescent. Often there is a focus to the point of hyperactivity on a specific activity such as a sport or schoolwork that takes on obsessive proportions. There is a marked phobia toward food and great alarm and shame at even a small weight gain. Body image distortion is such that these young women perceive themselves as fat even at alarmingly low weights. There is a lack of concern for their emaciated state. Bruch (1970) notes that anorectics do indeed experience hunger; in some cases they will binge and eat large amounts of food (bulimia) and then purge themselves by vomiting or using excessive amounts of laxatives. They may also focus their attention on the feeding of others.

Anorectics often show bizarre food preferences and cravings. They may entice others into eating by cooking gourmet meals, yet they will refuse to eat, priding themselves on their great sense of control. This behavior often infuriates their peers, which may enhance underlying feelings of depression and isolation. Sexuality—feelings of oneself as a sexual being—are often frightening and guilt producing. Sexual feelings and fantasies are denied and as the anorectic process continues, amenorrhea occurs; thus, in effect anorectics have even controlled the course of their own sexuality. (For further discussion, see Chapter 6.)

Male anorexia has received little attention, perhaps because of the emphasis on muscle development rather than thinness and the propensity for acting out rather than internalizing feelings in the young male. Crisp and Toms (1972) further suggest that anorexia in males is related to major gender identity problems and premorbid obesity. Data from the Bem Sex Role Inventory provide empirical support for observations of gender identification problems. A study by Kiecolt-Glaser and Dixon (1984) notes differences between preadolescent-onset anorexia and postadolescent-onset anorexia. Preadolescent-onset males are similar to female anorectics in that they tend to cope with feelings of inadequacy by striving for excellence and perfectionism. Postadolescent-onset males, however, tend to avoid competition or to withdraw from the challenges of life. These authors further suggest that the prognosis for postadolescent male anorexia may be relatively poor because later onset may reflect greater immaturity and regression. Morgan and Russell (1971) support the hypothesis that there is a significant difference in causation between early onset and later onset; those stressors occurring at a later date may be more difficult to reverse. It is also thought that in a majority of anorectic males, there is a preexisting developmental difficulty that influences the individual's ability to adapt successfully. Family dynamics of male anorectics have also been considered. These dynamics include overprotectiveness, rigidity, lack of differentiation among members, and avoidance of conflict. Children in this family system tend to remain dependent and eventually are unable to achieve a sense of autonomy and individuation.

Since there are few male anorectics, there has been little effort directed toward a systematic plan for assessment and intervention. It will be important to consider this clinical subgroup in the future; efforts to develop more information about the clinical picture and effective treatment modalities are necessary.

Bulimia (the binge and purge syndrome) is often discussed with anorexia because of similarities in eating patterns. The average bulimic client is somewhat older (between the ages of 18 and 29 years), tends to be more socially skilled than the anorectic client, and appears to be the ideal wife, mother, career woman; however, she recognizes that her eating patterns are disturbed, as are her feelings regarding self (Potts, 1984). Bulimic clients in general present a characteristic impairment of impulse control, low self-worth, and depressive affect. Potts (1984) maintains that bulimics binge several times a day, primarily in the late afternoon and evenings. They may ingest as many as 11,500 calories per binge. Laxatives, diuretics, fasting, and exercise are used to control weight gain; however, Johnson et al. (1982) state that vomiting constitutes the main method of purging. Garfinkel et al. (1980) report that bulimics as a group abuse drugs and alcohol; drinking in particular decreases abdominal discomfort and also masks feelings of diminished self-worth and alleviates the attending feelings of guilt. Depression and suicidal risk are also notable in the behavior pattern of most bulimics. Physiological alterations such as dehydration, hypernatremia, hypokalemia, and resulting cardiac arrhythmias, as well as renal impairment, may occur. (See also Chapter 17.)

Impulsive behaviors

In an attempt to separate and individuate, the adolescent may use inappropriate measures to achieve independence; antisocial behavior such as stealing, truancy, and running away may represent attempts to escape from tension-producing family situations, as well as being a method to achieve some measure of independence. Often parent-child relationships are characterized by rejection and ambivalence over the parenting role. Open communication between parent and child is not encouraged; the adolescent is not given the opportunity to work through the emotional conflicts that are experienced as part of adolescence. An adolescent's anger toward parents or care givers is expressed through stealing and running away—the motivation being to punish the parents for their lack of attention and love. In the case of stealing, the parents are often the focus of the punishment from the police or other authorities. Adolescents may feel that outside authorities will have an effect on parents when they themselves do not have any impact. Adolescents who run away may also feel that they are punishing their parents; unfortunately in some cases, parents may feel relief at having the responsibility removed. Impulsive behaviors such as those noted are used by adolescents to exert some measure of control, to separate from an untenable family situation, to express anger and frustration at parents, and to develop a sense of self-worth through their acts.

UNDERLYING DYNAMICS

The following section will present theories of child and adolescent mental health from a variety of perspectives. Each theory is recognized for its individual contributions; however, it is an underlying premise of this book that a holistic perspective must be considered in order to provide effective nursing intervention at all levels—primary, secondary, and tertiary.

Psychodynamic theory

Psychodynamic theory incorporates both the analytic viewpoint and those theories that are extensions or derivations of Freudian theory.

A primary characteristic of childhood disorders is the lack of appropriate ego functioning. Ego deficits may occur as a result of organic changes or faulty development during childhood. Freud states that fixation during a particular period of childhood will then determine the future level of functioning. Children with ego deficits are unable to control their impulses. Berman (1979) notes that their levels of tolerance of frustration are minimal. Immediate gratification of desires is necessary; aggressive acting-out behavior results when these children are placed in situations that create anxiety and frustration.

The lack of a sound ego prevents these children from forming relationships with others. Lack of ego boundaries causes them to fear engulfment from others while also desiring a warm caring relationship. These children have few problem-solving skills; thus they are unable to adapt to situations around them. They are unable to learn from their mistakes and move on to new experiences. Multiple stimuli generate panic rather than provide an opportunity for learning. These children may be insensitive to others and are unable to function within the accepted social norms. This behavior causes others to avoid and castigate them, which further forces them into a fantasy world and social isolation.

Blos (1962) describes the dynamics of adolescence as being crucial in the individuation of the self. The adolescent returns to former modes of adaptation in an attempt to renegotiate his or her role as an independent self—separate from the adult parents. Again, sound foundations in the early phases of life must be present for adolescents to successfully individuate from the parental system. As Blos further describes, adolescent behaviors such as anger, argumentative behavior, and resistance to authority serve as ways to facilitate separation. The importance of sound ego functioning is also supported by Erikson in his delineation of the eight stages of development. His description of the task of adolescence focuses on the need of the adolescent to define self in relation to environment, peers, parents, and life goals. For an adolescent to move along and complete further tasks, he or she must develop a sound sense of self.

Constitutional-biological theory

Temperament characteristics—characteristics that exist at birth—may influence a child's level of stress tolerance and shape the child's future life experiences. Thus the situations children find themselves in are influenced by their very temperaments. A quiet, shy child will select experiences that reflect a quality of interaction that is quite different from that of a child who is extremely active. Temperament in an indirect manner directs choice of peers, quality of interaction, and roles a child will play. These factors in turn have a relationship to the development of psychopathology.

The New York Longitudinal Studies (Chess et al., 1970) have demonstrated that certain temperamental characteristics were connected to the development of psychiatric disorders. Nine assessment categories were identified as a result of the study: activity level, rhythmicity, approach-withdrawal, adaptability, threshold of responsiveness, intensity of reaction, quality of mood, distractibility, and attention span and persistence. It was determined that there was not a direct correlation between temperamental characteristics and psychopathology; however, it was also determined that a child with vulnerabilities in one or more categories can become the target of parental frustration and irritability. Thus, one must consider not only the temperament of the child but also the attitude and response of the parents. Thomas et al. (1968) suggest that normal development results from a "goodness of fit" between the child's individual characteristics and temperament and the expectations of the family environment.

Individual differences in infants have been reported by Schaffer (1974) and Bridger and Birns (1968). Sucking behaviors in infants showed marked differences, as did startle responses. Consistent individual variation in heart rates in response to being touched was also noted. Bridger and Birns noted that an NIMH study provided empirical data that supported evidence that identical (monozygotic) twins are born with very different temperaments. Major differences were noted in the areas of attention span, physiologic adaptation, and level of calmness. The authors concluded that there was a strong indication of nongenetic factors affecting early congenital differences in temperament.

Bell (1971) in his research supports the aforementioned findings. He notes that there are congenital determinants of such childhood traits as assertiveness, sensorimotor capabilities, and sociability. Individual variations in these traits will affect the manner in which the parent responds. He concludes that these behaviors arouse a particular level of parental response that occurs within a response hierarchy and that reinforces certain parental behaviors once they have been elicited.

Chess et al. (1970) present data that support the genetic component in a longitudinal study of eight pairs of twins. Those characteristics that reflected the strongest genetic evidence were activity, approach-withdrawal, and adaptability. During the first year of study, the genetic influence seemed stronger than during the subsequent two years.

Although it is difficult to tease out prenatal factors that influence characteristics of children, Joffee (1969) notes that several risk factors increase fetal risk. These include low birth weight and maternal factors such as socioeconomic status, age, parity, ethnicity, nutritional state, cigarette smoking, and drugs. Methodological problems exist, however, that preclude accurate assessment of prenatal factors. It is important to note that factors in the external environment may potentiate characteristics present at birth.

Effects of sex differences on the development of childhood psychopathology were studied by Hutt (1974). She noted three aspects of male development: males experience an increased risk of and are more vulnerable to various dysfunctions; males are subject to greater phenotype variability; and males are slower in their development. Male infants seem to be more susceptible to postnatal complications. Cantwell and Tarjan (1979) support Hutt and suggest that dysfunctions such as childhood psychosis, learning disabilities, language disturbances, and behavioral disturbances occur to a greater degree in males than in females. Hutt (1979) suggested increased susceptibility may result in part from the extended developmental period experienced by males. Extended developmental periods would provide longer critical periods, increasing the amount of time stressors have to operate. Rutter (1970) further supports the premise of vulnerability in males. In his study of high-risk families (those having one parent with mental illness), he found that male children were more stressed by family dysfunction than females. A study of stresses experienced as result of short-term admissions of a parent into an institution also indicated a greater incidence of behavioral dysfunction in boys.

Sameroff and Chandler (1975) have developed three models to describe the relationship between constitutional-organic factors and the environment. The first model, the main effects model, states that an organic deficit will result in deviant behavior regardless of environmental influences. The interaction model suggests that deviant behavior is a result of the interaction between the child's constitutional-organic factors and psychosocial factors in the environment. However, this model does not emphasize the reciprocity of influence. Sameroff and Chandler suggest that a third model, the transactional model, considers the mutual influence child and environment have on one another. Neither factor exerts greater influence; each must be considered in concert. Thus, in the next section, the sociocultural and familial influences on the development of behavioral and emotional dysfunctions will be considered.

Sociocultural theory

Children exist within the context of their families; however, the influence of the larger society also impacts on their development and their behavioral responses. Thus, the community or cul-

tural context within which the child grows up will define various behaviors as abnormal. That definition of abnormal may vary depending on the age of the child. For example, crying, temper tantrums, and clinging behaviors may be age-appropriate until the age of five or six. These are unacceptable behaviors for the twelve-year-old and are likely to be indicative of a behavioral disorder. The people within the culture interpret behaviors and determine whether they are acceptable within the framework of that particular culture. As Looff (1979) notes, children are referred to mental health resources by those in the community such as nurses, teachers, local physicians, and guidance counselors, whose determinations are made by comparing presenting behaviors with culturally defined behaviors based on peer norms. A study of the Hutterites (Eaton and Weill, 1955) revealed that neurotic symptoms (for example, psychophysiological and depressive responses) were socially acceptable methods of tension relief in that culture. In another example of regional cultural influence, Looff (1979) indicates that in Southern Appalachia certain behavior patterns do occur with reasonable frequency while others do not. The children of Southern Appalachia rarely display symptoms of primary behavior disorders or impulse disorders. However, this population seems to reflect an increased occurrence of disorders based on sexual conflict, indicative perhaps of exaggerated sexual attitudes in this particular area. Looff further notes that verbal communication is a problem among these families, thus severely restricting their ability to discuss problems and solutions. He suggests that children from these families often have emotional problems that reflect nonverbal themes, a situation resulting from a lack of experience in verbally expressing difficulties.

It is also important to consider sociocultural influences on the development of strengths. The culture impacts on the shaping of the healthy aspects of the personality—in terms of developing effective methods of coping and basic ego strengths. Looff notes the strengths of the Southern Appalachian culture: the family is basically stable and organized; there is a remarkable sense of relatedness and trust with little sense of personal isolation; and there is an impressive capacity to deeply experience and differentiate feelings related to one's own experiences.

In considering the effects of society and class, one must be cautioned against assuming cause-and-effect relationships regarding the development of dysfunctions. When working with children and their families, nurses need to evaluate the following sociocultural factors: How does the culture influence the child's ability to master developmental tasks? What specific hopes, wishes, and fears emerge within the context of the culture? Consider, for example, the wish for thinness. Is it desired in the culture? Does it reinforce anorexia? Are there certain economic and geographic factors that may negatively influence development and behavioral response? What cultural patterns, if any, block potentially positive behaviors from generation to generation?

Several pertinent examples of societal pressure in today's culture bear mentioning at this point. The pressure to be thin and to have the perfect body has an impact on adolescent females and the development of anorexia and/or bulimia. McAnarney (1979) suggests society plays a role in the suicidal behavior of the adolescent. The pressures of society to achieve at all costs leave the adolescent feeling insecure and with few viable options.

As has been stated throughout, the child exists within the context of the larger society and within the context of the family. In the last section, the family will be discussed in relation to its impact on the developing child. (For further reference to the family, see Chapters 5 and 12.)

Lidz (1963) indicates that familial influences are the first imprint on the newborn child. These influences are so pervasive and consistent that they shape the child's life in such a way that they can be modified in later life but never truly altered.

Because every aspect of the child reflects the familial influence, certain family factors contribute to disturbances in childhood and adolescence. The ability to communicate in an open, honest manner, the ability to develop trusting relationships, and the ability to resolve conflict through effective coping strategies emerge out of early familial interaction.

Spitz (1951) noted that lack of human contact in the form of maternal deprivation and lack of stimulation were central factors in the development of disturbed behavior in the early stages of life, resulting in the "failure to thrive" syndrome. Kanner's early work (1955) suggests that infantile autism results from a disturbed parent-child relationship. According to Kanner, mothers of autistic children tend to be aloof and distant and to have little emotional attachment to their children; the relationship between mother and child exists primarily on an intellectual level.

Several family theorists suggest a strong reciprocal relationship among family members in the development of behavioral and emotional disorders in children and adolescents. For example, Laing (1964) notes that deficiencies in communication and parenting skills and disturbed family behavior patterns occur early in the family life cycle. In his work he described the distorted patterns of communication that characterize these families. He also described the concept of mystification, whereby family members have little, if any, specific identity. There is no sense of individual personality or spontaneity. The process of mystification includes many contradictions and inconsistencies, so much so that members are unable to determine what is actually so and what is not.

Watzlawick et al. (1967) discussed the concept of double-bind communication and its relationship to the development of schizophrenic behavior. In healthy families, double-bind communication does occasionally occur; however, in unhealthy families, double-bind communication is the primary mode. Eventually, a child is either immobilized or acts out inappropriately because either of two possible answers to a question, or ways of dealing with a problem, is incorrect. Serious impairment of cognitive abilities occurs, with resulting interference in thought processes.

Bowen (1978) describes family relationships in regard to the degree of differentiation between the two members of the parental dyad. Parents who are unable to define self clearly experience a fusion that influences their ability to relate to the child as well as to one another. Bowen suggests that for these parents to control tension and resolve conflict, two actions must take place: (1) the child is triangled into the parental dyad, and (2) the projection process occurs whereby the focus of the disturbance is placed on the child, taking the pressure off the parental dyad. Eventually, Bowen suggests, the child lives up to the distorted projections placed on him by the parents and dysfunctional behavior does occur.

Minuchin (1974) and his colleagues at the Child Guidance Clinic support the belief that family dynamics influences the development of psychosomatic illness. He notes that behavioral events and stressful interactions that occur among family members can be measured in terms of increases in the levels of hormones and other substances in the bloodstreams of family members as the events occur. Minuchin describes these families as being characterized by enmeshment, rigidity, and inability to effectively problem solve. For example, clients with eating disorders such as anorexia and bulimia experience difficulty in gaining control over and individuating self. Families of these clients are often characterized by a facade of ''normalcy,'' whereas beneath the facade exists little room for the development of a personal identity. Control over one's own body is perceived by the anorectic/bulimic as perhaps the singular form of control he or she has. Often the mother is viewed as controlling and chronically depressed while the father is seen as passive. Feelings and differences of opinion are not commonly expressed in this enmeshed family system. Thus one can begin to understand the complex relationship between parent and child and its effect on developing behavior patterns.

When parents are unable to maintain their own roles, role reversal may occur, which draws the child into a parenting position, as in the case of incest. Incestuous relationships occur in families where generational boundaries are not clear. Finkelhor (1978) states that in incestuous families, there is a breakdown in the marital dyad. The mother appears chronically depressed and withdrawn, while the daughter and father rely on one another to fulfill both physical and emotional needs. The relationship between father and daughter is perceived by them as a means of keeping the family together. Finkelhor suggests that the mother does not condone the relationship but indirectly supports it because it does in fact assuage her guilt over not meeting her husband's needs. Thus role reversal and weak generational boundaries permit an incestuous relationship. Machotka et al. (1967) further support the premise of weak generational boundaries in their study of incestuous families. These authors found that the mothers often were dependent individuals who sought to assume a dependent role with their daughters—in essence creating the relationship they would have liked to have had with their own rejecting mothers. Father and daughter are seen as being abandoned by the mother. Denial on the mother's part allows the relationship to continue. Through her weak, passive behavior she may actually become the cornerstone of the incestuous relationship. Fearing abandonment herself, the mother may choose husband over daughter, leaving the child victim to assume responsibility for initiating and maintaining the incestuous relationship. In some cases, the wife's initial response is to divorce the husband, which leaves the abused child feeling blamed for the incestuous behavior or for the family disruption that resulted when the incestuous secret was disclosed. Giarretto et al. (1977) state that the victim of incest often is left with the feeling that sex is offensive or that sex is used to replace feelings of rejection and abandonment. Dysfunction in the marital couple needs to be corrected; reassignment of roles is a key factor in the incestuous family. Each adult member is given the task of assuming responsibility for the incestuous behavior. The goals of family intervention are to maintain family unity, to help each member to assume responsibility for his or her own actions, and to develop more effective, mature coping behaviors.

Family dynamics—relationships between parents, relationships between parent and child, inconsistent parenting skills, inappropriate expectations of child and adolescent behavior, lack of adequate support systems for parenting role, lack of effective problem-solving skills, inability to express feelings directly, lack of knowledge regarding normal growth and development, undifferentiated self with a poor sense of worth, residual unmet dependency needs, isolation and alienation as a family unit—are factors that may operate at critical points throughout the family life cycle and exert a profound impact on the growth and development of children within the family system. To fully understand family dynamics, these factors must be considered in the assessment and implementation phases of the nursing process.

Holistic relationship of factors

Each theory previously discussed suggests a distinct etiological underpinning for the development of psychopathology in children and adolescents. Research has demonstrated, however, that a particular temperament may be present at birth, as well as a preexisting vulnerability, that influences the manner in which the newborn later uses those capacities and biases to interact within the context of his or her environment. Severe ego dysfunction in children may also have an organic base. Profoundly disturbed behavior may elicit disorganized and dysfunctional responses from a parenting system that does not know how to cope with the disturbed behavior of a child. In some instances, there is evidence of emotional disturbance in one or both of the parents, which in turn reinforces inappropriate behavior in the child or adolescent. There is a reciprocal relationship whereby children are actively involved in shaping their environments while the environments act to mold their responses. The degree to which children can mold their environments depends in part on constitu-

tional make-up, organic factors, sociocultural influences (including societal expectations), and family interrelationships. Thus, it is impossible and inappropriate to consider the development of psychopathology in children and adolescents as emerging from one single causative factor.

TREATMENT MODALITIES

Family therapy

As has been noted earlier in this chapter, children and adolescents exist within the context of a family system. Thus, regardless of whether a child is in residential treatment or outpatient therapy, the family should be considered as part of the treatment process. Goren (1984) notes that the family enters treatment because the child is ill, but the remaining family members consider themselves healthy. Family function will improve, it is thought, if the child's behavior is altered. The goal of family therapy, then, is to reframe the problem as reflective of the dynamics of the family system. Goren suggests that the focus of intervention is to enable family members to understand that symptomatic behavior of the child continues because it is supported in many ways by other members of the family. For example, a sibling of a "good" child may find that a satisfactory method of gaining parental attention is through acting-out behavior. Goren adds that altering the acting-out behavior will influence the "good" behavior of the other child because both participants are necessary for the interaction to occur. Identifying the process of interactional effects within the system will assist family members in understanding their influences on others' roles. Improved communication with clearly stated expectations and increased expression of feelings are also critical outcomes of family therapy. Within the therapy setting, the nurse acts as a role model in the direct expression of feelings as they relate to specific situations. Parents learn that rules, regulations, and consequences can be determined and maintained. Positive reinforcement is offered to support appropriate parenting behaviors. Smith and Murphy (1984) state that parents can learn how to *listen* to one another and their children, as well as how to spend more productive interactional time with their children. The family therapy setting provides an arena where aspects of normal growth and development can be identified and explored, providing anticipatory guidance for both parents and children by increasing their awareness of developmental tasks and behavioral changes. Finally, through treatment, family members learn to use their own strengths and capabilities to develop more effective problem-solving methods (Goren, 1984). (For further discussion of family therapy see Chapter 12.)

Individual therapy

Individual therapy can be done on a verbal or play level; the choice depends on the ability of the child to verbally express feelings and on the child's cognitive level. Axline (1969) states that play therapy as a treatment modality uses the child's natural medium of self-expression. Hostility toward a doll, for example, can be more readily expressed with no repercussions than can hostility toward a newborn sibling. The manner in which children respond to various games, the roles they choose to play (mother, father), and the media they use (clay, water, paints) are critical assessment data. Through play therapy children are permitted to experience and explore their feelings in a trusting, stable environment where they can begin to define their own senses of individuality. Thus, the individual setting—whether on a verbal level or a play level—can be used to explore relationships with peers and with family members.

Smith and Murphy (1984) support Axline's premises and suggest that play therapy is appropriate for children from preschool age through latency, particularly in cases in which behavior has regressed from a higher level of functioning. Adolescent individual therapy may be used as a means to explore developmental issues such as achieving independence and coping with emerging sexuality.

Milieu therapy

Jones (1953), who initiated the concept of therapeutic community, believed that mental illness resulted from an individual's inability to function effectively within the context of interpersonal relationships. Thus, relationships with staff members and other clients have an influence on an individual client, and that influence is reciprocal. Clients mature and learn through their experiences within the milieu. Community meetings are an integral part of milieu therapy. Issues of daily living are raised and problem-solving is explored. Milieu therapy within the context of residential treatment provides a structured environment where new coping skills can be tested and more effective communication skills can be developed. Smith and Murphy (1984) state that milieu therapy for children must provide basic rules to follow and consistent consequences for noncompliant behaviors. Inconsistencies may result in confusion for the child and regressive behaviors. Principles of behavior modification may be used to reinforce positive behaviors. Smith and Murphy add that development of rewards and consequences must be determined in relation to age and comprehension level of the client population. Consideration also must be given to the frequency and duration of the consequences and rewards.

Group therapy

Moss (1984) notes that some current literature supports the validity of child group therapy for a variety of clients and using different approaches. An open, unstructured group may be used for school-age and latency-age children; topics can be decided on by group members themselves. Younger children may use the group setting as a means to learn cooperative play and to view their behaviors as they relate to their peers (Smith and Murphy, 1984). Smith and Murphy also suggest that staff-directed, structured groups can be useful in assisting children in learning and practicing more effective methods of handling feelings and difficult situations. Staff members select a particular topic and develop a role play, puppet, or story-telling activity to deal with the identified issue.

Group therapy may be used for a variety of purposes: to increase object development, to correct family experiences, to improve interaction with peers, and to reduce ego dysfunction. Moss (1984) supports the belief that group therapy can be a productive treatment modality for children and adolescents with many different types of problems: psychoses, physical handicaps, victims of abuse, school behavior problems, and mental retardation. Consistency and structure are critical elements in the success of group therapy. Moss further notes that a diverse group enhances the potential therapeutic effect. For example, a withdrawn child gains when he or she reaches out to help a child who is hyperactive. The hyperactive child, on the other hand, profits from focusing attention on the interaction. The strengths of one child can be used to support another child, within the context of that child's limitations.

Child group therapy can be a useful means to reduce psychological and emotional dysfunction. Various techniques can be utilized by the therapist, such as role-playing, behavior modification, and activities to facilitate development of interpersonal skills and more appropriate behavioral responses. It is important to note that the success of child group therapy depend on parental support. Moss (1984) and Kaplan and Sadock (1981) identify the need for concurrent parent support groups. Through such a group, parents gain a better understanding of their child's problems and strengths. The group setting provides an opportunity to discuss their own feelings and to explore more effective methods of coping.

Somatic therapies

Pharmacological treatment is used with caution. Major tranquilizers may be given to reduce severe personality disorganization. Kaplan and Sadock (1981) suggest that the drug of first choice should be a common one so that side effects and dosage level are more well known. Behaviors should be specifically targeted so that effects can be monitored accurately. Lowest dosages possible should be used, and their dosages should be increased gradually until target symptoms are reduced or side effects result.

Tricyclic antidepressants may be used for childhood and adolescent depressions, although DSM-III does not list these as separate disorders. Judicious use of imipramine (Tofranil) has demonstrated success in the treatment of separation anxiety disorder. Lithium is not currently approved for use with children under twelve years of age. As yet its efficacy in the treatment of major affective disorders in childhood has not been proved (Kaplan and Sadock, 1981).

Methylphenidate (Ritalin) and dextroamphetamine (Dexedrine) have been used with reasonable success in the treatment of attention deficit disorders. Side effects are for the most part transient and decrease as the dose is adjusted. Tofranil has also been used, yet Kaplan and Sadock note that there tends to be a higher incidence of side effects.

There is a controversy over the use of electroconvulsive therapy (ECT). Bender (1947) states that children can significantly improve following electroconvulsive therapy and are then more amenable to concurrent therapies. Kaplan and Sadock (1981), however, believe that there is no justification for the use of ECT in childhood disorders.

NURSING INTERVENTION

PRIMARY PREVENTION

Primary prevention in the area of child and adolescent mental health focuses on assessment or screening for risk. To provide a comprehensive assessment, nurses must be aware of the criteria for mental health and of those factors that influence the child's ability to respond and adjust appropriately to environmental and internal stimuli. Bumbalo and Siemon (1983) suggest that there are three areas to consider when screening for risk: (1) environmental factors, (2) parental characteristics, and (3) characteristics indicative of increased vulnerability. Based on an expansion of these factors, principles can be derived to act as guidelines for the development of goals in primary prevention. These are:

1. Emotional difficulties in children and adolescents often arise from faulty or inconsistent child-rearing practices.
2. Surface conflicts may emerge from developmental transitions such as entry into school and development of sex characteristics.
3. Environmental factors such as poverty, lack of adequate support systems, major cumulative life stresses, and maternal employment influence coping abilities of children and adolescents.
4. Constitutional factors, or those characteristics within the child or adolescent, affect level of individual vulnerability.
5. Children and adolescents who have a secure sense of self are able to engage in satisfying relationships, learn new skills, and perceive the world without distortion.
6. Cultural factors influence each family's perception of child-rearing practices.

The goals for primary prevention of emotional disorders in children and adolescents include:

1. Providing knowledge of normal growth and development to parents
2. Minimizing the effects of factors that predispose children and adolescents to emotional disorders
3. Screening groups that represent high-risk parental systems—that is, abusive families, indulgent families, families with chronic illnesses, and families that engage in drug or alcohol abuse.

Nurses in schools and in community agencies are in key positions to observe children in their school environments and in family interactions. Children may not be symptomatic yet exist within the context of a family environment that presents a potential risk. An assessment should address the following areas*:

---

*Adapted from Murphy and Moriarity (1976).

1. Environmental factors
   a. Socioeconomic level
   b. Maternal employment
   c. Adequacy of housing, food, and clothing
2. Social support, resources, functioning
   a. Adequacy and availability of support systems
   b. Stability of family system (including number of major life changes)
   c. Characteristics of parental system
      (1) Abusive behaviors
      (2) Alcohol or drug abuse
      (3) Chronic illness (either physical or emotional)
      (4) Overindulgent, immature
      (5) Rejecting
   d. Cultural and spiritual factors influencing child-rearing practices
   e. Relationships existing among family members
      (1) Discipline practices
      (2) Consistency of approach to children or adolescents
      (3) Presence of maladaptive coping measures
3. Developmental level of child or adolescent
   a. Age-appropriate behaviors and intellectual functioning
   b. Sense of body image and personal identity (including major changes due to trauma or illness)
4. Level of vulnerability
   a. Primary vulnerability (congenital deficits or those acquired during the first six months of life, such as sensory deficits, developmental disabilities, or difficult temperament)
   b. Secondary vulnerability (which results from the individual's reaction to environmental stressors previously noted).
5. Knowledge of normal growth and development
   a. Awareness of transition periods as stressors (for example, entry into school, going away to college)
   b. Awareness of situational crises (for ex-

ample, illness in the family, loss of employment)

This assessment considers the child within the context of the family, with an emphasis on the three primary factors as noted by Bumbalo and Siemon (1983). Further data may be included for each individual situation. Bumbalo and Siemon also state that specific techniques such as children's drawings are good projective sources of information. Nurses may also use peer ratings and teacher ratings to assist in identifying children and adolescents at risk.

Primary prevention actually begins within the context of the family environment. Many theorists suggest that children learn behaviors through early parent-child interactions. Child-rearing practices are carried from one generation to the next. For example, there is literature to support the fact that parents who are abusive to their children were abused themselves. Methods of coping and problem solving are learned through family interaction, which suggests that unhealthy methods of coping are also transferred to children.

Parenting is perhaps the most important task an individual will confront in his or her lifetime—yet little has been done to help people to be more effective parents. Parent effectiveness programs such as P.E.T. are addressing this issue; however, parents who are struggling with such problems as low income, inadequate housing, and lack of support systems are not likely to be able to afford the time and money to take part in these programs. Active attention needs to be directed toward these at-risk populations to assist them in identifying the stressors they are experiencing in parenting and to actively explore problem-solving measures that are effective (for example, how to negotiate with large government agencies, such as departments of social services, in order to meet their needs).

Families need to learn appropriate means of communicating directly and honestly—to express feelings rather than to channel them in unhealthy directions such as abusive or psychosomatic behaviors. Through authentic expression of feelings, family members will develop sound feelings of self-worth—a key factor in healthy growth and development. Stress reduction techniques can be taught to individuals so they can be active managers of their lives rather than passive victims. Parents need to recognize that they too have feelings and needs that require attention and expression. When these needs are thwarted, the frustration is often directed toward other members of the family. Parents and prospective parents can be assisted in recognizing their own needs and the importance of meeting those needs through effective problem solving.

Nurses as health care providers are active in this area of promoting physical and mental health. Health education, family life curricula in school systems, anticipatory guidance in the prenatal and perinatal periods, and support groups for parents are necessary elements in effective primary prevention. It seems that how children feel about themselves as they develop into adults is the foundation for their behavior as prospective parents. The development of a healthy self-concept as a child and an adolescent is an essential component of a sound foundation for parenting.

SECONDARY PREVENTION

It is increasingly apparent that the role of nurses in hospitals, clinics, schools, and community agencies is being directed toward case finding and early diagnosis. Through observation of children and adolescents in activities at school, church, or elsewhere in the community, as well as within the context of the family environment, nurses have the opportunity to detect early signs of stress, such as extended clinging behavior following the birth of a sibling or possible behavioral problems such as attention or conduct disorders. Secondary prevention is involved in addressing the following objectives:

1. Early identification of disorders of childhood and adolescence
2. Seeking prompt and effective treatment to restore individuals and their families to optimum levels of functioning
3. Assessment of community resources avail-

able (for example, for abuse victims and their families)

4. Expansion of community resources as is appropriate

Case finding is most critical in the area of child and adolescent mental health. Nurses as members of the primary health care team are in contact with children and their families throughout the life cycle. A community health nurse, while providing health services to a person newly diagnosed as a diabetic, might observe that one of the person's children is experiencing difficulty relating to strangers. If this behavior occurs over an extended period of time, it may be an early sign of overwhelming stress. Nursery school, elementary school, and secondary school settings are fertile ground for observation of behaviors that may be indicative of problems. Settings where children and adolescents gather to participate in activities are also prime target areas for early case finding. Although nurses may not always function directly with children and adolescents, they may act as consultants to those individuals, such as teachers, who are in positions of direct-line activity.

Early assessments may be tentative and are subject to validation with the family, including the child (when age appropriate), and other health team members. The nature of the relationship between the nurse who has identified the early signs and the child or adolescent is a critical factor. A comfortable, accepting atmosphere permits the individual child or adolescent to explore his or her potential difficulty within the context of an environment that is supportive and trusting. Parents may be resistant to others entering the family system and identifying difficulties that their children may be experiencing. Again, the circumstances under which the client system (the family) and the nurse come together will set the tone for the relationship in the future. Often nurses who first identify early warning behaviors do not feel prepared to resolve presenting behavioral disorders. Nurses may then refer the family to mental health resources such as child guidance clinics, school psychologists, or independent nurse psychotherapists, depending on availability, financial status, and preference of the family. In any case, the goal of early identification is referral to mental health resources for appropriate intervention.

The focus of secondary prevention is best stated by the Report of the Joint Commission of Mental Health of Children (1969). The goals of secondary prevention are to improve the actual conditions or behavior and to prevent the possibility of its deterioration. Goals for the family include restoration of family system functioning by increasing effective parenting and prevention of deterioration in the future. The following principles of secondary prevention apply to family systems regardless of symptom picture:

1. The focus should be on the individual child or adolescent as he or she exists within the context of the family system.
2. Family system behavior represents the most effective level of functioning at that given point in time.
3. Individual symptoms and behaviors are defense mechanisms designed to maintain ego integrity and reduce anxiety.
4. Support and empathy are necessary to establish a relationship that provides for effective problem resolution.
5. Behavior of one individual within the family system affects all other members, and there is a reciprocal response.
6. Nursing interventions should be directed toward alleviating symptomatic behavior and assisting parents in developing more effective strategies of parenting.
7. Nurses must recognize their own emotional responses to parents and children (for example, their own frustration with parental responses and child-rearing practices).

Knowledge of these basic principles will facilitate nursing intervention with children, adolescents, and parents who are experiencing emotional or behavioral disorders.

Nursing process

The nursing process acts as a framework for therapeutic intervention.

ASSESSMENT

Bumbalo and Siemons (1983) suggest that there are three primary means to collect data: (1) use of self, (2) use of data from the child and family, and (3) other assessment techniques. As these authors note, assessment data are basically invalid unless a therapeutic climate has been established. Meaning can be attached to data that signifies the "who, what, and how" of the problem. Without this significance of meaning, there is little rationale for doing the assessment.

The family and the child or adolescent are major sources of data. Questions will depend on the nature of the problem and the age of the child. The information gathered should provide a profile of the course of development—where difficulties lie, as well as strengths, duration of problem, effectiveness of coping strategies, problematic family behavior, and family relationships. The third area of assessment may be the use of specific tools as adjuncts to the sources of information previously noted.

The assessment should include the following*:

I. Child or adolescent interview
   A. Developmental screening (Denver Developmental); used for infants through preschoolers
   B. Major areas to be considered for all age groups
      1. Gross motor skills
      2. Fine motor skills
      3. Communication skills
      4. Social interaction (self-concept)
   C. Relationships with peers, authority figures, parents, and other family members
   D. Play behavior (solitary; fantasy)
   E. Emotional state (including affect and mood)
   F. Perception of world and his or her place in it

---

*This assessment guide draws on concepts from Critchley (1979), Bumbalo and Siemons (1983), and Lourie and Reiger (1974).

   G. Perception of presenting problem (if age appropriate)
   H. Coping measures and effectiveness
II. Parent system interview
   A. Perception of presenting problem
   B. Perception of developmental functioning (including knowledge of normal growth and development)
   C. Duration and frequency of behavior
   D. Effectiveness of relief measures
   E. Responses of other family members to current functioning
   F. Previous developmental or behavioral difficulties of this child
   G. Situational crises occurring with or prior to present difficulty
      1. Trauma
      2. Separation from significant others
III. Family assessment (See Chapter 12 for comprehensive assessment tool)

The family assessment considers the family unit in light of current stressors, availability of support systems, previous successful coping strategies, significant nodal events in the family life cycle, family constellation, differentiation of roles, maladaptive coping styles (for example, history of alcoholism, drug abuse, or physical abuse), knowledge and experience relative to successful parenting (including parental expectations), and cultural and religious factors influencing child-rearing practices.

Bumbalo and Siemons (1983) note the importance of validating information collected through the assessment process. They suggest that practitioners may use one or more of the following measures to validate the data:

1. Observations of the child or adolescent in more than one setting
2. Input from a second observer (determine interrater reliability)
3. Videotaping in school, play, or other appropriate settings
4. Review of previous health records
5. Consultation with other health team members

6. Sharing observations with parents and child when appropriate
7. Use of specific tools, such as Achenbach Child Behavior Profile and Coopersmith Self-Esteem Inventories, that have established reliability and validity

Through the process of validation of information, nurses can determine whether enough data have been collected to make inferences or whether further assessment is necessary.

ANALYSIS OF DATA

As nurses assess the child or adolescent within the context of the family, they may begin to understand not only the presenting problem(s) but also the complex interrelationship between family dynamics, vulnerability, precipitating factors, and problem-solving measures. The analysis of data leads to the formulation of nursing diagnoses. The next two sections will present nursing diagnoses that are frequently made—first those related to the parenting system and then those specifically related to the child or adolescent.

▶Family nursing diagnoses

Children and adolescents exist within the context of their family environments—whether the environment be a single-parent family, a reconstituted family, a nuclear family, or an extended family. Behaviors of children and adolescents reflect the mood and dynamics of the family in the sense that what occurs within the family setting may be exhibited in symptoms displayed by the child or adolescent. For example, a member of a dysfunctional marital dyad may displace frustrations with his or her spouse onto a particular child, who in turn displays disruptive behavior in school. It is critical that nurses understand the interrelationships of parent and child within the context of the system of as a whole. Families who have autistic children or children with childhood-onset developmental disorders may experience a mixture of ambivalence, guilt, anger, and frustration. These feelings may be projected onto others in the environment, such as other children, friends outside the family, or the health care professional. Conflict may exist within the family as to which is the best method of working with the child. One or both parents may attempt to deny that a problem exists, stating that the child will ''outgrow'' the disruptive behavior. In an attempt to protect the child from outside stressors, the parents may refuse assistance from other family members and friends, thereby eliminating any possible relief from the daily care of the child. This may result in a further escalation of anger, guilt, and frustration in the parental system. The effect of these feelings may be felt in the husband's or wife's job performance, other siblings' school participation, the family's social activities, and other areas of the family system.

Parents may lack appropriate parenting skills or knowledge of developmental phases, which may then cause the imposition of unrealistic expectations on the child or adolescent. For example, it is important that parents of an adolescent recognize the ambivalence of that phase—of the desire to be independent yet still be taken care of. Undue pressure, whether verbal or nonverbal, from the parental system can increase feelings of helplessness, hopelessness, and lack of a secure identity. Lack of knowledge of age-appropriate behaviors may result in parental frustration and anger, which can then be projected onto the child and increase the probability of inappropriate behaviors. This process, in turn, becomes a vicious cycle in which both parent and child experience frustration and a loss of control. Further family system disruption may occur when parents do not share similar perceptions and expectations regarding child care. Inconsistent messages are transmitted to the child that may immobilize the child or may potentiate present disruptive behaviors. Children may learn to manipulate the dysfunctional parental system, which may further increase disruptive behavior.

Thus, family diagnoses may include alteration in knowledge level of age-appropriate behaviors and tasks; alteration in consistent parental approach; inadequate knowledge of effective parenting skills; alteration in ability to manage disruptive child behaviors; and increased guilt and frustration relative to the presence of a developmentally disabled child in the family. The nurse's role is to:

1. Facilitate open lines of communication and effective problem-solving techniques
   a. Identify unrealistic parental expectations
   b. Help parents to explore personal feelings regarding parenthood and their childhood experiences with their own parents
   c. Explore effective means of resolving inconsistent parenting approaches
   d. Support ego strengths of parental dyad
   e. Reinforce effective parenting behaviors as appropriate (for example, for promoting progressively more independent behavior on the part of an adolescent)
   f. Encourage parental verbalization of feelings of guilt, anger, and frustration (for example, the frustration involved in caring for a mentally retarded child on a day-to-day basis or the guilt of a working mother who is leaving her child in a day care center for the first time)
      (1) Validate those feelings as expected and situation-appropriate
      (2) Explore more effective methods of resolving these feelings
2. Act as a resource person
   a. Provide information on parent effectiveness programs, normal growth and development, and age-appropriate behaviors
   b. Facilitate access to further mental health treatment (for example, psychotherapy, family therapy)
   c. Mobilize support systems (other extended family members; clergy; close friends; church groups) and stress importance of support for one another in parental dyad
   d. Suggest "relief" options for parents of severely disturbed children (for example, periodic babysitting; special schools; day camps)
   e. Explore residential treatment as is appropriate and support parental decision regarding residential placement

Again, one must recognize that children exist within the context of the family—each member influences the others. Parents' behaviors are molded by their current situation and experiences as well as their experiences with their own parents—each factor contributing to the perception and actualization of parenting behaviors. We have noted specific disruptive or dysfunctional behaviors of children and adolescents that merit specific interventions. However, we must conclude that those specific interventions must exist within the context of the family as a whole system. (For further discussion of family therapy, see Chapter 12.)

▶ Nursing diagnoses of children and adolescents

Nursing diagnosis: Alteration in ability to attend to appropriate stimuli (behaviors associated with DSM-III diagnosis 314.01 or 314.00: attention deficit disorders with or without hyperactivity)

Planning: Establish goals for the client initially (depending on the age of the client, participation in goal setting will occur as necessary).

1. Long-term goal: Modify inappropriate responses to environmental stimuli.
2. Short-term goals
   a. Finish one project to completion.
   b. Organize school work in a manner that is meaningful.
   c. Sit in one spot for increasing periods of time (in class, during meals).

Implementation:

1. Evaluate neurologically; use appropriate psychological testing to determine accurate diagnosis.
2. Administer medication judiciously and monitor target symptoms.
3. Structure the environment to minimize stimuli, in school as well as home.
   a. Provide a predictable environment and experiences that can be managed with little frustration.
   b. Encourage participation of the child in setting the structure.
4. Educate parents to set limits and to recognize

that permissiveness can be destructive.

5. Encourage open lines of communication between parents and child.
6. Use behavior modification to control impulsive and inattentive behaviors and to reinforce appropriate behaviors.
7. Provide physical outlets for motor restlessness.

Nursing diagnosis: Inability of child to protect self from physical and/or conditional abuse secondary to ineffective coping skills of parents (behaviors associated with DSM-III diagnosis V61.20: parent-child problem)

Planning: Collaborate with child (as is age-appropriate) and parents in setting goals.

1. Long-term goals
   a. Achieve increased level of positive parenting skills.
   b. Learn to individuate self as a worthwhile human being.
   c. Develop trusting relationship with a significant other.
   d. Reach maximum developmental potential.
   e. Continue as an intact family system when possible.
2. Short-term goals
   a. Verbalize feelings in an open direct manner.
   b. Identify situations that precipitate abusive behaviors.
   c. Develop more effective coping skills.

Implementation:

1. Observe for signs of physical and/or emotional abuse in at-risk families.
2. Assess parental dysfunction and ability to achieve meaningful change in parenting skills.
3. Treat symptoms of physical abuse promptly.
4. Provide a warm, caring environment for the abused child or adolescent.
5. Explore alternatives for reducing environmental and social stressors (for example, suggest "time-outs" for the mother such as day care or periodic use of babysitters).

6. Mobilize support systems in the environment.
7. Provide education as to normal growth and development and age-appropriate behaviors.
8. Reinforce parental efforts to use more effective coping skills.
9. Reinforce child's behaviors that are indicative of increased self-esteem.
10. Prevent separation of family members unless parents are unwilling to change their destructive behaviors.
11. Report abusive behavior to appropriate authorities.

Nursing diagnosis: Increased anxiety level secondary to inability to manage separations (behaviors associated with DSM-III diagnosis 313.21: avoidant disorder of childhood)

Planning: Collaborate with the child (as is age-appropriate) and the parents in setting goals.

1. Long-term goals
   a. Resolve internal conflict that generates ambivalent feelings regarding separation (parents).
   b. Return to school setting (child).
   c. Experience decreased level of anxiety.
2. Short-term goals
   a. Verbalize feelings of anxiety and ambivalence.
   b. Identify situations in the past which generated similar feelings.
   c. Develop more effective interpersonal coping skills.

Implementation:

1. Do a physical assessment to rule out any physical problems.
2. Encourage the child's return to school on a day-to-day basis.
3. Explore the child's fears of leaving home.
4. Recognize parents' and child's anxiety as real.
5. Assist parents in recognizing the effect of their ambivalent feelings on the child.
6. Reinforce positive attempts by parents and child to manage the separation.
7. Mobilize other support systems in the en-

vironment that parents can use.

8. Incorporate school nurse, teacher, and other school officials in the treatment plan.

Nursing diagnosis: Alteration in self-esteem with self-destructive behaviors (behaviors associated with DSM-III diagnosis 309.0: adjustment disorder with depressed mood)

Planning: Nurse initially establishes goals for the client (client participation in the goal-setting process will occur when the client is able).

1. Long-term goals
   a. Increase feelings of self-worth as a competent and functioning individual.
   b. Decrease use of self-destructive behaviors.
2. Short-term goals
   a. Identify feelings of anger, loneliness, rage.
   b. Identify situations that precipitate use of self-destructive behaviors.
   c. Use non-self-destructive methods of coping with feelings.

Implementation:

1. Provide an atmosphere where the client can begin to develop a trusting relationship.
2. Observe for signs of self-destructive behaviors.
3. Complete a suicidal risk assessment (see Chapter 18).
4. Provide suicidal precautions (if on an inpatient unit, see Chapter 18).
5. Reinforce appropriate coping measures.
6. Explore with client the effects of self-destructive behavior on his or her parents.
7. Facilitate open lines of communication between parents and client.
   a. Assist parents in recognizing seriousness of self-destructive behaviors.
   b. Help client to note contagious effects of suicide and to be alert to such acts in the local community.
   c. Educate parents regarding developmental tasks of adolescence and age-appropriate behaviors.
   d. Assist parents in differentiating age-ap-

propriate behaviors from age-inappropriate behaviors (withdrawal, change in peer relationships, poor school performance, change in regular activities).

8. Administer medication judiciously.

Nursing diagnosis: Alteration in ability to individuate self from environment, secondary to diminished sense of ego boundaries (behaviors associated with DSM-III diagnosis 299.0x: infantile autism)

Planning: Determine goals for the client.

1. Long-term goals
   a. Develop ability to recognize physiological and emotional needs as separate from those of other people.
   b. Increase level of trust.
2. Short-term goals
   a. Learn ways to increase sense of self as separate from others.
   b. Experience reduced anxiety levels generated by contact with others.

Implementation:

1. Work on a one-to-one basis with child.
2. Use touching and physical contact cautiously.
3. Assist child in identifying own parts of body correctly.
4. Point out differences between self and nurse through touch and other appropriate measures.
5. Use photographs of child, drawings, and mirrors to reinforce own boundaries.
6. Use self-directed activities such as dressing and feeding to reinforce self as separate from others.

Nursing diagnosis: Alteration in ability to achieve satisfactory interpersonal relationships with significant others (behaviors associated with DSM-III diagnosis 299.0x: infantile autism)

Planning: Determine goals for the client.

1. Long-term goal: Increase ability to establish trusting relationships.
2. Short-term goals
   a. Respond to touch and eye contact in an appropriate manner.

b. Interact in simple sentences expressing own needs.

Implementation:

1. Work on a one-to-one basis with child.
2. Provide an accepting, warm environment.
3. Encourage interaction with child through use of favorite toy or other object.
4. Initially use eye contact as means of interaction, with reinforcement for appropriate responses to nurse.
5. Use other modes of relating, such as touching, smiling, hugging.
6. Reinforce child's attempts to relate to others as he or she feels comfortable.
7. Accept child's need for physical distance at times.

Nursing diagnosis: Alteration in ability to control self-mutilating behavior (behaviors associated with DSM-III diagnosis 299.0 [infantile autism] or 299.9 [childhood-onset pervasive developmental disorders])

Planning: Establish goals for the client.

1. Long-term goal: Reduce self-mutilating behaviors.
2. Short-term goals:
   a. Recognize situations that precipitate head-banging, picking behaviors.
   b. Verbalize anxiety, anger, other feelings.
   c. Use other effective methods of expressing needs (for example, punching bag).

Implementation:

1. Point out situations that stimulate self-mutilating behavior.
2. Protect child while head-banging occurs, through use of helmet or other devices as necessary.
3. Encourage the use of other body gestures that enable the child to explore the environment.
4. Recognize increased levels of anxiety and prevent use of self-destructive behaviors.

Nursing diagnosis: Alteration in ability to control impulsive and autoerotic behavior (behaviors associated with DSM-III diagnosis 299.9: childhood-onset pervasive developmental disorders)

Planning: Establish goals for the client.

1. Long-term goal: Decrease autoerotic and impulsive behaviors as responses to increased anxiety levels.
2. Short-term goals
   a. Recognize situations that precipitate impulsive and autoerotic behavior.
   b. Verbalize feelings that result in increased anxiety levels.
   c. Use other, more adaptive measures to gain satisfaction from environment and to reduce anxiety.

Implementation:

1. Identify situations that precipitate impulsive and autoerotic behavior (sudden changes in the environment; loud noises; new experiences; distasteful orders).
2. Intervene in such situations before anxiety levels increase to severe panic levels.
3. Assist the child in confronting new experiences, noises, and so forth, by approaching them cautiously with a familiar person (such as a nurse).
4. Encourage use of other, more adaptive movements within the environment (rocking chair; exercise).

Nursing diagnosis: Alteration in family generational boundaries, resulting in maladaptive sexual relationship between father and daughter (behaviors associated with DSM-III diagnosis V61.20: parent-child problem)

Planning: Establish goals with the client and family

1. Long-term goal: Reestablish appropriate family generational boundaries.
2. Short-term goals
   a. Increase family members' ability to share feelings.
   b. Reduce child's anxiety levels and guilt feelings regarding relationship.
   c. Increase use of adaptive means of meeting needs within the family system.

Implementation:

1. Provide structure for family therapy.
2. Encourage each member to identify and share feelings of anger, frustration (for ex-

ample, wife toward husband; mother toward daughter).

3. Assist family in recognizing the worth of expressing feelings openly.
4. Provide ego support for members as they explore family issues that may be painful.
5. Reinforce appropriate family boundaries (such as mother-father sexual relationship).
6. Report abuse to proper authorities.
7. Support family through legal proceedings, if necessary.

Nursing diagnosis: Alteration in ability to control adolescent acting-out behavior (behaviors associated with DSM-III diagnosis V71.02: adolescent antisocial disorder)

Planning: With the assistance of the nurse, the client will establish goals.

1. Long-term goals
   a. Decrease use of socially unacceptable behavior.
   b. Increase adaptive behavior within the family as a whole.
2. Short-term goals
   a. Recognize situations that arouse anxiety, anger, frustration.
   b. Relate current stressful situations to past situations that generated similar feelings.
   c. Develop more effective interpersonal coping skills.
   d. Recognize influence of maturational task on current behavior.
   e. Identify behavioral responses as occurring within the context of the family.

Implementation:

1. Assist adolescent in identifying situations that generate anger and anxiety.
2. Explore other means of expressing angry feelings (for example, jogging, racquetball).
3. Intervene in situations before anxiety levels become overwhelming.
4. Reinforce verbalization as a healthy, adaptive mode.
5. Support ego strengths of adolescent as a competent human being.

6. Assist adolescent in managing life situations in a manner that is positively directed toward achieving developmental goals.

Nursing diagnosis: Alteration in ability to differentiate self and develop sense of own identity (behaviors associated with DSM-III diagnosis 313.21: avoidant disorder of adolescence)

Planning: The client will establish goals with the assistance of the nurse.

1. Long-term goal: Integrate life experiences as an independent person into a holistic sense of self.
2. Short-term goals
   a. Identify separations as potentially anxiety-producing situations.
   b. Verbalize feelings of ambivalence regarding independent status.
   c. Develop effective modes of coping that will facilitate current and future individuation.
   d. Realistically perceive self as multidimensional (biological, intellectual, phychological, sociocultural, spiritual).

Implementation:

1. Support current ego strengths—what the client has accomplished in his or her life.
2. Positively reinforce decisions client has made regarding separation (going away to college; finding own apartment).
3. Assist client in viewing self within the context of family as an independent person.
4. Explore potential changes in family relationships as a result of separation.
5. Explore family's role in individuation process of the client.
6. Support effective methods of coping with separation (verbalization of feelings honestly; recognition of process of separation as a form of grieving).
7. Share with client the maturational tasks of this period.

Nursing diagnosis: Alteration in eating patterns (either self-starvation or gorging and purging) related to disturbance in self-image and conflicts about sexuality and control (behaviors associated with DSM-III diagnosis 307.10 [anorexia nervosa] or 307.51 [bulimia])

Planning: The nurse may initially establish goals, but as therapy progresses the client should enter into goal setting.

1. Long-term goals
   a. Develop a positive self-image (refer to Chapters 7 and 18 for a discussion of self-image).
   b. Work through conflicts of sexuality and control.
2. Short-term goals
   a. Verbalize feelings of anxiety, inadequacy, need to control.
   b. Identify life situations (which may include family dysfunction) that generate anxiety, inadequacy, need to control.
   c. Recognize a relationship between stressful life situations and food-related coping behaviors.
   d. Develop non-food-related coping behaviors.
   e. Decrease manipulative behaviors (control tactics).
   f. Increase interpersonal skills.
   g. Realistically perceive the five dimensions of self (biological, intellectual, psychological, sociocultural, and spiritual strengths and limitations will be put in perspective).
   h. Establish healthful habits of nutrition and elimination.

Implementation: People with anorexia nervosa most often come into contact with professional nurses only after the behavioral pattern of self-starvation has been well established and they have become so emaciated and malnourished that survival is threatened. If this is the case, they must be admitted to a medical or psychiatric unit of a general hospital as an emergency measure. The following are aspects of nursing intervention for clients with anorexia nervosa or bulimia.

1. Maintaining nutritional needs is usually the major concern. The clients, who are usually young women, are resistant to treatment and adept at thwarting efforts to improve nutrition. Close supervision is necessary to identify and circumvent evasive measures designed to avoid food intake or to purge food from the body. Clients should be weighed in clothes that do not permit the concealing of weights in the clothing or on the body. When clients refuse to eat, nasogastric (NG) tube feeding or intravenous feeding may be instituted in a nonpunitive manner. NG tubes should be removed immediately after feeding to prevent siphoning. Clients may have to be accompanied to the bathroom to prevent the purging of food.
2. Anorectic and bulimic clients have a strong need to maintain control. Although superficially compliant, such individuals use manipulation and evasiveness to achieve this end. Schlemmer and Barnett (1977) point out that this manipulation, which is constantly encountered in their treatment, appears to be an effort on the part of clients to control themselves and the environment. These authors recommend that in controlling behavior, nurses should set limits, when necessary, and consistently and firmly maintain the limits. Clients should be informed of the limits and their purpose, and infractions should not be overlooked. Inconsistency on the part of staff members in maintaining limits is noticed by clients and may be used as a weapon against the staff later. Anorectic and bulimic clients fear loss of control over their own behavior and seem to welcome staff intervention.
3. An anorectic or bulimic client has a distorted view of himself or herself and a distorted body image. Such a person has an underlying lack of self-worth, which may be masked by an air of superiority and a sense of helplessness and hopelessness. Displaying an accepting attitude, being available when needed,

consistently pointing out misperceptions, and verbally recognizing and reinforcing authentic communication of feelings and perceptions are important ways that staff members can enhance anorectic or bulimic clients' self-worth and increase their trust in others.

4. Opportunities should be provided, when possible, for clients to have control over their lives and environment. They need to be helped to understand that they do have control over, and responsibility for, weight gain and for the establishment of healthy patterns of eating and elimination. Incentives may be offered that are in the client's control to achieve. For example, privileges may be increased with weight gain and decreased with weight loss.

5. Clients' feelings should be explored as they gain or lose weight. Clients should also be helped to verbalize their feelings about their self-images and about their families (family dynamics, family roles, family alliances). Nurses should encourage clients to seek out a staff member when they are feeling stressed, to share their feelings with a friend or relative, and to participate in activities and hobbies that will help to decrease their anxiety.

6. Nurses should explore with clients the secondary gains associated with their altered eating patterns. Expectations that clients will participate in activities of daily living and in therapeutic modalities should be clearly stated. Clients should not receive any special privileges or dispensations because of their anorectic or bulimic behavior.

EVALUATION

Evaluation of child and adolescent behavioral and emotional dysfunctions occurs within the context of the family system. It reflects client and family participation in the achievement of goals. In cases where individual client behaviors are targeted, evaluation should reveal a positive change in behavioral symptomatology—for example, reduction in autoerotic activity, increased attention span, and reduction in impulsive behaviors. Outcome evaluation of the family system should reflect improved communication among members, more effective parenting skills, increased level of knowledge regarding normal growth and development and age-appropriate behaviors, and, finally, more effective coping strategies.

During the evaluation process, the nurse identifies goals that may need to be modified and goals that are to be met in the future. Referral sources outside the nurse-client relationship, such as community agencies and significant others in the network of the client and family, are important factors in the ongoing success of the therapeutic process. Reinforcement of behavioral change and of learning to identify and cope with potentially troublesome issues will enable clients to assume increased control over their situations. The ability to recognize the need for outside assistance also needs to be reinforced as part of the evaluation process.

Finally, evaluation must reflect an assessment of the nurse's own self. Intervention with the family may generate feelings of anger, protectiveness, and disgust. Caring for victims of abuse, for example, may arouse feelings of anger toward the parents, which may in turn block effective intervention. The nurse's careful assessment of his or her own responses throughout the nurse-client relationship and during the evaluation phase is critical to the success of therapeutic intervention.

TERTIARY PREVENTION

Tertiary prevention should include provision of ongoing services for those children and adolescents who do not show improvement as a result of secondary interventions. The chronicity of the behavioral dysfunction may require referral to other specialized agencies for further treatment. Children who display severe ego impairment may need residential treatment or perhaps a day treatment center. Adolescents may also need to be placed in residential treatment if impulsive, acting-out behaviors continue to disrupt the family system. In some cases where truancy or juvenile delinquent behavior occurs, adolescents come in contact with the police and court systems. Residential treatment may then be offered as an alternative to a sentence of confinement.

The role of the nurse in tertiary prevention is varied. Nurses may provide ongoing group, individual, and family therapy for clients who present chronic behavioral and/or physical dysfunction. In addition, nurses may identify children, adolescents, and their families who exhibit chronically disturbed patterns of functioning, yet have not received any form of treatment. Finally, nurses may act as resource persons who can provide referrals for various treatment modalities and act as a link between client and resource facility.

The goals of tertiary prevention are to prevent or reduce the residual effects of long-term impairment. Interventive techniques are designed to restore the client and the family system to their optimum level of functioning.

nosis. The diagnosis may specifically target a behavior, such as autoerotic activity or adolescent impulsive, acting-out behavior. Intervention is designed to reduce the target symptoms of the individual. However, particularly with children and adolescents, the parenting system needs to be addressed as well. The nurse may use behavior modification techniques with the child or adolescent client. At the same time the nurse may act as an educative-supportive person for the parents, providing information on normal growth and development and age-appropriate behaviors. Nurses may provide ongoing group, individual, and family therapy. They may also function as a vital link between client and other appropriate resources in the community.

Thus, nurses play a valuable role in the promotion of the mental health of children and adolescents, as well as assist in the maintenance of optimum levels of functioning in children, adolescents, and their families.

CHAPTER SUMMARY

The field of child and adolescent mental health has historically received little attention in undergraduate curricula. However, nurses are in key positions to assess and intervene with new parents and children in school, camp, and clinic settings. Nurses are able to observe families as they interact in the community health setting. Identification of behavioral disturbances can be made earlier and intervention initiated to reduce the incidence of major pathological disturbances.

Child and adolescent behavioral dysfunctions may be viewed within the context of the family system. Underlying dynamics reflect a holistic interrelationship of factors: biological, psychodynamic, familial, and sociocultural. Nursing assessment is directed toward collecting data relative to the above-noted factors and making a nursing diag-

SENSITIVITY-AWARENESS EXERCISES

The purposes of the following exercises are to:

- Develop awareness of the vulnerability of families to the development of childhood or adolescent emotional or behavioral disorders
- Develop awareness about the interrelationship of factors in the etiology of childhood and adolescent disorders
- Develop awareness about the subjective experiences of clients who are suffering from these disorders and of the experiences of clients' families
- Develop awareness about your own feelings and attitudes when working with clients who are suffering

1. Try to imagine that you are a child or adolescent who is experiencing one of the following disorders, and explain why you selected that particular disorder. Then describe what you think it would be like to suffer from that disorder.
   a. Attention deficit with hyperactivity
   b. Anorexia nervosa

c. An incestuous relationship with a parent
d. Infantile autism
e. Withdrawal and depression
f. Impulsive behaviors
2. Describe what you think it would be like to have a family member suffering from one of the disorders listed in exercise 1. Which disorder do you think would be easiest to tolerate in a family member? Why? Which disorder do you think would be hardest to tolerate? Why?
3. What might be some of your feelings and reactions as a nurse caring for clients and families who are suffering from emotional disorders of childhood and adolescence? Would your feelings and reactions vary with the disorders experienced by clients? Explain why.
4. Imagine that you are a community health nurse engaged in health supervision activities with new parents. What high-risk factors (biological, psychological, intellectual, sociocultural, spiritual) would you look for that might predispose children to the development of emotional and behavioral disorders?
5. Develop a plan for counseling parents about child-rearing that incorporates principles and goals for the primary prevention of disorders of childhood and adolescence.

REFERENCES

Axline, V.
1969 Play therapy. New York: Ballantine Books.
Bell, R.J.
1971 "Stimulus control of parent or caregiver behavior by offspring." Developmental Psychology, p. 41.
Bender, L.
1947 "Childhood schizophrenia: clinical study of one hundred schizophrenic children." American Journal of Orthopsychiatry 17:40.
Berman, R.
1979 "Ego differentiation." In Basic Handbook of Child Psychiatry, vol. 2. J. Noshpitz (ed.). Basic Books, Inc., Publishers.
Blos, P.
1962 On Adolescence. New York: The Free Press.
Blumenthal, S.
1983 "Teen suicides: a growing problem in the U.S." New York Times, August 7, 1983, p. 3.
Bowen, M.
1978 Family Therapy in Clinical Practice. New York: Jason Aronson, Inc.
Bridger, W., and B. Birns
1968 "Experience and temperament in human neonates." In Early Experience and Behavior. R. Newton and S. Levine (eds.). Springfield, Ill.: Charles C Thomas, Publisher.
Bruch, H.
1970 "Psychotherapy in primary anorexia nervosa." Journal of Nervous and Mental Disorders 130:51.
Bumbalo, J., and M. Siemon
1983 "Nursing assessment and diagnosis: mental health problems of children." Topics in Clinical Nursing 5:41.
Cantwell, D., and G. Tarjan
1979 "Constitutional-organic factors in etiology." In Basic Handbook of Child Psychiatry, Vol. II. J. Noshpitz (ed.). New York: Basic Books, p. 28.
Chess, S., A. Thomas, and H. Birch
1970 "The origins of personality." Scientific American 223:102.
Cline, F.
1978 "Adolescent suicide." Nurse Practitioner 3:44.
Coolidge, J.
1979 "School phobia." In Basic Handbook of Child Psychiatry, Vol. II. J. Noshpitz (ed.). New York: Basic Books, p. 453.
Crisp, A.H., and D. Toms
1972 "Primary anorexia nervosa or weight phobia in the male: report on 13 cases." British Medical Journal 1:334.
Critchley, D.
1979 "Mental status examinations with children and adolescents: a developmental approach." In Nursing Clinics of North America. Philadelphia: W.B. Saunders, p. 429.
Cytryn, D., and R. McKnew
1979 "Depressive disorders." In Basic Handbook of Child Psychiatry, Vol. II. J. Noshpitz (ed.). New York: Basic Books, p. 233.
Durkheim, E.
1951 Suicide. New York: The Free Press.

Eaton, J., and R. Weill
1955 Culture and Mental Disorders: A Comparative Study of the Hutterites and Other Populations. Glencoe, N.Y.: The Free Press.

Evans, D.
1982 "Explaining suicide among the young: an analytical review of the literature." Journal of Psychiatric Nursing and Mental Health Services 20:9.

Fagin, C. (ed.)
1972 Nursing in Child Psychiatry. St. Louis: The C.V. Mosby Co.

Feigelson-Chase, N.
1975 A Child is Being Beaten. New York: McGraw-Hill.

Finklehor, D.
1978 "Psychological, cultural, and family factors in incest and family sexual abuse." Journal of Marriage and Family Counseling, 5:41.

Fish, B., and O. Ritvo
1979 "Psychoses of childhood." Basic Handbook of Child Psychiatry, Vol. II. J. Noshpitz (ed.). New York: Basic Books, p. 241.

Garfinkle, P.E., et al.
1980 "The heterogeneity of anorexia nervosa: bulimia as a distinct subgroup." Archives of General Psychiatry 138:1036.

Giarretto, H., et al.
1977 Coordinated Community Treatment of Incest. Workshop sponsored by the Connecticut State Department of Children and Youth Services.

Gladston, R.
1979 "Disorders of early parenthood." In Basic Handbook of Child Psychiatry, Vol. II. J. Noshpitz (ed.). New York: Basic Books.

Goren, S.
1984 "Points of view." Journal of Psychosocial Nursing and Mental Health Services 22:51.

Haley, J.
1980 Leaving Home: The Therapy of Disturbed Young People. New York: McGraw-Hill.

Hart, N. and Keidel, G.
1979 "The suicidal adolescent." American Journal of Nursing 79:80.

Hutt, C.
1974 "Sex: What's the difference?" New Scientist 62:405.

Joffee, J.
1969 Prenatal Determinants of Behavior. Oxford: Pergamon Press.

Johnson, C., et al.
1982 "Bulimia: a descriptive survey of 316 cases." International Journal of Eating Disorders 2:3-16.

Jones, M.
1953 The Therapeutic Community. New York: Basic Books

Jones, V.
1980 Adolescents with Behavior Problems: Strategies for Teaching, Counseling, and Parent Involvement. Boston: Allyn & Bacon, Inc.

Kanner, L.
1955 "To what extent is early infantile autism determined by constitutional inadequacies?" Proceedings of the Association for Research on Nervous and Mental Diseases 33:378-385.

Kaplan, H., and B. Sadock
1981 Comprehensive Textbook of Psychiatry III. Baltimore: The Williams & Wilkins Company.

Kalb, C.
1979 "Conduct disorder." In Basic Handbook of Child Psychiatry, vol. 2. J. Noshpitz (ed.). New York: Basic Books, Inc., Publishers.

Kempe, C.H., and C. Helfer
1980 The Battered Child. Chicago: University of Chicago Press.

Kessler, J.
1979 "Reactive disorders." In Basic Handbook of Child Psychiatry. Vol. II. J. Noshpitz (ed.). New York: Basic Books, p. 173.

Kiecolt-Glaser, J., and K. Dixon
1984 "Post adolescent onset male anorexia." Journal of Psychosocial Nursing and Mental Health Services, 22:10.

Laing, R.
1964 "Mystification, confusion and conflict." In Intensive Family Therapy: Theoretical and Practical Aspects. I. Boszormenyi-Nagy and J.L. Frano (eds.). New York: Harper & Row Publishers, Inc.

Lewis, M.
1979 "Differential diagnosis." In Basic Handbook of Child Psychiatry J. Noshpitz (ed.). New York: Basic Books, p. 243.

Lidz, T.
1963 The Family and Human Adaptation. New York: International Universities Press.

Looff, D.
1979 "Sociocultural factors in etiology." Basic Handbook of Child Psychiatry, Vol. II. J. Noshpitz (ed.). New York: Basic Books, p. 87.

Lourie, R., and R. Reiger
1974 "Psychiatric and psychological examination of children." In American Handbook of Psychiatry, ed. 2. S. Arieti (ed.). New York: Basic Books, p. 3.

Machotka, P., et al.
1967 "Incest as a family affair." Family Process 6:98.

McAnarney, E.R.
1979 "Adolescent and young adult suicide in the U.S.—a reflection of societal unrest?" Adolescence 14:765.

Minuchin, S.
1974 Families and Family Therapy. Cambridge: Harvard University Press.

Morgan, H.G., and G. Russell
1971 "The value of family background and clinical features as predictors of long-term outcomes in anorexia nervosa: a 4-year follow-up of 41 cases." Psychological Medicine 5:355.

Moss, N.
1984 "Child therapy groups in the real world." Journal of Psychosocial Nursing and Mental Health Services 22:43.

Murphy, L.B., and A.E. Moriarity
1976 Vulnerability, Coping, and Growth. New Haven: Yale University Press.

Potts, N.
1984 "The secret pattern of binge/purge." American Journal of Nursing 84:30.

The President's Commission on Mental Health
1978 Task Panel Reports, vol. 3. Washington, D.C.: U.S. Government Printing Office.

Report of the Joint Commission on Mental Health of Children: Challenge for the 1970's
1969 New York: Harper & Row, Publishers, Inc.

Rutter, M.
1970 "Sex differences in children's responses to family stress." In The Child in his Family. E. Anthony and C. Koupernick (eds.). London: John Wiley, p. 58.

Sameroff, A., and M. Chandler
1975 "Reproductive risk and the continuum of caretaking casualty." In Review of Child Development Research, Vol. 4. F. Horowitz (ed.). Chicago: The University of Chicago Press, p. 187.

Sanger, E., and T. Cassino
1984 "Avoiding the power struggle." American Journal of Nursing 84:30.

Schlemmer, J.K., and P.A. Barnett
1977 "Management of manipulative behavior of anorexic patients." Journal of Psychosocial Nursing and Mental Health Services 15:11.

Shaffer, D.
1974 "Psychiatric aspects of brain injury in childhood: a review." Developmental Medicine and Child Neurology 15:211.

Smith C., and K. Murphy
1984 "Developing a children's inpatient psychiatric unit." Journal of Psychosocial Nursing and Mental Health Services 22:31.

Spitz, R.
1951 "The psychogenic diseases in infancy." In Psychoanalytic Study of the Child, vol. 6. R. Eissler (ed.). New York: International Universities Press, p. 255.

Teicher, J., and J. Jacobs
1966 "Adolescents who attempt suicide." American Journal of Psychiatry 122:1248.

Watzlawick, P., J. Bearen, and D. Jackson
1967 Pragmatics of Human Communication. New York: W. W. Norton.

ANNOTATED SUGGESTED READINGS

Brady, K.

1979 Father's Days: A True Story of Incest. New York: Dell Publishing.

This is an account of the devastating effects of an incestuous relationship by the victim herself. She explores her feelings at the time of the relationship as well as the subsequent effect on her life in the future.

Guest, J.

1976 Ordinary People. New York: The Viking Press.

This book explores the effects of an adolescent's suicide attempt within the context of the family. It provides an insightful portrayal of a subject that is timely.

Haley, J.

1980 Leaving Home: The Therapy of Disturbed Young People. New York: McGraw-Hill.

This text explores relevant issues confronting adolescents and their families as they seek to complete the tasks of that period. The author presents specific interventions and supports these with examples from his own experience.

Kiecolt-Glaser, J., and K. Dixon

1984 "Post adolescent onset male anorexia." Journal of Psychosocial Nursing and Mental Health Services 22:10.

The article summarizes literature to date on postadolescent anorexia in males in relation to etiology and symptomatology. The authors identify the need for long-term studies of the efficacy of various therapeutic approaches to male anorexia. They also describe the need for multicenter collaboration to provide data on prognostic features for this poorly defined subgroup.

McElvoy, E. (ed.)

1979 "Symposium on child psychiatric nursing." Nursing Clinics of North America, September, pp. 389-482.

This collection of articles explores a wide range of topics relevant to the practitioner of child mental health nursing. Areas included are legal rights of children, mental status exam of children, a systems approach to emotional disorders, child abuse, and behavioral aspects of physical disease.

Pothier, P. (ed.)

1984 "Focus on the child." Journal of Psychosocial Nursing and Mental Health Services, vol. 23, no. 2.

The March issue is devoted to issues in child and adolescent mental health. Topics addressed are child therapy group attachment, new roles of the school nurse, development of children's inpatient units, and the effects of chronic disability on well siblings.

Sanger, E., and T. Cassino

1984 "Avoiding the power struggle." American Journal of Nursing 84:30.

This article presents an overview of an inpatient program for anorectics based on a privilege/restriction formula. The authors describe assessment criteria, treatment modalities, evaluation of strategies, and discharge planning. It is a well thought out and logical article that provides clear-cut methods of addressing this relevant topic.

FURTHER READINGS

Fox, K.

1980 "Adolescent ambivalence: a therapeutic issue." Journal of Psychiatric Nursing 18:27.

CHAPTER 16

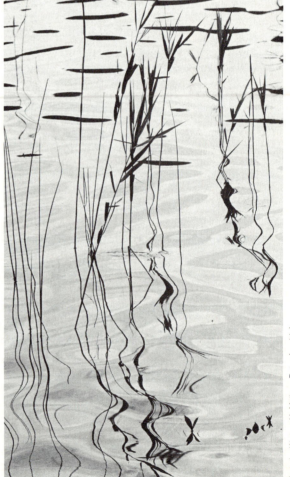

Photo by Werner H. Müller—Peter Arnold, Inc.

Coping through psychophysiological responses

CHAPTER FOCUS

This chapter focuses on psychophysiological responses to stress. It emphasizes the fact that such responses have many causes—including environment, genetic considerations, and interpersonal and intrapersonal factors—and that they all require equal weighting in the assessment process. Nurses as health care providers must begin to view the psychophysiological response as a two-way rather than a one-way process of interaction. Psychological factors such as anxiety, guilt, and shame affect the development of physiological responses. The reverse also occurs: a physiological response may then reinforce or intensify the feelings of anxiety, guilt, or shame. The two components act together to maintain a psychophysiological dysfunction.

The chapter includes a classification of dysfunctions. For each dysfunction, the underlying dynamics and the methods of expression of anxiety and communication of needs are described briefly. Specific etiological theories are presented in detail in a section devoted to that topic. Emphasis is placed on an *integrative* approach to the understanding of clients who express their needs through psychophysiological responses. The modalities of treatment described in this chapter reflect the fact that persons who exhibit psychophysiological responses to stress are seen more frequently in general hospitals than in psychiatrists' offices. This fact has implications for primary, secondary, and tertiary levels of prevention. Primary prevention deals with the identification of high-risk individuals or groups—for example, persons with type A personality (individuals who continually subject themselves to high levels of stress, such as high-powered business executives) and persons whose families used psychophysiological responses as appropriate methods of communicating needs. The chapter emphasizes the importance of parental counseling in relation to early interactional patterns within the family group and the significance of unmet needs and the eventual expression of those needs or feelings in later years. Secondary prevention directs attention to behavioral problems and appropriate nursing responses. Tertiary prevention involves the use of value clarification to help clients understand the origins of the stress they are experiencing. In addition, the use of adaptive methods to express needs should be encouraged by the nurse. The family and other significant social support systems are necessary components of tertiary care. Clients who communicate needs through psychophysiological responses should be assessed from a multifactorial frame of reference. Nurses must consider all relevant information to determine a nursing care plan that reflects the interaction of predisposing factors and precipitating events.

HISTORICAL PERSPECTIVES

Traditionally, the intricate interrelationship of physiology and psychology has been a question of interest and consternation. Cannon (1929) demonstrated that changes in organ secretion and muscle tension occur as a result of arousal of emotions. Selye (1956) suggested that stress causes the arousal of psychological and physiological responses and that the two responses combine to cause organ changes. Freud, in his study of conversion reactions, also noted the significance of the interrelationship of emotions and physiological responses.

We can no longer consider the dichotomy between mind and body appropriate when we assess an individual's health status. Nor can we predict that a stressor will lead to a certain set of responses. Each human being represents a complex interrelationship of internal and external factors. As we propose in the section on etiology that appears later in this chapter, cognitive, genetic, communication, learning, and psychoanalytic theories all must be used to explain psychophysiological responses, because experience, environment, personality type, and defense and coping strategies all combine to produce the responses. It is from such a perspective that nurses must work to determine an appropriate and comprehensive nursing care plan.

UNDERLYING DYNAMICS

Illness frequently is related to personality type and predetermined patterns of response to stress. Various physical symptoms may be related to the experience of stress in the environment. As we pointed out before, however, such a process does not operate in isolation from other significant factors. It is thus important to identify issues such as dependence, hostility, and self-esteem that arise as nursing problems in connection with the care of clients experiencing psychophysiological dysfunctions.

Dependence

Some clients are unable to express feelings of dependence and to feel comfortable being taken care of. Early patterns of interaction may have prohibited the expression of dependence needs. These needs then may have been translated into "words" that were expressed through the autonomic nervous system. Implicit messages from significant others and from society as a whole may prevent a person from acting out his or her dependence needs. For example, an active middle-aged man who experiences a heart attack may be unable to accept staying in bed. Denial of dependence needs is often a key issue in such a situation.

Hostility

Inability to express anger or resentment is another critical behavioral problem. Unacceptable hostile impulses and frustrations may be chronically repressed. This repression may be a response learned from early interactions with significant persons. Environmental factors may further accentuate the repression of these emotions. Expression of anger or resentment through psychophysiological responses may have been implicitly encouraged through the very same interactional patterns that prohibited the verbal expression of such emotions. Nurses need to remember that the development of a psychophysiological response is the result of a complex interaction among many factors.

Self-esteem

Self esteem is always a significant factor in a person's health status. When an individual is unable to communicate needs directly, there is a resulting loss of self-esteem. The degree of loss depends on the length of time such a pattern has existed, the repertoire of coping and defense mechanisms and their efficiency, the availability of active support systems, and the number and type of stressors operating at any given time. Loss of self-esteem may result from a client's inability to accept a less independent state. Increasing the client's ability to directly express needs will increase the likelihood that the client will feel better about himself or herself.

• • •

Through the process of exploring issues of dependence and anger, the client can identify his or her role in the interaction with significant others. With the support of others, the client can be assisted to deal with the anger and hostility associated with dependence. He or she can be helped to see that anger or resentment can be discussed during interactions with others.

It is important to reemphasize the complex interrelationship of factors that results in a psychophysiological response. Intrapsychic issues, life stresses, personality organization, environmental supports, and biochemical factors act in conjunction to *increase the probability* that a psychophysiological response will occur.

CLASSIFICATION OF PSYCHOPHYSIOLOGICAL DYSFUNCTIONS

Peptic ulcer

The client experiencing a peptic ulcer is not necessarily of any one personality type. Characteristically, there is a longing to be cared for and loved, which is repressed and replaced by aggressive behavior. In some cases, however, clients may be overly dependent or demanding—a situation that causes them to feel that they are being repudiated because of their dependent state. Thus, unconscious conflicts and negative responses from the environment for dependent behavior may be two factors forcing a client to maintain an independent stance. When the need for love cannot be met through a relationship, it may be converted into a wish to eat. The stomach then remains in a constant state of preparation for food. It is interesting to note that ulcer pains are relieved by food and exacerbated by hunger. In essence, food is equated with being loved (Cheren and Knapp, 1980).

No single factor is responsible for ulcer formation. Genetic predisposition to hypersecretion, relatively strong oral-dependent traits, increasingly high levels of stress in life experiences—these characteristics coupled with thwarted dependence needs encountered in later life and a limited repertoire of coping and defense strategies increase the probability of the occurrence of ulcers.

Individuals experience an exacerbation of ulcer symptoms when current sources of gratification are no longer available for whatever reason. Freedman et al. (1980) note that both men and women waiver in their need to be active and independent while also desiring to be taken care of. Women in particular present a profile that is typified by over-responsible and independent behavior. Internal conflict emerges as a result of the inability to express anger, frustration, and anxiety, which is then directed into the gastrointestinal system. Interestingly enough, when surgery is performed to relieve symptoms, the client substitutes other psychophysiological symptoms in response to stressful situations.

Ulcerative colitis

Ulcerative colitis may develop as a result of unmet dependence needs as well as feelings of guilt. The capacity for ego integration in a person with this condition is poor, and he frequently uses projection—diarrhea literally becomes a way of projecting unacceptable impulses onto the environment.

It has been suggested that genetic and autoimmune factors play a significant role in the onset of symptoms. Stressful situations cause a disequilibrium in the body's immune system that in turn facilitates the movement of anticolon antibodies. As a result of the increase in the number of antibodies in the colon, the bowel becomes increasingly irritable and hyperactive, leading to the onset of diarrhea.

As in the client with peptic ulcer symptoms, it seems that these individuals are dependent, unable to accept dependence, yet cannot express their unacceptance, so they exhibit passive-aggressive tendencies. Typical behaviors of ulcerative colitis clients include excessive intellectualization, hypersensitivity to rejection, limited affective responses, and distant social relationships with others. Aggressive feelings are again directed through the gastrointestinal tract. In this manner, anger is controlled (although ineffectively) and the threat of rejection is reduced.

The onset of ulcerative colitis is frequently associated with periods of emotional stress. Experiences relating to loss—of a body part, a relationship, or status, for example, with concurrent loss of self-esteem—are significant factors in the development of colitis. The response to loss is often characterized by hostility and depression. The inability to form a relationship of significance may result from the early mother-child relationship. In many cases the mothering figure was domineering, hostile, and rejecting. The child was left feeling helpless and unable to express rage. A nurse must be aware of genetic predisposition, personality pattern, strategies of coping, the degree to which stress is perceived as threatening, and the degree of unmet dependence needs to determine a nursing care plan that reflects the interrelationship of all factors (Kaplan and Sadock, 1981).

Asthma

Asthma has historically been identified as the "typical" psychophysiological response. Asthma's notoriety results in part from its relationship to a vital function—breathing. The influence of emotions on the functioning of the respiratory system is evidenced in such statements as "The scenery was breathtaking" or "The experience took my breath away." The etiology of asthma involves many factors—organic as well as psychological. Many personality types are seen among asthmatic clients. Some are aggressive-compulsive; others are hypersensitive to other people. Some asthmatic clients have an exaggerated dependence on the mothering figure that arouses conflict when the relationship is threatened. This situation does not result in a wish to be fed, as in the case of an ulcer client, but in the need to be protected. A recurrent theme of maternal rejection or attempts on the part of parents to make a child independent too quickly is often noted. The child is assumed to be mature; however, he is not mature, and, as he is forced to be mature, his insecure feelings about himself rapidly heighten. Dependent longings are viewed negatively. The child is not allowed to express feelings—particularly to cry. Thus an asthmatic attack can be viewed as being symbolic of the wish to reestablish a relationship with the mothering figure.

No single factor or theory can accurately account for the asthmatic response. Some theories suggest a strong correlation between stressful events—for example, seeing a picture of a dead parent or going to a place that the individual had frequented with the parent—and the onset of an asthmatic attack. According to this theory, hyperventilation occurs as a conditioned response to a conditional stimulation (the stressful event). Bronchial spasms and increased mucous secretions then occur, which may increase the individual's anxiety. The increase in anxiety then results in the asthmatic attack.

According to another theory, psychosocial stressors that threaten a person's current relationships activate familiar unpleasant feelings from past relationships with significant others. Fear of rejection and feelings of helplessness, lack of control, and dependence are generated, which have the *potential* to initiate an asthmatic response. Asthmatics respond to stress by regressing. When this defense is ineffective, the asthmatic attack occurs, which in effect discharges pent-up emotions such as anger, fear, or anxiety.

Obesity

To understand obesity, it is necessary to clearly identify two physiological processes—satiation and the act of feeding. The hypothalamus controls these processes. However, such physiological functions are also affected by parental influences, genetic predisposition, sociocultural determinants, amount of activity, psychological or physical stressors, and level of development. Within the family environment, the infant begins to develop an awareness of eating and hunger, as well as satiety of hunger. It is believed that satiety is not discriminated; thus it is not learned. In other words, the young child does not learn, through parental interaction and feedback, to eat to satisfy his hunger but rather to eat in an indiscriminate fashion.

Assessment of early family relationships is significant since a pattern leading toward obesity often develops in early childhood. Parents are often frustrated with their own lives and tend to live vicariously through the lives of their children. Parents frequently believe that they had difficult lives as children, and they are therefore determined that their own children will not experience the same frustrations they did.

However, feelings of resentment may be nonverbally transmitted to the child. The child may be viewed as an extension of the parent. As this view is perpetuated through infancy and early childhood, the child may be unable to develop an adequate sense of self. In adolescence, such an individual experiences difficulty in the accomplishment of a sense of identity. He becomes a passive, submissive person who has internalized feelings of resentment and hostility.

Instead of verbalizing feelings of affection, parents, particularly the mother, sometimes force food on a young child as a means of demonstrating love. The critical factor seems to be that often these children are not wanted. This message is transmitted to the child. Food then is equated with love and satisfaction. This dynamic can be demonstrated repeatedly in later, adult relationships. Forceful feeding rather than allowing a child to eat according to his hunger and satiety leads to his developing a distorted perception of his body. Bruch (1973) believes that the child who does not learn to respond to his own cues regarding hunger and satiety is unable to determine how much he should eat. Bodily distortion becomes an integral component of such an individual. By the time he reaches adulthood, the obese body image will have become a means to receive attention and praise. It may be the single factor that draws others close to him.

Characteristically, an obese person has poor ego strength, lacks a sound self-concept, and harbors repressed feelings of hostility toward the parental pair—particularly the mother. Because of the underlying low self-worth, the obese individual may experience difficulty in love relationships. Frustration results, and the excessive eating behavior is reactivated, as in past situations. Parents pushed food as a means of controlling anxiety and giving love; the obese client has internalized this mechanism, which is reactivated in an anxiety-provoking situation. Eating is equated with satisfaction and thus becomes a predominant defense.

Many factors can be involved in the development of obesity. For example, social factors such as class are relevant. It has been noted that members of lower-class families are more likely to become obese than are members of middle- and upper-class families. This situation may be caused by the frustration and hostility generated as a result of being unable to meet the most basic needs for survival.

An assessment of the strength of the need to eat as a means of maintaining personality integration is a necessary nursing measure. A weight-reduction program may be very anxiety provoking; it can cause a severe shift in the psychological equilibrium of a client.

Anorexia nervosa

The cluster of symptoms that characterize an anorectic client includes severe weight loss, absent or irregular menstrual periods, loss of sexual desire, and decrease in endocrine function with a resultant decline in growth rate. There is a mortality rate of 10% to 15% (Kaplan and Sadock, 1981). Anorexia nervosa occurs primarily in adolescent girls. The adolescent experiences a fear of being rejected by the mothering figure and often needs special attention to feel loved. Unconscious aggressive impulses take the form of envy and jealousy toward persons—often siblings—who receive such attention. Ambivalence is characteristic of the mother-daughter relationship. Hostility toward the mother exists, yet the daughter feels threatened by the thought of having to assume independence. The adolescent's cessation of eating may be a rebellion against parents. A feeling of loss of control and a sense of ineffectiveness and helplessness are also characteristic of the anorectic adolescent.

Several factors, then, interact to lead to anorexia: intrapsychic conflicts, overall personality traits, early parent-child interactions, past experiences, and present situations that reactivate feelings of dependence and helplessness. Current situations in an adolescent's life, such as the establishment of the first sexual relationship, may act as precipitants. Loss of the sense of one's childhood and of one's dependent status may also initiate the anorectic syndrome. The illness causes the family to shift its attention toward the anorectic child—an unconscious secondary gain for the child.

Minuchin and associates (1978) place a great deal of emphasis on the view that the syndrome involves the entire family even though the symptoms are expressed only through the adolescent member. They argue that anorexia encompasses the behavior of all family members. Overprotection in the form of excessive concern for psychobiological needs is apparent in such a family. The child develops the same excessive awareness of bodily needs. The child is also quite aware of her effect on the interactions in the family. There is a dependence on parental assessment, leading to inhibition of the development of independence and control over one's life. In addition, there is usually an excessive concern with eating and dieting. Members of the anorectic family are overinvolved in each other's lives, with a resultant loss of individuation. Conflict is negated by the use of the children—particularly through the use of the anorectic child's symptoms. In essence, the anorectic child is charged with maintaining the status quo of the family. When the status quo has been maintained, the symptoms are reinforced. This pattern continues even though family members may feel exploited. In a sense, everyone wins but also loses in such a situation. The anorectic child receives attention and feels in control, while other family members are able to avoid conflict once again. The dysfunction continues even though all members of the family are experiencing some level of discomfort. The ultimate goal of avoiding conflict is maintained.

Bruch (1973) delineates two types of anorexia nervosa. Primary syndrome anorexia is characterized by hyperactivity, continual seeking of perfection, preoccupation with food, and the pursuit of a thin body. The last aspect is often perceived as crucial in the anorectic person's search for identity. Food is frequently taken in only to be regurgitated—possibly because of overwhelming guilt for having eaten. The atypical syndrome is characterized by an overconcern for the actual function of eating. There is little evidence of the other characteristics.

The nursing assessment should reflect a consideration of all factors and their implications for client and family behavior. A comprehensive nursing care plan may be determined. There does not seem to be one specific therapy that has achieved success. The most important considerations are the predominant themes and the degree of starvation. (See Chapter 15 for an in-depth discussion.)

Migraine headaches

Clients who release anxiety through migraine headaches are best described as perfectionists who set exceptionally high standards for themselves and others. They are compulsive in their attention to detail and are not likely to delegate responsibilities. There is a characteristic repression of hostile impulses. Although they are of superior intelligence, they may not be as emotionally mature as their peers. They have a genetic predisposition to vasodilation. The onset of a migraine can often be related to a stressful event. The occurrence of a migraine frequently leads to episodes of vomiting, diarrhea, and vertigo. Clients are virtually immobilized until the persistent headache subsides. A lesser form of migraine is the "tension" headache, which is commonly experienced as a response to stress. When completing an assessment, a nurse should rule out the possibility of organic causes before attributing the headache to stress factors (Kaplan and Sadock, 1981).

Cardiovascular dysfunctions

Cardiovascular dysfunctions are frequently identified as being stress related. When stress becomes chronic, the cardiovascular system experiences changes in heart rate, blood pressure, and strength of contractions. As was stated in Chapter 7, these changes can then act as stressors in and of themselves, with resulting increases in anxiety levels.

Much emphasis has recently been placed on the type A personality as described by Friedman (1969). Such individuals are characterized as hardworking, competitive, and aggressive; they invest a great deal of energy in many commitments. These individuals usually occupy upper-level management positions. They frequently feel that their jobs or businesses cannot go on without them; they pay little attention to vacations or to time that could be spent pursuing personal or family interests.

It is imperative, of course, that nurses also consider other factors that are relevant to the increased incidence of cardiovascular disease (which includes coronary artery disease, angina, myocardial infarction, and congestive heart failure). Genetic and constitutional factors such as cholesterol levels are interrelated with personality factors, socioeconomic factors, and cultural factors.

Individuals who experience cardiovascular dysfunction are characterized as being controlled; they do not readily display emotions. Dependence needs and hostile impulses are repressed. Denial of dependence needs can take the form of not adhering to the cardiac regimen after myocardial infarction. In such a situation, the denial can be life threatening. Being controlled by hospital routine can be perceived as threatening, which may result in increased anxiety and further cardiac dysfunction.

Stressors in the environment—social, economic, cultural—may threaten an individual's sense of control, leading to increased incidence of cardiac dysfunction. An example of a stressor might be a change in job status that has social, economic, and cultural implications for the individual.

Nurses might care for a cardiac client who has excessive needs for dependence but is unable to express those needs verbally. Hospitalization and illness might permit an individual to give up some of his or her responsibilities—for example, to self, family, and job. It is often difficult for a client to make strides toward improvement if the secondary gains of illness are attractive.

Cardiac neurosis or "effort syndrome" is not characterized by structural changes in the cardiovascular system or by electrocardiogram changes. An individual with this condition does, however, experience shortness of breath, chest pain, rapid heart rate, dizziness, and several other symptoms of cardiac dysfunction. The condition seems to be related to an underlying conflict that involves unmet dependence needs and repression of hostile impulses. Personality factors, particularly immaturity, interact with stress occurring within the individual's interpersonal, social, and/or cultural spheres. It is important for the nursing assessment to include a physical examination to determine whether any physiological changes have occurred. If the results are negative, concern should be directed toward the identification of bio-psycho-social factors that may be precipitating the cardiac neurosis.

Essential hypertension

Bottled-up rage—a phenomenon that resembles the action of a pressure cooker—is the concept underlying the expression of tension through the cardiovascular system. The client's conscience will not permit the expression of angry impulses, even though dependent relationships are being threatened. His or her sense of guilt acts as a stop-gap measure. This mechanism continues until a pattern of repression of hostility is developed. The repeated vasoconstriction that results leads to irreversible changes in the cardiovascular system—particularly in persons who seem to be predisposed to hypertension. Characteristically, during early life experiences the individual was charged with an increased sense of responsibility. He or she was

not permitted the luxury of being angry, because of the implied message that a responsible individual does not show his or her anger. This behavior may have been learned from significant others in the environment and positively reinforced as a method of coping. The personality of the individual who has hypertension masks the intrapsychic conflict by displaying a calm, serene facade. This facade permits the individual to maintain relationships and thus to meet dependence needs. Socioeconomic, genetic-constitutional, cultural-ethnic, interpersonal, and intrapsychic factors interact to increase the probability that hypertension will develop. For example, a black American who is experiencing high levels of stress—perhaps as a result of divorce proceedings or loss of a job—may be prone to developing hypertension. No one factor is responsible alone for the development of hypertension, although the emotional component does seem to be significant (Kaplan and Sadock, 1981).

Arthritis

Clients who express their tension through the musculoskeletal system in the form of arthritis are often described as extroverts—jovial, happy, and interested in athletic activities. Arthritic clients may experience a chronic state of inhibited rebellious hostility, which is frequently related to strong dependence needs. One dynamic pattern suggests an overprotective parental influence, particularly on the part of the mother, which eventually causes a repression of hostile tendencies. Hostility is sublimated into physical exercise—particularly competitive sports. Arthritic individuals maintain control over their environments to prevent the expression of hostile impulses. Increased muscle tonus results from this prolonged inhibition of hostile impulses. The degree of inhibition is directly proportional to the degree of contraction of the muscle; the more repressed the hostile tendencies, the greater the contraction (Shontz, 1975).

Although personality factors and intrapsychic conflicts seem to play a significant role in the development of arthritis, genetic and constitutional factors, biochemical changes, and precipitating stressful events must also be considered. For example, stressful events cause changes in the levels of hormones and adrenocorticoids. These substances play a role in the development of collagen, a form of connective tissue. As hormone and adrenocorticoid levels change, there is a resulting change in the nature of the connective tissue formed, leading to arthritis. Stressors that precipitate the onset or reappearance of symptoms may be bio-psycho-social or cultural in nature. Often the stressor occurs in the form of a loss that is perceived as threatening to the dependence needs of an individual. Unresolved feelings of anger are then transferred to the musculoskeletal system. The interrelationship of genetic factors, intrapsychic conflicts, biochemical changes, and precipitating stressors—particularly those revolving around loss—must be an integral part of the nursing assessment.

Cancer

The correlation between psychological stress and the onset of neoplastic disease has been suggested by several research studies. There seems to be a complex set of interactions rather than a direct cause-and-effect relationship.

LeShan (1977) and Bahnson and Bahnson (1966) noted that the loss of a significant, intensely dependent relationship often occurs just before (within twelve months) the appearance of symptomatology. The loss may reactivate unmet dependence needs that were generated in the early mother-child relationship. Hostility, which the client cannot express openly, is aroused as a result of the loss. The loss may center around a personal relationship, a job, status in the community, or control over one's environment. As a result of responses that were learned in early parental interactions, the individual must repress his or her hostility in order to be ''the good person.'' The early mother-child relationship is characterized by an impoverishment of affection, by strong unresolved tensions, and by poor communication lines. The

child learns not to express feelings, not to expect much from anyone, and not to become angry.

As in the other psychophysiological responses, there is no single cause leading to the outcome. Biological factors, including changes in endocrine and metabolic function, occur as a result of stress. Genetic and constitutional predisposition may cause an individual to be more vulnerable to these endocrine and metabolic changes. A decreased immunological response resulting in a reduced antibody reaction may have occurred as a result of early infantile relationships. Stress in current life situations may act as a precipitant leading to a reduced antibody response in adult life. Greene (1966) suggested that anxiety and depression related to precipitating loss events such as death of a spouse or separation from spouse, children, or significant others were often factors in the etiology of cancer. This statement implies that, in such cases, early resolution of loss situations was not handled appropriately. Coping mechanisms were used to deny or repress the hostility, and feelings of dependence were generated by the unresolved loss situations.

Simonton (1980) suggests that the belief system cancer victims hold has a significant impact on their ability to cope with illness and sustain a longer survival rate. He notes that those individuals whose survival rates seem to be longer were more feisty and had a positive outlook on their own ability to effect some control over their illnesses. These individuals tended to be more assertive and, more aggressive, and were often characterized as ''difficult'' patients because they would not necessarily go along with the prescribed regimens. This is not to say that these individuals ignored the facts of their situations but rather that they accepted the challenge of their own illnesses and sought to be actively involved in their lives to the very last.

LeShan (1977) notes further that those individuals who are cancer prone tend to be negativistic in their outlook on life, do not feel validated as human beings with needs, rights, and wishes, and avoid conflict at all costs. There is a decided lack of assertiveness, and conformity is a priority. Approximation of genuine feelings is often never accomplished. In fact, the cancer-prone individual suppresses feelings rather than risk rejection. Life is charactetized by what ''ought'' to be done rather than what the individual desires to do. There is no real enthusiasm for life or a desire to be actively involved in what occurs in one's life. Hopelessness eventually results, with a concurrent sense of social isolation. These individuals often do not seek relationships with others, fearing intimacy and rejection. Thus, they tend to be socially distant, which in fact reinforces their feelings of helplessness and hopelessness.

Studies are not conclusive, however, concerning the impact of unresolved loss situations on the development of cancer. More definitive data need to be collected on what constitutes psychological stress as opposed to physiological (biochemical, genetic) risk factors and on the role of previous life events. Some evidence has suggested a relationship between stress and the development of leukemia and lymphoma (Greene, 1966). However, there is no consistent data indicating that the life stress theory is applicable to other types of neoplasms.

Consideration must be given to all factors—genetic and constitutional traits, intrapsychic conflicts, personality traits, past interpersonal experiences, and biochemical and autoimmune responses—and the interaction of these factors with precipitating events (life stress).

Accident-prone behavior

Freud suggested that there was a relationship between self-mutilating behavior and severe neuroses. This view emerged as an extension of Freud's belief that mistakes have meaning—for example, that the proverbial ''slip of the tongue'' does in fact have roots in the unconscious. He further proposed that individuals who are accident prone have an underlying need to punish themselves that is basically operative at the conscious level. Physical circumstances within the environment tend to influence the impulse to hurt oneself.

Freedman et al. (1980) note that individuals who are accident prone tend to place themselves in situations that reflect a high risk and that are likely to result in self-destructive behavior. These individuals have difficulty expressing aggressive drives directly and experience overwhelming feelings of guilt when confronted with their aggressive impulses. Freud supplies the basic rationale for the behavior: such an individual experiences self-punishment by virtue of the accident itself. In such a case, underlying dependence needs can be met in an acceptable manner because the person is in fact in the ''sick role.''

Sexual dysfunction

Sexual dysfunctions have historically been related to intrapsychic conflicts—particularly the repression of hostility. This factor retains considerable significance; however, biological, interpersonal, and sociocultural factors must be considered as well. Impotence, premature ejaculation, and retarded ejaculation are included among male sexual dysfunctions; female dysfunctions include preorgasmia, vaginismus, and dyspareunia. To determine a comprehensive plan of care, a nurse must consider all factors that may be relevant to a dysfunction.

Biological or organic factors play a part in the evolution of sexual dysfunctions. Organic causes may be natural in the developmental sense, such as aging, or they may be pathological, as in disease processes. Sexual functioning may be impaired as a result of chronic illness or degenerative disease. Diseases of the genitalia can alter sexual functioning, even to the point of total abstinence from coitus, depending on the degree of discomfort incurred as a result of sexual relations. Other disorders, such as diabetes, hypothyroidism, hepatitis, and cirrhosis, may also alter sexual functioning. Neurological impairment, including spinal cord trauma and diseases of the frontal and temporal lobes, may cause impotence or inorgasmia. Finally, drugs can have an effect on sexual performance—either a permanent one or a temporary one, depending upon the drug. Antihypertensive medications, estrogen, steroids, and anticholinergics may cause impotence. When administration of such a drug is stopped, sexual dysfunction usually disappears. However, in some cases, permanent dysfunction may result (Kolodny et al., 1979).

Intrapsychic conflict that generates anxiety may be detrimental to sexual functioning. Unconscious conflicts, particularly those surrounding the oedipal period, have been identified as being responsible for dysfunction. Castration anxiety is a common cause of impotence, according to the freudian school of thought. Incestuous wishes that are repressed in the oedipal phase may be reexperienced in later life, leading to guilt and the inability to perform sexually. Hostile impulses resulting from early conflicts may be precipitated by a current sexual relationship. The hostility is repressed; tension may be released through the penis in the form of impotence or through the vagina in the form of preorgasmia or what has been termed ''frigidity.''

Children often learn at an early age that sex and their bodies are ''dirty.'' This belief and other values and attitudes regarding sex are learned via an intricate network of experiences. Behavior in later life may reflect those early experiences. The original stimulus—for example, a parent telling a child that masturbation will lead to mental illness—is no longer necessary; the imprint from that original message will last a lifetime.

Fear may also play a significant role in the development of sexual dysfunctions. There is the fear of pregnancy for the female, as well as the fear of being found out and the fear of venereal disease. Situations may develop in which partners fear engaging in sex—for example, because visitors are staying in the house, the children are still awake and may come in or call out for the parents, or the partners are visiting in a friend's home. The environment must be as free of tension as possible so that each partner feels comfortable expressing himself sexually (Kaplan, 1974).

Interpersonal conflicts may indicate poor lines of communication between the partners. When one partner is distressed or angry at the other, the anger may be expressed through the sexual act or may inhibit the sexual act. Both partners need to feel that their wishes are being considered. Feeling as though one is a sexual object rather than an active participant in a relationship has deleterious effects upon sexual functioning. Innuendos regarding sexual competence—for example, comparison of the current partner with previous partners—lead to feelings of inadequacy and impaired sexual functioning. Sensitivity to one another's needs and respect for each other's bodies is a crucial interpersonal factor. Consideration of individual needs reduces the incidence of sexual dysfunction (Woods, 1984).

Sociocultural factors have a significant impact on the development of sexual attitudes and the sexual interaction that a couple experiences. Changes in attitude toward the role of the woman have had a significant effect on sexual functioning. The woman may no longer be considered the ''passive recipient'' of the sexual act. The male who has operated under the assumption that he is the dominant figure in the sexual relationship may perceive this change in mores as threatening. Much more emphasis has been placed on performance and competence. Anxiety has been generated, followed by a fear of failure. Sensitivity to one another's needs in a relationship has been replaced by the philosophy ''Do it more and do it better!'' This emphasis on function will surely lead to increased dysfunction.

Each of the factors mentioned must be considered in order to understand the evolution of sexual dysfunction. Again, no one theory is sufficient to explain a dysfunction, and it cannot be said that each type of conflict leads to one specific dysfunction. Precipitating events need to be considered in light of their interaction with bio-psycho-social factors. A brief description of each dysfunction follows (Masters and Johnson, 1970).

Impotence is the inability to achieve or maintain an erection. It results from an inhibition of the vasocongestive phase of sexual response. Men who have never had an erection are said to have primary impotence. Impotence that occurs in individuals who have experienced successful erections in the past is called secondary impotence. Impotence may be general—that is, it occurs in any and all sexual experiences. Or it may be situational—occurring only in certain situations. For example, a man may be potent with his wife yet unable to achieve erection while having a relationship with another woman, or vice versa. Impotence prior to old age is a devastating experience that may lead to a loss of self-worth and ultimately to failures in other areas of life.

Premature ejaculation is the ejaculation of semen before the partners reach a state in which mutual enjoyment is experienced. The man has not learned voluntary control over ejaculation; orgasm is reached quickly once he is sexually aroused. Although there is no real time limit for ejaculation, many men state that they are not able to delay ejaculation. Both partners can learn to be responsive to ejaculation; the man can begin to learn voluntary control, while the woman may also learn techniques to control ejaculation.

Retarded ejaculation is the opposite of premature ejaculation. This occurrence is normally associated with the aging process. In this dysfunction, the male is able to achieve erection but is unable to ejaculate.

Orgasmic dysfunction is the inability of the female to achieve orgasm. Orgasmic dysfunction may be situational or general. Women who have never achieved orgasm are said to have primary inorgasmia. These women may also be termed "preorgasmic." Women who have achieved orgasm through masturbation or intercourse but are presently unable to achieve orgasm are said to have secondary inorgasmia.

Dyspareunia refers to pain during intercourse. This situation may result from inadequate lubrication of the vagina.

Vaginismus refers to the development of spasticity in the pelvic muscles surrounding the opening of the vagina. The spasticity results in contractions, which lead to decreased probability of penetration.

Each dysfunction must be assessed in terms of the intricate relationship of many factors. Helen Singer Kaplan (1974) believes that the development of an erotic environment provides the atmosphere for the development of healthy sexual relationships. Feelings, needs, and concerns need to be openly expressed. Pressure to perform should not be the overriding principle. Couples should concentrate on making sexual experiences exciting, stimulating, and enjoyable for both partners.

• • •

Kolb (1977) states that there is strong support for the view that there is a close association between physical and psychological dysfunctions. Psychophysiological responses are commonly treated by a physician rather than a psychiatrist. In fact, psychiatrists often view clients with such responses as not being "sick" enough or at least not "mentally sick" enough to be treated. Often these persons are referred from physician to physician with little attention being given to their psychological needs. Such clients are typically found in medical and surgical units of general hospitals. It becomes the nurse's responsibility to accurately and comprehensively assess the needs of these clients to prevent further neglect of psychological dysfunction.

The Diagnostic and Statistical Manual of Mental Disorders no longer classifies psychophysiological dysfunctions as such but includes these disorders under the heading "Psychological Factors Affecting Physical Illness." This change in classification attests to the strong link between physical illness and psychological, social, and cultural factors.

ETIOLOGY

Psychological theory
PSYCHOANALYTIC-INTRAPSYCHIC THEORY

Franz Alexander (1950) claims that each physiological response specifically corresponds to an unconscious emotional conflict. For example, a client who has a need to be taken care of cannot accede to that need but must instead maintain the appearance of being independent. The tension or anxiety arising from the arousal of this unconscious conflict in a dependent individual is discharged through a peptic ulcer. Another client is unable to directly discharge his or her anger or hostility. The symptom that may appear is rising blood pressure. This ''specificity theory'' implies that there is a specific physiological response to each emotional conflict or emotional stimulus. The physiological response is under the control of the autonomic nervous system.

This theory assumes a one-to-one cause-and-effect relationship between particular conflictual issues and physiological responses. Little or no consideration is given to genetic predisposition, personal coping strategies, or past experience, to cite a few factors.

PSYCHODYNAMIC-INTERPERSONAL THEORY

Dunbar (1954) argues that clients have particular personality ''profiles.'' Such a theory implies that there is a definitive correlation between a particular personality type and a particular disease entity. To cite an example, this theory holds that the client who is most likely to develop peptic ulcers is the high-powered, goal-oriented, aggressive, long-term planner. The accident-prone client is an impulsive, unsystematic, and hostile individual.

Personality, however, cannot account in full as an explanation for the development of psychophysiological disorders. Friedman (1969) incorporates this fact into his description of the correlation between the type A personality and an increased incidence of coronary artery disease.

Stress and change theory

As has been noted in Chapter 7, stress created by change and loss has a profound negative impact on health. In a society that is characterized by rapid technological advances, less extended family support, and increasing numbers of single-parent families, the potential for stress-influenced illness is greatly enhanced. Change and loss are a functional component of the developmental cycle; as the infant becomes more mobile, individuation and separation become the primary focus. This individuation continues on through adolescence. Further change is required as individuals set out in their careers in marriage and in parenting. Healthy coping by the child and the parental dyad is a key concept. When coping is viewed as threatening and often impossible, individuals employ rigid, distorted, and, ultimately, maladaptive coping strategies. For individuals to respond to the instability that exists in human relationships, they must recognize the need for change, understand their responses to situations that require change, and initiate actions that assist them in establishing a sense of control, a feeling of equilibrium.

Conflict arises within the family system—among siblings, between the members of the parental dyad, and between parent and child. It also exists in the work environment; for example, staff members may be in conflict regarding the management of the time schedules, or nursing administration may be in conflict with nursing staff regarding the operationalization of the philosophy of the institution at the patient care level. Conflict can also exist on an intrapersonal level: Internal conflict generates feelings of helplessness, and a lack of an adequate solution is the overwhelming sense. When conflict continues, maladaptive methods of coping are employed, yet the conflict is never truly resolved.

Conflict may be a positive stimulus for change. As one might suspect, conflict occurs as a natural evolution from incompatible values, expectations, or beliefs. Viewed within the context of healthy collaboration, conflict resolution is seen as a productive end.

Conflict resolution that fosters growth and respects the rights and needs of both parties produces the most positive ends. Participants who choose to meet only their own hidden agendas and who behave in a hostile or passive-aggressive manner influence conflict resolution in a negative fashion. Conflict resolution can only occur when participants are willing to compromise and to reach a mutually determined end result.

Stress, change, and conflict are major concepts that need to be understood within the context of psychophysiological responses such as those that are addressed here. Intrapsychic conflict plays a major part in the development of these responses, as do genetic predisposition, personality traits, and familial influence.

Conditioned or learned response theory

Nurses need to consider how and if learning affects a response. Does the behavior result in dependence needs being met? Does it provide positive reinforcement from significant others in the environment? For example, does the onset of ulcer symptoms engender caring responses that the client cannot normally accept? Behavior may be learned from significant others such as family members. A child finds that one parent ''uses'' his or her ulcer pains to gain attention from others in the family. Others take care of the parent and perform the tasks that are part of that parent's responsibility. The child ''learns'' that such a technique is an effective way to be dependent while maintaining a facade of independence. This may be particularly true for men, since men generally are permitted neither to express emotions nor to be dependent—although this attitude does seem to be changing as society continues to emphasize the importance of sharing feelings openly. It is imperative that we recognize that the expression of tension through the autonomic nervous system may be a learned response that is well entrenched by the time a person reaches a point where he or she seeks treatment.

Biological theory

The discussion of psychophysiological disorders is not complete without the inclusion of Selye's

theory that pituitary-adrenal responses to stress lead to ''diseases of adaptation.'' Selye suggests that when sufficient stress occurs, anxiety arises, which in turn leads to the arousal of psychological and physiological responses. If coping strategies are unable to deal with the increased stress, a change in somatic functioning results. Selye further suggests that which organ is affected depends to a greater extent on physiology and genetic predisposition than on psychology. (For further discussion of this disorder, known as Selye's general adaptation syndrome, see Chapter 7.)

Family theory

The concept of family has become increasingly important over the last twenty years. The family transmits the mores and values of society to its members. The child is influenced by the manner in which parents communicate to one another and by the coping mechanisms they use to reduce stress and anxiety. The family structure provides an arena in which the offspring develop a sense of identity or a lack of identity. They learn to communicate with others, and they learn to relate in a healthy manner to others in their environment and in society as a whole. Satir (1972) points out not only that the family is charged with helping a child to accomplish these tasks, but that the child emerges as a mentally healthy adult as a result of their successful achievement. Satir therefore views the family as a complex, continuous interaction of individuals who assume various roles at various times, accomplish developmental tasks, cope with conflicts, and become active members in society. When discussing this concept of family, we often do not realize the full impact the family has on its individual members. As will be discussed later, adaptive behavior that clients use in response to stressors such as changes in body image, pain, immobilization, sensory overload or deprivation, and loss or change are greatly influenced by previous experiences with these stressors in the family setting. Parents act as role models for the handling of conflict situations. Communication patterns used by parents are adopted by children to be transmitted to future generations. As we know, this role modeling may be either positive or negative.

How is the concept of family related to the use of psychophysiological processes as modes of adaptation? How can it not be related? Minuchin (1978) believes that there is a "psychosomatogenic family." Reviewing what has previously been discussed, we see that the child's adaptation mechanisms, as well as his or her roles, are learned through the family process. Within the psychosomatogenic family, the child learns that his or her psychophysiological dysfunction serves as a source of concern for family members. This allows the family to focus on something other than family conflict. Minuchin feels that there is a particular type of family organization that submerges or denies outright conflict; conflicts are never resolved in such a family. As the psychophysiological dysfunction continues to mask the conflicts within the family, the child receives positive reinforcement for his or her symptoms, which in turn serves to maintain the ritual of conflict avoidance. Minuchin also discusses the question of physiological vulnerability. The child may have a particular physiological weakness that determines the organ of choice, but the operation of the family and its impact on its members is a crucial aspect of the dysfunction.

Ackerman (1966) supports the concept that a psychophysiological dysfunction in a child serves to control conflict within the family. The dysfunction maintains patterns of communication and prevents the occurrence of psychosis.

Holistic approach to wellness

A delicate interrelationship of genetic, intrapsychic, psychodynamic, cognitive, biochemical, spiritual, and familial factors must be considered before a psychophysiological response can be understood. This interrelationship operates in a multifactorial sense; that is, when several factors are present, there is an increased probability of a particular psychophysiological response. Precipitating stressful events, such as the perceived or actual loss of a relationship, act as catalysts. Individual coping strategies and personality traits also affect the development of psychophysiological responses. A nurse must consider multiple factors to determine a plan of care that is suited to a particular client and to his or her psychophysiological responses at the time.

TREATMENT MODALITIES

Medication

A primary goal of the nurse is to assess the meaning that a dysfunction holds for the client. Why does he or she choose to adapt to stress in this manner? However, it is often necessary to deal with the high levels of anxiety and the symptoms of depression that precipitate and exacerbate psychophysiological dysfunctions. Tranquilizers, antidepressants, and sedatives are the drugs most frequently indicated. They should be administered judiciously and according to the needs of each individual client. Medications are not replacements for therapy but should be used in conjunction with appropriate modes of intervention. Other types of medication, directed toward specific disease processes, are often indicated as well.

Individual and group therapy

There are various psychological modalities for the treatment of psychophysiological dysfunctions. Treatment plans are based on the theory that is most relevant to the client's situation. Psychotherapy is directed toward the long-term goal of initiating new adaptive measures. Intensive psychotherapy is successful in the treatment of most psychophysiological dysfunctions. However, the decision to engage in this interpretive form of therapy depends on the fragility of the client's ego. This type of therapy is not recommended for clients with ulcerative colitis or peptic ulcers, since the exacerbation of symptoms may be potentially life threatening.

Supportive one-to-one therapy is essential until

clients are able to accept themselves and their roles in their environments. They then will no longer "need" psychophysiological dysfunctions and will seek more realistic and self-satisfying modes of coping.

Anaclitic therapy may be used, but only in a well-controlled situation. This form of therapy involves the regression of the client to an earlier stage of development—a stage where he or she feels comfortable. The client then is gradually moved back through the developmental eras and helped to deal with feelings of dependence and/or guilt when appropriate.

Rest, diet, and other supportive measures, as well as medical intervention, are also used, as needed, in individual therapy.

Group therapy may be used as an adjunct to the supportive or psychotherapeutic one-to-one relationship. Initially, a client needs to feel comfortable with one helping person. He or she may then move into a group situation with greater self-confidence.

It is important to note that clients rarely seek psychiatric help for any of the dysfunctions discussed in this chapter. Frequently it is in the general hospital setting that nurses deal with clients who are experiencing stress-related dysfunctions. Society may, in fact, subtly condone the occurrence of such dysfunctions as ulcers or coronary artery disease as part of becoming successful— they are often seen as the mark of an aggressive, ambitious individual. Although therapy is important, it is more relevant for nurses to assist clients to gain an understanding of the interaction among dysfunction, stress, and life-style. In many instances, nurses can provide short-term supportive therapy that can enable a client to gain more control over his environment and to express needs in a more open, direct fashion.

Stress management techniques can be helpful in assisting clients in the identification of stressful situations and implementing strategies that will reduce the impact of stressors (see Chapter 7). Follow-up treatment in the form of family therapy can then serve to support the use of alternative methods of coping.

Family therapy

Proponents of systems theory view the individual as a subsystem that is in continuous interaction with many other subsystems in the environment. The underlying premise is that one cannot successfully treat an individual client without considering him or her as an integral part of the total system. Family therapy involves all family members or significant others in the client's environment. As was previously discussed, the goal of family therapy is to enable the *family,* not just the individual client, to resolve conflict and express needs directly, rather than force the client to use maladaptive behavior to maintain family patterns. (For further discussion see Chapter 12.)

NURSING INTERVENTION

PRIMARY PREVENTION

Primary prevention is a key concept in the area of psychophysiological dysfunctions. As Chapter 7 pointed out, it involves the identification of potential stressors and the education of individuals and families to enable them to develop healthy patterns of adaptation.

Nurses need to be aware of the following principles when developing goals for primary prevention of psychophysiological responses.

1. Psychophysiological responses are a means of coping with unconscious conflicts in order to maintain functional ability.
2. Change, loss, and conflict are major stressors in the current societal situation.
3. Anxiety occurs as a result of encountering stressful situations.

4. Behavioral responses are directed toward maintaining psychological equilibrium and reducing anxiety.
5. Awareness of feelings is limited during periods of increased anxiety.
6. Vulnerability to rejection and criticism is heightened during periods of increased anxiety.

Goals for primary prevention of psychophysiological disorders include:

1. Minimizing the effects of factors that predispose people to psychophysiological disorders
2. Identifying measures to prevent high-risk individuals from developing psychophysiological disorders

These goals can be implemented by identifying high-risk individuals and initiating family and marital counseling. (Refer to Chapter 7 for an in-depth discussion of change, loss, anxiety, and stress.)

It is important to identify high-risk groups, such as members of families in which one or both parents express needs primarily through psychophysiological behavior. This task may seem monumental, particularly since such clients do not usually seek psychiatric treatment. Nurses often see these clients in general hospital settings and physicians' offices. Assessment data should reflect the fact that the client is an integral part of his family and community system. Nursing intervention can be directed toward identifying the significance of early patterns of interaction within a family in which physical illness is directly affected by psychological factors. Since these issues are often quite emotionally charged, a client may deny that he or she has any difficulty expressing needs or feelings.

Through involvement with families on the community and school levels, the nurse is able to observe both children's and parents' responses to change. Indications as to the level of adaptability can be readily observed. Methods of maladaptive coping with stressful situations may be apparent in the parental dyad. Families in which parent-child relationships prohibit the expression of dependence needs, as well as the expression of anger,

guilt, fear, and anxiety, are a target population. Relationships that are founded on unrealistic expectations that can never be fulfilled set the stage for maladaptive coping strategies, as exemplified by the cancer-prone individual.

A major aspect of primary prevention is parental and family counseling. As has been noted elsewhere, children learn within the context of their environments, particularly from their parents and/or significant others. It is at this level, then, that we must direct our attention. Nurses can act as facilitators by assisting parents in the open expression of feelings—anger, frustration, and anxiety. Learning adaptive methods to exist in a society that promotes and expects change is a must. Those children who learn to be flexible, to use many different ways to handle change, and who are not threatened by change are the ones who will be most successful in confronting and resolving the issues that arise in society. Families need to be active participants in stress reduction measures such as biofeedback, progressive relaxation, and assertiveness techniques. It is through these measures that open communication is fostered and feelings are authentically experienced.

Parental education on an informal level may stimulate parents to become more aware of the role they play in influencing their children's methods of coping with stress—particularly the use of psychophysiological behavior. As was discussed in Chapter 7, the family is the target client system for nursing intervention. Nurses can enable clients to provide an atmosphere in which their children can feel safe and comfortable in sharing their needs to feel taken care of and to feel that they are whole, interdependent, unique beings. In such an atmosphere, expressions of anger, fear, and rage are dealt with in an open, honest manner. Providing open lines of communication may be difficult for a parent who has never experienced such a situation himself or herself. In spite of the significance of early parental interaction and direct lines of communication, it is important not to neglect the impact of genetic predisposition, personality factors, and precipitating factors that may interact to increase the use of psychophysiological responses as coping mechanisms.

Primary prevention is concerned with the identification of potential stressors and the education of the individual to deal with them. If a client has already developed a psychophysiological response as an adaptive measure, the focus of primary prevention shifts to the children of the client, with an increased emphasis on the influence of parental adaptive measures.

SECONDARY PREVENTION

Secondary prevention involves meeting the following objectives:

1. Early identification of cases of psychophysiological responses in the community
2. Obtaining cost-effective and prompt treatment that will assist clients in returning to their optimal levels of functioning
3. Assessment of available resources such as assertiveness training and stress management seminars
4. Participation with community groups and business organizations in developing expanded resources

Early identification of health deviations resulting from psychophysiological responses is particularly important. Many of these individuals do not actively seek help from health resources until symptoms are quite severe. At this point hospitalization for the physical symptoms is necessary. It is in this setting that nurses can become actively involved in assisting clients in identifying relevant stressors, assessing effective and ineffective coping strategies, and determining appropriate measures to resolve stressful issues. Nurses in occupational and community health are in key positions to identify and assess behavior patterns indicative of maladaptive coping measures. For example, the occupational health nurse may be the one individual that a young management trainee seeks out to discuss chronic intestinal problems that seem to be related to the beginning of the management program. These initial assessments are tentative and need to be further validated with the client and with other health care resources before further intervention is implemented. The goal of early identification in secondary prevention is the referral of the client to further mental health resources. In the case of persons with psychophysiological disorders, individual therapy is not usually cost effective or actively sought by clients. A supportive nurse-client relationship may be the primary vehicle for assisting the client in developing more effective coping strategies. These individuals are often resistant to therapy because they do not believe that it could be helpful. Nurses should refer these clients to resources that provide stress management techniques and support their efforts to communicate their feelings and needs more directly and to assume active control over their lives with all the responsibility that accompanies that control.

The focus of intervention in the secondary prevention phase is on resolution of internal conflict and identification and management of stressors. Through intervention, clients will be able to experience reductions in psychophysiological symptoms and to increase their levels of functional adaptation to both internal and external stressors. Nurses need to keep in mind the following principles, regardless of the symptom picture:

1. The focus must be on the client as a person rather than on symptoms.
2. Anxiety is an underlying concept whether it is observable or not.
3. The symptom is a mechanism of defense that is designed to control anxiety and preserve ego integrity.
4. Nursing intervention needs to recognize these behaviors as compensatory until clients are more able to develop effective adaptation measures.
5. Secondary gains may be powerful motivators relative to psychophysiological responses.
6. Clients are vulnerable to rejection and need to feel control over the environment.

7. Stress management techniques enable clients to manage their own stressors, including change and conflict. Knowledge of these principles will facilitate intervention.

Nursing process

The nursing process is the mechanism that provides the framework for therapeutic intervention.

ASSESSMENT

The assessment should reflect a comprehensive consideration of stressors, their impact, and the client's methods of coping. Although each disorder may impact on a different biological system, all clients share maladaptive coping strategies that prevent effective coping with their environments. The following areas should be assessed:

1. Presenting symptoms—systems involved (GI tract; respiratory tract; cardiovascular system)
2. Coping strategies—use of appropriate denial; general effectiveness; perception of precipitating event; past effectiveness of coping measures; level of communication of needs; origin of maladaptive coping strategies through past experiences
3. Emotional state—level of self-worth; degree of feelings of helplessness, hopelessness; feelings of frustration, anger, anxiety; degree of disruption incurred
4. Stimulus situations—stressful situations that create psychophysiological responses within the environment (social, work, school situations; within the context of familial relationships; client perception of stressors and methods of coping)
5. Support systems—available support systems (family, significant others; individuals within the context of other relationships with client)
6. Holistic health status—biological, psychological, intellectual, sociocultural, and spiritual status of the client. These factors may impede or facilitate wellness. Expectations

of unrealistic performance may, for example, generate angry feelings which are then repressed. These feelings are ultimately expressed through physical symptoms such as ulcerative colitis and asthma. In psychophysiological disorders, the primary mechanism of expressing feelings is through physical symptomatology.

ANALYSIS OF DATA

Nurses begin to understand their clients within the context of their relationships with family and significant others in their environment through a comprehensive health assessment. Following this assessment, nurses may formulate nursing diagnoses. Diagnoses reflective of internal conflicts relating to psychophysiological responses include dependence and hostility. These diagnoses are presented in Chapters 18 and 19 with appropriate plans of care and implementation. Physical symptoms must be addressed and acute conditions must be treated; however, the physical symptoms are not the focus. It is important for readers to refer back to Chapter 7 for an in-depth discussion of stress management techniques, which are critical to effecting change in psychophysiological responses.

Nursing diagnosis: Inability to express anger, secondary to repression of hostile impulses (behavior associated with all DSM-III diagnoses of psychological factors affecting physical illness)

Planning: With assistance of the nurse, the client will establish goals.

1. Long-term goals
   a. Work through the internal conflict that generates feelings of anger and anxiety.
   b. Increase the ability to express feelings.
   c. Increase the level of insight into external and internal forces which impact on behaviors.
   d. Increase self-esteem.
   e. Develop other methods to cope with life stressors.
2. Short-term goals
   a. Develop the ability to express angry feelings directly.

   b. Accept angry feelings without imposing guilt on client.

   c. Identify situations that precipitate feelings of anger.

   d. Relate past situations to present situations that aroused similar feelings.

   e. Realistically perceive the five dimensions of self (biological, psychological, intellectual, sociocultural, spiritual).

Implementation:

1. Recognize and support angry feelings as these feelings occur (angry feelings should not be taken personally).
2. Use more appropriate measures to express angry feelings (writing a letter and saving it to review when feelings are less intense).
3. Provide an atmosphere where clients can role play angry feelings in a safe, controlled environment.
4. Assist clients in recognizing in a realistic manner the effects of anger on others in the environment.
5. Act as a role model in expression of angry feelings.
6. Assist clients in operationalizing anger as a facet of a healthy, mature adult.

EVALUATION

Evaluation must reflect client participation in goal attainment and the impact of the client's family and significant others on the achievement of goals. The following areas must be considered:

1. The degree to which internal conflict has been resolved
2. The degree to which goals have been achieved and client functioning has improved—that is, decrease in physical symptomatology
3. Identification of goals that need to be modified or revised
4. Level of involvement in stress management techniques on an ongoing basis
5. Referral to support systems outside the nurse-client relationship
   a. Individuals within the client's network who will act as support systems
   b. Community agencies that provide services to assist clients in the management of their stressors (assertiveness training)
   c. Centers that specialize in treatment of specific psychophysiological disorders (for anorexia nervosa; for overeating)

TERTIARY PREVENTION

Tertiary prevention is directed toward the avoidance of further impairment of a client's physical, psychosocial, and emotional status. The nurse-client interaction continues, with the focus of intervention being placed on efforts to understand the client's need for the particular mode of adaptation.

Nurses are also concerned with how a client's perception of himself and his roles is related to the mode of adaptation. As mentioned previously, certain psychophysiological responses are perceived as status symbols or marks of success, as in the case of ulcers. The issue that arises is the extent to which such an adaptation mechanism impairs the individual in his or her current life situation. The primary focus of tertiary prevention then becomes one of clarification of values and life goals. The nurse does not step in and immediately imply that the client must change value systems and reorder priorities. Instead, nurses can facilitate the understanding of the relationship between stress, personal life-style, and a psychophysiological dysfunction. The client must then decide whether to commit himself or herself to the long-term process of change. Active support of the use of alternative methods of expressing needs and coping with stress becomes the focus of the nurse during this phase of prevention.

CHAPTER SUMMARY

Physical symptoms cannot be viewed simply as reflections of physiological dysfunctions. A delicate interweaving of physiological, psychological, and sociocultural factors can result in psychophysiological illness. This chapter has presented a discussion of the dysfunctions that have been traditionally identified as psychophysiological. Predominant behavioral problems have been identified, and nursing intervention has been presented in terms of the three levels of prevention—primary, secondary, and tertiary. Every day nurses in general hospital settings meet clients who exhibit physical illnesses that are related to psychological factors. These clients' cases are frustrating yet also most challenging! Such clients are not candidates for traditional therapeutic approaches. In fact, clients may be unwilling to acknowledge that they are experiencing any difficulty. Society compounds an already frustrating situation by subtly condoning a number of psychophysiological dysfunctions as being ''job-related'' or ''success-related'' hazards. The challenge for nurses, therefore, is to assess the physiological, psychological, and sociocultural components of dysfunctions. A nursing care plan must reflect a complete portrait of a client in the context of his own world. Nurses have the knowledge and skills to enhance a client's potential for change, through the use of short-term, flexible treatment measures. In the future, nurses will continue to be instrumental in assisting clients to assess their values, to identify and manage actual and potential stressors, and to develop alternative methods of coping .

- Develop awareness about your own feelings and attitudes when working with clients who are suffering from psychophysiological disorders.

1. Try to imagine that you are suffering from one of the following disorders and explain why you selected that particular disorder. Then describe what you think it would be like to suffer from that disorder.
   a. Asthma
   b. Ulcerative colitis
   c. Peptic ulcers
   d. Migraine headaches
   e. Cancer (select a particular site)
2. Describe what you think it would be like to have a family member suffering from one of the psychophysiological disorders listed in exercise 1. Which disorder do you think would be easiest to tolerate in a family member? Why? Which disorder do you think would be hardest to tolerate? Why?
3. What might be some of your feelings and reactions as a nurse caring for clients who are suffering from psychophysiological disorders? Would your feelings and reactions vary with the disorders experienced by clients? Explain why.
4. Imagine that you are a community health nurse engaged in health supervision activities with new parents. What high-risk factors (biological, psychological, intellectual, sociocultural, spiritual) would you look for that might predispose parents and/or their children to a psychophysiological disorder?
5. Develop a plan for counseling parents for child-rearing that incorporates principles and goals for the primary prevention of psychophysiological disorders.

SENSITIVITY-AWARENESS EXERCISES*

The purposes of the following exercises are to:
- Develop awareness about the vulnerability of client-families to psychophysiological disorders
- Develop awareness about the interrelationship of factors in the etiology of psychophysiological disorders
- Develop awareness about the subjective experience of clients who are suffering from psychophysiological disorders and of the experience of clients' families

*For other relevant exercises, refer to Chapter 7.

REFERENCES

Ackerman, N.
  1966 Treating the Troubled Family. New York: Basic Books, Inc., Publishers.
Alexander, F.
  1950 Psychosomatic Medicine. New York: W.W. Norton & Co., Inc.
Bahnson, C., and U. Bahnson
  1966 ''Role of the ego defenses: denial and regression in the etiology of malignant neoplasms.'' Annals of the New York Academy of Sciences 125:827-845.
Bruch, H.
  1973 Eating Disorders: Obesity, Anorexia Nervosa and the Person Within. New York: Basic Books, Inc., Publishers.

Cannon, W.

1929 Bodily Changes in Pain, Hunger, Fear and Rage, ed. 2. New York: D. Appleton Century Co.

Cheren, S., and P. Knapp

1980 ''Gastrointestinal disorders.'' In Comprehensive Textbook of Psychiatry, ed. 3. A. Freedman, H. Kaplan, and B. Sadock (eds.). Baltimore: The Williams & Wilkins Co.

Dunbar, H.F.

1954 Emotions and Bodily Changes. New York: Columbia University Press.

Freedman, A., H. Kaplan, and B. Sadock (eds.).

1980 Comprehensive Textbook of Psychiatry. Baltimore: The Williams & Wilkins Co.

Friedman, M.

1969 Pathogenesis of Coronary Artery Disease. New York: McGraw-Hill Book Co.

Greene, W.A.

1966 ''The psychosocial setting of the development of leukemia and lymphoma.'' Annals of the New York Academy of Sciences 125:794-801.

Kaplan, H., and B. Sadock (eds.)

1981 Comprehensive Textbook of Psychiatry. Baltimore: The Williams & Wilkins Co.

Kaplan, H.S.

1974 The New Sex Therapy. New York, Brunner/Mazel, Inc.

Kolb, L.

1977 Modern Clinical Psychiatry. Philadelphia: W.B. Saunders Co.

Kolodny, R., et al.

1979 Textbook of Human Sexuality for Nurses. Boston: Little, Brown & Co.

LeShan, R.

1977 You Can Fight For Your Life. New York: M. Evans & Co., Inc.

Masters, R., and V. Johnson

1970 Human Sexual Inadequacy. London: Churchill Press.

Minuchin, S., B. Rosman, and L. Baker

1978 Psychosomatic Families. Cambridge, Mass.: Harvard University Press.

Satir, V.

1972 Peoplemaking. Palo Alto, Calif.: Science and Behavior Books.

Schultz, S., and S. Dark

1982 Manual of Psychiatric Nursing Care Plans. Boston: Little, Brown & Co.

Selye, H.

1956 The Stress of Life. New York: McGraw-Hill Book Co., pp. 20-36.

Shontz, F.

1975 The Psychological Aspects of Physical Illness and Disability. New York: MacMillan, Inc.

Simonton, O., et al.

1980 ''Psychological intervention in the treatment of cancer.'' Psychosomatics 21:226-233.

Woods, N.F.

1984 Human Sexuality in Health and Illness, ed. 3. St. Louis: The C.V. Mosby Co.

ANNOTATED SUGGESTED READINGS

Dubovsky, S., et al.

1977 ''Impact on nursing care and mortality: psychiatrists on the coronary care unit.'' Psychosomatics 18 (August): 20-27.

This study explores the effects of psychiatric consultation on a group of critical care unit nurses. The study was prompted by research that suggested that the CCU milieu in general and nurses in particular affect patient outcome. This research showed that nurses can affect patient outcome directly by recognizing dangerous situations and indirectly by decreasing adverse physiological changes associated with the emotional climate of the ward.

The authors report that the psychiatric consultation resulted in an increase in the time the nurses spent in direct patient care and an increase in the importance assigned to and the enjoyment of that activity. There was also a significant increase in charting efficiency. Nurses seemed to become more acutely aware of situations that might trigger an arrhythmia, and they felt more comfortable with their own emotions.

The implications are striking: Nurses need to become more aware of their own responses to stressful situations in the CCU —for example, the impending death of a client resulting in depression and anxiety; increased workload; and excessive responsibility. Nurses must openly communicate their responses to these stressors to reduce the transmission of anxiety to the CCU client and thus to avoid or decrease the severity of any adverse physiological changes in the client that might result.

Herbert, D.J.

1976 ''Psychophysiological reactions as a function of life stress and behavioral rigidity.'' Journal of Psychiatric Nursing, May, pp. 23-27.

This study hypothesizes that disease occurs when a significant level of life stress is reached and that an individual's behavioral rigidity plays a role in the disease process. The hypothesis is supported by data collected from subjects. The important factor presented in this study that has not been discussed in other studies on life stress is the individual's ability to assume a flexible rather than a rigid approach to a problem. Nursing intervention can be directed not only toward the identification of life stressors but also toward assisting an individual to use a variety of methods of adaptation rather than be inflexible.

Minuchin, S., B. Rosman, and L. Baker

1978 Psychosomatic Families. Cambridge, Mass.: Harvard University Press.

This book applies family therapy techniques to the treatment of anorexia nervosa. The authors draw upon their clinical experience to suggest that the focus of therapy should be not on the individual but on the entire family. The therapist is viewed as an active agent for change who acts as a catalyst—with the catalytic activity resulting in new and healthier patterns of interaction. The book presents an eclectic model for treatment that can be used in any type of case involving psychophysiological dysfunction.

FURTHER READINGS*

Caplan, G.

1964 Principles of Preventive Psychiatry. New York: Basic Books, Inc., Publishers.

Flynn, P.

1980 Holistic Health. Bowie, Md.: Robert Brady Co.

Garfield, C. (ed.)

1979 Stress and Survival: The Emotional Realities of Life-Threatening Illness. St. Louis: The C.V. Mosby Co.

Hackett, T. and N. Cassem (eds.)

1978 Massachusetts General Hospital Handbook of General Hospital Psychiatry. St. Louis: The C.V. Mosby Co.

Kimball, C.

1970 ''Conceptual developments in psychosomatic medicine: 1939-1969.'' Annals of Internal Medicine 73:101-126.

LeShan, L.

1966 ''An emotional life-history pattern associated with neoplastic disease.'' Annals of the New York Academy of Sciences 125:780-793.

Menninger, K.

1963 The Vital Balance. New York: The Viking Press.

Nemiah, J.C.

1975 ''Denial revisited: reflections on psychosomatic theory.'' Psychotherapy and Psychosomatics 26:140-147.

Titchener, J.

1971 ''Families of psychosomatic patients.'' In The Theory and Practice of Family Psychiatry. New York: Brunner/Mazel, Inc., Ch. 37

*Other appropriate readings may be found in Chapter 7.

CHAPTER 17

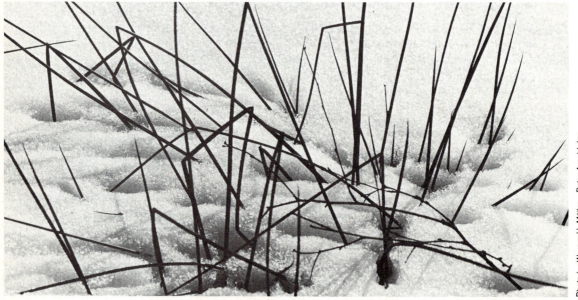

Photo by Werner H. Müller—Peter Arnold, Inc.

Coping through socially deviant behavior

CHAPTER FOCUS

Everyone lives within a social system, and every social system is based on a set of values and rules. These values and rules serve as standards to which members of society are expected to conform.

Some people try to cope with tensions and conflicts by acting out against society. These people behave in ways that deviate from society's standards. Such socially aberrant behavior often harms others and is condemned by society.

Various theories have been formulated to explain the etiology of socially deviant behavior. These theories fall into three major categories: psychological conflict, biological defect, and sociocultural conflict. It is probable that a combination of holistic health factors leads to the development of socially deviant behavior. Some type of socially aberrant behavior is known to all societies, but its form, meaning, and incidence are culturally influenced.

Persons who behave in socially aberrant ways are usually content with their behavior and may not seek treatment voluntarily. When treatment is instituted, a combination of therapies is usually indicated. The goals of therapy are to supplant the aberrant behavior with acceptable behavior and to facilitate an individual's reentry into society.

Although nurses may not directly participate in all treatment modalities, they do participate in all three levels of preventive intervention. When working with socially deviant persons, nurses need to be nondefensive, realistic, accepting, consistent, and firm. A nurse's insight into his or her own attitudes, values, and behavior is essential in helping socially deviant individuals confront their aberrant behavior. By clarifying their own attitudes and values, nurses can accept people who behave in socially aberrant ways, without condoning their life-styles.

Everyone lives within a social system, and every social system is based on a set of values and rules. These values and rules serve as standards to which members of society are expected to conform. However, any deviation from these standards is not necessarily socially deviant behavior. Schur (1971) restricts the definition of social deviance to behavior that violates social standards and thereby engenders anger, resentment, or the desire for punishment in a significant segment of society. For example, the violation of traffic regulations concerning double parking would not be regarded as a socially deviant act, but driving while intoxicated would be so regarded.

Social standards evolve to deal with problems that have arisen or to prevent the development of anticipated problems. Social standards also function to make more predictable and more controllable the behavior of members of society. When people try to cope with tensions and conflicts by acting out against society through the use of socially aberrant behavior, they often harm others and are condemned and stigmatized by society.

In his classic work on stigma, Goffman (1963) describes two types of socially condemned or stigmatized individuals: the discredited and the discreditable. Discredited people are those who, because their deviance is visible or known, are devalued by society. For example, the obesity of foodaholics is visible and generally makes them vulnerable to social disapproval. Discreditable people are those who, if their behavior were generally known, would be devalued and condemned by society. For instance, "secret" alcoholics are discreditable people. However, once their "secret" is exposed as a result of drunken driving, being discovered drunk on the job, etc., discreditable people become discredited people. Obviously, the families and social networks of discreditable people are often instrumental in ensuring that their secrets are not made public. A wife who calls her husband's place of employment and says that he is too ill to go to work, when in reality he is too drunk or too "hung over" to go to work,

is helping to keep her husband's alcoholism secret. Therefore, by preventing the visibility and exposure of his alcoholism, the wife is helping her husband to remain a discreditable, rather than to become a discredited, person.

Birenbaum and Sagarin (1976), while acknowledging that some social deviants are discredited and others are discreditable, go on to describe social deviants by life-style. Some deviants seek out others with similar behavior and become part of a deviant subculture. Such subcultures are characterized by values and perceptions that are at variance with society at large. Although subculture members never totally disassociate themselves from the larger society, their interactions tend to be predominantly with members of the subculture. Dependence on the subculture network becomes essential to survival, and relationships with family and friends in the larger society become minimally functional or completely nonfunctional. When the values and standards of the subculture are in direct opposition to those of society at large, so that peaceful coexistence is not possible, the subculture becomes a counterculture.* For example, drug addicts, juvenile delinquents, criminals, and prostitutes often belong to countercultures.

Other socially deviant individuals may choose an alternative life-style that runs counter to the values and rules of society at large, but they do not share this life-style with similarly oriented people. These social deviants tend to be "loners." Rapists and child molesters are examples of loners. Even when they do engage in socially deviant behavior in a group, as in gang rape, loners are not part of a subculture of like-deviants. The extent of their interaction and value sharing with others who use similar socially deviant behavior is too limited to be regarded as commitment to a counterculture.

The selection of a counterculture or a loner life-style depends not only on the type of socially deviant behavior being used but also on such factors as the need for a subterranean network in order

---

*Countercultures (counter-societies) will be further discussed in the section of this chapter dealing with antisocial behavior.

to make possible the continuance of deviant behavior, the need for acceptance, and the need to "belong." For example, whereas discreditable or "secret" prostitutes (such as housewives who earn extra money through prostitution) might eschew contact with other prostitutes for fear of calling attention to their sexually deviant behavior, discredited prostitutes can become part of the prostitute-pimp counterculture for the companionship and protection that it offers.

People who use socially deviant behavior to cope with anxiety and conflict are often content with their behavior and may not seek treatment voluntarily. When they are seen in mental health treatment centers, their behavior can be classified into one of the following DSM-III categories: conduct disorders, substance-use disorders, other psychosexual disorders, disorders of impulse control, and personality disorders (antisocial attitudes).

UNDERLYING DYNAMICS

Many people who behave in socially deviant ways have failed to internalize the social values and standards of society at large; they may habitually operate outside the norms of society. Socially deviant individuals tend to be egocentric and oriented toward the immediate present. They strive for satisfaction of immediate needs and are unwilling to tolerate delayed gratification. They often perceive other people as objects through which personal strivings may be satisfied. Interpersonal relationships tend to be superficial. Such people attempt to cope with the world and the people in it through alienation, anomie, manipulation, rationalization, blame placing, hostility, and poor judgment.

Alienation

Alienation can best be defined as a failure in reciprocal connectedness between a person and significant others. Alienation is the estrangement of self from others. Hobart (1965) and Halleck (1967) ascribe the following characteristics to alienated people:

1. Present oriented
2. Uncommitted to people, ideas, or causes
3. Possessors of poor self-images
4. Convinced that people do not understand them
5. Unable to communicate with others
6. Possessors of poor powers of concentration
7. Active in promiscuous but unsatisfyng sexual relationships
8. Users of marijuana or LSD

Alienation seems to arise from an interaction of several factors. Brown (1968) identifies these factors as urbanization, egalitarian disparity, a striving for success, and a lack of caring.

Urban life is marked by decentralized and depersonalized living. Work is a major source of economic gratification, social interaction, and personal esteem. With rising rates of underemployment and unemployment, however, many people are denied access to this primary source of life satisfaction.

Operating within this urban context is egalitarian disparity. There is a disjunction between actual behavior and idealized behavior. This is especially true for members of minority groups who are discriminated against and denied access to opportunities. The Glazer and Moynihan study (1963) has shown that all people do not have equal access to opportunity.

Coterminous with this egalitarian disparity is a need to succeed. Success is measured in terms of the possession of "things"—money, material goods, services, and education. In order to succeed, one must compete. If one is unable or unwilling to compete, success is usually unattainable.

Partially resulting from the aforementioned factors and certainly interrelated with them is a lack of caring. Modern society is technological. Technology often takes priority over people. Emphasis is on "doing," and succeeding is of paramount importance. Both men and women compete in this society. This competition often produces fatigue and irritability. There may be little time for meaningful interpersonal relationships. Within such a psychosocial context, alienation tends to develop.

Anomie

When prevailing social standards and values have little personal meaning, a state of anomie, or normlessness, develops. Anomie and alienation are closely related. McClosky and Schaar (1965) have found that alienation correlates positively with anomic responses. The loose social integration and impoverished interpersonal matrix associated with alienation provide a foundation for the development of anomie. Without significant interpersonal relationships, there is little internalization of social mores. A self-system of right and wrong does not develop. Freedom from norms not only means freedom from a socially sanctioned value system but also freedom from social constraints. An expectation usually develops that socially unacceptable behavior is required to attain desired goals (Clinard, 1974). Anomic responses are characteristic of many socially deviant persons.

Manipulation

Manipulation is the act of using the social environment for personal gain. Horney (1937) and Fromm (1947) refer to people who habitually manipulate as exploitative. People who are alienated and anomic tend to repeatedly use others to gratify their own needs and desires. Manipulation is a characteristic behavior of many socially deviant persons. Other people are perceived merely as means to ends. Socially deviant individuals usually manipulate others through force or guile. They can be domineering and ruthless, or they can be cunning and charming. Either approach is designed to allow them to use others. No one is exempt from being used. Family members, friends, and strangers are all fair game. Manipulative people feel little or no guilt about exploiting others and often be-

have as if they had a right to expect others to give them the good things in life.

Rationalization

Rationalization is a mechanism frequently used by socially deviant individuals. Rationalization is the process of constructing plausible reasons to explain and justify one's behavior. It allows a person to avoid looking at the actual reasons behind behavior. Underlying the rationalized explanation there is usually a shred of truth that is enlarged upon. For example, an alcoholic may tell himself that it is acceptable to drink three or four martinis at lunch: "Everyone has a drink at lunch. It relaxes a person." By accepting this explanation for his behavior, he denies the compulsive nature of his drinking; he denies the fact that he *must* have those martinis and that he becomes increasingly tense until he has had them.

Blame placing

Socially deviant persons tend to use the mechanism of blame placing in their interpersonal relationships. Responsibility for their behavior, and especially their misbehavior, can be placed on others. Such persons usually experience alienation in conjunction with the blame placing. They feel alienated from the persons they blame. Harkins (1965) states that blame-placing individuals often view others as personifications of cultural disjunctions that are at the root of their alienation.

By placing blame on other people, socially deviant individuals are able to avoid dealing with their roles in and responsibility for what happens to them. Blame is assigned to other people rather than to themselves. Blame placing is a way of manipulating the social environment. Clark (1963) points out that people tend to project blame when they feel powerless to control their social environments to the extent they consider necessary. Since being blamed is an extremely uncomfortable experience, even the threat of being an object of blame can often effectively control the behavior of many people. Scheflen and Scheflen (1972) observe that certain members of society have learned to use blame as a habitual way of solving problems. For these people, blame placing is a way of life.

Hostility

Hostility underlies all the interpersonal themes mentioned thus far. Hostility is a state of animosity. It is a response that endures; it builds up slowly and dissipates slowly. By reducing anxiety that is engendered by threats to one's security, hostility functions as a self-preservation mechanism. Hostility is expressed covertly in physical and verbal behavior that delivers some degree of injury or destruction to either animate or inanimate objects. Hostility is present in socially deviant behavior; the object of the hostility varies with the type of behavior. In some types of socially deviant behavior, such as rape, hostility is directed at others. In other types of socially deviant behavior, such as alcoholism and drug addiction, hostility is directed both at oneself and at others. In all types of socially deviant behavior, because conflicts and tensions are acted out in socially unacceptable ways, hostility is directed at society.

Impaired judgment

People who behave in socially aberrant ways usually evidence poor judgment. Many do not show any insight into their behavior, nor do they indicate any concern about the consequences of that behavior. They may not learn from experience. They express little remorse or guilt for the damage they do to themselves or to others. Although socially deviant persons can convincingly promise to repent and mend their ways, at the first opportunity they usually repeat the same behavior. The socially aberrant acts tend to be impulsive, and their perpetrators often take unnecessary risks of being caught. One explanation for this impulsiveness and poor judgment is that such persons tend to have a

low threshold for sameness; they are continually pursuing new sources of stimulation (DeMeyer-Gapin and Scott, 1977).

• • •

The dynamics of alienation, anomie, manipulation, rationalization, blame placing, hostility, and poor judgment interrelate. A hypothetical clinical situation will demonstrate this interrelationship.

A student nurse had established a therapeutic relationship with an adolescent male drug addict. Student and client had been interacting twice a week over a 12-week period. During one of these interactions the client lit up a reefer and began to smoke. Possession of any drug was grounds for being asked to leave the drug treatment center. When the student nurse reminded the client of the center's rules, he responded: "I've really been trying hard to get off drugs. I've just been so tense and pot helps me relax. It's harmless enough. It's even going to be legalized. Everyone smokes it. You or your friends might even smoke it. It's less harmful than cigarettes. Anyway, I promise I won't do it again. If you report me, I'll get kicked out of here and I won't be able to complete the program. You know if I'm sent out into the streets now I'll get hooked on drugs again."

The student nurse was faced with a dilemma: should she ignore the client's infraction of the drug center's rules, or, knowing that he might be made to leave the center for breaking the rules, should she report him?

This clinical situation demonstrates many themes common to people who behave in socially deviant ways. By smoking a reefer in front of the student nurse, the client was ignoring the center's rules (anomie) and was taking an unnecessary risk at being caught (poor judgment). The client had not learned from past experience and was repeating the same type of unacceptable behavior. The client's explanation that he was tense and needed to relax, that everyone does it, that marijuana is less dangerous than tobacco, and that marijuana might soon be legalized were rationalizations. Promising not to repeat the offense and reminding the student nurse that if she reported him he would be expelled from the treatment program were attempts at manipulation and blame placing. To the client's way of thinking, his expulsion from the treatment center would be a result of the student nurse's action and not a consequence of his misbehavior. The client would not accept responsibility for what might ensue. He placed the student nurse in a dilemma and showed neither concern nor remorse for the anxiety he caused her. Underlying his behavior were hostility and alienation. This clinical situation shows the interplay of themes that characterizes the behavior of socially deviant individuals.

TYPES OF SOCIALLY DEVIANT BEHAVIOR

People who behave in socially deviant ways are responding to and trying to cope with tension and conflict. However, the techniques they use for reducing tension and conflict are usually socially unacceptable. This situation results in ongoing opposition from society. We will examine four categories of aberrant behavior that represent major social problems: violent behavior, antisocial behavior, addictive behavior, and sexually deviant behavior.

Violent behavior

Violent behavior is behavior whose intent is to inflict physical harm on people or property (Brown, 1981a). Although forms of violent behavior include institutionalized violence (for example, war), mob violence, domestic violence,* criminal violence, and self-inflicted violence,† at this time

---

*Refer to Chapters 12 and 15 for a discussion of domestic violence.
†Refer to Chapter 18 for a discussion of self-inflicted violence as well as to the nursing process section of this chapter.

only criminal violence will be discussed.

For violent behavior to be considered criminal, it must conform to the definition delineated by the society in which it occurs. There are times when this delineation is relative. For example, in some societies, wife beating is not considered criminal behavior until it extends beyond the parameters established by that society. In the United States, police tend to be reluctant to become involved in instances of spousal violence, preferring to define such episodes as domestic disputes rather than as criminal violence. Furthermore, in the United States it is more socially acceptable for women to assault men than for men to assault women. It is also more acceptable for a small person to assault a big person than vice versa. Children in our society are admonished to "pick on someone your own size." These are all instances of ambiguous or unclear parameters delineating violent behavior. On the other hand, there are times when the violation of social norms clearly constitutes criminally violent behavior. For example, in many societies premeditated murder is unequivocally defined as a violent crime (Smith, 1981).

Contrary to popular opinion, people who engage in violent crime are usually not ex–psychiatric clients. Those discharged psychiatric clients who do engage in violent crime frequently have engaged in criminal violence prior to their treatment for psychiatric problems. Although a history of mental illness does not correlate with violent crime, a history of substance abuse, parental deprivation or abuse, intimidation of others, and/or an impulsive personality is associated with criminal violence (Burckhardt, 1981).

Criminal violence cannot be readily predicted. In fact, a previous history of violent behavior is the most consistently shared factor among people who engage in criminal violence. However, a combination of situational and personality factors seems to be implicated in criminal violence. Among these factors are:

Personality factors

1. Childhood history of bedwetting, arson, and cruelty to animals

2. Childhood history of intimidating other children
3. Impulsive personality
4. Coping behaviors of drug or alcohol abuse
5. Low self-esteem

Situational factors

1. Family history of social deviance
2. Dysfunctional family system
3. Unemployment
4. Job dissatisfaction
5. School-related problems (Roth, 1972; Rubin, 1972; Burckhardt, 1981)

Criminal violence may be viewed as a response to stress. This response consists of the following five phases:

1. Triggering phase: A stress-producing event "triggers" the cycle.
2. Escalation phase: Behavioral responses such as increased muscle tension, raised pitch and volume of voice, and emotional and physical agitation lead up to a violent outburst.
3. Crisis phase: A full-blown violent episode occurs.
4. Recovery phase: Assaultive responses decrease as the person returns to a base-line level of response.
5. Post-crisis depression phase: Emotional and physical responses become subnormal. This period may be characterized by apologies and other forms of reconciliatory behavior (Brown 1981b; Smith 1981).

While trying to ascertain what had occurred during a violent episode in the school locker room, a school nurse–teacher learned the following information: For the past two years, Tracy, now a junior in high school, had been extorting protection money from her classmates. One day while making a protection payment, a classmate referred to Tracy as a "butch." Tracy had long been in conflict about her sexual orientation. The word "butch" tapped into this conflict and triggered *the violent episode. She became red in the face, began trembling, and started screaming obscenities* (escalation phase).

Tracy's behavior became increasingly uncontrollable as she began kicking and slashing out with a Swiss Army knife. The victim of Tracy's extortion was cut on the face and shoulder. Following this violent outburst (crisis phase), *Tracy began to recover. Although she continued to curse her victim, Tracy's agitation gradually decreased. By this time school security guards were on the scene and Tracy let herself be led away. She appeared very subdued and mumbled an apology to the guards for "losing my cool and destroying school property"* (post-crisis depression phase).

Associated with the concept of violence as a response to stress are behavioral cues that may indicate impending violent behavior. These behavioral cues occur during the escalation phase of the five-phase assault cycle and include such indices of readiness for "fight or flight" as:

1. Verbal cues: sarcasm, obscenities, derogation, threats and statements about previous violent outbursts
2. Kinesic cues: angry facies, rigid posture, tremors, clenched fists, pacing and hyperactivity
3. Awareness cues: impaired sense of orientation, heightened level of reality testing, impaired degree of situational insight and ability to appropriately perceive, interpret, and respond to environmental stimuli (Clunn, 1981)

Rothenberg (1971) points out that although the open communication of one's anger is not condoned by society's norms and expectations, professional care-givers recognize that the expression of anger is an attempt to communicate. Violence and communication are often regarded as mutually exclusive. Therefore, the maintenance of open lines of communication is an important factor in the management of potentially violent individuals.

Criminal violence is not always a discrete behavior but is often a facet of the behavior pattern of people who engage in other types of socially deviant behavior (such as antisocial behavior, substance abuse, and rape).

Antisocial behavior

Delinquency and criminal activity are the most common types of antisocial behavior. People who display antisocial behavior are estranged from society and its predominant cultural themes. *Juvenile delinquents* and *criminals* often have grown up in environments in which socially approved role models and societal values, purposes, and goals are weak or absent. This is not to say that antisocial individuals have no standards or values. Quite to the contrary, antisocial persons usually belong to a counter-society—a society that runs counter to or against the established society in which it exists. This counter-society has its own role models, goals, and system of values and norms (Birenbaum and Sagarin 1976; Halliday, 1976).

Emerging from and reinforcing a counter-society is an anti-language. An anti-language contains special words that refer to the central activities of the counter-society—for example, words for "police" and "bomb." These anti-language words express meanings and values that are not shared with established society (Halliday, 1976).

Whereas antisocial behavior can be engaged in alone, it is usually engaged in with at least one other person. Antisocial behavior is essentially a group activity. It has a tradition. Antisocial persons are the bearers of this tradition, and anti-language is a major vehicle for socializing persons into the tradition. By conveying special "secret" meanings during verbal interaction, individuals establish ties of strong effective identification with significant others in the counter-society. These significant others serve as role models. Participants in a counter-society learn and pass on to others the rules, regulations, and modi operandi governing antisocial behavior. They learn how to engage in antisocial activities and how to avoid getting caught. They also learn about the social hierarchy of the counter-society and the rules governing loyalty to members of the counter-society (Yablonsky, 1963; Halliday, 1976).

In a sense, then, antisocial behavior can be viewed as adaptive. It helps a person obtain a positive self-concept and a sense of belonging and relatedness. It is an attempt to deal with frustrations, deprivations, and inadequacies. Antisocial behavior is adopted as a coping response when socially acceptable coping behavior has been thwarted (Birenbaum and Sagarin, 1976).

Addictive behavior

Some people compulsively use a substance or practice to cope with the stresses of daily living and to obtain a sense of well-being. The terms "addiction" and "dependence" are often used interchangeably, but they have distinct meanings. Dependence, also referred to as "habituation," is marked by *emotional withdrawal symptoms* when a practice or the ingestion of a substance is abruptly terminated. Addiction is marked by *physical withdrawal symptoms* in such a situation. Addictive or dependent behavior can be classified into two types: *substance abuse* and *practice abuse*.

SUBSTANCE ABUSE

In an attempt to cope with the stresses of daily living and to achieve a feeling of well-being, a person may use chemical substances. These substances may be introduced into the body through inhalation, ingestion, or injection. People who use chemical substances beyond the point of voluntary control are referred to as *substance abusers*. If certain chemical substances are used often enough, tolerance is encountered. Larger and larger amounts of the substance are then required to produce the desired effect. The following are some of the chemical substances on which people become dependent:

Narcotics. The term narcotics refers to opium and its derivatives. Users commonly call these drugs "hard stuff." Included in this group are heroin ("horse," "smack"), morphine ("white stuff," "morpho"), and codeine ("pop," "school boy").

Sedatives and depressants. These drugs have a quieting and sometimes sleep-producing effect. Bromides and barbiturates are frequently used. Alcohol, which is a central nervous system depressant, is so widely used and abused that it will be discussed separately. Users refer to barbiturates as "goof balls," "barbs," or "birds."

Tranquilizers. These drugs reduce anxiety without producing sleep. Diazepam (Valium) and chlordiazepoxide (Librium) have become increasingly abused, and there is growing evidence of tolerance and habituation.

Stimulants. These drugs produce mood elevation and a feeling of boundless energy. Included in this group are cocaine (''speed,'' ''coke'') and amphetamines (''pep pills,'' ''bennies,'' ''cart wheels'').

Hallucinogens or *psychedelics.* The effect obtained from these drugs is frequently referred to as ''tripping.'' A sense of unreality is experienced, and distortion in time, hearing, vision, and distance perception is produced. Actual hallucinations and delusions may occur. Pep reactions include hypersensitivity to visual and auditory stimuli, vacillation between withdrawal and extreme agitation or violence, and schizophrenic-like psychosis. LSD flashbacks may happen days, weeks, or months after a dose. Included in this group are D-lysergic acid diethylamide (''LSD,'' ''acid,'' ''cubes,'' ''royal blue''), mescaline (''mesc''), psilocybin (''God's flesh,'' ''mushrooms''), marijuana (''Mary Jane,'' ''tea,'' ''grass''), and phencyclidine (''PCP,'' ''angel dust'').

Solvents. Solvents include such substances as glue, gasoline, paint thinner, and lighter fluid. Their fumes are inhaled. The immediate effects are similar to those of alcohol intoxication. Thirty to forty-five minutes later, drowsiness, stupor, and sometimes unconsciousness occur. The user retains no memory of the episode. The majority of solvent inhalers are children between the ages of 10 and 15.

Because substance abusers do not necessarily restrict themselves to one category of drug, cross addiction is common. For instance, someone taking amphetamines during the day may take sedatives at night. Someone who drinks to ''steady his nerves'' may turn to tranquilizers when he is not ingesting alcohol. The substances that are most commonly used in combination are as follows: opiates and barbiturates; opiates and cocaine; opiates and marijuana; barbiturates and amphetamines; barbiturates and alcohol; marijuana, amphetamines, and hallucinogens; and tranquilizers and alcohol. These combinations are dangerous. Because they are both central nervous system depressants, alcohol and barbiturates used together may be life threatening.

Substance intoxication occurs when a person has ingested a toxic amount of a substance. If a person combines substances, adulterates substances, or experiments with new substances, it may be difficult to assess and treat substance intoxication. A person experiencing substance intoxication may appear disoriented, depressed, giddy, excited, inattentive, sleepy, or irritable. Body functions may be altered. (Table 17-1 summarizes the effects of chemical substances.) If substance intoxication is suspected, a physician should be summoned immediately. If the substance is known, nurses can make use of standing orders for antidotes. (Because of the danger of cross abuse, all medications should be administered judiciously.) Otherwise, nursing therapy involves the relief of symptoms or the administration of life-sustaining measures (for example, maintenance of an airway). In cases of alcohol or barbiturate abuse, abrupt withdrawal from the substance may precipitate convulsions (Desk Reference on Drug Abuse, 1970). It is especially important for nurses in general hospitals to keep this in mind.

Mr. Frink was admitted to his community hospital after he had suffered a stroke. He was placed in an intensive care unit, and his condition was closely monitored. He became increasingly restless, and muscle tremors began. Suddenly, he had a convulsion.

Mrs. Johnson was admitted to a hospital the day before gallbladder surgery. The next morning, when a nurse brought Mrs. Johnson her preoperative medication, he noticed that she was restless, shaky, and speaking rapidly. The nurse attributed Mrs. Johnson's condition to preoperative anxiety.

In both situations, delirium tremens was neither anticipated nor recognized, but it was present. These vignettes illustrate the importance of thorough history taking and of being alert for substance abuse.

Table 17-1. Usual reactions to chemical substances

Signs and symptoms	Sedatives and depressants	Stimulants	Narcotics	Hallucin- ogens	Tranquil- izers	Solvents
Behavioral						
Aggression	A*	A		A		
Depression	A	W				
Disorientation	A, W	A		A		
Euphoria		A	A	A		A
Drowsiness	A		A	A[1]	A	W
Hallucinations	A, W	A		A		
Inattentiveness	A		A			
Irritability	A	A				
Suspicion	W	A		A		
Restlessness	W	A	W	A		
Physical						
Slurred speech	A		A			
Gastrointestinal			A		A	
Respiratory	A	A	A			
Nasal			W[2]		A[3]	A
Lacrimation			W	A		A
Pinpoint pupils			A			
Dilated pupils	A	A	W	A		
Tachycardia		A	W	A	A	
Hypotension	A, W		A		A	
Skin rash	A	A			A	
Dangers						
Suicidal tendencies				A		
Convulsions	W					
Death[4]	W					A
Organ damage			A	A		A

*A, acute phase; W, withdrawal phase.
[1]Occasional.
[2]Runny nose.
[3]Nasal stuffiness.
[4]Death from overdose can occur with most substances.

Some evidence suggests that abuse of chemical substances may be harmful not only to the user but also to future offspring. For example, Kato et al. (1970) have found that the use of psychedelic drugs may cause chromosome changes in the user and may cause developmental anomalies in a fetus. However, other investigators believe that evidence relating chromosome damage to habitual use of psychedelics is inconclusive (Dishotsky et al., 1971; Leavitt, 1974).

People who use chemical substances in an attempt to cope with the stresses of daily living are usually engaging in illegal as well as socially aberrant behavior. Most of these substances are "controlled'' drugs. Under the Controlled Substances Act of 1970, unless these chemical substances are prescribed by a licensed physician, their possession is illegal.

▶ Alcoholism

One very common type of substance abuse is alcoholism. Alcohol is a central nervous system depressant. Because alcohol decreases inhibitions, it produces a transient feeling of well-being. People who are addicted to alcohol are referred to as *alcoholics*. Alcoholics compulsively use alcohol to cope with conflicts and tension. According to Roueche (1962), for the past 5000 years there have been people in most human societies who have used alcohol as an anesthetic for psychic pain.

Once alcoholics start to drink, they tend to become progressively unable to control their consumption of alcohol. However, Marlatt et al. (1973) have found that all alcoholics do not necessarily ''lose control'' and go on a drinking ''spree'' after only one drink. In addition, alcoholics do not all follow the same drinking pattern. Some alcoholics periodically go on drinking sprees and become noticeably intoxicated. Others drink consistently day in and day out. These alcoholics rarely show signs of intoxication but are continuously under the influence of alcohol. Authorities agree that the development of alcoholism usually occurs in three stages.

1. Social drinking. A person starts to drink socially in order to relax, to be less inhibited, and to be more convivial.
2. Escape drinking. Gradually, a person progresses from drinking to be sociable to drinking to escape stress and feelings of insecurity, inadequacy, and anxiety.
3. Addicted drinking. Ability to control the consumption of alcohol decreases, and the need to ingest alcohol increases. At this point, interpersonal relationships, work, and health are noticeably affected.

Alcoholism affects not only the life of the alcoholic, but also the lives of other family members. Members of an alcoholic's family usually assume one of four survival roles:

The family hero. Often this role is assumed by the oldest child in the family. By overachieving or becoming unusually responsible or successful, the hero makes the family proud.

The scapegoat. Often the second-born child assumes this role. By focusing the family's attention on his or her defiant or rebellious behavior, the scapegoat shifts the family's attention away from the alcoholic member. The concern that family members feel about the scapegoat's problems becomes a unifying element.

The lost child. This child characteristically appears withdrawn and assumes the role of a loner. The family views this child positively, as one member about whom there is no cause for concern.

The family mascot. Often the youngest child or the child that the family tends to overlook assumes this role. In an attempt to get attention, the mascot uses hyperactive, clowning, or obnoxious behavior.

In large families, several members may assume the same roles. Because family members tend to become entrapped in one role, so that role and role occupant become fused, all of these survival roles are potentially destructive. Family ''heroes'' may become workaholics and encourage dependency in family members. It is not uncommon for the spouses and children of family heroes to be substance abusers. Family ''scapegoats'' may eventually engage in criminal behavior or abuse drugs or alcohol. ''Lost children'' frequently demonstrate low self-esteem, psychosexual difficulties (sexual identity problems or promiscuous behavior), and suicidal behavior. Family ''mascots'' tend to experience difficulty coping with stress. Their maladaptive coping behavior may contribute to the development of ulcers or substance abuse. Many ''mascots'' marry ''heroes'' who will indulge their dependency needs. With treatment, the destructive aspects of survival roles can be prevented or reversed (Wegscheider, 1981).

Family members who try to cajole, beg, or intimidate alcoholics into sobriety soon become discouraged and frustrated. Alcoholics can only give up alcohol for themselves. Should an alcoholic decide to ''swear off the bottle'' for spouse or children, at the first argument he or she will return to drinking.

Even though alcohol reduces tension, awareness of deteriorating interpersonal relationships, knowledge of alcohol-associated physiological damage, and the realization that one may be drinking to cope with tension tend to increase an alcoholic's stress (Polivy et al., 1976). Since use of alcohol is an alcoholic's primary way of coping, a vicious cycle is perpetuated.

If alcoholism is allowed to progress, an alcoholic may develop delirium tremens (''d.t.'s''), a form of acute psychosis sometimes precipitated by abrupt abstinence from alcohol. It is characterized by delirium, gross tremors, irritability, hyperactivity, and hallucinations. While the hallucinations may be of any type, they are most often visual, in color, and threatening. A ''pink elephant'' is a popular stereotype of an alcoholic hallucination. Alcohol-induced hallucinations differ from those experienced during a schizophrenic episode (see Chapter 21). Unlike most persons with schizophrenia, alcoholics are usually aware that they are hallucinating. Prolonged alcoholism can also lead to Korsakoff's syndrome—a type of chronic brain syndrome characterized by amnesia, disorientation, confabulation, and peripheral neuropathy—or to Wernicke's syndrome—a type of encephalopathy characterized by amnesia, ophthalmoplegia, confabulation, and ataxia. Wernicke's syndrome sometimes culminates in coma.

These three disorders are usually seen only in chronic alcoholism. These syndromes seem to be related to the toxic effects of prolonged use of alcohol and the nutritional deficiencies (especially of thiamine and niacin) associated with chronic alcoholism. Alcohol consumption is especially harmful during pregnancy. Physical and mental birth defects are found more frequently in the babies of drinking women than in the babies of nondrinking women. Also, neonates of alcoholic mothers have to be monitored for symptoms of alcohol withdrawal, neurological difficulties, and respiratory distress.

▶ Compulsive tobacco smoking

In the wake of evidence that tobacco smoking is dangerous not only to smokers but also to non-smokers who inhale smoke-filled air, tobacco smoking is encountering increasing social disapproval. Theaters, restaurants, and some forms of public transportation are beginning to segregate smokers from nonsmokers; and many establishments completely prohibit smoking. Smoking is beginning to be perceived as socially deviant behavior.

Green (1977) identifies four types of smokers:
1. Habitual smokers—people who are psychologically dependent on tobacco and experience psychological withdrawal symptoms when tobacco is abruptly withheld
2. Positive-effect smokers—people who derive a stimulant effect from tobacco
3. Negative-effect smokers—people who derive a sedative effect from tobacco
4. Addictive smokers—people who are physically dependent on tobacco and experience physical withdrawal symptoms when tobacco is abruptly withheld

In addition, Reeder (1977) identifies the following sociocultural correlates in the development of adolescent smoking patterns:
1. A parent or older sibling who smokes. The influence is strongest where either both parents smoke or one parent and an older sibling smoke. The presence of two smokers in a family system increases fourfold the likelihood that an adolescent will begin to smoke.
2. Close friends of the adolescent who smoke. They may provide both role models and peer pressure.
3. Poor academic achievement. Adolescent smokers tend to have lower educational aspirations than do their nonsmoking peers. It may be that smoking serves as coping behavior to deal with the anxiety generated by poor academic performance.

Psychological withdrawal symptoms from smoking tobacco consist primarily of craving (which may persist for years) and restlessness. Physical withdrawal symptoms include a decrease in vital signs, lowered basal metabolism rate, increased salivation, and weight gain (Hammond and Percy, 1958; Larson et al., 1961).

Studies have shown that smokers have more antisocial tendencies than nonsmokers (Lebovits and Ostfeld, 1971; Nesgit, 1972). Smokers are more apt to attribute what happens to them to chance, fate, or the actions of others than are nonsmokers. Smokers tend to perceive the locus of control as existing outside themselves; they may not readily see occurrences as consequences of their own actions (Reynolds and Nichols, 1976).

Addictive smokers, also known as *smokaholics,* experience a compulsion to continue smoking. Over time, most smokaholics develop tolerance for tobacco (especially the nicotine in tobacco) and therefore increase the amount of their smoking (Windsor and Richards, 1935; Johnston, 1942; Finnegan et al., 1945; Van Proosdij, 1960). Many smokaholics cannot give up smoking without assistance.

▶ Chronic overeating

People who chronically overeat are sometimes referred to as *foodaholics*. Such people use eating to cope with the stress engendered by current or past problems. Obesity ensues, and this obesity can contribute to new problems (for example, alteration in self image, social rejection, self-rejection, hypertension, heart disease, arthritis). This feedback of problems creates additional stress and people again resort to eating to cope. An "avalanching spiral" is thus set into motion (Wick, 1976).

Wick (1976) has identified five typical patterns of overeating.*

1. Temporary, sporadic overeating
2. Phasic or impulsive eating
3. Continuous overeating
4. Repetitive, compulsive overeating
5. Eruptive, uncontrolled indulgence

Temporary, sporadic overeating is engaged in during periods of stress. Should stress become chronic, overeating becomes chronic. The purpose of this pattern of overeating is to restore a sense of inner balance. *Phasic or impulsive eating* is also

---

*Refer to Chapters 15 and 19 for discussion of the eating disorders anorexia nervosa and bulimia.

referred to as binge eating. Binge eating is precipitated by stress, and the purpose of binge eating is to release tension. *Continuous overeating* is often an eating pattern learned early in life from one's family members. An entire family may have this eating pattern and be overweight. Other continuous overeaters eat to avoid psychic pain. The purpose of this pattern of overeating is to maintain a sense of well-being. Since continuous overeaters tend to associate food with love, security, and nurturing, food is the route they take to maintain a feeling of well-being. *Repetitive, compulsive overeaters* seem never to achieve a sense of satiation. People who engage in this pattern of overeating are not in touch with their emotions. Anxiety, anger, etc., are interpreted as discomfit. This discomfit is then interpreted as hunger and a need to eat. The purpose that this overeating pattern serves is to give people something constant to hold on to in the face of threatening reality. The focus is on food rather than on real-life anxieties. *Eruptive, uncontrolled indulgence* is precipitated by food likes or food fantasies. People who engage in eruptive, uncontrolled indulgence in food are not tempted by disliked foods. However, in the presence of appealing food, such people cannot stop eating. During periods of indulgence, such people either are not receiving satiation signals or are ignoring them. The purpose of eruptive, uncontrolled food indulgence is to receive pleasure—to use food to create a pleasurable reality.

Foodaholics are well aware of the cardiovascular complications associated with obesity, such as heart disease and hypertension. Yet this knowledge is not an adequate motivator to keep them from overeating. Family members and friends who try to persuade foodaholics to lose weight for reasons of health or appearance soon become discouraged. In fact, family members may even negatively influence a dieter's efforts. Many family members consistently criticize an overeater's eating behavior and weight, while at the same time offering the overeater food; and they may not praise or otherwise reinforce controlled eating patterns (Stuart and Davis, 1972).

When diets are imposed on them, overeaters

often hide food and eat it surrepticiously. Food-aholics often diet in public and gorge in private. For foodaholics, life revolves around food: food that is low in calories and food that is high in calories, food that is permitted by a diet and food that is prohibited or restricted by a diet, food that will be consumed and food that will not be consumed, food that should have been eaten and food that should not have been eaten (Orbach, 1978). Overeaters experience a loss of control when they are around food; they cannot give up their habit without assistance.

• • •

The following substance abuse self-assessment guide* may help both nurses and clients to assess whether or not they have a problem with substance abuse. Do you . . .

1. Use substances (e.g., food, tobacco, drugs, or alcohol) to deal with personal problems (e.g., quarrels, disappointments, pressure situations)?
2. Lose time from your job or school because of your use of a substance?
3. Become very defensive or deny everything when criticized about your substance use?
4. Use drugs or alcohol routinely every day?
5. Have physical symptoms that may be related to your substance use (e.g., weight loss, weight gain, insomnia, confused thinking, lack of coordination, shortness of breath, "smoker's cough")?
6. Cause family members embarrassment, hurt, or concern by your substance use?
7. Need larger quantities of drugs or alcohol to obtain the same effect as when you first started using the substance?
8. Feel uncomfortable at or avoid social functions where drugs or alcohol are not available? Where tobacco smoking is not permitted? Where food will not be served?
9. Regret or feel guilty about the way you

overindulged in a substance (e.g., overate, got drunk)?
10. Break promises made to yourself or others about decreasing or controlling your substance use?
11. Avoid family and/or friends when you are high on drugs or alcohol, overeating, or smoking too many cigarettes?

"Yes" answers to one or more of these questions may indicate a problem with substance abuse and the need for prompt help.

PRACTICE ABUSE

In an attempt to cope with day-by-day stress and conflict and to achieve a sense of well-being, people may compulsively rely on or overuse a practice. People who rely on a practice beyond the point of voluntary control and who experience habituation (emotional withdrawal symptoms when that practice is abruptly terminated) may be termed practice abusers. Compulsive gambling and compulsive working are examples of practice abuse. Forrest (1979) points out that these practices usually start out as generative in regard to the physical and psychological well-being of the person. Initially, the person is able to exert control over the amount of time that the practice is indulged in and the practice offers the person a short-term "escape" from stresses of daily living. Over time, however, the practice becomes habituating. The practice encompasses the individual's entire experiential self. The increased dependence on the practice limits the person's ability to grow and change. What began as a generative practice evolves into a destructive practice.

▶ Compulsive gambling

Unlike people who occasionally gamble as a form of recreation and who usually frequent gambling spots with friends, compulsive gamblers bet excessively and uncontrollably and usually gamble in isolation. Bergler (1970) and Martinez (1978) identify some characteristics of compulsive gamblers: predisposition to risk taking; involvement with gambling to the exclusion of other interests; unrealistic optimism that is not altered by consis-

---

*Sources consulted in the preparation of this guide include The National Council on Alcoholism and The Freeport Narcotics Guidance Council.

tent losses; frequent fantasizing that they are prestigious, wealthy, or able to outsmart rivals; ability to derive an emotional ''high,'' or euphoria, from gambling; powerlessness to stop gambling when they are winning; and compulsion to bet beyond their means.

Compulsive gamblers view money as an avenue of adulation. The development of a winning system and the winning of money are perceived as evidence of intelligence, shrewdness, and success. When compulsive gamblers are gambling, their energy and attention are devoted to the challenge of the minute and the fantasies of winning (Livingston, 1974).

Goffman (1969) describes four stages of a complete gambling transaction:

1. ''Squaring off''—the decision to take a chance, the selection of a method of gambling, and the placing of a bet
2. ''Determination''—production of a result (for example, through the spinning of a roulette wheel or the dealing of cards)
3. Disclosure—realization of an outcome (calling of the numbers or dealing of the cards)
4. Settlement—payment of losses or collection of winnings

Compulsive gamblers usually do not want to stop gambling but do wish that the undesirable side effects of losing could be changed (Moran, 1970). While there are no physical withdrawal symptoms associated with the cessation of compulsive gambling, the psychological withdrawal symptoms of depression and guilt may be experienced (Hyde, 1978). Compulsive gamblers cannot give up their gambling without assistance.

▶ Compulsive working

Some people compulsively use work to control tension and to produce a feeling of well-being. *Workaholics* immerse themselves in work to the exclusion of other life activities. Immersion in work is one way of avoiding meaningful interpersonal relationships. Friedman and Rosenman (1974) and Jenkins (1975) describe workaholics as people who have an exaggerated sense of the work ethic and who suffer from environmental overbur-

dening. Workaholics work long hours and often take work home on evenings and weekends. They seldom take vacations; when they do vacation, they frequently bring work along or cut their vacations short in order to return to work. Workaholics are very competitive. Their setting of extremely high standards of productivity places workaholics in competition not only with others but also with themselves.

Workaholics have a ''type A'' behavior pattern. According to Friedman and Rosenman (1974), a type A behavior pattern consists of the following constellation of attitudes, actions, and emotional responses: competitiveness, achievement orientation, aggressiveness, restlessness, impatience, a constant sense of time urgency, drive, persistence, polyphasic thinking, rapid and explosive speech, and hurried motor movements. Recent research suggests that type A behavior is a significant predictor of coronary heart disease (Rosenman et al., 1970; Wardwell and Bahnson, 1973; Rosenman et al., 1975).

Workaholics cannot *not* work. Because they do not direct their tensions and conflicts against society, their compulsion to work cannot be accurately classified as socially deviant behavior. However, today's world is marked by unemployment and underemployment. Unions are trying to obtain shorter work weeks for employees. Management is exploring the possibility of early retirement for employees. Society is espousing the merits of leisure time. Although workaholics are not breaking society's norms, neither are they totally working within them. Workaholism may be a type of borderline socially deviant behavior.

• • •

The following practice abuse self-assessment guide* may help both nurses and clients assess whether they have a problem with practice abuse. Do you . . .

1. Compulsively engage in a practice to deal with your personal problems (e.g., quar-

---

*Sources consulted in the preparation of this guide include the National Council on Compulsive Gambling, and Forrest (1979).

rels, disappointments, pressure situations)?

2. Lose time from your job or school because of this practice?

3. Hear complaints from family members that your dependence on this practice is causing unhappiness at home?

4. Feel that dependence on this practice is ruining your reputation?

5. Feel regret or remorse because of this practice?

6. Experience a strong or irresistible urge to continue engaging in this practice?

7. Find yourself lying or sneaking in order to indulge this practice (e.g., understating the amount of money lost by gambling; making excuses for bringing work along on your vacation)?

8. Ever contemplate suicide because of the effect this practice has had on your life?

9. Find yourself so dependent on this practice that it takes priority over other aspects of your life (e.g., family responsibilities, job obligations, your reputation)?

10. Become very defensive or deny everything in the face of criticism about your dependence on this practice?

11. Experience depression, guilt, and/or anxiety when you try to give up this practice?

12. Break promises to yourself or others about decreasing or controlling this practice?

"Yes" answers to a majority of these questions may indicate practice abuse and the need for prompt help.

Sexually deviant behavior

Prostitution and rape are two types of socially deviant behavior that are of increasing social concern.* Underlying these behaviors are overt or covert hostility and aggression.

---

*Child molestation is a socially deviant behavior that is also of much social concern. Child molestation is discussed in Chapter 15.

PROSTITUTION

Persons who engage in coital or extracoital sex in return for money are engaged in prostitution and are referred to as prostitutes. Although much of the general public considers prostitution to be strictly an adult female activity, prostitutes may be children or adults, men or women, heterosexuals, homosexuals, or bisexuals (Masters, 1962; Chesser, 1971). Today many prostitutes are youngsters (16 years of age and younger) who have run away from home in an attempt to escape from intolerable home situations that often include alcoholism or drug addiction on the part of parents (Morgan, 1975; Thomkins, 1977).

People engage in prostitution for many reasons. Broken homes, parental promiscuity, and a social network that accepts prostitution can predispose people to prostitution. Economic incentives, opportunity for diverse types of sexual activity, and the expectation of a more leisurely and exciting life may attract people to prostitution. Economic difficulties, inducement by a pimp or by other prostitutes, or ready opportunity may precipitate entry into prostitution. By examining the reasons why people become prostitutes, Benjamin and Masters (1964) have divided prostitutes into two types: voluntary and compulsive. Voluntary prostitutes freely select prostitution as a way to support themselves, because of the advantages associated with it. Compulsive prostitutes enter prostitution because of a strong impulse to engage in sex for money. The classifications of voluntary and compulsive prostitutes are based on the *predominant* reasons people become prostitutes. These categories are not mutually exclusive, and most prostitutes have a combination of reasons. The attractive features of prostitution play an important role in the case of voluntary prostitutes. Predisposing elements play an important role in the case of compulsive prostitutes. A precipitating event or events usually increases the strength of attractive and predisposing factors (Benjamin and Masters, 1964; Gregg, 1976).

Prostitution, by definition, is an activity that necessitates the involvement of at least one other person, the client. Much of the research on prostitution has focused on female prostitutes and male clients. In the classic Kinsey report, *Sexual Behavior in the Human Male* (1948), it was found that 69% of white American men have had some type of experience with prostitutes.

Clients, like prostitutes, can be divided into voluntary and compulsive categories. Voluntary clients engage in sex with prostitutes for such utilitarian reasons as sexual unavailability of a mate due to distance or illness, limited opportunity (or no opportunity) to find a mate, and desire to prove one's "maleness" to male friends. Some voluntary clients engage in sex with prostitutes as an alternative to abstinence as a form of birth control: if one's mate refuses to use contraceptives, intercourse with the mate may be avoided and a prostitute sought instead.

Compulsive clients engage in sex with prostitutes for such psychophysiological reasons as inability to compete with others for a mate because of age or physical handicap; need for variety; sadomasochism or fetishism; and desire to avoid interpersonal relationships (Benjamin and Masters, 1964; Clinard, 1974; Donaldson, 1977).

An important aspect of prostitution is the prostitute-pimp relationship. Mutual exploitation is a predominant theme. Prostitutes turn their earnings over to their pimps and usually take their pimps as lovers. Pimps act as intermediaries between prostitutes and clients, drug dealers, police, and/or crime syndicate members. Pimps handle payoffs and protection money. From their relationship with pimps, prostitutes extract protection, the illusion of a caring figure, and a defense against loneliness. From their relationship with prostitutes, pimps extract money and the status symbols that money can buy. These status symbols plus the awareness of being a lover to a woman who has sexual relationships with many men increase the self-esteem of many pimps (Choisy, 1960; Benjamin and Masters, 1964; Donaldson, 1977).

In addition to the utilitarian nature of pimp-prostitute relationships, sadomasochism is a common theme. Pimps often viciously beat their prostitutes.

The prostitutes, who in most cases have isolated themselves from family and friends, tend to interpret these beatings as evidence that their pimps "care" about them. Sexual intercourse between pimp and prostitute frequently follows beatings (Choisy, 1960; Benjamin and Masters, 1964; Chesser, 1971).

Most prostitutes have antisocial tendencies that are developed and reinforced by their experiences in jail and by society's attitudes toward prostitutes. Risk taking is engaged in daily. They face the risk of arrest, the risk of bodily harm, and the risk of encountering clients who will make bizarre demands. Prostitutes display hostility toward society by being contemptuous of any work that society sanctions. Most prostitutes do not perceive prostitution as work. Instead they believe that by engaging in prostitution they are violating the work ethic—living off the workers of society and thereby outsmarting society (Benjamin and Masters, 1964; Chesser, 1971; Donaldson, 1977). "Sex for sale" is more than the sale of sex. By breaking with sexual mores and engaging in prostitution, prostitutes display their hostility toward society.

RAPE

Men who engage in forcible intercourse with an unwilling partner* are committing rape. Rapists not only act out their tensions and conflicts through forcible intercourse but also commit a crime. Rape is *not* an act of passion; it is an act of violence. Rape serves the nonsexual purposes of venting anger and hostility and exercising control and power. These themes—anger, hostility, control, power—are present in every rape, but in any given rape one theme or combination of themes may predominate (Brownmiller, 1975; Burgess and Holstrom, 1974).

Burgess and Holstrom (1974) identify three types of rapists. The "anger rapist" displaces his anger toward a significant woman or women onto the rape victim. He uses more physical force than

---

*See Chapter 18 for a discussion of the victim's reaction to rape.

is needed to subdue his victim. He brutalizes her. This type of rapist may also degrade his victim by forcing her to engage in oral sex, by masturbating on her, or by urinating on her. The victim selected by such a rapist is usually old or in some other way vulnerable.

The "power rapist" is the most common type of rapist. He uses only the amount of force necessary to subdue his victim. His aim is to get his victim into his power. He wants to gain control, demonstrate his power, and thereby "prove" himself as a man. Intimidation rather than physical force is used to gain control over his victim. Often, this type of rapist fantasizes that his victim will be sexually attracted to him because of the sexual prowess he will show during the rape. He will frequently ask his victim, while raping her, if she is enjoying the experience. This is the type of rapist who may ask his victim for a date at the conclusion of the rape.

The third type of rapist, the "sadistic rapist," seeks sexual gratification and an outlet for aggression through rape. Sexuality and aggression are blended together. This type of rapist receives his ultimate erotic excitement from the death of his victim. Instead of penetrating his victim with his penis, he may use an instrument. He may ejaculate at the moment of the victim's death, or he may have intercourse with the victim's dead body. In addition, there may be a ritualistic aspect to such a rape. The Boston Strangler and the Hillside Rapist are examples of sadistic rapists. Fortunately, this type of rapist is rare.

Selkin (1975) suggests that most rapists follow an identifiable pattern. First, a rapist selects a woman who is perceived as vulnerable (for example, old, living alone, or hitchhiking). Then he tests his potential victim. For example, a rapist may approach a woman, ask her for a match, make insinuating remarks, and then direct her to remove her clothes or tell her not to scream. In this way, he determines whether she can be intimidated. Next, he threatens her. He tells her what he wants her to do, that he will harm her if she does not submit, and that she will be spared if she cooperates.

EPIDEMIOLOGY

The exact incidence of socially deviant behavior is unknown. Hospitals usually treat only a small portion of the people who display socially aberrant behavior. Many such individuals are neither hospitalized nor treated by mental health practitioners but instead are sentenced to criminal justice institutions for their offenses against society.

An impressive amount of research has shown a correlation between socioeconomic environment and socially aberrant behavior. People who experience socioeconomic deprivation are often isolated from the mainstream of society. They may experience overcrowding, poverty, and scarcity of employment opportunities. They tend to have little access to information, goods, and services. Such an environment may lead to blocked aspirations and to the use of illegitimate means to achieve goals. A circular system of blocked aspirations and illegitimate ways of achieving goals may develop to maintain such people in a state of alienation and anomie. Drug addiction, alcoholism, gambling, prostitution, and violence are often commonplace in such an environment. Rather than being considered deviant, such behavior may come to be viewed as "adult" and to be considered part of a rite of passage from childhood to adulthood. Thus children who grow up in an environment of socioeconomic deprivation may be socialized into a system of deviant norms, a situation that may lead to a high incidence of socially aberrant behavior (Ashcraft and Scheflen, 1976; Clinard, 1974).

The incidence of socially deviant behavior is two to three times higher among men than among women. Chesler (1972) refers to various types of behavior as "male diseases." She points out that aggressive acts, sexual misbehavior, drinking, swearing, gambling, and even stealing are all part of an exaggerated stereotype of the male role. In order to be "masculine" in Western society, less powerful and secure men have to "prove" themselves by taking what more powerful and secure men either already have or can readily obtain. For example, the sociocultural environment surrounding the working-class male often equates risk taking, womanizing, and possession of money, cars, and clothes with ''machismo.'' Gambling may be a routine aspect of the life-style of many adult men. Such an environment tends to reinforce a gambler's self-image as ''action-seeker'' and to contribute to fantasies of power and prestige (Gans, 1962; Livingston, 1974). This is not to say that women do not behave in socially aberrant ways. For example, most prostitutes are women, and overeating occurs primarily in women. Orbach (1978) views overeating among women as a rebellion against culturally defined sex-role stereotypes. (For an in-depth discussion, refer to the sections on psychological and sociocultural theories in this chapter.)

Although many incidents of socially deviant behavior are not reported (for example, rape) or are recorded as crimes rather than as psychosocial disorders (for example, prostitution), the prevalence of two types of socially deviant behavior—drug addiction and alcoholism—has been estimated.

Drug abuse and addiction are found among all age groups. Drug use in general has increased in recent years. Moynihan (1984) estimates that 35% of the population has used illicit drugs. This represents a 31% increase in illicit drug use over the past 20 years.

Alcohol is the most commonly abused drug in the United States. Alcoholism ranks with cancer and heart disease as a major health problem. Yet alcoholism is one of our most neglected health problems. There are approximately 100 million persons aged 15 years or older who consume alcohol, and we know that many children younger than 15 drink. Of these users of alcohol, approximately 10 million are alcoholics. Violent behavior associated with alcohol intoxication is related to 64% of all murders, 41% of all assaults, 34% of all rapes, 29% of other sex crimes, and 60% of all cases of child abuse (Report of the National Council on Alcoholism, 1976). Alcoholism is therefore associated with many other types of socially aberrant behavior.

CROSS-CULTURAL CONTEXT

Socially deviant behavior must be viewed from a cultural perspective. Special attention should be paid to the fact that cultures define aberrant behavior in various ways.

Many anthropologists believe that violence is *not* universal. For example, adult violence is unknown among the Ifaluk of Micronesia (Burrows and Spiro, 1953). On the other hand, some societies have a high incidence of violence. The Yamana of Tierra del Fuego are almost continuously involved in brawls and interfamily murders (Gusinde, 1961).

Nash (1967) suggests a correlation between increased homicide rates and periods of social change. She has found that in response to social change among the Teklum, in Mexico, charges of witchcraft have increased, with an associated rise in homicide. Among the Teklum, murder is strictly a male activity. Both perpetrators and victims are men. Men who are murdered have usually been suspected of witchcraft. Most of this Indian community feel that these homicides are justified. This situation points to a correlation between social stress and social deviance. It also shows that while homicide might be perceived as a deviant form of behavior, members of a particular society might not always interpret it as troublesome.

In contrast to evidence suggesting that violence may not be a universal occurrence, the use of psychoactive substances is found in all societies. Each society decides which substances will be sanctioned and which will be condemned.

Even when socially acceptable drugs are used, certain rules must be followed. Persons who ignore the rules are considered just as deviant as those who use unacceptable drugs. This is best exemplified by a village in Rajasthan, India. In this village, members of different social castes approve of different intoxicants. Rajputs (members of ruler and warrior caste) regularly indulge in *daru* (alcohol), while Brahmins regularly use *bhang* (*Cannabis indica*). Each caste condemns the use of the other's drug. However, both Rajputs and Brahmins also have rules governing the use of their own drugs. Persons who break the rules are regarded as drug abusers (Carstairs, 1954). In the United States, many Indian tribes use peyote in religious ceremonies. The Native American Church uses peyote as a sacramental (LaBarre, 1960, 1964; Slotkin, 1967). Thus, the way a society views a drug and its use determines what constitutes drug abuse.

Alcohol is one drug that is known to most societies. However, the amount of alcohol that is imbibed and the frequency with which people become alcoholics is strongly influenced by culture. Defining alcoholism as the ingestion of 5 or more ounces of alcohol per day, DeLint and Schmidt (1971) found that the rate of alcoholism varies greatly from country to country. France has the highest incidence of alcoholism, and Norway and Finland have the lowest. With approximately 2% of its inhabitants developing alcoholism, the United States falls in the midrange of DeLint and Schmidt's international survey.

Bacon (1973) uses the concept of integrated drinking to explain why some societies have a lower incidence of alcoholism than do other societies. Integrated drinking refers to the incorporation of drinking alcoholic beverages into the lifestyle of a cultural group. Societies that have integrated drinking into their way of life usually have a high rate of alcohol consumption but not necessarily a high rate of alcoholism. In those cultural groups characterized by integrated drinking, the following factors seem to be associated with a low rate of alcoholism: indulgence of children's dependency needs, relatively strict toilet training practices, relatively permissive methods of socialization, acceptance of adult dependency (rather than an emphasis on independence) and family-oriented drinking and eating patterns.

Drinking patterns in the United States illustrate Bacon's concept of integrating drinking. Although Jewish Americans, Italian-Americans, and Chinese-Americans tend to drink alcoholic beverages more frequently than do people from other ethnic groups, these three groups have low incidences of alcoholism. This situation is probably related to many of the factors enumerated by Bacon. The factor most readily discernible is the family-oriented drinking patterns of these three ethnic groups.

In Jewish culture, the primary alcoholic beverage is the sweet wine served at family gatherings and especially on religious holidays. In Italian culture, drinking is usually limited to the wine served during meals and at social activities. Similarly, in Chinese culture, drinking is done within the family milieu. In these cultures, alcohol is viewed as a social beverage, and drinking patterns tend to be family oriented. Rarely do persons of Jewish, Italian, or Chinese heritage view alcohol as a way to escape from personal problems (Bell, 1970).

Prostitution is another type of socially deviant behavior that is found in many societies. The stigma attached to prostitution is related to other aspects of a social system. For example, in Latin societies such as those of Italy and Spain, prostitution must be understood in terms of a group of cultural patterns known as the Madonna complex. The Madonna—the mother of Christ—represents the ideal woman: loving, tender, forgiving, and asexual. In Latin cultures, the virginity of women prior to marriage and the fidelity of women after marriage are extremely important. "Decent" women need to be protected from sexual advances; protection is provided through patterns of chaperonage. In addition, the life of women revolves around the home. The home symbolizes femininity, safety, and asexuality. In sharp contrast, it is socially acceptable for Latin men to engage in premarital and extramarital sex. Boys first engage in sex during their teens, and the occasion is a time for boasting rather than secrecy. The life of Latin men revolves around the street, the bar, and the café, which represent the public domain, a domain that is closed to all women except prostitutes. Thus there is a clear dichotomy between the "decent" woman and the prostitute. The prostitute has violated cultural taboos and has assumed the prerogatives of masculine behavior (Buitrago-Ortiz, 1973; Martinez-Alier, 1974).

Some form of gambling is also found in many cultures. Even prior to the European colonization of the Americas, Indians engaged in dice matches (peach or other fruit stones were fashioned into dice). The form of gambling that is preferred by people is often influenced by their culture. For example, betting on cockfights is popular in Latin America and the Philippines, betting on jai alai is popular in Latin America and Southern Europe, betting on poker games is popular throughout the United States, betting on camel fights is popular in Turkey, and betting on scorpion races is popular in Arab countries.

While most societies outlaw some types of gambling (for example, cockfights are illegal in the United States), other forms of gambling may be sanctioned. For example, Mexico, Japan, Russia, and a majority of the states in the United States permit lotteries. Legal gambling casinos operate in such countries as Monaco, France, Germany, Puerto Rico, St. Martin, and the United States (Fleming, 1978).

Thus, some type of socially deviant behavior is known to all societies. The form it takes and the meaning it is given are related to other aspects of a social system. Socially deviant behavior is culturally influenced, and the incidences of particular types of socially aberrant behavior vary from society to society.

THEORIES OF SOCIALLY DEVIANT BEHAVIOR

It is probably true that people have always been trying to understand socially deviant behavior. In the 1600s, for example, Thomas Hobbes became concerned with the origins of social order and social disorder—a concern that has come to be known as the "Hobbesian problem of order." Hobbes believed that human beings are basically morally abject and that human nature causes people to pursue their own self-interests through any means, even through the use of socially unacceptable behavior. Hobbes maintained that only

through legitimized force, vested in government, could socially deviant behavior be controlled. John Locke disagreed with Hobbes. Locke believed that people are born with a "tabula rasa" (clean slate) and that they are molded by their experiences. Locke maintained that social order can be fostered and social deviance kept in check through a shared system of values and interests.

Concern and speculation about the causes of social order and social disorder persist. Why do people deviate from society's standards? Why do people act out tensions and conflicts in socially unacceptable ways? There are almost as many theories to explain socially deviant behavior as there are types of socially deviant behavior. These theories fall into three major categories: psychological conflict, biological defect, and sociocultural conflict. It is important to keep in mind that no definitive "cause" of socially aberrant behavior has been found. It is probable that a combination of factors leads to the development of deviant behavior. We will look at some of these factors and at how they are interrelated.

Psychological theories

The consensus of psychological theorists is that socially deviant behavior patterns and life-styles can be traced back to adolescence or even earlier. Superego formation or "conscience" is acquired through identification with the values of significant others, especially parents. Fundamental to the process of identification is a relationship built on trust and affection. In individuals who display socially deviant behavior, this identification process has not occurred or identification has been made with socially undesirable traits. When a parent of the same sex is absent, weak, or feared, a child may lack a warm and trustworthy role model. In the case of a weak or absent parent figure, there is little opportunity for a child to identify with the parent.*

---

*The generalization should not be made that all children of single parents are at risk for developing socially deviant behavior. Refer to Chapters 5 and 12 for a discussion of single-parent families.

In the case of a feared parent figure, a child often internalizes socially undesirable characteristics.

In either event, without a relationship of love and trust between child and parent (especially the parent of the same sex), a child is unable to effectively identify with parents and tends not to internalize socially approved roles or socially acceptable values. Such a child grows into adulthood with an inadequately socialized superego. Social acceptance and disapproval then prove to be ineffective motivators or constraints. Such individuals operate for pleasure. They are impulsive; they are unable to arrive at a successful compromise between society's standards and their own impulsive desires. This situation frequently places such individuals in direct conflict with society.

PSYCHOANALYTIC THEORIES

The psychoanalyst Freud (1930, 1959) identified three agencies of the mind: id, ego, and superego (see Chapter 6). He believed that human infants are dominated solely by the id. Only through the process of socialization do the ego and superego develop. The ego, through its appraisal of reality, and the superego, through its use of guilt, make people conform to social standards and thereby curb id behavior.

According to Freud, socially deviant individuals have defective egos. Their egos are unable to control and regulate behavior. Freud also held that people who display socially aberrant behavior have weak or immature superegos: these people feel little guilt or remorse about their behavior.

Some neo-freudian research supports Freud's ideas. This research relates the inability to internalize social expectations and controls through development of the superego to the emergence of violent behavior (Marmor, 1978; Eysenck, 1979).

INTERPERSONAL THEORIES

Another psychoanalyst, Horney (1937), criticized Freud for not recognizing the role that anxiety and inner conflict play in the development of socially deviant behavior. Horney saw quests for power, prestige, and possessions as attempts to find reassurance against anxiety. She also realized

that these quests are culturally specific and that they are not found in every society. She argued that in trying to obtain power, prestige, and possessions, some people become exploitative and manipulative.

More recently, psychoanalysts have found that the quest for power, prestige, and possessions is important in such socially deviant behavior as prostitution. Through the sale of sex, prostitutes and pimps are able to acquire money and improve their standard of living. Money is also symbolic of power and prestige. Choisy (1961) and Chesser (1971) suggest that a prostitute symbolically emasculates a client by taking both his erection and his money. However, not only do prostitutes use money to gain control over clients, but clients use money to exert control over prostitutes. Through the exchange of money for sex, clients make prostitutes purchasable items. Clients "thingify" and degrade prostitutes. Both prostitutes and clients have a need for power and prestige. The prostitute's sale of sex and the client's purchase of sex give each the illusion of power and prestige.

There are many ways in which human beings acquire and assimilate power, prestige, and possessions. They can be cooperative or competitive, egalitarian or authoritative, giving or exploitative. These orientations constitute basic character or personality patterns.

Fromm (1947) defined character or personality as the way human energy is "canalized" or directed in the process of living and relating to the world. Once energy is directed into a specific character orientation, behavior becomes fairly consistent or "true to character." Thus, personality orientation enables an individual to function in society, and personality orientation is itself molded by society. However, even within the same character orientation, individual differences exist. Because of constitutional differences, especially differences in temperament, no two people experience a situation in the same way.

Fromm's term "exploitative orientation" can be used to describe many socially deviant individuals. Such people perceive the source of good and bad to be outside themselves. The only way to obtain the good things of life is to take them—through manipulation, guile, and/or force. This orientation pervades an individual's life-style. Everyone and everything is subject to exploitation. People and things are valued only for their usefulness. Fromm believed that an exploitative orientation is so pervasive that it even affects one's facial expression and gestures. He asserted that hostility and manipulation underlie an exploitative life-style and that these characteristics may be reflected in a "biting mouth" and in aggressive, pointed gestures.

Some psychologists use Fromm's concept of exploitative orientation to explain the psychology of gambling. In gambling, winning and losing are matters of chance. Chance lies outside the control of gamblers. According to Bergler (1970), compulsive gamblers continuously rebel against logic, moderation, and morality. By gambling, compulsive gamblers are scorning socially approved rules for living and are relying on the rules of chance. Compulsive gamblers will use manipulation, guile, and force in order to continue gambling. These authors see gambling as an expression of hostility and aggression against those representatives of society (for example, parents, teachers, and clergymen) who have tried to inculcate socially approved rules for living.

When people gamble, there is always the possibility of getting rich without working. Compulsive gamblers are defying the work ethic. Chance determines how the die rolls, which card is dealt, or where the roulette ball stops. Compulsive gamblers thus are defying the idea that logic and reason prevail in the world (Lindner, 1950; Bergler, 1970).

No one psychological theory is adequate for explaining all types of socially deviant behavior or why different people display different types of such behavior. We cannot speak of a psychological "cause" for socially deviant behavior.

Biological theories

Biological theories purport that individuals become socially deviant because they are biologically predisposed to such behavior. On the basis of the cosmology of Empedocles, early scientists believed that people reflect the natural elements and that differences in temperament result from body structure, humors, and muscle tone. Phrenologists believed that it was possible to determine character traits by observing the protuberances on the external surfaces of people's skulls. These ideas pervaded the study of human behavior for more than 2,000 years.

Then, for many years, a link between biology and social deviance was discredited. Recently, however, improper nutrition, brain defects, and physiological malfunctions have been suggested as possible contributors to deviant behavior.

BIOCHEMICAL THEORIES

Diet, food colorings, sugar, and food allergies have all been related to the development of hyperactivity and/or violent behavior. For example, Bolton (1972) has found a relationship between violent behavior and hypoglycemia among Peru's Quolla Indians. Feingold (1975) contends that the increased incidence of hyperactivity among children is directly related to increased consumption of "junk foods" containing food additives. However, some researchers investigating the effect of additive-free diets on the incidence of hyperactivity have not substantiated Feingold's contention (Kolbye, 1976).

PHYSIOLOGICAL THEORIES

Some research indicates that early eating habits determine the number of fat cells an individual will have—that the number of fat cells becomes set early in a person's life and cannot be changed. Weight loss can only be accomplished by decreasing the size of fat cells. When people with large numbers of fat cells try to reduce, they experience energy deficits. Because it is very difficult for such people to curtail their eating, many of them may become compulsive eaters (Hirsch and Knittle, 1970; Nisbett, 1972).

Other studies indicate that neurological problems may cause socially deviant behavior. Mark and Ervin (1970) suggest that malfunctions in the brain may be responsible for such aberrant behavior. Brain mechanisms for controlling impulsive violence are believed to be located in the limbic system, especially in the amygdala. Removal of the amygdala in violent individuals, with ensuing control of violent behavior, has reinforced this theory.

At the 1979 annual meeting of the American Academy of Neurology, Pincus (1979), a neurologist on a research team, suggested that neurological disorders may contribute to violent behavior in juvenile delinquents. Pincus found that 96% of the violent delinquents studied had some neurological impairment, as compared to 22% of the nonviolent delinquents. The violent delinquents had such symptoms as memory lapses, dizzy spells, headaches, convulsions, and twitchy body movements.

GENETIC THEORIES

Genetic predisposition also may be involved in some types of socially deviant behavior. For example, it is postulated that violent behavior is part of the genetic composition of human beings and is similar to the innate aggressive responses seen in animals whose security (for example, territory, food, or offspring) is threatened. Although violence no longer has human survival value, human beings have not yet developed innate controls over violence (Montague, 1975; Marmor, 1978).

Research suggests that a genetic factor may be implicated in alcoholism. The blood samples of 80% of the alcoholics in a recent study showed elevated levels of the chemical 2,3-butanediol; only one member of the control group of social drinkers showed elevated levels of this chemical, and this social drinker subsequently developed alcoholism. These findings indicate that alcoholics metabolize ethanol differently than do nonalcoholics. Researchers believe that this enzyme defect may be genetically caused, although chronic alcohol consumption as a cause has not been ruled out. Researchers are optimistic that the presence of 2,3-butanediol might eventually serve as a marker for the screening of people with a predisposition for alcoholism (Alcoholics' Odd Blood, 1983).

Genetic research into other types of socially de-

viant behavior (for example, obesity, tobacco smoking) is also being conducted.

• • •

Although rapid advances in biochemistry, neurophysiology, and genetics are providing increasing amounts of evidence for a relationship between biology and socially deviant behavior, we cannot speak of a biological "cause" of such behavior. However, because people's perception of and response to the environment must be filtered through their brains and implemented by their total bodies, we should not negate the role of biology in social deviance.

Sociocultural theories

After observing behavior in many societies, Benedict (1934) theorized that although babies are born with a wide range of temperaments and personalities, each society sanctions only a certain few of these personality types. Only those personality types that conform to the society's cultural pattern are allowed to develop unimpeded. Since most personalities are malleable and responsive to socialization, the majority of persons in a society conform to the pattern and are accepted by the society. Those who do not conform are viewed as socially deviant.

URBANIZATION THEORY

Some years ago, Redfield (1947) developed a theory that deals with social deviance. He differentiated between "folk" and "urban" societies. A folk society is small, homogeneous, nonliterate, and isolated; it has a strong sense of community. An urban society is large, heterogeneous, literate, and nonisolated. While a folk society is characterized by a high degree of social integration and little deviant behavior, an urban society is characterized by a low degree of social integration and much deviant behavior. Redfield's theory would seem to explain the high crime rates in inner cities.

Travel and mass media have penetrated even the most remote parts of the world. As societies interact with one another, they tend to diversify and to take on each other's characteristics. As folk societies have disappeared, socialization has become less effective. Social integration has gradually weakened, and social deviance has increased. Mills (1950) believes that Redfield's ideas are important to the understanding of socially aberrant behavior.

While the folk-urban dichotomy continues to influence the study of social deviance, some anthropologists question the premise that social discord is absent in folk societies. Lewis (1951) found pervasive social conflict, mistrust, fear, and hatred among the villagers of Tepoztlan, in Mexico. Lewis' observations are especially significant, since Redfield's study of Tepoztlan (done before Lewis') had described tranquil, conflict-free people. It had been from his fieldwork in Tepoztlan that Redfield had derived many of his premises about the nature of folk societies.

SOCIAL STRAIN THEORY

Another theory that attempts to explain social deviance is social strain (or anomie) theory. Social strain theory originated with Durkheim (1938) and has been advanced by Merton and Nisbet (1961, 1971), Srole (1962), and Reich (1970). Social strain theory views people as basically moral and desirous of following the rules of society. This theory maintains that since people want to internalize society's rule system, only a major inconsistency in society can produce frustration, alienation, and socially aberrant behavior. For example, Orbach (1978) views overeating among women as a rebellion against culturally defined sex-role stereotypes. In order to fulfill the female sex-role stereotype, women are socialized to be appealing to men. Emphasis is placed on dependence, nurturing, sensualness, coquettishness, and physical attractiveness. This idealized image of femininity is imposed by significant others, the media, and the fashion industry.

Much of a woman's self-image reflects her dual social role of sex object and nurturer. Orbach states that many women find these two roles unrealistic and conflicting. For many women, it is impossible to be both a thin, demure, dependent sex object/lover and a reliable, well-organized giving wife/mother. For these women, fat symbolizes the sustenance necessary to fulfill the role of wife and mother.

Orbach goes on to explain that overeating also protects many women from the feelings of competitiveness and anger that women have been socialized to repress. Overeating diverts the energy associated with competitiveness and anger away from these feelings and toward the concern about obesity. Orbach suggests that being fat is one way that women rebel against the feminine stereotype.

▶ Sociocultural disjunctions

While society stresses certain values, roles, and standards of behavior, the social structure often makes it difficult for a person to act in accordance with them. There may be a disjunction between socially sanctioned goals and access to legitimized ways of achieving these goals, or the social situation may make the rules contradictory and meaningless. For example, while humanitarianism, honesty, and success are socially valued, many people find that they can succeed only through egocentric, aggressive, and cut-throat behavior.

Social strain theory speaks to the dilemma of people who have meager incomes but who, through the mass media, have been exposed to the revolution of rising expectations. These individuals often aspire to middle-class goals and life-style but are unable to achieve them. People with low access to legitimate means of achieving goals or high access to illegitimate means of achieving goals may develop socially aberrant behavior. For example, Bagley (1967) found a significant correlation between job opportunities and delinquency rates and between delinquency rates and services for children and adolescents.

▶ Community integration vs. community disintegration

Technology, once the American dream, has become the American idol. Progress and success are measured in terms of the possession of the biggest and fastest machines and the most machines. In this technocratic society, each person has become just another productive unit. Most people no longer directly participate in the production of their own food, shelter, or clothing. Piecework and mass production rob people of a sense of relatedness to nature and of a sense of accomplishment. This noninvolvement often results in a loss of the sense of self.

Fromm (1955) explains that in our age of technology, social structure and social relationships have become complex and impersonal. People often feel powerless, noncreative, and stripped of their uniqueness as individuals. Labor is often repetitive and meaningless, with workers taking little or no pride in workmanship. Rather than viewing themselves as the originators of their own acts, people often view their acts as alien to themselves. In modern society, alienation is pervasive; it characterizes the relationship of people to work, to things, and to other people.

There seems to be a correlation between social integration and social order, on the one hand, and social disintegration, alienation, anomie, and socially aberrant behavior on the other hand. Leighton (1959) points out that a community will almost certainly become disorganized if it is suffering from a disaster such as war, extensive flooding, or widespread fire; if it is experiencing pervasive poverty, either chronic or acute; if it is experiencing significant cultural change, as when ethnic groups are in conflict or are undergoing acculturation; if it is experiencing heavy immigration or emigration; if it is moving away from organized religion; or if it is experiencing rapid and extensive technological change.

Since it is not possible to directly measure the integration-disintegration balance of a community, specific sociocultural indicators are useful. By employing a set of indices, social disintegration can be operationally defined. A community can be characterized as disintegrated if it has many of the following sociocultural disjunctions:

1. A high incidence of ''broken'' homes (mal-functioning families). Little social control is exerted among family members.
2. Rapid social change. This leads to ambiguous standards of behavior.
3. A rapidly changing value system. This leaves people confused about the values around which to organize their lives.
4. Inadequate associations. There is little actual grouping of people around such common interests as religion, work, or recreation. Those groups that do exist are marked by low group cohesiveness.
5. Inadequate leadership. Leaders who live in the community are relatively ineffective in establishing meaningful, ordered social behavior.
6. Inadequate opportunities for recreation. Few opportunities exist for such group diversions as sports and hobbies. Recreation tends to take such individualistic forms as drinking and sexual promiscuity.
7. A high degree of hostility. There are many instances of physical and verbal abuse.
8. A high incidence of crime and delinquency. Criminal acts such as child abuse, robbery, physical aggression, and sexual assault are frequent.
9. Inadequate communication. Poor communication may be caused by such physically isolating factors as poor transportation systems or absence of telephones, or it may result from poor or nonexistent interpersonal relationships (Leighton, 1959; Detre et al., 1975; Halleck, 1978).

These disjunctions threaten the efficient functioning of a social system. Leighton (1959) and Yablonsky (1963) suggest that sociocultural disjunctions may result in inadequate socialization of children. Family patterns, kinship obligations, child-rearing practices, and economic activities may be disrupted. Value systems and role relationships may become confused, fragmented, or conflicting. Children may fail to learn socially sanctioned values, standards, and roles. Socially deviant behavior may develop. For example, Esselstyn (1967) found that violent behavior occurs predominantly among adolescents and young adults who live in urban slums, female-headed households, or middle-class homes in which adults are affectionally distant. In such situations, youths may become estranged from socially approved purposes and goals. Esselstyn concludes that violent behavior seems to be related to a system of socially deviant norms shared by population groups that are experiencing social disintegration.

Learning theory

Learning theory examines the psychosocial factors inherent in the process of learning socially deviant behavior. Learning theory holds that it is not the socioeconomic conditions of society that generate socially deviant behavior. Rather, social deviance is learned from role models and is reinforced by peer pressure and paternal and sibling influence. In environments where there is a high incedence of socially deviant behavior (for example, reform schools, prisons, disorganized communities), novices learn deviant behavior by associating with social deviants. Individuals observe that they and/or their role models are rewarded with prestige and material gains for their socially deviant behavior. With every occasion of reward for socially deviant behavior, the pattern of deviance is reinforced. However, learning theory does not explain why, among siblings reared in the same household, attending the same schools, and associating with the same people, one sibling develops socially deviant behavior while the others do not. Learning theory also does not explain why some people who as youths belong to gangs go on to become law-abiding adults (Birenbaum and Sagarin, 1976; Zillman, 1979).

Holistic health concepts

A holistic approach to social deviance that integrates the five dimensions of self (biological, psychological, intellectual, spiritual, and sociocultural) holds much promise for the understanding of and effective intervention in socially deviant behavior. Because these five dimensions of self are continuously interacting to produce human behavior, it is likely that socially deviant behavior also results from the interaction of psychophysiological, spiritual, and sociocultural factors (Grinker, 1971). For instance, physiological dysfunction may interfere with a client's ability to psychologically cope with spiritual or sociocultural stressors in a socially acceptable manner. Violent, sexually deviant, or addictive behavior may ensue.

Because a holistic health approach to social deviance takes into consideration the complexity of human behavior, it serves to facilitate awareness of the multiplicity and interrelationship of factors that contribute to the development of socially deviant behavior. This view is held by Wegscheider (1981) in her discussion of alcoholism. A poorly developed physical potential interferes with people's ability to enjoy life. This not only becomes a source of stress but makes people more vulnerable to other stressors. In addition, people may fear expressing their feelings. This fear may arise from the belief that particular feelings are wrong and from a concern about the ability to control one's emotions. Inability to express emotion may result in people manipulating others rather than relating in an open, compassionate manner. The intellectual or "mental" dimension of self is expressed in three ways: memories (past focus), ideas (present focus), and fantasy and imagination (future focus). Thus the intellect bridges the past and the future with the present, enabling people to get on with the business of living. The intellectual dimension of self also interprets the body's physical cues, channels the expression of emotion, regulates interpersonal relationships, and gives the spiritual domain an opportunity for expression. The spiritual dimension of self gives meaning to life. Wegscheider also includes one other dimension, the volitional. Well-developed volition, or will, enables people to establish goals, set priorities, engage in decision making, persevere in the pursuit of goals, and adapt to changing situational factors. Adaptation to changing situational factors means being flexible in the face of feedback and being able to discern which situations can be changed and which situations have to be accepted.

Well-functioning dimensions of self interrelate to give people a strong sense of self-worth. Conversely, defective development of any or all of the dimensions of self undermine feelings of self-worth. People who have low self-esteem utilize defenses to ward off further erosion of self-esteem, erosion that comes from the expectation of criticism and hostility from others (actual and projected). People turn to alcohol (or to other socially deviant behavior) as means of coping with the stress engendered by defective dimensions of self, as an anesthetic for emotions, as a way to end spiritual malaise, and as an attempt to boost faltering self-esteem. Once alcoholism (or other social deviance) develops, it contributes to further deterioration of the physical, emotional, social, mental, spiritual, and volitional dimensions of self. A downward ''spiral'' rather than a vicious cycle is set into motion.

A person's behavior is a product of interaction with others and the environment. Inadequate interpersonal relationships, biological dysfunction, socially undesirable personality traits, spiritual malaise, a poorly socialized superego, and the perception that society's norms are ambiguous, weak, or conflicting are all probably involved in the development of socially deviant behavior.

TREATMENT MODALITIES

Before we discuss specific therapies for persons who behave in socially aberrant ways, we need to consider the question of *when* to institute treatment. Because many socially deviant individuals come into conflict with society and are subsequently arrested, they are often considered criminals rather than persons in need of treatment. Factors that may precipitate the institution of treatment include the following:

1. Confrontation with the law
2. Impaired physical health
3. Medical emergencies
4. Psychiatric emergencies
5. Coercion by family, friends, or employer
6. Disenchantment with one's life-style
7. Desire to change one's life-style

Once a decision to begin treatment has been made, another question arises: *what type of treatment setting is appropriate?* Frequently, because of the medical problems associated with socially aberrant behavior (for example, malnutrition, venereal disease, infection, or personal injury), a general hospital may be chosen. Social deviants usually wish to have their medical problems treated and will cooperate with a medical regimen. Unfortunately, once the medical problems have been corrected, referrals are only infrequently made for psychosocial therapy.

Socially deviant individuals who are transferred to psychiatric treatment centers or who are remanded there by the courts are often poorly motivated to deal with their psychosocial problems. Since rationalization is a mechanism that is used frequently by such persons, they sometimes enter into treatment only half-heartedly. Ulterior motives may be operating. For instance, an addict may seek detoxification in order to reduce the severity of a habit rather than to kick it. A rapist may prefer the ambience of a treatment center to the environment of a jail.

Social deviants who are placed in psychiatric hospitals that also treat psychotic persons may resent being sent to a ''booby hatch.'' In all probability, they not only will try to keep themselves apart from psychotic individuals but also may ridicule, attempt to provoke, and exploit them.

Specialized treatment centers may be the best setting in which to treat persons who display socially aberrant behavior. In such centers, personnel are trained and experienced in working with specific types of socially deviant individuals. Very often, rehabilitated former offenders constitute part or most of the treatment team. This combination of professionals and former offenders is uniquely able to deal with the dynamics underlying much socially aberrant behavior.

Alternatives to hospitals and specialized treatment centers include such self-help groups as Alcoholics Anonymous, Gamblers Anonymous, Overeaters Anonymous, and Narcotics Anonymous. The support and intervention offered by these groups have proven effective in helping many socially deviant individuals. Of course, not everyone is a candidate for such a group. Social deviants whose behavior poses serious threats to society cannot safely be treated on a voluntary basis. Self-help groups usually provide a support system that functions 24 hours a day and 7 days a week to help sustain members through the periods of treatment, recovery, and rehabilitation.

Once a decision has been made to treat rather than to jail a socially deviant individual, any combination of the options mentioned may be used.

Laura was a middle-aged housewife. Her children were grown and had set up households of their own. She complained of feeling "edgy and jumpy." She would begin with one drink each morning to help her get started with her housework. By the time her husband, Jim, came home for dinner, she was usually drunk. Jim recognized that Laura drank too much, but he did not want to "humiliate" her by placing her in an alcohol treatment center. Instead he consulted their family doctor, who had been Laura's physician for many years. The doctor told Jim that Laura was very tense and anxious, and he prescribed Valium to help her relax. Laura took the Valium but cut down on her drinking very little.

One day, Jim came home and found Laura hemorrhaging from the mouth. She was rushed to their community hospital, where she underwent detoxification and was treated for esophageal varices, gastritis, and malnutrition.

After her medical problems had been corrected, Laura was sent to a treatment center for alcoholics. There she was helped to recognize that she was cross-addicted to alcohol and Valium. While at the center, weekly Alcoholics Anonymous meetings were held. At discharge, Laura was referred to AA for rehabilitation.

This situation demonstrates that a combination of medical, psychological, and social therapy may be indicated in treating socially deviant behavior. Once the decision to initiate treatment has been made, a number of settings may be used: general hospital, psychiatric hospital, specialized treatment center, and self-help groups. It is in these settings that the treatment modalities that facilitate recovery are instituted. We will now explore some of the most frequently used modalities.

Aversion therapy

Aversion therapy, or negative conditioning, makes use of learning theory to cause a person to stop behaving in a socially unacceptable way. Some unpleasant consequence is attached to the undesirable behavior. Aversion therapy is applied in a systematic manner. First, the unwanted behavior is identified. Next, its baseline frequency is established. Then, any environmental factors supporting the behavior are discerned.

A common type of aversion therapy for alcoholism involves the use of the drug disulfiram (Antabuse). Disulfiram remains inert in the body unless alcohol is ingested. Once an alcoholic beverage (or any medicine or food with an ethyl alcohol base) is taken, a physiological reaction similar to a severe hangover occurs. The reaction includes throbbing headache, dizziness, nausea, vomiting, facial flushing, heart palpitations, difficult breathing, and blurred vision. These symptoms last for 1 to 2 hours. Disulfiram must be taken regularly to be an effective deterrent to alcoholism. If people wish to drink, they can simply discontinue the use of disulfiram and thereby avoid its effects.

John's employer had given him an ultimatum: either stop drinking or be fired. John decided to enter a veteran's hospital. He had heard about disulfiram and requested it. While he was in the hospital he took the drug regularly. After he was discharged, he continued to take disulfiram. John's job performance and interpersonal relationships improved.

However, December came, and with it the office Christmas party. John decided to enter into the Christmas spirit–or should we say "spirits." He discontinued his use of disulfiram so that he would be able to "drink socially." He did not suffer any of the effects of disulfiram, but he did become intoxicated.

Thus there clearly are drawbacks to treatment with disulfiram. The use of the drug can be discontinued at any time. Disulfiram therapy requires self-motivation to be successful.

Aversion therapy is also used in treating compulsive gambling, drug addiction, smoking, and compulsive overeating. A combination of noxious stimuli and verbal imagery has been found to be most effective in cases involving these types of socially undesirable behavior (Hunt and Matarazzo, 1973; Elliott and Denney, 1975; Kingsley and Wilson, 1977).

Aversion therapy is based on the premise that aberrant behavior has been learned and therefore can be unlearned. Nurses are faced with an ethical question: who decides what behavior is "normal" and what behavior is "sick"? Although, ideally, socially deviant individuals participate in this decision, sometimes therapists do not include their clients in the decision-making process. As in any other type of therapy, nurses should be vigilant client advocates. They should be certain that aversion therapy is administered only with a client's informed consent. They should also be alert to any sadistic tendencies in attending therapists.

Aversion therapy has been criticized because it inflicts noxious stimuli on clients without providing opportunities for pleasurable reinforcement of positive behavior. In addition, critics argue, only overt behavior is dealt with: aversion therapists are not concerned with the dynamics underlying behavior.

Proponents of aversion therapy emphasize that such therapy often works in cases in which other types of therapy have failed. They maintain that noxious stimuli are administered only in an attempt to change behavior that both the client and society have defined as unacceptable. Proponents argue

that a short period of aversion therapy is preferable to a lifetime of socially unacceptable and inevitably self-destructive behavior.

The ultimate choice must be the client's. Nurses should ensure that candidates for aversion therapy have enough information to be able to weigh the advantages and disadvantages of negative conditioning and to compare it to other available treatments.

Drug therapy

Because of the addictive nature of much socially deviant behavior, the use of drugs as a treatment modality is extremely restricted. Many treatment programs are drug free: no drug, even aspirin, is permitted.

Some drugs have been found to have limited value in the treatment of specific types of acting-out behavior. In the discussion of aversion therapy, the use of disulfiram (Antabuse) for the treatment of alcoholism was mentioned. Two hundred fifty milligrams of disulfiram each day is an average maintenance dose. Disfulfiram must be taken daily. Many alcoholics will intentionally discontinue use of the drug so that they can return to drinking. Therefore, motivation for sobriety is very important. If disulfiram therapy is to be effective, concurrent psychotherapy is usually advisable.

People who take disulfiram need to avoid all substances containing ethyl alcohol, including not only alcoholic beverages but many medications, mouthwashes, and food preparations. Even inhaling alcohol fumes can cause a disulfiram reaction.

John had been discharged from an alcohol treatment program. He was taking disulfiram. One day he became violently ill; he had all the symptoms of a disfulfiram reaction. He telephoned a counselor at the treatment center and made an appointment for the next day. John swore that he had not been drinking, and the counselor believed him. After discussion and data collection that bordered on detective work, the counselor discovered that John had bought a new mouthwash and had begun using it the day before he became ill. The mouthwash had a high alcohol content. No one had thought to discuss such a potential problem with John before his discharge.

This vignette illustrates the importance of education. It is not enough to dispense medication; a medication's action and side effects, as well as any contingencies affecting the action, should be made known to a client.

Opiate-blocking drugs have been found to be useful in preventing the pleasurable, tension-reducing effects of narcotics. Methadone (Dolophine) and cyclazocine (WIN) are two opiate-blocking agents. Dolophine, the best known of these drugs, is a synthetic opiate. Like an opiate, it is an addicting drug. Treatment based on the administration of dolophine involves the substitution of a legal addiction (to Dolophine) for an illegal addiction (to narcotics). Dolophine has two functions. It enables addicts to stop opiate usage without the usual painful withdrawal symptoms, and it helps addicts stay off opiates because they no longer get "high" from them. Dolophine is administered orally. It is long acting and has to be taken only once a day. An average maintenance dose is 140 mg daily. This dosage level effectively eliminates withdrawal symptoms, blocks the pleasurable effects of opiates, and lessens the desire for narcotics.

Dolophine maintenance has been instrumental in the successful treatment of many "hard core" addicts—those who have not responded to other therapies. Many such addicts have been able to resume their normal social roles and to remain gainfully employed. However, because their addictive personality patterns have not been altered, many of these addicts may take nonopiate drugs along with Dolophine. As opponents of treatment through Dolophine maintenance point out, people using Dolophine are still addicted, even though their addiction is legal. Thus it is important that psychotherapy accompany Dolophine maintenance. Otherwise, addictive personality traits and socially

deviant patterns of coping and communicating may remain unchanged.

Group therapy*

One of the most commonly used treatment modalities for socially aberrant behavior is group therapy. The utilization of a group approach recognizes the need of socially deviant individuals for group identification.

Because socially deviant individuals demonstrate much hostile and aggressive behavior, they tend to threaten neurotic and psychotic persons. People who display socially aberrant behavior are better able to check one another's behavior than are outsiders. Therefore, socially deviant individuals may be treated more effectively in homogeneous groups than in heterogeneous groups. In a homogeneous group, limits are set by people who are experiencing or have experienced the same difficulties. Such a group setting permits socially deviant individuals to reveal their true selves without fear of retaliation. Authority, restraint, and controls arise from within the group. Because they may be deriving gratification from the group experience, socially deviant persons may begin to submit to group pressure. Satisfying group experiences may ultimately lead to the capacity to become integrated into groups. Rules and norms may be internalized, and, eventually, other people and society may no longer be perceived as antagonistic.

Family therapy†

Intervention with family members is essential to the treatment of socially deviant persons. The families of socially deviant individuals may mirror or facilitate and reinforce socially deviant behavior. It is thus necessary to work with these families so that they can serve as agents for socially acceptable behavior.

Intervention with the families of socially deviant

*Refer to Chapter 11 for further discussion of group therapy.
†Refer to Chapter 12 for further discussion of family therapy.

individuals should not be restricted to the efforts of psychiatric nurse–therapist. School nurse–teachers, occupational health nurses, and public health nurses have many opportunities to refer families in distress for treatment. Nurses in general hospitals also have prime opportunities for assisting members of distressed family systems. Staff nurses are often the first to see the destructive effects of socially aberrant behavior on network members. Socially deviant individuals are usually receptive to treatment for the physical problems associated with their behavior. For instance, very few alcoholics will refuse treatment for gastritis; few addicts will refuse treatment for infection; few juvenile delinquents will refuse treatment for traumatic injuries. Thus, nurses in general hospitals often see or hear about the devastation that is occurring within a socially deviant individual's family. Relatives and friends might confide to a receptive staff nurse just how difficult it is to live with the person.

Sharon had been admitted to her community hospital for cirrhosis of the liver. While she was hospitalized, some relatives and friends visited. Family members seemed annoyed with her. When a nurse asked if anything was the matter, the family denied having any problems. However, a neighbor confided to the nurse that Sharon's children (aged 15, 12, and 9) were "running wild." The neighbor said that Sharon was drunk most of the time and that the children were left on their own from the time they came home from school until their father came home from work. The children usually prepared their own meals and got themselves off to school. Any household chores that were done were done by the children. The oldest child, a boy, tried to keep an eye on the younger children but found it difficult. The younger children usually would not listen to him. In order to make ends meet, the husband/father was working at two jobs. Although some neighbors tried to help out and to keep an eye on the children, they often felt overwhelmed by the situation, believed that they were intruding, or felt imposed upon.

The nurse arranged an opportunity to talk with Sharon and her husband about how they were managing at home. Although Sharon denied that there were any problems, her husband later confided to the nurse, "I'm at my wits' end, and I'm thinking of divorcing Sharon and getting custody of the children." The nurse arranged for Sharon's husband to talk with the hospital's psychiatric clinical nurse specialist. Although Sharon refused to participate, her husband, her children, and some of the neighbors who had been helping the family entered into the therapy. In addition, the children began attending Alateen.

The behavior of socially deviant individuals can be very destructive to their families. At the same time, the behavior of family members can facilitate and reinforce a member's socially deviant behavior. For change to occur, the family should be part of the therapeutic process.

Social network therapy

A social network is a group of interconnected significant others, both relatives and nonrelatives, with whom a person interacts. Usually only a segment of a network is included in therapy. A small part of a network may be involved, as in couples therapy, or a somewhat larger part of a network may be included, as in family therapy. When a person's entire network is included in the therapeutic process, the process is known as social network therapy. In this type of therapy the support systems of society are utilized in the process of treatment (Speck and Attneave, 1973). Social network therapy involves the gathering together of client, family, and other significant persons into group sessions for the purpose of problem solving.

Every socially deviant individual has at least one facilitator in his or her social network. A facilitator may be a wife who calls the office and says her husband is sick when he is really drunk. A facilitator may be a child who assumes the role of parenting younger siblings and thereby enables the mother to spend more time gambling. A facilitator may be a father who closes his nose to the smell of alcohol on his adolescent son's breath. A facilitator may be a friend who suspects his "buddy" is a rapist but does not want to get him into trouble. Facilitators may be of any age, of either sex, and of any relationship to a socially deviant person. Facilitators make it easier for people to engage in socially deviant behavior.

Socially aberrant behavior involves other people. Many of the patterns of communication and coping that are apparent in a socially deviant individual may be subtly present in some of his or her network members.

Matthew was in his final year of a nursing program. His college performance had always been poor. At one point, he had been failing a course and had decided to withdraw from it and repeat it at a later time.

Each time Matthew was offered academic counseling he would refuse it. He would insist that his present academic performance was good. He would blame past academic difficulties on personality clashes between himself and his instructors, but he would always add that his present instructor was "really good—cares about students." Matthew would then recount in detail his current nursing experiences. He would sound enthusiastic, knowledgeable, and sincere. By the time he left his advisor's office, his advisor would be questioning her own judgment. Was she making too much of past performance? Was she overlooking Matthew's ability to change? It certainly sounded as though he now had the situation under control. He always promised to return if problems arose. Then the semester's grades would come in, and he would again be on probation.

During his senior year, which involved a work-study experience, Matthew demonstrated unsafe nursing practices. Both Matthew's instructor and the hospital staff were in agreement. When confronted with this inadequacy, Matthew talked about the head nurse's dislike of him and about how she had influenced the rest of the staff. Matthew rationalized that it was almost impossible to perform under such pressure. He also became enraged at the head nurse for not evaluating his performance

sooner. The head nurse insisted that she had spoken to him on several occasions. He accused her of lying.

Matthew's nursing instructor advised him to withdraw from the course before he failed it. He would then be eligible to repeat the course the following semester. The instructor also suggested that since he experienced so many personality conflicts he should consider psychotherapy. He became infuriated with the instructor. A few days later, Matthew's mother came to the university. She was enraged at the treatment her son had received, and she threatened to sue both the school and the head nurse. She explained that Matthew had worked very hard to get through the nursing program. "Even during the semester that he had to withdraw from that course, Matthew left the house at the same time each day so that his father would not suspect anything." Matthew had "conned" his father, and his mother had facilitated the deception.

When Matthew's mother realized that no amount of talk or threats would change the situation, she tried bribery. She said that if Matthew would be permitted to participate in the graduation ceremony, he would withdraw from the course and there would not be a lawsuit. This way no one, including Matthew's father, would have to know what had happened.

Matthew was obviously making use of deviant patterns of coping and communicating. He was charming, cunning, and manipulative; he engaged in rationalization and denial. Matthew's mother mirrored many of these mechanisms. Aberrant patterns of communicating and coping are often found in various members of a socially deviant person's network.

In addition, socially deviant individuals often precipitate problems in their social networks. For instance, a parent who feels guilty about a child's socially aberrant behavior may project this guilt onto a spouse. Conflict may develop between husband and wife. Couples therapy may be indicated. If one or both of a child's parents are socially deviant, the child may suffer role confusion and have difficulty finding role models who demonstrate socially acceptable behavior. Family therapy may be indicated. These are some of the problems that members of a socially deviant individual's social network might experience.

To date, therapy has focused on socially deviant individuals (individual therapy), on their relationships with spouses (couples therapy), or on their relationships with family (family therapy). Little has been done to implement a total social network approach. Yet social network therapy is essential to the treatment of socially aberrant behavior. Socially deviant individuals may not have internalized the standards of society. Since these values and ways of behaving are normally taught by family members and significant others, total network therapy includes both the family and these significant others. A social network is a microcosm of society. Social network therapy views the network as an open system.

Social network therapy should be designed to assist socially deviant individuals and their network members to cope with socially aberrant behavior. The purposes of network therapy can be summarized as follows:

1. To assess a socially deviant individual's communication patterns
2. To modify network patterns of communication (such as facilitating) that support a member's socially deviant behavior
3. To help a socially deviant individual's social network serve as a reference group for socially acceptable behavior
4. To facilitate a socially deviant individual's reentry into the community

In most cases, the client and the members of his social network should meet together, but there may be times when network members will attend therapy sessions without the client being present. Special organizations, such as Alanon and Alateen, have been designed to help network members cope with the destructive and unacceptable behavior of a socially deviant individual.

Allison, a 19-year-old student nurse, was receiving poor grades. She did not hand assignments in on time, and she frequently fell asleep in class. She developed a good relationship with one of her teachers, to whom she revealed that she had many family problems. Allison's father was an alcoholic, and her mother was schizophrenic. Allison had two younger brothers. The 16-year-old was "running around with a loose group and drinking." The 12-year-old seemed well adjusted. Allison was trying to hold the family together, straighten out her 16-year-old brother, and protect the 12-year-old. She had assumed the parenting role. Allison had not spoken about her situation with anyone except her teacher. She was afraid that if her classmates knew about her parents, they would not want to associate with her.

Allison's teacher referred her to Alateen, where she was helped to express her feelings of guilt and anger. She also learned that her situation was not unique and that many adolescents were in similar predicaments. Allison learned that although she could not change her family's behavior, she could change the way she reacted. She found the Alateen group very supportive.

Educational therapy

People who behave in socially aberrant ways usually have inadequate group identification and low self-esteem. Educational and vocational training programs offer opportunities for such persons to build self-esteem and to direct energy into socially acceptable channels (Winchester, 1972). Educational therapy also provides information that can facilitate personal and occupational adjustment.

Educational therapy should involve more than the teaching of subject matter. In an attempt to help socially deviant individuals reconstruct their lives, educational therapists should help clients to look at past failures in school and to ascertain what contributed to those failures. In this way, those experiences can provide opportunities for learning and growth. Educational therapy often also includes instruction in such personal matters as grooming, dress, and etiquette.

Lisa, an adolescent girl, had been admitted to a drug treatment center. She had been doing poorly in school and thought of herself as a "dummy." She planned to drop out of school as soon as it was legally permissible. The treatment team decided that Lisa was definitely a candidate for educational therapy. While at the drug center, Lisa not only attended daily classes but also received tutoring in subjects of special weakness. She was shown how to budget study time, how to take notes, and how to outline chapters. In addition, she was placed in a personal development group that included other adolescent girls. With the assistance of a nurse, the group regularly discussed clothing styles and experimented with hairstyles and cosmetics. By the time Lisa was ready to leave the center, she felt able to return to junior high school and was confident that she could at least pass her courses. She also felt more comfortable with her appearance.

Many socially deviant individuals are children, adolescents, and young adults. The preceding vignette shows how educational therapy can be designed to facilitate their social and academic reentry into society.

Meditation therapy

Transcendental meditation is one way of achieving relaxation and consciousness expansion. Clients are asked to focus their thoughts on a "mantra" (a word, a sound, or an image) and to relax. Some research on transcendental meditation indicates that it may be helpful in treating alcoholism and drug abuse. Studies have found that a large percentage of the people who practiced transcendental meditation over a 20-month period significantly reduced drug and alcohol consumption. Interviews with study participants indicated that because transcendental meditation reduced anxiety and tension and produced a sense of general well-being, the need for drug-induced experiences was diminished (Marzetta, Benson, and Wallace, 1972; Benson and Wallace, 1972). More research

is needed to determine the validity of meditation as a treatment modality for socially deviant behavior.

Milieu therapy

A therapeutic community* is a form of milieu therapy. A therapeutic community attempts to correct socially deviant behavior and to prepare residents for reentry into society. Every activity is designed to teach residents to live by society's standards and to function in a socially acceptable manner. A therapeutic community serves as a real-life reference group. As one resident of such a community explained,

We use a yardstick approach here. We figure that most of the people in society function at 24 inches. We try to bring ourselves up to 36 inches because we know when we leave here we'll slip back a little. But even with slipping back we'll be okay.

This "yardstick approach" explains why, in a therapeutic community for socially deviant persons, exacting behavior is expected and infraction of rules carries heavy penalties. Residents who do not clean their rooms may have to wear a sign that says "I'm a slob." Residents whose attitudes are manipulative or sullen may be verbally "blown away." Residents who run away from the therapeutic community and then want to return may receive a "haircut"—their heads may literally be shaved as a constant reminder of their immature behavior. These measures are taken to inculcate society's values and norms into people who have been operating outside society's rule system. Society may expect its members to function at "24 inches," but because socially deviant individuals start out with little or no social conscience, they have to be brought up to "36 inches."

Frequently, the staff of a therapeutic community for socially deviant persons is composed entirely of former offenders. Professionals may be only tangentially involved. The rationale for such a

---

*See Chapter 10 for a general discussion of milieu therapy and the therapeutic community.

staffing policy includes three elements:

1. Former offenders have experienced the problem and have overcome it. They therefore can serve as role models.
2. Since former offenders have used all the mechanisms common to socially deviant behavior, they can recognize and confront these mechanisms in newcomers.
3. Former offenders are considered peers by residents of a therapeutic community. Structure, challenge, confrontation, and discipline are more readily accepted when meted out by peers.

Many socially deviant individuals have become expert manipulators. Some are highly skilled at manipulating groups and have even been "gang" leaders. Most professionals do not have this kind of personal history. Professional education often focuses more on intervention with individuals than on intervention with groups. Many professionals have not learned confrontation techniques. Therefore, a former offender is often better able to deal with socialy aberrant behavior than is a health professional.

• • •

Socially deviant individuals may be treated in a variety of treatment settings and with a variety of treatment modalities. The goals of therapy are to supplant socially aberrant behavior with socially acceptable behavior and to facilitate reentry into society. Although nurses may not directly participate in all treatment modalities, they do participate in all levels of preventive intervention: primary, secondary, and tertiary.

NURSING INTERVENTION

The behavior of socially deviant individuals often challenges a nurse's value system. Frequently, such persons not only resist treatment but also attack the treatment process. They may try to "con" their therapists and "work" the system. In view of these difficulties, what qualities should nurses who work with these people possess?

First, nurses should be *nondefensive*. They should expect that socially deviant individuals may question, argue against, and reject society's values and standards. It is through socially aberrant behavior that such persons try to cope with tension and conflict. Once nurses understand the dynamics underlying socially aberrant behavior, they will find it easier to be less defensive.

Second, nurses should be *accepting, but firm*. Socially deviant individuals tend to resist treatment and do not readily ask for help. Often, the ways in which they try to communicate and cope alienate other people. Socially deviant individuals may try to charm, cajole, con, or dupe nurses. While it is necessary to set firm limits on such patterns of behavior, it is also important not to reject a person. Nurses can be accepting without condoning behavior; they can be firm without being punitive. Kimsey (1969) found that it is vital for therapists to assume a mature, "adult" role, rather than a peer role, if they are to teach impulse control and foster socially acceptable behavior.

Ruesch (1961) suggests that therapists find concrete ways to show concern and interest in socially deviant clients. Concern and interest may be demonstrated by treating somatic complaints or by alleviating stress-provoking situations. After such initial concrete demonstration of concern, therapists should be careful to avoid encouraging dependence. Socially deviant individuals often try to con therapists into doing things for them. Every effort should be made to encourage self-reliant behavior.

Finally, nurses need to be *realistic* about the course of therapy. In the treatment of socially deviant individuals, relapses are common. For instance, alcoholics may "go on the wagon" only to begin drinking a few months later. Drug addicts may undergo detoxification but later revert to drug abuse. Chronic overeaters may diet and lose weight only to regain it later. The course of recovery for socially deviant individuals is often marked by periods of improvement and relapse. Once nurses recognize that this pattern is not uncommon and that it is often a prelude to true recovery, they are less apt to respond with anger and disappointment. They may be able to help socially deviant individuals identify stressors that precipitate relapses to socially aberrant behavior and thereby prevent them.

PRIMARY PREVENTION

Socially aberrant behavior patterns can be traced back to adolescence or to even earlier periods. It is during these periods that a social conscience is developed. Social networks in general and family systems in particular are primary socializing agents. These agents form the matrix for the internalization or the noninternalization of society's rules and value systems. Rules and value systems influence and are influenced by the prevailing social climate. For example, during times of social strain, society may stress certain standards of behavior, but the existing social structure may make it difficult for a person to act in accordance with those standards. A contradictory rule system or a disjunction between socially sanctioned goals and access to legitimized ways to achieve the goals may result. This situation is known as social strain or anomie. When social networks and family systems operate within a milieu of social strain, children may either *learn* socially unacceptable behavior or *fail to learn* socially acceptable behavior. They may grow into adulthood without developing social consciences. The alleviation of conditions that produce crime (such as poverty, unemployment, and overcrowding) and the strengthening of family systems are essential elements in the primary prevention of social deviance (Minuchin, 1967; Rubin, 1972).

Only in recent years has socially aberrant behavior come to be viewed as a psychosocial problem. Emphasis is now being placed on treatment rather than on punishment. Such a wide range of disorders is included in socially aberrant behavior that

no one cause can be singled out. The consensus is that the etiology of social deviance is multifactorial and that a multifactorial approach therefore needs to be taken in primary prevention. Several factors may predispose a person to socially aberrant behavior:

1. A family history of social deviance
2. Loss of one or both parents (through death, noninvolvement, or separation)
3. Brutality by parents
4. Parental psychopathology
5. A disorganized sociocultural environment (characterized by overcrowding, poverty, inadequate housing, and poor job opportunities) (Roth, 1972; Rubin, 1972)

However, not everyone with such risk factors in their backgrounds develops socially aberrant behavior. What are the implications of this fact for primary prevention? The primary prevention of social deviance involves two goals:

1. To minimize the effects of predisposing factors
2. To find ways to prevent high-risk individuals from becoming socially deviant

Nurses can implement these goals by identifying high-risk individuals, initiating parental and family counseling, and modifying the social environment.

Identification of high-risk individuals

Reiner and Kaufman (1959) were among the first to point out that a high percentage of families known to social agencies display extreme degrees of social deviance in their family and community interactions. These families usually are disorganized. One or both parents may be absent. If parents are present, they may be only marginally functional.

Community health nurses and school nurse–teachers work with families and observe family interactions. As nurses become more intimately involved with families, they are better able to identify important risk factors. If nurses are not knowledgeable, they may fail to recognize risk factors or may be unable to make appropriate referrals for treatment.

Parental counseling

Early exposure to parental brutality has been associated with the development of socially aberrant behavior in children. From a feared parent figure, children often internalize socially unacceptable characteristics. In fact, parents who are child abusers* and who display identifiable social aberrations usually have histories of having been battered as children themselves (Rubin, 1972). In addition, Myrna Weissman (1972) has found that socially deviant individuals often had depressed mothers. Depressed women may be unable to express their anger appropriately and may instead direct it toward their children.

Public health nurses, school nurse–teachers, and child health nurses need to be alert for symptoms of maternal depression and signs of child battering. Intervention at an early stage may prevent the development of socially aberrant behavior.

Women who appear lethargic, apathetic, indecisive, hopeless, and helpless and who complain of anorexia, weight loss, insomnia, amenorrhea, and constipation may be suffering from *maternal depression*.† A nurse who recognizes this syndrome of maternal depression in a woman should refer her for therapy. Since a depressed person usually does not have the energy—physical or emotional—to ask for help or to initiate contact with a helping person, nurses need to enlist the support of family and social networks. Nurses should assess the potential of the woman and of her family to make the initial contact. If the family needs assistance, then help should be offered. In addition, nurses need to acquaint family and/or network members with the mother's depressed state, with her inability to handle anger, and with the possible need to protect children from misdirected angry outbursts. This

intervention should be carried out with the mother's knowledge and, when possible, approval. Since all therapeutic relationships should be structured on the basis of qualified confidentiality—the principle that only in the event of potential harm to the client or to others will confidential material be divulged, and then only to appropriate persons—the question of breach of confidentiality should not arise.

*Child abuse** should be suspected when a child repeatedly has fractured bones, soft-tissue swelling, welts, subdural hematomas, bruises, or abrasions. In most cases of child abuse, the degree and type of injury do not correspond with parental explanations of how the "accident" occurred.

Miriam and Jack were the parents of three children, aged 5 years, 3 years, and 3 months. The 3-month-old baby was a boy, Jackie Jr. Jackie physically resembled his father. Following the birth of Jackie, Miriam had bcome very depressed and was experiencing difficulty fulfilling her roles as wife and mother.

Jack's employment pattern had been sporadic, and the family was living on unemployment benefits, Jack was preoccupied with looking for a job. He offered little emotional support or child-rearing assistance to Miriam.

One day while Miriam was bathing Jackie, a public health nurse unexpectedly visited. Although Miriam hurriedly dried and dressed Jackie, the nurse noticed what appeared to be burns on Jackie's back. Miriam explained the burns by saying that she often smoked while bathing the baby: "Ashes from my cigarette must have fallen on his back."

Child abuse may develop when a parent has inadequate support in the parenting role. An abusing parent is usually isolated from a supportive social network and is not receiving support from the marital relationship. Such a parent may have unrealistically high developmental expectations for

---

*Child abuse is discussed in the next section of this chapter and in Chapter 15.
†Refer to Chapter 18 for a general discussion of depression and nursing intervention for it.

---

*Refer to Chapter 15 for further discussion of child abuse.

children and may become frustrated and angry when, at a young age, children cannot be toilet trained, for example, or feed themselves. In addition, many abusing parents have themselves been abused as children and have not personally experienced parental nurturing (Smith and Hanson, 1975).

Nurses who suspect battering need to assess parental attitudes. Accurate and well-documented records are also important. The name of anyone who has witnessed the abuse of a child should be noted in such records. Most importantly, suspected instances of child abuse should be reported to appropriate legal or social service agencies. Efforts need to be made to protect a child from further abuse. This may mean moving a child to a safe environment. In addition, abusing parents should be offered opportunities for treatment. Besides traditional psychotherapy, self-help groups composed of abusing parents are springing up in many communities (Collins, 1978). Since child-abusing parents often have low self-esteem, nonsupportive marital relationships, and unrealistically high developmental expectations of their children, treatment should focus on these areas. Ways should be explored to improve parental self-esteem, to develop a relationship of support and assistance between spouses, to educate parents about childhood growth and development, and to explore with parents alternative methods for coping with their children's disruptive behavior. The abused child is not the sole problem in the family relationship but represents a much larger problem: dysfunction in the family system.

Family counseling

Family disorganization predisposes a person to the development of socially aberrant behavior. Disorganized households are often characterized by insufficient income, food, fuel, and clothing. There may be instability regarding place of residence, time of meals, child-rearing practices, and interpersonal relationships. Because disorganized households may lack adequate space and furniture,

families may be unable to eat meals together. Minuchin (1967) emphasizes that disorganized families usually attempt to control and inhibit their children's annoying behavior rather than try to consistently guide children and teach them socially acceptable behavior. Bad behavior is punished, but good behavior is rarely rewarded. Children in such families may soon learn to respond to parental moods and parental discipline (external controls), but they may not learn to develop internal controls or social consciences. These children frequently react with aggression and display socially aberrant behavior.

Nurses need to help disorganized families on several levels. If such families are not already involved with social service agencies, referrals should be made. If disorganized families are involved with social service agencies, it is very probable that they are experiencing difficulties in their relationships with the agencies. The agencies may be handling the families in a way that provokes feelings of frustration, anger, alienation, and avoidance. Nurses should assist these families to communicate with the social service agencies, and vice versa.

Because the social deviance of one member is usually reflected in or facilitated by the rest of the family, families may need to learn more effective and socially acceptable ways to communicate. Parents may need to develop some sense of their own self-worth. Parents may also need to learn socially acceptable child-rearing practices.

Modification of sociocultural environment

Earlier in this chapter we discussed the correlation between community disorganization and socially deviant behavior. Inner cities experiencing widespread overcrowding and poverty and ethnic enclaves experiencing extensive occulturative pressure are examples of disorganized communities. Disorganized communities may be marked by broken homes, inadequate leadership, and frequent occurrences of violence, delinquency, and other forms of socially aberrant behavior. When neighborhoods begin to deteriorate, surrounding neighborhoods usually close their boundaries. Attempts may be made to keep ghetto residents in the ghetto. At the same time, there is usually a reduced flow of goods and services to the disorganized communities. The extent and condition of communication and transportation systems in ghetto areas may also be poor. Street maintenance, public transportation systems, and public telephones may be allowed to deteriorate. Buildings may fall into disrepair. Hallways, playgrounds, and streets may become extremely unsafe. In such disorganized communities, it is fairly common for abandoned buildings to become havens for youth gangs, "winos," and junkies (Freedman, 1975; Ashcraft and Scheflen, 1976).

Friends and relatives of persons who live in deteriorating communities are usually afraid to travel into the communities. At the same time, residents may not want to leave their neighborhoods. They may worry about what will happen to their apartments while they are away, or they may fear traveling on neighborhood streets after dark. Decreased interpersonal contact and bond servicing* erodes social networks. In addition, immigrants who live in inner-city ghettos usually have left supportive social networks in foreign lands and often find it difficult to develop new networks.

For residents of disorganized communities, scarcity of goods and services usually coexists with social isolation and alienation. Overcrowding, poverty, and scarcity of resources—all characteristics of disorganized neighborhoods—are inextricably associated with socially deviant behavior. Nurses, as concerned citizens and as client advocates, need to militate for social change. When budgets are streamlined, money for social services is usually cut. Yet this type of economizing usually contributes to further disintegration of already disorganized communities. Social changes that prevent neighborhood disintegration or im-

prove living conditions are essential components of primary prevention of socially deviant behavior.

A comprehensive approach to primary prevention of socially aberrant behavior is necessary. Since social deviance has many interrelated causes, only a multifactorial primary prevention program will be effective. Such a strategy has been used by one Eskimo community in Labrador, Canada.

In 1960 it became legal for Eskimos to buy and consume alcohol. Alcoholism, especially spree drinking, became a community problem. Community leaders developed a four-pronged attack on the problem. Bars were forbidden to sell alcohol for home consumption; people who wanted to buy liquor for home consumption had to place their orders 3 weeks in advance; educational programs about alcoholism were developed and implemented; and laws against public drunkenness were strictly enforced. This comprehensive program effectively changed both the community's accepting attitude toward alcoholism and the pattern of spree drinking (Wilkinson, 1970).

Such a multifaceted approach, encompassing a range of strategies, is necessary for an effective program of primary prevention.

SECONDARY PREVENTION

What is the secondary level of prevention for people who display socially deviant behavior? In the discussion of secondary prevention, two aspects will be stressed: case finding and direct intervention.

Case finding

Nurses—especially public health nurses, school nurse–teachers, occupational health nurses, and staff nurses in general hospitals—have unparalleled opportunities for case finding. Socially deviant individuals more readily seek help for phys-

---

*Refer to Chapter 8 for a discussion of bond servicing and interpersonal relationships.

ical problems, which may or may not be associated with their socially aberrant behavior, than for psychosocial problems.

CHILDREN

Rubin (1972) describes a childhood triad of behavior—firesetting, bedwetting, and cruelty to animals. When these types of behavior appear *in combination* and *consistently,* some degree of socially aberrant behavior may be present.

Johnny, a 7-year-old boy, was brought to the emergency room of a general hospital. Both his hands were severely burned. While taking a nursing history, the emergency room nurse discovered that this was not the first time that Johnny had "played with matches." Further exploration of his behavior revealed repeated enuresis and cruelty to animals. Both of Johnny's parents were concerned about his behavior.

Once Johnny's burns were treated, the emergency room nurse referred him and his parents to the hospital's clinical nurse specialist. The clinical nurse specialist suspected that Johnny's actions were indicative of early antisocial behavior. Although this community hospital did not offer family therapy, the clinical nurse specialist gave the family the names of three local agencies that did offer family therapy. He helped the family make the initial appointment. Three weeks later, he telephoned the parents to ascertain how they were managing. They confirmed that they had begun family therapy.

Separate and occasional appearances of any of the three types of behavior are often part of normal growth and development. However, when they appear in combination and consistently, they may indicate antisocial tendencies.

Nurses can be involved in early case finding and referral for treatment. Follow-up work to determine whether referrals are being acted upon, to reinforce the need for treatment, and to facilitate contact with appropriate agencies are also important nursing functions.

ADOLESCENTS AND ADULTS

The presence of the following cluster of behaviors in adolescents and adults may be indicative of emerging social deviance:
1. Violent outbursts against oneself and/or others
2. Repeated criminal behavior
3. History of poor work or school performance
4. Unsafe and aggressive automobile driving
5. Substance abuse or addiction
6. Repeated suicidal attempts (Bach-y-Rita, 1971; Roth, 1972)

In combination, these types of behavior express the interrelated dynamics of hostility, manipulation, alienation, anomie, poor judgment, and inability to learn from previous experience. These core mechanisms underlie and are manifested in most socially aberrant behavior. Once nurses recognize predictor or indicator behavior patterns, they can identify emerging social deviance and make appropriate referrals.

An occupational health nurse noticed that Mr. McCabe frequently called in sick on Mondays. His work performance during the rest of the week was sporadic. Mr. McCabe worked conscientiously in the morning, but in the afternoon he became lackadaisical about his work and irritable with his co-workers. During the past few months Mr. McCabe had experienced a number of minor industrial accidents. Each accident had occurred in the afternoon.

The occupational health nurse suspected that Mr. McCabe had a drinking problem. By observing his behavior and talking with him, the nurse confirmed this diagnosis. Mr. McCabe drank several beers with his lunch and took frequent afternoon work breaks for additional beers. He drank heavily on weekends "to relax and forget the rat race."

Mr. McCabe was told that if he did not seek treatment he would be fired. At the same time, he was assured that if he completed a treatment program his job would be waiting for him. The occupational health nurse helped Mr. McCabe find an appropriate treatment program.

This vignette illustrates how nurses may be able to identify incipient alcoholics (people who are still able to maintain some degree of control over their drinking behavior) and refer them for treatment. By involving alcoholics in treatment programs at this early stage, when they are still able to function in the community, nurses may prevent chronic alcoholism.

The Civil Service Commission (1971) has established a federal civilian employee alcoholism program. This program

1. defines alcoholism as an illness that directly affects job performance.
2. stresses that employees who are alcoholics should receive the same thoughtful attention and assistance received by employees suffering from other illnesses.
3. emphasizes that alcoholic employees have the same right to medical record confidentiality as any other employees have.
4. urges that alcoholic employees requesting sick leave for treatment be given the same consideration as employees requesting sick leave for other illnesses.
5. stresses that employee requests for counseling or referral to alcohol treatment programs should not threaten job security.
6. emphasizes that all information, referral, or counseling should be provided on a confidential basis.

In their role as client advocates, nurses in occupational health settings need to be aware of these guidelines and to be active in implementing them. These guidelines can be adapted and applied to intervention in other settings and in situations involving other types of socially deviant behavior.

Nursing process

The nursing process provides the framework for nursing intervention. The focus of this aspect of secondary prevention is twofold: (1) intervention into socially deviant behavior patterns and (2) supplanting socially unacceptable behavior with socially acceptable behavior.

ASSESSMENT

When they work with a client who copes with anxiety and conflict through socially deviant behavior, nurses have to begin their assessment with the identification of the problem given by the client or members of the client's social network. The following areas should be assessed:

1. Presenting symptoms—substance abuses and/or practice abuses that are creating problems for the client (or for members of the client's social network) even though the abuse behavior is serving as a defense against an emotional state that the client is experiencing
2. Emotional state—such feelings as anxiety, hostility, alienation, and/or anomie that are responses to a stimulus situation
3. Stimulus situations—stressful life situations that constitute threats to the client's security. Quests for power, prestige, and possessions are attempts to find reassurance against the anxiety aroused by threats to one's security. In trying to obtain power, prestige, and possessions, some people use maladaptive—socially deviant—coping behaviors.
4. Maladaptive coping behaviors—socially deviant behaviors of substance abuse and practice abuse and coping patterns of manipulation, rationalization, and blame placing that are used in relating to others, in attempting to satisfy needs, and in protecting oneself from hurt
5. Origin of maladaptive coping behaviors—identification of childhood experiences (e.g., inadequate interpersonal relationships, inadequate opportunity for superego socialization, or the perception that society's norms are ambiguous, weak, or conflicting) that contributed to the development of or learning of maladaptive coping behaviors
6. Holistic health status—biological, intellectual, psychological, sociocultural, and spiritual status of the client. These factors may facilitate wellness—e.g., in cultures where alcohol is viewed as a social beverage and

drinking patterns tend to be family oriented, rarely do people view alcohol as a way to escape from personal problems—or these factors may impede wellness—e.g., society may stress certain values and standards of behavior but the social situation may make it difficult to achieve these ideals in a legitimate way. In addition, many socially deviant behavior but the social situation may make it difficult to achieve these ideas in a legitiusers, respiratory disorders with tobacco smokers, cardiovascular disease with workaholics.

The following guide may assist nurses in making assessments*:

1. Behavioral observations
   a. State of consciousness
   b. State of orientation
   c. Thought and sensory functioning
   d. Motor activity
   e. Perception of time and space
2. Psychosocial observations
   a. Degree of anomie
   b. Ability to perform social roles
   c. Quality of interpersonal relationships
   d. Emotional state: depressed, alienated, hostile, anxious, etc.
   e. Coping behaviors: manipulation, rationalization, blame placing, etc.
   f. Threat to self-security† (intentional or inadvertent self-injury potential)
   g. Degree of self-awareness about the effect of socially deviant behavior on self and significant others
   h. Nature of social network: supportive, facilitative (of socially deviant behavior), uninvolved
   i. Purpose of substance or practice abuse: to escape problems; to achieve a sense of well-being; to avoid feeling emotional

pain (e.g., anxiety, loneliness, worthlessness, depression); to improve self-esteem; to punish self/others
3. Physical observations
   a. Vital signs
   b. Skin color and integrity
   c. Appearance of eyes
   d. Odor of breath
   e. Muscle tremors
   f. Elimination patterns
   g. Nutritional status
   h. Personal hygiene
   i. Speech patterns
   j. Sleep patterns
   k. Evidence of infection
   l. Known health problems
4. Contextual observations
   a. Substances or practices abused
   b. Alteration in life-style
   c. Changes in personality
   d. Changes in spirituality
   e. Deterioration in physical appearance
   f. Nature of stressors (e.g., sociocultural dysfunctions, social network dysfunction, physical problems)
   g. Motivation for behavior change (supplanting socially deviant behavior with socially acceptable behavior): eager to change behavior; ambivalent about changing behavior; resistant to changing behavior

ANALYSIS OF DATA

As nurses assess the presenting symptoms, emotional states, stimulus situations, maladaptive coping behaviors and their origins, and the holistic health status of the client, they begin to understand the client's (and often the social network's) perceptions of the presenting problem. The assessment also aids nurses in understanding the interrelationship among social network dynamics, predisposing and precipitating factors, and the client's socially deviant coping behaviors. At this point, nurses may be ready to formulate nursing diagnoses. The following are nursing diagnoses that

---

*Sources consulted in the preparation of this assessment guide include Morton (1979) and Schultz and Dark (1982).
†Refer to Chapter 18 for discussion of assessment of suicidal potential.

are frequently made in regard to clients who cope with anxiety and conflict through socially deviant behavior. Following each nursing diagnosis is a discussion of an appropriate plan of care and its implementation.*

Nursing diagnosis: Interaction theme of manipulation related to anxiety engendered by low self-esteem (behavior associated with DSM-III diagnoses of substance use disorder, other psychosexual disorders, impulse control disorder [intermittent or isolated explosive disorder, pathological gambling], personality disorder [antisocial], and conduct disorder)

Planning: The nurse may initially establish goals, but as therapy progresses the client should enter into goal setting.

1. Long-term goals
   a. Develop a positive self-image (refer to Chapters 6 and 18 for a discussion of self-image).
   b. Learn to relate to others in a nonmanipulative (trusting, cooperative) manner.
2. Short-term goals
   a. Express feelings of anxiety and inadequacy.
   b. Identify interpersonal situations that arouse feelings of anxiety and inadequacy.
   c. Develop self-awareness of manipulative behavior.
   d. Decrease the use of denial, blame-placing, intellectualization, and rationalization when confronted with problems.
   e. Develop more effective coping behaviors and interpersonal skills.
   f. Realistically perceive the five dimensions of self. (Biological, intellectual, psychological, sociocultural, and spiritual strengths and limitations will be put into perspective.)

Implementation: According to Sullivan (1953), low self-esteem† underlies all manipulative behavior. People with low self-esteem do not feel good about themselves and cannot feel good about others. This sense of worthlessness generates anxiety. Socially deviant individuals may not appear anxious because they channel their anxiety into exploitative behavior.

Nursing intervention in cases of manipulative behavior involves two goals: to increase self-esteem and to teach socially deviant individuals to rely on themselves. Nursing intervention should be based on an awareness that exploitation arouses anxiety and hostility in the people being exploited. These feelings may lead to rejection of socially deviant individuals. Nurses should work with the entire health team in recognizing and discouraging the use of manipulative behavior. If the health team is consistent in refusing to be used, a manipulative person will have to learn other ways of interacting with people.

The following are ways in which nurses can facilitate the learning of new, nonmanipulative behavior:

1. Practice nonreinforcement of any attempted manipulation.
   a. Identify manipulative behavior.
   b. Set limits on manipulative behavior.
   c. Communicate to clients what behavior is expected.
   d. Explain reasons for limits that have been set.
   e. Enforce these limits.
   f. Encourage clients to express feelings about the limits.
   g. Evaluate with clients the effectiveness of the limits.
   h. Assist clients to establish their own limits.
2. Help individuals acknowledge that they use and take advantage of others.
   a. Explore clients' preception of how needs are gratified.
   b. Discuss ways in which other people gratify their needs.
   c. Point out instances in which clients use rationalization and blame placing.
   d. Point out instances in which clients try to con people.

---

*Sources consulted include Clinard (1974) and Schultz and Dark (1982).

†At this point it may be useful to refer to Chapter 18 and the discussion of dynamics of low self-esteem.

3. Help individuals recognize that manipulation is not an effective way of coping or interacting.
   a. Point out instances of poor judgment and failure to learn from experience.
   b. Explore the damaging effects of manipulation on interpersonal relationships.
   c. Explore clients' feelings when they perceive that others may be trying to manipulate them.
4. Assist clients to develop alternative, constructive, and nonmanipulative ways to approach problems and needs.
   a. Discuss their behavior in a nonjudgmental and nonthreatening manner.
   b. Help clients to identify when they use denial, rationalization, and/or intellectualization.
   c. Encourage the expression of feelings.
   d. Help clients to identify the consequences of their behavior.
   e. Help them identify personal strengths and effective communication skills.
   f. Help them develop new skills and abilities.
5. Support clients while they test out their new, nonmanipulative approach to life.
6. Help them evaluate the effectiveness of this new behavior.
7. Remind them when they slip back into manipulative patterns.

When clients use ingratiation and charm, nurses or other team members may not recognize that they are being manipulated.

Mrs. Graff, who had been admitted to a hospital with drug-related hepatitis, was very charming and witty. She confided to one of the nurses, "You are the only one in this hospital who treats me like a person. All the other nurses try to avoid me. They don't like me very much." The nurse was flattered by this comment. Even though he did not approve of Mrs. Graff's drug abuse, he felt that of all the staff, he alone was able to relate to Mrs. Graff as a person. In an attempt to compensate for the reject-

ing attitudes of the other nurses, he tried to be available to Mrs. Graff and to comply with her requests. One day over coffee, several nurses began discussing Mrs. Graff's feeling of rejection. They discovered that Mrs. Graff had told each of them that the other nurses were avoiding her and that he or she was the only nurse who cared. Each had felt flattered and had responded by going out of the way to give Mrs. Graff extra attention.

Thus, when nurses fail to recognize manipulation, they may unwittingly reinforce it.

When nurses or other team members do recognize manipulative tendencies in clients, they sometimes respond defensively. They may begin to see manipulation in the actions of all clients, or they may reject or show hostility toward manipulative clients. If a staff member possesses manipulative tendencies, he or she may try to manipulate a client and rationalize that the client is "being taught a lesson" or "being given a dose of his own medicine." It is important for nurses and other health team members to be aware of these possible responses to manipulative clients. Such responses may reinforce a client's sense of low self-esteem and increase his or her need to engage in exploitive behavior.

Most nurses explain to clients that confidential material is shared with other health team members. This sharing minimizes client manipulation of staff and facilitates consistency in approach among staff members.

Nursing diagnosis: Dysfunction in relationships and life-style related to feelings of alienation and anomie (behavior associated with DSM-III diagnoses of substance use disorder, other psychosexual disorder, impulse control disorder [intermittent or isolated explosive disorder, pathological gambling], personality disorder [antisocial], and conduct disorder)

Planning: The nurse may initially establish goals, but as therapy progresses the client should enter into goal setting.
   1. Long-term goals
      a. Develop a sense of relatedness to others (sense of "belonging").

b. Internalize social norms.
2. Short-term goals
   a. Express feelings of alienation and anomie.
   b. Develop impulse control.
   c. Develop more effective interpersonal skills.
   d. Establish rapport in interpersonal relationships.
   e. Follow rules and regulations in the treatment setting.

Implementation: Alienation and *anomie* are frequent themes in the life-styles of socially deviant individuals. Alienation is a failure in reciprocal connectedness between an individual and the environment. Alienation is experienced as a sense of estrangement of self from others. Out of this loose social integration and impoverished interpersonal matrix anomie develops.

Srole (1956) uses a continuum to describe alienation and anomie. On one end is a sense of belonging. On the other end is a sense of alienation. Between these opposites are various degrees of distance between oneself and others. Personality factors interrelate with elements of societal dysfunction to produce anomie. Socially deviant individuals often are alienated and view society's rule system as something that exists to be broken.

The following are aspects of nursing intervention with alienated and anomic clients:

1. Nurses should be consistent in approach, and they should be consistent in setting and reinforcing limits. In conjunction with the rest of the health team, nurses should be consistent in sanctioning socially acceptable behavior and constraining socially unacceptable behavior. The message to a client should be clear: it is not you, but rather your behavior, that is unacceptable.
2. A structured setting, with opportunities for gradual increases in independence, facilitates the learning of socially acceptable behavior. Violation of rules should result in firm and consistent penalties. Step by step, socially deviant individuals should be taught to live within society's rule system. As their behavior becomes more acceptable and they demonstrate a sense of responsibility for their behavior, they should be allowed more opportunity for independence.

A unit for socially deviant male adolescents used a card system to reinforce socially acceptable behavior. The unit's environment was highly structured; strict adherence to routine and rules was required. When an adolescent was admitted to the unit, he had no privileges. Through the card system, privileges could be earned. Card 1 meant that an adolescent could use free periods (nontherapy periods) for activities of his choice. Card 2 carried grounds privileges: during free periods an adolescent could go outside unaccompanied by a staff member and could participate in sports, take walks, or lounge about. Card 3 carried weekend privileges: it allowed an adolescent to go home for weekends.

Just as cards could be earned for socially acceptable behavior, they could be lost for socially deviant behavior. If a card was taken away, a nurse would discuss the reasons for the penalty with the adolescent. The possibility of reearning the card and the behavior required to accomplish this were discussed. In this way, an adolescent was made aware of his socially disapproved behavior and of the penalty accompanying it. At the same time, the nurse did not reject the adolescent as a person.

---

3. Group therapy provides opportunity for socially deviant individuals to identify with and become integrated into groups. Within a homogeneous group, members can establish rapport with one another and develop a sense of "belonging." If they derive gratification from the group experience, socially deviant individuals may begin to submit to group pressure. Group members, all of whom are using or have used the mechanisms common to social deviance (e.g., manipulation, rationalization), can recognize and confront these mechanisms in one another. Structure, challenge, and confrontation are more readily accepted from one's peers than from an authority figure. Group members learn to fol-

low the rules and to internalize the norms of the group and, eventually, of society.

Because many socially deviant individuals have not internalized society's standards, nurses often find their own attitudes and values are under assault. For instance, a nurse who has been raised to be law-abiding and considerate of others may react to the alienation and anomie of a client with rejection, anger, derogation, or moralizing. Nurses should try, with the aid of peer supervision, to clarify their own values and attitudes.* In this way, they may gain greater insight into their own behavior and may be better able to intervene therapeutically in the cases of alienated and anomic clients.

Nursing diagnosis: Interaction theme of hostility related to frustration and anxiety engendered by threats to security (behavior associated with DSM-III diagnoses of substance use disorder, other psychosexual disorder, impulse control disorder [intermittent or isolated explosive disorder, pathological gambling], personality disorder [antisocial], and conduct disorder)

Planning: With assistance and/or guidance from the nurse, the client will establish goals.
1. Long-term goals
   a. Develop socially acceptable (non-hostile) ways of coping with frustration and anxiety.
   b. Decrease frustration and/or anxiety associated with threats to security.
2. Short-term goals
   a. Express feelings of hostility, frustration, and anxiety.
   b. Identify situations that arouse hostility, frustration, and anxiety.
   c. Identify the object of hostility.
   d. Develop impulse control (concerning harm to self and others and the destruction of property).
   e. Learn more effective coping behaviors and interpersonal skills.

Implementation: Hostility is a state of animosity. It develops slowly and dissipates slowly. Unlike anger, hostility does not generate measurable autonomic responses.*

When socially deviant clients are confronted with their behavior, they usually respond with evasiveness, denial, or anger. This response serves the dual purpose of venting hostility and focusing attention away from oneself.

Hostility functions as a coping mechanism by reducing anxiety associated with threats to security. If socially deviant individuals are confronted with their hostile feelings before they are ready to deal with them, they may become increasingly anxious, deny their hostility, and displace it onto people or objects in the environment.

Hostility is expressed *indirectly,* and it may be aimed at either animate or inanimate objects. Because hostility is not directly expressed, it is not easily depleted. Hostility underlies socially deviant behavior, and society is often the object of the hostility.

The following are ways to help clients deal with their hostility:
1. Help individuals realize that they feel hostile.
   a. Be alert for indirect expressions (clues) of hostility, and point them out to the client. You might say, "You sound upset about . . ." or "You seem annoyed with . . . ."
   b. Encourage the client to validate your assessment of hostility: "Yes, I feel annoyed" or "No, I'm not upset."
2. Help individuals identify and describe the objects of their hostility.
   a. Recognize anxiety-producing and frustrating situations that generate hostility.
   b. Because many socially deviant individuals have difficulty verbalizing their feelings, activity therapy can be used to facilitate the expression of hostility.
   c. Assist the client to gradually verbalize hostile feelings and the object of hostility.
3. Help individuals learn to express hostility in a socially acceptable manner.
   a. Explore with the client alternative ways

---

*Refer to Chapter 4 for a discussion of value clarification.

*Refer to Chapter 4 for a discussion of attitude clarification.

of dealing with hostile feelings. For example, activities such as gardening, tennis, and woodworking channel hostile energy into socially acceptable behavior.

b. Support the client in trying out new coping behavior.

c. Assist the client in evaluating the effectiveness of new coping behavior.

Because hostility is often unconscious, many people find it very difficult to express. Nurses can easily recognize overt hostility (such as sarcasm, vulgarity, or physical acting out) but may fail to recognize covert hostility (such as excessive politeness, obsequiousness, or ingratiation.) Nurses should also realize that what socially deviant clients initially identify as the objects of their hostility may not be what actually bothers them.

Hostility, like anxiety, can be communicated from person to person. A nurse may begin to feel hostile toward a client, or a nurse may become so caught up in a client's hostility that he or she begins to feel hostile toward the object of the client's hostility.

Many nurses are unaccustomed to acknowledging their own hostile feelings. They may fear the repercussions of dealing with their hostility. They may repress hostility, or they may try to diffuse it through griping. Occasionally, nurses may be fearful of hostile feelings in themselves or others. This apprehension may interfere with a client's expression of hostility.

Tony, a student nurse who was working with a socially deviant individual, began to realize that hostility was one of the client's predominant interpersonal themes. Although the student frequently assured the client that it was "all right to feel hostile" and encouraged him to talk about his hostile feelings, the client continued to deny any feelings of hostility. An instructor helped the student nurse look at his mode of intervention. Even though the student verbally encouraged the client to express hostility, his nonverbal communication (which included a very soft voice, hunched shoulders, and arms clenched

around himself) amounted to "I'm afraid of your hostility." Once this situation was pointed out, the student nurse was able to talk about his fear of expressed hostility. He said that his family had always repressed and denied hostile feelings.

With this newly gained insight into his own behavior, the student nurse's nonverbal communication no longer belied his words. The client then began to express his hostile feelings. The instructor was able to support the student nurse through the experience, and the student nurse was able to tolerate and understand the client's expression of hostility—even when it was verbally directed at him.

Thus, when nurses are unaware of their own feelings about hostility or are afraid of hostile feelings, they may be unable to understand or intervene in a client's hostility.

Nursing diagnosis: Social network or family dysfunction related to conflict or fear about a member's socially deviant behavior (behavior associated with DSM-III diagnoses of substance use disorder, other psychosexual disorder, impulse control disorder [intermittent or isolated explosive disorder, pathological gambling], personality disorder [antisocial], and conduct disorder)

Planning: With assistance and guidance from the nurse, clients will establish goals.

1. Long-term goals:
   a. Identify the most destructive conflict or fear about a network or family member's socially deviant behavior.
   b. Decrease the severity of this conflict, within the matrix of social network or family relationships.
   c. Increase the level of communication and interdependence among network or family members.
2. Short-term goals:
   a. Express feelings of anger and frustration about the network or family member's socially deviant behavior.
   b. Express feelings of anxiety and guilt about "causing" or facilitating the social-

ly deviant behavior of a network or family member.

c. Identify instances when feelings of anger and frustration that are generated by the socially deviant behavior are displaced onto other network or family members.

d. Develop more effective coping behaviors and communication patterns.

Implementation: The following are aspects of nursing intervention with the social networks of socially deviant individuals:

1. The primary role of a therapist should be to help modify the perceptual field of network or family members so that they will realize that change is possible. This may be accomplished through exploration of and intervention in the patterns of communication and coping that are evidenced during network or family therapy. When individual members alter their perceptions, it follows that their responses may also change. Consequently, the network or family as a whole may alter both its perceptual field and its reactions. Patterns of coping and communication may change. A network or family that in the past may have facilitated the socially aberrant behavior of a member may no longer tolerate the maladaptive interpersonal mechanisms used by the socially deviant member. As a consequence, the network or family member may change the mode of interaction with the social network or the family.

2. Social network or family members may need assistance to identify, describe, and deal with their feelings of anxiety, anger, frustration, and/or guilt that are related to the behavior of the socially deviant member.

   a. Be alert for the indirect expression of feelings (e.g., alluding to guilt; the use of sarcasm) or the displacement of feelings.

   b. Encourage network or family members to validate your assessment of feeling tones.

   c. Help network or family members to identify and describe the situations that generate these feelings.

d. Assist network or family members to learn to express these feelings directly and in a socially acceptable manner.

e. Encourage network or family members to examine how their own behavior aids or facilitates the social deviance of the network or family member.

f. Encourage network or family members to decrease behavior that has facilitated the social deviance of a member.

g. Support network or family members as they try out their new ways of coping and communicating.

h. Assist network or family members in evaluating the effectiveness of their new methods of coping and communicating.

Nursing diagnosis: Alteration in self-security (potential either for inadvertent self-injury or intentional self-injury*) related to disorientation, loss of impulse control, feelings of anger or hopelessness, and/or a desire for secondary gains (behavior associated with DSM-III diagnoses of substance use disorders, intermittent explosive disorder, and isolated explosive disorder)

Planning: The nurse may initially establish goals, but as therapy progresses the client should enter into goalsetting.

1. Long-term goals

   a. Develop a positive self-image (refer to Chapters 6 and 18 for a discussion of self-image).

   b. Develop impulse control.

2. Short-term goals

   a. Secure a safe environment.

   b. Express feelings of anger or hopelessness.

   c. Learn new coping behaviors to deal with feelings of anger or hopelessness.

   d. Develop insight about the consequences of one's anticipated behavior.

   e. Avoid secondary gains associated with self-injury.

   f. Realistically perceive the five dimensions of self. (Biological, intellectual, psycho-

---

*Refer to Chapter 18 for a discussion of suicide.

logical, sociocultural, and spiritual strengths and limitations will be put into perspective.)

Implementation: Several types of self-inflicted injury are commonly found among substance abusers: inadvertent injury, which generally occurs during either the acute phase or the withdrawal phase of substance abuse; intentional injury for secondary gains; and injury resulting from suicide attempts. (The acute phase is the period of maximal physical and/or behavioral effects caused by substance abuse. The withdrawal phase is the period of physical and/or behavioral symptoms caused by abrupt termination of substance abuse, especially if the body has become physically dependent on the substance.)

The following are aspects of nursing intervention with clients who have an alteration in self-security:

1. Nurses should be sure that substance abusers are treated in a protective environment. Every effort should be made to prevent them from injuring themselves. During the acute and withdrawal phases, substance abusers may be disoriented and restless. Protective measures such as side rails on beds, rounded corners on furniture, and padded rooms may be necessary.

2. During the treatment phase, it is not uncommon for substance abusers to intentionally injure themselves or to exaggerate their discomfort. Such behavior is usually designed to gain sympathy and to force the prescription of sedatives, tranquilizers, narcotics, or other drugs that reduce anxiety or produce pleasurable effects. Nurses need to be especially careful that addictive substances are not carelessly left within an addict's reach. Even cough medicines and alcohol-based mouth washes fall into this category.

3. There is a high incidence of suicide among substance abusers (Bell, 1970). Alternating moods of euphoria or omnipotence ("high") and severe depression ("letdown") usually accompany substance abuse. When coming out of the phase of depression, many addicts commit or attempt to commit suicide. Nurses therefore need to be alert for direct and indirect clues to suicidal intent. (Refer to the discussion of suicide in Chapter 18.)

Nursing diagnosis: Alteration in wellness related to poor health habits (behavior associated with DSM-III diagnoses of substance use disorder, other psychosexual disorder, impulse control disorder [intermittent or isolated explosive disorder, pathological gambling], personality disorder [antisocial], and conduct disorder)

Planning: With assistance and/or guidance from the nurse, the client will establish goals.

1. Long-term goals
   a. Understand the relationship between good health habits and high-level wellness.
   b. Develop health habits that promote high-level wellness.
2. Short-term goals
   a. Establish an exercise program.
   b. Establish a program of nutrition and hydration.
   c. Establish routines that promote rest and sleep.
   d. Establish routines of personal hygiene.
   e. Seek treatment for existent health problems.

Implementation: To determine the state of a socially deviant individual's health, a nurse should conduct a physical assessment. Nurses should help clients establish routines regarding exercise, diet, sleep, and hygiene. The following are aspects of nursing intervention for clients whose poor health habits jeopardize their potential for wellness:

1. Establishment of a diet that provides adequate nutrition and hydration is often necessary. Clients should be encouraged to eat well-balanced diets that are consistent with their cultural and spiritual orientations. Overweight clients should be counseled about low-calorie, nutritious foods. Malnourished clients may require dietary supple-

ments (e.g., fortified malts, vitamins). Unusual dietary practices, such as fad diets or diets composed almost solely of fast foods, should be evaluated for their level of nutrition. Clients should become knowledgeable about the basic four food groups and about the nutritional value (or valuelessness) of food additives and highly processed foods. Many socially deviant clients also need to develop skill in food purchasing, storage, and preparation.

2. Establishment of an exercise program not only promotes the physical fitness of socially deviant clients, but it also provides them with a socially acceptable way of coping with stress. By exerting control over their bodies through an exercise program, socially deviant clients can gain a sense of power that they had previously achieved primarily through the manipulation of others.

3. Promotion of rest and sleep are important with clients who up to now have looked to pills or alcohol to induce sleep. Quiet, relaxing, nonstimulating activities prior to bedtime; the establishment of a regular bedtime; and the ingestion of a light snack (e.g., milk and crackers) promote sleep. Clients should also be counseled to avoid drinking beverages containing stimulants. Herbal teas can be substituted for coffee or caffein-containing tea.

4. Teaching clients about personal hygiene may be necessary. A client's socially deviant lifestyle may have contributed to the development of an unkempt or slovenly appearance. Routines of bathing, shampooing hair, brushing teeth, and washing clothes may have to be re-established.

5. Seeking treatment for existent health problems may be indicated. Often, socially deviant individuals are in poor physical health. For example, hepatitis may develop in main line drug users, and avitaminosis may occur in alcoholics. Foodaholics may be overweight but undernourished. Rapists may contract venereal diseases. Narcotic users may never feel the pain of dental caries. Discussion of health problems associated with specific types of socially deviant behavior is an educative goal of nursing therapy.

For more than a year, Joanna had been using psychedelic drugs. In addition, after she had run away from home and joined a commune, much of her food supply had come from begging and scavangering. Joanna's physical examination revealed malnutrition and gonorrhea. A nurse talked with her about nutrition and sexually transmitted diseases. Joanna was unaware that untreated gonorrhea could cause permanent sterility. She was also surprised to learn that long-term patterns of poor nutrition could limit her body's ability to fight infection, affect the health of any children she might bear, and eventually shorten her life.

Thus, nurses can be instrumental in educating socially deviant clients about good health practices.

Nursing intervention aimed at assisting socially deviant clients to achieve a higher level of wellness should be begun when clients are first seen in detoxification or treatment centers.

A head nurse was orienting Gary to his nursing responsibilities on an alcohol detoxification unit. After giving Gary a tour of the unit and introducing him to the clients, the head nurse and Gary sat down and discussed the role of a nurse in a detoxification unit. Gary stated that he was aware that many of the clients would be malnourished and/or poorly hydrated and that at frequent intervals nourishing foods and fluids should be available to clients. The head nurse agreed and added, "Initially, bland foods are most easily tolerated. Because caffeine may increase tremors, only decaffeinated coffee and caffeine-free sodas should be offered."

Gary further recognized that clients' vital signs would have to be monitored and that clients would have to be observed for confusion, tremors, seizures, hyperactivity, and hallucinations. Gary knew that a safe environment should be provided in order to prevent self-injury and that seizure precautions should be instituted. Clients should also be supported through their hallucinatory experiences (see Chapter 21).

Gary was aware that because of the physiological effects of chronic alcoholism, these clients were at high risk for many ailments, including gastritis, gastrointestinal bleeding, cirrhosis, pancreatitis, esophageal varices, impaired renal function, and neurological disorders. Gary knew that besides closely monitoring clients and administering medication to minimize the effects of withdrawal or the complications associated with alcoholism, he would have to alert a physician to any newly developed symptoms or changes in a clients condition.

The head nurse thought that Gary's view of the role of the nurse was limited. The head nurse pointed out that not only clients' physical problems, but also their psychological, social, and spiritual concerns needed to be considered. The head nurse reminded Gary that clients who are withdrawing from alcohol may be disoriented, anxious, hostile, beligerent, or depressed. Nurses on an alcohol detoxification unit may have to reorient clients to time, place, person, and situation. Nurses also have to assess the degree of client anxiety, hostility, aggression, and depression and the lethality of any suicidal ideation and appropriately intervene. The emotional support of ex-alcoholics or pastoral counselors can be helpful. Nurses should be nonjudgmental of clients and should not try to reform or chastise them.

The head nurse also explained to Gary that clients who are experiencing severe withdrawal symptoms may have to be assisted with their personal hygiene. Other clients may have to be helped to develop routines of personal hygiene. In addition, the head nurse cautioned Gary that, because social network members often facilitate an alcoholic's drinking, during visiting hours nurses need to be alert to the possibility of visitors smuggling liquor to clients. The head nurse cited one instance in which a wife concealed whiskey in plastic bags in her satchel-type pocketbook. During visiting hours, the wife gave the whiskey to her husband. The head nurse pointed out that referral of social network members to such support groups as Al-anon and Alateen is important if nurses in detoxification units are to assist clients to reach their potentials for high-level wellness.

Thus, nurses can be instrumental in assisting socially deviant clients to improve their health habits, guiding clients as they learn about the process of wellness and supporting clients as they try to develop healthier life-styles.

Nursing diagnosis: Violent acting out related to stress, aggression, and poor impulse control (behavior associated with DSM-III diagnoses of conduct disorders, substance use disorders, disorders of impulse control, some psychosexual disorders, and child and adult antisocial behavior)

Planning: The nurse may initially establish goals, but as therapy progresses, the client should enter into goal-setting.

1. Long-term goals
   a. Learn to cope with stress and aggression in a nonviolent manner.
   b. Adhere to society's norms and expectations regarding nonviolence.
2. Short-term goals
   a. Identify and describe feelings of anxiety and anger rather than physically express them.
   b. Identify and describe the precipitating stressful life situation and the associated feelings.
   c. Develop more effective (nonviolent) coping behaviors.
   d. Avoid secondary gains associated with violent behavior.
   e. Develop impulse control.

Implementation: Clients who exhibit violent behavior often come into contact with professional nurses only after the clients have destroyed property or harmed others. The following are aspects of nursing intervention with violently acting-out clients:

1. Facilitate the nonviolent expression of feelings. Encourage clients to verbally identify and describe their anxious and angry feelings

and the situations that generate them. Help clients to physically, but nonviolently, expend the energy associated with these feelings through exercise, manual labor, etc. Nurses should also encourage clients to seek out staff members, friends, or relatives when they are feeling stressed and to share their feelings. Because clients may fear that they will lose control of their actions if they begin to express their anger, nursing staff members should reassure clients that they will be helped to control their behavior.

2. Provide a nonstressful environment. Since clients who feel threatened may perceive any stimulus as a "trigger" in the five-phase cycle of violence, environmental stimuli should be controlled. By lowering the volume of radios, phonographs, and televisions and by dimming lights, physical stimuli can be decreased. By modulating their voices, providing clients with a place to be alone, and taking care not to intrude on clients' personal space, nurses can decrease social stimuli. Remember that potentially violent individuals have a personal zone up to four times larger than that of nonviolent persons (Schultz and Dark, 1982).

3. Explore with clients the secondary gains associated with their violent behavior. Expectations that clients will participate in activities of daily living and in therapeutic modalities should be clearly stated. Clients should not receive any special privileges or dispensations because of their violent behavior.

4. Facilitate impulse control. Establish rapport with clients. Ideally rapport should be established before the occurrence of violent episodes. Be alert to behavioral cues of an impending violent outburst. Keep avenues of communication open. Remember that violence and communication are mutually exclusive. Inform clients of the consequences of violent behavior before it occurs. Carry out the consequences in a nonpunitive, matter-of-fact manner *immediately* after the violent episode. Similarly, give immediate feedback or rewards for nonviolent responses to stress. Gradually increase the amount of nonviolent behavior that warrants a reward, keeping clients informed of changes in the behavior-reward ratio. Relate to clients in a calm, nonpunitive manner. Should physical or chemical restraint be necessary to facilitate impulse control, carry out the procedure quickly and nonpunitively. Physical or chemical restraints should never be used as punishment. Other clients should not be permitted to participate in the restraining of a client. Neither should other clients be allowed to watch the procedure. After the situation is settled, provide an opportunity for other clients to express their feelings about the occurrence.

EVALUATION

The client, and, whenever feasible, the client's social network, should be included in estimating the client's progress towards attainment of goals. Any evaluation should encompass the following areas:

1. Estimation of the degree to which anxiety and conflict have been decreased
2. Estimation of the degree to which goals have been achieved and client functioning has improved (demonstrated by a decrease in socially deviant coping behaviors and the learning of socially acceptable coping behaviors)
3. Identification of goals that need to be modified or revised
4. Referral of the client to support systems other than the nurse-client relationship
   a. People in the client's social network who are willing to serve as a support system and who will not act as facilitators of socially deviant behavior
   b. Community agencies that help clients learn to live with socially deviant tendencies that may never be completely

eliminated (e.g., Alcoholics Anonymous, Gamblers Anonymous, Overeaters Anonymous)
   c. Centers that specialize in the treatment of specific socially deviant behaviors (e.g., drug or alcohol treatment centers, smokers' withdrawal clinics)

TERTIARY PREVENTION

Because social networks and communities change slowly, socially deviant individuals may be discharged from treatment centers and returned to the environments that contributed to the development of their unacceptable behavior. Following discharge from treatment centers, ongoing support in the form of *rehabilitative* or *after-care* services may be needed.

Although most people agree that tertiary prevention is a necessary part of treatment for socially aberrant behavior, after-care is not a major priority in the United States. Many people fear that they or their children will be seduced by former prostitutes, assaulted by former juvenile delinquents, or "turned on" to drugs by former addicts. Everyone supports the idea of rehabilitation, but few people want an after-care center located in their neighborhood.

A drug treatment center purchased a large house in a suburban community. The plan was to establish a drug-free day care program for former addicts. Community members, however, were concerned and angry; they did not want former addicts passing through the streets on their way to the day care center. Parents, clergymen, and educators feared that the former addicts would serve as antiestablishment role models, try to peddle drugs, or in some other way adversely influence children and adolescents. After three fires of suspicious origin occurred, the treatment center sold the house and dismissed the idea of establishing a day care program.

Limited tertiary prevention programs are available in the following settings.

Transitional services

Transitional services involve the gradual severing of ties with a treatment center. Socially deviant individuals spend ever-increasing amounts of time away from the center. They may start with an overnight pass, go on to weekend privileges, and finally work up to a week away from the center. Skills for community living and help in locating work and housing are provided. Once socially deviant persons are living in a community, many transitional programs encourage them to return to the treatment center for weekly, semi-monthly, or monthly "rap" sessions. At these sessions, problems of adjustment and daily living and ways of coping are discussed.

After-care centers

After-care centers are designed for socially deviant persons who have a place to live and an accepting, supportive family or social network but who are not yet ready to return to work. At a day center, some clients receive medication (such as methadone or Antabuse). All clients receive structure and organization. Social skills and activities of daily living are taught, and assistance is given in looking for a job and preparing for a job interview. Opportunities for socializing are provided. Many day care centers achieve a high degree of autonomy. A system of peer group control may develop, and members may actively set and reinforce rules. If a member experiences a crisis, other members may institute a 24-hour-a-day support system.

Night hospitals

Night hospitals are designed for socially deviant individuals who demonstrate a high degree of impulse control, judgment, and social conscience but who are not yet ready to function full time in the community. Clients work during the day and return to the treatment center each evening. Nightly supportive therapy sessions may be part of the program. Some prisons and drug treatment centers are experimenting with the night hospital approach.

Educational training

Depending on the age, interests, and abilities of socially deviant individuals, continued education, including college and vocational training (retraining in old skills or teaching of new skills), may be indicated. Education increases self-esteem and prepares clients to be as financially self-reliant as possible.

Self-help groups

Self-help groups support socially deviant individuals in their readjustment to community living and intervene in crisis situations. Such groups are composed of former socially deviant persons who have successfully learned to live by society's standards. Alcoholics Anonymous, Narcotics Anonymous, Gamblers Anonymous, and Overeaters Anonymous use a repressive-inspirational approach (see Chapter 11). Women for Sobriety attempts to teach women to live without alcohol. The Fortune Society helps former criminals learn to operate within society's standards, assists them to support themselves legitimately, and helps them to cope with the social stigma attached to imprisonment. A self-help group known as Scapegoat helps prostitutes leave their pimps, learn marketable skills, and find employment.

Voluntary rehabilitation groups

The purpose of voluntary rehabilitation groups is similar to that of self-help groups. What differentiates these groups from self-help groups is that most of the members of voluntary rehabilitation groups have not had socially deviant life-styles. The Salvation Army and the St. Vincent de Paul Society are examples of voluntary rehabilitation groups. Emergency aid in the form of financial assistance, housing, and food is usually available. In addition, counseling, assistance in finding employment and housing, work projects, and leisure time activities may be offered.

Family and social networks

Family and social networks are an essential part of tertiary prevention of socially deviant behavior. Counseling of family members and friends helps to decrease their feelings of guilt, frustration, and anger. Counseling also teaches network members how to avoid facilitating socially aberrant behavior and encourages them to remain involved with the socially deviant individual. Network members are helped to develop an honest, open, consistent, firm approach to the client and to identify and resist attempts at manipulation. Family and social network counseling may be done by professionals or by members of such self-help groups as Alanon, Alateen (for the network members of alcoholics), Gam-Anon, Gam-A-Teen (for the network members of gamblers), Families Anonymous and Straight (for network members of drug abusers), and Tough Love (for parents of children with antisocial behavior).

CHAPTER SUMMARY

Socially deviant or aberrant behavior includes a large number of seemingly disparate and incongruous ways of relating to people. Socially deviant persons are characterized by such deeply ingrained maladaptive personality patterns and restricted emotional responses that they develop life-styles that often bring them into conflict with society.

Many theories have been formulated to explain the etiology of socially aberrant behavior. These theories fall into three major categories: psychological conflict, biological defect, and sociocultural conflict. It is likely that a combination of holistic health factors leads to the development of socially deviant behavior. Some types of socially aberrant behavior are known to all societies, but its form, meaning, and incidence are culturally influenced and culturally relative.

Socially deviant individuals may be treated in a general hospital, a psychiatric hospital, a specialized treatment center, or a self-help group. Some of the most frequently used treatment modalities include aversion therapy, milieu therapy, individual therapy, and group therapy. A combination of therapies is usually indicated. The goals of therapy are to supplant socially deviant behavior with socially acceptable behavior and to facilitate reentry into society.

Although nurses may not directly participate in all treatment modalities, they do participate in all three levels of preventive intervention.

Primary prevention focuses on identification of and intervention for such high-risk individuals as depressed mothers and the victims of child abuse. Attempts are also made to rectify overcrowding, community disorganization, and other contributory social or environmental conditions. Secondary prevention involves case finding and application of the nursing process to socially deviant behavior. Secondary prevention is most effective when it involves a collaborative and consistent team approach. Nurses function as integral and important members of the mental health team. However, socially deviant life-styles are not easily changed. The course of recovery is often marked by relapses. Tertiary prevention of socially aberrant behavior requires that mental health workers, former socially deviant individuals, clients, and network members work toward a unified rehabilitative approach.

When working with socially deviant persons, nurses need to be *nondefensive, realistic, accepting, consistent,* and *firm.* Insight into their own values and behavior is essential in helping socially deviant individuals confront their unacceptable behavior. By clarifying their own attitudes and values, nurses can accept people who behave in socially aberrant ways, without condoning their life-styles.

SENSITIVITY-AWARENESS EXERCISES

The purposes of the following exercises are to:

- Develop awareness about the vulnerability of people to socially deviant behavior
- Develop awareness about the interrelationship of factors in the etiology of social deviance
- Develop awareness about the subjective experience of clients who use socially deviant behavior and of the experience of clients' families
- Develop awareness about your own feelings and attitudes when working with clients who use socially deviant behavior

1. Try to imagine that you use one of the following addictive disorders to cope with stress and conflict, and explain why you selected that particular addictive disorder. Then describe what you think it would be like to suffer from that disorder.
   a. Drug abuse
   b. Alcoholism
   c. Overeating
   d. Compulsive tobacco smoking
   e. Compulsive working
   f. Compulsive gambling
2. Describe what you think it would be like to have a family member who uses one of the following socially deviant behaviors: violent behavior, antisocial behavior, addictive behavior (specify which type), or sexually deviant behavior (prostitution or rape). Which socially deviant behavior do you think would be easiest to tolerate in a family member? Why? Which socially deviant behavior would be hardest to tolerate? Why?
3. What might be some of your feelings and reactions as a nurse caring for socially deviant clients? Would your feelings and reactions vary with the type of socially deviant behavior used by clients? Explain why.
4. Imagine that you are a community health nurse engaged in health supervision with new parents. What high-risk factors (biological, psychological, intellectual, sociocultural, and spiritual) would you observe for that might predispose parents and their children to social deviance?
5. Develop a plan for counseling parents about child rearing that incorporates principles and goals for the primary prevention of social deviance.

REFERENCES

"Alcoholics' odd blood suggests genetic disease"
1983 Science News (September 17) 124(12):180.

Ashcraft, N., and A.E. Scheflen
1976 People Space: The Making and Breaking of Human Boundaries. New York: Anchor Press.

Bacon, M.K.
1973 "Cross-cultural studies of drinking." In Alcoholism: Progress in Research and Treatment. P.G. Bourne and R. Fox (eds.). New York: Academic Press.

Bach-y-Rita, G., et al.
1971 "Episodic control: a study of 130 violent patients." American Journal of Psychiatry 127:1473-1478.

Bagley, C.
1967 "Anomie, alienation and the evaluation of social structures." Kansas Journal of Sociology 3:110-123.

Bell, D.S.
1970 "Drug addiction." Bulletin on Narcotics 22:21-32.

Bell, R.
1970 Escape from Addiction. New York: McGraw-Hill Book Co.

Benedict, R.
1934 Patterns of Culture. Boston: Houghton Mifflin Co.

Benjamin, H., and R.E.L. Masters
1964 Prostitution and Morality. London: Souvenir Press Ltd.

Benson, H., and R.K. Wallace
1972 "Decreased drug abuse with transcendental meditation: a study of 1,862 subjects." In Drug Abuse: Proceedings of the International Conference. Chris J.D. Zarafonetis (ed.). Philadelphia: Lea & Febiger.

Bergler, E.
1970 The Psychology of Gambling. New York: International Universities Press, Inc.

Birenbaum, A., and E. Sagarin
1976 Norms and Human Behavior. New York: Praeger Publishers.

Bolton, R.
1972 "Aggression and hypoglycemia among the Quolla: a study in psychobiological anthropology." Sterling Award paper in culture and personality. American Anthropological Association.

Brown, L.
1981a "Theoretical frameworks for understanding violent behavior." In Assessing Patient Violence in the Health Care Setting. K. Babich (ed.). Boulder: WICHE.

Brown, L.
1981b "A model for understanding the muddle between the legal and health care systems." In Assessing Patient Violence in the Health Care Setting. K. Babich (ed.). Boulder: WICHE.

Brown, W.N.
1968 "Alienated youth." Mental Hygiene 52:330-336.

Brownmiller, S.
1975 Against Our Will: Men, Women and Rape. New York: Simon and Schuster, Inc.

Buitrago-Ortiz, C.
1973 Esperanza: An Ethnographic Study of a Peasant Community in Puerto Rico. Tucson: University of Arizona Press.

Burckhardt, C.
1981 "Research on violence: principles and findings." In Assessing Patient Violence in The Health Care Setting. K. Babich (ed.). Boulder: WICHE.

Burgess, A., and L. Holmstrom
1974 Rape, Victims of Crisis. Bowie, Maryland: Robert J. Brady.

Burrows, E.G., and M.E. Spiro
1953 Atoll Culture: Ethnography of Ifaluk in the Central Carolines. New Haven, Conn.: Human Relations Area Files Press, Yale University Publications.

Carstairs, G.
1954 "Daru and bhang: cultural factors in the choice of intoxicant." Quarterly Journal of Studies on Alcohol 15:220-237.

Chesler, P.
1972 Women and Madness. New York: Avon Books.

Chesser, E.
1971 Strange Loves: The Human Aspects of Sexual Deviation. New York: William Morrow and Co., Inc.

Choisy, M.
1960 A Month Among the Girls. New York: Pyramid Communications, Inc.
1961 Psychoanalysis of the Prostitute. New York: Philosophical Library, Inc.

Clark, P.
1963 "Acceptance of blame and alienation among prisoners." American Journal of Orthopsychiatry 3:557-561.

Clinard, M.B.
1974 Sociology of Deviant Behavior. New York: Holt, Rinehart and Winston, Inc.

Clunn, P.
1981 "Nurses' assessments of violence potential." In Assessing Patient Violence in the Health Care Setting. Boulder: WICHE.

Collins, M.C.
1978 Child Abuser. Littleton, Mass.: PSG Publishing Co.

DeLint, J., and W. Schmidt
1971 "The epidemiology of alcoholism." In Biological Basis of Alcoholism. Y. Israel and J. Mardones (eds.). New York: John Wiley and Sons, Inc.

DeMeyer-Gapin, S., and T.J. Scott
1977 "Effect of stimulus novelty on stimulation-seeking in antisocial and neurotic children." Journal of Abnormal Psychology 86:96-98.

Desk Reference on Drug Abuse
1970 New York: New York State Department of Health.

Detre, T., D. Kupfer, and S. Taub
1975 "The nosology of Violence." In Neural Bases of Violence and Aggression. St. Louis: Warren H. Green.

Dishotsky, N., W. Loughman, R. Mogar, and W. Lipscomb
1971 "LSD and genetic damage." Science 172:431-440.

Donaldson, W.
1977 Don't Call Me Madam—The Life and Hard Times of a Gentleman Pimp. New York: New York: Mason/Charter Publishers, Inc.

Durkheim, E.
1938 The Rules of Sociological Method. New York: The Free Press.

Elliott, C., and D. Denney
1975 "Weight control through covert sensitization and false feedback." Journal of Consulting and Clinical Psychology 43:842-850.

Esselstyn, T.C.
1967 "The violent offender and corrections." Paper submitted to the President's Commission on Law Enforcement and Administration of Justice. Washington, D.C.: U.S. Government Printing Office.

Eysenck, H.J.
1979 "The origins of violence." Journal of Medical Ethics 5:105-107.

Feingold, F.
1975 Why Your Child is Hyperactive. New York: Random House, Inc.

Finnegan, J.K., P.S. Larson, and H.B. Haag
1945 "The role of nicotine in the cigarette habit." Science 102:94-96.

Fleming, A.
1978 Something for Nothing—A History of Gambling. New York: Delacorte Press.

Forrest, G.G.
1979 "Negative and positive addictions." Family and Community Health 2(1):103-112.

Freedman, J.L.
1975 Crowding and Behavior. New York: The Viking Press, Inc.

Freud, S.
1930 Civilization and Its Discontents. Joan Riviere (trans.). London: The Hogarth Press Ltd.
1959 Collected Papers of Sigmund Freud. Ernest Jones (ed.). New York: Basic Books, Inc., Publishers.

Friedman, M., and R.H. Rosenman
1974 Type A Behavior and Your Heart. New York: Alfred A. Knopf, Inc.

Fromm, E.
1947 Man for Himself. New York: Holt, Rinehart and Winston, Inc.
1955 The Sane Society. New York: Holt, Rinehart and Winston, Inc.

Gans, H.
1962 The Urban Villagers. New York: The Free Press of Glencoe.

Glazer, N., and D.P. Moynihan
1963 Beyond the Melting Pot. Cambridge, Mass.: The M.I.T. Press.

Goffman, E.
1963 Stigma: Notes on the Management of Spoiled Identity. Englewood Cliffs: Prentice-Hall.
1969 Where the Action Is. London: Allen Lane.

Green, D.E.
1977 "Psychological factors in smoking." In Research on Smoking Behavior: NIDA Research Monograph 17. M.E. Jarvik et al. (eds.). Washington, D.C.: U.S. Government Printing Office.

Gregg, G.
1976 "From masseuse to prostitute in one quick trick: a study by A. Velarde." Psychology Today 10:27-28.

Grinker, R.
1971 "What is the cause of violence?" In Dynamics of Violence. J. Fawcett (ed.). Chicago: American Medical Association.

Gusinde, M.
1961 The Yamana. New Haven, Conn.: Human Relations Area Files Press, Yale University Publications.

Halleck, S.L.
1967 "Psychiatric treatment for the alienated college student." American Journal of Psychiatry 124:642-650.
1978 "Psychodynamic aspects of violence." In Violence and Responsibility: The Individual, the Family and Society. R. Sadoff (ed.). New York: SP Medical and Scientific Books.

Halliday, M.A.K.
1976 "Anti-language." American Anthropologist 78:570-584.

Hammond, E.C., and C. Percy
1958 "Ex-smokers." New York State Journal of Medicine 58:2956-2959.

Harkins, A.N.
1965 "Alienation and related concepts." Kansas Journal of Sociology 1:78-89.

Hirsch, J., and J.L. Knittle
1970 "Cellularity of obese and non-obese adipose tissue." Federal Process 29:1516-1521.

Hobart, C.W.
1965 "Types of alienation: etiology and interrelationships." Canadian Review of Sociology and Anthropology 2:92-107.

Hobbes, T.
1965 Leviathan. Oxford: Clarendon Press.

Horney, K.
1937 The Neurotic Personality of Our Time. New York: W.W. Norton and Co., Inc.

Hunt, W., and J. Matarazzo
1973 "Three years later: recent developments in the experimental modification of smoking behavior." Journal of Abnormal Psychology 81:107-114.

Hyde, M.O.
1978 Addictions: Gambling, Smoking, Cocaine Use and Others. New York: McGraw-Hill Book Co.

Jenkins, C.D.
1975 "The coronary-prone personality." In Psychological Aspects of Myocardial Infarction and Coronary Care. W.D. Gentry and R.B. Williams, Jr. (eds.). St. Louis: The C.V. Mosby Co.

Johnston, L.M.
1942 "Tobacco smoking and nicotine." Lancet 2:742.

Kato, T., et al.
1970 "Chromosome studies in pregnant rhesus macaque given LSD-25." Diseases of the Nervous System 31:245-250.

Kimsey, L.R.
1969 "Out-patient group psychotherapy with juvenile delinquents." Disturbances of the Nervous System 30:472-477.

Kingsley, R.G., and G.T. Wilson
1977 "Behavior therapy for obesity: a comparative investigation of long-term efficacy." Journal of Consulting and Clinical Psychology 45:288-298.

Kinsey, A., et al.
1948 Sexual Behavior in the Human Male. Philadelphia: W.B. Saunders Co.

Kolbye, A.C.
1976 First Report of the Preliminary Findings and Recommendations of the Interagency Collaborative Group on Hyperkinesis. Washington, D.C.: Department of Health, Education and Welfare, U.S. Government Printing Office.

LaBarre, W.
1960 "Twenty years of peyote studies." Current Anthropology 1:45.
1964 "The peyote cult." Hamden, Conn: The Shoe String Press, Inc.

Larson, P.S., H.B. Haag, and H. Silvette
1961 Tobacco: Experimental and Clinical Studies. Baltimore: The Williams and Wilkins Co.

Leavitt, F.
1974 Drugs and Behavior. Philadelphia: W.B. Saunders Co.

Lebovits, B., and A. Ostfeld
1971 "Smoking and personality: a methodological analysis." Journal of Chronic Diseases 23(10/11):813-821.

Leighton, A.H.
1959 My Name is Legion. New York: Basic Books, Inc., Publishers.

Lewis, O.
1951 Life in a Mexican Village: Tepoztlan Restudied. Urbana, Ill.: University of Illinois Press.

Lindner, R.M.
1950 "The psychodynamics of gambling." Annals of the American Academy of Political and Social Science 269:93-107.

Livingston, J.
1974 "Compulsive gamblers: a culture of losers." Psychology Today 7:51-55.

Locke, J.
1967 Two Tracts on Government. Philip Abrams (trans. and ed.). London: Cambridge University Press.

Mark, V.H., and F.R. Ervin
1970 Violence and the Brain. New York: Harper and Row, Publishers, Inc.

Marlatt, G.A., B. Demming, and J.B. Reid
1973 "Loss of control drinking in alcoholics: an experimental analogue." Journal of Abnormal Psychology 81:233-241.

Marmor, J.
1978 "Psychological roots of violence." In Violence and Responsibility: The Individual, the Family and Society. R. Sadoff (ed.). New York: SP Medical and Scientific Books.

Martinez, T.
1978 Cited in Addictions: Gambling, Smoking, Cocaine Use and Others. Margaret O. Hyde. New York: McGraw-Hill Book Co.

Martinez-Alier, V.
1974 Marriage, Class and Colour in Nineteenth-Century Cuba. London: Cambridge University Press.

Marzetta, B.R., H. Benson, and R.K. Wallace
1972 "Combating drug dependency in young people: a new approach." Medical Counterpoint 4:13-37.

Masters, R.E.L.
1962 Forbidden Sexual Behavior and Morality. New York: Julian Press, Inc.

McClosky, H., and J. Schaar
1965 "Psychological dimensions of anomie." American Sociological Review 30:14-40.

Merton, R.K., and A. Nisbet
1961 Contemporary Social Problems: An Introduction to the Sociology of Deviant Behavior and Social Disorganization. New York: Harcourt, Brace and World.
1971 Contemporary Social Problems. Robert K. Merton and Robert A. Nisbet (eds.). New York: Harcourt Brace Jovanovich, Inc.

Mills, C.W.
1950 The Sociological Imagination. New York: Oxford University Press.

Minuchin, S.
1967 Families of the Slums. New York: Basic Books, Inc., Publishers.

Montague, A.
1975 "Is man innately aggressive?" In Neural Bases of Violence and Aggression. W. Fields and W. Sweet (eds.). St. Louis: Warren H. Green.

Moran, E.
1970 "Pathological gambling." British Journal of Hospital Medicine 4:59-70.

Morgan, T.
1975 "Little ladies of the night: runaways in New York." New York Times Magazine, November 16, pp. 34-38.

Morton, P.G.
1979 "Assessment and management of the self-destructive concept of alcoholism." Journal of Psychiatric Nursing and Mental Health Services 17:8-13.

Moynihan, D.P.
1984 "Drugs: where we've come from, where we're going." Newsday, Ideas section, June 24, p. 5.

Nash, J.
1967 "Death as a way of life: the increasing resort to homocide in a Maya Indian community." American Anthropologist 69:455-470.

Nesbitt, P.D.
1972 "Chronic smoking and emotionality." Journal of Applied Social Psychology 2(2):187-196.

Nisbett, R.E.
1972 "Hunger, obesity, and ventromedial hypothalamus." Psychological Review 79:433-453.

Orbach, S.
1978 Fat Is A Feminist Issue—The Anti-Diet Guide to Permanent Weight Loss. New York: Paddington Press.

Pincus, J.H.
1979 "Neurologic abnormalities in violent delinquents." Neurology 29(4):586.

Polivy, J., A.L. Schueneman, and K. Carlson
1976 "Alcohol and tension reduction: cognitive and physiological effects." Journal of Abnormal Psychology 85:595-600.

Redfield, R.
1947 "The folk society." American Journal of Sociology 52:298-308.

Reeder, L.G.
1977 "Sociocultural factors in the etiology of smoking behavior: an assessment." In Research on Smoking behavior: NIDA Research Monograph 17. M.E. Jarvik et al. (eds.). Washington, D.C.: United States Government Printing Office.

Reich, C.A.
1970 The Greening of America: How the Youth Revolution is Trying to Make America Livable. New York: Random House, Inc.

Reiner, B., and I. Kaufman
1959 Character Disorders in Parents of Delinquents. New York: Family Service Association of America.

Report of the National Council on Alcoholism
1976 Long Island Council on Alcoholism Fact Sheet. Garden City, N.Y.

Reynolds, C., and R. Nichols
1976 "Personality and behavioral correlates of cigarette smoking." Psychological Reports 38(1):251-258.

Rosenman, R.H., et al.
1970 "Coronary heart disease in the Western Collaborative Study: a follow-up experience of four and one half years." Journal of Chronic Diseases 23:173-190.

Rosenman, R.H., et al.
1975 "Coronary heart disease in the Western Collaborative Group Study: final follow-up experience of eight and one half years." Journal of the American Medical Association 233:872-877.

Roth, M.
1972 "Human violence as viewed from the psychiatric clinic." American Journal of Psychiatry 128:1043-1056.

Rothenberg, A.
1971 "On anger." American Journal of Psychiatry 129:90.

Roueche, B.
1962 Alcohol: Its History, Folklore, and Effects on the Human Body. New York: Grove Press, Inc.

Rubin, B.
1972 "Prediction of dangerousness in mentaly ill criminals." Archives of General Psychiatry 17:397-407.

Ruesch, J.
1961 Therapeutic Communication. New York: W.W. Norton and Co., Inc.

Scheflen, A.E, and A. Scheflen
1972 Body Language and Social Order—Communication as Behavioral Control. Englewood Cliffs, N.J.: Prentice-Hall, Inc.

Schultz, J.M., and S.L. Dark
1982 Manual of Psychiatric Nursing Care Plans. Boston: Little, Brown and Company.

Schur, E.M.
1971 Labeling Deviant Behavior: Its Sociological Implications. New York: Harper & Row, Publishers, Inc.

Selkin, J.
1975 "Rape." Psychology Today 8:70-76.

Slotkin, J.S.
1967 "Religious defenses (the Native American church)." Journal of Psychedelic Drugs 1:80.

Smith, P.
1981 "Empirically based models for viewing the dynamics of violence." In Assessing Patient Violence in the Health Care Setting. K. Babich (ed.). Boulder: WICHE.

Smith, S.M., and R. Hanson
1975 "Interpersonal relationships and childrearing practices in 214 parents of battered children." British Journal of Psychiatry 127:513-525.

Speck, R.V., and L. Attneave
1973 Family Networks. New York: Pantheon Books, Inc.

Srole, L.
1956 "Social integration and certain corolaries: an explorative study." American Sociological Review 21:709-716.

Srole, L., et al.
1962 Mental Health in the Metropolis: The Midtown Manhattan Study. New York: McGraw-Hill Book Co.

Stuart, R.B., and B. Davis
1972 Slim Chance in a Fat World: Behavioral Control of Obesity. Champaign: Research Press.

Sullivan, H.S.
1953 The Interpersonal Theory of Psychiatry. New York: W.W. Norton and Co., Inc.

Thomkins, S.S.
1977 "Youth for sale on the streets." Time (November 28) 110:23.

Ugarte, G., et al.
1970 "Relations of color blindness to alcoholic liver damage." Pharmacology 4:308.

Van Proosdij, C.
1960 Smoking. London: Elsevier.

Wardwell, W.I., and C.B. Bahnson
1973 "Behavioral variables and myocardial infarction in the South Eastern Connecticut Heart Study." Journal of Chronic Disease 26:447-461.

Wegscheider, S.
1981 Another Chance: Hope and Health for the Alcoholic Family. Palo Alto: Science and Behavior Books, Inc.

Weissman, M.
1972 "The depressed woman: recent research." Social Work 17:19-25.

Wick, E.
1976 "Overeating patterns found in overweight and obese patients." In Obesity: Etiology, Treatment and Management. M.V. Kline et al. (eds.). Springfield, Ill.: Charles C Thomas, Publisher.

Wilkinson, R.
1970 The Prevention of Drinking Problems. New York: Oxford University Press.

Winchester, H.V., Jr.
1972 "Educational therapy for adolescents in the short-term psychiatric hospital." Perspective in Psychiatric Care 10:37.

Windsor, A.L., and S.J. Richards
1935 "The development of tolerance for cigarettes." Journal of Experimental Psychology 18:113-120.

Yablonsky, L.
1963 The Violent Gang. New York: Macmillan, Inc.

Zillman, D.
1979 Hostility and Aggression. New York: Lawrence Earlbaum Associates.

ANNOTATED SUGGESTED READINGS

Ashcraft, N., and A.E. Scheflen
1976 People Space: The Making and Breaking of Human Boundaries. New York: Anchor Press.
The authors explore the use of space by people and the consequences of the human use of space. Within this context, such social problems as poverty, crowding, ethnic differences, scarcity of resources, deterioration of living conditions, and violence are examined.

Hyde, M.O.
1978 Addictions: Gambling, Smoking, Cocaine Use and Others. New York: McGraw-Hill Book Co.
Addiction is defined as a characteristic, habitual way of coping with life stressors. Within this framework such addictions as chronic overeating, compulsive drinking (alcohol, coffee, tea, and cola), compulsive gambling, drug abuse, compulsive working, cigarette smoking, and jogging are discussed. This book includes a list of associations and clearing houses that may serve as sources for further information.

Merton, R.K., and R.A. Nisbet (eds.)
1971 Contemporary Social Problems. New York: Harcourt Brace Jovanovich, Inc.
This book looks at the characteristics of social structure that generate social order and socially conforming behavior and that also have the potential for producing social disorganization and socially deviant behavior. Social disorganization and social deviance are viewed as untoward and tangential consequences of institutionalized behavior patterns of society. The book is divided into two parts: "Deviant Behavior" (juvenile delinquency, mental disorders, alcoholism) and "Social Disorder" (family disorganization, poverty, violence, race relations).

Wegscheider, S.
1981 Another Chance: Hope and Health for the Alcoholic Family. Palo Alto: Science and Behavior Books, Inc.
The author applies a holistic health approach to alcoholism—the etiology, the addiction spiral, and the treatment plan. In addition, the role of the "whole" counselor is explored. Although this book deals with holistic health and alcoholism, its holistic concepts can be applied to all socially deviant behavior patterns.

FURTHER READINGS

Drabman, R.S., and M.H. Thomas
1976 "Does watching violence on television cause apathy?" Pediatrics 57:329-331.

Halleck, S.L.
1974 "Legal and ethical aspects of behavior control." American Journal of Psychiatry 131:381-385.

Gove, W.R. (ed.)
1975 The Labeling of Deviance: Evaluating a Perspective. New York: John Wiley and Sons.

CHAPTER 18

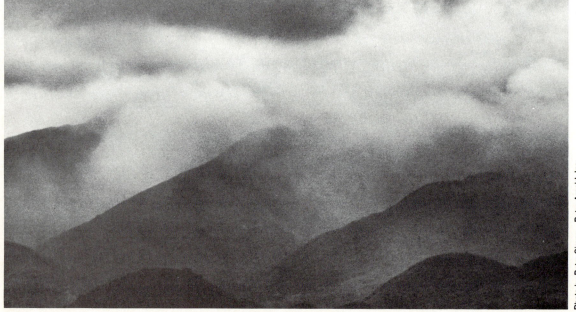

Photo by Peter Simon—Peter Arnold, Inc.

Coping through inwardly directed aggression

CHAPTER FOCUS

Depression is currently one of the most prevalent mental health problems in the United States. Discussion of depression as a disorder dates back to 1500 BC. The term is well known to many yet has several different connotations: mood disorder, change in affect, clinical syndrome, or cluster of behavioral symptoms.

Depression accompanies a significant proportion of physical illnesses, particularly those that are severe. Suicide is positively correlated with depression. Few individuals have not been touched by depression, at least in its mildest form, as a reaction to loss or change.

An understanding of depression begins with an understanding of the concepts of grief and loss. Depression may occur as a response to any form of loss—loss of function, body part, status or responsibility, or significant other. Depression, of course, is also experienced by persons who learn that they are going to lose their own lives. Phases of mourning will be discussed, and implications of healthy and maladaptive responses to loss will be identified.

The presentation of major theoretical constructs provides a framework for a thorough understanding of the complex underlying dynamics of depression. Predominant themes, coping mechanisms, and nursing interventions are discussed in relation to the manic-depressive response, involutional melancholia, and suicide.

GRIEF AND LOSS

Grief is a universal process that is generally taken for granted. According to Engel (1962), grief involves a series of subjective responses to the loss of a significant love object. Individuals may describe feelings of helplessness, loneliness, hopelessness, anger, sadness, and guilt. The frequency and duration of these responses depend upon several factors:

1. Amount of support received from the lost object
2. Degree of ambivalence toward the lost object
3. Anticipatory preparation
4. Extent to which the loss alters life-style
5. Other supportive relationships available to the bereaved

Mourning encompasses the psychological processes or reactions a person uses to assist him or her in overcoming a loss. In the case of the loss of a family member or friend, mourning includes the funeral ritual, the wearing of somber, dark colors, or the draping of purple or black cloth over doorways and windows. As we will discuss later, such rituals permit the survivors to acknowledge the loss of the significant person and to share the loss with others.

Loss can be defined as the relinquishing of objects, status, persons, or functions that are identified as supportive. Loss is very much a part of the life cycle. It is imperative that nurses direct their energies toward helping people respond in a positive manner to the crises caused by loss. Obstacles to mental health generally arise when a person attempts to avoid intense distress and the expression of related emotions.

What does a bereaved person feel or experience? Is there an empathic route a nurse might select that would facilitate a genuine involvement with such a client? John Bowlby (1973) believes that the grieving process is set in motion by a loss or separation that leads to a feeling of emancipation from the lost object. The individual experiences a varying array of feelings, ranging from numbness and anger to healing and resolution. Eric Lindemann (1944), in his extensive studies of grief, has described the grieving process in detail. The process is characterized by (1) somatic distress, including tightness in the throat, an empty feeling, a loss of appetite, and even a lack of muscular power; (2) a sense of unreality—that the loss has not actually occurred; (3) an accompanying sense of purposelessness, as well as an inability to maintain any patterns of organization; (4) feelings of guilt; and (5) feelings of hostility.

Bowlby divides the grieving process into four phases. Each phase is characterized by a predominant form of behavior. The first phase incorporates Bowlby's concept of denial. Individuals experiencing loss cannot believe what has occurred. They respond intellectually and appear to be in control; however, the emotional component is forced into the background. In modern society the emotional aspect is frequently not allowed to surface. Little emphasis is placed on attachment behavior. Rather, stoic behavior is encouraged, particularly on the part of men. After a death crying is considered acceptable in many instances, and it is recognized as a means of asking for support. Yet this aspect of the grieving process may be inadvertently negated as well. We are not able to tolerate the anguish of others; therefore, we cut off the grieving person through such casual statements as "Wasn't he ill for a long time?" or "It's better that she didn't suffer." The grieving person does not often hear "It's all right to feel relieved" or "I can understand you're feeling angry because you are the person who is left." What must nurses possess to intervene in this initial response to loss? The answer lies primarily in themselves. It is the listening ear, the willingness to sit, the ability to share in the intensity of grief.

During the second phase, the bereaved person begins to experience the sensation of the loss itself. The distress symptoms previously described, such as an empty feeling and a sense of helplessness and frustration, are characteristic of this period. It is difficult to speak of the loss without crying. A young woman described her feelings after the death of her father: "It was as though I couldn't even think of him or things we did without bursting out in tears. I would see his face in my mind's eye and just begin to cry, no matter where I was.''

"Rites de passage" provide an atmosphere in which bereaved individuals can share their loss with others. Through the process of a Christian wake or the shiva of Judaism, the family and friends of the deceased person can recount old times together. It is this genuine caring that supports the bereaved through a most crucial period, that of viewing the body and saying good-bye.

Mourning itself begins in the third phase, that of restitution. The ego does not feel whole; it is vulnerable at this point. The bereaved person may demonstrate a lack of concern or consideration for others. It is often difficult to acknowledge the happy times that had been shared with the deceased person or the positive aspects of one's own life. Ambivalence is frequently a part of this phase. On the one hand, there is the belief that the person who has died is at peace. On the other hand, there is a feeling of anger. "Why couldn't I have more time with him? He saw his grandchildren born, but I wanted him to see them graduate from college." There is always more to be wanted.

Catharsis, or talking, particularly in a repetitive fashion, is characteristic of this third, or restitution, phase of grief. Idealization of the deceased person occurs; the bereaved person cannot accept negative aspects of the person who has died. Such negative thoughts are repressed until a future time when they can be dealt with—or they may never be dealt with. There is an identification with the positive traits of the deceased person. In some instances, maladaptive behavior, such as the total introjection of the deceased individual's personality, occurs. Strong guilt feelings are usually the precursor of the process of introjection. In such a situation, the ambivalence, hostility, and intense sadness do not decrease. Instead, bereaved persons are more likely to assume the negative attributes of the dead person than the positive aspects, with little regard for their own sense of self.

Resolution does not occur within any particular time frame. Some theorists believe that 6 to 12 months is a realistic period of time; however, this phase may extend for as long as 2 years. The length of time required depends on the nature of the relationship between the bereaved and the deceased. How does a nurse *know* when a bereaved person is beginning to resolve a loss? There is a feeling of solitude, of renewed investment in other objects and relationships. The person who died is not forgotten but assumes a different yet always special place in the bereaved person's memory. The initial reinvestments may be quite similar to the investment in the lost object or person. Eventually this is no longer the case. Healthy resolution involves the incorporation of some aspects of the dead person into the bereaved person's ego structure, coupled with a drive toward new relationships. A point to remember: even after healthy resolution, significant dates or events, such as birthdays, Christmas, or the anniversary of the death, may precipitate intense feelings of loss.

As a result of healthy coping by means of the mourning process, individuals are able to remember both the pleasures and the disappointments of the lost relationship. The identity of the bereaved individual remains intact for them. They are able to reorganize thoughts and consider new patterns of problem solving. The behavior of the bereaved in this fourth phase is characterized by readiness to move forward, openness to new avenues, and reconciliation with the fact that the loss has occurred.

The four phases occur not only in response to the death of a loved one but also in response to any situation involving loss. As was discussed previously (see Chapter 7), research demonstrates that loss may be a critical precipitating factor in both physical and emotional illness. For example, LeShan (1966) concluded that "the most consistently reported, relevant psychological factor [in the development of neoplasms] has been the loss of a major emotional relationship prior to the first-noted symptoms." Greene (1966) and Bahnson and Bahnson (1966) reported similar findings. Loss of a relationship through divorce, loss through change in job status, loss of a body part or alteration in body function, and loss of a particular life-style as a result of marriage or the birth of a child are examples of changes that may precipitate the grieving process. The response to such a change, however, is often not recognized as grieving. A vague feeling of distress and sadness may occur, as well as somatic symptoms.

A young business executive had been experiencing feelings of lethargy, frustration, and helplessness in his work situation, and he described muscle spasms in his neck and back. A discussion with a nurse revealed that the young man's superior had recently been transferred. He had had a close relationship with the superior and had expanded his role within the company while working for this individual. By identifying the feelings he was experiencing as valid responses to the loss of a relationship and to the possible loss of some of his current responsibilities, the young man was able to accept the feelings as normal. Healthy coping with the loss was facilitated, and the experience could then be integrated into the self as a basis for future coping with loss.

What characterizes a maladaptive response to loss? Should a depressive response to loss be considered normal? A maladaptive response may frequently be characterized as depression, yet such a characterization is not always accurate. Denial may be operating at such an intense level that thoughts and feelings relating to the lost object are repressed. Reality is often rejected as being too painful to cope with. Restlessness, withdrawal, and disorganized patterns of behavior are predominant themes. Disintegration of ego functioning results. Why are some individuals able to make healthy adaptations while others develop depression or physical illnesses? There is no one answer to this question. Nurses must consider the individual as a system that is part of a larger system and that responds to that larger system. It must be remembered that diverse external and internal factors cause each individual to be unique and worthwhile.

Each individual responds to loss in a different manner. The life cycle of individuals is characterized by a series of losses, beginning with the loss of the breast or the bottle. Reactions to loss are based on many factors, including previous experiences with loss, our repertoire of effective coping measures, support relationships, and changes in daily living patterns necessitated by the loss.

The emotions experienced after a loss are quite likely to be the most intense of our lives. Nurses, however, do not always recognize that clients are frequently responding to loss situations. Nurses do not readily view illness as a loss situation, even though clients routinely lose the ability to function in their own environments, to wear their own clothing, and to determine their own schedules. Depression occurs as a result of such loss, but this behavioral response often goes unrecognized.

Loss of a significant object, relationship, status, or the like is a common human experience. Depression in its mildest form is a natural response to loss. In the following sections depression will be defined as it relates to the DMS-III category "Major affective disorders," and predominant themes, underlying dynamics, and intervention will be discussed.

DEPRESSION

"I'm depressed." How many times have you heard this statement? When you cannot find a solution to a frustrating situation, do you sit down with head in hands and stare at your toes? Things are just not working out well. Is this clinical depression? What is the difference between feeling low and overwhelming sensations of helplessness, anger, anxiety, and self-doubt? The human personality is dynamic; it constantly reflects the many changes that occur at its interfaces with the environment. Thus, depression, as one form of human coping response, cannot be pigeonholed.

During the past two decades depression, along with anxiety, has become one of the most prevalent disease entities. Interest in depressive states has also increased, perhaps as a result of increased coverage by the mass media of mental health in general. It has been widely publicized that significant persons in drama, art, and the professions have experienced depressive responses and have recovered—in the fullest sense of the word. There have been major new approaches to the treatment of depression, such as transactional analysis, family therapy, and milieu groups. Depression in some shape or form affects millions of people each year. According to Secunda (1973), 15% of the population of the United States between 18 and 74 suffers from significant depressive symptoms; only half of these people seek help. In a sense, depression occurs as frequently as the common cold. Some people develop depressive symptoms as an adaptive response, while other people respond through the autonomic nervous system. Still others are able to cope effectively. As has been mentioned previously, it is important that nurses realize that many variables may act to produce a depressive response. Intervention can then be directed toward identification of behavior that is indicative of a response to loss.

Phases of depression

For purposes of discussion, depression can be thought of in terms of three arbitrarily defined phases: depressive affect, mood disorder, and clinical depression.

Phases of depression

Mild (affect)	Moderate (mood disorder)	Severe (clinical syndrome)
- - - - →		- - - - - - - - - →

A depressive affect is characterized by feelings of sadness, dejection, and disappointment. Such feelings are transitory, usually being relieved within a period of 4 to 6 weeks. These feelings are related to the here-and-now and do not impair the everyday functioning of an individual. These "low" periods in the life cycle are related to a loss of some kind, such as a change in job status or function. The intensity of these transitory feelings can be correlated with the intensity of the grief response.

If this response continues and becomes distorted, other changes occur. A mood disorder is characterized by more intense feelings of self-doubt and dejection. A cluster of behavioral

changes occurs. Bodily function slows to a bare minimum. Great effort is required to accomplish everyday activities. A person becomes less kempt, and household tasks are often not completed. (In some instances, however, the opposite occurs. Obsessional impulses lead to continuous housecleaning and to other seemingly purposeless activities.) Eating habits change. Some individuals may drink and eat very little and therefore lose weight. Others eat very heavily, perhaps as a means of making up for the loss. Again, depending upon the individual, constipation or diarrhea may be present. Weakness and fatigue are common. Clients describe feelings of "aching all over" and joint weakness (Anthony and Benedeck, 1975).

Judy, a 25-year-old woman, came into a 24-hour emergency walk-in clinic at a large, urban hospital. She described herself as being a generally happy person; but during the past two weeks she had become increasingly dejected. She awoke early in the morning and was unable to fall back to sleep. Everyday activities became monumental tasks. She felt as though her whole body had come to a halt. Relationships with other people in her environment were also being affected. She no longer wanted to participate in social gatherings. She often found herself sitting alone, pondering her fate in life. She was prompted to come to the clinic by a co-worker who was concerned by her change in personality.

After several sessions at the clinic, Judy acknowledged that she had lost her mother a year ago. She had been coping "well" until recently, when she lost her cat. When discussing the two loss experiences, she said, "I never really cried it all out when Mom died." But the loss of the cat triggered the revival of the past loss. Judy began to experience again the angry and helpless feelings she had experienced when her mother died. These feelings had been repressed, only to surface later. Loss is one of the cornerstones of the dynamics of depression. Judy, in this hypothetical case history, not only felt the loss of her mother but also saw herself as no longer being important to anyone. These two factors acted as the foundation for the development of her depressive response.

The communication patterns of a person tend to be limited as he or she becomes more depressed. Most interactions with others are filled with self-deprecatory statements. A rigid, stereotypical pattern of responding to others develops. Feelings of low self-esteem manifest themselves: clients believe that they are incapable of succeeding. They believe that failures in life result from personal inadequacy, no matter what the circumstances might be. When this fact is pointed out to them, they hold fast to the belief that they, and they alone, are responsible. As in Judy's case, social interactions are diminished. The sense of low self-esteem becomes so strong that these clients believe that no one thinks much of them. The pattern then becomes cyclical. The clients isolate themselves, discouraging anyone from approaching them. Others perceive them as being cold, uncaring, even hostile. In their depressed state, these individuals are unable to perceive other people's needs. Energy is directed inward toward their own needs. Isolation continues to increase. They find themselves believing even less in their own worth; they believe that no one could possibly take an interest in them. Low self-esteem increases as isolation increases. A primary goal for nurses is to intervene in this cyclical pattern of interaction. Later in this chapter specific aspects of nursing intervention and rationale will be discussed.

The increasing symptomatology may reflect what had previously been termed a reactive depression. Historically, a reactive depression seemed to involve a precipitant. In contrast, severe depression was referred to as endogenous or psychotic depression. Severe depression, the last of the three major types of depressive responses, was also known as clinical depression. Many variables—psychological, chemical, genetic, familial—may singly or in any combination contribute to a depressive response. Hopelessness, powerlessness, and worthlessness are predominant themes. Individuals perceive reality in a grossly distorted fashion. Delusions and hallucinations occur. Feelings of low self-esteem are reinforced by the delusions. Individuals become trapped in the tangled web of a delusional system, unable to sift fact from fantasy. They form a shell to protect themselves as they retreat farther into isolation. Tasks of everyday living are perceived as overwhelming. All available energy is channeled into a hate campaign against the self. Concentration narrows; problem-solving capabilities are poor at best. Individuals often do not react to environmental stimuli. If they do react, it is in an inappropriate fashion. There is a marked decrease in bodily functioning and a vegetative state ensues. (As stated previously, the opposite may also occur— that is, agitated, purposeless, stereotypic behavior.) One of the primary characteristics of severe depression is its diurnal nature. Individuals awaken early in the morning, usually preoccupied with unpleasant thoughts. As the day progresses, the depressive pattern tends to lift. An overall assessment of severely depressed individuals reveals persons who perceive themselves as worthless; their movements and slouching posture reflect the low regard in which they hold themselves. (These characteristics will be discussed at greater length later in this chapter.)

In DSM-III, depressive episodes as well as manic episodes are categorized as major affective disorders. The disorders are divided into two groups: major depression and bipolar disorders. Major depression includes simple episodes or a recurrent process exclusive of manic episodes. Bipolar disorders include both depressive and manic episodes; the manic episodes are either single or multiple. Depression may or may not accompany the mania. This category of major affective disorders is further subdivided to reflect the status of the current episode—manic, depressed, or mixed. DSM-III describes each category as a distinct clinical entity.

It is interesting to note that in the past, the terms endogenous and exogenous were used to define depression. It was thought that endogenous depressions—those that seemed to be physiologically based—responded best to drug treatment. Exogenous depressions—those externally precipitated by loss, and/or other stresses—were thought to respond best to psychotherapy. Those categories are no longer appropriate and may, in fact, hinder comprehensive assessment and intervention. For example, stresses such as marital difficulties may result from, rather than precede, depression. If nurses are to consider the whole individual, the distinction between external and internal contributory factors is antithetical to that consideration. An understanding of the interrelationship of factors respects the holistic nature of individuals. Therefore, this description of depression is no longer adequate.

Manic depression

The manic-depressive reaction has become one of the most widely discussed depressive responses in Western society. It is characterized by mood swings; a manic-depressive person's moods range from profound depression to extreme euphoria, with periods of normalcy in between. It is important to point out that mania is considered to be the mirror image of depression. The psychoanalytic viewpoint suggests that mania is a defense against depression. DSM-III, however, notes that mania may be present as a bipolar disorder with no depressive symptoms.

Various theories regarding the development of the manic-depressive response have been proposed. Familial and genetic studies by Kallman (1953) indicate that genetic predisposition may be involved. Kolb (1977) suggests that a dominant X-linked factor accounts for the presence of manic depression in families whose members have had manic and/or depressive disorders. He notes that manic depression occurs twice as frequently in females as in males and that maternal relatives of a manic-depressive person are affected much more frequently than paternal relatives.

The roles of norepinephrine and the catecholamines in the origin of the depressive response will be discussed later in this chapter. Lowered levels of norepinephrine are apparent in a person experiencing a depressive response, and the converse is true in a manic response. Lowered intracellular sodium levels are also common during a manic response. We will discuss the implications of sodium levels further in the section on psychopharmaceuticals that appears later in this chapter.

The predominant themes in manic depression are similar to those encountered in the depressive response. Clients in the manic phase are outgoing; they easily involve themselves in relationships with others. They can be quite manipulative and controlling if a situation is not satisfactory in terms of their own interests. In order to feel important, they often attack the worth of others. Manic-depressive persons are unsure of their own worth. Nurses need to be eclectic in their approach to a manic-depressive client; their primary concern is to identify predominant themes and appropriate forms of intervention.

The mother-infant relationship and its impact on the development of the depressive response has been discussed previously. This factor plays a significant role in the dynamics of manic depression. The early dependence of the infant on the mother is pleasurable for the mother. However, as the child becomes autonomous, he or she begins to pose a threat to the mother figure. If the child is thwarted and labeled as bad each time he or she asserts independence, the child learns that in order to survive he or she must fulfill parental expectations, no matter what the price. The child then continually strives to gain parental affection by complying with each request, negating his or her own needs and wishes. Ambivalent feelings arise, as the child resents the mother while at the same time strongly desiring her attention. The following is an operational definition of manic depression:

Ambivalent feelings towards love object	→	Ego gives up	→	Punitive super-ego anger turned inward	*or*	Strong id ↓ Uncontrollable impulsive behavior

Such a child suffers from low self-esteem and the resulting inability to actively problem solve to meet his or her own needs. Since the parent-child relationship had been fraught with unreasonable demands, the child in later life is unable to experience a trusting relationship. The possibility of open, free lines of communication between self and others is never considered. Satir, in her book *Peoplemaking* (1972), points out that direct, honest communication among family members is necessary in order for positive feelings about oneself and one's capabilities to develop.

What are the onset and general course of manic depression? Can nurses be alert to clues in the environment? Published reports indicate that manic episodes usually occur in persons between the ages of 20 and 35 and that depressive episodes usually occur in persons between the ages of 35 and 50. Cyclothymia, hypomania, and depressive behavior are usually characteristic of the premorbid personality. The cyclothymic personality is characterized by alternating periods of high and low spirits (Fieve, 1975).

Manic-depressive behavior manifests itself in varying degrees. Responses can be entirely of one form—for example, all manic behavior. Responses may alternate with one another. For example, a first episode may be circular, a second depressive, and a third mainly manic. Following each attack, individuals return to their premorbid state; in some instances their condition is improved. This may be seen as flight into reality. An interesting point is the fact that the onset of mania is not necessarily linked directly to any precipitating event.

Manic-depressive behavior can be divided into three general categories or phases: manic, depressive, and circular.

The first category, mania, can be divided into hypomania and acute mania. Hypomanic behavior is characterized primarily by elation. The affected individuals are well liked by others; they are outgoing and often identified as the life of the party. Their energies seem boundless, and others often marvel at how much they can accomplish. Their behavior at this point is purposeful and goal oriented. But as the mood of elation increases, these clients become more grandiose in their responses to others. No task is beyond accomplishment. They allude to their personal achievements and capitalize on each opportunity to increase other people's awareness of them. Logic and rational thought processes are not always operational, although these individuals may seem to be in command of their faculties. Hypomanic clients frequently engage in projects requiring large sums of money that are rarely seen to fruition. The spending of money is no object (Dunner, Fleiss, and Fieve, 1976).

Mary K., a 34-year-old mother of three children, was admitted to a small, private psychiatric hospital. On admission, she was in a state of such hyperactivity that it required four people to assist her to her room. She was extremely hostile and was lashing out at all around her. Her husband described her as having progressed from being quite vigorous in her approach to tasks to being so aggressive in her actions that he could not control her. She had decided to build an addition to their house and had contacted four contractors. She had then ordered building supplies amounting to a total cost of $4,000. Flitting to another project, she had taken the children shopping to buy clothes for camp and in one afternoon had spent more than $5,000. It was at this point that her husband sought psychiatric help.

As the mood continues to escalate, attention span shortens. Clients speak rapidly yet coherently or write voluminous notes. Hypomanic clients have a great penchant for collecting items. They may save anything from bottle caps or old rags to scraps of paper. These collectibles may be hidden in body orifices, particularly the vagina and the anus. Nurses must be acutely aware of such a client's need to have these items. Intervention should include saving the items and, if need be, assisting clients to find alternative caches for them.

Creativity is a primary theme in the hypomanic phase. Designs are drawn in a large, bold hand.

There is much underlining for emphasis of pertinent points. It is obvious that the drawings correlate with the person's expansiveness.

Court (1972) notes that as clients move into the acute phase of mania, activity is accelerated to an even greater degree. Thought processes are characterized by flight of ideas; sentences are often incomplete, and pressured speech is common. It is difficult to engage in an interaction. This stream of verbiage often has at its base a central theme relevant to the client's needs—a theme that can be identified by a careful listener.

Motor activity increases to the point that clients spend most of their time in a constant flurry of motion. They involve themselves in everyone else's interactions and become quite irritating to other people. They often have suggestions about how this or that activity should be conducted. They may interfere in the personal lives of others, often giving advice. They have little time to sleep, eat, or groom themselves, and activity leads to physical exhaustion. However, there is little increase in sexual activity. Indiscreet sexual acts may occur, however, and the use of profanity may increase.

Inappropriate dress is quite common. Manic clients use heavy make-up, resembling that of a clown. Brightly colored baubles and beads accentuate every outfit. Clothing is usually mismatched and poorly fitting; often it is not appropriate to the climate. This type of behavior is observed in both men and women.

Ultimately, the acute manic phase may lead to complete physical and emotional exhaustion.

The most severe form of mania, delirious mania, is not frequently seen. Clients in this phase exhibit hallucinations and delusions, and may be dangerous to themselves and others. Activity is purposeless and continuous. Speech is accelerated to such a degree that thoughts are presented incoherently.

The second category of manic-depressive behavior—the depressive response—has already been discussed at length. It is important to note that one of the major clinical problems of the depressive phase of manic depression is the possibility of suicide, which will be the focus of discussion later in this chapter.

The third category of manic-depressive behavior is the circular response, which is characterized by alternating periods of manic and depressive behavior. Clients experience a period of manic behavior, followed by a period of "euthymia," or normal mood responses. This period may then be followed by depressive behavior. Clients are usually in a well-defined manic, depressive, or euthymic period. These recurrent periods or episodes may be separated by months to years of remission. It has been found that the longer the time between episodes, the smaller the chance that they will recur. Is it possible to experience a continuous series of mood swings? In some unusual instances, this has occurred, but it is not the common pattern.

In summary, there are both similarities and differences between manic depression and other types of depression. The influences of childhood on later life are significant in the understanding of any depressive state. Manic clients are often "the life of the party" or those who have the energy to accomplish everything. But is this pattern of response being used to escape from reality? Is the pain of loss so great? As in depression, a diminished sense of worth, a loss of dependence, and a fear of not being loved can be noted. Yet these feelings are hidden beneath a mask of pseudohappiness. Relationships are characterized by superficiality; manic-depressive persons manipulate their environments in order to continually receive the gratification and support they need. When anxiety increases, however, the mask no longer serves as an effective coping response. Individuals then turn to either the elative or the depressive response to preserve ego integrity.

AGE DETERMINANTS

Childhood

Spitz and Wold (1946) and Bowlby (1973) each suggest that the early mother-child relationship plays a critical role in a child's response to separation and loss. Separation anxiety occurs in the child prior to the establishment of object permanence. Inadequate preparation for separation can be stressful for the child and can ultimately lead to depression. Characteristics of prepubertal depression include school phobia and fear of loss of parents through death, along with feelings of sadness and dejection, as in adult depression. (See Chapter 15 for further discussion.)

Adolescence

Adolescence has been described as "initiation into mourning." An adolescent loses childhood and the dependent state that characterizes it; the implicit message is that he or she must grow up. Often the "all or nothing" principle operates in the development of independence. The adolescent believes that he or she must achieve independence immediately rather than accomplish it gradually over a period of time. Depression may result from a fear of failure—the fear of not being able to live up to the concept of self he or she has defined. Depression in an adolescent may resemble adult depression; however, a depressed adolescent frequently behaves impulsively, taking action against the environment. Restlessness, apathy, sulkiness, social isolation, grouchiness, and aggression characterize the depressed adolescent. His or her inability to gain approval or understanding may lead to feelings of rejection and to self-deprecation. He may then seek to run away to cope with feelings of inadequacy. Loss or lack of a significant other or a meaningful relationship often precipitates a depressive reaction. Suicide is the second leading cause of death among adolescents. The suicidal impulse may take the form of accident-prone behavior. Depression in adolescents, in whatever form it takes, needs to be recognized and assessed in order for appropriate nursing responses to be determined. (See Chapter 15 for further discussion.)

Old age

Changes in mood and affect are behaviors found in the elderly just as in other age groups. In this population, loss may occur more frequently, yet generalizations about reactions are inappropriate. Elderly people's responses to altered physical abilities, psychological loss, and changes in environment are influenced by the availability of support systems, previous coping styles, and current physical and physiological assets. Sudden changes in mood may indicate a decrease in the individual's ability to cope with current situations or may reflect physiological changes. Assessment of individuals who were content and well adjusted may reveal physiological factors as responsible for most alteration. Nursing intervention is directed towards alleviating anxiety by providing accurate information and responding to and correcting, if possible, those physiological alterations.

As in other groups, an extended grief response needs to be addressed as a depressive response. Symptoms indicative of depression that are not attributable to advanced age include: decrease in usual interaction with significant others and families, excessive fatigue, anorexia, and general apathy. A thorough understanding of these changes must include a recognition of the elderly person's response to the process of aging and to the prospect of dying and death. As this prospect becomes closer, elderly individuals may feel helpless and hopeless. A sense of social isolation follows; emotional investment in others may become increasingly difficult. This isolation may either precipitate or stem from a depression. Thus, it may be easy to assume that depression is a part of aging and allow it to go unnoticed or untreated. In some instances, medications such as tranquilizers and cardiotonics tend to enhance the depressive response.

Depressed elderly persons may express their feelings through overt angry responses or through physical behaviors. Feelings of confusion, paranoia, and memory loss may serve to compound their depressed behavior by further distancing them from others.

In an elderly person preoccupation with physical health may be present in conjunction with depression. The sense of self is vulnerable to the effects of both physical and emotional deterioration. Regression into the sick role requires that others respond in a concerned manner that, in turn, positively reinforces the self as being worthwhile and deserving. Nurses may respond to angry outbursts or episodes of hypochondriasis in a negative manner without consideration for their meaning in the larger context—that of a need for validation and support as individuals.

Suicide in the elderly is on the rise. It has been noted by Atchley (1980) that 25% of all suicides are in the over-65 age group. At particular risk are individuals who are socially isolated, individuals with changes in physical functioning that limit independence, and individuals who are terminally ill. The literature describes passive mechanisms of suicide or intentional death among the elderly. Examples of ''passive'' suicide include: lack of compliance with treatment or medication regimens that are life-sustaining; misuse of drugs—prescribed as well as others; refusal to eat; and engagement in activities or behaviors that increase risk to life.

In summary, depression cannot and should not be taken for granted in the elderly; all elderly individuals are not depressed. Accurate assessment of client strengths, coping abilities, support systems, and current physical and emotional capabilities is necessary in order to design and implement strategies of intervention.

SUICIDE

Suicide is the ultimate response to hopelessness, helplessness, and low self-esteem. It is the final escape from reality. For individuals who consider suicide, life has become so intolerable that previous mechanisms of dealing with stress are inadequate.

It is difficult to consider the possibility of ending one's life. It is also difficult to understand the dy-

namics of self-destructive behavior. Nurses who work with clients who have attempted suicide must understand their own feelings about and responses to such an individual. A relationship with a suicidal client can have a profound impact on a nurse. Health professionals devote much time and energy to the preservation of life. How can a nurse relate to a person who constantly deprecates himself or herself, finds no happiness in living, and simply wishes to die? Working with such a client is a frustrating, anxiety-provoking, discouraging experience. The client's negative perceptions may lead to negative responses by the nurse. A pattern may emerge in the interaction that increases the client's feelings of worthlessness.

In the past decade the trend toward the study of suicide (suicidology) and the development of suicide prevention centers and hot lines has been growing. The National Institute for Mental Health's Center for Studies of Suicide Prevention directs its efforts toward increasing the scope and amount of research being done in the areas of assessment of clues to suicidal behavior and the etiological factors in suicide. Suicidal behavior has many sources—biological, psychological, and sociocultural. A nursing care plan should incorporate all of these factors. An integrated concept of depression, and of suicide as a possible outcome of depression, is essential to the assessment process.

Freud believed that the instinct for life (Eros) and the instinct for death (Thanatos) exist in every human being. Self-destructive behavior results in hatred toward an internalized lost object. There is marked ambivalence, however, in a suicidal person. If the hatred becomes overwhelming, individuals literally have no choice but to kill themselves. Freud correlated suicide with the death instinct: Thanatos turned inward may cause individuals to take their lives.

Durkheim's (1951) sociological theory has been one of the fundamental constructs of suicide theory. He presents three basic forms of annihilative behavior: egoistic (finding life unappealing and killing oneself), altruistic (that which is demanded by society), and anomic (that which results from no longer feeling ties to the environment). This last form of behavior is engaged in by a person who feels powerless and alienated in a society that no longer has firm ground rules or structure.

Menninger, in his book *Man Against Himself* (1938), describes three basic components of the suicidal personality: the wish to kill (aggression), the wish to be killed (submission), and the wish to die (self-punishment). These components can be seen in overt acts or in the guise of addiction, frigidity, antisocial behavior, impotence, or a tendency to have serious accidents.

Schneidman and Farberow (1957) group individuals who attempt suicide into four general categories: those who commit suicide as a means of saving their reputations; those who regard suicide as a release—for example, the old and the chronically ill; those who commit suicide in response to hallucinations and/or delusions; and those who wish to hurt others in their environment.

Loss of self-worth and resulting helplessness and hopelessness are critical factors in the precipitation of suicidal behavior. Suicidal people perceive themselves as failures in every aspect of their lives. They place little or no value on their own existence. They seemingly have no hope for the future.

Wetzel (1976) points out that hopelessness, rather than depression, is positively correlated with suicidal intent. Wetzel found that when suicidal clients exhibited decreased hopelessness, depressive responses were no longer significant in the assessment of suicidal intent. Conversely, when depression was controlled but hopelessness continued to be a predominant theme, suicidal intent was high.

Attempts have been noted in the nursing literature to predict suicide and attempted suicide. Capodanno and Targum (1983) establish guidelines, similar to those of Hatton et al. (1977), that identify a set of potential predictor variables that may improve prediction of risk. They also note that the relatively low incidence of suicide makes it difficult to obtain pre-suicide data. The following are attributes of suicidal behavior that can be further developed by scale construction to improve prediction:

1. Perception of social environment as alien and hostile
   a. Significant others
   b. General environment
2. Hopelessness
3. Previous attempts
4. Family history
5. Biological markers
   a. Dexamethasone suppression test
   b. Reduced platelet MAO
   c. Elevated urinary cortisol levels

Papa's (1980) study on predictors of suicidal behavior contributes relevant information for nursing assessment. She considers the complex interaction of predictor variables such as hopelessness; locus of control; preference for inclusion, control, and affection; and stress from life events in relation to degree of suicidal intent. The focus is no longer on a single variable as a precipitating factor but on a relationship among or between variables. Two conclusions are noteworthy: that hopelessness and preference for affection are significantly related to suicidal intent; and that there are significant correlations between locus of control and hopelessness and between preference for affection and hopelessness. Papa indicates that the series of life events or the ''life process'' is such that individuals ultimately reach a point where there is an end to hope and suicide is the mechanism of resolution. In fact there is no one precipitating factor but rather a series of life events which may originate in childhood and continue throughout life. Nursing should consider the interrelationships of these variables in order to formulate more accurate assessment tools and to provide appropriate treatment for this population.

Demographic data

The suicide rate is highest among white males who have never been married. Divorced and widowed people have the next highest rate. The suicide rate increases with age. For women, however, the rate peaks at approximately age 55. There seems to be virtually no suicide among young children, although there is increasing evidence that accident-prone children may in fact be experiencing feelings of rage and helplessness. During adolescence the rate becomes markedly higher; suicide is the second leading cause of death among college students. Linden (1976) states that in the general population three times more males than females *commit* suicide but that females *attempt* suicide more frequently than males. Linden also points out that, generally, married people have the lowest suicide rates.

Although Linden states that suicide occurs predominantly among whites, there is evidence that suicide is increasing among blacks, particularly males. Farberow (1975) suggests that a history of rejection and abandonment in early mother-child relationships is often present in urban families. Abandonment may be a result of socioeconomic factors such as little or no income, poor shelter and clothing, and no means of support. In addition, feelings of low self-esteem may develop out of a continuing inability to meet one's most basic needs. A shortage of trusting relationships and feelings of hopelessness and alienation also serve as precursors to a suicidal act.

Familial determinants

Richman (1971) has identified several characteristics of families with suicidal problems: family fragility, family depression, intolerance for separation, symbiosis without empathy, closed family relationships, scapegoating, poor patterns of dealing with aggression, double-bind communicating, and inflexibility in responding to crisis. Since the family network has profound effects on a person's integrative functioning, it plays an important role in the development of any maladaptive response. But the role of the family is especially important in the case of a suicidal client. Oftentimes, it is a perceptive family that identifies clues to impending suicidal acts.

Sociocultural and spiritual context

American society is composed of various ethnic groups and subcultures. Each person is a unique being whose behavior reflects the environment from which he comes as well as biological and psychological factors. In this section the attitudes toward suicide held by several ethnic or cultural groups are discussed.

NAVAJO INDIANS

Suicide is not acceptable to the Navajo tribe, not because it is thought to be inherently bad, but because of its effect on the members of the family.

Webb and Willard, in Farberow's *Suicide in Different Cultures* (1975), point out the Navajo's belief that any death other than that resulting from old age is unnatural. A violent death is certain to bring misfortune to the family of the person who died. The usual precipitating event in suicide is bad feelings among kin; frequently, a person who commits suicide does so near his or her own residence and contaminates the family with a ghost. An intense fear of ghosts is an important element in the Navajo attitude toward suicide. Navajos believe that the dead person does not leave the situation but merely takes a new status—that of ghost. The Navajo's fear of the dead, coupled with their attitude toward violent death, clearly makes suicide unacceptable.

Suicidal behavior is found among the Navajo most frequently in men between the ages of 25 and 39. Use of alcohol is often noted as a variable.

Santora and Starkey (1982) note the impact of sociocultural, spiritual, and intrapsychic variables on suicidal behavior. Several tribes were studied and data revealed that victims were most typically young, single men who were in conflict with values, work, or significant others. The authors also note that little is known about the motives of the victims.

It is important to understand sociocultural variables. There is increasing conflict between values of the traditional cultures and the Anglo culture. There is a need on the one hand to integrate into the larger society while at the same time maintaining and preserving a distinct culture. This vacillation may serve as the basis for identity crisis, anomie, and social isolation—and ultimately, suicide.

SCANDINAVIAN-AMERICANS

Scandinavian-Americans, proud of their Viking heritage, do not look favorably on suicide. To kill oneself is a sign of weakness and an inability to cope with life's stresses. Survival of the fittest was a predominant theme among the Vikings, as was the idealization of the physically strong.

Scandinavian-Americans also carry with them the belief that suicide is a sin that cloaks the entire family with shame. Early Christian doctrine forbade the Church to give a eulogy for a person who committed suicide or sprinkle the traditional earth on the coffin.

Petterstol (in Faberow, 1975) sees a change of direction in Scandinavian-American attitudes toward suicide. There is still great concern for physical health, vigor, and life. However, there also is a more empathic attitude toward persons who have attempted suicide and toward the survivors of persons who commit suicide. The survivors themselves are ashamed and unsure of how they should respond to others. There are still strong taboos against taking one's own life.

ITALIAN-AMERICANS

For Italian-Americans, suicide is regarded as a grave sin; this belief is rooted in Catholic dogma. The family of an individual who commits suicide is dishonored; the avenues to certain occupations are closed to his or her survivors, and the body cannot be buried in consecrated ground. This attitude is so strong that physicians and members of the clergy will falsify death certificates. For example, mental illness might be listed as the cause of death, for this is acceptable to the Church.

According to Farberow (1975), an understanding of the family is of utmost importance to an understanding of the dynamics of suicide among Italian-Americans. The family is the primary support system. Individuals are encouraged to depend on others in their family constellation; the family provides nurturing in the form of love, help, and protection. With such a constant support system it may be difficult for individuals to feel worthless. Italian-Americans believe that each individual should be accountable for the welfare of others. Although the family is a support system, it often places great demands on its members. Since the family provides nurturance, it may also attach strings. Feelings of rage and helplessness may arise, leading to overt conflict and, in some instances, suicide.

Italian-Americans exemplify the characteristic ambivalence of persons who are considering suicide as a way of relieving overwhelming stress. Their ambivalence results from the strong doctrine of the Church and from an inability to escape the intricately woven net of family and Church. Members of third, fourth, and successive generations of Italian-Americans may no longer feel as constrained by Catholic dogma. Their concern for life, however, remains strong.

• • •

The people of the Orient do not normally disapprove of suicide. Suttee, or the suicide of a widow after her husband's death, was quite common in India until the last century. It was taught that this death would be a passport to heaven, would atone for any sins of the husband, and would even give distinction to the remaining family members. It must be noted that some aspects of Hindu philosophy encourage suicide for religious reasons. In China suicide is regarded as acceptable as a means of revenge because it not only embarrasses the enemy but permits the dead man to haunt him from the spirit world. Voluntary death has also been given a place of honor in Buddhist countries.

Suicide has been held in positive regard amongst all classes in Japan. Hara-Kiri, a ceremonial form of suicide, was taught as a means to avoid capture as well as to avoid disgrace and punishment in order to preserve one's honor. The suicide pact of lovers who choose to end their lives in this world and to go on to another is also not unusual.

Clinard (1974) states that the attitudes of Western European peoples toward suicide originated primarily in the philosophies of the Jewish and Christian religions. The Talmudic law looks upon suicide unfavorably and condemns the individual yet believes that comfort should be provided to the family. The Christian position against suicide has its roots in the beliefs that human life is sacred; individuals do not have the right to usurp God's authority and take their own lives; and that death is an entrance into a new life in which behavior in the old is important. The concept of life after death had a strengthening effect on the church's position against suicide.

Interestingly, early Christian teachings sanctioned suicide when it was connected either with martyrdom or protection of virginity. However, it was eventually disapproved for any reason and became a crime.

Throughout the Middle Ages, suicide was denounced. Augustine stated that suicide precluded repentance, and Thomas Aquinas maintained that it was unnatural and an offense against the community. Special treatment was provided for bodies of suicides—often they were not permitted in traditional graveyards. In some instances, the bodies were hung from gallows, burned, or thrown into the sewer.

During the Age of Enlightment, the belief that individuals should not transcend God's authority and take their own lives was challenged. David Hume, Montesquieu, Voltaire, and Rousseau spoke of the importance of choice, even on the issue of life and death. If one does not have control over all aspects of life, then who should?

At the present time both Catholics and Protestants oppose suicide; however, increasing consideration is being shown for individuals within the context of their lives and their motivations to commit suicide, and condemnation is decreasing.

Suicide as an act generates many questions for the care giver as well as for the client. One must confront one's own personal beliefs about suicide as a choice as well as about individual and societal responsibility.

EPIDEMIOLOGY

Are some people more prone to depression than others? If so, do these individuals have similar characteristics? Persons most likely to be depressed can be described as shy, perhaps oversensitive, self-conscious, and worriers. Reaching a level of perfection is their ultimate goal. The results of not achieving this end are self-deprecation and self-doubt—primary characteristics of depressed persons.

Statistics indicate that depression occurs more frequently in females than in males. However, this may not be an accurate assessment. The overt expression of depression by males is frequently frowned upon. Statistics also show that the incidence of depression increases with age in both men and women. Depression cuts across social classes. Neurotic depression, however, may be more common in the middle and upper classes, while psychotic depression may be more common in the lower class. To understand the prevalence of depression, nurses must consider socioeconomic factors, availability of mental health services, the attitude of each class toward mental health, and at what point treatment is sought.

General practitioners frequently treat depression either as a primary symptom or as a symptom that is secondary to a physical illness. According to Kolb (1977), less than 5% of persons who experience depression seek psychiatric care.

Depression affects all age groups, from childhood through senescence. Individuals may be born with a predisposition to depression; however, susceptibility to depression also depends on the many factors noted previously—familial, genetic, biological, and chemical—and on early life experiences.

THEORIES OF DEPRESSION

Psychoanalytic theory

Proponents of the psychoanalytic theory of depression believe that a depressive response has at its roots a significant loss, either real or imagined. Anger resulting from the loss is turned inward, and self-hate results. The original loss is repressed; however, subsequent losses reactivate the feelings associated with it. Freud, in "Mourning and Melancholia" (1917), postulates that the characteristics of the normal grieving process are similar to those of the pathological state of depression. Unlike individuals experiencing normal grief, however, those experiencing depression seem to be grieving over an inner loss that they are unable to resolve. It is this unresolved grief that depressed individuals carry with them.

Freud states that the initial lost love object is the parent. Individuals simultaneously feel both love and hate for the parent, yet it is the hatred that is incorporated or symbolically introjected into the self. The psychic mechanism of introjection serves as a basis for the development of the superego. For individuals who later suffer from pathological depression, the embryonic superego is punitive in that it never permits the acceptance of praise. Individuals never learn to value their own sense of self, a situation that is carried on throughout the life cycle.

The psychoanalytic literature suggests that such individuals' self-derogatory behavior is a sign that hostility toward the lost object has been internalized. They then become narcissistic. They believe that no one else cares enough about them to take care of their needs; therefore, they must care for themselves. By not becoming involved in any relationship, depressed individuals limit the social failures they might experience. Strong dependence needs become apparent. It is literally impossible to meet the needs of such persons; they never seem to be fulfilled. A cyclical pattern develops: Dependent individuals are disappointed in their attempts to gain recognition. They pull back from relationships in order to save face while at the same time chastising themselves for being so inadequate. The depressive response is adopted and promoted.

Melanie Klein (1934) suggests that the depressive response can be traced to the early mother-infant relationship. Feelings of rage and hostility characterize the infant's response to a lack of gratification of needs. A weakened ego state results; feelings of helplessness, sadness, and dejection arise as a result of tension between ego and superego. The introjective mechanism acts to internalize the persecutor. Klein points out that children need to feel fully assured that parental love is genuine. Without this assurance, sadness, dejection, lack of self-esteem, and a sense of loss result.

Rene Spitz and K.M. Wold (1946) and John Bowlby (1973) believe that the origins of depression can be found in the infant's responses to experiences of separation and loss. This "object loss theory," as it is commonly referred to, suggests that trauma results when separation from significant others occurs. Spitz and Wold, in their studies of mother-infant responses, point out a particular pattern of behavior that occurs following separation. (It is important to note that these authors argue that for the first 6 months of life a mother-infant relationship exists but that during the second 6 months of life the relationship is gradually severed.) Spitz and Wold describe infants reacting to separation as being withdrawn, stuporous, and anorectic; showing psychomotor retardation; and experiencing overall slowing of the normal growth and development process. They call this cluster of symptoms "anaclitic depression." Bowlby identifies similar patterns of response in older children. He proposes three phases:

1. Protest—crying, looking for mother
2. Despair—withdrawal from environment, apathy
3. Detachment—total lack of investment in any mothering figure

Bibring (1953), although psychoanalytically oriented, differs from other psychoanalytic theorists in his perception of the dynamics of depression. He suggests that depression is characterized primarily by a loss of self-esteem. This loss can be stimulated by inadequate fulfillment of needs for affection as well as by frustration of significant hopes and desires. Bibring's primary thesis is based on the assumption that all depressive reactions have one aspect in common—a sense of loss. He attributes much of the basis of depression to trauma during the oral phase. Bibring also postulates that attacks of the ego that result in feelings of loss can occur in any developmental phase. We know, for example, that during the toddler phase, children direct their energies toward increasing their mobility. Bibring believes that the inability to accomplish this task is viewed by the toddler as a personal failure, a loss. Nurses thus need to be alert to potential loss situations in any developmental phase. Primary prevention then can begin to make strides forward.

Cognitive theory

Cognitive theorists suggest that analysis of the depressive response too often becomes tangled in the web of the psyche. They point out that Freud's concept of hatred directed toward the introjected lost love object is difficult, if not impossible, to validate and that it seems to involve no actual connection between theoretical constructs and observable behavior.

Beck (1967) ascribes causal significance to illogical thinking processes. He believes that illogical thought patterns operate solely in relation to the self. These patterns generate self-doubt and self-deprecation. In essence, a person's thought processes determine his or her emotional reactions. Beck identifies a "primary triad" in depression—three major cognitive patterns that force individuals to view themselves, their environment, and their future in a negativistic manner.

First, individuals perceive themselves as unworthy and inadequate; they believe they are failures. They attribute their failures to some nebulous flaw, whether physical, emotional, or moral. Rejection of self occurs as a result of these perceptions.

Second, they view their interactions with the social world as being poor at best. They are particularly sensitive to any barriers placed in the way of the attainment of goals. Difficulties of any degree are interpreted as indicating total inadequacy on their part. (Depressed persons are programmed to respond with a sense of failure. A mildly depressed nursing student, for example, did poorly on one out of ten quizzes. She looked on this one quiz grade as an indication of total failure and considered dropping out of the nursing curriculum.)

Another facet of the negative interpretation of interactions is that of deprivation. Depressed persons perceive seemingly trivial events as serious losses. Beck gives the example of a depressed client on his way to visit his psychiatrist. The client felt he was losing valuable time by having to wait 30 seconds for the elevator. He then regretted the absence of companionship as he rode alone in the elevator. Then he discovered that he was not the psychiatrist's first patient, and he regretted not having the first appointment.

Other loss situations related to interactions with other people center around money or the comparison of others' possessions to one's own.

A young woman had just moved to a lovely new home in a new neighborhood. She had been quite upset over this move initially. Her husband held a very good job, and she was finally able to purchase the kinds of things she desired for herself, her children, and her home. Yet when friends bought items for their homes, she felt as though she were being deprived.

This woman, and the man in Beck's example, automatically interpreted their experiences negatively, even though more plausible explanations were available.

The third, and final, component in Beck's triad is depressed individuals' negative expectations of the future. Just as they hold negative interpretations of self and social relationships, so also do they perceive the future as being constantly overcast with large dark clouds. There are no silver linings for depressed individuals. Even short-range predictions are negative. Each day is viewed with trepidation: there is not a chance in the world that events will turn out positively. Thus the power of thought is clearly an overwhelming factor in depression. This factor is of great importance in the assessment of depressed clients and in the determination of nursing goals.

It is of value to posit a relationship among affect, motivation, and the cognitive triad. If individuals think they are worthless and base their behavior on this premise, mood will be negative. In addition, they will experience a loss of motivation —a primary characteristic of depression. They will consistently expect to meet with failure and humiliation; therefore, they will attempt nothing. Hopelessness and self-doubt will pervade thought processes. Depressed individuals envision themselves as being overwhelmed by tasks they had previously been able to cope with. It has been demonstrated that by changing such clients' thought patterns to a more positive track, a nurse can enhance their ability to actively solve problems.

Psychodynamic theory

Arieti (1974) describes depressed clients as those who have experienced a nurturing relationship that was later withdrawn. In its stead came a provisional relationship—a relationship based on the stipulation that the child must meet the expectations of the parents. In this relationship, praise and gratification were given, for example, when good grades or other symbols of prestige were achieved. Feelings of self-worth were not enhanced, since rewards were in the far distant future.

The failure to receive positive feedback can be perceived as a loss, even though the significant other may have been physically present. Again, the early beginnings of the inability to form relationships can be discerned. The expectations of an early significant relationship are not met; therefore, individuals believe that all other relationships

will fail. Little by little, they stop trying to interact with the environment.

It is important to see depression as a reaction or response. It is something individuals are doing rather than something that is happening to them. Depression is a behavioral interaction, a response to environmental stimuli.

Individuals who suffer from depression are often perfectionists whose few relationships are characterized by manipulation and control. They are unable to accept anything other than "black and white" solutions to problems. Underneath the veneer of a high-powered executive type may be the fear of total failure and powerlessness. The depressive response becomes apparent when individuals feel they have not met their own goals or those of significant others in the environment.

Biological theory

As they have in many emotional disorders, investigators have looked for an alteration in physiological functioning as a possible etiological factor. The study of electrolyte metabolism has indicated that in individuals suffering from depression there is a disturbance in the distribution of sodium and potassium from one side of a nerve cell to the other. Gibbons (1960), who worked with a group of 24 clients exhibiting depressive reactions, discovered that every client had an elevated sodium level within the nerve cells. During recovery from depression, the excess sodium was excreted.

These findings are consistent with what is known about the effect of the use of lithium compounds in the treatment of manic depression. Lithium interferes with sodium exchange at the cellular level. With the resolution of the mania, the tolerance of the body for lithium is lowered, and the lithium, along with the excess sodium, is excreted.

We need to be aware, however, that electrolyte changes may be a *result* of depression rather than a causative factor. Changes in diet and motor activity during depression could lead to electrolyte imbalance.

The biochemical theory described by Kicey

(1974) is worth noting. Her research suggests that the supply of norepinephrine at receptor sites is lowered when a person is depressed. There is an inhibition of the transmission of impulses from one neural fiber to another. The purpose of the monoamine oxidase (MAO) inhibitors is to increase the availability of active norepinephrine.

These are extremely simplified views of what are actually very complex biochemical operations.

Genetic and familial factors may play roles in the depressive response. Studies have shown that the incidence of affective disorders is higher among relatives of persons who have had such disorders than in the general population. One of the most striking results of genetic studies has been the division of affective disorders into unipolar and bipolar groups. This development may lead to the ability to predict the occurrence of affective disorders among family members. However, the role of genetics in the development of depression has yet to be definitively determined.

Recently, the biological theory of depression has gained support through the introduction of a diagnostic tool, the dexamethasone suppression test. The neuroendocrine disturbance indicated by an abnormal dexamethasone suppression test demonstrates a dysfunction in the limbic system and hypothalamus. A plasma cortisol level of 5 mEq/100 ml or greater indicates that the client has melancholia. In test results of depressed clients versus nondepressed clients, investigators noted that the test was abnormal almost exclusively for depressed clients. Researchers also found that abnormal results were not related to age, sex, psychotropic drugs, or severity of symptoms ("Testing for Melancholia," 1981).

The dexamethasone suppression test (DST) is the first test of its kind with practical and clinical application on a large scale. Since the depressive response may be elusive, a method which can determine biological alterations relating to depression can be an asset in diagnosis and treatment. The method, however, is not biologically specific to depression. Conditions which can generate a false positive are pregnancy, high-dose estrogen

therapy, Cushing's disease, marked weight loss, uncontrolled diabetes, major physical illness, trauma, fever, use of narcotics, and withdrawal from alcohol. False negative results may occur in clients who have Addison's disease, hypopituitarism, or are on corticosteroids. Although the test has significance for diagnosis of depressed clients, it is important for nurses to consider the above noted factors and to complete a comprehensive physical assessment and health history. All data must be considered in order to ensure accurate medical and nursing diagnoses and nursing intervention.

Sociocultural theory
LEARNING THEORY

Can a depressive response be learned? Is assuming a helpless position a viable adaptive mechanism for some individuals?

Seligman (1973) proposes that depression is learned helplessness. In his study with dogs, he found that the experience of having no control over what was happening interfered with the dogs' adaptive response. The dogs actually learned that they were helpless, that no matter what the situation was, their actions did not matter. They could not succeed. Seligman suggests that, in humans, the precursor to depression may be the belief that individuals have no control over their situation— that they are unable to effect any change in life experiences, to reduce suffering, or to gain praise. According to Seligman, if individuals have little success in mastering their environment, hopelessness, helplessness, and lack of assertiveness eventually become primary characteristics and the susceptibility to depression is heightened.

FEMINIST THEORIES

Published studies indicate that two to three times as many women experience depressive responses as men. There has been much investigation of the relationship between female hormones and the occurrence of depression. It is not unusual to hear a woman say she is "depressed" when she has her "period." In addition, depressive responses have been identified during times when changes in hormonal levels are marked—notably 2 to 3 days following childbirth, the general postpartum period, and menopause. However, there have been no data to validate these assumptions.

In previous sections of this chapter, we have discussed the various etiological factors in the manifestation of the depressive response. Common themes include powerlessness, helplessness, a sense of loss, and a negative view of self. These feelings are identical to those experienced by minority groups such as women, blacks, and the aged. Women, in particular, have assumed the depressive response as a natural part of their role.

According to Phyllis Chesler (1972), few women have been able to develop a true sense of identity outside of that of wife and mother. This fact can be seen vividly when the prestige levels of men and women in the male-oriented professional and business worlds are compared. Chesler proposes that "women are in a constant state of mourning, grieving for that which they never had or had too briefly." The concept of learned helplessness can be correlated with society's preconceived notion of how a woman is to respond. It is more acceptable for a woman to adopt a depressive response than for a male to do so.

Are women predisposed to depression? Dr. Pauline Bart (1971) studied depression in middle-aged women in relation to role loss. She suggests that women who have invested all their time and energy in their children and their homes are more likely to experience a depressive response than women who have not done so. These women are unable to find new roles for themselves. They have suffered the greatest loss—the loss of a purpose in life. Their self-doubt and low self-regard prevent them from seeing themselves as anything other than wives or mothers. The fear of attempting to adapt to new roles because they may fail in them becomes paramount. However, women who begin early to define roles outside of those of wife and mother will find it less difficult to adjust to the eventual loss of the nurturing role.

As a result of the women's movement, there has been increased recognition of rape and its implications for women.* Dr. Dorothy Hicks (1977) states that "rape is a violent crime that has nothing to do with sex except that the sex organs are involved." It is an act of aggression; the victim is assaulted and then left humiliated and isolated.

Courts in the United States have only recently become compassionate in their treatment of rape victims. The legal definition of rape can be traced back to the property rights of men. A woman belonged to her husband—if she were raped, *his* rights as property owner would have been violated. There was little, if any, consideration given to the woman.

Beginning in the early 1960s, the women's movement directed its attention toward consciousness-raising activities relating to rape. Feminists spoke out on rape as a political issue. Diane Russell (1975) proposed that the feminist movement might temporarily increase the amount of forcible rape. She believes the growing desire of women to be independent may threaten male egos, thus causing an increase in outwardly directed hostility. Susan Brownmiller (1975) addressed the theme of rape in much stronger tones: rape is the perpetuation of male domination over women by force. As a result of the efforts of these individuals and others, there has been an increased awareness of the crisis of rape and its impact on the victim. Myths surrounding rape, such as the belief that a woman "invites" an attacker or is responsible for the crime in some way, are slowly being dissipated.

Nurses may come into contact with rape victims in a variety of settings. A nurse may be the only person who has any type of sustained relationship with a rape victim. It is critical that the nurse recognize his or her own feelings as well as those of the client.

A woman who has been raped feels a sense of powerlessness, a sense of helplessness, and a sense of loss. She may feel unable to determine her life's course. She may also feel isolated from family,

---

*See Chapter 17 for further discussion of rape.

friends, and colleagues. She may be afraid to return to her home or to walk alone, whether it be day or night. The greatest assault, however, has been against the self. Her personal space has been violated by an aggressive act. Loss of her personhood, her self-esteem, results. The rape victim experiences a wide range of feelings, from anxiety and fear to profound depression. Rape victims should be allowed to grieve for the loss of self. A nursing assessment should identify loss of self-worth as a predominant theme, and intervention needs to address this sense of loss.

Burgess and Holstrum (1974) describe a two-phase response to rape—the rape trauma syndrome. The first, or acute, phase is characterized by disorganization. Feelings of embarrassment, anger, humiliation, fear, and self-blame are described by victims. Burgess and Holstrum identify two emotional styles characteristic of this phase. The first is the expressed style: the victim releases her angry, anxious feelings by talking, shouting, crying, or pacing. The second is the controlled style: the victim maintains a calm, subdued affect, acting as though nothing out of the ordinary has occurred. Burgess and Holstrum also describe the compounded reaction that can occur in women who have had previous psychological difficulties. This reaction is characterized by psychotic behavior, depression, acting-out behavior, and suicide.

The second, or reorganization, phase begins at a different time for each victim, depending on the availability of healthy coping measures, social support systems, and previous experiences with loss. This phase is characterized by change of residence, change of job, nightmares, fear of entering the house or apartment alone, fear of being followed, and sexual fears. Long-term studies indicate that rape victims benefit from extended follow-up counseling, which can frequently continue as long as 2 years after the rape.

The goal of nurses is to identify the feelings the rape victim is experiencing and to facilitate the grieving process as a normal response to loss. A nurse acts as a support person for the rape victim

during the medical and legal procedures that follow the rape. The nurse also assists the victim in her reintegration into the community by mobilizing significant support systems when appropriate (Clark, 1976).

Family theory

Individuals exist within many systems, one of the most powerful of these being the family. As has been noted in the discussion of psychodynamic theory, origins of depression may be related to inconsistencies in parent-child relationships resulting in lowered self-esteem. Family theory suggests that individuals who are depressed should be viewed within the context of the family process.

Exceptionally high expectations of self may be derived from the family. If praise and gratification are received only when appropriate behaviors are demonstrated, home becomes equated with meeting of parental expectations. Unrealistic expectations are brought from the family into current relationships, in which the individuals who are significant are expected to provide unquantifiable amounts of love. A cycle ensues: expectations are unrealistic; significant others cannot provide requisite amounts of love; and lowered self-esteem and depression result. Individuals continue to expect unrealistic praise and love, which are the bases for their tenuous self-worth. Often these individuals cannot develop their own reservoirs of inner resources and must continue their dependence on others.

It should be noted that depressed individuals may maintain a particular function in the family system. Other members may derive their roles from their relationship with the depressed individual. A sense of worth and personal identity may result from acting as a caretaker or as the over-functioning member. In essence, the over functioner cannot permit the under functioning member to change and assume a more independent role. Equilibrium is actually maintained through dysfunctional behavior. Energy resulting from other family conflicts or individual emotional distress may be directed toward the identified client or the overt symptom bearer—the depressed client. Whatever the issue, roles of family members are interrelated, with each member's behavior affecting others. An understanding of family relationships and dynamics is essential in nursing assessment and designing a plan of care (see Chapter 9).

Holistic approach to affective disorders

It is important to point out that *no one* theory is sufficient to explain depression. Any client is a complex, unique human being who cannot be understood through an assessment of only one factor. It would indeed be simple to say that biochemical changes or poor early relationships within the family system account for a depressive response. It would then be easy to develop a nursing care plan to facilitate the remediation of these problems. In reality, however, life is not that simple. A nursing approach based on one theory would not facilitate an understanding of the client as a total human being.

An integrated approach reflects the interaction of genetic, biochemical, cognitive, social learning, and object loss theories, as well as sex-role stereotyping. Akiskal and McKinney (1975) suggest that depression results from many variables, including biochemical responses, previous experiences, and learning and behavioral responses. According to these authors, a behavioral response such as social withdrawal is not an isolated factor but has direct impact on biochemical levels in the body. The reverse is also true: chemical imbalances may contribute to a person's perceiving situations in a distorted manner, thus leading to social withdrawal.

Nursing strategies must be based on an understanding of the various etiologic theories and their interrelationship with precipitating factors in order to be reflective of individual clients—their personalities, their expressions of needs, and their methods of adaptation—inclusive of physical, spiritual, and emotional modes.

TREATMENT MODALITIES
Psychopharmaceuticals

Antidepressants can be effective in the treatment of depressive states. These drugs produce the energy that a client needs in order to invest in his environment rather than retreat into isolation. Two basic categories of drugs are utilized—MAO inhibitors and tricyclic compounds. The drugs in each of these groups treat symptoms rather than underlying dynamics. The administration of medication is therefore not the total solution. Drugs must be utilized concurrently with a supportive relationship. Clients must receive active support from the environment once the medication has enabled them to move out of isolation.

MAO inhibitors inhibit the production of the enzyme monoamine oxidase, which is present in several vital organs, including the brain. This enzyme reduces the levels of norepinephrine, epinephrine, and serotonin, all of which serve to activate the body. MAO inhibitors counteract this reduction, thus permitting the reactivation of normal levels of these vital hormones.

Side effects and idiosyncratic responses must be considered in a comprehensive assessment of clients. The drugs in this group of medications can be lethal if they are not administered properly. The following points must be remembered:

1. These drugs are long-acting; they require three to four weeks to initially take effect.
2. There is a cumulative effect.
3. When switching from MAO inhibitors to tricyclics, wait one to two weeks so that synthesis will have occurred. When MAO inhibitors and tricyclics are given simultaneously, twitching, general restlessness, and even death can occur.
4. MAO inhibitors potentiate the actions of many other drugs, such as morphine, meperidine (Demerol), barbiturates, sedatives, tranquilizers, atropine derivatives, anti-parkinsonian drugs, antihistamines, and corticosteroids.

5. MAO inhibitors enhance the hypotensive effects of diuretics and will sensitize clients to procaine (Novocain) and other anesthetic agents.
6. Do not administer MAO inhibitors with amphetamines or ephedrine-like compounds, such as cold tablets or sinus aids.
7. Be alert to the ''Parnate-cheese'' reaction. Individuals receiving MAO inhibitors must avoid cheese, wine, yeast products, beer, yogurt, fava beans, chicken livers, and pickled herring. Otherwise, an increased level of tyramine, which is found in cheeses as well as these other products, results. Normally, tyramine is destroyed by MAO. However, this does not happen when the MAO inhibitors are in effect. The rise in tyramine levels leads to a hypertensive crisis. If the crisis is not controlled, blood vessels in the brain rupture, and death ensues.

The tricyclics are more widely used than the MAO inhibitors and have a higher success rate. The greatest difficulty encountered with the tricyclics is the premature removal of the client from the medication. Physicians often feel that the depression has lifted when the symptoms have been alleviated. In many cases, however, after a period of a month or more the client is again experiencing symptoms of the depressive response. Maintenance of an adequate dosage is the key to successful control of depression.

Tricyclics seem to affect the brain amine levels, although the specific response is not actually known. Unlike MAO inhibitors, tricyclics have little potential for causing hypertensive crisis. Most side effects can be regulated by adjusting the dosage as necessary.

Table 18-1, which is based on data of the Department of Drugs of the American Medical Association, lists the most common MAO inhibitors and tricyclics along with their trade names, dosage levels, routes of administration, and common side effects.

Nurses must act to support clients as barriers are let down through the action of medication. Leaving clients to function on their own because symptoms have been relieved can cause an exacerbation of those same symptoms. Another point to remember is that medication acts to lift the mood of clients to provide them with more available energy. This energy can then be turned toward self-destructive behavior.

Lithium carbonate is utilized primarily for the manic phase of manic depression. Marked reduction in manic behavior has been demonstrated after a period of 2 weeks. Lithium carbonate interferes with the elevated levels of norepinephrine and also affects the electrolyte balance within the brain, particularly sodium and potassium levels. Studies have shown that levels of intracellular sodium are low during the manic phase. Lithium increases the ion exchange factor, thus leading to higher levels of intracellular sodium and less impulsive behavior. Sodium regulation and the use of diuretics must be carefully monitored while a client is receiving lithium. Blood levels of lithium should be checked weekly, since the toxic dose is dangerously close to the therapeutic levels. Kidney function is of utmost importance, since the kidneys are responsible for a large percentage of the excretion of lithium.

Prior to the administration of lithium, the client must have a complete physical, which will provide a complete data base. It is critical to determine whether the client has a history of cardiovascular or kidney disease; the administration of lithium is contraindicated in those instances. There is a lag period of approximately 1 week between the initial administration and the subsiding of symptoms. Other tranquilizers may be used until the lithium takes effect. The nurse's primary role in the administration of lithium is the education of the client to the side effects and the results of misuse of lithium. It is imperative that the client continue to take lithium even though he or she is ''feeling fine.''

In their study of compliance with lithium regimens Kucera-Bozarth et al. (1982) reported that 45% of the sample reported compliance but actually were noncompliant based on lithium level cri-

Table 18-1. Antidepressants

Drug	Trade name	Method of administration	Usual daily dose (mg)	Side effects
Monoamine oxidase inhibitors				
Isocarboxazid	Marplan	Oral	10-30	Headaches, dizziness, blurred vision,
Nialamide	Niamid	Oral	12.5-200	dry mouth, postural hypotension,
Phenelzine dihydrogen sulfate	Nardil	Oral	15-75	increased appetite, nausea and vomiting, constipation or diarrhea, weakness, edema, tremors,
Tranylcypromine sulfate	Parnate	Oral	20-30	impotence, insomnia, dermatitis, nightmares
Tricyclics				
Imipramine	Tofranil	Oral	75-300	Palpitations, increased pulse rate,
		Intramuscular		postural hypotension, dizziness,
	Tofranil-PM	Oral		faintness, loss of visual
Amitriptyline hydrochloride	Elavil	Oral	50-200	accommodation, nausea and vomiting,
		Intramuscular		increased perspiration, constipation,
Desipramine hydrochloride	Norpramin Pertofrane	Oral	75-150	urine retention, aggravation of glaucoma, minor tremors, twitching
Nortriptyline hydrochloride	Aventyl	Oral	20-100	(NOTE: These symptoms are mild and can be controlled by reducing
Protriptyline hydrochloride	Vivactil	Oral	15-60	the dosage.)
Doxepin hydrochloride	Sinequan	Oral	25-300	

Adapted from American Medical Association Department of Drugs. 1973. AMA Drug Evaluations (ed. 2). Acton, Mass.: Publishing Sciences Group, Inc.

teria. The unreliability of self-reporting was further demonstrated by the fact that 9% reported noncompliance but were within compliance parameters based on serum lithium levels.

Noncompliant clients tended to be from lower socioeconomic backgrounds and were less likely to hold an internal health locus of control. Data of this nature is of particular importance since documentation of noncompliance among clients on lithium demonstrates compromise of the management of the disorder. Some clients may even show evidence of gross decompensation after missing only a few doses (Kucera-Bozarth et al., 1982).

Kucera-Bozarth et al. suggest that nurses consider this data in their assessment and intervention with these clients. Self-reporting cannot be relied upon for accurate prediction of compliance; thus the risks are increased of ineffective management of the disorder and exacerbation of inappropriate behaviors.

Individual and group psychotherapy

Individual psychotherapy is initially more fruitful than group psychotherapy. Depressed clients have difficulty seeing themselves as worthwhile people. Becoming part of a group may precipitate stress and be an overwhelming experience. These clients' greatest need is to be accepted as human beings. By relating to other individuals on a one-to-one basis, depressed clients can explore various ways to reach that goal. As they become more sure of themselves and cease to view trust as an unattainable goal, they will venture into a group setting. Groups may be strictly supportive, or they may be analytical and insight-directed. An effective group leader facilitates growth through interaction within the group setting. Each person needs to become what he or she is capable of becoming. This can be accomplished only when a group leader is warm, sincere, and most important of all, sensitive to the nature of the client's depressive behavior. Through the group process, depressed clients can learn alternative approaches to problems they are encountering. They may even find that the areas they considered problematic are no longer of primary concern. Whether the approach is individual or group, nurse-therapists must place top priority on the worth of human beings and the uniqueness of their responses.

The usefulness of the group approach with depressed women has been documented by Gordon (1982). She noted that depressed women who were exposed to a series of support groups on a regular basis were able to explore their feelings of inadequacy with regard to meeting society's demands, their feelings of anger in relation to dependency on their husbands, fears of being failures as wives and mothers, failure to be assertive, loneliness; the burden of responsibility for the care of elderly parents, and the need to express their feelings and get support. She also noted that many of these themes were reflective not only of depression but also of anxiety and anger.

Recommendations from this study suggest that further studies are necessary to determine the effect of structured group sessions with specific goals in this population. Replication is essential to substantiate the presence of relevant themes and evidence of cohesiveness.

Electroconvulsive therapy

Electroconvulsive therapy (ECT) was introduced by Ugo Cerletti and Lucio Bini in 1938. It is basically the administration of electricity via electrodes placed on the temples. Theories of the action of this therapy vary, and none seems to be widely accepted. One theory proposes that individuals who consider themselves worthless view the shock as a punishment that they deserve. Another theory holds that the shock rearranges brain cells, causing neurotransmission changes that, in turn, reduce the barriers to the understanding of the origins of the depressive response. Still another theory suggests that aggression is at last turned outward, through the tonic and clonic phases of the convulsion. Whatever the underlying dynamics, electroconvulsive therapy does seem to exert a profound effect on clients experiencing clinical depression.

The care of clients receiving electroconvulsive therapy parallels that of clients undergoing surgery. Prior to therapy, the nurse should explain the procedure thoroughly and simply. A complete physical, including spinal x-ray film, is required. A consent form must be signed. On the morning of the treatment, clients should eat or drink nothing. They should remove dentures, put on loosely fitting clothes, and void prior to the administration of the treatment. Tranquilizers may be given if anxiety levels are rising. Atropine may or may not be given to reduce secretions.

The client is placed on a stretcher in the treatment room, and a short-acting barbiturate is given intravenously, followed by a muscle relaxant. A rubber mouthpiece is inserted to maintain patent airway. The shock is administered, and a grand mal seizure results. Nurses in attendance allow the client's body to move with the tonic and clonic spasms, rather than holding him or her down. Restraining the body often causes fractures rather than preventing them.

Following the treatment, routine postoperative care is the primary nursing goal. Positioning the client on the side, with the head tilted, facilitates the maintenance of an open airway and reduces the possibility of aspiration.

Although clients may be alert and awake immediately following the treatment, assessment of vital signs every 15 minutes for the first hour is necessary. Since periods of confusion may occur after the treatment, clients need to be protected from injuring themselves. Nurses should orient clients to their surroundings, to enable them to feel in control of themselves and their environment to some extent.

Once clients are able to, they return to their own rooms. Nourishment is provided as well as an opportunity to rest. Electroconvulsive treatments are given in a series, ranging anywhere from 12 to 60.

Electroconvulsive therapy alone is not the solution to depression. As in other treatments, a client must be supported by a relationship with a significant other. Once the client's defensive barrier has been lowered, nurses need to be there to provide an atmosphere in which exploration of issues and problem-solving are priorities.

NURSING INTERVENTION

PRIMARY PREVENTION

Programs of primary prevention of depression are just beginning to be organized. Clinical research is providing nurses with steadily increasing amounts of data regarding the delicate interweaving of the etiological factors underlying loss and depression. Major goals of primary prevention are the promotion of positive feelings toward the self and the facilitation of a healthy adaptation to loss. The focus of this level of prevention is the promotion of open lines of communication and freedom of expression of feelings.

Nurses need to be aware of the following principles as they engage in activities of primary prevention of the major affective disorders:

1. Patterns of withdrawal and elation are a means of coping with unconscious conflicts

in order to maintain functional ability.
2. Loss is a fundamental theme in the origins of affective disorders because of its effect on feelings of self-worth and personal control.
3. Individuals exist within the context of relationships that have a reciprocal effect on all members of the relationship.
4. Awareness of feelings and social relatedness are decreased further during crisis situations.
5. Multiple variables are interrelated in their effect on coping strategies.
6. Crisis situations increase personal vulnerability and limit perceptions of internal control and sense of worth to self and others.

Goals for primary prevention of major affective disorders include:

1. Minimizing effects of factors that predispose individuals to affective disorders
2. Identifying high-risk populations

Nurses can implement these goals by assisting individuals in their ability to cope with loss and change through parental and family counseling and by identifying high-risk populations.

Coping with loss

Since loss is a fundamental theme in the origins of depression, primary preventive efforts need to be directed toward helping people to adapt to the various loss situations that occur throughout the life cycle. The crises of loss begin with the loss of the warm, uterine environment and end with the ultimate loss—the loss of one's own life. Programs such as those outlined in parent effectiveness training courses, health education curricula, and workshop presentations can identify potential loss situations and probable reactions to them. Individuals can learn to be managers of their lives rather than victims of circumstance. Loss situations can be turned into learning situations. Disappointments can be handled appropriately. Children can then be better equipped to react to crises in a healthy fashion in later life. Through positive appraisals from significant others, a child's self-esteem can be enhanced at particularly crucial times of development. The child will learn to be adept at using problem-solving faculties, a discovery that in turn reaffirms positive feelings of self.

Primary preventive programs are still new, yet they serve as the basis for the healthy development of tomorrow's generation.

Grieving is a healthy response to loss, whether it be of a love object, self-worth, status, or function. The resolution of this process ultimately leads to the investment of energy in new relationships and to positive feelings regarding the self. When grief is prolonged, however, and the loss is not resolved, anxiety arises. The depressive response is activated to contain and/or diminish the anxiety. (Hauser and Feinberg, 1976). Nursing intervention therefore needs to be directed toward facilitating healthy adaptation to loss. The following principles are important in such intervention:

1. The primary goal is to promote catharsis. Verbalization enables clients to work through feelings of anger, sadness, relief, and helplessness. Be particularly cognizant of nonverbal communication.

2. Recognize that ambivalence is common. There may be sorrow that the loss has occurred. Yet in the case of a client who is experiencing the loss of a relative, there may be a sense of relief that the process of dying is finally over. For example, a family may feel a sense of relief after the death of a loved one who has been chronically ill. These ambivalent feelings are quite common; however, they are also quite upsetting. Let the client know that these feelings are quite normal. Provide a setting in which these feelings can be shared.

3. Assess clients to determine what phase of the mourning process they have entered.

4. Assist clients in maintaining contact with highly valued objects or people. This is not the time for grieving clients to sell all belongings or give them away.

5. Support already existing coping mechanisms, such as denial. Denial is quite commonly utilized to deal with pain experi-

enced in a loss situation. If this mechanism is removed, the client will replace it with another, more pathological one. Do not reinforce denial, however; present reality as it can be tolerated.

6. Help clients to control their environments to prevent additional losses. Encourage them to participate as much as possible in the normal activities of daily living. They will then be able to feel as though their life-styles have not been irreversibly altered. They will see that they are still able to perceive events occurring in the environment accurately and that they can actively deal with them as necessary.

7. Be patient and tolerant of the wide range of behavior that can be exhibited by the grieving client. Anger toward the lost object that is released into constructive channels during this phase will not likely be turned inward upon the self at a later time.

8. Provide a private, quiet room for grieving clients in order that they may feel comfortable in their unique expressions of grief.

9. Assist the grieving person and family to review previous encounters with loss and methods of coping with them. Often individuals are unaware of their repertoire of coping mechanisms. The nurse can identify them with the client. The grieving person thus can be helped to develop a healthy approach to loss rather than to view it as a totally negative situation each time it occurs.

10. Allow enough space and time for the individual to grieve. Each person is unique in his or her responses, particularly in the response to loss. Healthy resolution may take as long as 2 years, depending on the extent and type of relationship with the lost object. Anniversaries, birthdays, a special song, or a type of food may cause a normal reactivation of sadness. It is important to point out that such a reaction is acceptable behavior and to encourage the sharing of feelings regarding the precipitating factor.

11. Since loss is inevitable in the developmental cycle, nursing intervention must involve anticipatory work, as was previously pointed out. Recognize that an individual is having a difficult time resolving a situation. There may be a continued state of denial; the person may be unable to progress to the awareness phase. Further supportive therapy is then necessary. In addition, nurses may want to consult resource people in the event that a depressive response is prolonged.

Identification of high-risk individuals

Community health nurses, family and pediatric nurse practitioners, and school nurses work with children and their families in a variety of settings. Through observation of family interaction— whether it be a marital dyad expecting the birth of a first child or a family visit to a well-child clinic— nurses can note predominant patterns of relating, personal and group coping strategies, and roles of various members. As nurses become more familiar with family structure and patterns of relationships, children who come from families where social withdrawal, elation, or self-destruction are characteristic behaviors can be identified.

Assessment of the family system should include recognition of:

1. Unrealistically high expectations of child in parent-child relationship
2. Unmet dependency needs in parenting figures
3. Contingency-based expression of love and gratification from parent to child
4. Lack of consistency of parental response in regard to giving gratification
5. Consistent lack of positive reinforcement for attempts and achievements
6. Consistent use of social withdrawal or elated behaviors as a means of coping
7. History of losses that have never been fully resolved

8. Overfunctioning or underfunctioning dyad in family system
9. History of suicidal behavior in present family system or family of origin
10. Consistent inability to express feelings of anger, apprehension, and dejection to others
11. Persistent perception of self, environment, and future in a negativistic manner
12. Persistent lack of role—appropriate definitions of self in various stages of the life cycle

These factors must also be considered in relation to biological, sociocultural, emotional, and spiritual factors that may predispose individuals to major affective disorders.

Parental and family counseling

Family members are often not cognizant of their impact on one another. As noted earlier, individuals exist within the context of relationships. Roles are maintained and behaviors learned through these relationships. Coping styles are often learned from parental role models. Facilitation of expression of feelings in an authentic and direct manner by nurses may enhance coping behavior in the developing family members and reduce the possibility of old conflicts and expectations being played out in new relationships.

Prenatal classes, well-baby clinics, and even physicians' offices are important target areas. The central goal at this level is to facilitate the mothering response, not just physically but emotionally as well. Mothers who are anxious and fearful are unable to meet their own needs, let alone attend to those of their infants. Parents who feel positive about themselves are more capable of allowing their children the room to explore their territory, to develop a sense of their own personal space—in other words, to be! Children need positive reinforcement on a continuous basis—not sporadically, when expectations are fulfilled. Mistrust begins to develop, as do feelings of low self-worth, when reinforcement is only sporadic. A child, as he or she grows up in such an anxious, uncomfortable environment, is not able to relate successfully to others in his or her social world. Relationships are characterized either by withdrawal or by aggressive, manipulative behavior. These responses tend to separate the individual from others even more.

Initial assessments are tentative and must be validated through consultation with other health care providers. Intervention should not be planned based on single observations. Health professionals such as community health nurses, family nurse clinicians, and occupational health nurses have the opportunity to observe and interact with clients and families on repeated occasions. Rapport develops between health care provider and client-family. Out of this relationship emerges a foundation of trust and accurate observation that can result in referral to a mental health resource—the goal of early identification in secondary prevention. It must be remembered that some clients find it difficult to enter into a relationship with a mental health resource person—whether the person be nurse-therapist, psychologist, social worker, or psychiatrist. These ambivalent feelings can be explored in a supportive relationship provided by the referring nurse. An empathic relationship can allay many fears as well as create an atmosphere that motivates the individual to enter further treatment. Nurses must also be careful not to move individuals too quickly into the mental health delivery system. Anxiety and inaccurate observations on the part of the referring nurse can be detrimental in themselves.

SECONDARY PREVENTION

Intervention in secondary prevention is based on the nursing process. In this section individual patterns of behavior will be addressed, with specific strategies of intervention being identified. However, it is important for nurses to consider these principles of action regardless of the presenting behavior or symptom:

1. The focus is client-centered rather than symptom-centered.
2. Behavior and/or symptoms are mechanisms of defense and attempts to maintain sense of self-worth.
3. Clients need acceptance and approval as vulnerability is increased.
4. Repressed hostility may be overtly expressed when pressure is increased.
5. Anger should not be provoked, since clients fear the impact of their own hostility on self and others.
6. Nurses and other staff members will have emotional responses to client behavior. These responses must be considered within the context of the current relationship as well as in relation to past experiences. Nurses cannot negate these feelings; rather they must learn how to use their feelings in a positive manner with the client.

These principles will guide nurses in their observations, data analysis, decision making, and determination of appropriate intervention strategies.

Nursing process

The nursing process acts as a guide for therapeutic intervention.

ASSESSMENT

Client identification of the problem is a key factor in the assessment process. Nurses need to begin at that point which the client deems appropriate. A mental status examination as well as information relating to social and family history provides a comprehensive base (see Chapter 9).
Specific areas of assessment include:

1. Presenting symptoms—slowed cognitions; retarded or agitated psychomotor activity; sleep disturbances; lack of energy; fatigue; verbal paucity
2. Emotional state—feelings of helplessness, hopelessness, lack of purpose and self-worth; anger; self-destructive feelings
3. Stress-producing situations—are these gen-

erated or potentiated by maladaptive coping strategies? (What changes or losses have occurred in past six months?)

4. Coping behaviors—how effective are they? (What coping strategies were used in the family and how effective were they?)

5. Available support systems and resources—friends, parents, others

6. Client strengths—what can and does the client do for self and/or others—i.e., regularly employed? Able to meet own personal hygiene needs? (What does client expect of self? Is this realistic?)

7. Holistic health status—biological, psychological, intellectual, sociocultural, and spiritual status of client. (These factors will influence client's wellness either positively or negatively, and in some instances, in both ways. For example, conflict between one's expectations of self and societal expectations may occur, generating guilt and ambivalence.)

ANALYSIS OF DATA

Careful assessment of data enables the nurse to have a *beginning* understanding of clients, the contexts in which they exist (families and other relationships), and their perceptions of the identified problems. At this point nurses may be ready to identify nursing diagnoses. (It is important to note that throughout the nurse-client relationship, data is gathered and nursing diagnoses reformulated as appropriate.) The following are nursing diagnoses and appropriate plans of care and implementation (based on Schultz and Dark, 1982).

Nursing diagnosis:

1. Interaction theme of dependency (see Chapter 19 for discussion) (behavior related to all DSM-III diagnoses of major affective disorders)

2. Interaction themes of powerlessness, helplessness, and hopelessness related to feelings of inadequacy and loss of control (behavior related to all DSM-III diagnoses of major affective disorders)

Planning: With assistance and/or guidance from the nurse, the client will establish goals.

1. Long-term goals
   a. Work through internal conflict *generating* feelings of helplessness, hopelessness, and powerlessness and creating feelings of inadequacy.
   b. Build relationships with others on assertive, decisive behaviors.

2. Short-term goals
   a. Verbalize feelings of helplessness, hopelessness, and powerlessness.
   b. Identify current situations that create the above feelings.
   c. Relate past situations that may have aroused similar feelings.
   d. Describe expectations of self in five dimensions—biological, intellectual, psychological, sociocultural, and spiritual, and determine their appropriateness to situations; develop a realistic perception of self.
   e. Develop more appropriate coping strategies and interpersonal skills.

Implementation:

1. Assist clients in manipulating their environments so that they can effect change. For example, suppose that a client describes feelings of being unable to change her role from strictly mother and wife to mother, wife, and interior decorator. The task seems overwhelming to her. Nurses can break down the overall goal into short-term, attainable goals. The client can experience success, and the pattern can be broken.

2. Recognize that helplessness may be a learned response. Provide situations in which clients can exert some control over their environments.

3. In response to behavior that indicates hopelessness, do not become ''Suzy Sunshine'' and try to talk clients out of their depression. Instead, work with them to develop experiences in which they will receive positive feedback.

4. Do not condemn the negative feelings of clients, since they have a right to those feelings. On the other hand, do not perpetuate those feelings by condoning them.

Nursing diagnosis: Interaction theme of anger/hostility related to sense of inadequacy and loss (behavior associated with all DSM-III diagnoses of major affective disorders)

Planning: With assistance and/or guidance from the nurse, the client will establish goals.

1. Long-term goals
   a. Work through internal conflict generating feelings of anger/hostility.
   b. Develop relationships that are based on appropriate expression of anger and hostility.
2. Short-term goals
   a. Verbalize feelings of anger and hostility in a constructive manner when it is appropriate to do so.
   b. Identify current situations that arouse feelings of anger and hostility.
   c. Relate past situations that may arouse similar feelings.
   d. Realistically appraise five dimensions of self—biological, intellectual, psychological, sociocultural, and spiritual.
   e. Develop more appropriate coping strategies and interpersonal skills.

Implementation:

1. Encourage clients to verbalize feelings of anger rather than to internalize them. Provide safeguards in the event that clients attempt to act out aggressive feelings against others or themselves.
2. Act as a role model. Let clients see that anger can be handled constructively, that it can be a healthy response to a situation. Show them that an angry retort by another person can be a positive learning experience.
3. Provide physical outlets for angry feelings. Gross motor activity, such as jogging, playing volleyball or tennis, and hammering or pounding copper, serve as useful releases for pent-up anger.

4. Be direct and honest in communication, since the client's interactions in the past have been laced with innuendo and misperception.
5. Do not be intimidated by clients, since they in fact fear their anger will destroy those around them. An empathic response by a nurse will help to alleviate anxiety.
6. Do not provoke clients into expressing anger by probing into emotionally charged areas. Depressed clients walk a veritable tightrope in their attempts to keep anger in check. A torrential outburst of anger may be a devastating event, emotionally draining them and making them more vulnerable to their own feelings and those of others.

Nursing diagnosis: Interaction theme of guilt relating to sense of inadequacy and loss (behavior associated with all DSM-III diagnoses of major affective disorders)

Planning: With assistance and/or guidance from the nurse, the client will establish goals.

1. Long-term goals
   a. Work through internal conflict that generates feelings of guilt.
   b. Relate to others in a manner that is not based on persistent expressions of inappropriate guilt.
2. Short-term goals
   a. Verbalize feelings about interpersonal relationships and behaviors without imposing excessive self-blame for their appropriateness or inappropriateness.
   b. Identify current situations that arouse feelings of guilt.
   c. Relate past situations that may arouse similar feelings.
   d. Realistically appraise five dimensions of self—biological, psychological, intellectual, sociocultural, and spiritual.
   e. Develop more appropriate coping strategies and interpersonal skills

Implementation:

1. Do not negate clients' guilt feelings, even though they seem totally unreasonable. Clients feel that they have done wrong and

should be punished for it. Some theorists have proposed that menial tasks assigned to depressed clients assist them in assuaging these guilt feelings. They perceive this treatment as being the punishment they rightfully deserve. However, at present such treatment is seldom considered appropriate, and it is not widely utilized.
2. Avoid closing off avenues of communication by refusing to listen to the constant degradation of self. Such a refusal will only serve to reinforce the client's already existing low self-esteem and self-doubt.
3. Encourage the client to accept the forgiveness of others and to look to the future instead of the past.
4. Explore alternatives to clients' self-inflicted punishment. Can they experience joy in any activities? If there is even the slightest kindling of interest in an activity, facilitate the client's participation in it.

Nursing diagnosis: Interaction theme of ambivalence relating to sense of inadequacy and loss (behavior associated with all DSM-III diagnoses of major affective disorders)

Planning: With assistance and/or guidance from the nurse, the client will establish goals.
1. Long-term goals
   a. Work through internal conflict that generates ambivalence.
   b. Develop honest, open social and intimate relationships.
2. Short-term goals
   a. Verbalize ambivalent feelings towards current and past significant others and relationships.
   b. Identify current situations that arouse feelings of ambivalence.
   c. Relate past situations that may arouse similar feelings.
   d. Realistically appraise five dimensions of self—biological, psychological, intellectual, sociocultural, and spiritual.
   e. Develop more appropriate coping strategies and interpersonal skills.

Implementation:
1. Recognize that opposing feelings are in existence within the depressed client. It is a frightening experience to feel both love and hatred toward another human being. The client does not know which feeling to attend to and is on the proverbial fence. On the one hand, it is very important to the client to feel close to another person; on the other hand, it is difficult for him (or her) to invest in a relationship. The response of the client resembles lack of interest but should not be taken as such.
2. Leave the door open for the initiating of a relationship. Do not ask if the client wants you to stay with him or her. The client is unable to make that decision. Instead, make a statement to the effect that you will come to see him or her at a designated time. You must be the positive, active force in the relationship. Leaving it up to the depressed client will result in no interaction at all. After a series of interactions, the client will begin to believe that you are truly interested in him or her. At this point, you and the client can develop a plan for increasing a feeling of worth.

Nursing diagnosis: Interaction theme of worthlessness relating to feelings of inadequacy and loss (behavior associated with all DSM-III diagnoses of major affective disorders)

Planning: With assistance and/or guidance from the nurse, the client will establish goals.
1. Long-term goals
   a. Work through internal conflict that generates worthlessness.
   b. Develop relationships that promote feelings of confidence and self-worth.
2. Short-term goals
   a. Verbalize feelings of low self-worth.
   b. Identify current situations that arouse feelings of guilt.
   c. Relate past situations that may arouse similar feelings.

d. Realistically appraise five dimensions of self—biological, psychological, intellectual, sociocultural, and spiritual strengths and weaknesses will be put into proper perspective.
e. Develop more appropriate coping strategies and interpersonal skills.

Implementation:

1. Accept clients as unique human beings with needs specifically their own. One of the most devastating factors in the depressed client's life has been a lack of praise and gratification for *being!* Nurses must start at this most basic of points in order to be effective in intervening with any of the other themes.
2. Define goals that are attainable so that clients can begin to achieve positive feedback in relation to their capabilities. Do not make situations so easy that success is achieved with little effort. This will only serve to reinforce feelings of worthlessness and the inability to function. Start with simple activities and move to complex.
3. Accept but do not condone the feelings of worthlessness exhibited. Avoid a power struggle. A shouting match between client and nurse as to the worth of the client will certainly not further any type of relationship.
4. Recognize clients' needs for privacy—do not "crowd" them. You must maintain a delicate balance: let clients know that you are concerned yet do not overwhelm them with your presence.
5. Attend to physical hygiene and nutritional needs. (These most basic needs must be met before you can move on to the development of a positive concept of self.)

Nursing diagnosis: Alteration in adequate nutritional intake and elimination relating to feelings of inadequacy and loss (behavior associated with all DSM-III diagnoses relating to major affective disorders)

Planning: The nurse will initiate goal-setting; however, as the relationship progresses the client will take responsibility for goal-setting.

1. Long-term goals
   a. Reach optimal level of nutritional status and eliminatory regularity.
   b. Develop an awareness of the relationship of good nutrition and elimination to increased feelings of self-worth.
2. Short-term goals
   a. Maintain adequate daily nutritional status.
   b. Plan meals and snacks that are nutritionally sound.
   c. Select times that are most pleasurable and will maximize good eating habits.

Implementation:

1. Monitor eating patterns and fluid intake. Calorie counts and intake and output need to be recorded.
2. Supplemental feedings may be necessary, i.e., high-protein foods.
3. Determine food preferences and have them available.
4. Provide fingerfoods for the hyperactive client.
5. Observe and record all bowel movements. Offer laxatives as necessary to prevent constipation.
6. Provide large amounts of fluid to prevent constipation.

Nursing diagnosis: Alteration in activity level (hyperactivity) relating to feelings of inadequacy and loss (behavior associated with DSM-III category 296.4-296.6, bipolar disorder)

Planning: The nurse will initially set goals; however, as the relationship progresses the client will assume responsibility for goal-setting.

1. Long-term goals
   a. Return to situation-appropriate levels of activity.
   b. Reestablish relationships with others within appropriate social contexts.
2. Short-term goals
   a. Maintain a balance between activity and sleep.
   b. Utilize physical energy in an appropriate manner to release tension.

Implementation:
1. Decrease environmental stimuli.
2. Note behavior indicative of increased restlessness and limit stimuli by removing the client to a quieter area.
3. Administer medications as necessary.
4. Discuss expectations of client behavior as soon as it is appropriate. Provide some sort of structured environment with well-defined expectations.
5. Encourage verbalization of feelings and seek more effective methods of coping through active problem solving.
6. Provide time for physical outlet of energy through structured activities—do not engage in extremely competitive activities.
7. Include time for a short nap or a rest period during the day while encouraging night time sleeping.
8. Observe sleep patterns and determine fatigue levels.
9. Provide a quiet atmosphere prior to bedtime, i.e., restful music, warm milk, reading.
10. Determine the client's level of responsibility for limiting his or her own activity levels.

Nursing diagnosis: Alteration in spontaneous verbal expression of feelings, relating to own sense of inadequacy and loss (behavior associated with all DSM-III diagnoses of major affective disorders)

Planning: Initially the nurse will set goals; however, the client will gradually assume that responsibility.
1. Long-term goals
   a. Verbalize thoughts and feelings relative to one's own life experiences, whether they be positive and/or negative.
   b. Take on the responsibility of resolving feelings by finding others to talk to, and develop a network of support.
2. Short-term goals
   a. Identify situations in which feelings can be shared in an appropriate manner.

b. Expand more fully a discussion of routine daily events.

Implementation:
1. Provide for opportunities in which verbalization can take place, i.e., a quiet atmosphere with little environmental stimuli.
2. Encourage expression of thoughts and feelings regarding events and/or people that are described by client.
3. Validate client's nonverbal messages so as to encourage expression of feelings.
4. Provide structured time that is just for client and nurse or client and significant others to talk.
5. Accept client's limited verbalizations while recognizing potential for increased expression of thoughts and feelings.
6. Assess family for overfunctioning members and subsequent disconfirmation of client's expression of feelings.

Nursing diagnosis: Alteration in ability to perform activities of daily living, relating to sense of inadequacy and loss (behavior associated with all DSM-III diagnoses of major affective disorders)

Planning: Initially the nurse will establish goals; however, as the client progresses, he or she will assume the responsibility.
1. Long-term goals
   a. Carry out activities of daily living on a regular basis.
   b. Develop an awareness of the importance of participating in self-care in relation to positive feelings of self-worth.
2. Short-term goals
   a. Establish and maintain adequate personal hygiene, i.e., bathing, dressing, and caring for clothing.
   b. Participate in keeping own personal space neat and clean.

Implementation:
1. Assist the client in bathing and dressing when he or she is unable to do so.
2. Encourage the client to take responsibility for personal hygiene as is appropriate, based on mood level.

3. Provide positive feedback for personal care as the client assumes increasing responsibility.
4. Structure times for getting up, bathing, and dressing so that client does not spend excessive time in bed.

Nursing diagnosis: Alteration in ability to protect self from self-destructive behaviors, relating to low self-esteem and lack of impulse control (behavior associated with all DSM-III diagnoses of major affective disorders)

Planning: Initially the nurse will set goals for the client; however, as the relationship progresses, the client will assume goal-setting responsibilities.

1. Long-term goals
   a. Work through internal conflict relating to feelings of poor self-worth and inadequacy.
   b. Acknowledge and accept hostile feelings and unrealistic expectations towards self and others.
   c. Decrease impulsive self-destructive behaviors.
   d. Develop an insight into self-destructive behavior and its relationship to feelings of poor self-worth, hopelessness, and personal inadequacy.
   e. Develop more appropriate methods of coping with suicidal feelings.
2. Short-term goals
   a. Increase ability to discuss feelings as they occur in response to specific situations.
   b. Identify stressors that initiate self-destructive behaviors.
   c. Identify ways in which life situations can be made less stressful.
   d. Identify unrealistic expectations of self and/or others.
   e. Identify and explore more effective problem-solving methods.

Implementation: The initial phase of implementation involves providing a safe environment and assessing suicidal potential. This is accomplished through an assessment that includes the following components (Hatton, et al., 1977).

1. *Demographic data.* The following information should be obtained: name, age, sex, race, education, religion, and living arrangements.
2. *Hazard.* What happened within the 2 to 3 weeks prior to entry into the health care system? Have there been any significant developmental or situational crises? Were there potential loss situations that might have precipitated the threat? The most crucial task is to identify the meaning the individual ascribes to such an event.
3. *Crisis.* What is the client experiencing internally? What are the psychological and somatic symptoms, and how severe are they? Be alert to the fact that as depression lifts, clients are more apt to attempt suicide, because they are able to view it as a way to resolve problems. Is the level of hopelessness elevated to such a degree that the suicide potential is great?
4. *Coping mechanisms.* It is important to determine how an individual usually approaches a problem. What makes the present situation different from others he or she has encountered? Is there a dependence on alcohol or drug abuse present that might alter the client's level of impulse control? Find out what the client perceives as helpful in reducing stress.
5. *Significant others.* Who constitutes the primary support system or systems in the client's environment? What does the client feel would be the reaction of significant others to his or her current behavior? Is this perception real or distorted? Contact may have to be made with these persons in order to obtain a complete data base.
6. *Social and personal resources.* What social resources, such as shelter, food, and clothing, are available? Personal resources include money, time, physical and mental abilities, and job. Clients are more able to cope with a crisis when such resources are available.

7. *Past suicide attempts.* Any past suicide attempts must be evaluated. Their seriousness, the methods used, and the resources available prior to those attempts should be determined. The current risk may be great if past attempts have been frequent and serious.

8. *History of psychiatric problems.* If the person has been hospitalized for emotional difficulties in the past, the risk of suicide should be considered great. Has the client made contact with any other psychiatric agencies? How did the client respond to them? Such information gives the nurse an idea of what alternatives have been explored and of what has been useful and what has not.

9. *Current medical status.* Is the client being treated by a health professional at the present time? If so, why is he or she now seeking out other people for support? Counseling is an emotionally charged process and may engender many feelings that a client feels he or she cannot share with the current therapist. The client may simply need another listening ear at this time. He or she then could be referred back to the original therapist. Does the client have any physical illnesses, acute or chronic, that may precipitate a stress response? If so, has this illness been going on for a long time? What were previous methods of coping, and were they effective? What has caused these coping mechanisms to be ineffective? Has there been any significant change in health status within the past 6 months? Has the client consulted a physician during that time? Often, a person's attempts at making needs known fall upon deaf ears. We need to be acutely alert for the underlying theme "Please help me."

10. *Life-style.* Is the individual's life-style fairly stable? Or does he or she move from one job to another, from one location to another, and from one group of friends to another? Such a life pattern offers no consistency, no certainty as to where a person might be or what he or she might be doing. Clients who have not had stable patterns of interaction with other people will be less able to cope with any significant crisis situations.

11. *Suicidal plan.* Four basic criteria are involved in the measurement of suicidal intent: method, availability, specificity, and lethality. Has the client selected a particular method? How available is that method? Assume, for instance, that a woman tells you she has four full bottles of barbiturates on the nightstand next to her and that she rattles them into the phone. This action alerts you to the fact that suicide could be readily attempted. If the individual has formulated a specific plan of action, right down to the exact time and place, then there is a marked increase in suicidal risk. How lethal is the method? Lethality can be expressed in terms of the time span between the suicidal act and death. The most lethal method is shooting; hanging is second. Slashing one's wrists is last. Ingestion of pills poses considerable danger, yet there is time to get help to an individual. Gunshot wounds and hanging have a more immediate effect. Assessment of a suicidal plan cannot be a one-time activity; the criteria must continually be reviewed if a nurse is to act effectively to prevent suicidal acts.

Hatton et al. (1977) have developed a system for rating suicidal risk; this system appears in Table 18-2. The types of behavior listed are not mutually exclusive, nor are they arranged in a hierarchy. The types of behavior are evaluated in terms of a hypothetical scale from 1 to 9. A rating of 1 to 3 indicates low risk. A rating of 4 to 6 indicates moderate risk, and a rating of 7 to 9 indicates high risk. All criteria are not necessarily relevant to all clients.

Particular groups are at risk because the nature and quantity of stressors they experience. Hankoff

Table 18-2. Assessing the degree of suicidal risk*

Behavior or symptoms	Intensity of risk		
	Low	**Moderate**	**High**
Anxiety	Mild	Moderate	High, or panic state
Depression	Mild	Moderate	Severe
Isolation/withdrawal	Vague feelings of depression, no withdrawal	Some feelings of helplessness, hopelessness, and withdrawal	Hopeless, helpless, withdrawn, and self-deprecating
Daily functioning	Fairly good in most activities	Moderately good in some activities	Not good in any activities
Resources	Several	Some	Few or none
Coping strategies/devices being utilized	Generally constructive	Some that are constructive	Predominantly destructive
Significant others	Several who are available	Few or only one available	Only one, or none available
Psychiatric help in past	None, or positive attitude toward	Yes, and moderately satisfied with	Negative view of help received
Life-style	Stable	Moderately stable or unstable	Unstable
Alcohol/drug use	Infrequently to excess	Frequently to excess	Continual abuse
Previous suicide attempts	None, or of low lethality	None to one or more of moderate lethality	None to multiple attempts of high lethality
Disorientation/disorganization	None	Some	Marked
Hostility	Little or none	Some	Marked
Suicidal plan	Vague, fleeting thoughts but no plan	Frequent thoughts, occasional ideas about a plan	Frequent or constant thought with a specific plan

*From Hatton, Corrine, Sharon Valente, and Alice Rink. 1977. Suicide: Assessment and Intervention. New York: Appleton-Century-Crofts.

and Einsedler (1979) have defined the following groups as being at risk:

1. *Alcoholics*—these individuals are characterized by poor impulse control, dependency, depression, and excessive use of denial. Often they drink and take drugs concurrently, which increases the possibility of an adverse reaction and death. The suicidal intent should be considered perhaps in a passive sense; however, over time the ultimate result remains the same—death.

2. *Elderly*—as noted previously, suicide in the elderly population represents 25% of the total of suicides committed. Those individuals are confronted with multiple life changes, including physical as well as psychological assaults on the sense of self. Previous coping strategies and available support systems are significant factors in determining depression and suicide risk.

3. *Adolescents*—during this time of rapid physical growth and psychological adjustment,

a person is particularly vulnerable. Suicide as a solution to conflicts is the second leading cause of death in this age group (for further discussion see Chapter 15).

4. *Police and physicians*—these individuals often deal with multiple serious problems on a regular basis. Society expects them to "take care of" and protect its members. This expectation can cause conflict and role confusion when the expectation is not met. Neither police officers nor physicians are expected, however, to experience stress or have difficulties of their own, lest they be labeled as "unfit." Stressors are allowed to build; isolation from significant others because of job responsibility and a sense of personal failure may lead to the suicidal act.

5. *Help-rejecting clients*—clients of this category are those who are unable to accept treatment or follow prescribed treatment plans. This type of client produces conflict for nurses as well as a sense of frustration, anger, and guilt. In a sense these clients are attempting to maintain a sense of control over their lives as well as prevent further loss of self-worth. Changes in life-style required by a treatment regimen may cause feelings of dependence and a lack of being a viable, active self. For example, a cardiac client with a lethal arrhythmia was advised to reduce his physical workload. The possibility of altering his productivity led to feelings of apprehension and uncertainty as to his own worth. He proceeded to return to work at his previous pace. Upon 3-month follow-up, his work schedule was noted by the clinical specialist. She was able to negotiate some changes in his work schedule, thus reducing both the risk of further heart damage and the loss of self-worth.

Responding to treatment plans also implies that one will indeed reach a higher level of wellness. In some cases, getting well may be threatening, since this change in role impacts on current relationships. It becomes important to determine the benefits of remaining in a "sick role" that could lead to self-destruction. Nurses also need to identify the risk to personal worth that is required by adhering to a prescribed treatment plan. The value of choice of a "good life" is a consideration for both the client and the health professional—particularly when life is at risk. The degree of helplessness is said to vary with the assumptions one has about causes of the uncontrollable events. Individuals who blame themselves are more likely to exhibit greater helplessness than those who blame external events or persons. Murphy (1982) suggests that learned helplessness results in cognitive, motivational, and emotional deficits. Cognitively, individuals expect uncontrollability. Lack of motivation ensues because of individuals' perceptions that things will not change, no matter what they do. Self-esteem is lowered and depressed affect results when individuals feel that events are beyond their control.

Murphy (1982) notes that there is considerable evidence that major life changes perceived and labeled as negative lead to increased risk for physical or psychosomatic illness. Learned helplessness seems to result when individuals are exposed to uncontrollable events and believe that nothing can be changed.

However, there are limitations to the theory. Further questions will need to be asked: When is helplessness adaptive or maladaptive; under what depressive conditions does helplessness exist; and during what situations do individuals seek causal information? Murphy concludes that psychiatric–mental health nurses have a vital role in determining expectations of control in their clients and in testing attributional theories. Strategies of intervention may then be designed to assist individuals in coping with situational and transitional events that generate feelings of helplessness.

Inpatient supervision of the suicidal client is a primary nursing objective. Measures that are critical in working with suicidal clients include:

1. Locating the client's room in an area central to the nurses' station
2. Removing sharp objects and other items which could be potentially dangerous

3. Remaining with clients if they are using items such as razors, lighters, etc.

4. Knowing where the client is at all times during the day—particularly at times when staff is busiest (e.g., change of shift and team meetings) or when there is a smaller staff (nights and weekends)

5. Checking periodically throughout the night at irregular times so that clients cannot identify a pattern in *your* behavior

6. Noting client behavior patterns and changes (e.g., decreased communication; sudden mood lift; increased frustration, dependency, or hopelessness; lack of interest in surroundings; subtle discussions of activities, such as with family, that no longer include the client)

7. Being alert to storing of medications

8. Observing relationships with other clients, i.e., those that may *reinforce* self-destructive behaviors or those individuals who may become confidants of the suicidal client

9. Maintaining lines of communication and interest—respecting privacy while at the same time not allowing the client to remain socially isolated

10. Identifying positive aspects of self and assisting the client in their integration into self

11. Reinforcing positive accomplishments

12. Assisting the client to deal with expression of angry feelings—promoting an atmosphere in which clients can test out more effective methods of coping with anger

13. Incorporating clergy (pastor, priest, rabbi) into the treatment plan at client's request

14. Examining client behavior within the context of current relationships and identifying stressors and strengths within those relationships (family, job, etc.)

15. Exploring alternative methods of coping with feelings should self-destructive feelings occur again

16. Identifying "lifeline" persons to contact when clients begin to feel they cannot control impulsive behavior

EVALUATION

Client, family, and/or significant others in collaboration with the nurse should review client progress toward goal attainment. The following areas need to be included in the evaluation process:

1. Degree of resolution of internal conflicts relative to affective disorders

2. Level and degree of goal attainment, i.e., improvement in client functioning demonstrated by use of more adaptive coping strategies

3. Identification of goals that need modification and revision

4. Designation of appropriate support systems other than the nurse-client relationship
   a. Available support systems within the context of current client relationships, e.g., friends, co-workers, clergy
   b. Community mental health centers which provide walk-in treatment, day/night hospitals
   c. Specialized services for treatment of affective disorders, e.g., mood clinics, suicide prevention centers and "hot-lines," and lithium clinics

TERTIARY PREVENTION

Continued research in the area of family dynamics and the interrelationship of etiological variables is an important concern of tertiary prevention. Nurses need to direct efforts toward modifying the environment to reduce the intensity of some of the stress factors that ultimately lead to depression.

What happens to an individual who has experienced loss? Where is the follow-up care? When symptoms disappear, the underlying dynamics may remain. A discussion of what significance the loss holds as well as its correlation with past losses can facilitate an individual's understanding of coping measures. Nurses need to be acutely aware of the need to provide follow-up care for clients who have experienced depressive responses, even though symptoms may have subsided. It is quite easy and comfortable for these clients to revert to maladaptive methods of coping when stress again becomes overwhelming. It is therefore of utmost importance that such a client, who may possess little self-worth, feels that there is always a link with someone who cares. Contact with family members and others in the community can help the client to develop a social network of support that can facilitate reentry into the community.

CHAPTER SUMMARY

Loss occurs throughout the life cycle. The grieving process can be a healthy, adaptive response to loss. Individuals develop a pattern of response to loss that is based on early childhood experiences. It is important to understand the significance of these early experiences with loss in order to facilitate the open sharing of feelings. Grief is a normal response. Nurses can encourage people to participate actively in the grieving process, whether the grief be for the loss of a person, status, self-esteem, a body part, or a bodily function. Through such active involvement, a person can lay a foundation for coping with future losses.

Recurrently unhealthy or maladaptive responses to loss situations may lead to a delayed grief reaction, depression, or even suicide. Nurses need to recognize that many variables may be responsible for the development of a depressive response. Several major theories of depression, manic-depressive reactions, and suicide have been presented. A nursing assessment must reflect an integration of these theories, since no one theory can explain depressive behavior.

Individual and group therapy, the administration of psychopharmaceuticals, and electroconvulsive therapy have been discussed as treatment modalities.

Nursing intervention has been discussed in terms of the three levels of prevention. Primary prevention is directed toward facilitating an individual's coping with loss. Secondary prevention involves the use of specific techniques in response to each of the predominant themes of depression. The goals of tertiary prevention are to minimize the effects of loss, through discussion of an individual's adaptive (or maladaptive) mechanisms, and to facilitate the reentry of the client into the community.

SENSITIVITY-AWARENESS EXERCISES

The purposes of the following exercises are to:

- Develop an awareness of the vulnerability of client-families to major affective disorders (mania, depression, suicidal behavior)
- Develop an awareness of the interrelationship of factors in the etiology of major affective disorders
- Develop an awareness of the subjective experiences of clients who are suffering from affective disorders
- Develop an awareness of your own feelings and attitudes that are aroused when working with clients experiencing major affective disorders

1. Try to imagine that you are experiencing one of the following disorders. Explain why you selected that particular disorder, and describe how you think it might feel to experience that disorder/behavior.
   a. Manic disorder
   b. Depressive disorder
   c. Self-destructive behavior
2. Describe what it would be like to have a family member or a significant other suffer from one of the major affective disorders. Which disorder do you think would be easiest to tolerate in a family member or significant other? Why? Which would be the hardest to tolerate? Why?
3. What might be some of your feelings and reactions as a nurse to clients who are suffering from major affective disorders? Helplessness; frustration; anger?
4. Examine your feelings toward clients who have attempted to take their own lives. Would your reaction vary from situation to situation? Why?
5. Imagine that you are a community health nurse engaged in health promotion and maintenance activities with new parents. What high-risk factors (biological,

psychological, sociocultural, intellectual, and spiritual) would you observe for that might predispose parents and/or their children to a major affective disorder?

6. Develop a plan for counseling parents about child rearing that incorporates principles and goals for primary prevention of major affective disorders.

REFERENCES

Akiskal, H., and W. McKinney
1975 "Overview of recent research in depression." Archives of General Psychiatry 32:285-290.

Anthony, J., and T. Benedeck (eds.).
1975 Depression and Human Existence. Boston: Little, Brown & Co.

Arieti, S.
1974 "Affective disorders: manic-depressive psychosis and psychotic depression." In American Handbook of Psychiatry. S. Arieti (ed.-in-chief). New York: Basic Books, Inc., Publishers.

Atchley, R.
1980 "Aging and suicide: reflection of the quality of life." In Epidemiology of Aging—Second Conference. S. Haynes and M. Feinleib (eds.). U.S. Department of Health and Human Services.

Bahnson, C.B., and M.B. Bahnson
1966 "Role of the ego defenses: denial and repression in the etiology of malignant neoplasm." Annals of the New York Academy of Sciences 125:827-845.

Bart, P.
1971 "Depression in middle-aged women." In Women in Sexist Society. V. Gornick and B. Moran (eds.). New York: Basic Books, Inc., Publishers.

Beck, A.
1967 Depression: Causes and Treatment. Philadelphia: University of Pennsylvania Press.

Beck, A., et al.
1979 Cognitive Theory of Depression. New York: The Guilford Press.

Bibring, E.
1953 "The mechanism of depression." In Affective Disorders. P. Greenacre (ed.). New York: International Universities Press.

Bowlby, J.
1973 Attachment and Loss: Separation, Anxiety, and Anger, vol. 2. New York: Basic Books, Inc., Publishers.

Brownmiller, S.
1975 Against Our Will. New York: Simon & Schuster, Inc.

Burgess, A., and L. Holstrum
1974 "Rape trauma syndrome." American Journal of Psychiatry 131(9):981-986.

Capodanno, A., and S. Targum
1983 "Assessment of suicide risk: some limitations in the prediction of infrequent events." Journal of Psychosocial Nursing and Mental Health Services 21(5):11-14.

Chesler, P.
1972 Women and Madness. New York, Doubleday & Co., Inc.

Clark, T.
1976 "Counseling victims of rape." American Journal of Nursing 76:1964-1966.

Clinard, M.B.
1974 Sociology of Deviant Behavior. New York: Holt, Rinehart and Winston, Inc., pp. 627-631.

Court, J.H.
1972 "The continuum model as a resolution of paradoxes in manic-depressive psychosis." British Journal of Psychiatry 120:133-141.

Dunner, D., J. Fleiss, and R.R. Fieve
1976 "The course of development of mania in patients with recurrent depressions." American Journal of Psychiatry 133:907.

Durkheim, E.
1951 Suicide. New York: The Free Press.

Engel, G.
1962 Psychologic Development in Health and Disease. Philadelphia: W.B. Saunders Co.

Farberow, N. (ed.)
1975 Suicide in Different Cultures. Baltimore: University Park Press.

Fieve, R.
1975 "Unipolar and bipolar affective states." In The Nature and Treatment of Depression. F. Flach and S. Draghi (eds.). New York: John Wiley & Sons, Inc., pp. 145-160.

Freud, S.
1917 "Mourning and melancholia." In The Collected Papers, vol. 2. London: The Hogarth Press Ltd.

Gibbons, J.L.
1960 "Total body sodium and potassium in depressive illness." Clinical Scientist 19:133-138.

Gordon, V.
1982 "Themes and cohesiveness observed in a depressed women's support group." In Issues in Mental Health Nursing, 4:115-125.

Greene, W.A.
1966 "The psychosocial setting of the development of leukemia and lymphoma." Annals of the New York Academy of Sciences 125:794-801.

Hatton, C., S. Valente, and A. Rink
1977 Suicide: Assessment and Intervention. New York: Appleton-Century-Crofts.

Hauser, E., and F. Feinberg
1976 "Operational approach to delayed grief and mourning process." Journal of Psychiatric Nursing 2:26-29.

Hicks, D.
1977 ''Not a sex act—a violent crime.'' Modern Medicine 1:15-21.

Kallman, F.J.
1953 Heredity in Health and Mental Disorders. New York: W.W. Norton & Co., Inc.

Kicey, C.
1974 ''Catecholamines and depression: a physiological theory of depression.'' American Journal of Nursing 74: 2018-2020.

Klein, M.
1934 ''A contribution to the psychogenesis of manic-depressive states.'' In Contributions to Psychoanalysis 1921-1945. London: The Hogarth Press Ltd.

Kolb, L.
1977 Modern Clinical Psychiatry, ed. 9. Philadelphia: W.B. Saunders Co.

Kucera-Bozarth, K., N. Beck, and L. Lyss
1982 ''Compliance with lithium regimens.'' Journal of Psychosocial Nursing and Mental Health Services 20(7): 11-15.

LeShan, L.
1966 ''An emotional life-history pattern associated with neoplastic disease.'' Annals of the New York Academy of Sciences 125:780-793.

Lindemann, E.
1944 ''Symptomatology and management of acute grief.'' American Journal of Psychiatry 101:141-148.

Linden, L., and W. Breed
1976 ''Epidemiology of suicide.'' In Suicidology: Contemporary Developments. E.S. Schneidman (ed.). New York: Grune & Stratton, Inc.

Menninger, K.
1938 Man Against Himself. New York: Harcourt, Brace & Co.

Murphy, S.
1982 ''Learned helplessness: from concept to comprehension.'' Perspectives in Psychiatric Care 20(1):27-32.

Papa, L.
1980 ''Responses to life events as predictors of suicidal behavior.'' Nursing Research 29(6):362-369.

Richman, J.
1971 ''Family determinants of suicidal potential.'' In Identifying Suicidal Potential. D. Anderson and L. McLean (eds.). New York: Behavioral Publications, Inc.

Russell, D.
1975 The Politics of Rape. New York: Stein & Day, Publishers.

Santora, D., and P. Starkey
1982 ''Research studies in American Indian suicides.'' Journal of Psychosocial Nursing and Mental Health Services 20(8):25-29.

Satir, V.
1972 Peoplemaking. Palo Alto: Science and Behavior Books, Inc.

Schneidman, E., and N. Farberow (eds.)
1957 Clues to Suicide. New York: McGraw-Hill Book Co.

Schultz, J., and S. Dark
1982 Manual of Psychiatric Nursing Care Plans. Boston: Little, Brown & Co.

Secunda, S.
1973 ''The depressive disorders: special report.'' In Department of Health, Education, and Welfare publication. Washington, D.C.: U.S. Government Printing Office.

Seligman, M.
1973 ''For helplessness: can we immunize the weak?'' Psychology Today 73:90-95.

Selkin, J.
1975 'Rape.'' Psychology Today 75:71-76.

Spitz, R., and K.M. Wold
1946 ''Anaclitic depression.'' In The Psychoanalytic Study of the Child. New York: International Universities Press.

''Testing for melancholia''
1981 Emergency Medicine, May, 1981, pp. 118-119.

Wetzel, R.
1976 ''Hopelessness, depression and suicidal intent.'' Archives of General Psychiatry 33:901-908.

ANNOTATED SUGGESTED READINGS

Cohen, S.
1977 ''Helping depressed patients in general nursing practice.'' American Journal of Nursing 77:1007-1009.
This article directs its attention toward depression as it is experienced in the general hospital setting. The presentation is in the form of programmed instruction, which proves useful for the beginning undergraduate student.

Fitzpatrick, J.
1983 ''Suicidology and suicide prevention: historical perspectives from the nursing literature.'' Journal of Psychosocial Nursing and Mental Health Services 21(5).
This article presents a comprehensive review of literature on nursing and suicide. Early studies on grief, general and specific nursing interventions, suicide as crisis and general health problem, and depression were major foci of the reviewed publications. Fitzpatrick concludes that suicidology and suicide prevention are of concern not only to nursing but to all health professions. She stresses the importance of continued research to develop a more thorough understanding of the nurse's role within the context of the health care team.

Seligman, M.
1974 ''Depression and learned helplessness.'' In The Psy-

chology of Depression: Contemporary Theory and Research. R. Friendman and M. Katz (eds.). Washington, D.C.: V.H. Winston & Sons, Inc.

Seligman proposes a direct correlation between lack of control over one's environment and depression: individuals who learn through repeated life experiences that they are unable to effect change eventually opt not to even attempt change. The inability to make changes in one's life and environment then leads to a sense of helplessness. Helplessness, in turn, becomes a learned lifestyle.

Swanson, A.

1976 "Communicating with depressed persons." Perspectives in Psychiatric Care 13(2):63-67.

Swanson suggests that therapeutic communication with the depressed person requires theory as well as practice. The key concept presented is the nurse's use of self to facilitate the client's perception of communication (or lack of it) with the external environment. Problematic verbal and nonverbal messages are identified, and attempts are made to match these two components of the communication process. This article is valuable in that the active role of the nurse in the communication process is emphasized as a mechanism for assisting the client to communicate needs in an adaptive manner.

FURTHER READINGS

Crary, W., and G. Crary

1973 "Depression." American Journal of Nursing 73:472-475.

Drake, R., and J. Price

1975 "Depression: adaptation to disruption and loss." Perspectives in Psychiatric Care 13:163-166.

Flack, F., and S. Draghi (eds.)

1975 The Nature and Treatment of Depression. New York: John Wiley & Sons, Inc.

Freedman, A.M., H. Kaplan, and B. Sadock

1976 Synopsis of Comprehensive Psychiatry, vol. 2. Baltimore: The Williams and Wilkins Co.

Jamison, K., et al.

1980 "Clouds and silver linings: positive experiences associated with primary affective disorders." American Journal of Psychiatry 137:198.

Malmquist, C.

1971 "Depressions in childhood and adolescence." New England Journal of Medicine 284:887-995, 995-1014.

Schmagin, B., and D. Pearlmutter

1977 "The pursuit of unhappiness: The secondary gains of depression." Perspectives in Psychiatric Care 15(2):63-65.

Stuart, G.

1981 "Role strain and depression: a causal inquiry." Journal of Psychosocial Nursing. 19:20.

CHAPTER 19

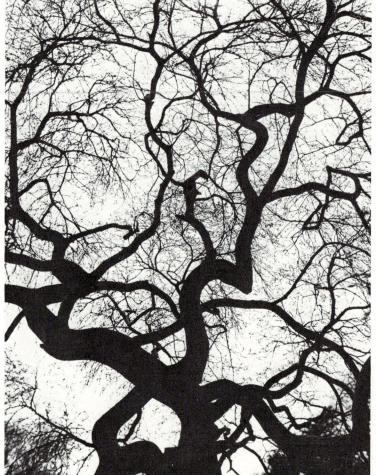

Photo by Michael Mather—Peter Arnold, Inc.

Coping through dependence, domination, and detachment

CHAPTER FOCUS

An understanding of human responses to stress is essential to the professional practice of nursing. Persons who experience ever-present anxiety and conflict and who try to cope with their anxiety and conflict through dependence, domination, or detachment are usually described as neurotic. Horney (1945) regarded such coping patterns as compromise solutions for neurotic conflicts. These neurotic conflicts may be manifested in anxiety disorders, somatoform disorders, dissociative disorders, and some types of eating disorders.

There are many persons whose modes of adapting to life and to their culture are not characterized by observable symptoms but who are more vulnerable to anxiety and have fewer options for coping than the average person. Many such people can be found among the clients requiring nursing services in any health care setting. It is important that the professional nurse be able to identify clients whose anxiety levels and coping responses are so significantly different from those of the average person that efforts to promote health are inhibited.

In keeping with the philosophy of professional nursing presented in this book, this chapter will focus on mental health maintenance (primary prevention) in persons coping with physical illness and injury, who may be more vulnerable to stress than the average person. Attention will also be given to aspects of primary prevention for families in which children may be at risk of developing neurotic coping patterns of dependence, domination, or detachment.

This chapter will, of course, also focus on secondary and tertiary prevention in anxiety disorders, somatoform disorders, dissociative disorders, and two types of eating disorders (anorexia nervosa and bulimia).

"Neurosis" and "psychoneurosis" have become commonly used terms in our society. Neuroses frequently figure prominently in works of literature and the cinema, in which they are subject to prevailing societal attitudes toward mental illness.

The nomenclature and diagnostic categories established by the American Psychiatric Association usually reflect the societal attitudes of the times. For instance, in 1934, psychoneuroses were included under the major diagnostic category of conditions "with psychosis." In 1947, psychoneuroses were removed from the psychosis classification, and they were placed in a catch-all category of "other diagnoses." In 1953, in a statistical report filed by the National Institute of Mental Health, psychoneuroses were classified as one of the "psychophysiologic autonomic and visceral disorders," and they were referred to as "psychoneurotic reactions." In 1966, psychoneurotic reactions were subdivided into three groups: anxiety reaction, psychoneurotic depressive reaction, and all other psychoneurotic reactions (McGrory, 1980).

The most recent revision of the American Psychiatric Association's *Diagnostic and Statistical Manual of Mental Disorders* (DSM-III) was in 1980. At that time, neuroses were eliminated as diagnostic categories and were included instead under the categories of affective disorders, anxiety disorders, somatoform disorders, dissociative disorders, and psychosexual disorders. However, the DSM-III states that the DSM-II terms for the neuroses are acceptable alternatives to the current DSM-III nomenclature. McGrory (1980) believes that these frequent changes in classifying the neuroses reflect confusion about the nature and treatment of the disorders.

We have attempted to avoid a disease orientation and to focus the mental health nursing process toward identifying and intervening in patterns or themes of behaviors that are distressing to clients and their families. However, diagnostic categories are frequently used in health care settings, and nurses should be familiar with those classifica-

tions. Therefore, along with nursing diagnoses, the associated DSM-III classifications are also included. Theoretical discussions are aimed at showing how the following DSM-III disorders are responses to conflict and stress:

Anxiety disorders
　Generalized anxiety disorder
　Panic disorder
　Phobic disorders
　Obsessive-compulsive disorder
Dissociative disorders
　Psychogenic amnesia
　Psychogenic fugue
　Multiple personality
Somatoform disorders
　Hypochondriasis
　Conversion disorder
Eating disorders
　Anorexia nervosa
　Bulimia

EPIDEMIOLOGICAL AND SOCIOCULTURAL ASPECTS OF NEUROSES

Although there are no definitive demographic studies available, it is believed that the neuroses are among the more prevalent functional disorders in our society. It is estimated that 15% to 20% of the population of the United States suffers from neurotic disorders (Colby and McGuire, 1981). However, reliable data on incidence are difficult to obtain for a variety of reasons. One factor may be that many people function effectively and successfully despite neurotic problems until or unless they are confronted with unbearable situational stress. Kubie (1974), for example, mentions that "a neurotic process . . . need never manifest itself in formal symptomatology." Another factor is that many people are treated by private physicians for a variety of complaints or seek assistance from private resources that may not be involved in any diagnostic data collecting system.

There are, however, many indications that substantial numbers of people are seeking help in coping with psychological stress. Among these indications is the extensive use of minor tranquilizers. Diazepam (Valium), for example, is currently one of the most frequently prescribed pharmaceuticals in the United States. The rapid growth in the popularity of such short-term group modalities as encounter sessions, assertiveness training classes, and EST (Erhard Seminar Training) also indicates a widespread need for help in coping with life's problems. The growing number of self-help books dealing with a wide range of psychological problems and the many works of fiction dealing frankly with neuroses also suggest that many people are interested in finding ways to function more comfortably.

The relationship between culture and mental disorders has long been recognized (Dunham, 1976). Interpersonal psychiatrists (for example, Horney and Sullivan) incorporated sociocultural concepts into their theories of neuroses and other psychiatric disorders. Some of the research that has been done during the past quarter-century has been concerned with the relationship between social status and the incidence of mental disorders. Hollingshead and Redlich (1958), in an extensive study of social stratification and mental disorders, found a much higher incidence of neuroses in the upper and middle classes than in the lower classes.

Other researchers have looked at the incidence of neuroses in relation to geographic locale and gender. Dohrenwend and Dohrenwend (1974) found the incidence of neuroses to be higher in urban areas than in rural areas. McGrory (1980) reported that neurosis is the most frequent diagnosis of women who are treated as out-patients and that 3,718 (per 100,000 population) more women than men are admitted to state psychiatric hospitals with a diagnosis of neurosis. This statistic led McGrory to contend that it is primarily women who are affected by the long-standing confusion in categorizing, understanding, and treating neuroses.

According to David (1976), a summary report of the World Health Organization's Expert Committee on Mental Health found that the incidence of neuroses and personality disorders in the developing countries was "difficult to ascertain." The report indicated that there is evidence that more than 40 million people in the developing countries suffer from "serious untreated mental disorders" but that reliable statistics on the incidence of neuroses in developing countries are not readily available.

Cultures may differ considerably in the traits they seek to encourage in their people. In Japan, for example, strong group identification and social conformity are emphasized. In contrast, in the United States individuality, competitiveness, and personal freedom are considered important. The group orientation of the Japanese involves rather strict rules and formalities for social behavior, even within the immediate family. Child-rearing practices in Japan promote group identification through direct teaching, role modeling, and the use of the group as the punisher of persons who engage in undesirable behavior. The admonition "People will laugh at you," given by the Japanese mother to her child, tends to induce feelings of shame in the child, which help to reinforce group identification. A culturally specific neurosis, termed *Taijin Kyofu*, appears in Japan. It is manifested as a phobic fear that one's gaze can hurt other people and a corresponding reluctance to meet with others (Nakakuki, n.d.).

The advances in science and technology of the last quarter-century have had a profound impact upon the people of many cultures. Technological advances have taken much of the drudgery out of the struggle for survival that prior generations experienced. These advances have often been accompanied by changes in long-established social mores and values. In the United States, changes in the status of women and in religious practices are but two examples. When a culture is in a state of transition, or when an individual who is sensitive to stress moves from one cultural environment to another, a form of culture shock may occur (see Chapter 4). In the United States, values and life-styles have been undergoing rapid change during the past two decades. The stress that such change has induced has caused increasing feelings of helplessness and alienation in many people.

THEORIES OF NEUROSIS
Psychological theories
PSYCHOANALYTIC THEORIES

According to Freud (1936, 1960, 1969), neuroses originate during the period of psychosexual development (see Chapter 6). Neuroses are related to innate drives or instincts, particularly libidinal (sexual) and aggressive drives, and to the struggle to express these drives in a socially acceptable manner. Neurotic anxiety is generated by these libidinal and aggressive impulses.

The eventual outcome of psychosexual development depends upon the experiences of the early years. The child who experiences repeated trauma, or in whom excessive fears are generated during developmental sequences, may develop a neurotic character structure (Drellich, 1974).

In Freudian theory intrapsychic conflict is viewed as a universal experience. The basic conflict is between the unconscious fantasies, wishes, and so on that are seeking overt expression and the forces (ego defense mechanisms) that are striving to prevent overt expression and keep such fantasies out of awareness. The drives or instincts most frequently involved are libidinal and aggressive drives. Such thoughts or fantasies, termed ''drive derivatives'' in Freudian terminology, are considered primitive, since they have their roots in early developmental years. The overt expression of such primitive fantasies and wishes represents a danger to the person. The danger may come from external reality, or it may result from a conflict with the individual's moral standards and values. For example, acting out aggressive or sexual wishes impulsively against another person may result in punishment or pain. Such action may also result in feelings of shame and guilt.

One of the functions of the ego is to keep unacceptable thoughts or fantasies out of awareness to prevent their overt expression. Covert or disguised expression takes place primarily through dreams, humor, and sublimation.

Drellich (1974) points out that when the two forces (unconscious fantasies and wishes versus ego defense mechanisms) are in balance, there is little interference with a person's daily functioning or personality. In a neurosis, however, there is an imbalance between the two forces. The degree or intensity of inner turmoil is greater. The person with a neurotic character has less variety of defenses and fewer options for gratification of unconscious strivings than does the ''normal'' person. Available defenses or compromise solutions are used more frequently and more rigidly than in the nonneurotic personality. Anxiety is aroused when unconscious wishes threaten to become conscious. Additional defenses are then needed to control anxiety.

INTERPERSONAL THEORIES

One interpersonal theorist, Karen Horney, viewed cultural conditions as being as important as biological or psychological factors in the development of neuroses. Horney (1937) proposes that it is not only individual experience but also the specific cultural environment in which individuals live that generates neuroses. For instance, Horney points out that rigidity is only symptomatic of neurosis when it deviates from culturally acceptable behavior. Horney gives as an example the cultural context of Western folk or peasant society, in which ''rigid suspicion'' of anything new or different was often the norm and she states that such behavior should be regarded as ''normal rigidity'' and not as evidence of neurotic rigidity.

Therefore, according to Horney (1937, 1939, 1945), it is to both the cultural context and the individual experiences of early developmental years that we must look for the origins of neurotic conflict.

The young child who consistently or frequently experiences feelings of fear, distrust, and conditional love with parents and other significant people may well acquire enduring attitudes of fear and distrust of significant people in the environment. The child may also experience helplessness, confusion, and rage in a world perceived as frightening. Since the young child is dependent upon the care-giving people in the environment, the ways in which he or she can cope with such traumatic experiences are limited. During childhood, submitting, rebelling, or withdrawing may be the only alternatives available for coping with noxious situations and with the rage, helplessness, and other emotions such situations arouse. Whether the child surrenders, fights back, or withdraws into the self depends upon the particular situation and the innate characteristics of the child. Surrendering, fighting back, or withdrawing may begin in early life as a conscious effort to cope with a confusing or frightening situation. When such experiences repeatedly occur, the child's response may become automatic or unconscious. Over a period of time, the child develops attitudes about the self and other people that become internalized and part of neurotic conflict (Portnoy, 1974).

According to Horney's theory, the conflicts in neurosis center around meeting the basic interpersonal needs that we all share. The needs for affection, attention, approval, and recognition from others and the opportunity for expressing aggression and sexuality are some of the familiar human needs. In meeting such needs, everyone at times experiences distress, anxiety, guilt, and conflict within themselves and between themselves and others.

People are pulled or driven by a compelling need or striving to move toward others, to become dependent upon others. This striving is blocked, however, by an equally compelling need or striving to move against others (to dominate them) or to move away from others (toward detachment).

Trapped between such powerful and opposing forces in meeting fundamental needs, the individual is immobilized and unable to function unless some adaptive compromise can be achieved. Such a compromise can be achieved, and the conflict somewhat defused in its ability to generate unmanageable anxiety, if the person accedes to one aspect of the conflict in all interpersonal situations

and forces opposing aspects out of awareness.

For example, one compromise solution is to move toward others by being compliant, submissive, and dependent—in a sense, to seek protection of others as a means of containing fears and anxiety and maintaining self-esteem. Another compromise is to move against others by gaining power or domination over them. A third compromise solution is to move away from others—to become detached and, when possible, to limit interpersonal interactions (Horney, 1945).

Such compromise solutions represent defensive maneuvers that serve to control anxiety and to enable an individual to function despite underlying conflict. It must be emphasized, however, that both the compromise and the conflict are unconscious. Once a particular compromise solution has been adopted, and the other aspects of the conflict repressed, the compromise becomes a part of the personality structure of the individual; it is used compulsively and indiscriminately in every interpersonal situation, whether it is appropriate or not (Horney, 1945).

The compromise solutions discussed thus far have been in relation to conflicting attitudes toward other people. However, neurotic conflicts also involve attitudes about the self. The use of a number of compromise solutions to cope with underlying conflicts brings about an alienation from the self and a lack of genuine self-awareness or self-understanding. Such a situation also results in some inflexibility or rigidity in behavior.

One form of inflexibility or rigidity that can be observed in some people is compulsive behavior. This kind of behavior can be interpreted as an unconscious extension into the external world or an effort to maintain internal order. Whereas a little compulsive neatness and organization lends order to our lives, carried to extremes it can be a burden to others who have to comply with rigid demands and prescribed methods of carrying out various endeavors.

For example, a noncompulsive student who shares a dormitory room with a highly compulsive student runs into difficulties in trying to maintain harmony. Frustration of the compulsive person's need to maintain strict order in the surroundings, or in ways of accomplishing certain tasks, arouses anxiety that may be expressed as overt anger. The presence of anxiety when compulsive needs are frustrated is a clue that compulsivity is an ego defense mechanism.

The need to maintain unity within the self despite feelings of anxiety, helplessness, insecurity, and inferiority can also lead to a compromise solution that is designed to counteract and force out of awareness the existence of internal conflict. People who have a compulsive craving for perfection and admiration may come to view their actual selves as unreal and may create instead an *idealized image*. These people then try to live up to this idealized image and to receive affirmation from others that the self and the idealized image are one and the same (Horney, 1945; Portnoy, 1974).

The particular qualities that are incorporated into an idealized image depend upon the ideals, beliefs, and needs of an individual. For example, people may regard themselves as intellectually or morally superior to others. Although the attitude may initially arise as a fantasy, the idealized image may be internalized as an unconscious defense and thus come to be regarded as the real self. Like other compromise solutions, the idealized image is compulsively adhered to and defends against any efforts on the part of others to point out discrepancies between the way people see themselves and the way others see them. Although the idealized image serves the defensive purpose of reinforcing feelings of self-worth and denying conflicts, it also tends to alienate people from themselves. In addition, such a compromise solution prevents the experiencing of pride in genuine achievements, a situation that can lead to new conflicts. Additional defense mechanisms may then be necessary to cope with them.

BEHAVIORAL THEORIES

Behavioralists such as Skinner (1953) and Wolpe (1974) view neuroses as conditioned or learned responses to a painful stimulus. Urbanization, social insecurity, and overcrowding are ex-

amples of aspects of the environment that frequently serve as stimuli for anxiety. Because a stimulus produces anxiety and this anxiety, in turn, engenders more anxiety (neurotic anxiety), when the stimulus is again encountered, a reflex arc is established where conditioned responses become self-perpetuating and circle back upon themselves (Wolpe, 1974).

Since anxiety functions at a primitive or subcortical level of the brain, behavioralists hold that logical reasoning and the development of insight are ineffective in controlling anxiety. Behavioralists explain that neuroses and neurotic anxiety are due to a disturbance in the arousal and inhibition of the central nervous system. This aberrant arousal-inhibition system leads to abnormal neural synopsis and pathological reflexes and cognition. In turn, pathological thoughts and actions become established as learned patterns of behavior (Beech and Perigault, 1974). Therefore, the only effective intervention into neuroses, according to behavioralists, is the elimination of old patterns of neurotic behavior, primarily through desensitization* (Marks, 1976).

Biological theories

Biological theories look at the role of biological factors in the etiology of neuroses. Family studies have not established a clear genetic basis for neurosis. For example, twin studies on phobia have shown that one twin may be phobic while the other is not (Marks, 1969). Yet twin studies on anxiety neurosis indicate that under conditions of severe stress the genotype is expressed. One research team found that 65% of monozygotic (MZ) twins and 13% of dyzygotic (DZ) twins studied had symptoms of anxiety, but that 50% of the MZ twins and only 2.5% of the DZ twins studied evidenced anxiety neuroses. The researchers explained this apparent genetic loading by hypothe-

---

*Desensitization is discussed in the treatment modalities section of this chapter.

sizing that under moderate stress conditions the response is one of adaptive anxiety, but that under conditions of severe anxiety, symptoms of anxiety neurosis are elicited (Slatter and Cowie, 1971).

Biochemical imbalance or disorder has also been explored as an etiological basis for neuroses. The lactate hypothesis purports that alkalosis, hypocalcemia, and increases in both blood lactate and epinephrine stimulate the anxiety that is present in neurosis. However, Ackerman and Sachar (1974) believe that, although lactate infusions seem to stimulate anxiety in some types of neurotic disorders (e.g., phobias), a conditioned response by people to their own "internal" somatic symptoms of dyspnea, diaphoresis, tachycardia, etc., is probably also involved. Thus, to date, a definitive relationship between a person's biochemistry and the development of anxiety neurosis has not been demonstrated.

Yet among the Polar Eskimo in northern Greenland, where the calcium content of the diet is low, the anthropologist Anthony Wallace (1961) has noted the incidence of *piblotoq* (a culturally patterned form of hysteria) to be high, especially in the winter months. Wallace also points out that in the past century, along with an improved diet that has provided better calcium intake, there has been a dramatic decrease in the incidence of hysterical disorders among Western Europeans.

Some neurophysiologists have tried to explain the etiology of neuroses by looking at the relationship between the functioning of the central nervous system and behavior. For example, with an increase in corticofugal inhibition of afferent stimulation there is a decrease in self-awareness and body functioning. Via conditioning a feedback loop is set up, and a person reacts to stress with cognitive and physical disturbances that are manifested as conversion disorder or dissociative disorder (Bendefeldt et al., 1976). Such a neurophysiological explanation for the neuroses parallels biological explanations for the instinctive behavior of threatened animals. One animal pattern of instinctive behavior in response to danger is displayed by the frenzied motor reactions of birds that

are looking for a way out of an enclosed area. This "flight" or escape behavior may be compared to human tremors and dissociative disorders. Another pattern of instinctive behavior is demonstrated by frightened animals that become immobilized and "freeze in their tracks." This behavior pattern is sometimes referred to as the sham-death reflex and it parallels conversion disorders of blindness, deafness, and paralysis in human beings (Kretschmer, 1937; Ludwig, 1972).

Still other neurophysiological explanations are being sought for hypochondriasis and bulimia. In hypochondriasis, a disorder in the limbic or reticular activating system may permit impulses that usually are not consciously registered to be discerned and to cause discomfit. This explanation may prove to be similar to the gate control theory explaining phantom limb pain* (Slater and Roth, 1970). In bulimia, there may be a disorder in the central nervous system where the signals of satiation and craving for sweet foods are integrated.

The etiology of neuroses appears to be complex. Although biochemical, genetic, and neurophysiological factors are being investigated, a relationship between biology and neuroses has not been definitely demonstrated. Future research may more clearly indicate what role biological factors play in the etiology of neuroses.

Sociocultural theories

Sociocultural theories of neuroses examine the way that sociocultural factors contribute to people's vulnerability to neurosis and influence neurotic symptoms and patterns of behavior. Leighton and Murphy (1965) point out that there are several ways that culture can increase vulnerability to neuroses; chief among these are (1) childrearing practices that promote feelings of shame and guilt, (2) role stress, and (3) socially unrealistic expectations. In addition, such social stressors as unemploy-

---

*Refer to Chapter 7 for a discussion of the gate control theory and phantom limb pain.

ment, acculturative pressures, and marital discord may significantly weaken people's social support systems and function either as predisposing or precipitating factors in the development of neuroses. Horney (1939) views the person with neurosis as a "stepchild of (his or her) culture."

Because childrearing is very much influenced by cultural practices and social institutions, some social scientists have looked to sociocultural factors for an explanation of the higher incidence of neurotic behavior among women than among men. Chesler (1972) sees sex-role stereotyping and the crossing of sex-role stereotype lines as neurotigenic factors. Women are raised to be submissive, dependent, shy, and passive. According to Chesler, when women exhibit such "malelike" behaviors as competition, anger, and possessiveness, they are labeled "neurotic." Similar behaviors in men are perceived by society as "normal."

Yet, sex-role stereotyping may contribute to neurotic conflicts in both men and women. For example, Díaz-Guerrero (1955) holds that rigidly defined sex-roles among Mexicans engender among women frustration of their aggressive and sexual drives and among men guilt about the absence of such frustration. The frustration of Mexican women and guilt of Mexican men is strong enough to lead to the development of neuroses in both sexes, although neuroses are more common in Mexican women. The finding of Fabrega et al. (1967) that Mexican men are less apt to admit to neurotic symptoms when these symptoms are present than are Mexican women, because neurotic symptoms are not consistent with *machismo,* may partially account for the lower incidence of recorded neuroses among Mexican men.

Other social scientists see the diverse and often conflicting societal sex roles that women are expected to fulfill as contributing in the following ways to their greater vulnerability to neuroses:

1. Women who are not employed outside the home have only their families as a major source of societal gratification. In contrast, most men have two sources, work and family. Dissatisfaction with one area may be compensated by satisfaction in the other area. Unemployed women often have no alternative source of gratification.
2. Many women find housework frustrating, unchallenging, and lacking in prestige.
3. The homemaker role is unstructured and accomplishments may not be readily visible. For example, one client told a nurse, "When my children were young, I used to make all their clothes. It was a help financially but it also gave me a sense of having accomplished something at the end of the day. Otherwise, I washed dishes and clothes and they got dirty again. I prepared meals and they were eaten in 15 minutes."
4. Women experience greater job discrimination than do men. Women, more often than men, hold jobs that are beneath their educational preparation, skills, and abilities. In addition, working wives usually also have to assume the majority of the household responsibilities along with their employment responsibilities.
5. The diversity and conflicting nature of the sex-roles that women are expected to assume (roles as wife, mother, employee, etc.) may create overburdening and role stress for women (Chesler, 1972; Grove and Tudor, 1978; McGrory, 1980).

Still other social scientists believe that society and culture may foster the development of neuroses through factors that promote or engender feelings of anxiety, helplessness, insecurity, hostility, and/or emotional isolation in both men and women. For instance, Horney (1939) and Marcuse (1972) point to the contradictions in Western society that create confusion, conflict, and a sense of helplessness. The emphasis upon humility and brotherly love, for example, conflicts with the emphasis upon achievement, success, and competition.

Kubie (1974) observes that the ability to change is an essential ingredient of mental health. He notes, however, that many factors in Western culture not only inhibit the freedom to change but also reinforce the compulsive aspects of the human personality. Since compulsivity, or ''obligatory repetition,'' is so prominent a feature in neuroses, the reinforcement of this quality by society can be deemed neurotigenic. Kubie suggests that educational practices that emphasize ''drill and grill'' contribute to the loss of freedom by encouraging the automatic repetition inherent in neurotic processes.

In addition to contributing to people's vulnerability to neurosis, sociocultural factors also influence the symptoms and behavior patterns that are evidenced in neurotic disorders. In looking at the mental health status of individuals from non-Western societies or of Americans with non-Western cultural backgrounds, nurses can either erroneously look for manifestations of neuroses common in the United States or they can try to understand the indigenous or culturally patterned disorders of these clients. Among the non-Western types of neuroses that appear to be culturally patterned are those that are hysteria-like and those that are phobia-like.

Latah (found in Southeast Asia and Indonesia), *imu* (found in northern Japan), *saka* (found among the Wataita tribe of Kenya), and *pibloktoq* (found among Polar Eskimos in northern Greenland) are culturally specific forms of hysteria. Despite the distinctly different geographical areas and cultural groups in which they are found, *latah, imu, saka,* and *pibloktoq* manifest similar symptomatology. Victims become frightened; they may become agitated or violently excited; they scream obscenities, and they may engage in compulsive imitative behavior (echopraxia) or in compulsive imitative speech (echolalia). Victims may engage in compulsive imitation until they are exhausted. Although men occasionally display these culturally specific forms of hysteria, women are primarily affected (Aberle, 1961; Winiarz and Wielawski, 1936; Harris, 1957; Wallace, 1961; Suinn, 1970).

Definitive explanations have not been found for these culturally patterned forms of hysteria, but it has been noted that they tend to appear in cultures that are characterized by a low level of technolog-

ical development and by a dominance-submission relationship between men and women, with women assuming the submissive role. It has been suggested that, since women are primarily affected and much of the behavior manifested in these disorders is an exaggeration of behavior that is ordinarily acceptable for men (e.g., violence, obscene language), these culturally specific hysteria-like disorders reflect ambivalence about the submissive female role (Yap, 1952; Aberle, 1961; Harris, 1957).

After studying the Polar Eskimo, Parker (1962) suggests that those individuals who develop hysteria-like symptoms inappropriately use the interaction techniques that they acquired during socialization. Thus, their interaction techniques do not attract the attention of their social networks and sought-after nurturance and affection are not forthcoming. Parker concludes that, among the Polar Eskimo, hysteria-like symptoms function to attract the attention of the Eskimo's social environment and to place the Eskimo, once again, in the ''bosom'' of the social network. Parker also identifies the following characteristics that describe societies with a high incidence of hysterical behavior:

1. Socialization of children tends to be non-repressive of dependency needs and sexual drives, and there is relatively high satisfaction of dependency needs.

2. A cooperative social organization plus a communistic value system contribute to a world view that the social environment is basically nurturent and that in times of crisis aid will be forthcoming.

3. The female role is characterized by passivity and submissiveness, and it has lower status than the male role.

4. Religious practices provide socially acceptable situations and role models for the demonstration of hysteria-like behavior.

Pattison and Wintrob (1981) in their discussion of ''possession behavior/neurotic,'' also contend that in many cultures ''symbolized behaviors'' are a socially acceptable way of expressing personal and interpersonal conflict without evoking retribution from members of the family or the community.

Culturally specific phobia-like disorders also shed some light on the role of sociocultural factors in the etiology of neuroses. For example, among the Japanese there is a high incidence of *taijin kyofu,* which is a phobic fear *(kyofu)* of meeting people *(taijin).* Japanese who suffer from this phobia experience feelings of inadequacy, and they fear that their presence can harm and cause discomfort to others. Specifically, victims of *taijin kyofu* fear that their gaze can be harmful and bothersome; therefore, they avoid looking at people. In addition, victims of this phobia fear that they will blush, stutter, emit foul-smelling body odors, look ugly, or otherwise do things that will produce discomfort and harm in the people with whom they are interacting.

If *taijin kyofu* is to be understood, it must be considered within the context of Japanese culture. Japanese mothers tend to be nurturing and soothing to their children. Infancy and childhood are characterized by ready gratification of needs and little need frustration. Furthermore, Japanese mothers use much eye-to-eye communication, unaccompanied by speech, as a primary mode of mother-child interaction. Such eye-to-eye communication may convey pleasure, displeasure, sadness, frustration, etc. Therefore, Japanese children have first hand experience with the Japanese proverb, "The eyes speak as eloquently as the mouth." This factor may partially explain why the eyes are the locus of their neurotic disorder. In addition, Japanese children are reared to be group-oriented and to conform to the many rigid social rules and formalities of Japanese society. Individuals who violate these rules and formalities are met with social ostracism and humiliation. "Saving face," the avoidance of shame and humiliation, is a primary guideline for social interaction. Shame, as opposed to the Western idea of guilt, is an important concept in this Japanese neurosis. When victims of *taijin kyofu* avoid being among people, they also avoid the possibility of experiencing shame and humiliation (Nakakuki, n.d.).

In the United States today the technocratic nature of our society and the permeation of technology into our daily lives seem to be contributing to the development of a new phobia: compuphobia. Compuphobia, the fear of working with computers, is experienced by many people. This phobia has three aspects: (1) the general fear of using computers, which may stem from a person's quantitative or linguistic anxieties, (2) the fear of failing when working with computers, which may arise from a person's anxiety about loss of control, especially in the area of work, and (3) the fear of being replaced by technology (Suinn, 1983). This third aspect of compuphobia seems to relate to anxiety engendered by a sense of inadequacy, helplessness, and loss of control.

Thus, there is much evidence that sociocultural factors not only contribute to people's vulnerability to neurosis but also contribute to the pattern that symptoms and behavior take.

Holistic health concepts

The etiology of neuroses appears to be complex and multifactorial. An holistic health approach to neuroses integrates the five dimensions of self and looks at how these five dimensions are continuously interacting to promote healthy behavior or to contribute to neurotic behavior. For example, conflict between one's social behavior and one's cultural values and/or spiritual standards may generate neurotic anxiety and guilt. In addition, physiological and psychological symptoms are found in all neuroses and the form that these symptoms take varies from person to person and from society to society. Thus, it is likely that neurotic disorders arise from the interaction of psychological, physiological, intellectual, spiritual, and sociocultural factors. Sloman (1976) states that neuroses seem to develop when the symmetry among interacting etiological factors becomes so disrupted that a person cannot adaptively cope. Then maladaptive or neurotic coping behaviors emerge.

Nursing strategies should be based on an understanding of the holistic health status of clients and on the way that holistic health factors may facilitate healthy coping behavior or contribute to neurotic coping behavior. In this way, nurses will be able to adapt nursing intervention to the psychological, intellectual, physiological, spiritual, and sociocultural needs of their clients.

CHARACTERISTICS OF NEUROSES

Anyone who has worked in one of the health professions for any length of time soon becomes aware that it is more difficult and challenging to provide needed health services to some individuals than it is to others, regardless of the health problems involved or the complexity of the services required. Every professional nurse has, from time to time, encountered the helpless, dependent client whose demands upon staff time and attention seem excessive and disproportionate to the client's needs. Also familiar is the client who rejects the dependent role necessitated by a particular health problem and who defies medical orders and staff efforts designed to promote recovery. Such a client is often frustrating to nurses providing health services. Less frustrating, perhaps, but still of concern, is the detached individual who resists involvement with staff in the meeting of health care needs.

Nurses generally recognize the hypochondriac, the compulsive hand washer, or the severely phobic client as a person who is suffering from severe psychological distress. There is an awareness that the behavior or symptoms represent coping mechanisms essential to the individual's ability to cope. There is often less recognition that consistent interpersonal patterns of dependence, domination, or detachment are indicative of a similar type of psychological distress, or that such interpersonal patterns also represent unconscious coping mechanisms needed to control anxiety in a stressful situation.

It is important for the professional nurse serving clients who display such patterns to be aware that they represent unconscious efforts to cope with stress. Such interpersonal patterns may become exaggerated when a client is confronted with a health problem and placed in a dependent role in the health service structure.

In general, people who use neurotic coping patterns are functioning members of society. Many such individuals pursue careers in business, the professions, or the arts and often are highly successful in our competitive industrial society. Since there is little or no impairment in intellectual functioning, the achievement of educational and other goals is not impaired. Indeed, some neurotic traits may provide the impetus needed to achieve positions of dominance in society. A mild degree of compulsivity, for example, can be a definite asset in certain fields of endeavor requiring precision and attention to detail. A neurotic coping pattern thus may be helpful for an individual.

Neurotic individuals remain in contact with reality, in contrast to psychotic persons, who experience delusions and hallucinations (see Chapter 21). Even when such symptoms as phobias or compulsions are being experienced, there is an awareness that the behavior is in response to some internal force that cannot be resisted.

Some characteristics of persons with neuroses can, under certain circumstances, be interesting and charming. For example, the dramatic flair and histrionic features often associated with the hysterical personality are frequently regarded as attributes in such professions as the performing and creative arts. In addition, such characteristics can lend a certain richness to the lives of friends and relatives.

It should be kept in mind that each of us responds to experiences in an infinite variety of ways. Each person has innate and learned interests, attitudes, strivings, and ideals, as well as a multitude of other motivating forces. These may be expressed in innumerable ways at different times and under differing circumstances. Everyone needs relief from anxiety from time to time and makes use of defense mechanisms and other coping measures for this purpose. Neurotic behavior differs from normal behavior only in the degree of anxiety experienced and in the extent to which defense mechanisms are needed or available to help a person cope with it. The degree to which people are neurotic varies with circumstances, with their biological and psychological status, and with the culture in which they live.

There may be no overt symptoms or specific complaints on the part of clients with character neuroses. Vague expressions of dissatisfaction with life, concerns about developing lasting and meaningful relationships with others, or complaints about job satisfaction or working relationships may be the only problems mentioned even by those who seek psychiatric help. Family members or coworkers who have long associations with such people may be aware of certain inflexibilities or peculiarities in their personalities. They may even regard such people as being, in modern parlance, "uptight" and as having "hangups" in certain areas.

Some of the inflexibilities revolve around the ways in which such people relate to others. Their constant assumption of the submissive, dependent role or the dominant role can be frustrating to family, friends, and coworkers who are themselves more flexible. But such fixed attitudes and patterns in relations with others represent unconscious solutions to underlying conflict. People who compulsively utilize such inflexible behavior are aware of neither the underlying conflict nor their own inflexibility. They can readily justify or rationalize to themselves and to others their actions in any situation.

Underlying dynamics
DEPENDENCE ON OTHERS

Individuals who function on a submissive, dependent level in relations with others have excessive needs for attention, affection, and approval. To such people, acceptance by other people is essential to maintaining security. In order to achieve these ends, they may view other people as superior and adopt their attitudes and opinions. Since they

consider the approval of others to be essential to the maintenance of self-esteem, dependent people may function in a manner that is in accord with other people's beliefs and judgments rather than their own. Such traits may initially cause a hospitalized client to assume the "good patient" role, since submissiveness and dependence are often encouraged in health agencies. However, excessive demands for attention and approval and an inability to tolerate criticism or anything perceived as rejection will soon become apparent.

Each of us has a friend, relative, neighbor, or classmate who needs to be coaxed and pleaded with to join some group activity and who becomes hurt and upset when such urging is not sufficiently forthcoming. Each of us knows people who are often anxious and who become excessively tense and emotional when they are involved in a "fender-bender" automobile accident or another type of minor crisis. We are all familiar with people who need frequent emotional support, confirmation of any proposed activity, and approval of even minor achievements. Most of us are also flattered when our advice is sought in relation to the solution of problems or when we are effusively praised for our superior knowledge or experience. We may not often recognize the underlying needs being expressed, although we may tend, at times, to become skeptical when our advice is ignored, or to become annoyed or angry when demands exceed our ability or willingness to comply with them.

Such submissive, dependent behavior does not, of course, resolve the underlying conflict. The dependent role itself may lead to resentment, anger, or despondency.

DOMINATION OF OTHERS

People who cope with interpersonal relationships by dominating other people have underlying feelings that everyone is hostile to them. The strong need to maintain control over other people may be expressed in a variety of ways. Taking command in any situation may serve to threaten other people and thus maintain control. Overt expressions of anger when orders are challenged or not carried through can be effective in maintaining control and, in addition, can serve as outlets for anxiety. At other times, particularly in circumstances in which such direct methods would be ineffective, forms of subtle manipulation may be employed. Such manipulation may take the form of flattery, excessive concern about the plight of others, or efforts to make others feel obligated (Horney, 1945).

As in the case of the dependent person, such behavior is motivated by anxiety and conflict. Although the dependent aspects of the conflict are forced out of awareness, and partially maintained there by the dominating behavioral patterns, the dependence needs are still present. Situations, such as hospitalization, that place the person who distrusts others in a dependent role can be particularly threatening for such an individual.

In such a situation, there is often an inability to admit to oneself or others any feelings or fears, since to do so could be overwhelming. There is a strong need to prove to oneself and to others that one is strong and right, in order to maintain equilibrium and contain anxiety. Efforts to establish anything other than a superficial relationship usually fail, since relationships tend to be regarded as dangerous.

Although such methods of relating with other people tend to distort human relationships, the feelings and attitudes about the self are even more distorted. The vignette that follows may serve to demonstrate this point.

Mr. H. was admitted to a hospital in the small community where he lived; the diagnosis was peptic ulcer. Married and a father of two children, Mr. H. was in his late thirties and held an important position in a bank. While in the hospital, he continued to carry on business on the phone and through visits from employees of the bank.

During the visits Mr. H. on several occasions shouted at a co-worker and made disparaging remarks about his intelligence in front of hospital staff and the other client in the room. At other times, Mr. H. was heard to flatter the co-worker and then send

him off on a personal errand. When the charge nurse attempted to set limits on such business activities, Mr. H. became very angry and threatened to report her. Efforts to explain to Mr. H. that his own recovery was not being helped by the business activity and that the other client in the room was very ill and needed a quieter atmosphere only served to increase Mr. H.'s anger.

When the supervisor appeared to discuss the matter with Mr. H., he became very conciliatory and expressed concern about the other client. He flattered the supervisor about the way in which she ran the unit and expressed interest in her personal likes and dislikes. The next day he sent her tickets to a play they had discussed. The unit staff received a large box of candy.

Mr. H. continued to conduct business from the hospital room. When the subject was raised with him again, Mr. H. explained to the staff that his position was very important and that he was unable to rely upon the people under him. He attempted to convince the staff that he rested easier knowing that things were under control at the bank.

Since all of the nursing staff members were becoming frustrated in working with Mr. H., a group meeting was held to work out a plan of care. Underlying anxiety was identified as one of the major problems, and a plan of care that emphasized emotional support and health teaching through a one-to-one relationship was developed and implemented. However, Mr. H. initially thwarted any efforts to establish anything other than a superficial discussion. He said that he regarded talking about his experience as "sentimental hogwash." He resisted just as adamantly any interest in health teaching, and responded to the nurse's efforts to open any avenue of communication with sexually seductive remarks.

In a supervisory session with a mental health nurse, the staff nurse mentioned the frustration and humiliation she was experiencing in working with Mr. H. After a review of the content of the interactions, the nurse was able to identify Mr. H.'s responses as "distancing maneuvers" related to anxiety about the nurse getting too close psychologically. Once this nursing diagnosis had been formulated, the staff nurse was able to utilize an approach that encouraged the client to take the lead in discussing areas of concern to him. This ap-

proach was less threatening to the client and more effective in meeting some of the nursing care objectives.

DETACHMENT FROM OTHERS

The characteristics of people who resolve neurotic conflicts by becoming detached from others are in sharp contrast to those of dependent, submissive people. Detached people have strong needs to maintain independence and self-sufficiency. They have a strong drive to keep a distance between themselves and others and to avoid becoming emotionally involved. Intellectualization and a superior manner are two of the means used to accomplish this end. Although such people do not like being taken for granted, they often prefer being alone. Superficial relations with others may be amicable, but any effort to place such people in a dependent position or a position in which there must be submission to others' expectations arouses uneasiness, rebellion, and further emotional withdrawal.

As might be predicted, illness is bitterly resented by people with such strong needs for detachment from others (Horney, 1945). Any question about their personal life is likely to be regarded as a shocking intrusion, and attempts to give advice of any kind are apt to be perceived as attempts to dominate and to be met with resistance. Any health problem that results in dependence upon a health agency is likely to be resented and highly emotionally unsettling (Horney, 1945).

Symptoms of neuroses

Neurotic conflicts are believed to originate during childhood. The onset of symptoms usually occurs in late adolescence or early adulthood, although it may occur at any point along the life span, during periods of developmental or situational crisis. Developmental crises are the periods of vulnerability encountered as a person moves from one developmental stage to the next (see Chapters 6 and 13). Situational or incidental crises

occur when people are confronted with stressful events of such unusual intensity or duration that customary methods of coping are no longer effective. In the crisis state, additional defensive mechanisms are brought into play. For the individual who is particularly sensitive to stress, such defensive measures may include neurotic symptoms. People are especially vulnerable to emotional crises when stressful events coincide with crisis points in development, such as adolescence or old age. Health problems that involve admission to a hospital or dependence upon a community health agency for treatment and rehabilitation are examples of stressful situations that may lead to development of conditions that are even less adaptive than the three personality patterns just discussed—symptom neuroses.

As we noted earlier, the ways in which neuroses are expressed are determined by culture. It is interesting to note that even within the same culture, the ways in which neuroses are expressed vary from one period to another, much as fashions in clothing and other aspects of life change. This is not to imply that neurotic symptoms are as whimsical as dress styles. Rather, such symptoms reflect many aspects of our constantly changing environment, and our relationship to it. As lifestyles change, the ever-creative human being utilizes whatever resources are available to achieve both healthy and neurotic ends.

Neuroses are classified according to observable symptoms. The primary symptom in a neurosis gives the neurosis its name. Symptoms represent, to a great extent, either direct manifestations of anxiety or defense mechanisms utilized to control anxiety.

ANXIETY DISORDERS*

Anxiety disorders are overt manifestations of anxiety; they are classified according to the physiological and psychological effects the anxiety has

---

*Refer to Chapters 7 and 13 for further discussion of anxiety and stress.

upon an individual. Although anxiety is a prominent feature and one of the motivating forces in all neuroses, the anxiety neuroses differ from the other symptom neuroses in the degree of anxiety and in the lack of any stable defense mechanisms or symptom formation to counteract the anxiety. This form of neurosis may be chronic, or it may occur in acute attacks.

▶ Generalized anxiety disorder

Experiences of chronic anxiety closely resemble the physiological and psychological responses to fear. The emotional responses are often described as feelings of apprehension, awe, and dread and fear of impending disaster. In the chronic form, anxiety neurosis is exhibited through such character traits as timidity, indecisiveness, self-doubt, inability to concentrate or organize activities, and aggressive outbursts. Vague fears and feelings of inferiority may be verbalized. Insomnia and nightmares may occur.

The physiological symptoms of muscle tension, chronic fatigue, restlessness, palpitation, and somatic complaints are common. Since a sustained high level of anxiety has an effect upon the autonomic nervous system—and, indeed, upon the functioning of all body systems—psychosomatic and other physiological disorders may coincide with chronic anxiety or be precipitated by it (see Chapter 16).

▶ Panic disorder

The most dramatic form of anxiety neurosis is the acute anxiety attack, which, as its name implies, comes on suddenly and overwhelms people with a terrifying anxiety that is akin to panic. The sudden onset, without apparent cause, often occurs when people are alone and away from home. Although they are acutely aware of the anxiety and its physiological aspects, the reason for the occurrence is not known to them. The source is, of course, within the self, internal and unconscious, although it may be associated with or triggered by environmental stress.

An attack may last from several minutes to several hours. The emotional response is accompanied by rapid breathing and heart rates, muscle tension, and restlessness. Palpitation, trembling, profuse perspiration, faintness, and dizziness as well as nausea, vomiting, and diarrhea may convince sufferers that they are having heart attacks or even that they are going to die.

To an observer, the face is flushed, and the pupils are dilated; pulse rate and respiratory rate are very rapid. The person is extremely restless and perspires heavily. The ability to answer questions or follow directions may be very limited. Since many of these symptoms also occur in some physical illnesses, the possibility of such an illness should be ruled out before a diagnosis of acute anxiety attack is made.

Anyone who has experienced the anxiety that occurs when one awakens from a nightmare can understand the distress of an acute anxiety attack. The following vignette may help to clarify some aspects of such an attack and of anxiety neurosis in general.

Mary J., a young college student who was enrolled in a social work program was very shy and retiring in class. She rarely participated in classroom discussion, and when called upon to express an idea or opinion, she became very tense, restless, and obviously uncomfortable. She readily acceded to the opinions and decisions of other students in the class, even on controversial issues about which she privately expressed different opinions. When course assignments required that she speak before the group or participate in panel discussions, her obvious level of anxiety made other students uncomfortable. Mary's achievement on written assignments and examinations indicated that she was intellectually mastering the material, and she was receiving fairly high grades.

During the course of the semester Mary became very dependent upon the teacher, constantly seeking approval and guidance outside of the classroom. When the teacher was unable to spend as much time with her outside of class as Mary demanded, or when the suggestion was made that she discuss in class some of the points she brought to the teacher, Mary reacted with an outburst of anger at the teacher. The outburst was followed shortly by submissive and conciliatory actions, including excessive praise and compliments.

Mary, who had an older brother and a younger sister, described her family as being religious and very strict. High moral standards and demands for achievement had been stressed throughout her life. Failure in either area had been severely punished. Mary believed that her parents favored her brother because he was a boy and her sister because she was prettier and more like the mother. The mother and the younger sister often went on vacations together and shared many other activities—a practice that at times left Mary with the feeling of being alone and abandoned. Mary often expressed envy of her college classmates, whom she described as being more independent and having more fun than she did.

When Mary was placed in a social agency for field work practice, she continued to seek out the former teacher and even attempted to have the teacher intervene on her behalf with her agency supervisor, whom she described as being very difficult and impossible to please. Mary described her efforts to memorize all of the procedures and techniques the agency used, and she expressed the wish that she could exchange places with the clients she was serving. The agency supervisor described Mary as being disorganized and unable to plan or conduct even the simplest interview.

Mary experienced an acute anxiety attack in her car while driving to the agency one day. Following the attack, she became so fearful of leaving her immediate neighborhood that she had to temporarily withdraw from the program and seek professional help in coping with her anxiety.

▶ Phobic disorders

A phobia is a persistent pathological fear. The object of a phobia can be almost anything in the environment to which fear can be attached. Some of the more common phobias currently found in Western culture involve closed spaces, open spaces, heights, and various means of travel. A number of phobias have been given Greek names —for example, claustrophobia and agoraphobia.

Phobias are believed to occur far more commonly than statistics indicate (Kolb, 1977); they are often associated with anxiety reactions and other forms of neurosis.

A phobia represents a transfer of internal anxiety to some object in the environment. Two major mechanisms, projection and displacement, are combined in a complex and unconscious process to accomplish this end. The mechanism of projection transforms an internal psychic threat into a fear of some object in the environment; displacement serves to transfer the emotional investment—the anxiety—to the selected object. These maneuvers have the effect of changing anxiety into a more manageable form—fear. The feared object can then be avoided, thereby further controlling the anxiety. Although the avoidance may inhibit one's lifestyle, it does serve to maintain functioning in other spheres. Thus, as in other neuroses, the containment of anxiety and the preservation of functioning are the primary gains.

Fear of an elevator—to cite one fairly common type of fear—is not necessarily a pathological experience. Many of us have qualms when we step onto an elevator. But this mild fear differs from that of a phobia. Instead of having a pathological origin, it often stems from having been stuck in an elevator between floors; it is relatively easily overcome, and we get on the elevator. People with a phobia are unable to do so; they avoid riding an elevator even if they reside on an upper story of a tall apartment building and become, in effect, prisoners of their apartments.

For the person who is trapped in such a phobic pattern, many needs, such as shopping for food and other necessities, must be met by other people, and many of the onerous chores of living can thus be avoided. These kinds of effects and the additional attention often given the phobic individual by family and friends provide the secondary gains that are typical of many of the neuroses. Such secondary gains may serve to reinforce the phobia.

It is interesting to note that the object of a phobia may change to meet changing conditions in the environment. For example, the pathological fear of being bitten by a horse, described by Freud in 1903 in ''The Analysis of a Phobia In a Five Year Old Boy,'' would not serve as a containment for anxiety in current society, in which horses are relatively rare. But it may well have been a very prevalent phobia in an era when the horse was the major means of land travel and transport. An airplane or bus phobia would serve the same psychodynamic purpose today.

Phobic disorders that begin after puberty (usually in late adolescence or early adulthood) in persons who live in a highly industrialized, mobile society such as that of the United States, often involve less specific phobic objects than those discussed so far. *Social phobias* (interpersonal phobias) occur in the interaction with one other person rather than with a group of people or a crowd. Some therapists view social phobia as a stage in the development of agoraphobia. However, opponents of this view point to the fact that, unlike the social phobias, which have equal sex distribution, agoraphobia is found more frequently in women than in men (Gray, 1978). Agoraphobia, the fear of open spaces, in current terminology refers to the fear of entering public places. Manifestations of this phobia can vary in degree from an inability to leave one's own home to the somewhat less restrictive inability to travel any distance from one's own neighborhood without experiencing overwhelming anxiety. Agoraphobia is currently one of the most prevalent forms of phobia (Marks, 1969).

The fear of being promoted in one's work (fear of success), which may be manifested as acute anxiety attacks or depression, and an abnormal fear of contracting a disease such as cancer are also common in modern society.

It should be noted that not everyone who experiences phobic fears succumbs to the inhibiting restrictions. Some individuals attempt, by sheer force of will and repeated exposure, to overcome their phobias. For example, a person who has a fear of heights may attempt to master this phobia by becoming a mountain climber. (This is not to imply that all mountain climbers are phobic.) But it is probable that a phobic person does not derive

the same quality of joy and pleasure from mountain climbing as the nonphobic person. This effort at mastering a phobia is termed ''reactive courage.''

▶ Obsessive-compulsive disorder

The most observable symptom that characterizes an obsessive-compulsive reaction is the repetitious performance of ritualistic acts. When one observes a person with this disorder, one is struck by the persistence in the performance of behavior that, in itself, is useless or that is made useless by the repetition. For example, washing one's hands or flushing a toilet are perfectly reasonable acts unless they must be repeated some magical number of times, as occurs in a compulsion. The observer of such a compulsive person is also struck by the intensity and concentration with which such acts are performed and by the obvious tension and discomfort of the performer.

Not available to the eyes of the observer are the obsessive thoughts or impulses that keep recurring despite the individual's efforts to banish them. The life of the obsessive-compulsive person is beset by such thoughts.

As in all neuroses, the compulsive behavior represents an effort to control or contain anxiety arising from unconscious conflict. The intrusion of the obsessive thoughts into consciousness signals the danger that repression may not be completely effective in keeping the conflict out of awareness. The obsessive thoughts, which represent the expression of a part of the conflict as an unacceptable idea or impulse, increase the anxiety and further threaten the ability to function.

The compulsive behavior also serves as a mechanism for banishing obsessions and controlling guilt and anxiety. The conflicts in this disorder frequently concern one's views of good and evil—particularly aggressive and sexual thoughts and impulses that come into conflict with internalized standards and beliefs. The ritualistic behavior expresses, at least symbolically, aspects of the underlying conflicts and the self-punishing efforts at controlling guilt. The hand-washing compulsion is clearly an effort to wash away something, although the ritualistic aspects and magical quality indicate that it is a far more complex process. The ritualistic behavior may appear meaningless or useless to the observer and sometimes is also so regarded by the performer. However, it cannot be interrupted or prevented without extreme anxiety or even panic being aroused.

Compulsive behavior may consist of a single act, carried out some magical number of times, or it may involve complex rituals, but the repetitive nature of the behavior remains in both instances. In addition to hand washing, which is frequently seen, compulsions take many forms having to do with aspects of living and working. Complex rituals in bathing and dressing are very common.

In the milder forms of obsessive-compulsive behavior, a single compulsive act may serve to contain anxiety and enable a person to reestablish character defenses and to return to the premorbid state. In the more severe forms, anxiety is not contained, increasingly more elaborate rituals develop, and steadily greater portions of the individual's life are devoted to carrying them out. The more severe forms are quite resistant to treatment and may become chronic.

An obsessive-compulsive neurosis can begin at any period of life, although it most often appears in adolescence. The onset is usually associated with developmental or family crisis or situational stress.

The following vignette illustrates a severe form of obsessive-compulsive neurosis.

Jane M., a young woman of 24, was brought to a mental health clinic by her husband, who said that she had developed such elaborate rituals for getting dressed each morning that she was unable to get to work on time. The rituals included repeated hand washing and a pattern of dressing and undressing that took several hours to accomplish. These activities were interfering not only with Jane's life but also with her husband's, since he was unable or unwilling to leave home until she was ready to leave also.

Jane's compulsive behavior began shortly after their marriage. It started with an inability to throw away dirt after she swept the kitchen floor. The hand washing started shortly after that incident, and the other rituals soon after that. At the time of the visit to the clinic, Jane was unable to do any of the housework because of her preoccupation with dirt. As a consequence, her husband had assumed these chores. The history revealed that Jane had refused to have sexual relations with her husband after the first month of marriage.

Jane had always done well in school and had graduated from college with honors. She was currently employed as an accountant. Her employer thought highly of her work and, despite the current difficulties, continued to employ her.

Jane was the only child in a middle-class family that she described as being very strict and upright. Her mother took great pride in maintaining her home in an immaculate condition, and was completely unable to understand Jane's current inability to do the same. Although the parents had always placed demands upon Jane to excel in school and to conform to their precepts, they were also very proud of her and rewarded her for her achievements.

During the course of treatment at the clinic, Jane was very consistent in arriving on time. However, the hand-washing ritual increased to the point that, even though she arrived at the clinic on time, she would be late for appointments. She also developed an additional ritual that symbolically expressed her anxiety and ambivalence. This ritual consisted of repeatedly walking up to the front door of the clinic and then retreating back to the sidewalk.

Psychotherapy and the administration of anti-anxiety drugs were combined in the treatment. Although Jane made some progress, the therapy was not completely effective in eliminating the symptoms.

This vignette hints at some additional features of obsessive-compulsive disorder. For example, the hand-washing ritual results in painfully chapped hands. The obvious embarrassment and discomfort that accompany the activity—particularly when it is done in a public rest room—are evidence of the self-punitive, masochistic nature of the symptom. The treatment of the husband—and, to a lesser degree, the therapist (in keeping the therapist waiting for each appointment)—demonstrates the sadistic nature of the behavior. Such sadistic and masochistic traits, although unconscious rather than deliberate, are common features of the disorder. They may represent a reenactment of earlier experiences in the life of the neurotic person. The secondary gains that the symptoms provide Jane are fairly obvious. The concern and attention of her husband and the avoidance of the boring chores of housework, which were taken over by the husband, may well have served to reinforce the symptom picture.

DISSOCIATIVE DISORDERS

Dissociative disorders represent a form of psychological flight from the self in which a part or all of the personality is denied, or dissociated. The most frequently occurring form of dissociative reaction is *amnesia,* in which a part or all of a person's past life is forgotten or, more accurately, forced out of awareness through repression. In partial amnesia people are unable to recall or remember a significant portion of their experience. Total amnesia is characterized by failure to recall any aspects of past life, including such vital information as name, place of residence, names of family and friends, and occupation.

Amnesia comes about in response to extremely anxiety-provoking situations experienced by persons who exist in chronic states of anxiety. The precipitating events often are traumatic situations that involve loss of or rejection by a loved one. Amnesia may be preceded by dream-like or trance states, referred to as *fugues,* during which a person may travel distances from home, act out impulsively, or engage in childish behavior. The defense mechanisms that are involved in amnesia are repression and denial.

To the casual observer, the person with amnesia appears normal and often seems quite calm. Intellectual functioning in spheres other than those involved in the amnesia remains normal, and there is little overt evidence of anxiety.

Typically, people with amnesia come to psychiatric attention when they are brought to an emergency room or psychiatric hospital by the police, who have found them wandering aimlessly during the trance-like state or to whom they have appealed for help because of their memory loss.

Although in popular fiction persons with amnesia sometimes take up new lives and live them for years, amnesia is usually an emergency response from which people recover in a relatively short time. A psychiatrist may use hypnosis to treat the disorder. During a hypnotic trance, people may be able to provide information about themselves that has been repressed, although it will not usually be available when they come out of the hypnotic state into a conscious state. In some instances the therapist may suggest to clients that they will be able to recall certain facts when they come out of the trance.

MULTIPLE PERSONALITY

Multiple personality is a disorder characterized by a primary personality that is usually shy and introverted and two or more alter or secondary personalities, each exhibiting values, behaviors, and sometimes ages and sexual orientations that differ from each other and from the primary personality. At any given time, the personality that is "out" (dominant) controls the person's behavior (Coons, 1980). Popularized reports of actual case histories of multiple personalities include *The Three Faces of Eve* and *Sybil*.

Amnesia is always present initially in the primary personality and may be experienced as "blackouts," "fainting spells," or "blank spells." Secondary personalities may have varying degrees of awareness of or interest in one another. A personality that has total awareness and memory of *all* coexisting personalities is said to have "memory trace." A personality that is aware of the thoughts, feelings, and behavior of at least one other personality is said to have "co-consciousness." The personality that has memory trace is often very helpful in psychotherapy. In addition to these characteristics, people with multiple personality disorder may experience headaches, conversion disorders, brief psychotic episodes, and difficulties with interpersonal relationships. Drug abuse and suicide are also common in people with multiple personality disorder (Coons, 1980; Greenberg, 1982).

During their childhood, people with multiple personality disorder have usually suffered severe physical and/or sexual abuse. Often one parent is abusive while the other parent, although aware of the child abuse, remains a passive onlooker. The victimized child is coerced by threats of severe punishment into not divulging the abuse to others. In order to cope with the physical and psychological stress engendered by the abuse, the child utilizes defense mechanisms of dissociation, repression, and amnesia. Dissociation may begin with the creation of imaginary playmates (a normal and not uncommon occurrence in childhood) who later evolve into alter personalities. As imaginary playmates (conscious level of functioning) or alter personalities (unconscious level of functioning) the purposes served are fundamentally the same—to help the primary personality cope with the loneliness, trauma, and hostility of life and to act out impulses (often of a hostile or sexual nature) that are not sanctioned by the primary personality (Coons, 1980; Greenberg, 1982).

Recent studies using electroencephalography indicate that there is as drastic a variation in the brain waves of the primary and secondary personalities inhabiting a multiple personality's body as there is from one ''normal'' person to another. This finding indicates that each personality of a multiple personality has a functionally different brain and a separate reality from the other personalities (Hale, 1983).

The goals of psychotherapy are for each of the pesonalities to become aware of and to communicate with the other personalities about the traumas that contributed to the disorder and, ultimately, for all of the discrepant personalities to become fused or integrated (Greenberg, 1982).

SOMATIFORM DISORDERS

▶ Hypochondriasis

Hypochondriasis is a morbid preoccupation with the state of one's health. Such concern can range from a series of minor complaints to the conviction that one has some serious disease.

Hypochondriacs are frequently seen in acute health care settings. Their repeated visits with the same, or similar, complaints often arouse anger or indifference on the part of health professionals. People's persistent beliefs that they have a physical illness should, of course, always be taken seriously and evaluated medically.

Hypochondriasis represents an unconscious transformation of internal conflicts into physical symptoms, which are more acceptable to the individual and to others than is a psychological disorder. As in other forms of neurosis, the symptoms represent attempts to contain anxiety and maintain integration of the personality. It should be kept in mind that the symptoms seem very real to the person experiencing them and that they may result in as much physical discomfort as they would if they were real. Attempts to reason such symptoms away, or to explain them on a logical basis, will at best be rejected and at worst result in increased anxiety and the need for additional defense mechanisms to cope with it. The less adaptive defense mechanisms that might then develop could take a psychotic form, since the false belief that one has a physical disorder is a delusional idea. The individual who entertains such a belief is on the borderline between neurosis and psychosis. Fenichel (1945) observed that hypochondriasis may be a transitional state between neurosis and psychosis.

▶ Conversion disorder

Hysterical neurosis may be viewed as psychological flight from overwhelming anxiety. Such flight is somewhat comparable to physical flight from a feared object or incident. Psychological flight may take the form of a *conversion disorder*. In such a disorder, unconscious conflict and the attendant anxiety are transformed, through several defense mechanisms, into a physical symptom in a body part. As in a phobia, the conflict is changed, through condensation, displacement, and projection, from an internal phenomenon into a physical symptom. The symptom is usually expressed as impairment of one of the senses or as paralysis of a limb or other body part. A symptom such as hysterical blindness or paralysis of a hand or a forearm may symbolically express some aspect of the underlying conflict and may, temporarily, eliminate the anxiety.

Conversion disorders produce self-limiting symptoms that serve as emergency responses to situations that generate overwhelming anxiety. Such reactions occur most often in persons who have chronic anxiety levels, and they occur more often in persons who tend to believe in magic and mysticism than in persons who do not hold such beliefs.

A young woman was brought into an emergency room of a general hospital from a family court session, with the complaint that she had suddenly become blind. Physical examination revealed no pathology that could account for the symptom. The examining physician was struck by the complete absence of any anxiety or other emotional response to what could be presumed to be a terrifying experience. Following a psychiatric consultation, a diagnosis of conversion disorder was made and the woman was admitted to the psychiatric unit, where, after a few days of supportive treatment, she recovered her sight and was discharged to an outpatient clinic.

The woman had become blind during the family court session moments after her husband had refused to consider a reconciliation and had demanded a divorce and custody of their children. The couple had been having marital difficulties for several years following their immigration to the United States from Puerto Rico.

The blindness symbolically expressed, in part, the woman's unwillingness or inability to "see" or accept the abandonment by her husband.

The total lack of observable anxiety is a common feature of conversion disorder. Termed "la belle indifférence," this feature often serves as a clue that the problem is a psychological one rather than a physical one. Hysterical paralysis of an arm

or a hand, which may be found in battle neuroses and other situations that involve an underlying conflict centering around aggression, is another clue that a problem is psychological rather than physical. Such symptoms rarely conform to the neurological pathways that they would normally follow if there were a physiological basis for their occurrence.

EATING DISORDERS*

▶ Anorexia nervosa

Anorexia nervosa is a condition that is not usually included among the neurotic disorders. We have included it in this chapter because it has many features in common with neuroses. Anorexia nervosa resembles a neurosis in that, apart from the symptom formation, there is little interference with intellectual functioning and reality testing and in its compulsive nature. Kolb (1977) cites a compulsive drive to be thin as a prominent feature of this disorder.

Anorexia nervosa is characterized by excessive dieting, which is often carried to the point of severe malnutrition and emaciation. In some instances the disorder results in death. The condition appears to involve a disturbance in body image, since, even in an emaciated state, the individuals tend to perceive themselves as overweight. Anorexia nervosa often has its onset in adolescence; it may have been preceded by an overweight condition. Although it can occur in men, the majority of people with this disorder are young women. Such women are often highly intelligent, well-educated people, some of whom are found in the health professions. The equation of thinness with beauty in modern culture and the focus upon diet foods and activities may influence, somewhat, the incidence of this condition, but these factors cannot account for the severity and persistence of the disorder (Dikowitz, 1976; Kolb, 1977; Bruch, 1978; Boskind-White and White, 1983).

---

*Refer to Chapters 15 and 17 for further discussion of eating disorders.

The origins of anorexia nervosa are believed to lie in the early developmental stages, in which disturbances in the mother-child relationship result in ambivalent feelings toward the mother. A wish to remain a child is sometimes fostered by the mother. Resistance to food and to attempts at treatment are prominent features of this condition.

▶ Bulimia

Bulimia is an eating disorder that is characterized by binge eating (often done in secret) and by self-induced purging. The foods that are compulsively consumed during binges are usually high in calories and sweet (e.g., ice cream, pastries). Purging is usually accomplished through self-induced vomiting and the use of laxatives. Gastrointestinal disorders and severe dental problems (gastric acid regurgitated with vomitus destroys tooth enamel) often are consequences of long-term purging.

Bulimia is differentiated from anorexia nervosa in two respects: (1) people suffering from bulimia, unlike those suffering from anorexia nervosa, are aware that their eating behavior is abnormal, and (2) because of their pattern of binging and purging, bulimic individuals do not experience the severe weight loss that is associated with anorexia nervosa. Similarities between bulimia and anorexia nervosa include the following: (1) depressive symptoms are associated with both conditions, and (2) both bulimia and anorexia nervosa are found predominantly in Caucasian, adolescent females from the upper-middle or upper socioeconomic strata of society (Powers, 1980; Spitzer et al., 1981; Boskind-White and White, 1983; Herbert, 1983).

TREATMENT MODALITIES

The therapeutic modalities used in the treatment of neuroses include many of the measures employed in the treatment of the other emotional disorders. The most frequently employed modalities in the treatment of neuroses are individual psychotherapy, family therapy, group psychotherapy, behavior therapy, and administration of psychopharmaceuticals. The therapeutic milieu and recreational, occupational, and other activity therapies are included in the brief-hospitalization modality.

Individual psychotherapy
PSYCHOANALYTICALLY ORIENTED PSYCHOTHERAPY

Psychoanalysis is a type of individual psychotherapy developed by Freud for the treatment of neurosis. It has been adopted as a therapeutic modality by analysts in all of the schools of psychoanalytic thought, including those of Horney, Sullivan, and Fromm. Psychoanalysis is a long-term and intensive form of therapy that is oriented toward the restructuring of the personality. Emphasis is placed upon growth of the ego and resolution of unconscious conflicts. Psychoanalysis may last over a period of two or more years, with sessions being held as often as three times a week.

Psychoanalytically oriented psychotherapy is a modified form of psychoanalysis in which the goals are more limited. The method of treatment is much the same as that in psychoanalysis, but the objective is symptom reduction or change in areas of the personality that are troubling to the client. Psychoanalytically oriented psychotherapy may extend over a period of a year or more. It is often the method of choice for clients who are unsuitable for analysis or unwilling or unable to undergo analysis but who could benefit from a limited form of therapy.

SHORT-TERM PSYCHOTHERAPY

Short-term, or brief, psychotherapy is another type of individual psychotherapy. As the name implies, it is a brief form of psychotherapy designed for people in emotional crisis. Such a crisis can arise in a neurotic person as a result of any form of situational stress perceived as a threat or danger. As had been noted earlier, almost anything can precipitate a crisis response in a vulnerable individual. Sifneos (1972) describes two forms of brief psychotherapy. In the first, anxiety-provoking (or dynamic) psychotherapy, the goal is to achieve some change in the client's problem-solving ability and interpersonal relationships, rather than simply symptomatic relief. These clients are carefully selected. In the second, anxiety-suppressive (or supportive) psychotherapy, the aim is the reduction of anxiety through the interpersonal techniques discussed in connection with the nurse-client relationship (see Chapters 9 and 10). Supportive psychotherapy is often used as a crisis intervention measure, in combination with brief hospitalization and other forms of therapy, in the treatment of clients who have the more disabling forms of symptom neuroses.

Family therapy*

Oftentimes, when a person develops a neurotic disorder, the client and the client's family become involved in family therapy. Family systems theory views the neurotic disorder of a family member as evidence of dysfunction within the family system. The family system becomes unbalanced, anxiety is generated in a family member, and that family member develops a neurotic disorder. For example, multigenerational family therapists describe neurotic individuals as people with a low level of self-differentiation. Family therapy focuses on resolution of unresolved emotional attachments with one's parents, differentiation of self from one's family of origin, and identification and modification of one's role in the family triangle (Beal, 1978). Structural family therapists assume that neurotic disorders are a result of the anxiety engendered by dysfunctional family transactional patterns. Structural family therapy focuses on helping family members establish new transactional patterns or scripts. Interactional family therapists believe that neurotic disorders are related to

the anxiety and confusion produced by vague and ambiguous rules regulating family interaction. Interactional family therapy focuses on clarifying these rules.

Group psychotherapy*

People suffering from neurotic disorders usually benefit from insight-oriented group psychotherapy. Psychoanalytically oriented group therapy is perhaps the most effective and the most common type of group therapy used in the treatment of the less maladaptive forms of neuroses. The therapist is either an analyst or a person who is skilled in both analytic method and group process. The group is usually limited to about eight members, who are carefully screened by the therapist. The long range goal is to work through basic conflicts that provoke anxiety and that interfere with clients' ability to function. Group therapy with people who are experiencing neurotic disorders tends to be conducted in an out-patient rather than an in-patient setting.

Desensitization

Desensitization therapy, a form of behavior modification, seeks to extinguish maladaptive behavior. There are two types of desensitization therapy: in vivo and fantasy. In vivo desensitization requires that a client be exposed to the real life situation or object that produces anxiety. Exposure to the anxiety-producing event can be done in steps (a client is gradually exposed to anxiety-producing situations of increasing intensity) or all at once (a client is suddenly put in the anxiety-producing situation). The latter method is referred to as implosion or flooding. Fantasy desensitization, on the other hand, requires that a client actively imagine being exposed to the situation or object that generates anxiety. Muscle relaxation techniques may

---

*Refer to Chapter 12 for an in-depth discussion of family dysfunction and family therapy.

*Refer to Chapter 11 for an in-depth discussion of group therapy.

be used as aids in both in vivo and fantasy desensitization (Marks, 1976). Desensitization therapy is most frequently used to treat clients with phobias, anxiety disorders, and sexual perversions.

Psychopharmaceuticals

Minor tranquilizers, or anti-anxiety agents, are widely used in the treatment of neuroses and other anxiety states, either alone or in combination with other therapeutic modalities. Baldessarini (1977) points out that two of these drugs—diazepam and chlordiazepoxide—are among the most commonly prescribed drugs in the United States. Although the current era has been described as the "age of anxiety," human beings have, throughout recorded history, used a variety of substances to help them cope with the noxious feelings of anxiety. Such substances have included alcohol, opium derivatives, and barbiturates. Research is continuously being conducted in an effort to find chemical substances that are more effective and less toxic in controlling anxiety. The following substances are among the drugs most commonly used in the treatment of neuroses at the present time.

Benzodiazepines (the most effective and least toxic of the minor tranquilizers)

Generic name	Trade name	Daily dosage
Chlordiazepoxide	Librium	15-100 mg
Diazepam	Valium	5-60 mg
Oxazepam	Serax	30-120 mg
Clorazepate	Tranxene	15-60 mg

Glycerol derivatives (related to muscle relaxants)

Generic name	Trade name	Daily dosage
Meprobamate	Miltown, Equanil	200-1200 mg
Tybamate*	Solacen	750-3000 mg

Diphenylmethane (antihistamine)

Generic name	Trade name	Daily dosage
Hydroxyzine	Atarax, Vistaril	100-400 mg

---

*Not widely used—effective only in some severe neuroses.

Barbiturates

Generic name	Trade name	Daily dosage
Phenobarbital	Luminal	60-150 mg
Butabarbital	Butisol	60-150 mg

Tricyclics

Generic name	Trade name	Daily dosage
Imipramine pamoate	Tofranil-PM	75-300 mg

PHARMACOLOGIC ACTION

All of the minor tranquilizers are central nervous system depressants. The degree to which central nervous system depression occurs depends upon dosage and varies according to the particular drug group. The barbiturates and the antihistamines have a greater sedative effect than the benzodiazepines and the glycerol derivatives. The benzodiazepines are among the safest and most effective in the treatment of anxiety. They also have anticonvulsant and muscle relaxant properties and produce little effect on autonomic functions such as blood pressure. All of these drugs can produce physiological addiction, but the benzodiazepines are less addictive than the others and have fewer side effects. The side effects of the minor tranquilizers, which are often dosage related, are daytime drowsiness and sedation, decreased mental acuity, and decreased coordination. Overdoses produce muscle weakness, lack of coordination, sleep, and coma (Baldessarini, 1977). Because the tricyclic drugs have a sedative as well as an antidepressant action, imipramine has often proved more effective than tranquilizers in treating some phobias, such as the social phobias and agoraphobia (Gray, 1978). The actions and side effects of imipramine are further discussed in Chapter 18.

CONTRAINDICATIONS

Since the minor tranquilizers are central nervous system depressants, they should not be used in combination with other central nervous system depressants such as the phenothiazines and alcohol. They are also contraindicated in pregnancy, particularly in the first trimester, and, because of the potentially addicting effect, in people known to be addicted to alcohol or other drugs.

Clients should be alerted to the possible side effects of anti-anxiety medications, and they should be cautioned against the use of other sedatives such as sleeping pills and alcohol. They should also be alerted to the possible dangers involved in driving a car or operating tools or machinery that require alertness and attention—especially in the early weeks of administration, when side effects are most apt to appear. Withdrawal symptoms, which can occur if the administration of a drug is suddenly ended, can be avoided through a gradual decrease in dosage over approximately a week's time. Nurses in health care settings are responsible for the administration of medication and the assessment of client responses, including side effects. Nurses are also responsible for health teaching in relation to dosage and side effects.

NURSING INTERVENTION

PRIMARY PREVENTION

The practice of nursing brings members of the profession into contact with persons of all ages and various states of physical and mental health. This professional contact in the community offers nurses the opportunity to participate in the primary prevention of neuroses.

Nurses should keep the following principles in mind when they engage in activities of primary prevention of neuroses:

1. Interpersonal patterns of dependence, domination, and detachment are means of coping with unconscious conflicts in order to maintain the ability to function.
2. Neurotic conflict cannot be resolved by rational decision.
3. Anxiety is present whether or not there are overt symptoms.

4. A behavioral response in any situation is aimed primarily at maintaining psychological security and keeping anxiety under control.
5. During periods of crisis, anxiety increases and regression may occur.
6. Awareness of feelings and interpersonal behavior is low during such periods.
7. Such periods are characterized by excessive vulnerability to criticism, rejection, or desertion.

The *goals for primary prevention* of neuroses include

1. Minimizing the effects of factors that predispose people to neurotic disorders
2. Finding ways to prevent high-risk individuals from developing neuroses

Nurses can implement these goals by identifying high-risk individuals and by initiating parental and family counseling.

Identification of high-risk individuals

Community health nurses and school-nurse teachers work with families and observe family interactions. As nurses become acquainted with family members, they are able to identify those children who are asymptomatic but who come from families where people relate to others through dependency, domination, or detachment. Family members should be assessed as to:

1. Level of interpersonal dependency
   a. Characteristically relates to others in a helpless or vulnerable manner
   b. Persistently and/or indirectly expresses dependency needs
   c. Persistently and/or repeatedly needs attention and approval from others
   d. Consistently is hypersensitive to anything that may be perceived as rejection, criticism, or neglect
   e. Excessively complies with the wishes of others
2. Level of interpersonal domination

a. Characteristically relates to others by taking command of the situation and projecting an image of competence
b. Consistently views the world as a hostile, threatening place where it is difficult to trust others
c. Habitually is unable to admit to one's self or to others feelings of apprehension, fear, and anxiety
d. Repeatedly responds to anxiety-producing situations with angry outbursts or with sarcasm; perceives any questions of a personal nature (including a health history) as prying and is resentful; resists advice, suggestions, and health teaching

3. Level of interpersonal detachment
   a. Characteristically relates to others with indifference, disinterest, or an air of superiority
   b. Persistently uses intellectualization to cope with anxiety
   c. Excessively is needful of privacy and much value is attached to privacy and to being alone
   d. Habitually perceives questions of a personal nature (including a health history) as an intrusion of privacy and responds with evasion, withdrawal, or anger

In addition, nurses should be aware of holistic health factors, including the family environment, that may predispose people to neurotic disorders. For example, because neurotic coping behavior may be learned, Aldrich (1981) points out that parents who cope with conflict and anxiety by becoming preoccupied with their health may predispose their children to hypochondriasis.

Parental and family counseling

Since some theorists believe that neurotic symptoms are learned behaviors for coping with conflict and anxiety, nurses should help families learn more adaptive coping behaviors. Families should be taught stress reduction techniques (e.g., meditation, progressive relaxation, and physical exercise)

as well as ways of expressing feelings of anxiety, fear, and apprehension directly and authentically.

A child born into a family in which one or both parents use neurotic coping patterns is in a vulnerable state. Poverty or other environmental stressors that contribute to a chronic crisis situation may cause a child to experience difficulty in accomplishing the tasks of normal development. Identification of and preventive intervention for such families are particularly pertinent in the prenatal and perinatal periods, during developmental crises in the child, in family developmental crises, and in situational crises.

Practitioners of family nursing have long been active in promoting physical and mental health in prospective parents. Natural childbirth, health education, anticipatory guidance, and genetic counseling, as well as the support of persons who are learning the role of parent, are but a few areas of concern that have been extensively studied. Much of this effort, however, has focused on the normal family or on prospective parents who are relatively mentally healthy. Less attention has been given to persons whose character structures suggest the need for intervention in periods of family crisis. For example, a prospective parent who has excessive dependence needs may be unable, without ongoing support, to meet the dependence needs of an infant and, later, the developing child. A person who copes by means of patterns of domination may be unable to allow a toddler the degree of freedom necessary to develop autonomy, or an adolescent the degree of independence essential to the development of identity. Identification of such prospective parents before their children are born and supportive follow-up care during their children's early developmental years are aspects of primary prevention of neurosis.

SECONDARY PREVENTION

Although professional nurses have traditionally been involved in the treatment of the more severe psychiatric disorders, such as the psychoses, changing patterns of health care and the expanding role of the nurse in community health and mental health are placing increasing demands upon the profession to participate in secondary prevention in the neuroses. Such prevention involves meeting the following objectives:

1. Early identification of cases of neurosis in the community
2. Obtaining prompt and effective treatment to restore the individual to optimum mental health
3. Assessment of available community resources for referral
4. Participation with community groups in expanding needed resources

Early identification, or case finding, is important in neuroses since many individuals suffering from them do not seek professional help until or unless the symptoms severely inhibit the ability to function. The professional involvement of nurses in many aspects of community life brings them into contact with families and individuals. Nurses thus have opportunities for case finding that may not be available to other health professionals. A nurse may be the first health professional to come into contact with a person with a neurotic disorder. In such an instance, the nurse may be concentrating primarily on family health or social problems that may or may not be related to the neurosis. A community health nurse, for example, providing services to a family in a home, may be the first health professional to learn of a phobia in a mother that is undermining the mental health of the entire family. A school nurse may be the first to recognize an anxiety disorder in a parent that is interfering with a child's learning or to recognize school phobia in a child. An industrial nurse may be the first to recognize symptoms of an underlying neurosis that is contributing to alcohol abuse in an employee.

Such early assessments are tentative and should be validated through consultation and, when possible, through referral of clients to other health professionals, before further intervention is planned. The amount of consultation and the manner in which it is carried out depend upon the circumstances and on the way in which a client and a nurse come together. A community health nurse will have an opportunity to discuss a plan of action with a supervisor, may be able to consult with a mental health nurse, and will have opportunities for repeated visits to a client's home. A school nurse may be able to refer parents and children to a school psychologist. An industrial nurse may have the services of a physician or a psychiatrist available.

The objective of early identification in secondary prevention is the referral of the client to a mental health resource for treatment. Many neurotic clients, however, are highly resistant to any form of psychiatric intervention. In such a case, the person's right to refuse treatment must be respected. For persons who are reluctant to accept treatment or who are ambivalent about becoming involved, a supportive nurse-client relationship, with the limited goal of providing emotional support while the client is in a crisis, may be effective in motivating the individual to accept further treatment.

The focus of this aspect of secondary prevention is on intervention into clients' patterns of dependency, domination, and detachment; alleviation of symptoms associated with the neurotic process; and restoration of functional patterns of client behavior. Nurses should keep the following principles in mind regardless of the symptom picture:

1. The focus should be upon the client as a person who is suffering, and not upon the symptom.
2. Whether or not it is observable, underlying anxiety is present and should be assessed.*
3. The symptom is a defense mechanism designed to contain anxiety and to preserve ego integrity.
4. Nurses and other staff members may have emotional responses to client behavior. For example, nurses may experience anxiety or become frustrated with clients. Occasion-

---

*Refer to Chapter 7 for a discussion of anxiety and its assessment.

ally, nurses may also need to separate out their own problems and conflicts from those of their clients. Nurses should not try to deny their own feelings and conflicts. Instead, they should acknowledge these feelings and conflicts and work them through in supervision or counseling. In this way, a nurse's personal growth may be enhanced.

5. Nurses should protect the client's right to the symptom and, when necessary, should serve as an advocate for the client during interaction with other staff members.

6. Nursing interventions and activities should permit the client to carry out demands of the disorder, such as an obsessive-compulsive ritual.

7. The client needs acceptance and approval, and he or she is vulnerable to any form of rejection.

8. If the disorder is characterized by indecisiveness, any pressure to have the client make decisions should be avoided.

9. Although the client is in contact with reality and able to think logically, the client may be out of touch with his or her own feelings.

10. Repressed hostility may be overtly expressed when the client feels pressured or frustrated.

11. Since the client fears his or her own hostility and anger, and anxiety increases when these feelings become overt, actions that may arouse anger should be avoided.

12. Any attempt to rationally explain symptoms or underlying dynamics should be avoided. Such attempts would be met with resistance and increased anxiety.

Knowledge of these principles will facilitate intervention with clients who are experiencing neurotic disorders.

Nursing process

The nursing process provides the framework for therapeutic intervention.

ASSESSMENT

When they work with clients who cope with anxiety and conflict through dependence, domination, or detachment, nurses need to begin their assessment where the client identifies the problem. Utilizing the concepts of Horney (1945) and Dean (1979), the following areas should be assessed:

1. Presenting symptoms—phobias, compulsions, hypochondriacal behavior, etc. that are creating problems for the client even though they are serving as defenses against an emotional state that the client is experiencing

2. Emotional state—such feelings as helplessness, anxiety,* or anger that are responses to a stimulus situation

3. Stimulus situations—stressful life situations that are characterized by a threat to one's security and the frustration of one's attempts to satisfy needs (These stressful life situations are engendered by maladaptive (neurotic) coping behaviors.)

4. Maladaptive coping behaviors—neurotic symptoms and coping patterns of dependency, domination, and detachment that are used in relating to others, in attempting to satisfy needs and in protecting oneself from hurt

5. Origin of maladaptive coping behaviors—identification of childhood experiences that contributed to the development of or learning of maladaptive coping behaviors

6. Holistic health status—physical, intellectual, emotional, sociocultural, and spiritual status of the client (These factors may either facilitate wellness (e.g., a culturally approved belief in spirit possession may permit expression of personal and interpersonal conflict through "possession behavior"), or these factors may impede wellness (e.g., a conflict between one's social behavior and

---

*Refer to Chapter 7 for a discussion of assessment of anxiety levels.

one's cultural values and/or spiritual standards may generate neurotic anxiety and guilt). In addition, many neurotic disorders involve physical as well as emotional manifestations (e.g., clients who compulsively wash their hands may have excoriated hands; anorexic clients may have amenorrhea, malnutrition, etc.)

ANALYSIS OF DATA

As nurses assess the presenting symptoms, emotional states, stimulus situations, maladaptive coping behaviors and their origins, and the holistic health status of clients, nurses begin to understand the client's (and often the family's) perceptions of the presenting problem. The aforementioned assessments also aid nurses in understanding the interrelationship between family dynamics, predisposing and precipitating factors, and clients' maladaptive coping behaviors. At this point, nurses may be ready to formulate nursing diagnoses. The following are nursing diagnoses that are frequently made when caring for clients who cope with anxiety and conflict through dependency, domination, and/or detachment. Following each nursing diagnosis is a discussion of an appropriate plan of care and its implementation.*

Nursing diagnosis: Interaction theme of dependency related to dependence-independence conflict and feelings of inadequacy, anxiety, and/or hostility (behavior associated with all DSM-III diagnoses of neurotic disorders)

Planning: With assistance and/or guidance from the nurse, the client will establish goals.

1. Long-term goals
   a. Work through the dependence-independence conflict and sense of inadequacy that are generating anxiety and/or hostility.
   b. Learn to relate to others in a nondependent (assertive) manner.

---

*Sources consulted include Dean (1979), Jorn (1982), and Schultz and Dark (1982).

2. Short-term goals
   a. Verbalize feelings of anxiety, inadequacy, and/or hostility.
   b. Identify interpersonal situations that arouse feelings of anxiety, inadequacy, and/or hostility.
   c. Relate current stressful interpersonal situations to situations in the past that aroused similar feelings.
   d. Develop more effective coping behaviors and interpersonal skills.
   e. Realistically perceive the five dimensions of self. (Biological, psychological, intellectual, sociocultural, and spiritual strengths and weaknesses will be put in perspective.)
   f. Build self-esteem (refer to Chapter 18 for a discussion of self-esteem).

Implementation: Nearly everyone is placed in a somewhat dependent role when confronted with a health problem requiring professional assistance. The decision to seek such assistance indicates that people recognize that they have a problem with which they are unable to cope without assistance. The health agency and the type of services required may foster feelings of dependence. Health professionals, to whom a particular health problem may be an everyday occurrence, and who are familiar with its course and treatment, may automatically assume an authoritative manner toward a client without fully comprehending the emotional response of the client toward the situation. In addition, many people experience a degree of regression when they are ill and feeling helpless. These and many other factors increase a client's feeling of dependence when coping with a health problem.

The following is a realistic approach for dealing with overly dependent behavior.

1. Initially, meet the client's dependency needs. Trying to force a client to be independent will only increase client feelings of anxiety, inadequacy, and hostility.
2. Identify the degree of the client's dependency and potential for independent function-

ing. Use your own observations as feedback, and obtain the client's perceptions of how he or she functions with peers and authority figures and in structured, unstructured, competitive, and noncompetitive situations.

3. Help the client develop the necessary skills for independence. Teach the client to write out lists, schedules, strategy plans, etc., that aid in organizing tasks. Help the client learn assertiveness techniques.

4. Assist the client to increase self-esteem (refer to Chapter 18).

5. Include the client in a plan to gradually progress from having things done for him or her to accepting assistance with tasks to taking independent action to accomplish tasks. Support the client during this transitional period.

Excessive compliance with the demands of others and excessive praise of—or unrealistic expectations about—the abilities of staff members may be subtle forms of manipulation, which communicate feelings of helplessness and a need for emotional support. As the client's self-esteem increases and ability to problem solve improves, he or she will be able to function more independently both with staff members and with significant others.

Nursing diagnosis: Interaction theme of domination related to dependence-independence conflict and feelings of inadequacy, anxiety, and/or hostility (behavior associated with all DSM-III diagnoses of neurotic disorders)

Planning: With assistance and/or guidance from the nurse, the client will establish goals.

1. Long-term goals
   a. Work through the dependence-independence conflict and sense of inadequacy that are generating anxiety and/or hostility.
   b. Learn to relate to others in a nondomineering (trusting, cooperative) manner.

2. Short-term goals
   a. Verbalize feelings of anxiety, inadequacy, and/or hostility.
   b. Identify interpersonal situations that

arouse feelings of anxiety, inadequacy, and/or hostility.

c. Relate current stressful interpersonal situations to situations in the past that aroused similar feelings.

d. Develop more effective coping behaviors and interpersonal skills.

e. Realistically perceive the five dimensions of self. (Biological, psychological, intellectual, sociocultural, and spiritual strengths and limitations will be put into perspective.)

f. Build self-esteem (refer to Chapter 18 for a discussion of self-esteem).

Implementation: The individual who copes with experiences by attempting to dominate other people seems, on the surface, to be the exact opposite of the overly dependent person. But this facade is misleading. During stressful situations such a person is just as vulnerable to anxiety and its disruptive forces as a dependent person. Instead of depending upon others to bolster self-esteem, the person who copes by domination must take command of the environment and project an image of competence. An underlying view of the world as a threatening, hostile place makes it difficult, if not impossible, for such a person to place the degree of trust in others that is often necessary during a health crisis. In addition, the dependent role necessitated by admission to a hospital can arouse anxiety, unconscious dependency needs, and the underlying conflict of which such needs are a part. An inability to admit to oneself or others such feelings as apprehension, fear, and anxiety makes it difficult for this type of person to deal with these feelings when they emerge. The need to be dominant may also result in conflict with physicians, nurses, and other health care providers in their professional roles of authority figures.

Although overt evidence of anxiety may not be discernable in such clients, many other clues may be detected that suggest an underlying struggle to maintain equilibrium. Consistent disregard for or defiance of medical orders or a prescribed treatment plan may indicate that the need to preserve psychological equilibrium is of higher priority than the threat to physical well-being. For example, the refusal of a person with diabetes to adhere to a prescribed diet, or of a person with a coronary occlusion to accept restrictions on activity, frequently results in annoyance and frustration for nurses and other health professionals.

Hostility, whether expressed overtly through angry outbursts or covertly through sarcasm or being late for appointments, may indicate underlying anxiety. Resentment of questions about personal life and habits and resistance to accepting advice, suggestions, or health teaching may be indications of the need to remain in control in order to contain anxiety and preserve psychological integrity.

Professional nurses, who are confronted daily with the more extreme manifestations of disorders, may respond with frustration and even anger to a client who refuses to follow a treatment plan or to accept advice or instruction. Such a response to a client's behavior on the part of a nurse may itself be a clue that a client is experiencing psychological distress or anxiety.

The following is a realistic approach for working with clients who try to dominate others.

1. Assist the client to recognize the means used to dominate people or situations. Help the client to differentiate between assertiveness and domination.
2. Help increase the client's self-esteem (refer to Chapter 18).
3. Consistently adhere to previously established limits regarding time, focus, etc., for nurse-client interactions.
4. Encourage the client to express feelings of anxiety, inadequacy, or hostility.
5. Explore with the client the relationship between interpersonal situations and his or her thoughts, feelings, and actions.
6. Help the client find outlets for self-assertiveness that are nondomineering.

Nursing diagnosis: Interaction theme of detachment related to dependence-independence conflict and feelings of inadequacy, anxiety, and/or hostility (behavior associated with all DSM-III diagnoses of neurotic disorders)

Planning: With assistance and/or guidance from the nurse, the client will establish goals.

1. Long-term goals
   a. Work through the dependence-independence conflict and sense of inadequacy that are generating anxiety and/or hostility.
   b. Learn to relate to others in a nondetached (interdependent) manner.
2. Short-term goals
   a. Verbalize feelings of anxiety, inadequacy, and/or hostility.
   b. Identify interpersonal situations that arouse feelings of anxiety, inadequacy, and/or hostility.
   c. Relate current stressful interpersonal situations to situations in the past that aroused similar feelings.
   d. Develop more effective coping behaviors and interpersonal skills.
   e. Realistically perceive the five dimensions of self. (Biological, psychological, intellectual, sociocultural, and spiritual strengths and limitations will be put in perspective.)
   f. Build self-esteem (refer to Chapter 18 for a discussion of self-esteem).

Implementation: People who cope with stress by becoming detached from other people are especially vulnerable when they experience physical illness or injury, which of necessity may bring them into closer contact with other people than can be tolerated. The need to feel self-sufficient or even superior may result in conflict with professional authority. Medical orders, a treatment plan, or the requirement that the routine of a health agency be adhered to, may be perceived by the detached person as coercion and responded to with uneasiness and rebellion.

Nurses working with detached clients should do the following:

1. Assist the client to recognize the detached ways (e.g., intellectualization, air of superi-

ority) that he or she uses to relate to people.

2. Encourage the client to express feelings of anxiety, inadequacy, or hostility.
3. Help the client increase self-esteem (refer to Chapter 18).
4. Explore with the client the relationship between situations that generate anxiety, inadequacy, or hostility and his or her detached behavior.
5. Encourage the client to respond more authentically to situations that provoke anxiety, inadequacy, or hostility. Redirect client attempts at intellectualization to expressions of his or her feelings about situations. As the client begins to feel more secure about expressing feelings, he or she will become increasingly open to interdependent relationships with others.

The need for privacy, which is of great importance to the detached individual, may be violated in several ways in the health care setting. A medical or nursing history often probes into aspects of life regarded as private and personal. Resistance and evasion in responding to such questions, and accompanying signals of anxiety or withdrawal, can alert the questioner to the client's distress. Sharing a room in a hospital with one or more other clients may be particularly distressing; it may increase the use of defense mechanisms to control the discomfort and maintain some degree of privacy. Intellectualization and an air of superiority may be employed to keep other people at a distance. Indifference and disinterest in others and even in one's own condition may be clues to detachment. Conversely, people who furnish many clues that they prefer to be alone may become angry if they feel that they are being ignored or taken for granted. Such inconsistent messages demonstrate the very human need such clients have for contact and acceptance by other people. They also indicate the incompatability of the needs and strivings of individuals who cope through detachment. (This incompatibility also characterizes the situation of persons who cope through domination.)

Nursing diagnosis: Alteration in activity (either immobilization or hyperactivity) related to a panic level of anxiety* engendered by underlying conflicts (e.g., social role conflict; sex conflict) and a precipitating stressful life situation (behavior associated with DSM-III diagnosis 300.01, panic disorder)

Planning: The nurse may initially establish goals but, as therapy progresses, the client should enter into goal-setting.

1. Long-term goals
   a. Work through the conflicts that are arousing anxiety.
   b. Learn to effectively cope with stressful life situations so that a panic level of anxiety is not generated.
2. Short-term goals
   a. Identify and describe feelings of anxiety.
   b. Identify and describe the precipitating stressful life situation and the associated feelings.
   c. Relate the precipitating stressful life situation to situations in the past that aroused similar feelings.
   d. Re-evaluate the potency (in terms of stress) of the precipitating stressful life situation.
   e. Develop more effective coping behaviors.

Implementation: Panic disorder comes on suddenly and lasts from several minutes to a few hours. People may be immobilized by anxiety, or they may place themselves in danger by attempting to run away from it, perhaps into a busy street. Although the ability to perceive what is happening is severely restricted, they may also overreact to external stimuli. The physiological symptoms may convince them that they are having a heart attack or experiencing some other physical disorder.

A major aspect of nursing intervention is the protection of the client. Lipkin and Cohen (1973) note the importance of staying with the client until the anxiety level subsides. As they point out, a

---

*Refer to Chapters 7 and 13 for further discussion of intervention into anxiety.

nurse can prevent the client from taking any action that might be dangerous. More importantly, the calm, accepting manner of the nurse can provide some sense of security. Communications with people in panic should be brief, clear, and concrete and should be made in a calm, slow manner. If they are able to do so, clients should be encouraged to talk about the feelings they are experiencing. Any probing or pressure should be avoided. Since the source of anxiety is unconscious, any suggestions about the possible cause will only increase the anxiety (Lipkin and Cohen, 1973). Comfort measures such as loosening tight clothing, giving hot or cold fluids, and providing calm, quiet surroundings are also important in supporting the client in a panic state.

Anxiety disorders are often associated with phobias. For example, a person with agoraphobia—an abnormal fear of leaving one's home—who travels even a short distance from home alone may experience an acute anxiety attack.

Nursing diagnosis: Alteration in behavior (disproportionate fear of and avoidance of an object or situation) related to displaced anxiety about control, aggressiveness, sex, self-esteem, etc. (behavior associated with DSM-III diagnoses 300.23 [social phobia] and 300.29 [simple phobia])

Planning: With assistance and/or guidance from the nurse, the client will establish goals.

1. Long-term goals
   a. Work through the conflicts about sexuality, aggressiveness, control, self-esteem, etc., that generate anxiety.
   b. Decrease phobic behavior to a degree where the client can effectively function in society (phobic behavior may never be completely eradicated).
2. Short-term goals
   a. Verbalize feelings about anxiety, sexuality, control, inadequacy, aggressiveness, etc.
   b. Identify life situations that generate anxiety and conflict.
   c. Relate current stressful life situations to situations in the past that aroused similar feelings of anxiety.

   d. Recognize a relationship between stressful life situations and phobic behavior.
   e. Learn more effective coping behaviors to deal with feelings about sexuality, anxiety, aggressiveness, control, inadequacy, etc.
   f. Become desensitized to the feared object or situation.
   g. Avoid secondary gains associated with the phobic behavior.

Implementation: Many aspects of nursing intervention for the phobic person have already been discussed in the section on panic disorder. Focusing upon the client as a person and not on the phobia is an important aspect of the nurse-client relationship. Protecting the client's right to the symptom and supporting the client's efforts to avoid contact with the feared object help to contain the underlying anxiety. A phobic person is aware of the irrationality of the symptom and very often is able to discuss it and to examine the impact it is having upon his or her life. The degree to which a phobia is disruptive of a person's life depends upon the nature of the fear. The fear of flying in an airplane may be far less inhibiting than the fear of riding in an elevator, when one lives on an upper floor of a high-rise building. The degree of disruption in a person's life may also be related to the degree to which one is motivated to give up the symptom or to seek professional help. A nurse must be alert to the secondary gains that may result from a phobia. A client who has a bus phobia may be able to avoid some boring chores and to obtain additional attention from others, who must provide the needed services. At times a nurse may be able to modify a phobic person's environment slightly, and with the cooperation of family and friends, limit some of the services provided that tend to reinforce the symptom. In a hospital setting, it may be possible, through careful study of the situation, to limit secondary gains that reinforce the symptom, while at the same time permitting the client to avoid the feared object. Although such a plan can be more easily carried out in the controlled environment of a hospital, the benefits will be greater when it is carried out in the home, where the problem originated.

Plans for such environmental manipulation, especially the nonreinforcement of secondary gains, should be made with the client and appropriate family members and friends when the client appears to be ready for such a step and agrees to participate in the planning.

A community health nurse had met several times with Mrs. M, the mother of three children, in her home. Because of a phobia, Mrs. M was unable to leave her home even when accompanied by her husband and children. She eventually had reached the point where she was motivated to contact a nearby mental health clinic. During each of the past two visits by the community health nurse, a plan to leave the home in the company of the husband and the nurse had been agreed upon by the client. But it had to be canceled each time because the client had an anxiety attack and could not follow through. During a supervisory meeting with a mental health nurse, the community health nurse expressed her frustration with Mrs. M and mentioned that she believed the client was enjoying her disability. After examining this idea for evidences of secondary gain in the situation, both agreed that the perception was valid. Together they developed a plan for intervention. In a subsequent meeting between the community health nurse and the client, the client agreed to the plan and with the nurse began to examine aspects of her lifestyle that might be subtly reinforcing the symptom. Several factors were identified. The husband regularly brought Mrs. M a variety of magazines and books, in addition to doing all of the shopping for the family, which the client admitted had always bored her. The husband also was very good about buying the foods and delicacies she preferred and about keeping her informed about affairs of the community. Many small comforts were provided by a friend who visited regularly and shared Mrs. M's interest in fashion and design. In the next session, in which both the husband and the friend participated, everyone agreed upon a plan that would eliminate all but necessities from Mr. M's shopping list. The friend's visits would be suspended for a time. The nurse would continue to hold regular sessions and would be available by phone for crises that might ensue from the plan. Several small crises did arise, but the husband and the friend, with the support of the nurse, held firmly to the agreed-upon plan. The client was eventually able to keep an appointment at the mental health clinic.

Nursing diagnosis: Sensorimotor dysfunction (e.g., blindness, deafness, or paralysis) related to stress engendered by an underlying conflict about social roles, hostility, etc. (behavior associated with DSM-III diagnosis 300.11, conversion reaction)

Planning: The nurse may initially establish goals but, as therapy progresses, the client should enter into goal-setting.

1. Long-term goals
   a. Work through the conflict that is contributing to sensorimotor dysfunction.
   b. Develop coping behaviors other than sensorimotor dysfunction to deal with conflict.
2. Short-term goals
   a. Verbalize feelings of anxiety, hostility, guilt, etc.
   b. Identify the underlying conflict.
   c. Recognize a relationship between the underlying conflict and the sensorimotor dysfunction.
   d. Learn new coping behaviors to deal with feelings of anxiety, hostility, guilt, etc.
   e. Avoid secondary gains associated with the sensorimotor dysfunction.

Implementation: Conversion reactions are among the most dramatic events found in psychiatry. For the client they represent emergency defenses against situational crises that are intolerable and from which temporary relief is achieved by the symptom. To the viewer, the client who is suddenly struck blind in the face of hardship appeals to the sense of drama and symbolism that we all share. Who among us has not had fantasies that, through some magical act of omnipotence, we can reject unpleasant reality? Vicarious pleasure may, indeed, be one of the responses of staff members to a client who has a conversion symptom. Staff members may pay much superficial attention to such clients when they are first admitted to a psychiatric unit. This situation can be detrimental to a client because it derives from the needs and curiosity of the staff and because staff members may later experience vague feelings of guilt and wish to avoid the client. It is thus particularly important that nurses who work with persons experiencing conversion reactions understand their own responses. Nurses should also:

1. Protect the person's right to the symptom. The absence of anxiety, which is often the case in conversion reactions, may tempt staff members to prematurely convince the client with a conversion symptom that medical evidence does not support the existence of the symptom. Staff members may also be tempted to interpret the meaning of symptoms to a client. When successful, such efforts can result in psychosis.
2. Hysterical symptoms usually indicate an immature personality. Feelings and responses are often acted out in a hystrionic fashion, which masks low self-esteem. Establishment of a therapeutic milieu, in which the client can be encouraged to achieve gratification in activity therapies and in which appropriate and reasonable limits can be maintained, is an important nursing measure.
3. Focus interactions on the client's feelings rather than on conversion symptoms. Recognition of the symptom as a way of coping with conflict should be encouraged. Clients should also be encouraged to participate in activities of daily living and in occupational and recreational therapies, since such participation helps to focus the client's attention away from the physical symptom. A conversion symptom should be dealt with in much the same way as a delusion—that is, by accepting the client's need for the symptom and by neither denying nor confirming its existence.

4. Explore with clients their stressful life situations and their ways of dealing with conflict and stress. When the stressful life situation involves the family, family therapy may be necessary.
5. Help clients to identify possible secondary gains from their conversion symptoms and to explore ways of avoiding these secondary gains. Families should be assisted to decrease any behavior that enables clients to experience secondary gains. Do not give clients special dispensations or privileges because of their conversion symptoms. Clearly state the expectation that they will participate in activities of daily living and in therapeutic modalities.

Nursing diagnosis: Obsessional thoughts and ritualistic behavior related to anxiety and/or guilt about sexuality, aggressive impulses, etc. (behavior associated with DSM-III diagnosis 300.30, obsessive-compulsive disorder)

Planning: With assistance and/or guidance from the nurse, the client will establish goals.

1. Long-term goals
   a. Work through the conflicts that are generating anxiety and/or guilt.
   b. Decrease obsessional thoughts and ritualistic behavior to a degree where the client can effectively function in society. (Obsessional thoughts and ritualistic behavior may never be completely eliminated.)
2. Short-term goals
   a. Verbalize feelings of anxiety and guilt.
   b. Identify life situations that generate anxiety and/or guilt.
   c. Recognize a relationship between stressful life situations and obsessional thoughts and ritualistic behavior.
   d. Learn nonritualistic coping behaviors to deal with anxiety and guilt.
   e. Improve self-esteem (refer to Chapter 18 for a discussion of self-esteem).
   f. Eliminate self-mutilating behavior and alleviate any existing injuries (e.g., chapped hands, sores, cuts).

Implementation: In working with an obsessive-compulsive client, a nurse must set realistic goals. This form of neurosis tends to be chronic and quite resistant to almost any form of therapy. Unless the onset is recent and the symptom limited, any expectation of results other than some reduction in the level of anxiety and the severity of symptoms is unrealistic in most cases. Obsessive-compulsive behavior can be a source of frustration to the nurse who works with such a client. Setting unrealistic goals only increases the frustration the nurse experiences.

Many aspects of nursing intervention discussed in relation to the person who is detached are relevant to intervention for the obsessive-compulsive client. There is difficulty in establishing an interpersonal relationship, since the obsessive-compulsive client has difficulty feeling close to other people. Frequently, such a client finds it difficult to express thoughts and feelings. Underlying hostility and a need to control the environment pose problems for both the client and the nurse.

The following is a realistic approach for dealing with obsessive and ritualistic behavior:

1. In establishing a nurse-client relationship, a calm, quiet approach is important. After a statement of interest and availability, it is important to wait for clues from the client before proceeding with further verbal communication. It is necessary that communication move at a pace that is comfortable for the client. The focus of interaction should be the person, not the symptom, and any form of pressure or prying should be avoided. In early stages of therapy, calling attention to clients' symptoms or trying to prevent clients from performing compulsive or ritualistic acts will only increase their anxiety. Initially, only harmful rituals should be limited by substituting safe behavior for dangerous rituals. For example, picking the nap off a piece of wooly or fluffy material could be substituted for picking at one's own skin.

2. Any level of nursing intervention for obsessive-compulsive clients should take into ac-

count the fact that they are tense and anxious. They have little tolerance for frustration, and their strong need to control the environment may conflict with the established routines of a health agency. Efforts to make a client comply with fixed routines may result in increased anxiety and possibly in overt expressions of anger. Initially, extra time may need to be alloted to accommodate a client's ritualistic routines. As the client's anxiety decreases (as a result of verbalization, environmental support, and other interventions), the client will have less need for ritualism and/or will be more amenable to verbal instructions about participating in activities of daily living.

3. Since clients are struggling to contain underlying hostility, situations that increase frustration or provoke anger may be detrimental to the progress of their treatment. Demands made and limits imposed on the client should be reasonable, and their purpose should be made clear. It should be kept in mind that obsessive-compulsive people are ambivalent; they have difficulty making even minor decisions or choices. Pressuring such people to make decisions should be avoided.

4. To protect clients' rights to their symptoms, it is necessary to allow time for rituals to be performed. This approach acknowledges the importance of their behavior to clients. Protecting clients from the criticism or ridicule of other clients, as well as staff members, is frequently necessary. In the event that limits must be set on ritualistic behavior, they should be clear, concise, and reasonable; and the limits should be consistently enforced. For example, a nurse and a client could mutually agree that the client would only focus on or indulge in obsessive thinking or ritualistic behavior for 10-15 minutes of every hour. For the rest of the hour, the client would engage in other thoughts and behaviors. The amount of time alloted for symptomatic behavior should gradually be

decreased, and the client should be helped to learn more adaptive ways for handling anxiety.

5. At times, ritualistic symptoms interfere with or threaten the health of the client. Such situations range from dermatitis of the hands, as a result of compulsive hand washing, to malnutrition, as a result of rituals concerning food. Appropriate measures must be taken in such instances to maintain physical health.

Nursing diagnosis: Somatic complaints and rumination about one's health related to anxiety and dependence-independence conflict (behavior associated with DSM-III diagnosis 300.70, hypochondriasis)

Planning: The nurse may initially establish goals but, as therapy progresses, the client should enter into goal-setting.

1. Long-term goals
   a. Work through the dependence-independence conflicts that are generating anxiety.
   b. Develop ways other than somatic complaints and rumination to cope with anxiety and stress.
2. Short-term goals
   a. Verbalize anxiety, dependency needs, and the anger that ambivalence about dependency needs may generate.
   b. Identify life situations that generate anxiety and dependence-independence conflicts.
   c. Recognize a relationship between stressful life situations, somatic complaints, and rumination.
   d. Develop nonsomatizing coping behaviors to deal with anxiety.
   e. Decrease the amount of time and attention devoted to rumination and somatic complaints.
   f. Avoid secondary gains associated with somatic complaints.

Implementation: Hypochondriasis is one of the more severe neuroses; it can result in regression to a psychotic state. Hypochondriasis appears in an immature person who has an underlying depend-

ence-independence conflict. Strong dependency needs are thwarted by fear and distrust of others. The individuals are often self-centered or narcisistic; they are often preoccupied with the body and its functions. Chronic anxiety is expressed in the form of physical symptoms. Hypochondriacal symptoms differ from psychosomatic symptoms in that the hypochondriacal symptom, although very real to the person affected, has no physical basis. The psychosomatic symptom is caused by a disease process.

Persons with hypochondriasis often come to the attention of nurses in acute health care settings such as clinics, emergency rooms, or general hospitals. Although the symptoms are very real to the client and the suffering is as great as, or greater than it would be in a physical illness, nurses and other staff members often respond with impatience, anger, or frustration when such a client rejects medical findings that indicate that no underlying disease is present. Family and friends often respond with similar contempt and rejection. Such responses only increase clients' anxiety and their need for the symptoms.

A common feature of hypochondriasis is strong resistance to any challenge to the validity of the physical complaint or to any form of referral for psychiatric therapy. The symptom (or symptoms) represents a strong effort to maintain ego integrity and the ability to function. Nursing intervention that is designed to provide support during crisis situations can prevent regression to a less adaptive level of functioning. Some principles of nursing intervention for hypochondriacal clients are as follows:

1. Recognize the underlying dependency needs of clients.
2. Accept clients as they are and adapt nursing intervention to meet their dependency needs.
3. Recognize negative staff responses to clients and protect them from subtle forms of rejection, isolation, or derogation.
4. Provide staff members an opportunity for ventilating and sharing feelings and responses.

5. Identify social networks within the family and community that can provide support when necessary.
6. Attempt to enlist the cooperation of family members and other persons in the client's social network who can provide support without reinforcing secondary gains.
7. Make use of discussion groups in health care settings, such as prenatal or child care clinics, for sharing problems of coping with children or with daily living. Health teaching and anticipatory guidance can offer support for the hypochondriacal client, who is often isolated in the home.
8. Make clients aware of the resources available for crisis intervention when it is needed.
9. Refer clients to family therapy resources when they and their families can accept this form of intervention, and when such resources are available.

Nursing diagnosis: Alteration in personality development (the development of one primary and one or more secondary personalities) related to chronic anxiety and severe physical and/or sexual abuse as a child (behavior associated with DSM-III diagnosis 300.14, multiple personality)

Planning: The nurse may initially establish goals but, as therapy progresses, the client should enter into goal-setting.
1. Long-term goals
   a. Communication and cooperation among all the personalities
   b. Fusion or integration of all the personalities into one whole person
2. Short-term goals
   a. Recognize the existence of secondary personalities.
   b. Learn about the traumas and repressed painful feelings that contributed to the development of secondary personalities.
   c. Develop new coping behaviors to deal with anxiety and such other painful feelings as loneliness and hostility.

Implementation: It may take one or more years for all of a client's secondary personalities to re-

veal themselves to a therapist. Since fusion or integration of the personalities is dependent on communication and cooperation among those personalities, it is important to facilitate personality revelation. Jorn (1982) emphasizes the role that trust plays when working with clients who have multiple personalities. Implementation of goals is based on each personality of a multiple personality developing trust in the therapist.

1. As each personality develops a trust relationship with the nurse, that personality will share with the nurse its feelings, conflicts, traumas, and needs.
2. The nurse then helps the client to understand that he or she has a multiple personality and encourages the client to work toward the goal of personality integration. In order to achieve client participation in and commitment to the treatment plan, trust between nurse and client is essential.
3. Next, the nurse works with each secondary personality on a cognitive level. Each secondary personality must not only trust the therapist, but it must also have some degree of trust in the primary personality. At this point, each secondary personality will tell the primary personality what it knows about past experiences and feelings of which the primary personality is unaware. Such revelation by secondary personalities to the primary personality is the beginning of personality fusion or reintegration.
4. As the primary personality becomes aware of past experiences and feelings that had previously been reposited in secondary personalities, the nurse will help the client to verbalize painful feelings and to mobilize support from friends, relatives, clergy, etc.

Although it is not rare, neither is multiple personality disorder as common as most of the other neurotic disorders. Therefore, many nurses may not be knowledgeable about working with clients with multiple personalities. Nurses who are not theoretically and experientially prepared to work with clients suffering from this disorder should refer their clients to therapists or mental health centers that specialize in the treatment of multiple personality disorder.

Nursing diagnosis: Alteration in memory (either partial or complete) of one's past life related to chronic anxiety and a precipitating traumatic event (behavior associated with DSM-III diagnoses 300.12 [psychogenic amnesia] and 300.13 [psychogenic fugue])

Planning: The nurse may initially establish goals but, as therapy progresses, the client should enter into goal-setting.

1. Long-term goals
   a. Work through conflicts that are generating chronic anxiety.
   b. Develop coping behaviors other than memory loss to deal with conflict and stress.
2. Short-term goals
   a. Verbalize feelings of anxiety, especially those surrounding the precipitating traumatic event.
   b. Identify life situations, both current and past, that generate anxiety.
   c. Recognize a relationship between stressful life situations and loss of memory.
   d. Learn more effective coping behaviors to deal with anxiety.
   e. Avoid secondary gains associated with memory loss.

Implementation: People suffering from partial memory loss may not recognize their friends and relatives and they may forget large areas of their past lives. When memory loss is complete, people may wander great distances from their homes and have no memory whatsoever of their previous existences. This condition is referred to as a fugue state and is usually a means of escaping from an intolerable situation. Intervention into memory loss related to chronic anxiety and a precipitating traumatic event is similar to intervention in acute crisis.* In addition to crisis intervention, the following approaches may be initiated:

---

*Refer to Chapter 13 for a discussion of crisis intervention.

1. Because the alleviation of dissociative symptoms makes clients more amenable to therapy, measures should be initiated to help clients regain some memory. The longer amnesia persists, the more difficult it is to overcome. Gray (1978) suggests that physical stimuli such as smelling salts or cultural/spiritual stimuli for "believers," such as faith healing, can help clients emerge, at least partially, from their dissociative states. As soon as clients have regained some memory, any activity, even walking or talking, will reinforce their renewed level of awareness. In these ways, nurses can facilitate the recovery of memory. However, nurses should not tell clients about their past lives. Provision of such information (which amnesic clients are denying or repressing) can escalate client anxiety and precipitate psychosis. It should also be remembered that the gain from measures that help clients regain memory will only be temporary unless underlying conflicts are resolved.
2. The nurse-client relationship should focus on the client's feelings (especially those surrounding the precipitating event) and on stressful life situations. Family dynamics, family roles, and feelings about and among family members may need to be explored. Thus, rather than focusing on a client's amnesia, the conflicts and stresses that engendered anxiety, the way the client copes with anxiety, and the learning of more effective ways of coping should be the focus of the nurse-client relationship.
3. Clients should be helped to identify the secondary gains associated with their amnesia. Ways to avoid these secondary gains should then be explored. Family members should be assisted to decrease any behavior that enables the client to experience secondary gains. Expectations for client participation in the treatment program should be clearly stated. Nurses should not allow clients to use their memory loss to get special privileges or to gain dispensations.

Nursing diagnosis: Alteration in eating patterns (either self-starvation or gorging and purging) related to disturbance in self-image and conflicts about sexuality and control (behavior associated with DSM-III diagnoses 307.10 [anorexia nervosa] and 307.51 [bulimia]). Nursing intervention for these nursing diagnoses is discussed in depth in Chapter 15.

EVALUATION

The client and, whenever feasible, the client's family or significant others (e.g., housemate, very close friend) should be included in estimating the client's progress towards attainment of goals. Any evaluation should encompass the following areas:

1. Estimation of the degree to which neurotic conflicts have been worked through
2. Estimation of the degree to which goals have been achieved and client functioning has improved (demonstrated by a decrease in neurotic coping behaviors and the learning of more effective coping behaviors)
3. Identification of goals that need to be modified or revised
4. Referral of the client to support systems other than the nurse-client relationship
   a. People in the client's social network who are willing to serve as a support system
   b. Community agencies that help clients learn to live with neurotic disorders that may never be completely eliminated (e.g., phobia clinics)
   c. Centers that specialize in the treatment of specific neurotic disorders (e.g., anorexia nervosa centers; centers for the treatment of multiple personalities)

TERTIARY PREVENTION

Relatively little attention has been given to the long-range effects of neuroses upon the personality and the ability to function. The level of maladaptive functioning that occurs in neuroses does not produce the severe psychological crippling that is seen in schizophrenia, for example, and the other psychoses. Except for individuals with hypochondriasis, which is sometimes a stage preliminary to schizophrenia, persons who have neuroses often function satisfactorily in society, although they may require some psychiatric intervention in times of crisis.

However, everyone arrives at the so-called golden years with the personality characteristics and coping patterns that have developed over a lifetime. The sociocultural and physiological problems that beset people in the older age group may be made more severe by any neurotic coping patterns that, under less stressful circumstances, have been used to maintain the ability to function. When confronted with the loss of family and friends, who earlier provided needed support, and with decreasing economic status, a neurotic individual is often less able to cope with the problems of aging than the average person. Many such individuals can be found, somewhat isolated, in single-room dwellings and health-related facilities, where they are often viewed as problem clients by staff members and other residents.

Tertiary prevention should include the provision of mental health centers where crisis intervention and individual and group psychotherapy are available for such persons and for others who may be similarly isolated in the community. In addition, tertiary prevention should include the identification of individuals in the community who have chronically displayed neurotic symptoms, such as obsessive-compulsive behavior or phobias, and the provision of psychiatric services for them.

CHAPTER SUMMARY

A neurosis can be defined as a personality organization characterized by excessive anxiety and unconscious conflict. Although such a disorder involves little or no distortion of reality or impairment of intellectual functioning, the use of various defense mechanisms and compromise solutions to maintain functioning and to control anxiety results in rigidity of the personality and the development of interpersonal patterns of dependence, domination, or detachment. When a neurotic person experiences stress, symptoms that are more pathological may appear.

Neurotic conflicts have their origins in the early developmental years—during the long period in which a child depends upon significant others for nurturing and enculturation. Neurotic behavior differs from normal behavior only in degree, and a neurosis can be understood only in relation to the culture in which a child is reared.

Neuroses are believed to be among the most prevalent psychiatric disorders in Western culture, although no reliable demographic studies are available. Whether neuroses exist in all cultures is not clear at this time.

Treatments for neuroses include individual, family, and group psychotherapy, administration of psychopharmaceuticals, and behavior therapy. Primary prevention includes early identification of and intervention with persons who experience chronic anxiety states and who display interpersonal relationship patterns that indicate that maladaptive coping patterns could develop during a crisis. Adapting nursing intervention to meet the needs of such clients during health-related crises is another important aspect of primary prevention.

The role of the nurse in secondary prevention depends, to some extent, upon the type of neurosis and the setting in which the nurse intervenes. A fundamental aspect of nursing intervention, however, is a supportive nurse-client relationship. Collaboration with other health professionals and utilization of available therapies are other important measures. Tertiary prevention includes collaboration with community groups in securing and utilizing resources for rehabilitation.

SENSITIVITY-AWARENESS EXERCISES

The purposes of the following exercises are to:

- Develop awareness about the vulnerability of client-families to neuroses
- Develop awareness about the interrelationship of factors in the etiology of neurotic disorders
- Develop awareness about the subjective experience of clients who are suffering from neurotic disorders and of the experience of clients' families
- Develop awareness about your own feelings and attitudes when working with clients who are suffering from neuroses

1. Try to imagine that you are suffering from one of the following disorders and explain why you selected that particular disorder. Then describe what you think it would be like to suffer from that disorder.
   a. Anxiety disorder
   b. Obsessive-compulsive disorder
   c. Multiple personality
   d. Amnesia
   e. Anorexia nervosa or bulimia
   f. Conversion disorder (select one symptom)
   g. Phobic disorder (select one phobia)
   h. Hypochondriasis
2. Describe what you think it would be like to have a family member suffering from one of the neuroses listed in Question I. Which disorder do you think would be easiest to tolerate in a family member? Why? Which disorder do you think would be hardest to tolerate? Why?
3. What might be some of your feelings and reactions as a nurse caring for clients who are suffering from neuroses? Would your feelings and reactions vary with the neurotic disorders experienced by clients? Explain why.
4. Imagine that you are a community health nurse engaged in health supervision activities with new parents. What high risk factors (physical, emotional, intellectual, sociocultural, and spiritual) would you watch for that might predispose parents and/or their children to a neurotic disorder?
5. Develop a plan for counseling parents about child-rearing that incorporates principles and goals for the primary prevention of neuroses.

REFERENCES

Aberle, D.F.
1961 " 'Arctic Hysteria' and *Latah* in Mongolia." In Social Structure and Personality: A Casebook. Y.A. Cohen (ed.). New York: Holt, Rinehart, and Winston.

Ackerman, S.H., and E.J. Sachar
1974 "The lactate theory of anxiety: a review and reevaluation." Psychosomatic Medicine 36(1):69-72.

Aldrich, C.K.
1981 "Hypochondriasis, part 2." Postgraduate Medicine 69(6):149-156.

Baldessarini, R.J.
1977 Chemotherapy in Psychiatry, Cambridge, Mass.: Harvard University Press.

Beal, E.W.
1978 "Use of the extended family in the treatment of multiple personality." American Journal of Psychiatry 135(5):539-542.

Beech, H.R., and F. Perigault
1974 Toward a theory of obsessional disorder. In Obsessional States. H.R. Beech, ed. London: Methuen.

Bendefeldt, F., L.L. Miller, and A. Ludwig
1976 "Cognitive performance in conversion hysteria." Archives of General Psychiatry 33(10):1250-1254.

Boskind-White, M., and W.C. White
1983 Bulimarexia: The Binge/Purge Cycle. New York: W.W. Norton & Company.

Bruch, H.
1978 The Golden Cage, The Enigma of Anorexia Nervosa. Cambridge, Mass.: Harvard University Press.

Chesler, P.
1972 Women and Madness. New York: Avon Books.

Coelho, G.V. (ed.)
1974 Coping and Adaption. New York: Basic Books, Inc. Publishers.

Colby, K.M., and M.T. McGuire
1981 "Signs and symptoms: Zeroing in on a better classification of neuroses." The Sciences (November), pp. 21-24.

Coons, P.M.
1980 "Multiple personality: Diagnostic considerations." Journal of Clinical Psychiatry 41(10):330-336.

David, H.P.
1976 "Mental health services in the developing countries." Journal of Psychiatric Nursing and Mental Health Services 14(1):24-29.

Dean, P.R.
1979 "The neurotic process: an overview and its application to nursing." Journal of Psychiatric Nursing 17(12):35-37.

Díaz-Guerrero, R.
1955 "Neurosis and the Mexican family structure." American Journal of Orthopsychiatry 112:411-417.

Dikowitz, S.
1976 "Anorexia nervosa." Journal of Psychiatric Nursing and Mental Health Services 14(10):28-37.

Dunham, H.W.
1976 "Society, culture and mental disorder." Archives of General Psychiatry 33(2):147-156.

Dohrenwend, B.P., and B.S. Dohrenwend
1974 "Psychiatric disorders in urban settings." In American Handbook of Psychiatry (ed. 2), vol 2. G. Caplan (ed.). S. Arieti (ed. in chief). New York: Basic Books, Inc., Publishers, Ch. 29.

Drellich, M.
1974 "Classical psychoanalytic school. A theory of neuroses." In American Handbook of Psychiatry (ed. 2), vol. 1. S. Arieti (ed. and ed.-in-chief). New York: Basic Books, Inc., Publishers, Ch. 37.

Fabrega, H., A. Rubel, and C. Wallace
1967 "Working class Mexican psychiatric out-patients." Archives of General Psychiatry 16:704-712.

Fenichel, O.
1945 The Psychoanalytic Theory of Neuroses. New York: W.W. Norton & Co., Inc.

Freud, S.
1936 The Problem of Anxiety. New York: W.W. Norton & Co., Inc.
1960 Group Psychology and the Analysis of the Ego. New York: Bantam Books, Inc.
1969 A General Introduction to Psychoanalysis. New York: Pocket Books.

Fromm, E.
1962 The Art of Loving. New York: Harper & Row, Publishers, Inc.

Gray, M.
1978 Neuroses: A Comprehensive and Critical Review. New York: Van Nostrand Reinhold Company.

Greenberg, W.C.
1982 "The multiple personality." Perspectives in Psychiatric Care 20(3):100-104.

Grove, W.R., and J.F. Tudor
1978 "Adult sex roles and mental illness." American Journal of Sociology 78(4):812-835.

Hale, E.
1983 "Inside the divided mind." New York Times Magazine (April 17) VI, p. 100+.

Harris, G.
1957 "Possession 'hysteria' in a Kenya tribe." American Anthropologist 59:1047-1051.

Herbert, W.
1983 "Behavior: Modeling bulimia." Science News 123(20):316.

Hollingshead, A.B., and F.C. Redlich
1958 Social Class and Mental Illness: A Community Study. New York: John Wiley and Sons, Inc.

Horney, K.
1937 The Neurotic Personality of Our Time. New York: W.W. Norton & Co., Inc.
1939 New Ways in Psychoanalysis. New York: W.W. Norton & Co., Inc.
1945 Our Inner Conflicts. New York: W.W. Norton & Co., Inc.

Jorn, N.
1982 "Repression in a case of multiple personality disorder." Perspectives in Psychiatric Care 20(3):105-110.

Kolb, L.C.
1977 Modern Clinical Psychiatry (ed. 9). Philadelphia: W.B. Saunders Co.

Kretschmer, E.
1937 "Instinct and hysteria." British Medical Journal 4002:574-578.

Kubie, L.
1974 "The nature of the neurotic process." In American Handbook of Psychiatry (ed. 2), vol. 3. S. Arieti and E. Brody (eds.). New York: Basic Books, Inc., Publishers, pp. 3-16.

Leighton, A.H., and J.M. Murphy
1965 Approaches to Cross-Cultural Psychiatry. Ithaca, N.Y.: Cornell University Press.

Lipkin, G.B., and R.G. Cohen
1973 Effective Approaches to Patients' Behavior. New York: Springer Publishing Co., Inc.

Ludwig, A.
1972 "Hysteria: A neurobiological theory." Archives of General Psychiatry 27:771-777.

Marcuse, H.
1972 Counterrevolution and Revolt. Boston: Beacon Press.

Marks, I.M.
1969 Fears and Phobias. New York: Academic Press.
1976 "The current status of behavioral psychotherapy: Theory and practice." American Journal of Psychiatry 133(2):154-159.

McGrory, A.
1980 "Women and mental illness: A sexist trap?" Journal of Psychiatric Nursing and Mental Health Services 18(10):17-22.

Nakakuki, M.
n.d. "Japan's homegrown neurosis." In Psychiatric Perspectives: Roche Reports, Frontiers of Psychiatry.

Parker, S.
1962 "Eskimo psychopathology in the context of Eskimo personality and culture." American Anthropologist 64:76-96.

Pattison, M., and R. Wintrob
1981 "Exorcism and possession in America." Journal of Operational Psychiatry 11(3):231-235.

Portnoy, I.
1974 "The school of Karen Horney." In American Handbook of Psychiatry (ed. 2), vol. 1. S. Arieti (ed. and ed.-in-chief). Basic Books, Inc., Publishers.

Powers, P.S.
1980 Obesity: The Regulation of Weight. Baltimore: The Williams and Wilkins Co.

Schlemmer, J.K., and P.A. Barnett
1977 "Management of manipulative behavior of anorexic patients." Journal of Psychiatric Nursing and Mental Health Services 15:11.

Schultz, J.M., and S.L. Dark
1982 Manual of Psychiatric Nursing Care Plans. Boston: Little, Brown & Co.

Sifneos, P.E.
1972 Short Term Psychotherapy and Emotional Crisis. Cambridge, Mass.: Harvard University Press.

Skinner, B.F.
  1953 Science and Human Behavior. New York: Free Press.
Slatter, E., and V. Cowie
  1971 The Genetics of Mental Disorders. New York: Oxford University Press.
Slatter, E., and M. Roth
  1970 Clinical Psychiatry. Baltimore: Williams and Wilkins.
Sloman, L.
  1976 ''The role of neuroses in phylogenetic reference to early man.'' American Jounral of Psychiatry 133(5): 543-547.
Spitzer, R.L., A.E. Skodol, M. Gibbon, and J.B.W. Williams
  1981 DSM-III Case Book. Washington, D.C.: The American Psychiatric Association.
Suinn, R.M.
  1970 Fundamentals of Behavior Pathology. New York: John Wiley & Sons, Inc.
''The fear of using computers is common''
  1983 Part II. Newsday (July 9), col. 1, p. 5.
Wallace, A.F.C.
  1961 ''Mental illness, biology and culture.'' In Psychological Anthropology. F.L.K. Hsu, (ed.). Homewood, Ill.: The Dorsey Press, Inc.

Winiarz, W., and J. Wielawski
  1936 ''*Imu*—A psychoneurosis occuring among Ainus.'' Psychoanalytic Review 23:181-186.
Wolpe, J.
  1974 ''The behavior therapy approach.'' In American Handbook of Psychiatry (ed. 2), vol. 1. S. Arieti, (ed.). New York: Basic Books, Inc., Publishers, Ch. 43.
Yap, P.M.
  1952 ''The *Latah* reaction: Its pathodynamics and nosological position.'' Journal of Mental Science 98:515-564.

ANNOTATED SUGGESTED READINGS

Colby, K.M., and M.T. McGuire
  1981 ''Signs and symptoms: Zeroing in on a better classification of neuroses.'' The Sciences (November) pp. 21-23. *The authors address the longstanding difficulty of classifying neuroses and then they describe their research project, which is designed to develop a new diagnostic classificatory system. The authors' approach utilizes a natural-language analyzing algorithm to identify key ideas (themes or class-defining properties) that distin-*

guish neurotic individuals from a non-neurotic control group. The objective of their research project is to develop a taxonomy that is based on property classes that are qualified by the efficacy of different treatment modalities.

Dean, P.R.
  1979 "The neurotic process: An overview and its application to nursing." Journal of Psychiatric Nursing 17(12):35-37.

  The author delineates a psychodynamic model of the neurotic process that progresses from the identification of a "hurt," to the current life situation precipitating the hurt, to the behavioral patterns that create the life situation and, lastly, to the childhood experiences in which the behavioral patterns developed. The author then discusses how this model can facilitate the utilization of the nursing process with neurotic clients.

Gray, M.
  1978 Neuroses: A Comprehensive and Critical View. New York: Van Nostrand Reinhold Company.

  The author gives an overview of the etiology, classification, and history of psychiatric disorders as a foundation for his holistic approach to neuroses. Separate chapters are devoted to the discussion of each neurotic disorder (the history, classification, etiology, diagnosis, differential diagnosis, course and prognosis, and treatment). An additional chapter is devoted to an in-depth discussion of various somatic and psychotherapeutic treatment modalities.

FURTHER READINGS

Cain, A.H.
  1970 Young People & Neurosis. New York: J. Day Co.
Mitchell, R.G.
  1983 "Breakdown: anxiety states & phobias, part 5." Nursing Times (Feb.) pp. 16-22.
Schrieber, F.R.
  1973 Sybil. Chicago: Regency Press.
Takiesungiyama, L.
  1983 "Shame & guilt: A psychocultural view of the Japanese self." Ethos 2(3):192-209.
Thigpens, C.H., and H.M. Cleckley
  1957 The Three Faces of Eve. New York: McGraw-Hill Book Co.

CHAPTER 20

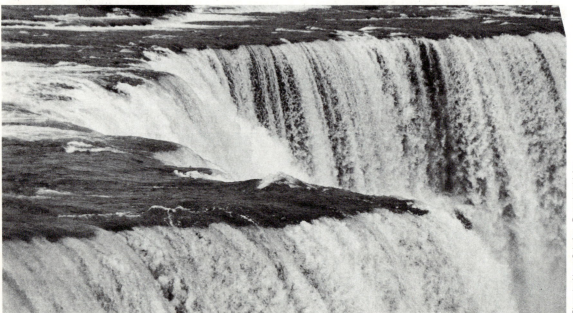

Photo by Horst Schafer—Peter Arnold, Inc.

Coping with emotional turbulence through primitive defenses

CHAPTER FOCUS

Borderline personality disorder is a relatively new diagnosis of mental illness that is receiving a great deal of attention today. Characterized by themes of anger, erratic and self-destructive behavior, and severely disordered interpersonal relationships, the syndrome is believed to be increasing in our society. In fact, it has even been suggested that this disorder is "a metaphor for our unstable society" (Sass, 1982, p. 12).

In terms of etiology, borderline personality disorder (also referred to as "borderline syndrome," "borderline pathology," and "borderline personality organization") is viewed as a developmental arrest in the separation-individuation phase of the first year of life.

Until recently, most of the theoretical work on etiology and the treatment methods based on clinical experience have been presented by psychoanalysts who have treated borderline clients. For this reason, the focus of this chapter is necessarily influenced by a psychoanalytical viewpoint. While nurses in various psychiatric settings increasingly are interacting and intervening with borderline clients, to date very little material on the disorder has appeared in the nursing literature.

As with other forms of mental illness, nursing intervention with clients diagnosed as having borderline pathology is focused on therapeutic response to behavior. Material on nursing intervention that is quite relevant to manifestations of borderline pathology but that is also covered in detail in other chapters (for example, substance abuse and other addictive behaviors in Chapter 17; suicidal behavior and self-derogation in Chapter 18; brief psychotic episodes in Chapter 22) will not be repeated here. Seven major problems that the borderline client experiences will be reviewed in conjunction with the nursing process. These include five primitive defenses that Kernberg views as core underlying dynamics (splitting; primitive idealization; projective identification; rapidly shifting ego states; omnipotence of self with devaluation of others) and two recurring themes in the lives of borderline clients (the inability to tolerate aloneness; chronic boredom). This work is based on theoretical and clinical concepts from the literature and the author's [H.M.A.] clinical practice in intervening with borderline clients in inpatient and outpatient settings.

It is generally agreed that long-term treatment is necessary for meaningful changes in the personality organization and life-style of the borderline client. Most often this will be carried out by clinical nurse specialists and clinicians from other disciplines who are treating clients on an ongoing, outpatient basis. Long-term goals build on short-term goals, however, and the frequent hospitalizations and many crises that these clients experience make an understanding of the condition and its treatment important for all professional nurses working in psychiatric settings.

HISTORICAL ASPECTS AND DEFINITIONS OF "BORDERLINE PERSONALITY DISORDERS"

Borderline personality disorder, borderline personality syndrome, and borderline personality organization are various terms used to denote a condition that is capturing the attention of many writers and workers in the mental health fields. Thus, borderline personality is becoming increasingly familiar to nurses working in a variety of psychiatric settings. The category is controversial—some writers suggest that it is a "catch-all" or "wastebasket" term to cover a very large group of individuals who don't quite fit into the more conventional diagnostic categories (Klein, 1977; Freed, 1980; Lynch and Lynch, 1977). Many others insist that it is a definite, recognizable syndrome (Arieti and Chrzanowski, 1975; Adler, 1975; Capponi, 1979; Freed, 1980; Gunderson and Singer, 1975; Rinsley, 1977). Currently the latter group seems to be in the majority and the designaton is not only an accepted one (for example, it is now included in DSM-III), but it seems to be one of the most frequently discussed disorders in mental health journals today. There is a proliferation of books, workshops, panels, conferences, and "popular press" articles

on the subject. Certainly, borderline disorder is more precisely defined than it has been, even in the fairly recent past. Wolberg, writing in 1973, pointed out that most of the material on the borderline client had been written in the past five or six years (Wolberg, 1973). While it may be receiving a good deal of attention and interest and while much of the clarification, description, terminology, and analysis are just evolving, the syndrome itself is probably not a new one, nor is it simply a contemporary development of new psychiatric thinking. It is quite probable that terms such as Freud's "narcissistic neuroses" (which he considered unanalyzable), Wilhelm Reich's "impulsive character disorder," Helene Deutsch's "as-if personality," and the later designations of "psychotic character," "pseudoneurotic schizophrenia," "ambulatory schizophrenia," "latent schizophrenia," and "nonpsychotic schizophrenia" all included a good number of people who would now be diagnosed as suffering from borderline personality disorder (Capponi, 1979; Mack, 1975). The earlier descriptions of pathology seem to parallel many of our current delineations of borderline personality. It can be seen from these early terms that at first the concept was used to characterize something that lay between schizophrenia or psychosis and neurosis. For example, Laplanche and Pontalis' definition (1973, p. 54) of "borderline case" states: "Term most often used to designate psychopathological troubles lying on the frontier between neurosis and psychosis, particularly latent schizophrenias presenting an apparently neurotic set of symptoms." Many modern writers affirm that there is such a thing as borderline or latent schizophrenia but that it is discrete from borderline personality disorder. Later contributions from a variety of theorists tend to place borderline personality disorder on a continuum, not simply between neurosis and psychosis but one that requires differentiating the diagnosis from several other pathologies (see Fig. 20-1). In 1975, Chrzanowski noted that while borderline pathology may still be considered something of a hybrid concept and that the state is often classified as early, ambulatory, transient, or latent forms of schizophrenia, this tendency is changing. He states: "In recent years, greater emphasis has been placed on the relatively specific pathology of borderline states compared to conceptualizations of either a continuum ranging from neurosis to psychosis and vice versa or to a halfway station between moderate and severe mental illness" (Chrzanowski, 1975, p. 147).

Perhaps, as many writers have suggested, a more appropriate word would be "border*land*." For example, Green states: "So the contradiction emerges. Our clinical experience tells us that the border of insanity is not a line; it is rather a vast territory with no sharp division: *a no-man's land* between sanity and insanity" (Green, 1977, p. 16).

The borderland has been explored by many and the condition is differentiated from other forms of mental illness mostly in terms of *degree or severity of illness*. Papers have been written distinguishing borderline disorders from schizophrenia (Chrzanowski, 1975; Gunderson and Kolb, 1978); depression and other affective disorders (Gunderson and Kolb, 1978; Kibel, 1978); character disorders (Chrzanowski, 1975; Boyer and Giovacchini, 1967; Kibel, 1978); narcissistic personality (Adler, 1981; Grotstein, 1979; Kohut, 1971); neurosis (Kibel, 1978); and psychosis (Giovacchini, 1979; Kernberg, 1977; Kibel, 1978; Masterson, 1973, 1974; Pine, 1974).

Thus, borderline personality disorder can be viewed as "bordering" on several other psychopathological conditions (see Fig. 20-1), and the reason for so much confusion about the term becomes apparent.

Some definitions of the disorder that may help to clarify the concept include:

> The borderline condition represents a degree of psychopathology that differs, on the one hand, from neurotic and character disorders, and, on the other hand, from the psychoses. Thus, borderline patients have ego impairment of a severity that lies midway between these and other conditions (Kibel, 1978, p. 342).

> . . . patients with stable character structures who demonstrate the immature defenses stressed by Otto F. Kernberg*—splitting, primitive idealization, projection and projective identification—and the core conflicts related to primitive hostility and fear of abandonment (Adler, 1975).

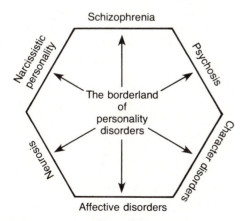

Schizophrenia

Narcissistic personality

Psychosis

The borderland of personality disorders

Neurosis

Character disorders

Affective disorders

Fig. 20-1

---

*Kernberg is considered one of the leading authorities on borderline pathology. See later parts of this chapter for discussion of some of his concepts and of those "immature defenses" mentioned here.

Borderline people typically are harrowed by a sense of aloneness, and in their relations with others are tortured by alternating horrors of abandonment and engulfment. In order to relieve their exhausting inner despair, these patients exhibit a strong tendency to act impulsively and to defend with denial, projection and splitting (Maltsberger and Buie, 1975, p. 126).

. . . nonpsychotic character disorders who suffer from severe developmental failure, and who possess the potential for slipping in and out of psychosis . . . the ego of the borderline can be said to be preoccupied primarily with problems of a preoedipal nature centering around symbiosis and object relatedness (Leboit and Capponi, 1979, p. 5).

Chrznowski (1975, p. 147) described the borderline client as having a common denominator in these three aspects:

1. An inhibition to display overt anger and aggression
2. A tendency to maintain a certain amount of social distance
3. A tendency toward intense transference phenomena

The definitions all make serious attempts at the difficult task of illuminating the controversial concept of borderline personality disorder but one is still left with a rather vague, and sometimes conflicting, understanding of the syndrome.

Gunderson and Singer (1975) presented an excellent overview of the literature on borderline personality disorder in which they were able to abstract six descriptive features of the disorder. They are

1. *Intense affect,* usually depression or, more often, anger
2. A history of *impulsive behavior* (self-mutilation, drug abuse, alcoholism, gambling)
3. A certain amount of *superficial social adaptiveness* (more of a mimicry)
4. *Brief, psychotic episodes* characterized by intact reality testing in the face of a poor sense of or relationship to reality
5. *Primitive personality organization* as revealed by psychological tests and loose thinking

6. Severely *disordered interpersonal relationships* vacillating between transient, superficial states and intense, dependent relationships. Relationships are marred by devaluation of others, manipulation, and a tendency to be demanding.

Kernberg would add another characteristic: *a negative and indistinct sense of self;* and Singer has noted that these individuals suffer from *rapidly shifting ego states* (Singer, 1979). Finally, many writers have pointed to another prevalent and important characteristic of the borderline personality: the greatly *diminished ability to use sublimation* as a defense mechanism. This difficulty in sublimating is an important factor in two recurring themes—*the inability to tolerate aloneness* and *chronic boredom.*

A similar listing of characteristics is found in DSM-III (coded on Axis II—301.83), which provides a detailed description of the disorder as a basis for making the diagnosis:

. . . the following are characteristic of the individual's current and long-term functioning, are not limited to episodes of illness, and cause either significant impairment in social or occupational functioning or subjective distress.

A. At least five of the following are required:
1) impulsivity or unpredictability in at least two areas that are potentially self-damaging, e.g., spending, sex, gambling, shoplifting, overeating, physically self-damaging acts
2) a pattern of unstable and intense interpersonal relationships, e.g., marked shifts of attitude, idealization, devaluation, manipulation (consistently using others for one's own ends)
3) inappropriate, intense anger or lack of control of anger, e.g., frequent displays of temper, constant anger
4) identity disturbance manifested by uncertainty about several issues relating to identity, such as self-image, gender identity, long-term goals or career choice, friendship patterns, values, and loyalties, e.g., ''Who am I?'', ''I feel like I am my sister when I am good''
5) affective instability: marked shifts from normal mood to depression, irritability, or anx-

iety, usually lasting a few hours and only rarely more than a few days, with return to normal mood

6) intolerance of being alone, e.g., frantic efforts to avoid being alone, (being) depressed when alone

7) physically self-damaging acts, e.g., suicidal gestures, self-mutilation, recurrent accidents or physical fights

8) chronic feelings of emptiness or boredom

B. If under 18, does not meet the criterion for Identity Disorder (Diagnostic and Statistical Manual [DSM-III], p. 322).

UNDERLYING DYNAMICS

Otto Kernberg prefers the term *borderline personality organization* to describe these clients. He views the organization as a pathological one and has described some of the primitive and pathological defense mechanisms* that are frequently used. These include (1) splitting, (2) primitive idealization, (3) projective identification, (4) denial of ego states, and (5) omnipotence of self with devaluation of others (Kernberg, 1977).

Splitting

Splitting is the failure to synthesize the positive and negative experiences and ideas one has of oneself and other people (or things). It is a normal developmental style when the infant is attempting to differentiate *self* from the rest of the world. Mother is seen as a separate, distinct person (object) who is powerful and *good* (brings food, comforts) but also as *bad* (doesn't come when she's needed). One way of conceptualizing this is to note the infant's self-protecting (keep the "bad" away from the "good") perception of mother as the "good mother" and the "bad mother," or "the good breast" and the "bad breast." Things become, in this *either-or* and *primitive* point of view,

*The reader is referred to Chapter 7 for a review of defense mechanisms in general.

"good-bad" or "black and white"—there is no "gray" or ambiguous area tolerated. Since in reality, life is a mixture of good and bad, positives and negatives, this primitive defense, if overused in later life, can lead to rather severe problems in ego development and a decrease in the ability to function in a healthy manner. One's sense of identity and one's sense of others and other things tend to shift rapidly. There is a lack of integration and the contradictory images of the world cause one to relate to *part objects* rather than *whole* (and therefore a mixture of "good" and "bad") persons, situations, or institutions. In healthier development, one's sense of identity and one's sense of the *other* are based on a synthesis of different characteristics of any personality. Being able to tolerate a certain sense of ambivalence in relating to the other (an imperfect human being or situation) is one of the important hallmarks of mental health.

Gerry is a 24-year-old young woman who has a long history of serious mental and emotional difficulties. She has been hospitalized several times, usually for brief periods only, and she has had two superficial suicide attempts and one serious attempt. After three years of intensive psychotherapy with a clinical nurse specialist (Anna), Gerry is just beginning to notice and to understand how "I do a number on people in my own head." In one recent session, her therapist pointed out that she seemed to be strongly degrading and expressing rage toward her mother, whom she "hated" and who was "no good for anything," and that last week she was experiencing very strong loving feelings toward her mother, praising her highly and wanting to be "close with her." Also in this particular session in which she was vehemently degrading her mother, Gerry told Anna that she loved Anna, wanted to be just like her, that she was sure that Anna was the "best therapist in the world" and that everything would be OK in her own life if Anna were only her mother. Gerry said that she has "a lot of trouble remembering any of the good" about people whenever she feels angry with them. She also remembered, with Anna's help, how she hates herself and feels like a bad person —"a piece of garbage" whenever she gets depressed. Gerry has a great deal of difficulty remembering or acknowledging any of her own good points when she is experiencing one of her frequent bouts with depression.

Primitive idealization

Primitive idealization is a derivative of *splitting* and in the clinical example described above, it is quite evident that Gerry uses primitive idealization in her reaction to her therapist ("things would be perfect if you were my mother—you do everything just right").

Primitive idealization is a defensive maneuver in which the person tends to see the external object (often the therapist, perhaps a new lover or friend) as *all good* and powerful and necessary for protection against all-bad objects. The idealized external object is also seen as all good in order to protect it from one's very bad and dangerous self-image. This mechanism is not like the higher level defense mechanism of *reaction-formation,* where the other person is protected out of concern or regard for the individual's welfare. With primitive idealization, it is mostly derived out of a more basic need-fulfilling motivation ("I need the other to survive"). The object (friend, lover, therapist) can protect or serve by (1) protecting against bad objects in the world, and (2) serving as a recipient for omnipotent identification; the person using this mechanism can "share" in the chosen one's greatness as a direct gratification of narcissistic needs.

Projective identification

Projective identification is a lower, or more primitive, level of the defense mechanism known as projection, and it is characterized by:
1. A tendency to experience impulses that are, at almost the same time as they are experienced, projected onto another person
2. A fear that this other person who serves as the recipient of the projection will act under the influence of that projected impulse and do harm
3. The felt need to control this person who is under the influence of this dangerous projection

This mechanism serves to externalize all-bad self and object images, but it leads to the perception of dangerous, retaliatory persons as populating one's world—persons whom one had better control (through manipulation, devaluation).

Gerry, in the course of her therapy, began to experience angry feelings toward her therapist and to experience therapy as "difficult," "no fun anymore," "not helping me at all." Partly she wanted to run away from this situation where she felt very dependent on her therapist, yet she also felt unimportant —not counting for much with the therapist. Using the mechanism of projective identification, she began to suspect and verbalize that Anna wanted "to kick me out of therapy," that Anna was "tired of working with me." Gerry began to increase the number of phone calls to Anna, much past the pattern of contact they had both agreed on and with which they had been working for some time. Calls began to come at unusual times; demands for attention outside of the parameters of their working relationship increased. Gerry took comments or statements of Anna's out of context, interpreting and using them in such a manner as to "prove" negative feelings toward herself on Anna's part. Indeed, Anna began to experience a sharp increase in her feelings of frustration in working with Gerry (see discussion of countertransference, Chapter 9). In working with her supervisor, Anna was able to identify these negative countertransference feelings and the signs of projective identification in Gerry. This helped Anna to regain her perspective and begin to work more constructively with Gerry.

Denial of ego states

This is typically a "mutual denial" of two different and emotionally independent ego states or "areas of consciousness." This denial reinforces splitting. The person may be aware that two ego states are experienced with completely opposite perceptions, thoughts, and feelings. However, this awareness has no emotional impact. This awareness is not helpful in influencing present feelings toward an object at all. For example, a person may calmly convey a cognitive awareness of the situation while denying its emotional implications. As Kernberg states: "The patient is aware of the fact that at this time his perceptions, thoughts, and feelings about himself or other people are completely opposite to those he has had at other times; but this memory has no emotional relevance, it cannot influence the way he feels now" (Kernberg, 1977, p. 31). Again, there is a lack of integration in the person suffering from borderline pathology.

Omnipotence of self with devaluation of others

This is also linked to splitting. A highly inflated, grandiose, and omnipotent self relates to a depreciated, devalued representation of others. Underneath the feelings of insecurity and harsh self-criticism, the borderline person often experiences grandiose and omnipotent trends. There may be an unconscious belief that one has the right to expect to be treated as a special and privileged person. If another person no longer provides the narcissistic gratification or protection that is sought, that person is usually dropped. Devaluation of the other person is also used defensively and intrapsychically to control and protect oneself from this potentially dangerous person. Kernberg notes that the devaluation of significant people in the person's past (for example, the parents) can have very serious detrimental effects on superego development and integration. This is because devaluation of one's internalized object relations interferes with healthy identifications.

• • •

For a schematic representation of underlying dynamics, see box on p. 622.

CLASSIFICATION OF BORDERLINE PERSONALITY DISORDERS

Based on a thorough and systematic inquiry into the borderline syndrome, Grinker et al (1968) have defined four subgroups of the disorder. These are descriptive of clustering symptomatology:

1. *Group I:* "the psychotic border"—characterized by inappropriate and negativistic behavior. Members of this group tend to be angry, withdrawn, depressed, and hostile.
2. *Group II:* "the core borderline syndrome"—negativistic, chaotic feelings and behavior is evident. Individuals seem unstable, labile, and vaccillating emotionally. There is a high potential for acting out.
3. *Group III:* "the adaptive, affectless, defended 'as if' person." This person is schizoid, obsessional, detached and withdrawn and has a bland and superficial adaptiveness with an "as if" quality to interpersonal interactions.
4. *Group IV:* "the border neurosis"—characterized by childlike, clinging behavior, anxiety, and depression

Donald Klein (1977) has noted the similarity of the classification of Grinker et al (1968) to some groupings he has made and, based on his own research, he believes that in some cases, specific medications are effective within each group. (See discussion of pharmacological treatment below.)

EPIDEMIOLOGY AND SOCIOCULTURAL CONTEXT

Millman et al (1982) state (with no apparent validation) that the disorder is more common in women than in men. And it has been noted by a Harvard Medical School professor that "some psychiatrists believe the disorder affects as much as 7 to 10 percent of the population of the United States and 25 percent of those who receive any kind of psychiatric or psychological treatment" (Louis Sass,

---

A SCHEMATIC REPRESENTATION OF THE UNDERLYING DYNAMICS OF BORDERLINE PERSONALITY DISORDER

Etiology	Effects on the Psyche	Behavioral Results

A. Abundance of interolerable rage (perhaps an inborn, higher level of aggressive feelings)
 B. "Mothering failure"* in early life
  1. Failure to synthesize the "good" and the "bad"
  2. Failure to separate-individuate
  3. Failure to develop adequate sublimation—unable to derive pleasure from anything that is not a direct sensual pleasure (no pleasure, for example, in work performance)
	Negative, indistinct self-image; rapidly shifting ego states with use of denial; use of splitting, projective identification; primitive idealization, omnipotence of self with devaluation of others	Severely disordered interpersonal relations; brief, psychosis-like episodes; impulsive, self-destructive behavior; dependency on excessive use of drugs and alcohol and on promiscuity; poor work history

*For further discussion of these etiological factors, see etiology section in this chapter. Briefly, (1) is related to Winnicott's concept of the *good enough mother* (the mother who is not perfect but who is predominantly able to meet her infant's needs); (2) is related to Mahler's idea of the maternal failure to facilitate the toddler's developmental task of separation-individuation; and (3) can be related to Winnicott's views on the transitional object as a precursor to development of *sublimation*—the ability to substitute something for the original object.

New York Times Magazine, August 22, 1982, p. 12).

However, these unsupported statements and the general lack of epidemiological references in the literature point to the fact that an epidemiological approach to the problem of the borderline syndrome has not been taken at this time. Kaplan and Sadock (1981, p. 488) note that "no systematic studies of borderline pathology have been carried out."

In spite of this, the study by Grinker and his associates (1968) and another by Lazar (1973), concerning patients applying for therapy at the Columbia University Psychoanalytic Clinic, raise some important questions about the syndrome and its interaction with our present culture. These questions are:

1. Is the syndrome becoming more prevalent because of our particular culture's characteristics, such as the chaos of urban living, the increase in existential anxiety, and some profound changes in social structures and family life?
2. Do shifts in diagnostic categories (that is, the increase in diagnoses of "borderline") reflect real population changes or are they more apt to be due to increased attention by professionals to certain phenomena or diagnoses? (Mack, 1975, p. 17)

Freed (1980) suggests that our society is an

etiological factor. To support her belief she cites a discussion of "the new narcissism" by Reiner (1979) and Christopher Lasch's book *The Culture of Narcissism* (1978). She points to such deep and pervasive disorders as "a sense of irrelevance in society, alienation, narcissistic "deification of the isolated self," "lifeboat ethics," social pressures and stresses, massive traumas (. . . the Holocaust, terrorism, the Viet Nam war, nuclear war, violence in families), inhuman environments in which people live, and widespread discrepancies between values and beliefs" (Freed, 1980, pp. 552-553). Chessick, writing in 1977, agrees with this view and lists ten features of Western culture that may be contributing to problems in interpersonal relating and to the development of borderline pathology.

THEORIES OF BORDERLINE PERSONALITY DISORDER

An inborn, overabundance of aggressiveness that may have a biological basis is postulated by several theorists as an important factor in the borderline personality. Most of the investigation and theorizing, however, has been focused on early childhood development. The disorder is considered a *preoedipal* or *pregenital* disorder (see Chapter 6 for a review of the psychosexual stages of development according to Freud) and a *mothering failure* during this period is related to development of the syndrome. Five theorists who have added the most clear and cogent ideas to our present understanding of the condition include Melanie Klein, Margaret Mahler, D.W. Winnicott, Otto Kernberg, and James Masterson. Some relevant points that they make will be reviewed here and Mahler's theory of the preoedipal stages of development will be treated with some depth. All five theorists focus on object-relations and human development. Object-relations is the term used to designate the way an individual (subject) relates to his world (object). Of course, the first object-relationship is with the mothering one.

Melanie Klein's extensive contribution to the theory of object-relations will not be reviewed here* but it includes a view of the infant, very early in life, as defensively needing to deny the terror associated with a potential loss of the good object (mother). The child needs to deny the complexity (good and bad qualities together in one object) of the object and this is done by splitting it into *either* all-good *or* all-bad. Depending on chronology, this is seen as a normal developmental stage in object-relations (Rinsley, 1977).

Otto Kernberg believes that the defects in ego functioning and most specifically in interpersonal relating, grow out of the interaction of the mother-child dyad. He sees them originating in the period toward the end of the first year of life. Kernberg cites early relationship problems with the mothering one as leading to an inability to internalize good interpersonal relating. This in turn affects the child's self-concept—the superego and ego-ideal are negatively influenced and borderline pathology may be the result. Specifically, a synthesis of "good" and "bad" introjects† does not take place—there remains a split. The world is then something of an "either-or" situation. The person has defects in the ability to relate to *whole* (and therefore mixtures of "good" and "bad" qualities in) other persons. Trusting, meaningful, *reciprocal* interpersonal relationships are inhibited and feelings of loneliness, emptiness, and depression result. The split is also in the image of the "self," as well as the "other." The image of a good, acceptable self is protected from the image of a bad, aggressive (and therefore dangerous) self, just as the image of a good other (mother) is protected from the dangerous other (mother). This is a nor-

---

*The reader is referred to *Introduction to the Work of Melanie Klein,* second edition, by Hannah Segal, for a more detailed explanation of some of Melanie Klein's theories of infant development.

†An introject is a mental image of someone or something that becomes incorporated into one's ego system. The process of *introjection* is opposite to that of *projection.* An introject becomes emotionally invested for the individual and is involved in the process of *identification* and superego development.

mal developmental stage but when inadequate mothering occurs and continues into the first year or two of life, the child fails to separate from the mother in a healthy way and an integrated self concept does not evolve. The roots of the primitive defense mechanisms that Kernberg describes can be seen. Extreme, idealized images and an extremely sadistic superego to punish the ''bad self'' and a continued excessive use of splitting in later life are some of the results. Extreme dependency and desires to merge with powerful others are never worked through adequately and in fact are reinforced to become pathological factors in adult life. The development of healthy sublimation and other coping mechanisms is retarded because of energy being expended to control the good-bad conflict, anxiety, and frustration. The individual is in an intolerably painful position: the use of splitting and the feelings of rage tend to isolate the person, wreck interpersonal relationships, and cause feelings of aloneness and abandonment. The individual feels what Masterson has termed the ''abandonment depression'' (see below for further discussion of this concept). Dependency and lack of development of sublimation (for substitute pleasures, interests, distractions) offer no solution to the powerful loneliness and emptiness and can lead to escape through alcohol and drugs. A failure to separate-individuate leads to a continuing need-fear dilemma as far as merging with the significant other is concerned, and this too may be defended against by seeking oblivion through drug and alcohol abuse.

D.W. Winnicott proposes a specific maternal task—the provision of a ''holding environment''—to provide the matrix that can facilitate normal development in the infant. Winnicott has been called ''the analyst of the borderline'' (Green, 1977, p. 24). Winnicott, originally a pediatrician and later a renowned psychoanalyst, had long been interested in the maturational processes of childhood development. He believed that a necessary component of healthy development is a *maternal preoccupation* of the mother with her newborn infant. This preoccupation is necessary for the baby to form a healthy symbiotic attachment to its mother. Failure to enter into a symbiosis with her would lead to serious withdrawal—autism, childhood schizophrenia, or later schizophrenia depending on the degree and timing of the withdrawal. The mother, and to some extent the father who protects the symbiotic dyad, *is* the *facilitating environment* for healthy development. The *True Self* of the human organism, according to Winnicott, begins to have life through the mother's preoccupation. His term ''the good enough mother'' is relevant to the development of schizophrenia *and* borderline pathology.

Winnicott describes this good enough mothering: ''The 'good enough mother' meets the omnipotence of the infant and to some extent makes sense of it. She does this repeatedly. A *True Self* begins to have life through the strength given to the infant's weak ego by the mother's implementation of the infant's omnipotent expressions'' (Winnicott, 1965, p. 145).

''Good enough mothering'' implies imperfect mothering, which is all any human mother can expect to provide. This fact of imperfection is not only realistic, it is necessary to provide an optimal level of frustration so that the infant can encounter the reality principle of life. But the encounter should be a gradual one; the frustration should not be more than the baby can tolerate. It should be, in the words of Winnicott (1965, p. 57): ''here and there, now and then, but not everywhere all at once.'' If needs could be met without any frustration, it would be impossible for the child to gradually learn self-reliance. The *transitional object* helps to bridge the gap between extreme dependency and self-reliance. The transitional object is an important part of childhood development. The teddy bear or the favorite blanket substitutes for the absent and needed mother. The baby is beginning, in a sense, to sublimate through a primitive substitution of one object for another. It soothes and makes separation (frustration) tolerable.

Thus the small failures of mothering that must

naturally occur facilitate growth and lead to a strengthening of the baby's ego. It is only when there are profound failures in mothering that borderline pathology develops. Specifically, these failures are seen as occurring in the separation-individuation stage of preoedipal development. Some discussion of this and Margaret Mahler's theory will follow.

Margaret Mahler's theory of human development has gained considerable attention in recent years as a basis for understanding the development of borderline personality syndrome. Much of the present treatment approach to the disorder has also evolved from Mahler's work. Basing her theory on her many years of therapeutic work with children and direct observation of mother–child dyads, Mahler has delineated the phases and subphases of preoedipal development. Mahler's theory incorporates an ego-psychology* and an object-relations focus.

The infant does not develop in a vacuum—it needs human contact and relationship to grow in complexity. The child grows normally, in a matrix of the *average expectable environment* (Hartmann, 1958). That is to say that the environment does not have to be a perfect one but that the frustrations should not be overwhelming. Severe failures in mothering may prevent the child from adequately negotiating with its environment and from successfully navigating through the preoedipal developmental stages. These stages are the autistic stage (birth to one month), the symbiotic stage (one month to five months), the separation-individuation stage (five months to two and one half years). The separation-individuation stage has been defined further by Mahler into four subphases and it

is these phases that are important to our understanding of borderline pathology. Depending on the particular preoedipal stage where developmental arrests occur, serious pathology may result. Just as failure to resolve the oedipal crisis is seen as resulting in psychoneurotic problems (see Chapter 19), a failure along the continuum of development from birth to the oedipal period results in an arrest in differentiation of both ''self'' and ''object'' (other). Ego functioning related to these important differentiations will also be arrested (Masterson, 1977, pp. 476-477). For example, a failure to form a symbiotic bond with the mother is postulated as the defect leading to pathological *early autism*, whereas failure to work through the symbiotic phase and begin to separate-individuate leaves the individual stuck in symbiosis manifested by the various forms of schizophrenia (see Chapter 21 for further discussion). A brief description of Mahler's phases and subphases follows.

1. *The autistic phase.* The infant lacks cognitive awareness of any mothering agent. This is termed *normal autism* and it gradually changes as the child becomes aware of needs that cannot be satisfied by oneself. To be stuck in this phase would imply pathological autism. At approximately one month (and it must be remembered that all of Mahler's age estimates are approximate), the infant begins to be aware of the mothering one and enters into the next stage, the symbiotic phase of development.

2. *The symbiotic phase.* From one month to approximately five months of age, the child participates in what Mahler describes as the ''symbiotic orbit.'' This is a ''magic circle'' of the mother-infant world in which all parts of mother, including her voice, gestures, clothing, and even the space in which she comes and goes, are joined with the infant.

3. *The separation-individuation phase.* The third phase begins when the infant starts to psychologically ''hatch'' from the symbiotic orbit, to see and experience itself as separate

---

Ego-psychology is a direct outgrowth of Freudian psychology and includes in its ranks such theorists as Heinz Hartmann, Ernst Kris, Rudolph Lowenstein, and Anna Freud; *object-relations* is a school of psychoanalytic thought that is strongly influenced by people such as Melanie Klein, Donald Winnicott, W. Ronald Fairbairn, and Harry Guntrip. The reader is referred to their various works (see reference list) to gain a deeper understanding of their ideas.

from the mother. Mahler views the infant's *psychological birth* as occurring here. This happens over a period of time (five months to two and one half years) and evolves through four distinct subphases. The subphases of the separation-individuation phase are:

a. Differentiation (five months to nine months). Maturation of partial locomotor functioning brings the first tentative moves away from mother and interest in her as a separate being begins. Differentiation of a primitive but distinct body image seems to occur at this time.

b. Practicing (from nine months to about fourteen months of age). During the second subphase, the child is able to move away from mother and return to her (crawling at first, later through upright locomotion). Investigation of the environment and practicing locomotor skills become very important to the child and *elation* is a common theme.

c. Rapprochement (from approximately fourteen months to approximately two years of age or more). This is a stage that is characterized by a rediscovery of mother, now as a separate individual. The narcissistic inflation of the subphase of practicing, when the child is in love with the world, is replaced by the realization of separation and vulnerability. The *rapprochement crisis* occurs now and this is seen as a very important developmental event. *Ambivalence* is the significant theme here. The child wants to be united with and, at the same time, separate from mother. This phase and its inherent crisis are seen as extremely significant in the development of borderline pathology. Mahler believes that the collapse of the child's belief in its own omnipotence combined with the mother's emotional unavailability leads to a hostile dependency on the mother (Akhtar and Byrne, 1983, p. 1014).

d. Consolidation of individuality and emotional object-constancy. The fourth subphase of separation-individuation begins toward the end of the second year and it is seen as open ended. A degree of object constancy* is accomplished and separation of self and object representation is established. "Mother is clearly perceived as a separate person in the outside world, and at the same time has an existence in the internal representational world of the child" (Mahler et al, 1975, p. 289).

Of course, the battles of one's separation-individuation task continue throughout one's lifetime and it is an ongoing process. But within healthy psychological development, a firm beginning is established with this fourth and final subphase. Failure to attain object constancy in the process of separation-individuation is the *core problem of the borderline* states. Object constancy and clear ego boundaries are necessary for a strong sense of self-identity to develop.

James Masterson (1977) designates the rapprochement subphase as *the* most critical one in the development of borderline personality disorder. Rapprochement occurs after the child has practiced separating and has begun to assert the self and to individuate. The child now needs to return to the mother, to sort of "check in" with her. Some children get confusing messages from a mother who may not have resolved her own separation-individuation. The mother is threatened by the child's

---

*Object constancy occurs when the child is able to maintain a mental and emotional representation of mother within. This definition has important implications for treatment goals for many borderline clients who enter a treatment situation at the level of need gratification. The therapeutic task becomes one of raising object-relations to the level wherein the image of the object (for example, the therapist) is retained regardless of need state. This is a significant indication that the individual has synthesized the "good" and "bad" object representations, incorporated a healthy ambivalence, and can relate to a whole object (person). It also means the individual has become less dependent on the environment and is moving toward greater autonomy (Blanck and Blanck, 1979, p. 35).

efforts to separate and may react by rejecting the child at this period. According to Masterson, two messages may be given: *regression is rewarded* and *separation-individuation is punished by withdrawal* of the mother. This reinforces a maintenance of ''split-object relations'' in the child. Masterson terms these split-object relations:

1. The rewarding part unit. Feelings associated with the rewarding part unit are those of receiving unconditional love, feeling gratified, and being taken care of.
   a. The child maintains an image of the mother (part-object representation) that provides approval, support, and other rewards for regressive clinging.
   b. The child maintains a self-image (part-self representation) (as being good and passive and compliant.
2. The withdrawing part unit. Feelings associated with this withdrawing part unit are rage, helplessness, and depression. The child feels that attention and concern from the parent must be paid for through conforming. The rapprochement stage is not adequately resolved and object constancy is not achieved.
   a. The child maintains an image of a maternal part-object that is hostile and attacking and that withdraws supplies in the face of any efforts on the child's part to separate-individuate.
   b. The child maintains a part-self object that is bad, guilty, inadequate, and helpless.

Masterson points to an *abandonment depression* in the individual as what is being defended against by the primitive and pathological defenses of the borderline client. Abandonment depression is a major personality feature of the disorder (Lynch and Lynch, 1977, p. 74). The dilemma is one of striving for autonomy versus fear of abandonment, and the depression implies a helpless ''giving up.''

Masterson (1976), in his own work with borderline clients, found that many of the mothers and fathers of these clients suffered from borderline personality disorder themselves.

FAMILY DYNAMICS AND ETIOLOGY

Zinner and Shapiro (1975, p. 105) believe that the primitive regressive defenses such as splitting occur as a family norm in the families of clients exhibiting borderline pathology. They point to a relationship between severity of the disorder in an individual and the following three variables within a family.

1. The parents' capacity to experience themselves, as separate from a particular child (the ''identified patient''—see Chapter 12)
2. The parents' own dependence on such primitive defenses as projective identification, which leads to a necessary collusion on the part of the child (in the case of projective identification, for example, the child must serve as a container for the projection)
3. The level of maturity of the parents' own object-relations (that is, self-object differentiation).

Zinner and Shapiro have also pointed out the four choices posed by the family group to the borderline adolescent:

1. To preserve good ties to family by repudiating one's own maturation
2. To choose autonomy with a persisting ''bad'' self-object relation with one's family
3. To oscillate between the two choices, while remaining in a state of conflict, anxiety, and uncertainty
4. To choose developmental progression—growth toward autonomy

Zinner and Shapiro see this fourth option as open to the borderline adolescent within a conjoint family therapy situation that provides a growth-enhancing ''holding environment'' that allows for separation of individuals.

TREATMENT

While some work has begun on the pharmacological, family and group therapy approaches most of what has been written to date, has focused on psychoanalytically oriented therapy for borderline clients. The following section will review some of the concepts relevant to the treatment of these individuals. The long-term goals for *any* treatment modality involving borderline clients have been well defined by Freed (1980, p. 554):

1. To heal the "split": to bring about integration of "good" and "bad" images; to work toward eliminating the need for excessive use of splitting mechanisms and patterns
2. To accept primary (healthy) ambivalence rather than fight it
3. To develop normal repression through bringing primitive idealization and projective identification within reality contexts
4. To develop a mature level of dependence through the experience of the therapeutic relationship
5. To develop increased mastery of the environment, impulse control, and frustration control, and frustration tolerance
6. To develop an ability to use realistic planning and healthy coping behavior through the problem-solving process
7. To increase self-esteem and improve the self-image through a reduction in self-defeating behavior and through a realistic recognition of achievements
8. To accept one's separateness and wholeness
9. To improve ability to relate to others; to permit closeness without fusion, separation without abandonment, and individuality within a social or family context
10. To use the therapeutic experience as part of relationship and trust building

Psychopharmacological treatment

Donald F. Klein, one of the foremost experts in psychopharmacology in this country, believes (1975, 1977) that a psychiatric diagnosis that considers observable affects rather than the more abstract structural defects or drives is a more useful method of defining the appropriate drug treatment for clients who have been termed "borderline." He has had a long-term interest in the diagnostic use of drugs in psychiatry. Comparing the four subtypes of Grinker et al. (1968) (see p. 621) to some groupings of his own, he has suggested specific medications as being helpful.

In studies carried out by Klein (1977) and his associates, they found that Group I individuals (who are characterized as angry, withdrawn, depressed, and hostile) were best treated with monoamine oxidase inhibitors.

Group II individuals, who are described as labile, vacillating, and emotionally unstable, seem to be improved by lithium carbonate for mood swings and phenothiazines for both anxiety with impulsivity and for depression with withdrawal. (See Chapter 18 for a discussion of monoamine oxidase inhibitors and lithium carbonate and their actions; see Chapter 21 for a discussion of phenothiazenes.)

Group III individuals, characterized by schizoid, detached withdrawal, do not display clearly understood responses to medications. An exception to this was in a case where depression in a relatively well-integrated person was found. For this individual, antidepressant medications were found useful.

Group IV of Grinker's classification, which Klein closely compared to neurotic depressives and which are described by Grinker and his associates as characterized by clinging anxiety and depression, responded well to imipramine. (See Chapter 18 for a discussion of imipramine.)

Psychotherapy

Although one writer (Mendelsohn, 1982) has outlined an "active, short-term" approach to treatment for the borderline client, psychotherapy for these individuals is almost always seen as a long-term situation. Therapy is a combination of supportive approaches and psychoanalytically oriented psychotherapy. Boyer (1982), who uses these methods, has outlined six principles for effective treatment of the borderline client:

1. Initially, the client's negative reactions to the therapist should be discussed in a here-and-now focus without attempts to relate them to the past.
2. The therapist should point out defensive maneuvers when they occur.
3. Limit-setting to control acting out of transferential feelings is important. (For a discussion of the phenomenon of transference, see Chapter 9.)
4. While positive responses toward the therapist are encouraged, any tendency to see the therapist as *all good* or *all bad* should be pointed out.
5. Distortions about the therapist's interventions or about real life events need to be clarified.
6. Any bizarre or psychoticlike fantasies about the therapist need to be worked through to facilitate the client's reexperience of actual childhood events.

Most of those who have written on the topic of psychotherapy for borderline syndrome agree that a *modified form of psychoanalysis* or *psychoanalytically oriented* psychotherapy is the treatment of choice. This involves parameters and techniques beyond a more conventionally structured psychoanalytic situation. Two important concepts related to this are Winnicott's "the holding environment" (1965) and "the transitional object" (see p. 624). The *holding environment* implies that the therapeutic relationship, in a sense, provides a climate of "good enough mothering" while encompassing an "empathic awareness and response to adult strengths and self-esteem issues," rather than the therapist's omnipotent wish to save the patient (Adler, 1977).

The *transitional object* is particularly relevant in matters of technique and in the necessary management of potentially self-destructive anxiety in the client. For an individual who has not adequately achieved object constancy and who has difficulty maintaining contact with an effective memory of the therapist during inevitable absences (for ex-

ample, the therapist's vacation or unexpected illness), such times can become desperate ones and contributes to escalating anxiety. There is an increased risk of acting-out behavior as a coping mechanism. Some transitional objects that have been used by therapists or by clients on their own include the therapist's business card, a picture of the therapist, a copy of the monthly bill, and the client's own efforts to keep a journal of thoughts and feelings during the therapist's absence. Adler and Buis (1979) postulate that intense, painful aloneness is a theme in the lives of borderline clients. They see this aloneness as an intrinsic aspect of the disorder related to the inability to remember positive images of the significant, sustaining people in their lives *or* being overwhelmed by negative images and memories of these significant others. The developmental defect or arrest is in the rapprochement subphase and implications for treatment include the therapist's use of transitional objects (from those of an abstract, symbolic quality to actual ones, depending on the client's situation) during absences.

Relaxation therapy

Relaxation therapy that is adapted to work with borderline clients is seen by Glantz (1982) as a useful adjunct to psychoanalytic treatment. Deep and rhythmic breathing exercises are taught to the client. This therapy helps the client (1) to discover previously unrecognized anxiety that could be worked with in therapy and (2) to reduce anxiety to a level where difficult material can be discussed.

Relaxation therapy is begun only after a trusting relationship with the therapist has been well established; the timing for introducing it is a crucial factor. Relaxation therapy is used after the therapist has observed the dissociated ego states (for example, immersion in angry, hostile feelings or pervasive feelings of affection) and the repetitive alternation between two ego states with a concomitant denial of one while in the other. During these times the client's memory is affected and when angry, for example, there is no memory of pleasant feelings or events for the object of this anger. It is not used when the client is immersed in a particular ego state; it is used while the client is in the "zone of fear that lies between the two states" (Glantz, 1982, p. 345).

Family therapy

Family therapy for borderline clients involves moving the family structure from lower level defensive patterning to a higher level of patterning (Mandelbaum, 1977, p. 437).

The same issues and problems arise within a family setting as do within the individual treatment of the disorder. Use of primitive defenses such as splitting and issues of separation-individuation are all present and must be dealt with. While problems are similar, there may be (particularly in the case of the borderline adolescent) more opportunities for change. There may be another chance within the family of origin to resolve failures thus reconciling good and bad images and to reach a point where ambivalence can be tolerated. Feelings of closeness and love need to be experienced without the threat of loss of identity, without risking merger and fusion. Separation and growth toward autonomy can be worked on through the individual and supported through working with all of the family members.

Group therapy

Borderline clients who present severe weaknesses in ego functioning and object relations development may benefit from group therapy. As an adjunct to individual therapy, group therapy is recommended by numerous therapists as providing the kind of mutual support and mutual control that severe borderline clients need (Freed, 1980, p. 357). Freed notes that there are several advantages to group therapy that are specific to borderline pathology:

1. Group therapy helps the client learn to listen to others, to explore and begin to understand the communication of others.

2. There is much opportunity for reality testing within the group.
3. There is the possibility of a corrective emotional experience without the forced (and threatening) closeness of a one-to-one relationship.
4. Reactions can be somewhat diluted within the group. For instance, clients may not feel narcissistically devastated by any criticism when others in the group are hearing similar comments.
5. Defensive mechanisms like splitting and projective identification are ideally handled in the group situation.
6. There are opportunities for dealing with maladaptive behavior with the goal of learning new ways within the protective atmosphere of a group.
7. A supportive, working group can enhance the formation of trust and the kind of closeness that can help foster individuation in each group member.

In conducting group therapy sessions with borderline clients, the basic principles of group therapy apply (see Chapter 11). Some principles adapted from Kibel (1978) that are specific to the disorder include:

1. Clarification of the here-and-now relationships within the group is important to foster increased understanding of distortions and of the tendency to distort through projective identification, splitting, and primitive idealization. The client needs to distinguish what is "inside" (defensive distortions) from what is "outside" (the reality situation).
2. Improved reality testing in all areas needs to be fostered and supported.
3. The mutual support and mutual control of the group is facilitated by the leader's directing major interventions toward the group as a whole. The threat of closeness with, or harm from, the leader is also diluted through this process.
4. Aggressive drives are channeled through verbalization and problem solving.

5. The degree of confrontation of individuals needs to be modified from that for a group of neurotic clients since there is the danger it may serve as a narcissistic blow.

Hospitalization

Hospitalization, when it is necessary for the borderline client, should be brief. This is to prevent a negative therapeutic reaction activated by a tendency to regress in situations of dependency. Hospitalization most often occurs at times of crisis in the client's life and often around issues of dependency on significant others (for example, the breakup of a relationship). Hospitalization may be precipitated by threats of suicide. Regressed, suicidal individuals need a setting that provides Winnicott's ideal of a "holding environment." This implies an empathetic, nurturing yet appropriately limit-setting situation.

Borderline clients tend to repeat with the staff the interaction patterns they have employed in the past. This is the basis for a major problem—the development of negative countertransference by staff members. (See Chapter 9 for a discussion of countertransference.) Manipulation of others is a common life-style theme of borderline clients. Most often this manipulation serves unconscious needs but the staff may interpret it as conscious, willful behavior and may respond with decreased empathy, increased anger, and withdrawal. Adler (1977) points out that hospitalization is a special problem because the chaotic behavior of borderline pathology can activate in the staff members themselves repressed, primitive defenses, such as splitting and projective identification. He emphasizes the importance of this potential and advocates continuing vigilance for the danger signals of countertransference.

Wishnie (1975, p. 43) lists three factors necessary for brief hospitalization to be effective as a therapeutic modality for borderline clients:

1. *Rapid identification* of the client as suffering from borderline pathology
2. *Clear limit-setting*—goals, limits and what

can be expected from the hospitalization all need to be defined
3. Administrative support of *consistency* from the staff members through education, supervision, and communication

NURSING INTERVENTION

PRIMARY PREVENTION

Since the genetic roots of a borderline syndrome are believed to be in a disturbed, preoedipal period of development (roughly, before three and a half years of age), primary prevention of the disorder naturally encompasses some sort of therapeutic intervention with the mother-infant dyad and the family. Bowen (1976) (see Chapter 12) has pointed out that mental illness results from a multigenerational transmission of disorder so that treatment of the parent becomes a means of primary prevention for the child. Grinker and his associates (see below) point out that maternal depression is an outstanding feature in the families of borderline individuals. Family therapy can be viewed as primary prevention. Minuchin (1976) points to the enmeshment patterns of a pathological family system. This includes overresponsiveness and overinvolvement but also distancing maneuvers. Such a pattern can activate abandonment depression and seriously disturb issues of separation-individuation.

In addition to *treatment* of the parents as a primary prevention method, *education* of parents about their roles in fostering healthy object relations with the child is a means of primary prevention. Some work has been done on the need for and methods used to facilitate healthy parent-infant interactions (Brazelton and Als, 1979; Field, 1982). *Interaction coaching* is a term used to describe this. An intuitive and natural sensitivity of a mother to her child's needs is not present in everyone. Interaction coaching is an attempt to modify disturbed mother-infant interactions with the goal of improving the ''fit'' between them.

If primary prevention is to be possible, it is necessary that high risk families be identified. Grinker and his associates (1968), in their research study of borderline pathology, have delineated ten recurring qualities that they found in the nuclear families of borderline individuals:

1. A highly discordant marital relationship
2. Relationships within the family that reflect chronic, overt conflict or competition
3. Parenthood rejected outright or conflict over parenthood
4. A lack of provision of nurturing care for the children
5. The mother's affect is predominantly negative
6. The marital couple is unable to achieve mutuality of purpose and their conflicting demands remain unresolved
7. Family goals do not include support of its members
8. Father's affect remains predominantly negative
9. The couple engage in mutual devaluation and criticism
10. The husband and wife are unable to achieve reciprocal role relationships

To summarize, some important points under ''primary prevention'' would include

1. Identification of parent-child dyad and families at high risk for producing borderline offspring
2. Therapeutic intervention with, and support of, high-risk parents and family units
3. Education and interaction coaching aimed at facilitating healthy relationships within the nuclear family
4. Education of parents about the needs of the toddler for healthy separation-individuation

SECONDARY PREVENTION

Most writers agree that the borderline syndrome is a rather long continuum that includes varying degrees of pathology. The range is from severely impaired ego functioning, with severely disordered interpersonal relationships, to minimal impairment with relatively high functioning. It is important to remember that, because of the chaotic nature of the individual's inner and outer life, the course of treatment may also be chaotic.

Nursing process

This section focuses on secondary prevention through nursing intervention into clients' patterns of impaired ego functioning and object-relations development, alleviation of symptoms associated with borderline personality syndrome, and restoration of functional patterns of client behavior. It is important to assess an individual's level of functioning and coping in general.

Nurses, in establishing therapeutic nurse-client relationships with borderline clients, may be helped by the following guidelines (adapted from Masterson's four-stage guide for treating the borderline client [1974]):

1. In the initial phase of treatment, the client is defending against abandonment depression and needs assurance that this relationship will not intensify the terror of abandonment. The client's defenses may include acting-out behavior (see Chapter 17 for a discussion of acting out) and other forms of ''testing.'' When the client becomes more comfortable with the relationship, the second phase of the therapeutic relationship is begun.

2. In this ''working through'' phase, the abandonment depression is dealt with. The client's depression may deepen somewhat during this second phase but the relationship provides a structure that makes it easier to cope with. Through the use of therapeutic communication techniques, the principles of psychiatric nursing, and the use of self as a therapeutic tool, the nurse helps the client to get in touch with the anger that is underlying the depression. There is the possibility of working through some of the feelings of hopelessness, rage, and loneliness that are

the core of the developmental arrest.

3. The client begins to develop some ability to integrate ''good'' and ''bad'' images of people through a consistent, nonexploitative relationship with the nurse. The client's development of an internalized sense of identity and object representations is facilitated while healthy separation-individuation is encouraged by the nurse. Examples of this would be allowing for and discussing ''differences'' between nurse and client and supporting the client's decision-making processes.

4. In the termination phase of the relationship, the client may experience regressive feelings and may need to be reminded of the differences between separation and abandonment. The goal is for the client to realize his or her potential for a separate but related life with others.

An understanding of potential problem areas and of the possibilities for healing within the context of the nurse-client relationship is important in working with borderline clients. The nursing process serves as a conceptual framework for this work.

ASSESSMENT

Based on some of the theoretical constructs of ego psychology and object relations development as discussed earlier in this chapter, the following areas can be assessed when working with the borderline client:

1. Presenting symptoms. Brief, psychoticlike episodes; impulsive self-destructive behaviors; disordered, chaotic interpersonal relationships; drug and alcohol abuse; promiscuity; poor work history. These are the behavioral manifestations of the core problem—abandonment depression that is based on developmental defects (failure to synthesize ''good'' and ''bad''; failure to separate-individuate; failure to develop *sublimation* adequately).

2. Emotional state: Feelings of rage, depression, helplessness, anxiety, and boredom in response to stimulus situations. An under-

standing of the tendency for the individual to rapidly ''shift'' emotional states is also important here.

3. Stimulus situations. Stressful life situations are often part of a vicious cycle wherein the person's self-defeating behavior perpetuates a life of poor functioning, disordered interpersonal relationships, and many painful crises.

4. Maladaptive coping behaviors. Coping patterns based on primitive defensive organization—splitting, projective identification, primitive idealization, omnipotence-devaluation in relating to others. These primitive defenses are attempts to satisfy and protect oneself but they are unsuccessful in that they perpetuate a painful, unsatisfactory life-style of disordered interpersonal relations and inadequate functioning in the world.

5. Origin of maladaptive coping behaviors. Identification of childhood experiences that contributed to the development or learning of maladaptive coping behaviors, to the continued reliance on primitive defenses, and to severe difficulties in separation-individuation.

6. Holistic health status. Physical, intellectual, emotional, sociocultural, and spiritual status of the client. These factors may either facilitate wellness (for example, an intact, nuclear family that is motivated to change through their desire to help the ''identified client,'' may well facilitate the client's growth through participation in family therapy), or these factors may impede wellness (for example, a seriously physically disabled borderline client who must necessarily be very dependent on others may find it extremely difficult to work through and resolve issues of separation-individuation.

ANALYSIS OF DATA

With some understanding of presenting symptoms, emotional state, stimulus situations, maladaptive coping behavior and their origins, and the holistic health status of these clients, the nurse will get a clearer and more empathetic understanding of the predicament these clients and their families face. This empathetic understanding is a prerequisite to formulating nursing diagnoses. The following section will focus on nursing diagnoses which may be made for borderline clients. A discussion of short-term goals, long-term goals, and implementation of planning will be included with each diagnosis. *Helplessness, dependency* and *feelings of worthlessness* as themes have been covered in Chapter 18; *manipulation, aggressive behavior* and *acting out through substance abuse* were discussed in Chapter 17; approaches to *psychotic behavior* are found in Chapter 21. Since these are all important themes of the borderline personality, it will assist the nurse to review the principles discussed in these chapters. Nursing diagnoses based on themes of splitting, primitive idealization, projective identification, rapidly changing ego states, omnipotence of self with devaluation of others, boredom, and inability to tolerate aloneness will be discussed.

Since the borderline client is coping with the effects of an early developmental arrest with hopes of growing toward greater autonomy, the treatment of this disorder tends to be a long-term undertaking. Therefore, the long-term goals (as outlined under the nursing diagnoses that follow) will most often be undertaken or accomplished by clients working with a clinical nurse specialist (or other therapists) in an outpatient setting. The short-term goals support these long-term goals, however, and they are consistent with the work of the professional nurse working in a psychiatric setting.

Nursing diagnosis: Defects in perceptions related to an impairment in ability to synthesize contradictory images of self, others, and situations— splitting (behavior associated with DSM-III diagnosis 300.83: borderline personality disorder)

Planning: With assistance and guidance from the nurse, the client will establish goals.

1. Long-term goals
   a. Synthesize and integrate contradictory images of self and others in order to accept self and others as wholes.
   b. Accept ambivalence of self and ambivalence in the world.
   c. Develop and strengthen an observing ego.*
2. Short-term goals
   a. Develop awareness of splitting mechanisms and patterns when they are used.
   b. Identify interpersonal and environmental situations that trigger the use of splitting mechanisms and patterns.
   c. Identify difficulties in interpersonal relationships and in the ability to function that are related to the reliance on splitting mechanisms and patterns.
   d. Develop more effective coping behaviors and interpersonal skills.

Implementation: Splitting can be defined as a defense mechanism that helps the individual cope with anxiety by keeping two opposite affective states separate—"bad" and "good" images cannot be integrated because of an early developmental arrest. At a very early age, it is a normal protective mechanism for keeping the "bad" mother image from contaminating the "good" mother image. However, in normal development, this becomes unnecessary and the representations merge. Some ways in which the nurse may help the client who has not been able to accomplish this, to "heal the split," follow:

1. Point out the client's tendency to see only one aspect of self, others, and situations as it occurs within the course of the nurse-client relationship (for example, "You seem to have a great deal of difficulty remembering anything good about yourself when you get depressed"; "Today, it sounds like you are not able to accept anything positive about your mother—that's different from yester-

---

*Strengthening an *observing ego* implies that there is (1) an increasing awareness of one's own behavior and its effects on self and the environment and (2) a decreasing tendency toward harsh, judgemental (punitive superego) reactions to oneself that only serve to escalate defensive, self-defeating behaviors. Instead, one is able to work toward realistic behavioral changes that will enhance separation-individuation.

day, when you said you felt very close to her'').

2. Relate specific occurrences of the client's splitting to any particular stimulus situations.

3. Support the development of active self-observation by the client when he or she is experiencing strongly positive or negative feelings (an ''observing ego'').

4. Respond verbally to the client's splitting in a manner that helps to integrate contradictory reactions (for example, ''It sounds like you're saying that you like some of the things your mother does when she's being helpful but sometimes you get angry with her when she tries to take over too much; I guess you have a mixture of feelings toward her, which is very natural'').

5. Remember, as a nurse, the importance of self-awareness to avoid identifying with the client's negative or positive split. The goal is for the client to accept self, others, and the world as a necessary mixture of good, bad, and indifferent.

Nursing diagnosis: Distortions in perceptions with disturbed interpersonal relationships, related to protection of self from dangerously perceived introjects—projective identification (behavior associated with DSM-III diagnosis 300.83: borderline personality disorder)

Planning: With assistance and guidance from the nurse, the client will establish goals.

1. Long-term goals
   a. Synthesize and integrate negative and positive images of self and others to relate to self and others as whole persons.
   b. Accept ambivalence in the self and ambivalence in the world.
   c. Relinquish dependency on projective identification as a defense and develop normal repression.
   d. Develop and strengthen an observing ego.

2. Short-term goals
   a. Develop awareness of any distortions of others and their motives in interpersonal situations.

b. Identify interpersonal and environmental situations that trigger the use of projective identification as a defense.
   c. Identify difficulties in interpersonal relating and in ability to function related to reliance on projective identification as a defense.
   d. Develop more effective coping behavior and interpersonal skills.

Implementation: Projective identification is a lower level or more primitive defense mechanism than projection. Projective identification serves to externalize (get rid of) all-bad, potentially dangerous images of the self and all-good, potentially nurturing images of the self. However, its use leads to a view of the world as full of dangerous, powerful, and retaliatory persons whom one must control. In projective identification, attributes, tendencies, strengths, and weaknesses may be projected into the person (1) to externalize and thus ''control'' the dangerous introject or (2) to achieve symbiosis with a powerful and good externalized introject. The end result is a severe distortion of reality that can disorder interpersonal relationships and impair one's ability to function in life.

A *consistent clarification* to reduce distortions as they appear in the nurse-client relationship is an appropriate and therapeutic nursing response. *Self-awareness* and a *nondefensive,* objective stance on the part of the nurse is crucial, because part of projective identification includes the client's unconsciously motivated efforts to manipulate the person to react in harmony with the projection (see Chapter 17 for a discussion of the nursing responses to manipulation). To summarize:

1. Observe the client for tendencies to overreact in interpersonal situations or to distort perceptions of others.

2. Explore the client's perception in situations of possible overreaction or distortion.

3. Clarify situations whenever possible—provide additional input, examples of modifying circumstances, other view points; use the communication technique of ''reasonable doubt''; be a bridge to reality in this situation

(for further discussion of communication techniques, refer to Chapter 9).

4. Support the development of active self-observation by clients when they suspect any hint of overreacting or distorting in interpersonal situations (an ''observing ego'').

5. Remember the importance of self-awareness to minimize any manipulation by the client aimed at inducing you to react in harmony with the projection.

Nursing diagnosis: Interaction theme of *primitive idealization* related to (1) the protection of self from dangerously perceived internal images and projections and (2) the gratification of needs through identification with an ''all-good'' and powerful other (behavior associated with DSM-III diagnosis 300.83: borderline personality disorder)

Planning: With assistance and guidance from the nurse, the client will establish goals.

1. Long-term goals
   a. Work through exaggerated and debilitating fears of living in the world.
   b. Tolerate a probabilistic world and the possibility of ambivalent, negative, or indifferent feelings from others or toward others.
   c. Begin to relate to others on a more realistic level that incorporates healthy ambivalence.
   d. Develop a mature level of dependence on others rather than immature dependence.
   e. Develop a mature level of interdependence with others.
   f. Develop and strengthen an observing ego.

2. Short-term goals
   a. Verbalize feelings of loss, inadequacy, and fear.
   b. Identify interpersonal situations that arouse fears of possible attack from the environment or from a harshly critical superego (review the concept of superego in Chapter 7).
   c. Relate current stressful situation to situations in the past that aroused similar feelings.

d. Develop more effective coping and interpersonal skills.
   e. Realistically perceive self (biological, psychological, intellectual, sociocultural, and spiritual strengths and weaknesses will be put in perspective).
   f. Realistically perceive strengths and weaknesses of others.
   g. Build self-esteem (refer to Chapter 18 for a discussion of self-esteem).

Implementation: Expressions of idealistic admiration for the nurse that are exaggerations or unrelated to any real situation are indications that a client is using primitive idealization as a defense. It will be helpful to remember the following points:

1. Allow the client to verbalize and explore the nature of fears about self and the world.
2. Clarify any distortions about you, the nurse, in an objective and dispassionate manner.
3. Use the communication techniques of ''reasonable doubt'' in response to the client's exaggerated claims about your attributes. (This is not to be confused with a ''becoming modesty''—the goal is not to confess the ordinary nature of your *self* so much as it is to help the client to see and tolerate an imperfect, human *you*. This should be done in combination with the acknowledgement of any realistic appraisal of your good qualities. Again, it is apparent that self-awareness on the part of the nurse is crucial.)
4. Explore with the client incidents, situations, and interpersonal relationships outside of the nurse-client relationship wherein a tendency to use primitive idealization is evident.
5. Explore with the client a more realistically based appraisal of self.

Nursing diagnosis: Interaction theme of *omnipotence of self with devaluation of others* related to protection of self from self-derogating introjects and projections (behavior associated with DSM-III diagnosis 300.83: borderline personality disorder)

Planning: With assistance and guidance from the nurse, the client will establish goals.

1. Long-term goals

a. Work through exaggerated and debilitating fears of living in the world.
b. Tolerate a probabilistic world.
c. Develop a realistic sense of self and others.
d. Accept oneself and others as separate, whole people.
e. Develop a mature level of dependence on others.
f. Develop a mature level of interdependence with others.
g. Develop and strengthen an observing ego.
2. Short-term goals
a. Verbalize feelings of grandiosity and inadequacy.
b. Identify interpersonal situations that arouse defensive feelings of grandiosity of self or devaluation of others.
c. Relate current stressful situation to situations in the past that aroused similar feelings.
d. Identify current difficulties in interpersonal relations and in ability to function related to viewing the self as omnipotent and others as devalued.
e. Develop more effective coping skills.
f. Realistically perceive self (biological, psychological, intellectual, sociocultural, and spiritual strengths and weaknesses will be put in perspective).
g. Realistically perceive strengths and weaknesses of others.
h. Build self-esteem in a reality-based context.

Implementation: Feelings of insecurity and a harsh, punitive superego underlie the more obvious statements and actions of grandiosity. Devaluation of others is part of the same matrix of low self-esteem but it is more likely to appear on a more subtle level. In this case, it is important for the nurse to maintain an equilibrium that will lead to a nondefensive approach. Limit-setting that points out the reality of a situation in an objective manner may be necessary whenever grandiosity leads to testing behavior, manipulation, and acting out. A helpful technique in dealing with a client's *devaluation of others* is to relate it back to the client. ''Do you ever have any of these same complaints about yourself?'' This may lead to an exploration of the underlying fears and harsh judgements about the self.

Nursing diagnosis: Psychic disequilibrium related to rapid alterations in perceptions and feelings about self, others, or situations—*rapidly shifting ego states with mutual denial** (behavior associated with DSM-III diagnosis 300.83: borderline personality disorder)

Planning: With assistance and guidance from the nurse, the client will establish goals.
1. Long-term goals
a. Synthesize and integrate contradictory inner images in order to relate to self and others as whole persons.
b. Accept a probabilistic world and healthy ambivalence in self and others.
c. Develop a consistent sense of self-identity.
d. Develop and strengthen an observing ego.
2. Short-term goals
a. Develop a trusting relationship with the nurse.
b. Develop awareness of phenomenon of rapidly shifting ego states in self.
c. Verbalize the subjective experience of rapidly shifting ego states in self.
d. Develop awareness of the use of denial in relation to rapidly shifting ego states.
e. Identify stressful situations that seem to trigger rapid shifts in ego states.
f. Identify difficulties in interpersonal relating and in ability to function that are related to this phenomenon.

Implementation: When experiencing this phenomenon, the client may or may not be aware (on

---

*The phenomenon of rapidly shifting ego states with mutual denial is engendered by the underlying defect in synthesizing contradictory internal images of the self and others. There may be intellectual awareness of two opposing ego states, but there is denial of the emotional relevance of one while immersed in the other.

an intellectual level) that perceptions, feelings, and thought about self and others are quite opposite to those held previously. However, even when this intellectual awareness is present, the emotional relevance of it is denied in the current situation. Confrontation about the client's use of denial as it occurs can help bring the problem into focus while it is still fresh in the mind, but at a point in time when the client is able to be fairly calm, it can also help to do some tracking of behaviors and experiences just prior to immersion in the ego state. Exploration of the phenomenon as it operates within the self should also be included (for example, what may have happened to trigger the shift from one state to the other; was there a threat to the self-system and, if so, what was it? Is this reaction to this particular stressor an identifiable pattern in the client's life?)

Nursing diagnosis: Psychic disequilibrium related to extreme fears of abandonment, impairment in separation-individuation process, and inadequately developed ability to sublimate—*the inability to tolerate aloneness* (behavior associated with DSM-III 300.83: borderline personality disorder)

Planning: With assistance and guidance from the nurse, the client will establish goals.

1. Long-term goals
   a. Accept one's separateness and wholeness; tolerate closeness in interpersonal relationships without the need for fusion.
   b. Work through issues of separation-individuation with growth toward object constancy (see p. 626 for discussion of object constancy) in one's inner life.
   c. Develop an increased ability to sublimate.
   d. Develop the ability to be in comfortable harmony with one's aloneness.
2. Short-term goals
   a. Develop a trusting relationship with the nurse.
   b. Explore any underlying feelings of anger.
   c. Explore fears of separation and aloneness.
   d. Identify difficulties in relating interper-

sonally and in ability to function that are related to fears of abandonment and inability to tolerate aloneness
   e. Explore difficulties in sublimating the need for contact with others through substitute activities, interests, etc.
   f. Develop alternative ways of sublimating through substitute activities, interests, etc.
   g. Increase tolerance for times of "being alone."

Implementation: The inability to tolerate aloneness is a long-term treatment issue and would be more apt to arise with the clinical specialist who is involved in ongoing, individual therapy with a borderline client. Short-term goals are relevant and appropriate to the professional nurse working in a psychiatric setting. Consistency and trust in the nurse-client relationship are important features in helping the client deal with fears of abandonment and the underlying rage that is being defended against. The nurse will need "skill, empathy and the capacity to tolerate rage, confusion and disappointment" (Adler and Buie, 1979, p. 441) in helping the client to grow and develop a tolerance for inevitable periods of aloneness.

The client's feelings of panic over aloneness can be manifested through a profound sense of emptiness, painful restlessness, and boredom and feelings of anger that may be displaced onto the nurse. When feelings of panic over isolation and aloneness escalate, this is generally the time of greatest danger for suicide attempts in the borderline client. Nurses in inpatient units and in outpatient settings must be aware and vigilant at this time to protect the client (a discussion on nursing intervention for suicidal clients can be found in Chapter 18).

A failure to accomplish object constancy is a core problem underlying the difficulties borderline clients have with aloneness. The use of transitional objects (see above discussion) may prove useful at times of separation from the therapist such as vacations or illnesses. Examples include structured telephone contacts and the client's keeping a journal of thoughts and feelings to evoke memories of the therapist.

Verbal acknowledgement of the client's efforts toward successful mastery of these difficult periods can serve as a positive reinforcement and stimulate further growth in this area.

Exploration and, at times, concrete assistance from the therapist may be necessary in developing new interests, hobbies and vocations that can encourage healthy sublimation and increased ability to cope with aloneness.

Nursing diagnosis: Psychic disequilibrium related to denial of feelings and inadequately developed ability to sublimate—*chronic feelings of boredom* (behavior associated with DSM-III diagnosis 300.83: borderline personality disorder)

Planning: With assistance and guidance from the nurse, the client will establish goals.
1. Long-term goals
   a. Increase awareness of underlying feelings and be able to cope with them in a healthy manner.
   b. Develop meaningful interests, hobbies, or vocation—increased ability to sublimate.
2. Short-term goals
   a. Explore feelings of boredom.
   b. Explore underlying feelings (anger; emptiness; fear; hopelessness).
   c. Identify times when there is a greater tendency to feel bored.
   d. Identify activities that help to decrease feelings of boredom.
   e. When appropriate, relate any tendencies to "act out" with self-destructive behavior to attempts to cope with boredom.

Implementation: Chronic feelings of boredom are an especially painful part of the borderline syndrome. It is also a difficult symptom to alleviate. Some suggestions for working with this problem include:
1. The client's awareness and verbalization of underlying (denied) feelings may be the most important aspect of dealing with chronic boredom. It is possible that the release of energy associated with even a partial resolution of conflict can provide the stimulus to the client's own successful efforts to counteract boredom.
2. Boredom implies a sort of hopelessness in the person who suffers from it. Therefore, patience on the part of the nurse is crucial. Clients who are experiencing chronic feelings of boredom tend to take a help-rejecting stance in response to any assistance toward constructive coping with it.
3. Helping the client develop a reality-based, problem-solving approach to the problem of boredom is more helpful than supplying pat suggestions for dealing with it. However, concrete direction in the form of client teaching or referral to outside sources can be beneficial and is often necessary in helping the client develop new interests in life.

EVALUATION

The client and, whenever feasible, the client's family or significant others should be included in estimating the client's progress toward attainment of goals. Evaluation should encompass the following areas:
1. Estimation of the degree to which conflicts around separation-individuation and defects in achieving object constancy have been dealt with (this would include *awareness* of conflicts and problem areas and beginning efforts toward working them through)
2. Estimation of the degree to which goals have been achieved and client functioning has improved (demonstrated by decreased disorder in interpersonal relationships; increased ability to function in society; decreased reliance on addictive behavior and increased inner harmony)
3. Identification of goals that need to be modified or revised
4. Referral of the client to support systems other than the nurse-client relationship
   a. People in the client's social network who

are willing to serve as a support system
   b. Clinics or individuals for ongoing individual psychotherapy
   c. Community agencies or self-help groups that help clients learn to live with disorders that may never be completely eliminated (for example, Recovery, Inc.)
   d. Centers or organizations that specialize in the treatment of specific problem areas for some borderline clients (for example, Alcoholics Anonymous, Gamblers Anonymous)

TERTIARY PREVENTION

Borderline personality syndrome is a disorder that usually requires long-term treatment. Because of the chaotic life-style with poor impulse control, low frustration tolerance, and a tendency to act out internal conflicts, many borderline clients will need much in the way of supportive, rehabilitative services. Hospitalization, when it is necessary, is generally brief and is specifically recommended to prevent the tendency to regress that is a common feature of borderline pathology. Follow-up care *after* hospitalization is important. A more severely disturbed individual may benefit from a structured day hospital or partial hospitalization setting and from re-training through vocational rehabilitation programs. In those cases where acting out has taken the form of substance abuse or other addictive behaviors, referrals to such self-help groups as Alcoholics Anonymous, Narcotics Anonymous, Gamblers Anonymous, or Overeaters Anonymous should be explored. For the borderline client who suffers from debilitating, chronic anxiety, a group such as Recovery, Inc., which uses a form of self-monitored behavioral modification, can be very helpful. The client whose dysfunctional interpersonal relations have gravely affected marital and family harmony should be referred for marital or family therapy. During any brief psychoticlike episodes, it may be necessary for the client to be placed on a temporary regimen of major tranquil-

izers to prevent the deterioration of self-esteem to which one is vulnerable at these times.

CHAPTER SUMMARY

Borderline personality disorder is a DSM-III diagnostic category used to describe an ever increasing number of clients. Borderline syndrome or borderline personality organization are terms also used to describe the condition. Much of the work on etiology and treatment methods has been carried out by psychoanalysts, but, more often, intervention with this group is carried out by social workers and nurses working in inpatient units and outpatient settings. It is a condition that can be viewed as being on a continuum of degrees of pathological functioning. Severely disordered interpersonal relationships, difficulties in functioning as evidenced by poor school and vocational histories, lack of impulse control demonstrated by addictive behaviors, and a general tendency to act out inner conflicts are some of the common features of the syndrome.

Behavioral symptoms of borderline pathology include a reliance on primitive-level defense mechanisms such as splitting, projective identification, and primitive denial; the dysfunctional interpersonal modes of primitive idealization and omnipotence of self with devaluation of others; and the subjective experience of rapidly shifting ego states with mutual denial, chronic boredom, and an inability to tolerate aloneness.

The etiology of borderline syndrome is believed to be rooted in the rapprochement subphase of the developmental phase of separation-individuation. Because of problems in the interaction of the mother-child dyad, a developmental arrest is believed to occur that interferes with the person's ability to synthesize the ''good'' and ''bad'' qualities (or contradictory images) of self and others. The important developmental task of object constancy is not adequately mastered. Excessive reliance on splitting has its genesis here and most of the behavior and the other defenses are derivatives of this reliance on splitting.

Some theorists have pointed to profound sociocultural changes (such as the changes in values, family life) as being closely related to the increase in borderline pathology.

Primary prevention of the syndrome would focus on therapeutic intervention with the parents *before* the rapprochement crisis and interaction coaching of mother-child dyads to improve the "fit."

Secondary prevention includes individual therapy as the treatment of choice, with adjunct services from family and group therapy for some clients. Treatment tends to be long-term. Tertiary prevention may encompass vocational rehabilitation, self-help groups, and structured treatment settings such as day care. Since the chaotic lifestyle and disordered interpersonal relationships of the borderline client may damage family and marital relationships, therapy in these areas needs to be considered, too.

SENSITIVITY-AWARENESS EXERCISES

The purposes of the following exercises are to:

- Develop awareness about the subjective experiences of clients who are suffering from borderline personality disorder and the experience of clients' families in relating to them
- Develop awareness about the interrelationship of factors from the past and in the present in perpetuating the syndrome
- Develop awareness about your own feelings and abilities when working with clients who are suffering from borderline disorder

1. Try to imagine what it would be like to experience one of the following (and explain why you selected that particular problem area and what you think it would be like to experience it):
   a. Rapidly shifting states of thinking, feeling, perceiving; rapid and complete swings from one emotional state to the other (for example, angry and rageful to loving and affectionate)
   b. A need to see someone you are close to as *only* good, caring, comforting, brilliant
   c. A need to see someone you are interacting with as bad, disgusting, frightening
   d. Recurring periods of *extreme* anxiety, bordering on panic, in response to the absence of someone with whom you are close (Try to imagine that this person has left temporarily and you are alone and that you have a great deal of difficulty remembering that person's qualities, voice, and even picturing his or her face in fantasy.)
   e. Chronic feelings of boredom with little or no desire or ability to engage in creative or even distracting activities
2. Describe what you think it would be like to relate to a close friend or family member who experiences several of the problem areas listed above.
3. What might be some of your feelings and reactions as a nurse caring for clients who are suffering from borderline personality disorder? Would some of the problem areas outlined above be more difficult to deal with than others? Might some (for example, the client's need to see you as all-good, caring and loving, and very bright) be fairly "easy to take"? (Explain your answers.)
4. What do you think might be some of the difficulties in establishing and maintaining a consistent, trusting relationship with a borderline client?
5. As a community health nurse engaged in health supervision with new parents, develop a plan of counseling parents about child rearing that incorporates principles and goals for primary prevention of borderline personality disorder.

REFERENCES

Adler, G.

1975 "The usefulness of the 'borderline' concept in psychotherapy." In Borderline States in Psychiatry. J. Mack (ed.). New York: Grune and Stratton, pp. 29-40

1977 "Hospital management of borderline patients and its relation to psychotherapy." In Borderline Personality Disorders: The Concept, the Syndrome, the Patient. P. Harticollis (ed.). New York: International Universities Press, Inc., pp. 307-323.

1981 "The borderline-narcissistic personality disorder continuum." American Journal of Psychiatry 138:46-50.

Adler, G., and D. Buie

1979 "The psychotherapeutic approach to aloneness in the borderline patient." In Advances in Psychotherapy of the Borderline Patient. J. LeBoit and A. Capponi (eds.). New York: Jason Aronson, Inc., pp. 433-448.

Akhtar, S., and J. Byrne
    1983 "The concept of splitting and its clinical relevance."
        American Journal of Psychiatry 140(8):1013-1016.
Arieti, S., and G. Chrzanowski (eds.)
    1975 New Dimensions in Psychiatry: A World View. New
        York: John Wiley and Sons, Inc.
Blanck, G., and R. Blanck
    1979 Ego Psychology II. New York: Columbia University
        Press.
Bowen, M.
    1976 "Theory in the practice of psychotherapy." Family
        Therapy. P.J. Guerin (ed.). New York: Gardner Press,
        Inc.
Boyer, L.
    1982 "Borderline personality disorder: Psychoanalysis." In
        Therapies for Adults. H. Millman, J. Huber, and D.
        Diggins (eds.). San Francisco: Jossey-Bass Publishers,
        pp. 336-341.
Boyer, L., and P. Giovacchini
    1967 Psychoanalytic Treatment of Characterological and
        Schizophrenic Disorders. New York: Science House.
Brazelton, T., and H. Als
    1979 "Four early states in the development of mother-infant
        interaction." In The Psychoanalytic Study of the Child,
        34. New York: International Universities Press.
Capponi, A.
    1979 "Origins and evolution of the borderline patient." In
        Advances in Psychotherapy of the Borderline Patient. J.
        LeBoit and A. Capponi (eds.). New York: Jason Aron-
        son, Inc., pp. 61-147.
Chessick, R.
    1977 Intensive Psychotherapy of the Borderline Patient. New
        York: Jason Aronson, Inc.
Chrzanowski, G.
    1975 "Recent advances in concepts and treatment of border-
        line cases." In New Dimensions in Psychiatry: A World
        View. S. Arieti and G. Chrzanowski (eds.). New York:
        John Wiley and Sons, Inc., pp. 145-220.
Diagnostic and Statistical Manual of Mental Disorders
    1980 The American Psychiatric Association.
Fairbairn, W.
    1952 Psychoanalytic Studies of the Personality. London:
        Tavistock. Reprinted as An Object-Relations Theory of
        the Personality. New York: Basic Books, 1954.

Field, T.
    1982 "Interaction coaching for high-risk infants and their
        parents." Prevention in Human Services, vol. 1, no. 4.
Freed, A.
    1980 "The borderline personality." Social Casework 61(9):
        548-558.
Freud, A.
    1936 The Ego and Its Mechanisms of Defense. London: Ho-
        garth Press.
Glantz, K.
    1982 "Borderline personality disorder: Relaxation technique
        as an adjunct to psychodynamic treatment." In Ther-
        apies for Adults. H. Millman, J. Huber, and D. Diggins,
        (eds.). San Francisco: Jossey-Bass Publishers, pp. 342-
        346.
Green, A.
    1977 "The borderline concept." In Borderline Personality
        Disorders: The Concept, the Syndrome, the Patient. P.
        Harticollis (ed.). New York: International Universities
        Press, Inc., pp. 15-44.
Grinker, R., Sr., B. Werble, and R. Drye
    1968 the Borderline Syndrome. New York: Basic Books.
Grotstein, J.
    1979 "The psychoanalytic concept of the borderline organi-
        zation." In Advances in Psychotherapy of the Border-
        line Patient. J. LeBoit and A. Capponi (eds.). New
        York: Jason Aronson, Inc., pp. 149-183.
Gunderson, J., and J. Kolb
    1978 "Discriminating features of borderline patients."
        American Journal of Psychiatry, 135:792-796.
Gunderson, J., and M. Singer
    1975 "Defining borderline states." American Journal of
        Psychiatry, 132:1-10.
Guntrip, H.
    1961 Personality Structure and Human Interaction: The De-
        velopment Synthesis of Psychodynamic Theory. New
        York: International Universities Press.
Hartmann, H.
    1958 Ego Psychology and the Problem of Adaptation. New
        York: International Universities Press.
Hartmann, H., E. Kris, and R. Lowenstein
    1946 "Comments on the formation of psychic structure."
        The Psychoanalytic Study of the Child 2:11-38. New
        York: International Universities Press.

Kaplan, H., and B. Sadock
1981 Modern Synopsis of Comprehensive Textbook of Psychiatry, 3rd ed. Baltimore: The Williams and Wilkins Co., p. 488.

Kernberg, O.
1975 Borderline Conditions and Pathological Narcissism. New York: Jason Aronson, Inc.
1977 "The structural diagnosis of borderline personality organization." In Borderline Personality Disorders: The Concept, the Syndrome, the Patient. P. Harticollis (ed.). New York: International Universities Press, Inc., pp. 87-121.

Kibel, H.
1978 "The rationale for the use of group psychotherapy for borderline patients on a short-term unit." International Journal of Group Psychotherapy, 28(3):339-364.

Klein, D.
1975 "Psychopharmacology and the borderline patient." In Borderline States In Psychiatry. J. Mack (ed.). New York: Grune and Stratton, Inc., pp. 75-91.
1977 "Psychopharmacological treatment and delineation of borderline disorders." In Borderline Personality Disorders: The Concept, the Syndrome, the Patient. P. Harticollis (ed.). New York: International Universities Press, Inc., pp. 365-383.

Kohut, H.
1971 The Analysis of the Self. New York: International Universities Press.

Laplanche, J., and J.B. Pontalis
1973 The Language of Psychoanalysis (translated by D. Nicholson-Smith). New York: W.W. Norton & Co., Inc.

Lasch, C.
1978 The Culture of Narcissism. New York: W.W. Norton & Co., Inc.

Lazar, N.
1973 "Nature and significance of changes in patients in a psychoanalytic clinic." Psychoanalytic Quarterly 42: 579-600.

LeBoit, J., and A. Capponi
1979 Advances in Psychotherapy of the Borderline Patient. New York: Jason Aronson, Inc.

Lynch, V., and M. Lynch
1977 "Borderline personality." Perspectives in Psychiatric Care 15(2):72-87.

Mack, J.
1975 Borderline States in Psychiatry. New York: Grune and Stratton.

Mahler, M., F. Pine, and A. Bergman
1975 The Psychological Birth of the Human Infant. New York: Basic Books, Inc.

Maltsberger, J., and D. Buie
1975 "The psychiatric resident, his borderline patient and supervisory encounter." In Borderline States in Psychiatry. J. Mack (ed.). New York: Grune and Stratton, pp. 123-134.

Mandelbaum, A.
1977 "The family treatment of the borderline patient." In Borderline Personality Disorders: The Concept, the Syndrome, the Patient. P. Harticollis (ed.). New York: International Universities Press, Inc., pp. 423-438.

Masterson, J.
1973 "The borderline adolescent." In Adolescent Psychiatry, vol. 2. S. Feinstein and P. Giovacchini (eds.). New York: Basic Books, pp. 240-268.
1974 "Intensive psychotherapy of the adolescent with a borderline syndrome." In American Handbook of Psychiatry. S. Arieti (ed.). New York: Basic Books, pp. 250-263.
1975 "The splitting defense mechanism of the borderline adolescent: Developmental and clinical aspects." In Borderline States in Psychiatry. J. Mack (ed.). New York: Grune and Stratton, pp. 93-101.
1976 Psychotherapy of the Borderline Adult. New York: Brunner/Mazel, Inc.
1977 "Primary anorexia nervosa in the borderline adolescent —An object-relations view." In Borderline Personality Disorders: The Concept, the Syndrome, the Patient. P. Harticollis (ed.). New York: International Universities Press, Inc., pp. 475-494.
1978 New Perspectives on Psychotherapy of the Borderline Adult. J. Masterson (ed.). New York: Brunner/Mazel, Inc.

Masterson, J., and D. Rinsley
1980 ''The borderline syndrome: The role of mother in the genesis and psychic structure of the borderline personality.'' In Rapprochement: The Critical Subphase of Separation-Individuation. R. Lax, S. Bach, and J. Burland (eds.). New York: Jason Aronson, Inc., pp. 299-329.

Mendelsohn, R.
1982 ''Borderline personality disorder: Short-term psychoanalytic therapy.'' In Therapies for Adults. H. Millman, J. Huber, and D. Diggins (eds.). San Francisco: Jossey-Bass, Inc., pp. 354-357.

Millman, H., J. Huber, and D. Diggins
1982 Therapies for Adults. San Francisco: Jossey-Bass, Inc.

Minuchin, S.
1976 ''A conceptual model of illness in children.'' Archives of General Psychiatry 32:1031-1038.

Pine, F.
1974 ''On the concept 'borderline' in children: a clinical essay.'' The Psychoanalytic Study of the Child 29:341-368.

Reiner, B.
1979 ''A feeling of irrelevance: The effects of a nonsupportive society.'' Social Casework 60(4).

Rinsley, D.
1977 ''An object-relations view of borderline personality.'' In Borderline Personality Disorders: The Concept, the Syndrome, the Patient. P. Harticollis (ed.). New York: International Universities Press, Inc., pp. 45-70.

Sass, L.
1982 ''The borderline personality.'' *New York Times Magazine,* August 22, 1982:12-67.

Segal, H.
1964 Introduction to the Work of Melanie Klein (ed. 2). New York: Basic Books, Inc., Publishers.

Singer, M.
1979 ''Some metapsychological and clinical distinctions between borderline and neurotic conditions with special consideration to the self experience.'' International Journal of Psychiatry 60:489-499.

Winnicott, D.
1965 The Maturational Processes and the Facilitating Environment. New York: International Universities Press, Inc.

Wishnie, H.
1975 ''Inpatient therapy with borderline patients.'' In Borderline States in Psychiatry. J. Mack (ed.). New York: Grune and Stratton, Inc., pp. 41-62.

Wolberg, A.
1973 The Borderline Patient. New York: Intercontinental Medical Book Corp.

Zinner, J., and E. Shapiro
1975 ''Splitting in families of borderline adolescents.'' In Borderline States in Psychiatry. J. Mack (ed.). New York: Grune and Stratton, Inc., pp. 103-122.

ANNOTATED SUGGESTED READINGS

Adler, G., and D. Buie
1979 ''The psychotherapeutic approach to aloneness in borderline patients'' In Advances in Psychotherapy of the Borderline Patient. J. LeBoit and A. Capponi (eds.). New York: Jason Aronson, Inc., pp. 433-447.
This is an exploration of the borderline client's difficulties in coping with aloneness. It includes a discussion of some of the developmental and psychodynamic aspects involved in an individual's reactions to aloneness. Issues in the clinical treatment of borderline clients, including the use of transitional objects *(such as tape recordings of sessions, a postcard from a vacationing therapist) are reviewed. The importance of such themes as rage and regression are also dealt with.*

Akhtar, S., and J. Byrne
1983 ''The concept of splitting and its clinical relevance.'' American Journal of Psychiatry 140(8):1013-1016.
Splitting is a central defense seen in borderline clients. The literature on the concept of splitting is reviewed here and several clinical manifestations of this primitive defense are described. These manifestations include (1) the inability to experience ambivalence, (2) impaired decision making, (3) oscillation of self-esteem, (4) ego-syntonic* impulsivity, and (5) intensification of affects. Differential diagnoses of personality disorders and treatment issues are explored.

Kibel, H.
1979 ''The rationale for the use of group psychotherapy for borderline patients on a short-term unit.'' International Journal of Group Psychotherapy 28(3):339-358.
This article focuses on three topics: the borderline client; milieu therapy for the borderline client; and group therapy within that milieu. The author focuses on descriptions and treatment recommendations for the more severely disturbed borderline client. Theoretical concepts (for example, the work of Kernberg) are reviewed and specific goals and methods for treating the client in group therapy are discussed. The topics of brief hospitalization and the problems it presents are addressed as they relate to these clients.

Lynch, V., and M. Lynch
1977 ''Borderline personality.'' Perspectives in Psychiatric Care 15(2):72-87.
The authors present a brief but well-developed overview of some of the outstanding theorists on borderline pathology (Gunderson and Singer, Kernberg and Masterson) and their important concepts (object splitting; abandonment depression). Masterson's four-stage guide for intervening with abandonment depression is included.

Mack, J. (ed.).
1975 Borderline States in Psychiatry. New York: Grune and Stratton.
This small but comprehensive book is a compilation of articles dealing with several facets of the borderline syndrome. Contributors include many well-known theorists and clinicians. There are chapters on such topics as differential diagnosis, inpatient treatment, psychopharmacology, adolescent and family treatment, as well as an informative historical perspective on borderline personality disorder.

Sass, L.
1982 ''The borderline personality.'' The New York Times Magazine, August 22:12-15, 66-67.
A well-written, comprehensive yet concise overview of the borderline syndrome, including intrapsychic, familial, and sociocultural aspects. The author is a clinical psychologist. Differing theoretical viewpoints on etiology, differential diagnosis, and effective treatment are reviewed. There is some clinical case material presented.

Singer, M.
1979 ''Some metapsychological and clinical distinctions between borderline and neurotic conditions with special consideration to the self experience.'' International Journal of Psychoanalysis 60:489-498.
This article is concerned with the experience of self in the borderline client. The importance of maintaining intact (inner) self representations and the corresponding cohesive ''sense of self'' in severe borderline pathology is explored for its implications in treatment. Therapeutic problems that arise because of a loss of the self experience are explored and there is some discussion of primitive defense mechanisms.

---

*See glossary.

CHAPTER 21

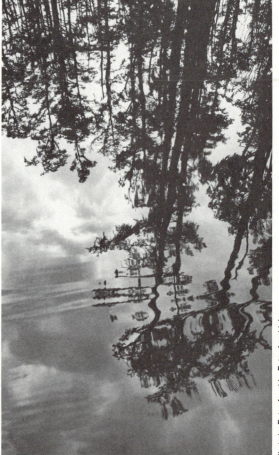

Photo by Peter Arnold—Peter Arnold, Inc.

Coping through withdrawal from reality

CHAPTER FOCUS

Schizophrenia is the most perplexing of all the psychopathies. More has been written about its etiology, course, and treatment than about any other emotional disorder.

Schizophrenia is more properly called a syndrome than a disease. It can involve any of several combinations of symptoms, disturbances, and reactions. Some writers and investigators have suggested that it would be more accurate to refer to the schizophrenias rather than to a single entity. The condition has probably always been with mankind, at least since man became a social animal.

Because of the complexity of schizophrenia, many theories of its etiology have been proposed and many treatment modalities have evolved and are still evolving. This chapter will summarize several of the etiological theories, including the psychodynamic, sociological, and biological views. Current and past treatment methods will be reviewed as well as the many dimensions of primary, secondary, and tertiary prevention.

Nursing intervention for schizophrenic individuals is based not on a reaction to a diagnostic category but on a therapeutic response to specific types of behavior. These forms of behavior, while maladaptive, are not unexplainable and awesome derivatives of madness, as they have been thought of in the past. They represent an individual's attempts to deal with a threatening environment and a disintegrating sense of self.

HISTORICAL ASPECTS

There are ancient tomb writings that graphically describe what was most likely schizophrenia. Undoubtedly, many of the witches who were burned at the stake in medieval times for being possessed by the devil were suffering from schizophrenia.

The syndrome was termed ''dementia praecox'' by Morel, a contemporary of Sigmund Freud. Dementia praecox, as Morel used it, meant youthful (precocious) insanity. It was thus distinguished from the dementias of later life, such as senility. Kraepelin, who has been called the ''Great Classifier'' of mental disturbances, used the term when he set about developing his taxonomy. Another contemporary of Freud, Eugen Bleuler, reacted to the primary symptom of dementia praecox—a splitting off of the emotions ordinarily connected to thoughts—by inventing the term ''schizophrenia.'' The word comes from the Greek ''schizo'' (to split) and ''phren'' (mind). Schizophrenia is the term now in popular use.

SOCIOCULTURAL ASPECTS OF LABELING

The label ''schizophrenia'' has caused some difficulties. A minor difficulty is the confusion many people experience over the meaning of the word. Many have understood the word to mean ''having more than one personality.'' This is really a description of another psychological disturbance—a severe psychoneurotic condition of the dissociative type called *multiple personality* (see Chapter 19). *The Three Faces of Eve* and *Sybil* are both accounts of persons with the disorder of multiple personality. *Dr. Jekyll and Mr. Hyde* is a fictional account of a person with multiple personality.

The difficulty in the average person's understanding of the term schizophrenia is inconsequential when compared to the problems it has caused for most of the people who suffer from the disorder. These problems are inherent in the process of labeling. The fear and utter hopelessness associated with schizophrenia, which have grown throughout the history of the disease, remain with us even after more effective treatments for controlling the symptoms have evolved. Schizophrenia is still the most dreaded of all psychiatric disorders (Grinker, 1969). Being told that one is schizophrenic is akin to receiving a diagnosis of cancer. Yet, if one were to compare the prognosis for successful adaptation to life, a diagnosis of schizophrenia is more hopeful than one of *sociopathy*. (See Chapter 17.)

Another problem with the label of schizophrenia is that, as defined by Bleuler, it suggests ''OK, here it is—live up to it!'' In other words, expectation of pathological behavior tends to elicit pathological behavior. Through the expectations and interpretations of other people, symptoms that had been dormant or even nonexistent may be manifested. Any of a therapist's biases or distortions may be projected onto a client during a therapeutic relationship; the effects of such projection should never be underestimated. It is particularly important to remember this point, in view of the studies (such as Sarbin, 1972) that have shown that many persons who have been labeled schizophrenic do not demonstrate one or more of the cardinal symptoms of schizophrenia. It has also long been known that anyone—schizophrenic, neurotic, or normal—who is under sufficient stress may demonstrate any of these symptoms.

Another problem arising in connection with the use of diagnostic categories has to do with cultural differences between the labeler and the person who gets labeled. For example, it is well known that in Great Britain, where the average citizen is more reserved than the average American, the label most frequently given at the time of admission to psychiatric facilities is manic-depressive psychosis. In the United States, where dynamic, gregarious characters are more common and withdrawal is less acceptable, the most frequent diagnosis upon admission to state hospitals is schizophrenia.

The economic factor is also important in the diagnosis of schizophrenia. Psychiatrists are reluctant to give their private clients that label on admission. Upper- and middle-class clients admitted to psychiatric units in general hospitals are less apt to be called schizophrenic than the lower-class patients of the state hospital systems.

Much of the discontent with the diagnostic term schizophrenia is reflected in one prominent psychiatrist's statement:

The term schizophrenia should be abandoned. It has no priority, it misleadingly implies an understanding of a supposed basic disorder, and its two main subdivisions (process and reactive) are defined by responses to therapy, which is absurd! (Altschule, 1970)

The validity of labeling people with psychiatric terms has been questioned by many. For example, Laing (Boyers and Orrill, 1971) and Szasz (1961) have both pointed out that such labeling has served a purpose for society—it has allowed society to explain away as ''sick'' any behavior that deviates from accepted norms.

A nurse working with psychiatric clients usually has an aversion to putting people into pigeonholes. Nurses are aware that such a practice can be destructive. However, there is another side to this question, and other factors need to be examined. Some would argue that it is not the label itself but the stigma attached to it that causes the damage. They see the label as a potentially *helpful* device. For example, proponents of the medical model of the etiology of schizophrenia suggest that we say to a client: ''You have a biochemical disorder called schizophrenia. We have medications and other treatments to help you control your symptoms. We will work together.'' Proponents of the medical model thus believe that confronting the client with the disorder, in the same way in which a diabetic person must be confronted with the metabolic disorder, is more helpful than shrouding the term ''schizophrenia'' in mystery. They accuse the ''radical therapists''* of not providing any real help to a person trying to cope with schizophrenia

when they deny that it is a disease, as Szasz does, or define it as ''the only way to be sane in an insane world,'' as Laing views it. Whichever side of the debate you agree with, an understanding of terms and diagnostic categories is necessary if you are going to be able to read the enormous amount of literature about the schizophrenic experience. With this point in mind, we will review several classification systems, along with the underlying dynamics and common symptoms of the schizophrenic syndrome.

UNDERLYING DYNAMICS

The schizoid personality*

The development of schizophrenia often follows a predictable course. The first stage of this course is the assumption of the schizoid personality. The schizoid personality is characterized by a tendency toward isolation and withdrawal, a bland affect, vagueness in communicating, and an overuse of the defense mechanism of projection. There seems to be an emptiness or poverty of personality, and the individual may appear rather eccentric to other people. While most schizophrenic processes may be shown to have developed in persons who have schizoid personalities, it does not follow that everyone who demonstrates a schizoid personality will necessarily develop schizophrenia.

The preschizophrenic state

The next stage of the process is the preschizophrenic state. This stage, which may last 1 or 2 years, is characterized by excessive daydreaming, an aloof and withdrawn attitude, and indifference to others.

THE NEED-FEAR DILEMMA

The individual has low self-esteem and a basic feeling of rejection combined with a fear of relat-

---

*R.D. Laing is considered one of the ''radical therapists'' because of his beliefs, for example, that schizophrenia is a liberating experience. Thomas Szasz is also counted among the radical therapists because of such views as his denial of schizophrenia as a disease.

---

*DSM-III coding: Axis II, 301.20, schizoid personality.

ing to others. This fear is a factor in the conflict that has been termed the "need-fear dilemma" (Burnham et al., 1969). The preschizophrenic person seems to suffer from an inordinate *need* for interpersonal closeness and an inordinate *fear* of that closeness. Since we all suffer from the need-fear dilemma, it is the adjective *inordinate* that sets the preschizophrenic person's experience apart from that of everyone else. Leopold Bellak (1958) has illustrated this dilemma by citing the philosopher Schopenhauer's parable of the porcupines:

On a cold winter day the porcupines move close to each other in order to take advantage of the warmth from their body heat. As they move closer and closer, they hurt each other with their quills. The porcupines had to move back and forth to find the best distance between each other in order to get the maximum body warmth while minimizing the hurts from their quills.

We only have to think of the instances when the need-fear dilemma has operated in our own lives. For example, we fall in love and experience fear because the loved one now has the power to hurt by leaving. An expectant mother experiences the need-fear dilemma: her desire for the new baby is combined with a fear of the baby's power to hurt her by becoming sick or dying.

THE "AS-IF" PHENOMENON

Feeling rejected by others leads to increased and painful isolation from others, which leads in a circular fashion to increased feelings of rejection. Gradually the person's whole existence takes on an "as if" quality (Laing, 1960). One may go through the necessary actions related to job, family, and friends in a mechanical way—acting *as if* one was an interested worker, a loving husband and father. But there is little emotional involvement in the action.

INAPPROPRIATE AFFECT

The person's affect may be inappropriate. A few preschizophrenic persons may be depressed or euphoric, but most seem to have a bland affect. The bland, shallow affect that accompanies the preschizophrenic and schizophrenic states may be an indication of a withdrawal into the individual's inner world.

There is not always a clear line of demarcation between the preschizophrenic state and the schizophrenic state. Often an insidious development from one stage to the next occurs. With some individuals, however, there *is* a dramatic shift. Usually, when there is a florid and sudden psychotic "break with reality," the prognosis is better than it is when the break is gradual.

The schizophrenic state

The symptoms of many emotional problems can be viewed as unconscious attempts to make the best of a bad situation; so can the symptoms of schizophrenia. They are unconsciously mediated attempts to halt the destructive process of the disease. It is useful to divide the symptoms of schizophrenia into primary and secondary groups. (The difference between primary and secondary symptoms becomes clear if we consider some examples from pathophysiology. In the physical disorder of rheumatic heart disease, the primary symptom is the stenosed mitral valve of the heart. Secondary or accessory symptoms include orthopnea, decreased renal function, and fatigue. In cirrhosis, a fibrotic, nodular and therefore inefficient liver is the primary symptom. Secondary symptoms include jaundice, bone demineralization, cholesterol lesions of the skin due to high serum levels, and a tendency toward bleeding. In both rheumatic heart disease and cirrhosis, the secondary symptoms result from the primary symptom and are ways the organism compensates for the primary symptom.)

PRIMARY SYMPTOMS

The primary symptoms of schizophrenia were delineated by Bleuler and are usually remembered as *Bleuler's four A's*. They are: autism, an associative looseness, ambivalence, and affective indifference or inappropriateness.

▶ Autism

The term autism refers to thought processes that are not used by the normal person in conscious thinking. They are similar to the thought processes of very young children or to those found in dreams. The ego judgments of time and place, of possible and impossible, are not used, and there is a strong element of unreality. In a case of autism that is so extreme that it leads to a break with reality, an individual might construct a private inner world, complete with characters. A person may then live in this dream world, which could become a nightmare. Cameron (1963) has termed this phenomenon the *pseudocommunity*.

Autism is a compensating maneuver of the ego. It may be an attempt to deal with the pain of failing to relate to other people (Mendel, 1976). Autism is closely tied to the ability to think abstractly. When this function is impaired, as is often the case in schizophrenia, autism results. Words, objects, events, and even people may take on private, symbolic meaning for a schizophrenic person, and communication may therefore become difficult. Autism may be manifested in personally symbolic communication, concrete thinking (inability to think abstractly), or associative looseness, another of Bleuler's A's.

▶ Associative looseness

Associative looseness is characterized by verbalizations that are very difficult and sometimes impossible to understand. Associative looseness may seem similar to the *flight of ideas* that is seen in the manic phase of manic-depressive psychosis (see Chapter 18). Flight of ideas, however, is different in that even though it involves rapid jumping from one topic to another, there is some connection between one phrase or idea and the next. In associative looseness, the connection between one phrase and another is apparent to the speaker but

not the listener. Associative looseness may be diagramed as follows:

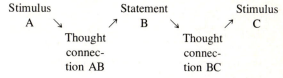

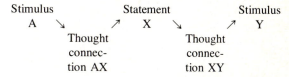

The logical sequence of A to B to C makes the normal thought processes easy to understand and follow. The esoteric or autistic connections of thought that characterize associative looseness make conversation difficult or impossible. Consider the following sample conversations:

Both persons normal

Person 1: "I'm late because the phone was ringing." (A)
Person 2: "Did you answer it in time?" (AB)
Person 1: "Yes." (B)
Person 2: "Who was it?" (BC)
Person 1: "My mother." (C)

One person schizophrenic

Person 1: "I'm late because the phone was ringing." (A)
Person 1: "Are you engaged?" ("ringing" is associated with getting a ring and being engaged.) (AX)
Person 1: "Excuse me?" (X)
Person 2: "I cannot teach you." (The association is that one is dismissed or "excused" in class by a teacher.) (XY)
Person 1: "I don't understand you." (Y)

Loose association is not limited to individuals who are suffering from schizophrenia. Anyone may at times demonstrate this dysfunctional communication—especially under conditions of stress.

You may have witnessed this symptom if you have taken part in a lengthy telephone conversation in which the other person's way of communicating was unclear to you. Perhaps that person was upset about something, and you slipped into agreeing with some points along the way because of your reluctance to admit that you did not quite understand all of what was being said. At the end of the conversation you may have been disturbed to find yourself agreeing with a point when you were not at all sure that you actually did agree. At that point you may have been embarrassed to admit that you had not been "tuned in." It is quite possible that one reason you found yourself in this uncomfortable position was that the person you were listening to was demonstrating loose association.

▶ Ambivalence

We all experience ambivalent feelings at times. The difference between this "normal" ambivalence and that experienced by a schizophrenic individual lies not so much in the frequency or even the intensity of the ambivalence. It lies in the effect the ambivalence has on behavior (Mendel, 1976).

A schizophrenic person may experience a powerful combination of conflicting emotions of love and hate toward his significant others. These strong and opposing emotions neutralize each other, leading to psychic immobilization and difficulty in expressing *any* emotion. The result is often inactivity and *apathy,* an extreme, defensive "blunting" of the emotions. Apathy is always a defense against possible pain—it has been described as the defense mechanism of the concentration camps (Frankl, 1959). Apathy is evident when a person is indifferent to what might be expected to cause emotional arousal. Affective indifference is part of another of Bleuler's four A's.

▶ Affective indifference or inappropriateness

A schizophrenic person often displays indifference or apathy or expresses feelings that do not fit a situation, such as laughing loudly after being notified that one's mother has just died.

The term "inappropriate" may be misleading. Mendel (1976) maintains that if we were to understand the purely personal logic and thought processes of a schizophrenic individual, the behavior would not seem inappropriate. He suggests that a better term would be "socially inappropriate."

SECONDARY SYMPTOMS

The secondary symptoms of schizophrenia can be viewed as disturbances in thought, speech, mood, behavior, sensation, and perception.

▶ Anxiety

Anxiety, of course, is more than a secondary symptom. It is the basis for all emotional disturbances, and in that sense it might be considered the most primary, or fundamental, of all symptoms. However, it is a secondary symptom in schizophrenia because much anxiety is generated by the trauma and the social consequences of being schizophrenic. In addition, anxiety can occur in response to other secondary symptoms. For example, the experience of hallucinating can be very anxiety-producing. Anxiety often occurs at various points in the natural history of schizophrenia, such as hospital admission and discharge, initial diagnosis, and exacerbations of symptoms.

▶ Depression

Because depression is in itself a psychiatric entity or category, nurses sometimes lose sight of the fact that schizophrenic clients can be and usually are depressed. Like anxiety, depression can occur in response to the schizophrenic experience. To feel that one is a failure in interpersonal relationships can be extremely depressing. In addition, schizophrenia is usually a chronic condition, and depression often accompanies chronicity.

▶ Social withdrawal

Shyness, isolation, fear of others, and withdrawal can be expressed in degrees. The extreme situation would be characterized by *mutism* and *stupor.*

▶ Loosening of external ego boundaries

Inappropriate identification, depersonalization experiences, and gender identity confusion can occur as a result of a loosening of external ego boundaries. External ego boundaries are those mental processes that help us differentiate between our inner subjective thoughts and stimuli that are coming from the outer environment.

Inappropriate identification. A client, involved in a therapeutic relationship with a nurse, might begin to dress like the nurse, verbalize a decision to become a nurse, use identical phrases, and so on. This behavior can vary in severity; an extreme example would be clients who are unable to distinguish their wants and needs from those of other people or to make their own decisions.

Depersonalization. Depersonalization results from feelings of change in self or environment. These feelings may be relatively mild—expressed by such phrases as ''I don't look like I usually do'' or ''Somehow the room has changed—it seems completely different.'' The feelings and experiences may, however, be more extreme; believing that one has been ''transformed'' or that one has entered another dimension of the universe would be examples. The delusion* that one is someone else would be an even more extreme situation. Delusions of this kind and others often follow current cultural trends and facts. For example, it is not likely that a person would have the delusion of being Napoleon, as is often portrayed in comic situations. Today, clients are more apt to believe that they are the President, the Godfather, Martin Luther King, Marilyn Monroe, or Elvis Presley reincarnated. The most common delusions of this kind are for a male to believe he is Jesus Christ and for a woman to believe she is the Virgin Mary. Many factors are operating within such delusions; feelings of evil versus good and of power versus impotence are among them.

Gender identity confusion. Sexual identification might become weak or confused. Instead of a comfortable acceptance of one's sexual orientation (heterosexual, homosexual, or bisexual), a labile, primitive, guilt-ridden stance in relation to sexuality might develop. In some instances this situation may be characterized by a wish to become a member of the opposite sex or by a fear that such a transformation might occur spontaneously and magically. In extreme cases there may be delusional and symbol-laden beliefs that one is actually half male and half female.

▶ Loosening of inner ego boundaries

Inner ego boundaries are the borders between the repressed unconscious of an individual and conscious mental life. They help us to differentiate ''real'' from ''unreal.'' Defective inner ego boundaries can lead to the *attribution of supernatural powers to self and others.* Symptoms of this phenomenon include ideas or delusions of reference, ideas or delusions of control, and religiosity.

Ideas or delusions of reference. Ideas or delusions of reference occur when individuals believe that others are referring to or communicating with them through newspapers, television broadcasts or books (even books published many years ago) or in passing conversations. A mild form of this condition would be to believe that the people across the hall are talking about you (something that perhaps most of us have experienced). An extreme form is the belief that the headline of this morning's paper is actually a coded message about oneself.

Ideas or delusions of control and influence. Ideas and delusions of control or influence are demonstrated when there is a belief in the ability to control and influence other people through supernatural means. The belief that others can influence one's own mind or control one's behavior is another example. The following letter illustrates such a delusion.

Dear Sir:

My name is _____. I am writing to you in hope of some answers. My wife, three sons, and myself are being bugged by some kind of electronics, which I believe is in your field. I went to electronics

---

*A delusion is a belief that is contrary to fact.

experts for consultation, and they told me it would cost about $3,000 for them to help me. I don't have that kind of money, so I'm writing to you and pray that you can help me and my family. Here are some of the things that are taking place: (1) Using some kind of transmission to our heads, they can jam our memory so we can't think straight. (2) The equipment they're using can induce personality changes, such as increased friendliness or aggression. (3) They can keep us awake or make us sleep. (4) They can put words in our mouth, and make us say things we don't want to say. (5) At times I hear a high ringing noise in my ears that causes great pain. (6) It affects us mainly on our heads. (7) It appears that I can hear voices from the liquid in my stomach. (8) The frequency they use affects our equilibrium and causes pain to our spinal column.

I would appreciate any help you can give me.

Thank you,

———————————
(name and address)

Religiosity. Religiosity is a difficult symptom to assess in another person, since religious belief and degree of commitment are exceedingly personal and variable. It has been pointed out that it is extremely difficult for people to agree on the line of demarcation between normal and pathological religious investment (Field and Wilkerson, 1973).

An individual in a preschizophrenic state that is becoming steadily more severe may seek out religion to compensate for the cruelty of an increasingly alien world and to provide structure and guidelines for behavior. Religion and God thus become good parents, substituting for the real, "bad" parents (Arieti, 1955).

Field and Wilkerson (1973) view the schizophrenic's use of religiosity as a restitutive attempt to deal with two major pathological processes that are operating in the disorder—tendency toward withdrawal and lability of affect. They suggest that religious preoccupation helps support and rationalize this withdrawal and that it also helps to stabilize or control emotions.

▶ Autistic thinking and acting

Symbolic distortions and neologisms. Schizophrenic individuals may exhibit any of several forms of symbolic distortions: Overuse of generalization and universal pronouns (for example, "They" said . . .), vagueness, and inaccurancy are all relatively common patterns of communication. Neologisms are words that are invented to describe people, things, and events. They have completely personal meanings, and they may be egocentrically symbolic in nature. In extreme disorders of communication it may be necessary to "decode" the verbalizations of a client. This requires the establishment of a trusting relationship and may take a fairly protracted period of time.

Concrete thinking. Symbolic distortion often has its roots in another autistic form of thinking—concrete thinking. Concrete thinking involves the fairly consistent use of literal interpretation of others' communication; it is a regression to an earlier form of thinking. A person who thinks such a way has great difficulty in thinking abstractly. The belief that this symptom is frequently associated with schizophrenic thought disorders has led to the use of a "proverb test" in the diagnosis of schizophrenia. The individual is asked to give the meanings of some common proverbs, such as "A new broom sweeps clean" or "A rolling stone gathers no moss." Inability to give the abstract meanings of the proverbs is viewed as evidence of concrete thinking and becomes one of the factors in a diagnosis of schizophrenia.

Primary process thinking. Primary process thinking, a Freudian term, is an early, prelogical form of thinking that incorporates such elements as concrete thinking, the post-hoc fallacy,* and paralogical or paleological thinking. Dreams are examples of a type of primary process thinking that is considered normal experience. During a psychotic experience, a person may seem to be dreaming while in a waking state.

Paralogical or paleological thinking. Paralogical thinking is a term that has been adopted by clinicians (Von Domarus, 1944) to denote a type

———————————
* "After this; therefore because of it." The post-hoc fallacy is also an element in Sullivan's concept of *parataxic distortion* (Arieti, 1967).

of logic that accepts identity based upon identical predicates—in contrast to normal logic, which only accepts identity based upon identical subjects. Arieti prefers to designate this type of thinking, which is a frequent correlate of schizophrenia, as "paleologic," from the Greek word for ancient, "palaios." This form of thinking is illogical according to normal logic, but it is really a logic of its own (Arieti, 1955, 1967). The following is an example of normal, or Aristotelian, logic:

All men are mortal.
Socrates is a man.
Therefore, Socrates is mortal.

Compare this with the following example of paralogical or paleological thinking:

The Blessed Mother Mary is a virgin.
I am a virgin.
Therefore, I am the Virgin Mary.

For a more detailed examination of this complex and interesting phenomenon, see *Language and Thought in Schizophrenia,* edited by J.S. Kasanin, *Interpretation of Schizophrenia,* by Sylvano Arieti, or *The Intrapsychic Self,* also by Sylvano Arieti.

Stereotypical actions, echopraxia, echolalia. Stereotypical actions involve the persistent repetition of a motor activity. A "normal" example of this is thumb twiddling or finger tapping. Such actions are often much more bizarre when used by a psychotic client; they may include posturing, intricate hand gestures, or facial grimacing. A stereotypical action is used to control anxiety, but it may also have symbolic, personal meaning. Echopraxia, which is also characterized by persistent movement, is the imitation of someone or something a person is observing; it thus involves the element of loose ego boundaries. Echolalia is the pathological repetition of the words or phrases of another person.

Lack of social awareness. A withdrawn, self-preoccupied person may exhibit some degree of social insensitivity and crudeness. An example

would be engaging in such activities as nose picking and masturbation in public places, with little or no awareness of the impact on other people. The activities of daily living (ADL), such as body cleanliness, grooming, and proper attire, may be completely neglected. In a very extreme situation, there may be bizarre, repulsive behavior, such as coprophagia, the desire to eat feces. In fact, the habitual ingestion of various objects (for example, knives and spoons) is a symptom of the extreme or regressed stage of schizophrenia, which is not often seen today. This behavior is sometimes symbolic for the schizophrenic person. Before the advent of psychotropic drugs, it was not as rare an occurrence as it is now.

Somatic preoccupations. A person who is either preschizophrenic or schizophrenic may exhibit an excessive amount of concern about body functions and health. This behavior may be demonstrated in varying degrees—from vague fears about one's health, to hypochondria, to the extreme situation wherein the person suffers from bizarre somatic delusions. The following are some somatic delusions that have been expressed by schizophrenic clients:

1. Complete body infestation by worms
2. Body infestation by snakes
3. Electrical wiring throughout the body
4. Electrical wiring of the brain
5. Depletion of energy and life force by others and through the eyes
6. Exposure of one's inner thoughts, to be read as if in a book, through the eyes
7. One side of the body being female, the other male
8. One side of the body being clean and healthy, the other filthy and diseased

It is evident that these delusions, like most other secondary symptoms of schizophrenia, may serve more than one purpose for a person with a threatened and crumbling ego. Symbolic statements, expressions of guilt, projection of blame onto others and outside forces, and rationalization of weaknesses and fear of others are a few explanations that are possible.

CLASSIFICATIONS OF SCHIZOPHRENIA

Classic

Several systems for categorizing schizophrenia have been devised. The oldest one—the classic one—was first described by Kraepelin. It included several types, four of which are still in use today: *catatonic, paranoid, hebephrenic,* and *simple*. Before Kraepelin devised this classification system, all the types of schizophrenia were considered to be one disease and were seen as that particular kind of madness that strikes at a young age—dementia praecox. Three of these four types (catatonic, paranoid, and hebephrenic) can be shown to involve specific patterns of defensive reactions to the threat of the ego-disintegrating schizophrenic process.

CATATONIC SCHIZOPHRENIA

Catatonic schizophrenia (DSM-III: schizophrenia, catatonic; see Appendix A for other DSM-III codings) is associated with motor disturbances. There are two stages to this type of schizophrenia: *catatonic excitement* and *catatonic stupor*. Someone who is in the excited stage may exhibit a frenzied overactivity that is in many ways similar to the extreme state of mania that is part of manic-depressive psychosis (see Chapter 18). There is, however, more personality disorganization evident in this schizophrenic condition than in mania. Before the antipsychotic drugs were available, a person in the excited stage of catatonic schizophrenia was in danger of dying from exhaustion.

In catatonic stupor, the motor disturbance is underactivity, which can occur in varying degrees. In severe cases, a person may exhibit the symptom of cerea flexibilitas, or "waxy flexibility." The phrase describes a situation wherein the person's arms, legs, or any other body part can be moved about by another person and will remain in any position in which they are placed. The childhood game of "statues" is a little like this situation—it is as if the person has relinquished voluntary move-

ment. Catatonic stupor was a fairly common occurrence in psychiatric wards before the availability of the major tranquilizers; there was an ever-present danger of such conditions as leg ulcers, because of the impaired circulation that results from remaining in any one position too long. Hypostatic pneumonia was also a danger, as were accidental burns from radiators that were leaned against during the stuporous phase.

Hallucinations and delusions may be present in catatonic schizophrenia; the delusional system may be persecutory or mystical and magical. Catatonia, of all of the four Kraepelinian types, is most often the one to come on and clear up suddenly—it is thought to have the best prognosis of the four. Denial is the defense mechanism that is pathologically overused—the individual denies reality and the environment through complete withdrawal or through frenzied overactivity that shuts out the world and everyone in it.

PARANOID SCHIZOPHRENIA

The defense mechanism being used in a pathological manner by a paranoid schizophrenic person is projection. Fear, insecurity, or a hostile and threatening inner world is projected or blamed on the outside environment and on other people. Delusions are often persecutory or grandiose, and suspicion is a predominant theme. The paranoid schizophrenic (DSM-III: schizophrenia, paranoid; see Appendix A for other DSM-III codings) often appears more organized and better able to function within a psychosis than the catatonic schizophrenic, but the prognosis is considered less favorable.

HEBEPHRENIC SCHIZOPHRENIA

Hebephrenic schizophrenia was thought to represent massive regression to a primitive, childlike state. The word comes from the name for the Greek goddess of youth—Hebe. It was seen as a more extreme condition than the previously mentioned types of schizophrenia, with rapid disintegration of the personality. Hebephrenic schizophrenia was considered to have the poorest prognosis of the four types. Hallucinations and delusions are common, and it is described as childishness, silly giggling, and bizarre facial grimacing. Speech may be garbled—a person may exhibit "word salad," an unintelligible jumbling of words and phrases. Sometimes complete disorganization and dissociation from the self take place, and the person believes he or she is someone else. (Hebephrenia is not a term used in DSM-III. Schizophrenia, disorganized type, is used to describe the classification.)

SIMPLE SCHIZOPHRENIA

There is no predominant pattern of defensive reaction in simple schizophrenia—only the primary symptoms of schizophrenia appear. Loose association and poor attention span are usually present. Persons with simple schizophrenia are seen less often in psychiatric units and hospitals than in jails, skid rows, and isolating jobs. Such persons sometimes become "neighborhood eccentrics." Some heroin addicts may actually be simple schizophrenics, since heroin can have an encapsulating effect on a person's life. Simple schizophrenia is often described as a "poverty of personality." (Simple schizophrenia is not coded in DSM-III.)

The newer types

Kraepelin's classification system has been enlarged and refined throughout the years. Several additional types of schizophrenia have been delineated.

SCHIZOAFFECTIVE SCHIZOPHRENIA*

Schizoaffective schizophrenia includes a pronounced affective element—there is much similarity to manic-depressive psychosis. The underlying thought disorder that characterizes schizophrenia is present, along with a marked lability of mood.

---

*Termed "schizoaffective disorder" in DSM-III.

PSEUDONEUROTIC SCHIZOPHRENIA

Pseudoneurotic, borderline,* latent, residual, ambulatory, nonpsychotic—these are all terms that have been used by various writers and clinicians to describe approximately the same state. An affected person seems to have moderately severe neurotic problems, but there is actually an underlying schizophrenic process. Sometimes treatment that is traditionally used for neurotic symptoms (for example, psychoanalysis) will uncover the schizophrenic process.

CHILDHOOD SCHIZOPHRENIA†

There is some debate in clinical circles as to whether early infantile autism and childhood schizophrenia are the same thing. However, most writers do distinguish between the two disorders. While the etiology of early *infantile autism* (DSM-III) is not known, several theorists believe that it has a definite organic basis.

Childhood schizophrenia, which has also been termed "pathological symbiosis," it is thought to involve a pathological fusion of mother and child. Each is dependent upon the other, and independence in one is a threat to the other.

CHRONIC, UNDIFFERENTIATED SCHIZOPHRENIA

Reflecting the fact that no one ever fits into neatly delineated categories, the term "chronic, undifferentiated schizophrenia" has come into common use in recent decades. A sort of wastebasket term, it is probably the most common diagnosis for schizophrenia in large psychiatric facilities. "Burned-out schizophrenia" is another term used to describe chronicity in schizophrenia. While it means that the condition has become chronic, it

---

*See Chapter 20 for contemporary beliefs about the differentiation of borderline schizophrenia and borderline personality disorder

† For further discussion of childhood schizophrenia, see Chapter 15.

also implies that the rather dramatic, florid aspects of the process are not especially evident. There may be an element of docility in an affected person's approach to life. For this reason, many clinicians feel that such a person is more amenable to rehabilitation than someone who is actively psychotic.

Process schizophrenia and reactive schizophrenia

A recently devised way of categorizing schizophrenia is to describe it as either "process" or "reactive." This broad system looks at schizophrenia in terms of the parameters of premorbid adjustment, timing and quality of onset of symptoms, progress, and prognosis.

PROCESS SCHIZOPHRENIA

A person with process schizophrenia has had a relatively poor premorbid adjustment. In terms of ability to form and maintain interpersonal and sexual relationships, to function at school or in an occupation, or to master the environment, there has been very little success. The onset of symptoms is early (most commonly at or just after puberty), and the onset of the schizophrenic condition tends to be slow and insidious rather than sudden and dramatic. The precipitating events in the environment are not particularly obvious. This disorder is characterized by a steady, progressive worsening rather than an abrupt, florid exacerbation followed by remission. The prognosis for a person with process schizophrenia is considered to be poorer than that for a person with reactive schizophrenia.

REACTIVE SCHIZOPHRENIA

A person with reactive schizophrenia probably has made a fairly adequate—in some cases, a rather good—premorbid adjustment. There is usually evidence of accomplishment in the areas of social, sexual, educational, and occupational adjustment. Perhaps the person has graduated from high school or college, for instance. The events that lead to

diagnosis or hospitalization are fairly obvious, and the onset tends to be abrupt and dramatic. Often, remissions will follow acute exacerbations—there is a periodic quality to the course of the disorder. There is often evidence that one has developed insight into the effects of one's behavior on the quality of life. The prognosis for an improved adjustment to life is much more promising in reactive schizophrenia than in process schizophrenia.

Orthomolecular psychiatry

A group of psychiatrists has adopted a system for categorizing schizophrenia that is based on the principles of orthomolecular medicine, a term that was coined by the biochemist and double Nobel laureate Linus Pauling. Orthomolecular medicine involves the provision of "the proper quantities of nutrients for the individual" (Pfeiffer, 1975). Orthomolecular psychiatrists believe that in schizophrenic persons, the blood (and therefore the brain) contain abnormal levels of histamine: *histapenic schizophrenics* have abnormally low levels, and *histadelic schizophrenics* have abnormally high levels. Histapenic schizophrenics comprise 50% of all schizophrenics, and histadelics comprise 20%. The remaining 30% are *mauve factor schizophrenics,* so called because of an abnormal factor that is excreted in the urine in greater frequency than is the case with normal persons (Pfeiffer, 1975). Orthomolecular psychiatrists have characterized persons who have schizophrenia-like clinical pictures as *facsimile schizophrenics.* Facsimile schizophrenia can result from such conditions as brain syphilis (dementia paralytica), pellagra, thyroid hormone deficiency, amphetamine psychosis, vitamin B_{12} deficiency, or wheat gluten sensitivity.

Persons with histapenic schizophrenia are apt to be excessively affected by inner stimuli and thus to have misperceptions of place, time, self, and other people, which result in confusion and distortion. They often hallucinate and suffer from delusions. There is hyperactivity and a high pain threshold.

Histadelic schizophrenia is characterized by suicidal depression, obsessive rumination, and loss of contact with reality. Hallucinations and delusions are much less frequent, but there is difficulty in thinking and an inability to concentrate. Frequent headaches may be a symptom.

In mauve factor schizophrenia, the classical symptoms of schizophrenia are often present, but insight and affect are better than in the other two types. This condition is sometimes called *pyroluria* because pyrroles are found in the urine. Other symptoms may include white spots on the fingernails, stretch marks on the skin, memory problems, sweet breath odor, constipation, photosensitivity, impotence, and intolerance for barbiturates. The illness is viewed as stress-induced (Pfeiffer, 1975).

EPIDEMIOLOGY AND SOME SOCIOCULTURAL ASPECTS OF THE SCHIZOPHRENIC SYNDROME

While schizophrenia can strike at almost any age, the usual range for onset is 15 to 45, and especially 25 to 35. For some unknown reason, significantly more schizophrenic persons are born in the first quarter of the year than in any other quarter (Cancro, 1970; Kety, 1978). Schizophrenia is a major health problem. Of all of the hospital beds in the country, roughly 50% are located in facilities designed for the treatment of mental illness, and 50% of these are occupied by schizophrenic clients (Henley, 1971). Many more schizophrenics function with varying degrees of success outside of hospitals. It has been estimated that as many as 4,000,000 people in the United States may suffer from schizophrenia. Estimates range from 0.85% to 2% of the population (Trotter, 1977).

Schizophrenia is found in all cultures throughout the world and in all socioeconomic groups. However, the distribution is not equal: there is a definite correlation between poverty and the incidence of schizophrenia. The possible reasons for this are complex and debatable. Various workers cite eco-

nomic, sociological, and genetic factors. For one thing, schizophrenia depletes financial resources, as any debilitating and chronic disorder does. Roman and Trice (1967) found, in their synthesis of several studies of the etiology and epidemiology of schizophrenia, that one generalization was possible—the positive correlation among life in the lower socioeconomic strata, excessive psychological stress, and schizophrenia. Certainly, the effects of poverty are felt in many areas of living. Poor people generally do not receive proper nutrition and health care, and they lack adequate living space. They also have little opportunity for socialization and self-actualization. These conditions may increase the chances that a person will develop a schizophrenic psychosis. Finally, there is an element of subjectivity inherent in the act of diagnosing: many clinicians are reluctant to condemn their middle-class clients with the label of schizophrenia, even when they believe the condition to be present.

Sociocultural factors must be considered integral parts of the schizophrenic process. For example, which etiology is accepted depends on culture. The Awilik Eskimos may attribute a case of catatonia to the machinations of a vengeful ancestral spirit (Carpenter, 1953) while a Washington psychiatrist may proclaim it to be the result of an escalation of multigenerational psychopathology.

Treatment also is related to sociocultural forces. In Israel, where a premium is placed on being a productive citizen, even the most passive, chronic psychotic is considered capable of some personal and social regeneration and is treated accordingly. Communal philosophy in China fosters the development of self-help groups for people, and reintegration into family and community groups is an important goal of treatment (Howells, 1975).

The content of delusions and hallucinations is shaped by sociocultural trends and current events. Presidential assassinations, moon landings, or the popularity of a movie star are all possible influences.

The severity of and prognosis for a case of schizophrenia depend in large part upon a socioeconomic or cultural group's reactions to the disorder. Since medieval times, ambulatory schizophrenics in the village of Gheel, Belgium, have easily made the transition from hospital to community because of the villagers' acceptance of them.

Anthropologists have pointed out that the incidence of mental illness seems to increase during the social unrest that accompanies periods of change and acculturation (Carpenter, 1953). Sometimes, according to medical anthropologist Edward F. Foulks (1975), schizophrenia may even be helpful to an individual or to society during times of social upheaval. The hallucinations and delusions of an individual can help to explain catastrophic events to the people or provide guidelines for change when social change is required. Foulks describes a New York Seneca Indian, called Handsome Lake, whose stress-induced hallucinations in the mid–eighteenth century told him of a new and useful code for his people to adopt. His society was in a period of rapid change and therefore of social disorganization with its potential for destructive trends. Thus, through his hallucinatory experience, Handsome Lake was able to assume the role of prophet or shaman.

The syndrome of schizophrenia has a long history in the development of mankind and a wide incidence throughout the world. Symptoms of the syndrome can be viewed as restitutional; they are extreme exaggerations of the defense mechanisms we all use. Useful definitions of schizophrenia acknowledge the complexity of the syndrome and of the etiological factors surrounding it. While several systems of classification have been devised and are used by clinicans and writers, it remains crucial to recognize and remember the concept of individuality in the treatment of schizophrenic clients. Mendel and Green (1967) have pointed this out succinctly:

Obviously, the patient does not have a diagnosis; we, the physicians, have the diagnosis. When the diagnosis and the patient do not fit we must feel free to abandon the diagnosis and return to the patient.

THEORIES OF SCHIZOPHRENIA

The exact etiology of schizophrenia is unknown. There are, however, many theories about the origin of the disorder, and several of them will be reviewed here.

Genetic theories

Many studies concerned with the genetic basis of schizophrenia have been carried out, with various results. Some early studies reported a concordance as high as 76% (Slater, 1953) or 86% (Kallman, 1938) for monozygotic twins as compared to 14% to 15% for dizygotic twins. Other studies have reported lower degrees of concordance. Possible explanations for this variability in findings in studies of twins include the use of differing statistical methods, research designs, and diagnostic criteria.

More recently, adequately controlled studies of schizophrenic persons were carried out in Denmark. These studies, which involved schizophrenics who had been raised by adoptive families, showed a significant incidence of schizophrenia in the biological parents (Kety, 1978). This incidence was close to that described in earlier studies, which had shown an expectation of 16.4% that children of one schizophrenic parent would become schizophrenic (versus 0.85% for the general population) and an espectation that ranges from 38% to 68% when both parents are schizophrenic (Jackson, 1960).

Both early and recent studies show that nonschizophrenic relatives of schizophrenic persons have significantly more of the conditions, such as eye-tracking disorders, that are associated with schizophrenia than the general population (Holzman et al., 1974).

Most theorists, whether they are concerned with organic, psychodynamic, or sociocultural bases for schizophrenia, do agree that a genetic factor is operating. There is no conclusive evidence as to the mode of genetic transmission—schizophrenia, like many other disorders, seems to be polygenetic.

At least one aspect of the genetic controversy that needs to be refined is the differentiation of genetic factors from perinatal and prenatal influences.

Biochemical and physical theories

PRENATAL AND PERINATAL INFLUENCE THEORY

Prenatal and perinatal influences have been cited as factors in the etiology of schizophrenia. Explanations include a possible alteration of the fetal oxygen supply, passage of endocrine and toxic substances across the placental barrier, and the effects of maternal emotions on fetal endocrine balance and nervous system.

Birth trauma of one sort or another has been suggested as an explanation for schizophrenia. Significantly more prenatal and perinatal complications have been found in the histories of schizophrenics than in those of nonschizophrenics (Taft and Goldfarb, 1964), and stillbirth rate, rate of premature births, and incidence of serious congenital malformations in offspring have been found to be higher in schizophrenic mothers (Campion and Tucker, 1973). Some investigators suggest that some sort of trauma present at or before birth is the agent that interacts with a genetic predisposition to result in schizophrenia.

Recently, a group of researchers in California has suggested that subtle brain abnormalities occurring in the first trimester of pregnancy help to trigger chronic forms of schizophrenia (Greenberg, 1983). They found a high incidence of minor physical anomalies (which are known to develop during the first trimester) and evidence of neurological impairment among the schizophrenic males they studied. They propose an interaction model incorporating *functional* and *organic* defects as etiological factors in some forms of schizophrenia.

ANATOMICAL OR PHYSIOLOGICAL DEFECT THEORIES

One physiological defect that has been identified as a possible etiological factor is an abnormally responsive autonomic nervous system. One group of researchers, who verified this finding in a large-scale study, found an overresponsive autonomic nervous system to be especially evident in schizophrenics who had suffered complications at birth. The researchers hypothesized that this overreactivity combines with a genetic predisposition for schizophrenia and results in expression of the disorder (Trotter, 1977).

In the past, anatomical and physiological defects have been hypothesized as the basis of schizophrenia. Until recently there has been no evidence to support these hypotheses. Now, however, investigators have announced findings that they view as a breakthrough in our understanding of the physical basis of schizophrenia. *Amphetamine psychosis* is a condition that closely mimics the schizophrenic process and symptomatology. In this disorder, amphetamine stimulates the release of dopamine (a neurotransmitter catecholamine), and a possible flooding of the brain with dopamine may occur. Also consistent with the anatomical or physiological defect theory are aspects of another disorder—Parkinson's disease. In this disease the problem is that the individual's brain lacks many of the dopamine-producing cells, resulting in a scarcity of the substance. Treatment with L-dopa alleviates symptoms of parkinsonism. Another fact linking schizophrenia to a physiological defect is that antischizophrenic drugs, which are believed to act on the neurotransmitters in some way, possibly reducing the level of dopamine or blocking its transmission, also produce side effects that mimic the symptoms of Parkinson's disease.

Another etiological model (Stein and Wise, 1971) suggests a possible deficiency in the level of the enzyme that converts dopamine to norepinephrine, and yet another model (Potkin et al., 1978) postulates decreased activity of the enzyme monoamine oxidase, which is involved in the degradation of chemicals such as dopamine. In addition, it was discovered through autopsy studies that the brains of schizophrenics contain about twice the normal number of receptor sites for dopamine. They theorize that schizophrenics are overstimulated with their own brain signals and thus are flooded with strange thoughts, hallucinations, and misperceptions (Science News, Vol. 112, p. 342, 1977).

The *dopamine hypothesis* was the second hypothesis to be derived from attempts to understand the physical bases of schizophrenia. The first was the *transmethylation hypothesis,* which was derived from the study of psychotomimetic drugs such as mescaline. Mescaline, which is a methylated catechol, produces symptoms that mimic schizophrenia. It was theorized that a transfer of a methyl group to neurotransmitters or their precursors changes them into psychotomimetic substances. Methylated catecholamines and methylated indoles were looked for, but so far there has been no definitive evidence of elevated levels in schizophrenic persons. The difficulty of separating the effects of diet, drugs, stress, and environmental conditions has complicated the picture. It seems likely that excess dopamine is a fundamental factor in schizophrenia. Currently, the dopamine hypothesis is the most widely accepted biochemical theory.

In 1972, Murphy and Wyatt of the National Institute of Mental Health reported their findings that people with schizophrenic disorders have a low activity of the enzyme monoamine oxidase (MAO) in their blood platelets. Further investigations revealed a wide range of MAO activities in the disorder (Maugh, 1981). In 1981, Schildkraut (as cited by Maugh) reported that different ranges of MAO activity appear to be characteristic of certain subgroups of schizophrenia. Specifically, schizophrenics who do *not* hallucinate have normal range levels of MAO activity, whereas there is a below normal level in schizophrenics who do hallucinate. Many in this latter grouping exhibit paranoid symptoms. An above-average level of MAO activity was observed in those schizophrenics who were characterized as asocial, depressed, markedly introverted, and exhibiting bizarre behavior.

Edelstein and his associates (1981) have estimated that 24-40% of schizophrenic-like, psychotic individuals may have a ''lithium-responsive'' type of illness. This conclusion was based on earlier work with individuals diagnosed as schizophrenic and who have an above-average *lithium ratio*. These people responded very well to lithium therapy. This lithium ratio has been described as a defect in the transport of sodium and lithium ions across the membrane of red blood cells. This can be quantitatively measured—the ratio of the concentration of lithium in the red blood cells to that in the plasma is determined. The defect leads to a higher than normal ratio and this condition responds to lithium therapy (Maugh, 1981).

TOXIC SUBSTANCE THEORIES

A theory suggested by Heath et al. (1958) concerned a toxic or abnormal protein, called *taraxein,* in the blood of schizophrenics. When injected into nonschizophrenics, it produced behavior and symptoms similar to those of schizophrenia. This substance has been isolated by three different researchers, but it is not generally considered to be the fundamental factor in schizophrenia. The dopamine hypothesis seems more widely accepted as the biochemical basis for schizophrenia.

It has been hypothesized that food might contain a toxic substance—specifically, the protein gluten that is found in wheat. A research team found that when wheat was removed from the diet of schizophrenics, their symptoms improved dramatically. While the research team cautioned that this is not a simple cause-and-effect situation, it concluded that wheat gluten is a pathogenic factor in schizophrenia (Singh and Kay, 1976).

It has been suggested that a slow viral infection process may be responsible for the subsequent development of schizophrenia. This theory has received support because of the discovery that the organic brain syndrome known as Jakob-Creutzfeldt disease may be of viral origin and because of the fact that individuals suffering from herpes encephalitis have a clinical picture that is very similar to an acute schizophrenic episode (Wynne et al., 1978).

ORTHOMOLECULAR THEORY

Mescaline psychosis has been used as a model by the proponents of the orthomolecular theory of schizophrenia. Osmond and Hoffer studied mescaline psychosis and saw similarities to the delirium associated with the vitamin-deficiency disease pellagra (Pfeiffer, 1975). They noted that earlier findings had shown that vitamin B_3 (in the form of niacin or nicotinic acid) not only cured the physical symptoms of pellagra but also provided complete relief from the mental symptoms. They hypothesized that perhaps schizophrenia, with symptoms that are also similar to mescaline psychosis, represents an abnormally high requirement for vitamin B_3. They began treating people with megadoses of the vitamin—usually 3 gm combined with 3 gm of vitamin C and trace mineral supplements.

The orthomolecular psychiatrists prefer to designate the disorder in the plural—the schizophrenias. They have categorized them as histadelic schizophrenia, histapenic schizophrenia, and mauve factor schizophrenia. The histapenic schizophrenics are the ones who are treated with vitamin B_3. Vitamin therapy is not the sole treatment; a combination of vitamins, psychotropic drugs, and psychotherapy is used. Young schizophrenic persons, whose symptomatology is still labile, are viewed as the most likely candidates for the treatment.

The theory is not widely accepted in established medical circles, and conflicting claims are made by proponents and skeptics.

Perceptual and cognitive disturbance theories

SENSORY INPUT DYSFUNCTION

Several theories have been postulated and explored concerning a possible defect in the schizophrenic's ability to perceive and organize experi-

ence effectively. The defect in controlling incoming stimuli from the environment results in overload. According to those theories, a schizophrenic person has an ineffective barrier between inner self and the parade of events he or she is exposed to in the environment. One theorist (Cameron, 1963) has termed this situation "overinclusiveness" and has described it as a failure to weed out irrelevant material, with a resultant flooding of the ego. The person is unable to organize perceptions appropriately. Such theories are consistent with several studies of the effects of sensory deprivation, which indicate that chronic schizophrenics tolerate sensory deprivation much better than nonschizophrenics.

Another way of looking at sensory input dysfunctions and schizophrenia is to view the schizophrenic as being deficient in the ability to modulate sensory input. Two manifestations of this defect are possible—the overresponsiveness of the acute stage of schizophrenia and the underresponsiveness of the chronic schizophrenic (Epstein and Coleman, 1971).

LEARNING THEORY

One hypothesis concerning schizophrenia holds that the disorder is learned. According to this theory, an overresponsive autonomic nervous system, a genetic predisposition for schizophrenia, and a harsh environment all combine to encourage a person to learn to avoid stress by displaying schizophrenic symptoms—hallucinations, delusions, withdrawal, isolation from others, and so on (Trotter, 1977).

Psychodynamic theories

Harry Stack Sullivan did a good deal of his work with schizophrenic persons. His "interpersonal" theory of psychiatry pointed to an unhealthy relationship between the schizophrenic and his parents. His view of schizophrenia was more hopeful than Freud's; he believed that a later, more satisfying relationship could do much to erase the harm of the early, unhealthy ones.

Heinz Hartmann, a follower of Freud and the

father of ego psychology, believed that schizophrenia is a defect in the capacity to neutralize the instinctual drives (Hartmann, 1964). He saw this as resulting in an interference with object relations* and the development of healthy defenses. He postulated a vicious circle of increasing frustration, mobilization of more aggression, and the incapacity to neutralize *instinctual drives*, leading eventually to schizophrenic symptom formation (Pao, 1979).

Fairbairn, an object-relations theorist, pointed to a crystallization of the conflict ''to love or not to love,'' which he viewed as derivative of the infant's conflict of ''to suck or not to suck.'' He saw the schizophrenic as stuck in the *schizoid position* or early oral stage of psychosexual development (Pao, 1979).

Margaret Mahler et al. (1975)† in outlining the preoedipal period of childhood point to the *symbiotic phase* as the crucial one in the subsequent development of the various forms of schizophrenia. The child with a pathological symbiotic orientation has not been able to grow adequately beyond that stage. The mother is viewed not as a separate being but as ''fused with the self.'' The child is unable to integrate the mother's image as a whole object and, therefore, a split good object–bad object is perceived. There is a disabling alternation between the desire to incorporate the good and the desire to expel the bad.

Generally, the psychodynamic theorists argue that the roots of schizophrenia are in the oral stage of psychosocial development—the stage in which a child develops an ability to trust other people. These theorists believe that schizophrenia originates in problems in the mother-child relationship that develop during this period. There is a faulty development of the ego. In particular, the defense mechanism of repression is ineffective, a situation that constitutes the underlying psychodynamic problem. Clinicians have long noted that the

---

*See Chapter 20 for more discussion of object relations.

†See Chapter 20 for an outline discussion of Mahler's theory of preoedipal development.

schizophrenic's unconscious seems very close to the surface. Since the defense mechanism of repression is weak and ineffective, unconscious material threatens to flood the ego and thus stimulates the psychotic symptoms as defense mechanisms. Freud viewed schizophrenia as a regression to a state of infantile narcissism with a withdrawal of the libido from the external world to the internal self. Freud did not work with many schizophrenics —most of his patients were neurotics. In fact, he was rather pessimistic about the value of psychotherapy for schizophrenics.

Carl Jung viewed schizophrenics as centripetal (inner-directed) in their relationships with the world rather than centrifugal (outer-directed).

Sylvano Arieti, a contemporary American authority on schizophrenia, sees schizophrenia basically as a defensive reaction to severe anxiety that originates in childhood and recurs in later life. It is a restitutive attempt to make the best of a bad situation.

Eric Berne's transactional analysis system defines schizophrenia as a situation in which the ''child ego state,'' rather than the ''adult ego state,'' is in command of the ego functions. The child is frightened and ''not OK.'' In the schizophrenic person the ''parent ego state'' participates sporadically, mostly in a harsh and oppressive manner. Berne believed that the only way to proceed with psychotherapy for a schizophrenic is to engage the child ego state and obtain its cooperation.

Family systems theories

Family systems theorists have identified communication patterns and family relationship patterns (see Chapter 12) that may be etiological factors in schizophrenia. Murray Bowen (1976, 1977), a leading family systems theorist who did his original work with schizophrenic clients, argued that a *multigenerational transmission* may be operating in the disorder. He postulated that in some families, a process that is based on the defense mechanism of projection is passed down from one generation to the next. If two people who are neurotic marry and have a child, their neuroses may "mesh" in such a way as to produce a more severe neurosis in the child. If this child eventually marries a neurotic person, once again neuroses will mesh to produce an even more severely impaired offspring. Bowen views schizophrenia as a severe emotional disorder. Whereas others see neurosis and schizophrenia as discrete entities, he considers schizophrenia to be on a continuum with neurosis and other emotional disorders. According to Bowen's theoretical system, schizophrenia is a product of several generations of escalating impairment, with increasing use of a *family projection process* and decreasing levels of differentiation between family members. As a treatment goal, Bowen stresses increased differentiation of each family member from the family system, as opposed to unhealthy "fusion" among family members. He sees a tendency to fuse or merge with others operating in all families. This is the "undifferentiated family ego mass." If this tendency is strong enough and pervasive enough, it can be pathological for individual family members, who lose their sense of self.

Thus, some family systems are viewed as being pathological to the point of being *schizophrenogenic*. That is, the family system itself fosters schizophrenia. The person who is identified as the client is simply the carrier of the family's illness.

Certain *family configurations* have been singled out by Lidz (1973) as being schizophrenogenic. According to Lidz, the *skewed family pattern* is most often seen in the development of male schizophrenics. While the mother is most apt to be termed schizophrenogenic, the father, through his ineffective role modeling and inability to counteract the actions of his wife, plays an equally important role. The mother is described as domineering and egocentric. She is unable to differentiate her own feelings and anxieties from those of the other members of the family—particularly those of her son. In the beginning she has great difficulty relating to her infant son. This situation leads to overprotection and then to symbiosis. Eventually, she

begins to use her son to make up for her own failures and disappointments in life.

In the *schismatic family pattern* there is usually overt conflict between the spouses—the father is dominant and perhaps overtly paranoid. He tends to downgrade his wife and her role as mother and wife. Both spouses undercut each other and the child is competed for and used as a pawn in the conflict between the parents. Lidz believes that this pattern is more apt to produce schizophrenia in a girl than in a boy. There is overprotection, great concern about morality, and intrusiveness into the child's sexual behavior during adolescence.

There are some similarities between these two patterns—overprotection, a poor relationship with the parent of the same sex, and parental failure to establish proper and healthy boundaries between self and child. The child is unconsciously used by the parent of the opposite sex to fulfill needs and make up deficiencies.

Other patterns that family theorists see as particularly important in the development of schizophrenia include emotional divorce, coalition across generation boundaries, vagueness in communicating, tangentiality, double-bind communication, family myths, and mystification (see Chapter 12).

Existential theories

The existential psychologist Binswanger believed that the great philosopher Kierkegaard referred to schizophrenia when he described sickness of the mind as "the sickness unto death" (May, 1958). Existentialists point to altered perceptions of time, space, and causality as essential ingredients in the creation of the schizophrenic's world. Themes that existential psychologists and psychotherapists mention when they discuss schizophrenia include emptiness, nothingness, and painful internal vacuum. The schizophrenic's defect resembles a hole that requires constant filling; there is constant fear of annihilation. This need for constant filling and the fear of nonexistence are cited as reasons for obesity in some schizophrenics and latent schizophrenics. It has been suggested by clinicians, existential and otherwise, that a certain percentage of obese individuals should not attempt to reduce, since doing so may prescipitate a schizophrenic break with reality.

The internal emptiness or lack of identity of the schizophrenic leads to strained interpersonal relations; the whole existence takes on the "as if" quality described earlier in this chapter. R.D. Laing, considered to be an existential psychiatrist, believes that schizophrenia is not an illness but a way of being in the world. He views it as a potentially growth-promoting state, a change to correct a developmental problem. He sees the submerging into a psychotic state as beneficial, with a higher and more insightful level of development being the eventual compensation. His Kingsley Hall experiment allowed individuals to enter psychotic states, in a tolerant and drug-free atmosphere. This philosophy of treatment is not shared by more conventional therapists, who see the potential for residual damage to the personality inherent in each psychotic break.

Sociocultural theories

R.D. Laing also suggests that schizophrenia may be the only way to be sane in an insane world. Thus he implicates society in the etiology of schizophrenia.

Other theorists, notably Thomas Szasz, have proposed that schizophrenia is not a disease or a psychological disorder at all but rather a construct that has been invented by society to serve some of its needs—for example, to explain behavior that is deviant from the mainstream and to segregate persons who, in their deviance, make us uncomfortable. Proponents of this view remind us of the historical beginnings of care for the mentally ill, when the so-called mentally ill included what was considered the dregs of society—beggars, paupers, the physically disabled, and the diseased. They were an embarrassment to the more privileged classes, so they were warehoused in large institutions—at first mixed in with criminals. Szasz and theorists who agree with him maintain

that the "treatment"—the warehousing of people—existed first and that it then became necessary to have the "patients" to fit the treatment. The furtherance of the modern mental health industry, which does indeed provide financial support and security for many workers, is pointed to as one of the purposes the mentally ill serve for society.

One facet of society that has been implicated in the etiology of schizophrenia is poverty: poverty and schizophrenia are strongly correlated. Several explanations for this are possible. One that has been postulated is that poverty is an etiological agent through the medium of increased stress. Crowded living conditions, poor nutrition, inadequate or nonexistent prenatal care, and lack of meaningful recreation are only some of the concomitants of poverty that increase stress in everyday living. In their review of the massive literature on schizophrenia and social class, Roman and Trice (1967) hypothesized that a combination of child socialization patterns and patterns of environmental stress and social disorganization is related to the high incidence of schizophrenia in the lower social strata. One well controlled study comparing schizophrenics with normal persons found that schizophrenics experience significantly greater stress in dealing with life events than do nonschizophrenics (Serban, 1975). An animal study that incorporated increasingly stressful conditions resulted in the delineation of three groups of animals—those that remain relatively disease-free, those that suffer from various psychosomatic disorders, and those that exhibit behavior that could well be described as psychotic (Stroebel, 1969).

Holistic health concepts

An interesting example of the interweaving of theories is provided by Ernest Hartmann (1982) in his article "Toward a Biology of Mind." This may be an answer to what Dr. Hildegard Peplau (1983) has called a "lack of convergence of theories that are biogenetic and those that are sociopsychological explanations."

Ernest Hartmann cites the wealth of evidence

that supports a theory of increased brain dopamine activity as a correlate of schizophrenia. The evidence is based on the ability of amphetamine and similar drugs* to induce schizophrenia-like processes, whereas the antipsychotic major tranquilizers all appear to be dopamine receptor blockers. His view is that the dopamine plays a role in the biology of psychosis, that it may be related to unneutralized psychic energy (or, the unneutralized aggressive energy that Heinz Hartmann [1964] earlier postulated as the genesis of schizophrenia). Ernest Hartmann (1982) also states that the excess dopamine is responsible for the psychotic symptoms rather than schizophrenia as a whole, and he goes on to say that "clearly, the dopamine-blocking drugs reduce psychotic manifestations in schizophrenia, but do not cure an underlying schizophrenic defect."

His explanation reaches toward a "clear synthesis of available theories explanatory of the etiology and causation of schizophrenia," (Peplau, 1983) for what Hartmann is saying implies a holistic approach to understanding the etiology and treatment of schizophrenia.

STRESS-DIATHESIS THEORY

While environmental stress is considered to be the most important etiological factor by many—just as genetic predisposition, metabolic disorders, psychodynamic weaknesses, and family dysfunction each have their advocates—current psychiatric opinion favors a multifactorial etiology or a stress-diathesis model for the genesis of schizophrenia. The disorder is considered to be the final outcome of many complex factors. Eisenberg (1973) describes the stress-diathesis model as follows:

Psychobiological stress acts on an individual with a genetic predisposition to psychosis and eventually leads to abnormal metabolic processes that cause disorders of

mood and thought. Predisposition probably varies on a continuum.

Within this etiological model, psychobiological stress and genetic predisposition both vary on a dynamic continuum. An individual with a strong genetic predisposition might succumb to moderate or even minimal stress—for example, the stress of adolescence (the process schizophrenic described earlier). A person with relatively little genetic predisposition might react to severe stress with a psychotic break (the reactive schizophrenic). This model for stress and genetic predisposition is compatible with Murray Bowen's view that schizophrenia exists on a continuum with neurosis and other psychological disorders (Bowen, 1976). While some theorists disagree and consider schizophrenia and neurosis as discrete and unrelated phenomena, Karl Menninger (1963) also views neurosis and schizophrenia on a continuum of mental health and mental illness.

SCHIZOPHRENIA AND PSYCHOPHYSIOLOGICAL COMPLEMENTARITY

Carrying the continuum model a step further, Bahnson and Bahnson view all the human individual's disorders, psychological and physiological, as being on a continuum—a continuum of psychophysiological complementarity. This particular construct seeks to identify alternate forms for the discharge of energy associated with stress experienced by the human organism. As the degree of stress increases, an individual becomes more vulnerable to physical or psychological disorders. Which type of disorder is chosen depends on habitual patterns of response. The extreme manifestation of disorder in a person who tends to somatize is cancer, while in an individual with a tendency toward emotional lability it is schizophrenia. The Bahnsons point to various studies that demonstrate an inverse relationship between cancer and schizophrenia (Bahnson and Bahnson, 1964). This approach represents an attempt to develop a monistic theory rather than a false splitting of "mind" and "body" (Bahnson, 1969, 1974).

---

*Another example is PCP or "angel dust," which has been used as an animal model in the study of schizophrenia (Herbert, 1983a).

INTEGRATION OF THEORIES

The exact etiology of schizophrenia is not known. The many theories that have been postulated focus on such areas as genetic endowment, biochemical abnormalities, anatomical differences, psychodynamic defects, family dysfunction, and social disorganization. The schizophrenic syndrome is a complex disorder, and the most generally accepted view is that it is a multifactorial disorder incorporating many or all of the holistic health elements that have been discussed in this section.

TREATMENT

History

The treatment of schizophrenia has a history as long as the history of the disease itself. In ancient times, treatment was quite enlightened; it involved music, poetry, and dance therapy; rest; and "talking therapy." In ancient Greece temples were set aside for such treatments. In medieval times, when madness was thought to indicate possession by evil spirits or to be evidence of the practice of witchcraft, treatment took the form of exorcism and burning at the stake. After this period, but before any scientific approach to mental illness had evolved, treatment consisted of segregation from society in places like Bedlam in England or the prototype of the modern mental hospital, the Hôpital Général in France. In these large institutions people were kept in crowded, filthy conditions, and they were watched over by keepers who were at best apathetic and often cruel. Even at the beginning of the twentieth century, families of schizophrenics were told to forget about their hospitalized relatives. There was little hope for improvement.

When psychiatrists began to treat schizophrenia, their approach was mainly somatic. *Prefrontal lobotomy* is a brain operation that was used on many schizophrenics before the discovery of the phenothiazine drugs. In this procedure the tracts between cortex, subcortex, and basal ganglia are severed. It often resulted in a mitigation of aggressive, violent behavior, but it also left the patient* in a fairly deteriorated condition—docile, unmotivated, and demonstrating regressive, crude behavior. Thousands of lobotomies were performed on schizophrenics during the 1940s and early 1950s.

Hydrotherapy was a much less destructive modality. The purposes of hydrotherapy included sedation of the overactive patient (continuous tub baths and wet sheet packs) and production of tonic effects (needle spray and alternate jet showers). The wet sheet packs did seem to have a highly sedating action, and before effective psychotropic drugs were available, some patients would ask to be put into the packs when they realized that tension and anxiety were building up.

Isolation from others in seclusion rooms was a common treatment. There is a legitimate rationale for reducing environmental stimuli and allowing the hyperactive patient to calm down. Unfortunately, the seclusion rooms were sometimes used as punishment in the manner of solitary confinement in prisons. Seclusion also became the easiest way to treat excited patients; some were kept in the same small, bare seclusion rooms for long periods—sometimes for years.

Insulin coma therapy, or *insulin shock,* was used, for the most part, in the 1940s and early 1950s. The patient was given insulin to induce coma; he became somnolent and pacified in the hypoglycemic state. There appeared to be some successes with the treatment, particularly in cases of young schizophrenics who had just experienced their first psychotic breaks. There were also some very real dangers attached to insulin coma therapy, and some fatalities resulted—one reason why it is no longer used as a treatment for schizophrenia. The apparent remissions that sometimes occurred were later attributed to the intensive and intimate

---

*In this section the term "patient" is used because of the historical content.

nursing care required during the coma period—care that was described as a healthier and more loving re-parenting (Schwing, 1954). Perhaps some of the remissions were ones that would have occured in any group of young schizophrenics undergoing their first psychotic breaks.

Electroconvulsive therapy

Electroconvulsive therapy is sometimes called *electric shock therapy* or *electrostimulative therapy,* which is the currently preferred term. The rationale for using this treatment in cases of schizophrenia was originally based on a misconception. It was thought that schizophrenia and epilepsy do not occur together and that convulsions perhaps prevent schizophrenia (Rowe, 1975). This view was later shown to be untrue, since schizophrenia and epilepsy can occur in the same person. While the reason for the treatment was inaccurate, the treatment was helpful in some cases. Today electroconvulsive therapy is considered useful for schizophrenics who are in severe, life-threatening catatonic stupors (Redlich and Freedman, 1966) or for severely depressed and suicidal schizophrenics (Goldfarb and Goldfarb, 1977; Mendel, 1976; Redlich and Freedman, 1966; Rowe, 1975). It also seems to be helpful for extremely confused and agitated postpartum psychosis clients. A woman who is suffering from postpartum psychosis is actually experiencing an acute schizophrenic reaction.

Psychotropic drugs

The somatic treatment most widely used for schizophrenia today is the administration of psychopharmaceuticals. The major tranquilizers, which came into widespread use in the early 1950s, are called *antipsychotic drugs,* or *antischizophrenic drugs* by some. In some ways, ''tranquilizer'' is a misnomer, since the action of such a drug is to decrease the severity of psychotic behavior more than it is to sedate. In fact, the tranquilizers will stimulate or energize persons who are withdrawn and apathetic and calm those who are hyperactive—in other words, these drugs tend to normalize levels of activity. Chlorpromazine was the first of the phenothiazine drugs to be used. Other drugs were developed from the prototype. Some common phenothiazines that are used today include chlorpromazine (Thorazine), promazine (Sparine), butaperazine (Repoise), triflupromazine (Vesprin), trifluoperazine (Stelazine), perphenazine (Trilafon), prochlorperazine (Compazine), fluphenazine (Prolixin), and thioridazine (Mellaril). Haloperidol (Haldol), chlorprothixene (Taractan), and thiothixene (Navane) are not phenothiazines but are examples of some other major tranquilizers or antipsychotic drugs. Haldol is a butyrophenone, and Taractan and Navane are thioxanthenes.

A psychotropic drug that was used in India for several centuries, *Rauwolfia serpentina,* is used today to make the calming agent reserpine (Serpasil). However, the use of reserpine as a psychotropic drug is infrequent—it is more often used to lower blood pressure.

While it must be remembered that any drug can demonstrate a paradoxical reaction in any one person, some of the major tranquilizers tend to be sedating and some tend to be activating (see Table 21-1).

Characteristics specific to some of these drugs are as follows:

Haldol is believed to be especially helpful in decreasing the severity of hallucinations and delusions. It is also the drug of choice in *Gilles de la Tourette's syndrome,* a physiologically based disorder that is characterized by bizarre choreiform movements and the compulsive and uncontrollable utterance of obscene words—coprolalia. The syndrome is believed to be related to excess dopamine in the brain, and antipsychotic drugs are thought to somehow block the transport of dopamine.

Prolixin, in the form of Prolixin Enanthate, is a long-lasting phenothiazine. Intramuscular injections can be given in dosages that will last for 1 to 3 weeks, with an average of 2 weeks' duration. For this reason, Prolixin is believed to be an especially

Table 21-1. Sedating and activating tranquilizers*

	Daily dose	
	Outpatients	**Inpatients**
Sedating tranquilizers (used with overactive clients)		
Chorpromazine (Thorazine)	50-400 mg	200-1600 mg
Thioridazine (Mellaril)	50-400 mg	200-800 mg
Chlorprothixene (Taractan)	30-60 mg	75-600 mg
Promazine (Sparine)	Range: 25-1000 mg	
Activating tranquilizers (used with withdrawn clients)		
Trifluoperazine (Stelazine)	4-10 mg	6-30 mg
Prochlorperazine (Compazine)	15-60 mg	30-150 mg
Perphenazine (Trilafon)	8-24 mg	16-64 mg
Haloperidol (Haldol)	2-6 mg	4-15 mg
Thiothixene (Navane)	6-15 mg	10-60 mg
Fluphenazine (Prolixin)	1-3 mg	2-20 mg
Butaperazine (Repoise)	Range: 30-50 mg	

*Data adapted from Dimascio, Alberto, and Richard I. Shader. 1970. Clinical Handbook of Psychopharmacology. New York: Science House.

appropriate drug for persons who, for various reasons, resist taking their medication or are unreliable self-medicators. Among schizophrenics, failure to take drugs is one or the main reasons for readmission to hospitals.

Dosages of *Mellaril* should not exceed 800 mg per day. In high doses, Mellaril can cause pigmentary retinopathy and eventual blindness. Any complaints of decreasing visual acuity from clients who are taking phenothiazines should be investigated immediately, and this is particularly important for those who are taking Mellaril.

The major tranquilizers are relatively safe drugs for long-term use, and they are not addicting. Minor or moderate side effects occur fairly frequently; serious and life-threatening side effects are rare (see Table 21-2).

Psychotherapy

Forms of psychotherapy representing all of the schools of psychology have been used in the treatment of schizophrenic clients. Many clinicians believe, as Freud did, that psychoanalysis is not the treatment of choice for schizophrenics because of its goal of freeing unconscious conflicts. They argue that the psychodynamic defect in schizophrenia is an impaired ability to repress and that the unconscious is all too close to the surface. It is the threat that unconscious material will flood the ego that stimulates the psychotic symptoms as defenses.

Some notable clinicians, however, have worked with schizophrenics in a psychoanalytic manner: Harry Stack Sullivan (1953), Gertrud Schwing (1954), John Rosen (1953), Marguerite Sechehaye (1956), Harold Searles (1965), and Frieda Fromm-Reichmann (1950) are examples. All have written about their work. A well known psychiatric nurse who works within the psychosis of a client is June Mellow. She calls her in-depth approach *nursing therapy*. Mellow helps the client to relive the original mother-child symbiotic attachment, but the new emotional experience is a corrective one (Mellow, 1968).

Table 21-2. Side effects of the major tranquilizers

Side effects	Nursing intervention
Minor	
Menstrual irregularities	Inform client of possibility
Changes in libido	Inform client of possibility
Increased weight, increased appetite	Nutritional counseling
Constipation	Increased ingestion of bulk-producing foods; exercise; laxatives as needed
Dry mouth	Rinse with water; give sugarless gum (however, not advisable for elderly clients because of increased danger of choking—the phenothiazines can effect the swallowing reflex)
Postural hypotension	As a preventative, client should learn to sit up gradually from a lying position; to combat, have have client lie down with feet elevated
Photosensitivity	Use sun hats and sunscreening lotions during the summer months
Allergic rash	May require an order to change to another drug
Contact dermatitis in staff members dispensing the drug in liquid form	Use of rubber gloves when the drug is being dispensed
Moderate	
Extrapyramidal symptoms: drugs act on limbic area of brain to promote muscular dysfunctions (see Table 21-3)	Extrapyramidal symptoms, if they persist, require drugs to counteract them; such drugs as benztropine (Cogentin), procyclidine (Kemadrin), trihexyphenidyl (Artane), and biperiden (Akineton) may be used; these drugs, however, are not without side effects of their own (e.g., constipation); the automatic prescribing of one of these is not an advisable practice, since extrapyramidal symptoms are sometimes transitory and thus may disappear after a few days
Serious	
Agranulocytosis (often is manifested as a sore throat or high fever)	Stop giving the drug immediately; notify a physician when a client complains of a sore throat or has a fever; total and differential white cell counts are done, and in some cases reverse isolation may be used
Drug-induced jaundice (begins like influenza)	Periodic liver function tests should be carried out when clients are receiving phenothiazines

Continued.

Table 21-2. Side effects of the major tranquilizers—cont'd

Side effects	Nursing intervention
Tardive dyskinesia. Although one of the extra-pyramidal symptoms, it is included here because unlike the other extrapyramidal symptoms it can become irreversible. It is a disfiguring and disabling syndrome characterized by involuntary twitching of the face, tongue, arms, and legs. Abnormally low levels of acetylcholine are believed to be responsible. Signs of such emotional disturbances as euphoria, unstable moods, and manic interactions with people have been associated with the worst cases of tardive dyskinesia and several groups of researchers have suggested that this syndrome may be related to extensive use of the drugs. The terms used to describe the syndrome—"iatrogenic schizophrenia" and "tardive dysmentia"—point to the need for a close monitoring of major tranquilizers and to the strict avoidance of any inappropriate use (Herbert, 1983b).	Some success has been reported recently at M.I.T. with the treatment of tardive dyskinesia. Researchers used lecithin, a natural food substance and a major source of choline, which is a precursor of the neurotransmitter acetylcholine

Table 21-3. Extrapyramidal symptoms

Akinesia	Akathisia	Dyskinesia	Pseudo-parkinsonism
Usually has slow onset	Usually has slow onset (most often occurs in middle-aged people)	May have sudden onset (most often occurs in younger people)	Slow onset (most often occurs in older people)
Reduced physical activity	Restlessness, pacing	Torticollis	Shuffling gait
Listlessness	Jittery movements	Carpal spasms	Masklike facies
Apathy (often not recognized)	Fine hand tremor	Opisthotonos	Increased salivation
Development of painful muscles and joints	Facial tics	Oculogyric crisis	Stooping posture
	Insomnia		"Pill rolling" tremor Cogwheel rigidity

Therapists who do work in this manner with schizophrenic clients point out that the clinician must be a healthy, well integrated person in touch with thoughts, feelings, and reactions. The ethical practice of psychoanalysis mandates that the therapist be analyzed as part of the training process. Psychoanalysis is not an economical form of treatment, since one therapist can treat only a limited number of clients and there are many schizophrenics in need of help. Psychoanalysis is a specialized and expensive form of therapy. In comparison to the number of schizophrenics in need of treatment, there are *very* few psychoanalysts willing and able to treat them in this manner. Aside from this fact, as was mentioned before, many clinicians and writers believe that psychoanalysis, with its goal of uncovering unconscious conflicts, is not a useful or even safe treatment for schizophrenics, whose faulty use of repression may be the basic defect of the disorder.

Several mental health workers point to relationship or supportive therapy as the most appropriate form of psychotherapy for schizophrenics. Such therapy can be long term, and it can be crisis oriented at intervals when necessary. It can be modified over time to match the needs and the growth of the client. Rather than attempting to uncover the unconscious, the goal of relationship or supportive therapy is to gain insight into the effects of one's behavior on one's life and to encourage the development of ego strengths through the realization of successful changes in behavior. Mendel and Green (1967) describe this type of treatment and suggest that while the beginning stages of a relationship may require frequent meetings with the client, the number of meetings may gradually decrease. Eventually—perhaps after several years, in some instances—once-a-year phone calls to "check in" with the therapist may be sufficient.

Mendel and Green take the "as if" phenomenon, described earlier, and turn it around to use it therapeutically. For example, they suggest encouraging a person who feels unable to get up and face the world and a daily job as other people do, to act "as if" that was possible. After acting this way for a period of time, the client gains some ego strength from the realization of being able to accomplish this task every morning.

In relationship therapy, the nurse lends ego strength to the client in order to provide support while they both work toward the goal of developing the client's own ego strength. The nurse-client relationship in psychiatric nursing is ideally suited to relationship therapy.

Family therapy

Therapy that involves the families of schizophrenics is focused on clarifying mystifying forms of communication, such as double-bind communicating and tangentiality, which were discussed in Chapter 12. Family therapy is also concerned with strengthening appropriate boundaries between family members. For instance, one approach to decreasing the debilitating hold of a mother and a son's symbiotic relationship might be to improve the relationship between the two spouses and the relationship between the son and his father. Insight into communication and relationship patterns within the family is encouraged, and alternate patterns are explored.

The initial and primary goal of the family therapist, according to Murray Bowen (1977), is to decrease the level of anxiety within the family system, since it is this anxiety that fosters development of the various types of pathological behavior. Bowen's definition of a mental health professional is "someone who helps decrease anxiety."

Pittman and Flomenhaft (1970), have described a marital configuration that is characterized by an unequal relationship between the spouses. One spouse's incompetence is required and encouraged by the other spouse, in order to verify his or her own competence. This "doll's house marriage"— the name comes from the situation portrayed in Ibsen's play *The Doll's House*—usually involves a childlike wife and a masterful husband, although the roles can be reversed. Each spouse needs this system of relating to maintain inner equilibrium and the equilibrium of the marriage. Pittman and

Flomenhaft view this type of unequal relationship as common in a potentially schizophrenic population; they suggest that one or both spouses may be latent schizophrenics maintaining stability through the marriage. With the development of crises such as severe financial difficulties or the addition of children to the family, such individuals may come into a treatment situation. It is then that the tendency of a therapist to push for too much and too rapid change can precipitate a psychotic break. The great importance that the therapist places on individual growth may foster an attempt to promote more change than is necessary, thus destroying the family and precipitating illness in one or more family members. Pittman and Flomenhaft suggest that the therapist work with caution and develop an ability to tolerate a certain degree of inequality within a marriage, which may be the wiser choice for some couples.

Group therapy

As in the case in individual psychotherapy, few clinicians advocate psychoanalytically oriented group therapy for schizophrenics. Group therapy should be focused not on probing the unconscious but rather on the development of insight into behavior. A more comfortable adjustment to life is a legitimate goal of group therapy for schizophrenic clients. Group therapy can promote socialization—or resocialization for a regressed schizophrenic—and can provide opportunities for a client to become more outer-directed. Concern for other people can be positively reinforced, a development that can lead to increased self-esteem. Sharing of experiences and problems can provide the reassurance that comes from knowing that others have lived through similar situations. Support from a peer group during periods of crisis and attempted change can help to make experiments with new behavior less frightening.

The leader in group therapy for schizophrenics—particularly withdrawn schizophrenics—needs to take a more active role than the leader of another type of group might take, especially in the beginning stages of the group. But the same principles of group dynamics apply (see Chapter 11). Besides psychotherapy groups, various activity therapy groups, such as dance, music, and poetry groups, are helpful. *Remotivation groups* are often used to bring severely regressed schizophrenics back to a here-and-now orientation; such groups constitute a particularly useful tool for psychiatric nurses.

Certain self-help community groups are available for discharged schizophrenics; giving a client information about them would be an appropriate and helpful referral. Recovery Inc. is one such group—its method is a type of self-mediated behavior modification combined with peer group support. Schizophrenics Anonymous is another self-help group that is available in many communities.

Milieu therapy

Since disorganization in living is a major aspect of the schizophrenic experience, milieu therapy can provide schizophrenic clients opportunities to learn or relearn interpersonal skills and to become competent in the activities of daily living. Milieu therapy can also provide opportunities for satisfying recreation. An ideal milieu for schizophrenics is one that provides the structure that is so badly needed in a disorganized life.

Milieu therapy of a specific kind has been used in combination with regressive electroconvulsive therapy, a procedure that induces confusion, amnesia, and a decreased ability for self-care. A milieu is set up to recapitulate a family situation, with the goal being a healthy reparenting of the schizophrenic client. This treatment, however, has not gained wide acceptance.

Brief hospitalization versus institutionalization

Many clients believe that much of the apparent deterioration in chronic schizophrenics is due not to the disease process but to the effects of long-term institutionalization. Some of the dangers of institutionalization have been pointed out by Mendel and Green (1967) in their excellent book on the treatment of chronic schizophrenics:

1. The client loses a ''place'' in the family and community. It is not so unusual for people who are discharged after many years of hospitalization to go back to their ''roots'' and find, for example, that a parking lot or a highrise has been built where the old neighborhood stood.
2. The fact that the person has failed in a developmental task is reified. Secondary guilt is an accompaniment of this realization.
3. The role of the person as a passive receiver of treatment is reinforced instead of the role of active participant in the individual's own treatment plan.
4. The person's energy and resources (for example, financial) go toward adaptation to the hospital rather than toward adaptation to living in society.

Mendel and Green argue that short-term hospitalization should be viewed as a coping mechanism or safety valve to be used when a person's anxiety approaches unbearable heights. They suggest that the person's knowing the hospital is there when needed may help to reduce anxiety.

Cancro (1970) has outlined criteria on which the decision to hospitalize a schizophrenic person should be based:

1. Safety—the person is endangering self or others.
2. Crisis times—coping mechanisms are strained, and anxiety is high in the person or the family (death in the family or divorce are possible examples).
3. Stabilization of treatment and observation of the client (for example, stabilization of a medication regimen or administration of electroconvulsive therapy) may be necessary.

• • •

Many forms of treatment are used to help schizophrenic clients live more comfortably in the world. While a few specially trained clinicians provide psychoanalytical therapy for schizophrenics, psychoanalysis is a comparatively rare form of treatment in schizophrenia, and the value and safety of it for schizophrenics are questioned by many clinicians. Supportive individual and group therapy, in combination with psychotropic drugs and, if possible, family therapy, seems to be the treatment of choice for schizophrenic clients.

NURSING INTERVENTION

PRIMARY PREVENTION

Primary prevention of schizophrenia includes modification of the environment and strengthening of coping abilities. It is only in recent years that much has been attempted or even written as far as prevention of schizophrenia is concerned. This is probably because there has never been agreement on the etiology of the disorder. Since the consensus is that it is of multifactorial etiology, a multifactorial prevention program must be developed. Some work has begun. Clinicians have identified high-risk groups—this process is termed *vulnerability research*. Basically, it is the selection and study of children who are at risk of developing schizophrenia. This determination is based on the presence of the following factors:

1. Genetic predisposition
2. History of deprivation of some kind in the prenatal or neonatal period
3. Evidence of excessive disorganization in the family
4. A disordered sociocultural environment such as that found in poverty-stricken inner-city areas or that occurring after a massive natural or man-made disaster (Garmezy, 1971).

Through study of the vulnerable children, a group of children classified as ''invulnerables'' has been delineated. These are people who, through every indication, should have developed schizophrenia but did not—in fact, many excelled in various life tasks. The goal of researchers is to try to determine what factors helped to prevent these children from becoming schizophrenic and then to use this information to help prevent other children from developing the disorder.

Several areas have in the past been defined as providing possible approaches to the prevention of schizophrenia. *Premarital counseling* has been employed to help ensure a strong base for the future family or, in some instances, to prevent marriages from taking place. Most marriages are the result of ''falling in love,'' which is an interweaving of the unconscious and often neurotic needs of two people. Later, it is the projection of these needs by one spouse onto the other that contributes to many marital problems. Some insight into the potential hazards may help to minimize marital discord or at least set a pattern for individual self-awareness and open communication between the spouses. Perhaps people need lessons in how to be married—it is not something that we know instinctively.

Marital counseling has been used for marriages that are showing signs of strain because of discord or dysfunctional family members. Alleviation of anxiety between married persons may prevent the conflict from being projected onto a child, a situation that can, according to family theorists, result in a schizophrenic reaction.

Family therapy that is instituted in the preschizophrenic stage of a child or adolescent's disorder may prevent a full-bown schizophrenic break. Alleviating anxiety within the family system, fostering insight into disordered patterns of communicating and relating, and encouraging the learning of new patterns are all parts of the family therapist's goal.

Prenatal care and *neonatal care* should be optimal in order to prevent the possible damage to fetus and infant that is significantly correlated with the incidence of schizophrenia.

Genetic counseling may be appropriate for families that are at extremely high risk of having schizophrenic offspring because numerous family members have the disorder. However, the exact mode of genetic transmission is unknown.

Child-rearing counseling can help alleviate such problems as ''poor fit'' between mother and child as far as stimulus barriers are concerned. A mother who enjoys giving and receiving stimuli might have a child with a low tolerance for stimuli, or vice versa. Developmental stages and the mother's need for rest, recreation, and time away from her children are also important aspects of this type of counseling. Just as people may need lessons in how to be married, preparation in parenting might prevent potentially harmful family discord.

There is rather extensive documentation in the literature that the children of schizophrenic women are at ten to fifteen times greater risk for developing the disorder than is the general population (Siefer and Sameroff, 1982, p. 87). The symbiotic phase of preoedipal development (which occurs approximately from one month to five months of age) is believed to be the crucial one in the subsequent development of schizophrenia. Mahler (1975) found that the most deeply disturbed schizophrenic children were never able to establish a healthy symbiosis with their mothers. Searles (1965) pointed out that, if they were able to establish it, they were never able to resolve it in a healthy way.

The infant's psyche takes shape in harmony and counterpoint to the mother's own particular ego and lifestyle. Spitz (1965) has called the mother *the auxiliary ego of the infant*. The important factor is whether or not the mother provides a healthy or pathological object for this adaptation of the infant. Strong ego boundaries can only be established by the mother at the phase-appropriate time. During the symbiotic phase, it is healthy for the mother to be preoccupied with her infant (Winnicott, 1965) in order to protect the child from inappropriate stimuli. Thus, the mother serves as a replacement for the earlier, inborn stimulus barrier and protects the child from undue stress and strain (Mahler, 1975). Mahler suggests that an infant who later become schizophrenic is unable to invest in its mother or to use her to establish affective-tension homeostasis and, instead, must resort to maintenance mechanisms that are pathological (schizophrenic) and lead to isolation and withdrawal (Pao, 1979). These are maladaptive mechanisms but they help the baby to cope in the absence of ''mutual cuing.''* The lack of mutual cuing in the mother-child dyad is perhaps where efforts at primary prevention may best be focused. Field (1982) agrees and suggests that early intervention to facilitate healthy interactions between mother and child may be helpful. ''Interaction coaching'' is the term used to describe attempts to modify disturbed mother-infant interaction. Efforts are directed toward improving the ''fit'' or mutual cuing between the two. Field's set of interventions that are aimed at modulating arousal and improving the level of information processing in high-risk infants include:

1. Appropriate games for the age level
2. Coaching mothers through an earpiece microphone
3. Replaying videotapes for her viewing

Using ''infant gaze'' as the dependent variable in 14- to 18-week-old infants, the data suggested that mothers of high-risk infants can be taught other ways of interacting. The goal is a more harmonious relationship for mother and child. Field states:

The problem relates to finding the optimal level of stimulation since low levels do not seem to arouse or elicit responses from infants while high levels eventuate in gaze aversion or fussiness.

Field also points out that infant gaze avoidance and irritability and parental overactivity and overcontrol were revealed in a retrospective analysis of the harmonics of infants later diagnosed as schizophrenic.

Mutual cuing is defined by Mahler (1975, p. 290) as ''a circular process of interaction established very early between mother an infant, by which they 'empathically' read each other's signs and signals and react to each other.''

To summarize, primary prevention of schizophrenia through intervention at or before the symbolic phase (Arnold, 1983) would include:

1. Identification of parent-child dyads and triads at high risk for producing schizophrenic offspring
2. Therapeutic intervention with, and support of, the high-risk mother and family unit; both pre- and postpartum
3. Education and interaction coaching aimed at facilitating a healthy symbiosis in high-risk mothers
4. Support of the sensitivity-facilitating preoccupation of the low-risk mother

The preceding material on possible avenues for preventive intervention makes it obvious that there is an important role for nurses in the prevention of schizophrenia, whether they work in the community, in maternal and child-focused agencies, in psychiatric settings, or in traditional hospital settings.

Traditionally the allocation of funds for research into the etiology and treatment of schizophrenia has been sparse—this area is sometimes called the stepchild of research in this country. Perhaps one of the reasons for this situation is that chronically ill schizophrenics have very little political power, they have neither the personal nor the financial resources to mount much of a protest movement. As concerned and informed citizens and as advocates of their clients, nurses can make their voices and their votes count. Social changes that lead to improved living conditions and to the availability of optimum health care for all people may be viewed as primary preventive measures for all mental illnesses, including schizophrenia. The reason for the strong correlation between poverty and schizophrenia is unclear, but that there is a strong correlation is undisputed.

SECONDARY PREVENTION

What constitutes nursing care for the schizophrenic client? Just as no person fits exactly into any of the diagnostic categories, there is no exact set of rules or techniques that nurses use to intervene in cases of schizophrenia. It is best to deal with the behavior manifested rather than with the client as a psychiatric category. According to Freud, all behavior has meaning and the psychotic behavior of the schizophrenic is a form of communication.

The two areas that nurses can be particularly helpful in are interpersonal relationships and communication—these are usually the two areas that the schizophrenic has the most problems with in life. A well known psychiatric nurse, Marguerite Holmes, believes that in the nurse-client relationship, the nurse should concentrate on learning about and understanding the way the client is experiencing the world. The client will then have been *heard* and *understood,* and because this communication will have taken place, may be able to move toward changing behavior.

> The skills required of the nurse then, are that she be able to (a) help the patient accept and appreciate his own inner experiences, which means that she has to be able to tolerate sharing in some of these experiences, and (b) meet the patient in real encounter (Holmes, 1971).

Many things can happen to the nurse and the client through their attempts to relate to each other in a meaningful way. An important development is that the client may be able to increase trust in other people. One relationship is rarely, if ever, the remedy for many years of social withdrawal, but one relationship can lead to another.

Bleuler's "four A's"—his delineation of the primary symptoms of schizophrenia—were reviewed earlier in this chapter. While they may be helpful as a mnemonic device, they are basically a negative concept, since they focus on pathology. There is a danger in this. Expectation of pathological responses is a powerful stimulus for the production of pathological responses in people. A more helpful way of viewing the interaction between the nurse and the schizophrenic would be to focus on *four A's of therapeutic intervention* (Arnold, 1976). Unlike Bleuler's four A's, which

are concepts that are often projected onto the client, the therapeutic four A's apply to both partners in the relationship. The therapeutic four A's are as follows:

1. Acceptance. Crucial to the relationship is the nurse's acceptance of self, of the client as he or she is in the present stage of development, and of the world as *he* or *she* sees it.
2. Awareness. Before nurse and client can begin to communicate effectively, the nurse must be aware of his or her own thoughts, feelings, and actions. This self-understanding, combined with an awareness of the client's verbal, nonverbal, and symbolic communication, is an essential part of the therapeutic relationship.
3. Acknowledgement. The existence of a person whose communication is not acknowledged is disconfirmed. People need to know that they have been heard, and they need to know whether they have been understood.
4. Authenticity. Most important of all of the elements of a therapeutic relationship, whether they begin with "A" or not, is authenticity. The tool of a psychiatric nurse is *self*. The self can only be a useful tool if it is real. Because of the nature of their disorder, it is not unusual for schizophrenic clients to have a history of many hurtful relationships. For this reason they tend to be very sensitive interpersonally and can quickly detect any signs of dissembling or deceit.

Nursing process

Many approaches to the etiology and treatment of schizophrenia have been discussed. Psychiatric nursing is based on an eclectic theoretical approach and on appropriate responses to behavioral problems. This section will deal with secondary prevention through nursing intervention into clients' patterns of underactivity and withdrawal, overactivity and anxiety, autistic behavior, feelings and thoughts of unreality, low self-esteem, depression, and suicide. The nursing process will provide guidelines for our interventions.

ASSESSMENT

In using the nursing process to intervene with the schizophrenic client, the nurse should assess the following areas:

1. Presenting symptoms, or patterns of behavior—underactivity and withdrawal, overactivity and anxiety, verbal hostility and physical aggression, suspicion and fear of interpersonal relationships, autistic behavior (symbolic communication, inappropriate behavior, ritualistic behavior), feelings and thoughts of unreality (depersonalization, loose ego boundaries, delusions, hallucinations), low self-esteem, and suicide.

2. Emotional state—feelings of anger, fear, anxiety, helplessness, apathy. An understanding of the tendency toward a crippling ambivalence and the subjective experience of the "need-fear dilemma" is important here.

3. Stimulus situations—stressful life situations that threaten the self-system and engender an increased tendency to withdraw inwardly.

4. Maladaptive coping behaviors—coping patterns based on withdrawal from interpersonal relations and control of the environment and one's inner life through magical level thinking. Coping behaviors may also be influenced by thought and perceptual disorders. The behaviors are an attempt to maintain a cohesive sense of self in the face of overwhelming anxiety, but they are maladaptive in that they lead to further problems in relating and functioning in the world.

5. Origin of maladaptive coping behaviors—identification of childhood experiences that contributed to the development of or learning of maladaptive coping behavior.

6. Holistic health status—physical, intellectual, emotional, sociocultural, and spiritual status of the client. These factors may either facilitate wellness (e.g., a benevolent, protective marital relationship may shield the

client from some of the stresses of life) or these factors may impede wellness (e.g., difficulties in concentrating can be exacerbated by poor nutrition and amplify any tendency toward a thought disorder).

ANALYSIS OF DATA

A clear and comprehensive assessment of presenting symptoms, emotional state, stimulus situations, maladaptive coping behavior and its origin, and the holistic health status of the schizophrenic client can assist the nurse who is formulating a nursing diagnosis. The following section focuses on behavioral problems and nursing responses to these problems. Following each nursing diagnosis will be an appropriate care plan and its implementation.

Nursing diagnosis: Underactivity and withdrawal related to fears of interpersonal relating and of functioning in the world (behavior associated with DSM-III diagnoses 295.1x through 295.6x, schizophrenic disorders; and 297.10, 297.30, 298.30, 297.90, paranoid disorders; and 295.40, 298.80, 295.70, 298.90, psychotic disorders not elsewhere classified)

Planning: With assistance and guidance from the nurse the client will establish goals.

1. Long-term goals
   a. Work through some of the fears of relating to other people.
   b. Increase confidence in ability to function in the world.
2. Short-term goals*
   a. Verbalize feelings of anxiety, inadequacy, helplessness.†
   b. Identify interpersonal situations that arouse feelings of anxiety, inadequacy, and helplessness.

---

*Because the degree of underactivity and withdrawal varies, short-term goals may need to be modified. (For example, in the case of a mute client, short-term goals as stated here would be intermediate or long term.)

†This should be encouraged at a rate and to a degree that are not overwhelming to the client or threatening to the self-concept. In other words, it should be facilitated but not "pushed."

c. Relate current stressful interpersonal or mastery situations to situations in the past that aroused similar feelings.

d. Identify any effective coping behavior used during these past situations.

e. Develop more effective coping behavior and interpersonal skills.

f. Realistically perceive the five dimensions of self (biological, psychological, intellectual, sociocultural, and spiritual strengths and weaknesses in perspective).

g. Build self-esteem in a realistic manner (see Chapter 18).

h. Meet needs for adequate rest, exercise, food, personal hygiene, and leisure activity.

Implementation: Years ago, before psychotropic drugs and under conditions of inadequate care, withdrawal could progress to the point that some people actually became ankylosed into a fetal position. Conditions have improved, but the tendency toward withdrawal is always present. The "good patient," who makes no trouble for the staff, and the "unpleasant" one, whose behavior feeds into a pattern of mutual withdrawal between client and staff, are examples of clients whose interpersonal isolation may be reinforced by the hospital experience. Remotivation groups and activities such as art, exercise, and dance are important therapeutic interventions. The nurse's encouragement and support of the client's efforts to participate in unit activities can make a crucial difference.

The withdrawn schizophrenic may be neglectful of personal hygiene. Direction given in a way that protects self-esteem, as well as positive reinforcement of any efforts through praise, can help facilitate learning.

One way that withdrawal may be manifested is through varying degrees of mutism. Intervention for a nonverbal client requires an attitude of patience and quiet optimism on the part of a nurse. The communications from the nurse to the client should be simple and precise, and they should be phrased so as to require an answer from the client. Excessive detail and the introduction of many topics may be overwhelming and should be avoided. Orientation as to the proposed length of time for the interaction and the schedule of future interactions should be part of each exchange. Asking for a description of actions and events is probably less threatening to the nonverbal client than asking for thoughts or feelings (Oden, 1963). While fear is most often involved in the client's need to be mute, a need to control interpersonal situations may also be present. For this reason it is important to avoid making the client's mute behavior part of a power struggle with the nurse.

Nursing supervision and maintenance of physical health are necessary in the treatment of many withdrawn clients. Since subjective reports of physical condition are not always reliable in the case of a preoccupied, autistic schizophrenic, the nurse needs to be vigilant in observing the state of health. Nutrition, regular exercise, rest, and necessary medical examinations may all be neglected by the schizophrenic who copes with the world through withdrawal and isolation. While the nurse may take on a "mothering" role for the withdrawn client as an appropriate intervention, the fostering of excessive dependence in the client should be avoided. The good mother is one who allows her child to grow and leave the dependent state.

Nursing diagnosis: Overactivity related to anxiety, fears of interpersonal relating and of functioning in the world (behavior associated with DSM-III diagnoses 295.1x through 295.6x; schizophrenic disorders; 297.10, 297.30, 298.30, 297.90, paranoid disorders; and 295.40, 298.80, 295.70, 298.90, psychotic disorders not elsewhere classified)

Planning: With assistance and guidance from the nurse, the client will establish goals.

1. Long-term goals
   a. Work through some of the fears of relating to other people.
   b. Increase confidence in ability to function in the world.

2. Short-term goals*
   a. Verbalize feelings of anxiety, inadequacy and helplessness (facilitate but do not force).
   b. Identify interpersonal situations that arouse feelings of anxiety, inadequacy, and helplessness.
   c. Relate current stressful interpersonal or mastery situations to situations in the past that aroused similar feelings.
   d. Identify any effective coping behavior used during these past situations.
   e. Develop more effective coping behavior and interpersonal skills.
   f. Realistically perceive the five dimensions of self (biological, psychological, intellectual, sociocultural, and spiritual strengths and weaknesses in perspective).
   g. Build self-esteem in a realistic manner (see Chapter 18).
   h. Meet needs for adequate rest, exercise, food, personal hygiene, and leisure activity.

Implementation: Some clients may block out harsh reality through frenzied overactivity. As in the case of the withdrawn, underactive client, nursing intervention may be necessary for maintenance of physical health. Many of the principles used in working with the manic client will apply here (see Chapter 18). Exercise and games that do not involve a great deal of concentration may help dissipate the tension and energy associated with the state of anxiety. The need for adequate rest and nutrition may be ignored. The same is true of the symptoms of physical illness—one young schizophrenic man was developing a serious case of pneumonia, but his hyperactivity belied his temperature of 105°.

Sometimes the frenzied behavior and rapid speech can prove overwhelming to the staff mem-

ber assigned to work with the overactive client. For this reason it may be necessary to plan staff involvement on a rotating basis, which will help ensure a therapeutic approach rather than one that is influenced by negative countertransference.

Anxiety is often a part of the schizophrenic experience. The times when a client is particularly vulnerable to acute anxiety attacks are as follows:

1. On admission to a psychiatric facility (and particularly on first admission—depression is more apt to accompany subsequent readmissions)
2. When the client begins to participate in any new activity, such as group therapy
3. When the staff member or therapist the client is accustomed to working with goes on vacation, is transferred, or resigns
4. Just before discharge from the hospital (Many hospitalized schizophrenics express feelings of ambivalence and anxiety about being discharged. The hospital may seem less threatening and more accepting than the outside world, the client may feel overwhelmed by the thought of increased responsibility.)

In working with an anxious client, a nurse must remember that anxiety can interfere with the client's hearing and comprehension; a nurse may have to repeat much of what he or she says. Complete but concise directions are best. The nurse's support of the client through his or her presence as the client begins to participate in new activities or try out new behavior may help ease discomfort. Adequate preparation, with opportunities for the expression of concerns, will help a client during the anxiety-provoking predischarge period or when a trusted staff member is leaving.

Underactivity and overactivity, besides being indications of a client's psychological state, may be extrapyramidal symptoms resulting from the use of psychotropic drugs. The client should be evaluated for appropriate medication.

Nursing diagnosis: Interaction theme of verbal hostility related to anxiety, anger, frustration, dis-

---

*As in the case of underactivity, short-term goals may need to be viewed as intermediate or long term, depending upon the degree of overactivity in the client.

appointment, or threats to the self-system (behavior associated with DSM-III diagnoses 295.1x through 295.6x, schizophrenic disorders; 297.10, 297.30, 298.30, 297.90, paranoid disorders; and 295.40, 298.80, 295.70, 298.90, psychotic disorders not elsewhere classified)

Planning: With assistance and guidance from the nurse, the client will establish goals.

1. Long-term goals
   a. Work through any feelings of anxiety, anger, frustration, disappointment, and fear.
   b. Learn to relate to others in a manner that is not hostile and that allows for appropriate expression of anger.
2. Short-term goals
   a. Verbalize feelings of anxiety, anger, frustration, disappointment, and fear.
   b. Identify interpersonal situations that arouse these feelings.
   c. Relate current stressful interpersonal situations to situations in the past that aroused similar feelings.
   d. Identify any effective coping behavior used in the past under similar circumstances.
   e. Develop more effective coping behavior and interpersonal skills.
   f. Realistically perceive the five dimensions of self (biological, psychological, intellectual, sociocultural, and spiritual strengths and weaknesses in perspective).
   g. Build self-esteem in a realistic manner (see Chapter 18).

Implementation: It is not unusual for a nurse working in a psychiatric setting to witness a client's verbal hostility. The nurse may also be the recipient of such hostility. Verbal hostility may be displaced anger that the client actually feels for someone else. Quite often the nurse is viewed as a less threatening object for displacement of feelings. However, there are times (such as when maintenance of the therapeutic milieu interferes with the wishes of the client) when angry feelings are indeed felt toward the nurse. In dealing with verbal hostility, a nurse must keep certain important facts in mind.

The expression of anger serves a purpose. It substitutes a more comfortable feeling for feelings of anxiety, and it provides relief from the tension that comes from being frustrated or disappointed or from a threat to self-esteem (Hays, 1963). Also, verbally expressed anger may be viewed as a more mature form of behavior than the *physically* expressed anger that previously may have resulted in many unpleasant situations for the client. Jurgen Ruesch, who is an expert in the field of human communication, views communication as a continuum. Acting out one's feelings—a primitive form of communicating—is situated on one end of the continuum. Verbalizing one's feelings—a more developed form of communicating—is situated on the other end. Interestingly, Ruesch views psychosomatic illness as being situated in the middle, between acted-out feelings and verbalized feelings (Ruesch, 1957):

Acted-out	Psychosomatic	Verbalized
feelings	illness	feelings

Continuum of communication

The client who is able to express feelings of anger and hostility is demonstrating a healthier, more mature form of communicating. It is important to remember, however, that it may be necessary at times to intervene in order to protect the self-esteem of a client who is the recipient of the angry feelings.

When a client expresses anger toward the nurse, the *nondefensive stance* is the most therapeutic way of dealing with the behavior. If the nurse becomes defensive in reacting to hostility, he or she may lose complete control of the situation. The nurse's defensive reaction tends to escalate the defensive behavior of the client, and little real communication takes place. If the nurse instead remains nondefensive, he or she may be able to disarm the client and defuse the situation. The vicious circle of escalating feelings will then be broken, and nurse and client can explore the situation together in an authentic learning experience.

Nursing diagnosis: Interaction theme of physical aggression related to anxiety, anger, frustration, disappointment, or threats to the self system (behavior associated with DSM-III diagnoses 295.1x through 295.6x, schizophrenic disorders; 297.10, 297.30, 298.30, 297.90, paranoid disorders; and 295.40, 298.80, 295.70, 298.90 psychotic disorders not elsewhere classified)

Planning: With assistance and guidance from the nurse, the client will establish goals.

1. Long-term goals
   a. Work through any feelings of anxiety, anger, frustration, disappointment, or threats to the self-system.
   b. Learn to express feelings verbally rather than resorting to a physical "acting out."
2. Short-term goals*
   a. Protect client, self, and others from harm.
   b. Identify feelings of anxiety, anger, frustration, disappointment, or threats to the self-system.
   c. Verbalize these feelings.
   d. Relate current stressful interpersonal situations to situations in the past that aroused similar feelings.
   e. Relate difficulties in interpersonal relationships and in the ability to gain satisfaction from the environment to the reliance on physical aggression as a mode of expressing feelings.
   f. Identify any effective coping behavior used in the past under similar circumstances.
   g. Develop more effective coping behavior and interpersonal skills.
   h. Realistically perceive the five dimensions of self (biological, psychological, intellectual, sociocultural, and spiritual strengths and weaknesses in perspective).

---

*Goal a implies that the locus of decision making is no longer with the client (e.g., the client is exhibiting assaultive behavior). Goals b through h are appropriate after the threatening situation has been resolved. They may, depending upon the status of the overactive, anxious client, be interpreted as intermediate or even long-term goals.

Implementation: The optimal way to deal with physical aggression is to prevent it from happening in the first place. Careful observation of the levels of tension and anxiety and early, judicious use of medication may do much in this area. If a client must be restrained because of physical aggression, chemical restraints are much more acceptable and protective of self-esteem than any physical restraint. The use of seclusion or "quiet" rooms, where threatening environmental stimuli can be controlled, is preferable to such devices as camisole restraints. It is best to work with a client in a way that will encourage communication of a need for sedation before the tension becomes unbearable.

When a situation has reached the point where a client is clearly exhibiting signs of assaultiveness, some points are helpful to remember:

1. A unit should have a preplanned way of dealing with such incidents; all staff members should know what it is.
2. The self-esteem of the client should be protected, through the nurse's attitude and communication.
3. Since anxiety is contagious, a calm attitude the nurse's part may also help to soothe the client.
4. Nurses should avoid smiling at the client. A suspicious, paranoid person may feel he or she is being laughed at.
5. A sufficient number of staff members should be available to deal with the problem physically. Even the frailest of psychotic clients can exhibit tremendous strength under conditions of panic. But a nurse should *not* automatically use all staff members present at the scene to surround the client at close quarters. Sometimes the very sight of a number of staff members in the background will quiet an assaultive client, while a feeling of being surrounded can be a threat that increases panic.

Nursing diagnosis: Psychic disequilibrium related to suspicion and fear of interpersonal relationships (behavior associated with DSM-III diagnoses 295.1x through 295.6x, schizophrenic disorders; 297.10, 297.30, 298.30, 297.90, paranoid disorders; and 295.40, 298.80, 295.70, 298.90, psychotic disorders not elsewhere classified)

Planning: With assistance and guidance from the nurse, the client will establish goals.

1. Long-term goals
   a. Work through some of the fears of relating to other people.
   b. Develop an increased ability to trust other people.
2. Short-term goals
   a. Verbalize feelings of anxiety, inadequacy, helplessness.
   b. Verbalize suspicions and fears of other people.
   c. Learn to clarify any doubts, suspicions, or possible misinterpretations of other people's communications or actions.
   d. Identify situations that arouse feelings of suspicion.
   e. Relate current stressful situations to situations in the past that aroused similar feelings of fear and suspicion.
   f. Identify any effective coping behavior used during these past situations.
   g. Increase self-esteem in a realistic manner* (see Chapter 18).
   h. Realistically perceive the five dimensions of self (biological, psychological, intellectual, sociocultural, and spiritual strengths and weaknesses in perspective).

Implementation: A client who is habitually suspicious of other people requires a thoughtful and consistent nursing approach. The following are some helpful points:

1. A matter-of-fact attitude is better than one that is overly warm. While a nurse's warmth may be an asset with other clients, in this situation it can arouse even more of the client's feelings of suspicion ("Why is she pretending to be my friend?" "What does she really want?").
2. In situations in which an apology may be appropriate (for example, a nurse is delayed because of another client or a necessary procedure and thus is late for a scheduled appointment) it is best to offer the apology in a matter-of-fact way and to avoid overdoing it. Profuse apologies may elicit increased suspicion.
3. Physical contact should be avoided—it can be interpreted by a paranoid client as a sexual advance or threat.
4. Too much eye contact can be threatening, while too little can arouse suspicion.
5. The nonverbal behavior of a nurse is important—smiling, as mentioned earlier, may be misinterpreted by a suspicious client.
6. A nurse should speak clearly and concisely and with sufficient loudness. There should be no chance for a client to misinterpret what is being said. The use of the communication technique of *consensual validation* may be helpful.
7. A nurse should never hide medications in the food of *any* client but particularly that of a client who has difficulty trusting others.
8. In situations in which the nurse is taking notes while talking with the client, the nurse should be prepared to let the client read them at any time he or she seems concerned.
9. The *need to control* and the *fear of being controlled* often characterize a suspicious client. Nurses should avoid power struggles or situations wherein nurse or client is required to be dominant or submissive. The client should be allowed as many opportunities for decision making as possible. But a nurse should avoid a situation wherein efforts to provide such opportunities result in his or her being manipulated or feeling controlled by the client.
10. A nurse must always be aware of, and allow

---

*Goals *g* and *h* may be intermediate or long term, depending upon the particular client's status.

for, the *need-fear dilemma* of the client. The client should be allowed to set the pace for the closeness of the relationship and to backtrack whenever the degree of closeness becomes threatening.

11. Nurses should be as honest as possible about their own feelings when asked about them by clients. A suspicious person is usually very sensitive in interpersonal situations and may ''test'' in this way to see if the nurse really can be trusted.

Nursing diagnosis: Symbolic, dysfunctional communication related to thought disorder and to fears of interpersonal relating (autistic behavior associated with DSM-III diagnoses 295.1x through 295.6x, schizophrenic disorders; 297.10, 297.30, 298.30, 297.90, paranoid disorders; and 297.40, 298.80, 295.70, 298.90, psychotic disorders not elsewhere classified)

Planning: With assistance and guidance from the nurse, the client will establish goals.

1. Long-term goals
   a. Work through some of the fears of relating to other people.
   b. Increase ability to communicate effectively and directly with other people.
2. Short-term goals
   a. Identify difficulties in communicating with others.
      (1) Increase awareness of the tendency to use symbolic forms of communication.
      (2) Increase awareness of the difficulties others have in understanding one's symbolic communication.
   b. Identify interpersonal situations that elicit increased reliance on symbolic communication.
   c. Relate current stressful interpersonal situations to situations in the past that tended to elicit increased reliance on symbolic communication.
   d. Relate difficulties in interpersonal relating, in the ability to function, and in the ability to gain satisfaction from the environment to the reliance on symbolic forms of communication.
   e. Develop more effective communication and interpersonal skills (e.g., seeking clarification, asking for validation).
   f. Realistically perceive the five dimensions of self (biological, psychological, intellectual, sociocultural, and spiritual strengths and weaknesses in perspective).*

Implementation: The verbalizations of schizophrenics are often quite difficult to follow. Loose association of thoughts, the use of neologisms, a tendency to use pronouns in unusual ways, and paleological thinking all are elements in a way of communicating that is disguised, confusing, and ineffective in facilitating interpersonal relationships. Decoding this communication pattern and helping the client to learn clearer ways of communicating with others are important nursing problems. Some particularly helpful communication techniques include consensual validation, asking for clarification, exploring content, and asking for amplification (Hays and Larson, 1963).

The most important aid in communicating with a schizophrenic client is the attitude of the nurse who wants to learn to decode the client's communication system and who conveys this interest to the client. Autistic communication may be used as a defense against threatening interpersonal closeness. As trust grows within a therapeutic relationship, however, the client may begin to translate this personal language for the nurse.

It is essential that the nurse let the client know when he or she does not understand—the nurse should not let things slip by because of the fear of alienating the client by asking for clarification frequently. The client may be testing the nurse to see if he or she is interested enough to ask for this clarification. Also, a nurse who does not ask for clarification may reinforce a client's ineffective way of communicating with others.

---

*Goal f may be intermediate or long term, depending upon the particular client's status.

It is important to avoid fostering the notion that either the nurse or the client can read the other's mind. Such notions are not at all uncommon among schizophrenics. Responding to hints, inferring meanings that are not obvious or intended, offering interpretive statements, and finishing the other person's sentences are all examples of communication techniques that are not therapeutic.

Nursing diagnosis: Dysfunctional social behavior related to anxiety, lack of social awareness, fears of interpersonal relating, magical level thinking (autistic behavior associated with DSM-III diagnoses 295.1x through 295.6x, schizophrenic disorders)

Planning: With assistance and guidance from the nurse, the client will establish goals.

1. Long-term goals
   a. Work through some of the fears of relating to people.
   b. Increase level of social awareness.
   c. Increase interpersonal skills.
2. Short-term goals
   a. Verbalize any feelings of anxiety and any fears of interpersonal relating.*
   b. Increase awareness of effects of behavior in interpersonal situations.
   c. Identify interpersonal situations that tend to elicit dysfunctional social behavior.
   d. Develop more effective coping behavior and interpersonal skills.
   e. Increase self-esteem in a reality-based context (see Chapter 18).
   f. Realistically perceive the five dimensions of self (biological, psychological, intellectual, sociocultural, and spiritual strengths and weaknesses in perspective).

Implementation: For regressed schizophrenic clients who are hospitalized, masturbation in public is one possible form of dysfunctional social behavior; *ritualistic* or *stereotypical* behavior is another. The implementation of a helpful, cooperative nurse-client plan should include the following:

*Depending upon the level of regression, this goal may be an intermediate or even long-term one.

1. Nonjudgmental acceptance of the client
2. Awareness of the purpose the behavior serves on the part of both client and staff (usually the behavior is used to help decrease anxiety or to communicate something)
3. Expectations on the part of the staff that the client can control behavior
4. Protection of other people from the client's behavior, when necessary
5. Substitution of activities for the behavior (helpful in some cases)

Some types of behavior of regressed schizophrenics, while serving very real purposes, may get them into trouble in social situations. For example, a client who is very anxious may masturbate openly in a crowded day room. Masturbation, besides providing relief from tension for a psychotic client, may be a substitute for interpersonal relatedness and a way of maintaining reality contact (Gibney, 1972). This statement suggests several possible elements of nursing intervention:

1. The rest of the client population may need to be protected from a scene that could be anxiety provoking. The needs of the entire group are important to consider.
2. The client's need to masturbate and for increased social awareness can best be served by suggesting, in a nonjudgmental way, that a more private place be found.
3. A nurse can respond to the message that the client may need or wish greater interpersonal contact by increasing his or her efforts to relate to the client and by encouraging the client to relate to others in the unit.
4. Masturbation that has become compulsive may indicate severe regression.

Another form of socially inappropriate behavior, ritualistic or stereotypical behavior, was demonstrated by a young schizophrenic girl who felt compelled to touch other females or stroke their hair. The behavior may have had its roots in an exceptionally strong symbiotic relationship with her mother. She would make such statements as "My mother is my only reason for living." The touching and stroking aroused anger among other clients—particularly those who felt threatened by physical closeness. She was sometimes assaulted. At best, her behavior alienated her from many of the ward residents. The nursing staff members used a firm but gentle approach. They conveyed their expectations that she could indeed control her behavior. After a student nurse taught her how to crochet as a possible substitute activity for her hands, she was able to decrease the touching significantly, resorting to it only when anxiety was extremely high.

An elderly and chronically ill woman greeted every morning with her ritual of placing a cloth packet of salt she had made on her head and facing the east for 15 minutes. Her need for this strange but harmless ritualistic behavior was accepted by the nursing staff. After this ritual she would go about her business of the day. One burly, middle-aged man controlled his anxiety by twirling about the room like a ballet dancer. Staff members responded by accepting his need for this behavior, but they also focused on developing his ability to control it at times. Eventually, the frequency of the behavior decreased to a point where the success of his placement in the community was ensured. His substitute behavior was an unspoken slogan that he would recall during times of increased anxiety.

Nursing diagnosis: Distortion in perception of self (depersonalization and/or loose ego boundaries) related to escalating anxiety and threats to the self-system (behavior associated with DSM-III diagnoses 295.1x through 295.6x, schizophrenic disorders; and 295.40, 298.80, 295.70, 298.90, psychotic disorders not classified elsewhere)

Planning: With assistance and guidance from the nurse, the client will establish goals.

1. Long-term goals
   a. Work through some of the conflicts that are generating the underlying anxiety.
   b. Develop a clearer, more consistent sense of self.
   c. Increase the ability to cope with stress without the use of psychotic defenses or severe distortions of reality.
2. Short-term goals

   a. Recognize the relationship between escalating anxiety and the subjective experience of depersonalization and other manifestations of loose ego boundaries.
   b. Verbalize and explore feelings about current inner conflicts, current stressful situations in life.
   c. Recognize and differentiate inner (intrapsychic) stimuli and outer (environmental) stimuli.
   d. Increase self-esteem in a reality-based context (see Chapter 18).
   e. Realistically perceive the five dimensions of self (biological, psychological, intellectual, sociocultural, and spiritual strengths and weaknesses in perspective).*

Implementation: Feelings of strangeness and estrangement or thinking that one's body or objects in the environment have changed are all highly anxiety provoking. They are also anxiety based. Such situations are examples of anxiety feeding upon itself. A nurse can combat this escalation by explaining the phenomenon to the client. By explaining that depersonalization is a by-product of increased anxiety, the nurse can remove the unknown, frightening quality and interrupt a vicious circle. Things that are unknown or unexplained are always frightening to the person experiencing them. Depersonalization increases with increasing anxiety, and it is a part of the phenomenon of loose ego boundaries.

No clear concept of self, getting one's needs and desires "mixed up" with other people's, difficulty in forming opinions on any subject, and problems in differentiating internal stimuli from environmental stimuli are all manifestations of loose ego boundaries. The phenomenon can be thought of as a dynamic continuum on which manifestations range from indecisiveness and lack of clarity about one's own feelings to having a delusion that one has been transformed into someone else.

---

*This goal may be, depending upon the degree of regression in the client, an intermediate or even long-term goal.

Sometimes loose ego boundaries will result in mild or intense identification with another person. For example, expressing a desire to be a nurse, stating that one really is a nurse, wearing the same sort of clothes, copying a hairstyle, and so forth may all be indications that a client is identifying with the nurse. Saying things like "You'd like to go down to the music room" when wanting to go there oneself is also an indication. It is important that a nurse use correcting, clarifying statements such as "Did you mean that *you* would like to go to the music room?" Differences between the nurse and the client should be pointed out whenever appropriate.

Nursing diagnosis: Delusional* thinking related to escalating anxiety, threats to the self-system, and fears of interpersonal relating (behavior associated with DSM-III diagnoses 295.1x through 295.6x, schizophrenic disorders; 297.10, 297.30, 298.30, 297.90, paranoid disorders; and 295.40, 298.80, 295.70, 298.90, psychotic disorders not elsewhere classified)

Planning: With assistance and guidance from the nurse, the client will establish goals.

1. Long-term goals†
   a. Work through some of the conflicts that are generating the underlying anxiety.
   b. Work through some of the fears of relating to other people.
   c. Increase the ability to cope with stress without the tendency to severely distort, misperceive, misinterpret, and exaggerate.

2. Short-term goals
   a. Recognize the relationship between escalating anxiety and the increased tendency to severely distort, misperceive, misinterpret, and exaggerate.
   b. Identify any difficulties in interpersonal relating and in functioning in the world that are related to the tendency to severely distort, misperceive, misinterpret, and exaggerate.
   c. Verbalize and explore feelings about current stressful situations in life.
   d. Increase self-esteem in a realistic manner (see Chapter 18).
   e. Realistically perceive the five dimensions of self (biological, psychological, intellectual, sociocultural, and spiritual strengths and weaknesses in perspective).*

Implementation: More extreme feelings of unreality that are based in loose ego boundaries include delusions and hallucinations. In responding to these experiences of the client, the nurse can act as a bridge to reality.

Delusions are ideas that are contrary to culturally accepted facts. Delusions can be persecutory, grandiose, of control or of influence, somatic, or religious. There is a kernel of truth somewhere in a delusion, although, if it is a long-standing delusion that has been embellished through the years into a complex delusional system, it may be difficult to find. A delusion may be difficult to dispel. If a delusion is just beginning to form and is still rather fluid, it may be possible to intervene in order to prevent its adoption by the client. In the case of a rigid delusional system, however, some researchers suggest that the best way to work with it is to help the client see the importance of not verbalizing the delusional beliefs so that he or she can function acceptably in society.

The difference between these two approaches to the treatment of delusional beliefs can be illustrated by a comparison of the cases of clients with

---

*Because of the inevitable denegrating connotations that the term delusional can elicit, it is not a helpful term to use with a client in planning care (an exception might be a client, recovering emotional health, who has accepted that he or she *has* been delusional and refers to the experience in direct terms. Less threatening terminology for most clients would be *distortions, misperceptions, misinterpretations, exaggerations.*

†For a client who has been delusional for many years, these long-term goals may never be achieved (see implementation section for different approaches to delusional clients based on this point).

---

*May be a long-term goal in the case of many clients.

whom a student nurse worked. One client was an elderly woman who had had numerous admissions to the hospital. She usually remained in the hospital for 3 to 4 months and then was able to function quite adequately in the community for several months. Her delusion was complex and quite fixed. Among other things, she believed that pigeons carried secret messages about her to the Nazis and that they, in collaboration with a Puerto Rican political group, carried out experiments on human beings in the apartment beneath her—no matter where she lived. When she was less anxious and ready for discharge, she was able to keep quiet about these beliefs. But they never really left her, and she would start to talk about them more as her anxiety began to increase.

In contrast to this woman, the other client the student was involved with had experienced her first psychotic break and was exhibiting obsessive-compulsive behavior and indications of low self-esteem. She washed her hands constantly after touching anyone or anything in her unit, and she dusted off any chair she intended to sit on. One day she greeted the student in an excited, worried state: "Don't touch me! I have all of these worms growing inside of me and you might catch them!"

By spending time with her and asking for details and clarification, the student learned the basis for this belief. The client had been eating almost constantly (probably because of a combination of anxiety and the appetite-increasing effects of thorazine), and an aide in the unit had jokingly said, "You must have a tapeworm, you eat so much!" Interpreting this remark concretely and in the light of her low self-esteem, she began to believe that she had worms growing inside of her. The student was able to explain what the aide really meant, and the client was able to accept the explanation.

In responding to a delusion that is already formed, a logical, rational confrontation is usually not helpful. In fact, in the cases of some clients it may stimulate a defensive argument. Usually it is best to respond to what is at the "core" of the delusion and to the feelings associated with it (Donner, 1969). For instance, at the core of a delusion of grandeur one might expect to find feelings of low self-esteem and powerlessness. Most likely at the core of a persecutory delusion are projected feelings of hostility toward other people. The following are some points to consider in responding to the client who is experiencing delusions:

1. Collect data before formulating a response; in the beginning, noncommittal responses may be necessary. In some situations you may only suspect that a client is making a delusional statement. It is easy to make a judgment when the client says she is the Virgin Mary and that she is being controlled from the planet Mars, but a client who tells you she has 16 children may be telling you the truth. Then again, she may not be, since this is a fairly common sort of delusion. Give the client the benefit of the doubt until you know whether he or she is suffering from a delusion, but remain fairly noncommital in your responses.

2. In responding to the client's delusion, convey your acceptance of a need for the belief while letting the client know you do not agree with the delusion.

3. Do not argue with the client about the belief—incorporating *reasonable doubt* as a communication technique is more effective.

4. If possible, connect the belief to the client's feelings (for example, "It's possible to misinterpret things when anxiety is very high" or "Things can seem like they're out of control when you're frightened").

5. Respond to the core of the delusion. If low self-esteem is at the core, try to help the client build self-esteem in a realistic way. An individual who thinks that there is a complex and well-controlled plot against him or her may need to express anger appropriately in everyday situations.

Nursing diagnosis: Severe distortions in sensory perceptions (hallucinations) related to escalating anxiety and threats to the self-system (behavior associated with DSM-III diagnoses 295.1x through 295.6x, schizophrenic disorders; and 295.40,

298.80, 295.70, 298.90, psychotic disorders not elsewhere classified)

Planning: With assistance and guidance from the nurse, the client will establish goals.

1. Long-term goals*
   a. Work through some of the conflicts that are generating the underlying anxiety.
   b. Increase the ability to cope with stress without the reliance on hallucinations.
2. Short-term goals†
   a. Verbalize the *content* of any hallucinations (important especially in the case of *command hallucinations*).
   b. Identify the times and situations when the tendency to hallucinate increases.
   c. Recognize the relationship between escalating anxiety and an increased tendency to hallucinate.
   d. Identify any difficulties in interpersonal relating and in functioning in the world that are related to the reliance on hallucinating as a defense.
   e. Verbalize and explore feelings about current stressful situations in life.
   f. Increase self-esteem in a reality-based context (see Chapter 18).
   g. Realistically perceive the five dimensions of self (biological, psychological, intellectual, sociocultural, and spiritual strengths and weaknesses in perspective).

Implementation: Hallucinations are false sensory perceptions. They can be auditory, visual, tactile, olfactory, gustatory, or kinesthetic. The majority of schizophrenic hallucinations are auditory. In fact, the occurrence of auditory hallucinations is correlated so strongly with schizophrenia that some suggest that it be considered a fifth "A" to be tacked on to Bleuler's original "four A's". (Hofling et al., 1967).

Hallucinations are seen in conditions other than schizophrenia such as those associated with very high fevers and toxic conditions. The nursing intervention is the same.

Approaches to hallucinations depend upon the need that the hallucinations are serving and upon the length of time the client has been experiencing them. If a client has been hearing voices for a short time, it is important to know *what* the voices say, since they could be *command hallucinations* (commands to commit suicide or homicide, for example). It is helpful to know if the hallucinations are frightening, degrading, or kind and helpful to the client. The therapeutic response in each situation would be different.

In the case of a person who has hallucinated over a long period of time, a nurse might not be as concerned with content as with *when* the client tends to hallucinate. This information is useful if the nurse intends to distract the client back to reality or to attempt to decrease anxiety and thus the need for hallucinations. Also, continually focusing on content that is already well known might reinforce the hallucinations.

In general, the following points are helpful in the treatment of the hallucinating client:

1. An accepting approach will encourage the client to share the content and the times of hallucination. It is important to accept the client and the need for the hallucinations and to accept the fact that while you do not share these perceptions, the client does indeed experience them.
2. Determine the content of the hallucinations in order to prevent possible injury to client or to others from command hallucinations.
3. When discussing hallucinations, phrase your comments in such a way as to avoid reinforcing the hallucinations. For example, "What do the voices *seem* to be saying when you get anxious?" rather than "What are the voices telling you to do?"
4. Respond to and reinforce the aspects of reality that the client reacts to. Connect the hallucinations to anxiety as an explanation that might prevent the escalating sequence of in-

---

*For a client who has relied on (comforting) hallucinations for years, these long-term goals may never be achieved.

†Depending upon the degree of regression in the client, short-term goals may be intermediate or even long-term goals.

creased anxiety, increased hallucination, increased anxiety.

5. Be alert for times of hallucinating. Arieti (1975) has identified a ''listening pose'' that a schizophrenic who is hallucinating may assume.

6. Distract the client at times of hallucinating. Bring the client back to reality through interpersonal involvement and activities.

7. In cases of clients who have hallucinated chronically, instructions to ''talk back'' to voices, telling them to ''shut up,'' have sometimes helped, since they can give the client a feeling of control over these symptoms and thus decrease anxiety. This technique *must* be used with a clear message that the voices are not awesome realities but symptoms of anxiety.

Schizophrenia is often accompanied by *anhedonia,* the inability to experience pleasure. The schizophrenic is quite apt to be depressed. The symptoms of the disorder, its incapacitating effects, the inhibition of personal growth, and the drain on financial resources are some of the reasons for depression. As in any chronic illness, depression is part of the process of the individual's acceptance of the disorder. In addition, low self-esteem is the common denominator of *all* emotional illnesses.

The therapeutic response to depression in the schizophrenic is the same as that for any depressed client (see Chapter 18). Realistic emotional support, activity, and gradually increasing interpersonal involvement are all helpful. Since depression can produce symptoms of psychomotor retardation, nurses must allow clients enough time to react to questions or statements and to verbalize. Like any depressed person, a depressed schizophrenic may attempt suicide. But factors other than depression may also lead to suicide attempts. Suicide attempts by schizophrenic persons are sometimes bizarre and are often quite unpredictable. A suicide attempt may occur in response to a hallucinated voice, or it may be a response to a delusional system. Since a break with reality af-

fects an individual's judgment, the impossible—for example, ''flying'' out of a window of a tall building—may seem possible. A suicide attempt might be precipitated by loose ego boundaries. For example, a young, very psychotic man reacted to the successful and just-completed suicide of his roommate by jumping out of a window after him. He was badly injured, but he lived. His explanation of why he jumped was that the crumpled body lying on the ground was really *him* and that he was jumping to put himself back together again.

Since the suicides of schizophrenic persons are so unpredictable, with few if any ''clues'' being given, it is particularly important for nurses to be vigilant. A vague, subjective uneasiness about the possibility of the client committing suicide may be an important clue and should not be dismissed lightly.

EVALUATION

The client, and, whenever feasible, the client's family or significant others should be included in estimating the client's progress toward attainment of goals. Evaluation should encompass the following areas:

1. Estimation of the degree to which there has been effective coping with any disorders of thought, mood, feeling, sensation, perception, and behavior. This would include *awareness* of tendency to use withdrawal from interpersonal relationships and from reality and beginning efforts toward modifying this.

2. Estimation of the degree to which goals have been achieved and client functioning has improved (demonstrated by decreased disorder in interpersonal relationships; increased ability to function in society; decreased reliance on withdrawal mechanisms, and increased self-esteem and increased interpersonal and social involvement)

3. Identification of goals that need to be modified or revised

4. Referral of the client to support systems other than the nurse-client relationship

a. People in the client's social network who are willing to serve as a support system
b. Clinics or individuals for ongoing individual, supportive psychotherapy
c. Community agencies that help clients learn to live with disorders that may never be completely eliminated (e.g., Recovery, Inc.; Schizophrenics Anonymous)
d. Centers or organizations that focus on rehabilitation for the schizophrenic client and on specialized treatment of specific problem areas (e.g., vocational counseling, family therapy, family support groups, day hospitals, medication administration and supervision)

TERTIARY PREVENTION

While an individual may experience one schizophrenic break, recover, and perhaps never have another, schizophrenia is most often a chronic disorder.

According to Mendel and Green (1967), two elements that are most needed in the lives of chronic schizophrenics and that can be fostered through supportive relationship therapy are *organization* and *structure*. A chronic schizophrenic's whole life is unstructured and disorganized; the ordinary activities of daily living seem overwhelming. The goals of relationship therapy are to foster remission, to prevent complications, and to support the functioning of the schizophrenic client. Mendel and Green transform the "as if" phenomenon, a symptom that appears in the preschizophrenic state, into a concept that can be used as a therapeutic aid for the chronic schizophrenic. They suggest that a therapist say to a client, "OK, so you *don't* feel like you have the ability to get up, get dressed, and go to work every morning—act *as if* you can." After the client has done so for a number of mornings, ego strength will be gained from having accomplished something that seemed overwhelming.

Mendel and Green also advocate long-term involvement between a helping professional and the chronic schizophrenic. In some cases the amount of this involvement may be decreased, during times of low anxiety and adequate functioning, to a monthly or even yearly "check in" with the therapist. Of course, at times of developmental or situational crises, involvement would be increased again.

The schizophrenic, the community, and tertiary prevention

What was probably one of the most ideal communities for discharged schizophrenics ever to be devised existed at one time in the village of Gheel, Belgium. This town is situated near a shrine to St. Dymphna, the patron saint of the mentally ill, and a psychiatric hospital dedicated to her. During the Middle Ages and later, people from all over the world came to the shrine and hospital, hoping for saintly intervention in their illness. After treatment at the hospital they were often discharged into the town. Some lived in the village while they awaited admission to the hospital. The villagers were quite accepting of them; eccentric behavior was tolerated, and individuals were allowed to participate in the community to the degree that they were able.

Unfortunately, in the United States today there are few such friendly and accepting communities. An exception is *Fountain House* (Rehab Brief, 1982), a "club for former mental patients." Fountain House was started in the early 1940s by a small group of former "patients" from a New York State psychiatric hospital. Their goal was to achieve successful deinstitutionalization* through cooperative efforts. The club has grown tremendously and the Fountain House concept has provided a model for other, similar efforts. For example, Plymouth House (on the grounds of Pilgrim State Hospital in Brentwood, New York) used the

---

For in-depth discussion of deinstitutionalization, see Chapter 14.

Fountain House model and offers its services not only to discharged clients but to those still hospitalized who choose to take advantage of them.

There are four primary beliefs in the Fountain House concept:

1. People with emotional disabilities, even severe ones, have productive potential.
2. Work is important for all people.
3. Everyone needs social relationships.
4. All people need adequate housing.

The staff of Fountain House continually conveys four basic messages to the members:

1. Fountain House is a club and its participants are members, not clients.
2. Members are made to feel that their participation is expected, and that staff anticipate their arrival with pleasure.
3. Members are wanted as contributors to the club.
4. Members are needed by the club, staff, and other members.

Various community and professional and volunteer services are also provided. While more research needs to be done into the effectiveness of the Fountain House model, it does hold out some hope for successful adjustment to the community and for improvement in living for some schizophrenic clients.

However, a discharged schizophrenic too often faces a harsh, intolerant, and unwelcoming community situation. *After-care* of mental illness has not been a major priority in our country; it can only be described as inadequate. We have the knowledge of what is required to provide optimum after-care services for chronic schizophrenics, but most often only lip service is paid to the ideals. Services that are available to a limited degree include the following:

1. *Transitional services*—a concept that includes a gradual lessening of the client's dependent ties with the hospital. Clients are given lessons and help in tasks of everyday living. Particularly in the case of a client who has been institutionalized for a long time, many skills may not have been learned or they may have been long since forgotten. Helping a client to arrange for suitable living accommodations is another transitional service.

2. *Day care centers*—for the client who has a supportive, accepting home environment but who cannot yet function in a job. This service provides structure to the day, opportunities for socialization, and a chance to learn some skills. In addition, medication may be supervised in such a center.

3. *Night hospitals*—for the client who can function in a job but has no suitable living arrangements. Perhaps, as is so often the case with the chronic schizophrenic, there are no family ties. The client may also benefit from supportive therapy within the night hospital. For instance, group therapy sessions may be held in the evening as part of the hospital's program.

4. *Halfway houses and foster homes*—for the client who does not have a family or whose family can no longer support him or her. Such a client needs some supervision in such areas as diet, medication, recreation, and activities of daily living. Some foster homes in a community may be excellent; others may be deplorable. A system of inspection before placement is therefore crucial to the protection of the client's welfare.

5. *Rehabilitation, vocational training, and sheltered workshops*—retraining in old skills and training in new skills in order to help the client function to the maximum of potential and strengthen self-esteem.

6. *Token economy programs*—for severely regressed schizophrenics. These programs, which have been used in some psychiatric inpatient and outpatient facilities, involve a form of behavior modification. Tokens that can be exchanged for goods (cigarettes, food, or clothing) or privileges are given in return for participation in certain activities. For example, a token may be given for making one's bed in the morning or for attending

group therapy sessions. Such a program can be useful if it is carried out in a way that protects the dignity of the client. Unhappily, this is not always the case.

Working with family and client

An important aspect of the tertiary care of schizophrenics is the supervision of medications. Failure to take prescribed drugs is one of the most common reasons for readmission to hospitals (Van Putten, 1974). A drug like prolixin, which can be given in two-week intervals, is very often useful. But the most important aspect of tertiary care is the continuing and regular involvement of the community mental health nurse with the client's family. Some hospitals provide ''crisis teams'' of hospital personnel—people the client has known while in the hospital.

Three important guidelines for a community mental health team to provide and monitor services such as medication supervision and psychosocial intervention are:

1. Services should extend over decade-length periods, since schizophrenia is so often a lifelong disturbance.
2. Since the clinical course of schizophrenia tends to be episodic, services should include a crisis-oriented component.
3. Services may be provided over decades, yet they need to be provided *precisely* enough to fit a widely fluctuating severity in the condition. This implies that the client must be enabled to take a role in regulating the medication (self-regulation through education) (Hansell, 1978).

Education of families is often as important as education of clients. A study at the University of Southern California School of Medicine reported that when families are taught to talk out their problems and to use the problem-solving method, identified clients are more likely to remain free of schizophrenic symptoms (Newsday, 1982).

Home visits at times of increased anxiety for the client may prevent rehospitalization. It is essential that a nurse engage the family of the chronic schizophrenic, along with the client, as part of the treatment team. It is especially important to avoid arousing any feelings of guilt in family members, since such feelings can lead to a withdrawal from involvement with helping professionals and perhaps to a withdrawal from the client. Family members can be helpful in alerting professionals to increasing anxiety in the client, and they can assist in the supervision of medications. In addition, they can help modify environmental stress in the client's life and facilitate the client's necessary acceptance of his or her illness.

CHAPTER SUMMARY

Schizophrenia is a disorder of thought, mood, feeling, sensation, perception, and behavior. It is characterized by a disturbed ego, no clear concept of self, and inadequate ways of communicating with and relating to other people. Schizophrenia is a major health problem. It affects 0.5% to 2% of the population of the United States, and there is some evidence that the incidence is increasing (Kramer, 1978).

Schizophrenia was originally called ''dementia praecox'' (dementia of the young); its incidence seems to be highest among young adults, but it can occur at any age. ''Schizophrenia,'' the term invented by Bleuler, means ''split mind''; it refers to a splitting apart of some of the functions of the mind. For instance, thoughts and feelings that normally go together may be split apart.

The disorder occurs in all cultures and all socio-economic groups, but for complex reasons it is strongly correlated with poverty.

Several systems for classifying schizophrenia are in existence. Some writers believe that schizophrenia is actually several disorders and therefore refer to ''the schizophrenias.''

The etiology of schizophrenia is unknown, but several theories have been postulated. These include genetic, biochemical, intrapsychic, interpersonal, family, communication systems, sociological, and adaptation theories. An eclectic or multifactorial approach to the etiology of schizophrenia is most widely accepted.

Treatment for schizophrenia includes somatic approaches (particularly the use of drugs), psychotherapy, group and family therapy, and occupational and recreational therapy. Primary prevention at this time is limited mainly to the identification of high-risk groups. Secondary prevention currently focuses on the belief that much of the deterioration in the condition of a schizophrenic may result from institutionalization rather than from the disorder itself. A more active treatment approach has provided a much better prognosis for recovery. However, schizophrenia is often a chronic disorder. Tertiary prevention of schizophrenia involves a cooperative, rehabilitative effort from health workers, client, and family. Providing support and helping to add structure and organization to the client's life are very important.

In working with a schizophrenic client, a nurse helps most by assisting in the improvement of *communication skills* and *interpersonal skills.* *Therapeutic use of self* in an authentic relationship with the client is the most important component of nursing intervention.

SENSITIVITY-AWARENESS EXERCISES

The purposes of the following exercises are to:

- Develop awareness about subjective experience of clients who are suffering from schizophrenic disorders
- Develop awareness about the subjective experience of the families of clients who are suffering from schizophrenic disorders
- Develop awareness about your own feelings and attitudes when working with clients who are suffering from schizophrenic disorders
- Develop awareness about the interrelationship of factors in the etiology of schizophrenia

1. Try to imagine what it is like to experience one of the following symptoms:
   Auditory hallucinations
   Delusional thinking
   Depersonalization
   Loose ego boundaries
   Tardive dyskinesia
   Mutism
   Explain why you selected that particular symptom. Then describe what it would be like to experience it.
2. Describe what you think it would be like to have a family member who is suffering from chronic schizophrenia. How do you think you might cope with this? Which schizophrenic symptom do you think it would be most difficult for you to accept in a family member?
3. Imagine that you are a community mental health nurse engaged in health supervision activities with new parents. What high risk factors would you observe for that might predispose children to developing a schizophrenic disorder?
4. Develop a plan for teaching and counselling parents about parent-child interaction that incorporates principles and goals for the primary prevention of schizophrenia.

REFERENCES

Altschule, M.
   1970 In The Schizophrenic Reactions: A Critique of the Concept, Hospital Treatment and Current Research. R. Cancro (ed.). New York: Brunner/Mazel, Inc.
Arieti, S.
   1955 Interpretation of Schizophrenia (ed. 1). New York: Basic Books.
   1967 The Intrapsychic Self. New York: Basic Books.
   1975 Interpretation of Schizophrenia (ed. 2). New York: Basic Books.
Arnold, H.
   1976 "Working with schizophrenic patients, four A's: A guide to one-to-one relationships." American Journal of Nursing 6:941-943.
   1983 "Is schizophrenia preventable? A psychoanalytic view." A paper presented at the Annual Nurse Scholar Series, First Endowed Hildegard E. Peplau Lecture, Rutgers College Alumni Association, April 15, 1983.

Bahnson, C.B.
1969 "Psychophysiological complementarity in malignancies: Past work and future vistas." Annals of the New York Academy of Sciences 125(3):827-845.
1974 "Epistemological perspectives of physical disease from the psychodynamic point of view." American Journal of Public Health 64(11):1036.

Bahnson, C.B., and M.B. Bahnson
1964 "Cancer as an alternative to psychosis: A theoretical model of somatic and psychological regression." In Psychosomatic Aspects of Neoplastic Disease. D.M. Kissen and L.L. LeShan (eds.). Philadelphia: J.B. Lippincott Co.

Bellak, L.
1958 "The schizophrenic syndrome: A further explanation of the unified theory of schizophrenia." In Schizophrenia: A Review of the Syndrome. L. Bellak (ed.). New York: Logos Press.

Bowen, M.
1976 "Theory in the practice of psychotherapy." In Family Therapy. P.J. Guerin (ed.). New York: Gardner Press, Inc.
1977 Workshop in Family Therapy, Mercy Hospital, Rockville Center, N.Y.

Boyers, R., and R. Orrill (eds.)
1971 R.D. Laing and Anti-Psychiatry. New York: Harper & Row, Publishers.

Burnham, D.L., A.I. Gladstone, and R.W. Gibson
1969 Schizophrenia and the Need-Fear Dilemma. New York: International Universities Press.

Cameron, N.
1963 Personality Development and Psychopathology: A Dynamic Approach. Boston: Houghton Mifflin Co.

Campion, E., and G. Tucker
1973 "A note on twin studies, schizophrenia and neurological impairment. In Annual Review of the Schizophrenic Syndrome. R. Cancro (ed.). New York: Brunner/Mazel, Inc.

Cancro, R. (ed.)
1970 The Schizophrenic Reactions: A critique of the Concept, Hospital Treatment and Current Research. New York: Brunner/Mazel, Inc.

Carpenter, E.
1953 "Witch-fear among the Aivilik Eskimos." The American Journal of Psychiatry 110(3):194-199.

Donner, G.
1969 "Treatment of a delusional patient." American Journal of Nursing 12:2642-2644.

Edelstein, P., et al.
1981 "Physostigmine and lithium response in the schizophrenias." American Journal of Psychiatry 138:1078.

Eisenberg, L.
1973 "Psychiatric intervention." Scientific American 229(3):117-127.

Epstein, S., and M. Coleman
1971 "Drive theories in schizophrenia." In the Schizophrenic Syndrome: An Annual Review. R. Cancro (ed.). New York: Brunner/Mazel, Inc.

Field, T.
1982 "Interaction coaching for high-risk infants and their parents." In Prevention in Human Services, I (4). New York: The Haworth Press, pp. 5-24.

Field, W.E., and S. Wilkerson
1973 "Religiosity as a psychiatric symptom." Perspectives in Psychiatric Care 11(3):99-105.

Foulks, E.F.
1975 "Schizophrenia held useful for evolution." New York Times, December 9.

Frankl, V.
1959 Man's Search for Meaning: An Introduction to Logotherapy. New York: Washington Square Press.

Fromm-Reichman, F.
1950 Principles of Intensive Psychotherapy. Chicago: University of Chicago Press.

Garmezy, N.
1971 "Vulnerability research and the issue of primary prevention." American Journal of Orthopsychiatry 41: 101-116.

Gibney, H.
1972 "Masturbation: an invitation for an interpersonal relationship. Perspectives in Psychiatric Care 10(3): 128-134.

Goldfarb, C., and S. Goldfarb
1977 "Multiple monitored electroconvulsive treatment." In Current Psychiatric Therapies, vol. 17. J.H. Masserman (ed.). New York: Grune & Stratton, Inc.

Greenberg, J.
1983 "Fetal brain damage linked to schizophrenia." Science News 124(11):164.

Grinker, R., Sr.
1969 "An essay on schizophrenia and science." Archives of General Psychiatry 20:1-24.

Hansell, N.
1978 "Services for schizophrenics: A lifelong approach to treatment." Hospital and Community Psychiatry 29(2): 105-109.

Hartmann, E.
1982 "Toward a biology of the mind." In The Psychoanalytic Study of the Child, 37. New York: International Universities Press.

Hartmann, H.
1964 "Contributions to the metapsychology of schizophrenia." In Essays on Ego Psychology by Heinz Hartmann. New York: International Universities Press.

Hays, D.R.
1963 "Anger: A clinical problem." In Some Clinical Approaches to Psychiatric Nursing. S. Burd and M. Marshall (eds.). New York: Macmillan, Inc.

Hays, J.S., and K.H. Larson
1963 Interacting with Patients. New York: Macmillan, Inc.

Heath, R., et al.
1958 "Behavioral changes in nonpsychotic volunteers following the administration of tarexein, the substance obtained from the serum of schizophrenic patients." American Journal of Psychiatry 114:917-920.

Henley, A.
1971 "Schizophrenia: Current approaches to a baffling problem. Public Affairs Pamphlet No. 460. New York: Public Affairs Committee, Inc.

Herbert, W.
1983a "Schizophrenia clues in angel dust." Science News 123(26):407.
1983b "Mental illness from psychiatric drugs?" Science News 124(14):214.

Hofling, C.K., M.M. Leininger, and E. Bregg
1967 Basic Psychiatric Concepts in Nursing (ed. 2). Philadelphia: J.B. Lippincott Co.

Holmes, M.J.
1971 "Influences of the new hospital psychiatry on nursing." In The New Hospital Psychiatry. New York: Academic Press, Inc.

Holzman, P., et al.
1974 "Eye-tracking dysfunctions in schizophrenic patients and their relatives." In Annual Review of the Schizophrenic Syndrome. R. Cancro (ed.). New York: Brunner/Mazel, Inc.

Howells, J.G.
1975 World History of Psychiatry. New York: Brunner/Mazel, Inc.

Jackson, D.
1960 The Etiology of Schizophrenia. New York: Basic Books, Inc., Publishers.

Kallman, F.J.
1938 The Genetics of Schizophrenia. New York: Augustin.

Kasanin, J.S. (ed.)
1944 Language and Thought in Schizophrenia. New York: W.W. Norton & Co. Inc.

Kety, S.
1978 "Heredity and environment." In Schizophrenia: Science and Practice. J.C. Shershow (ed.) Cambridge, Mass.: Harvard University Press.

Kramer, M.
1978 "Population changes in schizophrenia, 1970-1985." In The Nature of Schizophrenia: New Approaches to Research and Treatment. L.C. Wynne, et al. (eds.). New York: John Wiley & Sons, Inc.

Laing, R.D.
1960 The Divided Self. Chicago: Quadrangle Books.
1965 "Mystification, confusion and conflict." In Intensive Family Therapy: Theoretical and Practical Aspects. I. Boszormenyi-Nagy and J.L. Framo (eds.). New York: Harper & Row.

Lidz, T.
1973 The Origin and Treatment of Schizophrenic Disorders. New York: Basic Books.

Mahler, M., F. Pine, and A. Bergman
1975 The Psychological Birth of the Human Infant. New York: Basic Books, Inc.

Maugh, T.
1981 "Biochemical markers identify mental states." Science 214(2):39-41.

May, R.
1958 "The origins and significance of the existential movement in psychology." In Existence: A New Dimension in Psychiatry and Psychology. R. May, et al. (eds.). New York: Simon & Schuster, Inc.

Mellow, J.
1968 "Nursing therapy." American Journal of Nursing 68(11):2365-2369.

Mendel, W.
1976 Schizophrenia: The Experience and Its Treatment. San Francisco: Jossey-Bass.

Mendel, W.M., and G.A. Green
1967 The Therapeutic Management of Psychological Illness: The Theory and Practice of Supportive Care. New York: Basic Books.

Menninger, K.
1963 The Vital Balance. New York: The Viking Press, Inc.

Newsday
1982 "Health watch: Handling schizophrenics at home." Newsday (June 21, 1982) Part II:7.

Oden, G.
1963 "There are no mute patients." In Some Clinical Approaches to Psychiatric Problems. S. Burd and M. Marshall (eds.). New York: Macmillan, Inc.

Pao, P.
1979 Schizophrenic Disorders: Theory and Treatment from a Psychodynamic Point of View. New York: International Universities Press.

Peplau, H.
1983 "Some dimensions in the concept of prevention." A paper presented at the Annual Nurse Scholar Series, First Endowed Hildegard E. Peplau Lecture, Rutgers College Alumni Association, April 15, 1983.

Pfeiffer, C.
1975 Mental and Elemental Nutrients: A Physician's Guide to Nutrition and Health Care. New Canaan, Conn.: Keats Publishing, Inc.

Pittman, F.S., and K. Flomenhaft
1970 "Treating the doll's house marriage." Family Process 9(2):143-155.

Potkin, S.G., et al
1978 "Are paranoid schizophrenics biologically different from other schizophrenics?" New England Journal of Medicine 298(2):61-66.

Redlich, F.C., and D.X. Freedman
    1966 The Theory and Practice of Psychiatry. New York: Basic Books, pp. 480-481, 512-513.
Rehab Brief
    1982 "Fountain House: a club for former mental patients." Rehab Brief 5(2). National Institute of Handicapped Research. Washington, D.C.: Office of Special Education and Rehabilitation Services Department of Education.
Roman, P., and H.M. Trice
    1967 Schizophrenia and the Poor. Ithaca, N.Y.: Cayuga Press.
Rosen, J.
    1953 Direct Analysis: Selected Papers. New York: Grune & Stratton, Inc.
Rowe, C.J.
    1975 An Outline of Psychiatry (ed. 6). Dubuque, Iowa: William C. Brown Co., Publishers, p. 246.
Ruesch, J.
    1957 Disturbed Communication: The Clinical Assessment of Normal and Pathological Communicative Behavior. New York: W.W. Norton & Co., Inc.
Sarbin, T.
    1972 "Schizophrenia is a myth, born of metaphor, meaningless." Psychology Today 6(June):20-27.
Schwing, G.
    1954 A Way to the Soul of the Mentally Ill. New York: International Universities Press.
Searles, H.F.
    1965 Collected Papers on Schizophrenia and Related Subjects. New York: International Universities Press.
Sechehaye, M.A.
    1956 A New Psychotherapy in Schizophrenia. New York: Grune & Stratton, Inc.
Seifer, R., and A. Sameroff
    1982 "A structural equation model analysis of competence in children at risk for mental disorder." In Prevention in Human Services, I(4). New York: The Haworth Press, pp. 85-96.
Serban, G.
    1975 "Stress in schizophrenics and normals." British Journal of Psychiatry 126:397-407.
Singh, M., and S. Kay
    1976 "Wheat gluten as a pathogenic factor in schizophrenia." Science 191:401-402.
Slater, E.
    1953 Psychotic and Neurotic Illnesses in Twins, London: Her Majesty's Stationery Office.
Spitz, R.
    1965 "Innate inhibition of aggressiveness in infancy." In The Psychoanalytic Study of the Child, 20. New York: International Universities Press, Inc.

Stein, L., and C.D. Wise
    1971 "Possible etiology of schizophrenia: Progressive damage to the noradrenergic reward system by 6-hydroxydopamine. Science 171:1032-1036.
Stroebel, C.F.
    1969 "Biological rhythm correlates of disturbed behavior in the rhesus monkey." In Circadian Rhythms in Nonhuman Primates. F.H. Rohles (ed.). New York: S Karger.
Sullivan, H.
    1953 The Interpersonal Theory of Psychiatry. New York: W.W. Norton & Co., Inc.
Szasz, T.S.
    1961 The Myth of Mental Illness. New York: Dell Publishing Co., Inc.
Taft, L.T., and W. Goldfarb
    1964 "Prenatal and perinatal factors in childhood schizophrenia. Developmental Medicine and Child Neurology 6:32-34.
Trotter, R.J.
    1977 "Schizophrenia: A cruel chain of events." Science News #2 (June 18, 1977), p. 394.
Van Putten, T.
    1974 "Why do schizophrenic patients refuse to take their drugs?" Archives of General Psychiatry 31:67-72.
Von Domarus, E.
    1944 "The specific laws of logic in schizophrenia." In Language and Thought in Schizophrenia, Collected Papers. J.S. Kasanin (ed.). Los Angeles: University of California Press.
Winnicott, D.
    1965 The Maturational Processes and the Facilitating Environment. New York: International Universities Press, Inc.
Wynne, L.C., et al
    1978 The Nature of Schizophrenia: New Approaches to Research and Treatment. New York: John Wiley & Sons, Inc.

ANNOTATED SUGGESTED READINGS

Kasanin, J. (ed.)
    1944 Language and Thought in Schizophrenia. New York: W.W. Norton & Co., Inc.
    A compilation of the works of several well known authors, this classic book describes and analyzes various aspects of the thought and communication processes in schizophrenia. For example, the schizophrenic's tendency to use paralogical thinking is examined.
Koontz, E.
    "Schizophrenia: Current diagnostic concepts and implications for nursing care." Journal of Psychiatric Nursing and Mental Health Services 20(9):44-48.

The focus of this article is schizophrenic disorders and their classification in DSM-III (Diagnostic and Statistical Manual of Mental Disorders, third edition). There is some comparison of DSM-III with the earlier edition (DSM-II). This is a clear and concise introduction to the manual as it applies to schizophrenia.

Lidz, T.
1973 The Origin and Treatment of Schizophrenic Disorders: New York: Basic Books.
This book presents a unified theory of schizophrenia that views disorders in the family system as the primary causative factor. Family settings (schismatic or skewed) are described, the thought disorder is examined, and appropriate family treatment is discussed.

Mendel, W.
1976 Schizophrenia: The Experience and Its Treatment. San Francisco: Jossey-Bass Publishers.
The most prominent etiological theories are reviewed, including the genetic, the physical, and various psychological theories. Mendel's own comprehensive theory is described as well as his suggested method of treatment for the schizophrenic client.

Mendel, W., and G. Green
1967 The Therapeutic Management of Psychological Illness: The Theory and Practice of Supportive Care. New York: Basic Books.
Mendel and Green describe helpful long-term treatment methods for the chronic schizophrenic client. Emphasis is placed on helping the client remain in the community through supportive relationship therapy.

Reed, L.
1979 "Approaches to the aftermath of schizophrenia." Perspectives in Psychiatric Care 17(6):257-259, 282.
The author believes that the schizophrenic client can assume an active role and responsibility for control of the disorder. Confronting troublesome issues and making reasonable plans are ways to enable the client to reach a more satisfying level of functioning in life. The need to separate the disorder with its symptoms from the client's reactions to it is emphasized. Some clinical examples are presented.

Schroder, P.
1979 "Nursing intervention with patients with thought disorder." Perspectives in Psychiatric Care 17(1):32-39.
This well written article points to the need for nurses to be aware of the differences in thought processes that schizophrenic clients may experience. This includes a different type of logic, autistic associations, the use of denotative rather than connotative meanings for words, and, in general, more concrete thinking. Helpful ways of intervening are included, as well as clinical examples to illustrate.

Snyder, S.
1974 Madness and the Brain. New York: McGraw-Hill Book Co.
This book traces the breakthroughs in research into brain function and the effects of various chemicals on the brain. Snyder attempts to shed some light on the mystery of schizophrenia by explaining how schizophrenic symptoms and the effects of psychotropic and psychotomimetic drugs are related.

FURTHER READINGS

Moser, D.H.
1970 "Communicating with a schizophrenic patient." Perspectives in Psychiatric Care 8(1):36-45.

Shershow, J.C. (ed.)
1978 Schizophrenia: Science and Practice. Cambridge, Mass.: Harvard University Press.

CHAPTER 22

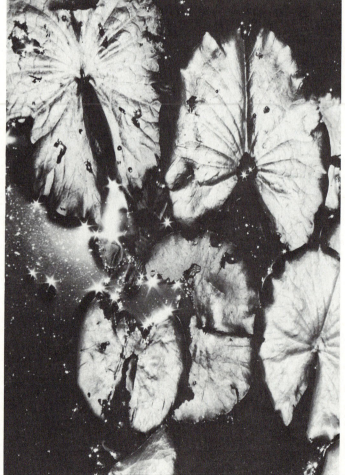

Photo by Horst Schafer—Peter Arnold, Inc.

Coping with impaired brain function

CHAPTER FOCUS

Mental disorders have historically been attributed to a variety of natural and supernatural forces. In our own era, many people, including prominent research scientists, have come to believe that most, if not all, psychiatric disturbances are the result of altered physiological processes within the central nervous system. Such a belief has even been attributed to Freud, the father of dynamic psychiatry.

The neuropsychiatric conditions to be discussed in this chapter—the organic brain dysfunctions—have long been known to have their etiology in disturbances in central nervous system functioning. Research in neurophysiology during the last quarter-century has led to increased knowledge of neuronal functioning and to a better understanding of the complex metabolic processes of the central nervous system. This advancement in knowledge has made possible the improvement in treatment for many conditions, including organic brain dysfunctions, although treatment of organic conditions has not always kept pace with the expanding knowledge. Wells (1978) points out that in the early stages of organic brain dysfunction, when treatment could be most effective, the proper diagnosis often is not made.

Organic brain dysfunction, in either the acute form or the chronic form, may occur at any point in the life cycle, although it is more common in the later years of life. The organic brain disorders are believed to be among the most prevalent of psychiatric disorders. There is some evidence that the incidence of the acute form of organic brain dysfunction is increasing as more complex medical treatments become possible with advances in medical technology and that it may even be endemic in acute health care settings. Since nurses are frequently the health professionals having the most direct and continuous contact with persons experiencing organic brain dysfunction, they are often in the best position to identify early manifestations and to set in motion the early treatment measures that are essential to a client's health—and at times, survival. This chapter will focus on the symptoms and etiology of organic brain dysfunction and on the therapeutic modalities that are used in the treatment of these conditions. In addition, attention will be given to primary, secondary, and tertiary prevention in both the acute and the chronic forms of organic brain disorders.

CLASSIFICATIONS OF ORGANIC DYSFUNCTIONS

Psychiatric disorders* are frequently broadly classified as either *functional* or *organic*. The functional disorders include the mood, thought, and personality disorders that have been discussed in previous chapters; they are believed to have their origins in psychogenic or psychological processes. The term "functional," in this context, refers to psychosocial or psychodynamic functioning, rather than to biological functioning. The symptoms of functional disorders are viewed as defensive responses to stress and anxiety; they differ from symptoms of organic conditions in that disturbances in cognitive functioning either are not present or are secondary to such symptoms as delusions or hallucinations. The term "organic" refers to psychiatric conditions, both chronic and acute, that are known to have their origins in disturbances in neurophysiology or brain tissue functioning. Disturbances in cognitive functioning characterize these disorders.

Current research strongly suggests that there is some neurophysiological contribution to the etiology of such disorders as schizophrenia (see Chapter 21) and the affective disorders (see Chapter 18). These findings therefore cause some confusion in the use of the terms "organic" and "functional" in the classification of psychiatric disorders.

Organic brain dysfunction is usually classified as either *acute* or *chronic*. Factors that cause alterations in normal brain functioning may produce an acute, temporary dysfunction that responds readily to appropriate therapy and the normal physiologi-

cal reparative processes, leaving no residual effects. For such conditions the terms "acute" and "reversible" are used. In some instances of organic brain dysfunction, there are residual deficits that result from diffuse alterations of neuron structure or from some continuing interference with neurophysiological processes. The terms "chronic" and "irreversible" are often used to categorize this type of dysfunction. The terms acute and chronic can be misleading, however, since some brain dysfunctions can progress from acute to chronic, often depending on the etiology of the disorder and the effectiveness of treatment. In addition, chronic disorders of unknown origin can appear with a gradual or insidious onset, without an acute phase. Chronic disorders may also be classified as mild, moderate, or severe, depending on the degree of cognitive dysfunction.

The neuropsychiatric disorders associated with impaired brain function may also be classified according to etiology. Organic brain dysfunction has been associated with systemic disorders; infections; chemical, drug, and alcohol intoxication; nutritional deficiencies; intracranial trauma and neoplasms; neurological disorders; iatrogenic disorders; and genetic factors. Organic syndromes of unknown etiology are termed *primary,* signifying the absence of any known etiology. Organic disorders of known etiology are termed *secondary,* to indicate an association with some known pathophysiological process.

CHARACTERISTICS AND UNDERLYING DYNAMICS

The clinical manifestations that make up the syndrome, or symptom complex, that results from

---

*See Appendix B for the many codings for organic mental disorders.

organic brain disorders are disturbances in attention, comprehension, memory, orientation, and judgment. Emotional instability, or lability of affect, may also be present. These disturbances in cognitive or intellectual functioning are always indicative of brain dysfunction.

Acute brain syndrome

Symptoms of delirium or an acute confusional state generally have an acute onset that is associated with some underlying pathophysiology. These symptoms are indicative of a serious level of brain dysfunction, and they require immediate treatment of the underlying pathology, often as a life-saving measure.

Difficulty in focusing attention and in comprehending incoming stimuli are often the most prominent features in acute brain dysfunction (Seltzer and Sherwin, 1978). The difficulty in focusing or maintaining attention will be reflected in an inability to grasp an idea or a simple communication. There will be difficulty in comprehending the facts of a situation and in responding to questions or other verbal communication. Even when grasped or understood, information or ideas will not be retained. There may be a lack of clarity or a fuzziness in thinking and an inability to recall or remember pertinent information. Difficulties in focusing attention also lead to an inability to screen out irrelevant stimuli so that anything going on readily distracts the person's attention. Persons who are experiencing delirium often convey their confusion and lack of comprehension through facial expressions and other forms of nonverbal communication.

In a health care setting, a person with an acute brain dysfunction may have difficulty in comprehending and cooperating with monitoring and treatment activities. People who are regaining consciousness after general anesthesia often display a similar difficulty in sustaining attention and a similar distractibility. They also may experience the fluctuations in levels of consciousness that may appear in acute brain dysfunction. Disturbances in levels of consciousness may vary from a clouding of consciousness, in which the individual is not fully conscious and responsive, to intermittent periods of stupor or coma.

Emotional instability may or may not be present in acute brain dysfunction. Some people respond with sustained fearfulness, apprehension, irritability, and restlessness. In others, such emotions may alternate with periods of calm and lethargy. Other symptoms may appear, often in association with the underlying pathophysiology. Hallucinations and delusions, for example, may appear in dysfunction that is associated with withdrawal from alcohol or drugs.

Chronic brain syndrome

The onset of symptoms in chronic brain dysfunction is usually insidious in those cases termed senile or presenile dementia, in which the causative factor is unknown. Some chronic dysfunctions may, however, directly follow an acute phase, when the causative agent has resulted in irreversible brain tissue damage, as in some cases of prolonged anoxia or when a disturbance in neurophysiology persists. Although chronic brain syndrome may occur at any age, the majority of cases appear in the geriatric population and are of unknown etiology.

The prominent symptoms of chronic organic brain dysfunction are disturbances in intellectual abilities—particularly memory, orientation, and judgment. Disturbances in attention are reflected in the distractibility that is often present. Fluctuations in emotional tone—that is, lability of affect—are often present. Additional neurological symptoms may also occur, depending on the kind of neurophysiological impairment.

The extent to which chronic organic brain dysfunction disrupts a person's ability to function in society varies considerably. Some people are able to adapt to the deficit and continue to function adequately. Others may be so severely impaired in functions of daily living that they are unable to care for themselves. Disturbances in memory, for example, may be so mild as to be imperceptible to anyone other than the affected person or a close family member. Forgetting where one put down one's eyeglasses or reading material or not remembering the names of people recently met are lapses of memory that most of us experience from time to time. More serious defects in memory, such as a tendency to forget appointments or details of important events, may be compensated for by such special efforts as note taking and association tricks. In severe memory loss, there may be difficulty in recalling what, if anything, one had for breakfast or in the ability to recognize friends and family members. In chronic brain syndrome, memory of recent events is often more impaired than remote memory or memory of earlier phases of life.

Severe memory disturbances are apt to be accompanied by disturbances in orientation—in the ways in which we relate to and in our environment. Disturbances in orientation may involve time, place, or people. Disturbances that involve time are usually of a gross nature, such as an inability to distinguish night from day or to identify the season, the year, or even the decade. The hour of the day or the day of the month may, however, be unknown to a client who is shut off from ongoing events. Many of us, when on vacation, may ignore the clock or the calendar. People from cultures that are not highly time oriented may pay little attention to precise times, days, and dates. It is important, therefore, that an evaluation of time orientation take into account an individual's circumstances.

Disturbances in orientation to place may vary from a recognition of where one is (but an inability to recall how one got there) to an inability to accurately perceive one's present location. The former type is often seen in persons who have suffered head injuries followed by a period of coma. A period of amnesia or total loss of memory of events immediately preceding the trauma often occurs. Disorientation in relation to place may also appear spontaneously and for no known reason in persons who suffer from chronic organic dysfunction.

Disorientation in relation to other people is an inability to accurately perceive or comprehend the identity of persons who are in the immediate envi-

ronment. In a hospital setting, a person may mistake health care providers for family members. A nurse may be perceived as a mother, for example. In an extreme case of this form of disorientation, there may be a lack of recognition of a close family member.

Disturbances in judgment are manifested by impairment of the ability to perceive, interpret, and respond appropriately or effectively to situations in the environment. Judgment will usually be impaired to the degree or extent to which the other cognitive functions are impaired. Behavioral manifestations may vary from mild peccadilloes that embarrass family and friends to a failure to observe social mores or to use economic and other resources prudently. In some instances, impaired judgment is so extreme that a person can endanger his or her own life or other's lives through imprudent acts. Goldfarb (1974) uses the phrase "disorientation to situation," which may more accurately describe the disturbances in judgment noted here.

Certain communication and speech patterns may be found in chronic brain disorders. Among them are circumstantiality, confabulation, and (to some extent) recall and association difficulties.

Circumstantiality is the name given to a speech pattern in which a person has difficulty in screening out relevant from irrelevant material in describing an event. There is a tendency to include every detail, often in sequential order. While a raconteur may delightfully embellish a story with interesting details that bring it to life, circumstantiality often has the opposite effect, arousing impatience in the listener that may cause him to tune out or lose interest. In a busy health care setting, there may be a tendency on the part of health care providers to complete a story for a person who displays circumstantiality or to intervene in other ways. This tendency may arouse anxiety and anger. If the person is under stress and vulnerable to any additional frustration, pressure to get to the point of the story or omit unnecessary detail may increase confusion or even result in a catastrophic anxiety reaction.

Circumstantiality may, at times, cause the individual who is affected to lose the point of a story or a question, as one association leads to another and the main thread is forgotten. Often the person, realizing that the main point has been lost, will say so and ask to have a question repeated.

The following vignette illustrates circumstantiality in an older woman who has mild to moderate brain dysfunction. In the situation described here, pain and fear played an important role.

Mrs. M., who lived alone in her own home, phoned a niece and told her that she had hurt her foot and did not know what to do. The niece took her aunt to the emergency room of the local hospital for treatment. Mrs. M. was in pain from the injured foot, and she was very anxious about what would happen if she were unable to walk for any length of time. When asked by a nurse to tell her what had happened, Mrs. M. responded: "I was going to the department store to buy a shower gift for my neighbor's daughter. She's getting married to a very nice boy, and my neighbor across the street is having a shower, and all the people on the block are invited. I am all alone, you know, and have to do everything for myself, and the girl's family has been very good to me. So I wanted to get something nice for the shower. I was reading the paper last night and saw an ad for a coffee pot on sale. I don't have too much money, you know, so I rushed out early this morning to buy it before they were all gone. I don't have anyone to drive me, so I have to do everything for myself. It's awful to be alone." Prodded a bit by the nurse, Mrs. M. continued to explain how, in her rush to get on the bus, she had turned her ankle as she stepped off the curb.

Although Mrs. M. was able to arrive at the appropriate end point in her description of the event, she also included many ramifications that were irrelevant to the immediate situation in the emergency room. The story had been told in the same detail, and almost identical language, earlier, when Mrs. M. told the niece about the accident. The astute observer will also note an underlying theme of dependence, or fear of dependence and helplessness. These emotions and the uncertainty they in-

dicate may have a higher priority of concern for Mrs. M. than the physical injury and pain in this situation.

Another symptom of brain dysfunction that may be demonstrated in speech patterns is difficulty in recalling words, ideas, or events and in making associations with other words, ideas, or events. Difficulties in *recall* and *association* are not uncommon, nor are they limited to persons with brain dysfunction. Who among us has not forgotten words or things that, in retrospect, we should have remembered? When memory is impaired by brain dysfunction, however, the ability to recall or make associations may inhibit communication ability. The symptom may be severe in the more extreme forms of chronic brain syndrome. In Pick's disease, for example, in which cerebral insufficiency is related to damage to the areas of the brain having to do with speech and association, there may be an inability to name such commonly used items as pencils. An affected person may, however, be able to state the purpose for which such an item is used. Even in such a situation, the association loss may be selective; the amount of loss depends on the familiarity and value to the individual of a particular object or idea. For example, Mrs. L. was unable to recall the word for a wristwatch when she was asked to name this commonly used item during an examination, but she could readily identify coins by their monetary value.

Confabulation is a commonly observed phenomenon in chronic brain syndrome, one that is often seen in residents of nursing and adult homes and psychiatric hospitals. In confabulation, an individual who cannot recall specific aspects of an event will often fill in the gaps in memory with relevant but imaginary information. For example, a man whose recent memory was being tested responded to a question about what he had eaten for breakfast by saying a soft-boiled egg and toast, when, in fact, he had been given oatmeal and coffee cake. Confabulation is occasionally viewed by health care providers as a wish-fulfilling fantasy, as a deliberate attempt to deceive, or as evidence of severely impaired memory. It is often none of these, but represents a face-saving device or ego defense mechanism in which the person copes by filling in gaps in memory with substitutions. Thus, confabulation can represent a strength: it can be an attempt to cope with and adapt to an intolerable situation. A recognition of the defensive nature of confabulation can serve a useful purpose in the provision of needed emotional support for such clients.

Factors that influence coping ability

Disturbances in cognitive abilities always reflect a disturbance in brain tissue functioning, which to some degree influences a person's ability to cope with life's experiences. However, the degree to which such dysfunction is disorganizing to a person is influenced by a variety of factors. Although the extent of neuronal damage or dysfunction may be a factor in some instances, other factors may be of even greater significance as a person attempts to cope with the stress of life. Among these factors are the developmental era in which an organic dysfunction begins and the psychodynamic and sociocultural forces that have an influence on the functioning of everyone.

DEVELOPMENTAL FACTORS
▶ Acute brain syndrome

The age of onset of organic dysfunction, particularly when it is early in life, may have a profound influence on the ability to cope with life. A young child who has not yet mastered language and logical thinking will respond to brain dysfunction quite differently from the way an older person, who has mastered these developmental tasks, responds. In a hospitalized child, the failure to focus attention and the irritability or apathy that may be symptomatic of acute organic dysfunction can be confused with the psychological coping process of regression, which often accompanies the stress of illness and separation from home and family. In an older person the symptoms of acute brain dysfunction may mistakenly be attributed to a degenerative

process associated with aging. Conversely, deficits in the sensory apparatus, particularly those involving sight and hearing, may be mistaken for a disturbance in comprehension, especially when such deficits are severe enough to promote a level of isolation that leads to illusions or hallucinatory experiences. Culture shock (see Chapter 4), which many people experience when first admitted to a hospital, may also influence adaptive responses to the hospital setting. This is particularly true when there is a language barrier or when there is a marked cultural difference between the client and the health care providers. Severe pain, apprehension, and anxiety may also distort or be mistaken for symptoms of acute brain dysfunction. The picture is further confused when an organic dysfunction is superimposed upon a functional psychiatric disorder. Because symptoms may be distorted by such factors, a history of an individual's patterns of functioning and ways of coping with stress, prior to the onset of the medical problem underlying the acute brain dysfunction, is an important aspect of nursing assessment and intervention. Taking such a history will be discussed later in this chapter in the section on nursing intervention.

▶ Chronic brain syndrome

The characteristics of chronic brain dysfunction will, of course, be affected by the age of onset. Up to this point we have focused primarily upon the older adult, because the largest number of people with chronic brain syndrome is in this age group. However, since chronic cerebral dysfunction can occur at any age, it is important to mention its effects on the child and the young adult. If organic dysfunction has its onset in the early adult years, the individual has already mastered the language and the learning tasks necessary for adaptation to his or her culture. The person has educational and living experiences to fall back on in coping with the deficit, in addition to a variety of coping measures to rely on. The young child, in contrast, must learn language and must negotiate the developmental crises upon which personality and cultural adaptation are founded. A child must also master the knowledge, skills, and other requirements essential to adapting to the people and mores of a complex culture.

Organic brain disease can occur at any point during the developmental process, from conception to the end of life. When the onset is in the prenatal or perinatal period, the child may fail to master language and may be so impaired in the ability to function or learn that severe mental retardation may be the result.

Onset later in childhood also may have a profound effect on the child and the family. The memory disturbance makes learning difficult, and the shortened or altered attention span increases the learning difficulties. Such a child has a very low tolerance for frustration, and is often restless and hyperactive. The following excerpt from a history illustrates some of the aspects of such brain damage in a child:

Thomas was brought to a mental health clinic by his parents when he was six years old. He was of average size for his age and physically well developed and well nourished. He did not respond to any questions or directions and was extremely restless and hyperactive. He had a very pained facial expression, and he exhibited stereotypical movements of the hands: he would hold them in front of him and shake them up and down. He had been excluded from all schools, even those for emotionally disturbed children. The mother reported that he had frequent, severe temper tantrums at home, in which he would break anything in sight. He required constant and direct supervision. The family was very devoted to him and willing to make any sacrifice to get help for him and to care for him at home.

The parents described Thomas' early development as normal. He was a very happy, responsive child whose language development was normal. The father, who was a professional photographer, had taken many movies of the son from birth until the onset of the present symptoms when he was three years of age. A review of these movies tended to confirm the parents' assessment of Tommy's early development. Between the ages of two and three, he developed an acute infectious illness, from which he appeared to have an uneventful recovery. But shortly following the illness, language development stopped and his personality changed from that of the happy, responsive child he had been to the hyperactive, anxious, and unresponsive child he was upon admission to the clinic. Neurological, psychological, and other testing measures confirmed a diagnosis of organic brain dysfunction.

In the young adult, the symptoms closely resemble those in the older adult, although the social and psychological impact may be more devastating in the young adult. Cognitive defects inhibit learning of new material, thus often interfering with career plans. Even previously mastered knowledge and skills are affected. For example, a computer programmer may no longer be able to function in that field. In severe cases, the memory defect may be so embarrassing in relationships with peers that it promotes isolation and withdrawal. In instances in which the functional deficit is mild or moderate, a young adult may be more resilient in compensating for and adapting to the cognitive defect than an older person is.

Disturbances in cognitive functioning that result from organic brain dysfunction may, of course, be superimposed upon such functional disorders as the thought and mood disturbances. Depression* and elation frequently accompany organic brain disease. Goldfarb (1974) points out that such mood disorders are functional disturbances secondary to brain dysfunction. He notes that they are often the "emotional responses to the organic deficit and to the loss of an important part of the self." Depression often represents a grief and mourning process similar to that which occurs after the loss of a body part. Such depression responds to appropriate therapy. Depression, particularly in the elderly, may be mistaken for brain dysfunction. Anger, apathy, and depression are often misperceived by health care providers as organic dysfunction.

---

*See Chapter 18.

Mrs. S. had been active all of her life, participating in running a small store that she and her husband owned. When her husband died, Mrs. S. was in her early seventies. The store was sold, and she moved to a small apartment near her only son, in a community far removed from the one in which she had lived for many years and where she knew many people. Alone much of the time, and isolated from old friends and acquaintances, Mrs. S. became severely depressed. She was taken to a mental health center, where she was diagnosed as having chronic brain syndrome. After a few weeks, Mrs. S. was transferred to an adult home, where she came to the attention of a community mental health nurse. Working with Mrs. S. over a period of time, the nurse became aware that her cognitive abilities were intact but that she was depressed and lonely. Her mental state was exacerbated by a physical infirmity that was not being treated and was somewhat immobilizing. The immobilization increased her feelings of helplessness and abandonment. Working with the son and community agencies, the nurse was instrumental in having Mrs. S. transferred to a health-related facility that was more suitable to her needs. Her medical and psychological problems were treated there. In the new setting, where she felt more safe and secure, Mrs. S. made excellent progress and began to take part in and enjoy social and other activities.

SOCIOCULTURAL FACTORS

Many sociocultural factors influence each of us in our ability to cope with the normal stresses of life. The psychosocial needs for love, approval, acceptance, status, recognition, and achievement are important to the mental health of everyone. Economic security and the availability of family, friends, and other social support systems are essential to meeting these needs.

For the individual with organic brain dysfunction, many factors may combine to limit the ability to satisfy these normal human needs. In an older person, as Goldfarb (1974) points out, organic brain dysfunction often occurs at a time of sociocultural stress. Loss of family and friends through marriage, death, illness, and change of residence frequently coincides with physical ailments that contribute to organic dysfunction. Forced retirement from productive employment conflicts with one's need to be a useful, constructive member of society. In addition, retirement often leads to economic insecurity and isolation from friends and coworkers.

Although these factors are especially pertinent to older persons, a young person with some cognitive deficits may suffer very similar deprivations. Work and earning capacity can be limited by the disability, and isolation from family and peers often occurs.

All of these factors influence a person's ability to cope. The person who can maintain close ties with family and friends and who experiences little disruption in life-style may cope more effectively to the disability.

PSYCHODYNAMIC FACTORS

Stress and emotional responses to it can be disruptive of anyone's ability to function (see Chapter 7). For an individual with some organic brain dysfunction, such emotional factors as anxiety, anger, hopelessness, and depression may cause greater disorganization of behavior than would be the case for a person with normal brain functioning. This exacerbation of symptoms may be erroneously attributed to cerebral damage (Goldfarb, 1974). For example, an individual with a mild degree of organic brain dysfunction, when confronted with interpersonal, economic, social, or other crises, frequently experiences increased fear, anxiety, anger, frustration, and feelings of helplessness. These emotions in turn may cause restlessness, inattention, and difficulty in comprehension and memory. All of these symptoms are characteristic of organic dysfunction, but easily become exaggerated under emotional stress. Thus, assessment on the basis of cognitive function alone, without the level of anxiety and coping responses to it being taken into account, may easily lead to an inaccurate assessment of the degree of brain dysfunction and to an overlooking of the strengths of a client.

Clients with organic brain dysfunction are often quite aware of their disability and of their emotional responses to pressure, stress, or assaults upon their self-concept and security. Such individuals may mention that they become very nervous and confused when pressured. They also frequently respond with embarrassment and anger when deficits in memory or other cognitive abilities are pointed out to them.

• • •

Thus, many factors in addition to the cognitive dysfunction influence the coping abilities of persons who have organic brain syndrome. The following brief case summaries point up some of the differences in the ways people cope.

Mrs. M., who is in her mid-seventies, has lived alone in a single-family dwelling since the death of her husband, which occurred when she was 60. She has no children, but she maintains close family ties with her four siblings and their children. Although she had to drop out of school after the eighth grade to help support her immigrant family, Mrs. M. is fluent in and able to read and write both English and the language of her ethnic group. She is in good physical health, and she is economically secure. Mrs. M. is able to do her own housework, shopping, and cooking. She also maintains a small yard and flower garden, and takes great pride in her home. Always socially active, Mrs. M. continues to entertain family and friends and participates in various social and religious activities with them.

Mrs. M. has several complaints that she associates with aging, which shows a degree of insight. She complains of having trouble remembering things. If one observes her carefully, however, one finds the memory defect to be selective and related to new material or to areas that have little value for her. For example, she cannot remember where her favorite nephew's wedding will be held, although she has heard the plans many times and in detail. But she has no need to remember, since she will be taken there and brought home by a family member. She can, however, remember in detail the previous day's soap opera episode in order to recount

it to a friend who missed the broadcast. In the retelling and in other social interactions, her speech is somewhat stereotypical and circumstantial.

She also complains that she becomes very nervous and upset when she is under any pressure or when she is confronted with a problem in her home that requires maintenance from service people in the community. But she is very effective in using problem-solving techniques and in appealing to appropriate family members or friends for assistance. And she meets the need to feel useful by doing minor alterations and repairs of clothing for family members and close friends.

Mrs. G., also a widow, is in her late seventies. In many ways, her situation is similar to that of Mrs. M. She is also economically secure and owns her own home. Although she has several married children and a large extended family, her home is at some distance from any of them, so any immediate support or contact with her family is limited. In addition Mrs. G. speaks little English, and since she does not live in a neighborhood where her language is spoken, her community contact is more limited.

She is a strong-willed woman, however, and for several years had been able to manage her affairs and care for herself fairly effectively. Gradually, however, her family began to notice changes in her ability to function. Her memory had become progressively poorer. She would forget where she had put her money and other things, and whether or not a tenant had given her a check for the rent of an apartment. She also began to make errors in judgment, such as renting the apartment to a second family after she had already rented it and giving to strangers articles of furniture that she needed. When Mrs. G. began to lose weight, a daughter suspected that she had been forgetting to prepare meals or eat an adequate diet. A physical check-up revealed no disease, but the physician convinced the family that Mrs. G's cognitive difficulties were making it impossible for her to continue living alone. At this point, she moved into her daughter's home.

Although immediately following the change she became somewhat disoriented during the night, when she would awaken and think she was still in her own home, Mrs. G's condition has become more stable. She continues to have some defects in memory, but in the protective and supportive environment, with adequate nutrition and the presence of family members, the cognitive defects have become less disabling.

Mrs. A. was also a widow in her late seventies who was economically secure and in good physical health. She lived in a stable ethnic community throughout her lifetime and had many relatives and friends nearby. Within a period of three years Mrs. A. lost both her husband and her only daughter, and her grandsons married and moved away. Much of Mrs. A.'s social activity prior to their deaths had centered around the husband, the daughter, and the daughter's family. The husband had been retired for many years; he did all the shopping for the family and made all of the major decisions. Although he was several years older than Mrs. A., he had, over a period of time, kidded her about her forgetfulness. A few months after the husband's death, Mrs. A.'s neighbors began phoning a son, who lived some distance from his mother, with complaints about Mrs. A.'s behavior. They described her as confused and said she was harassing them about not paying rents, which they had indeed paid. The son and his wife visited Mrs. A. and hired someone to stay with her, but her condition continued to deteriorate. She became increasingly disoriented to time, confusing the night with the day and summer with winter, often appearing outside on very cold days clad only in a sweater. She also began to confuse her neighbor's children with the grandsons, who were grown and married. She began to cook large pots of food for the deceased husband and daughter, which she stored in the refrigerator to await their arrival. She continued to harass the tenants about the rents and, at times, to confuse them with people from her youth. On one occasion, she left home, saying she was going to visit her mother. She was found some distance from her home, and in a very confused state, by the police. They took her to a psychiatric hospital, where she was admitted with a diagnosis of chronic brain syndrome. In the hospital her general health and cognitive abilities deteriorated until her death about six months later.

EPIDEMIOLOGY AND SOCIOCULTURAL ASPECTS

Organic brain dysfunctions are the most ubiquitous of all mental health problems. Acute forms occur with regularity in many health facilities as complications of physiological and traumatic disorders and their treatment. The chronic forms constitute one of the major mental health problems. Despite, or perhaps because of, this prevalence, definitive data about the incidence of organic brain dysfunction are not currently available. The multiplicity of etiological factors that may contribute to organic dysfunction, however, suggests a very high and possibly increasing incidence and also is an indication of some of the problems involved in gathering demographic data.

When acute confusional states occur as complications of medical conditions, data are often not compiled on such complications or, when collected, are related to specific underlying diagnoses. In addition, delirium often goes undiagnosed by physicians, although nursing staffs are often more aware of the symptoms and record them in their notes (Butler, 1975a and b; Heller and Kornfeld, 1974).

The incidence of organic dysfunctions of both acute and chronic nature is highest in people over 65 years of age. Persons in the older age groups are more susceptible to the major health problems (cancer, cardiac and respiratory diseases, and so on), with which organic dysfunctions are often associated. There is also empirical evidence that susceptibility to delirium is high among persons who experience illness and injury in the later years of life. Many individuals with some degree of chronic organic impairment are living in the community and do not come into contact with any data collection system. In some instances, a diagnosis of chronic brain syndrome is made purely on the basis of behavioral assessment. Butler (1975a and b) terms chronic brain syndrome a "wastebasket" diagnosis that is made when anyone starts acting "senile."

The diagnosis of chronic brain syndrome frequently arouses feelings of hopelessness in physicians, nurses, and other health professionals and leads to a lack of interest in the active treatment of such disorders in the elderly (Butler, 1975a and b). Such responses may have contributed to the historical paucity of research in this area of psychiatry (Wells, 1978). There is, however, a growing interest in the neuropsychiatric conditions associated with impaired cerebral functioning, and there has been an increase in the amount of research into the causes and treatment of such conditions (Wells, 1978).

Organic brain disturbances occur in all social classes and ethnic groups. Many sociocultural factors contribute, directly or indirectly, to the incidence of organic brain dysfunction. Poverty, with its concomitant poor housing, overcrowding, and malnutrition, may increase the incidence of infectious and other diseases, which can be complicated by organic brain disorders of either an acute or a chronic nature. Leighton (1974) notes that "societal malfunction" or "social disintegration" increases the frequency of organic disease, in part through malfunctioning of the health care network and the resulting disruption of preventive and treatment services.

Spector (1979) points out that lead poisoning is a serious health problem among black and Hispanic Americans. When untreated, it results in chronic brain dysfunction. Many victims of lead poisoning live in old houses in which lead-based paints had been applied to exterior and interior surfaces. Current legislation has fairly well eliminated the use of lead in paints for most purposes, and many states have directives for preventing inhalation of lead when old paint is removed. In some older dwellings, however, lead paint remains on walls, where it becomes a source of lead poisoning as a result of flaking, paint removal efforts, and children chewing on painted surfaces.

Social stress and the competitive pressures of highly industrialized society are experienced by people of all classes, ages, and ethnic groups. Pressures on the adolescent to achieve in school, on the adult in many work situations, on the older

person forced into retirement and often into isolation, and on minority group members who are excluded from the job market and meaningful participation in other aspects of life are commonplace.

The ways in which people cope with social stress often contribute, directly or indirectly, to organic disease. Social pressures contribute significantly to drug and alcohol abuse, as people increasingly turn to such chemicals in an effort to cope with the pressures of modern life. Suicide attempts may also result in brain damage, depending on the particular method employed and other factors.*

Prejudice, another source of social stress, may contribute indirectly to organic brain dysfunction in a variety of ways, including the failure to provide early or preventive treatment of disorders that can lead to chronic organic dysfunction when they are untreated. Raskus et al. (1979) note "the sense of futility" of health professionals toward treatment of emotional disturbances in older people. Butler (1975a) speaks of the "profound prejudice against the elderly which is found to some degree in all of us." To be elderly and from a minority ethnic group places the person in "multiple jeopardy." (Butler, 1975b).

The technological era in which we live may contribute to the incidence of organic dysfunction. Environmental pollution from industry and other sources is an ever-present danger. Advances in medical technology, which have been so effective in prolonging life and functioning ability, have also contributed to the increase in the incidence of organic dysfunction. Heller and Kornfeld (1974) discuss the delirious states associated with cardiac and general surgery, intensive care units, and treatment of renal diseases.

High-speed transportation, another aspect of our advanced technology, has increased the incidence of head injury—through automobile and other accidents. While improved treatment has decreased

---

*Sociocultural aspects of alcohol and drug abuse are discussed in Chapter 17; sociocultural aspects of suicide are discussed in Chapter 18.

mortality from head trauma, organic dysfunction is an increasingly common sequela of severe head injury (Tuerk et al., 1974).

ETIOLOGY

Acute confusional states

"Acute confusional state" is a term used by Seltzer and Frazier (1978) to describe the acute brain dysfunction that often accompanies physical illness and injury. Many other diagnostic terms are also used, among them "delirium," acute delirious states, "acute brain syndrome," and "toxic psychosis." The following are some major causes of an acute confusional state, but it should be borne in mind that any condition that interferes with complex biochemical or metabolic functions may result in temporary or permanent brain dysfunction.

SYSTEMIC DISORDERS

Among the systemic disorders that may be associated with an acute confusional state are chronic heart and lung diseases, hepatic and renal insufficiencies, acute forms of diabetes, and severe anemias. The specific etiological factors that such systemic disorders produce vary with the underlying pathological process. Among these factors are hypoxia, which is particularly prevalent in chronic heart and lung disorders and in severe anemias, and hypoglycemia, which often occurs in severe diabetes. Disturbances in acid-base and electrolyte balances and in the water-sodium balance may be present in any of these physical ailments and in many others. Toxic substances in the blood that accompany renal and hepatic dysfunction can also contribute to brain dysfunction. Uremic toxins may cause such neurological symptoms as seizures and asterixis—a characteristic flapping tremor of the hands—in addition to acute brain dysfunction (Seltzer and Frazier, 1978).

INFECTIOUS DISORDERS

Acute confusional states frequently occur in systemic infectious disorders such as typhoid fever,

malaria, pneumonia, and infectious hepatitis. Central nervous system infections such as meningitis and encephalitis may also cause delirium. In the systemic infectious conditions, brain dysfunction is believed to be associated with the high temperature and level of toxicity that are symptomatic of the diseases. The debilitating effects of such an illness may also be a contributory cause. Encephalitis may be followed by a chronic syndrome. Immunization against the communicable diseases of childhood and effective treatment of syphilis with penicillin have nearly eliminated the encephalitis often associated with these diseases. Antibiotic treatment of viral and bacterial encephalitis has also been effective in preventing chronic brain dysfunction as a result of these diseases.

CHEMICAL INTOXICATION

Chemical intoxication is becoming an increasing hazard in industrial societies. The presence of numerous chemical additives in foodstuffs and the chemical pollution of our air, water, and soil have received wide attention because of their potential for the production of cancer and birth defects. There has, however, been far less attention paid to the potential hazard of such chemicals to the normal physiological processes of the central nervous system and the rest of the body.

Two chemicals that have long been associated with brain dysfunction are carbon monoxide and lead, although other chemicals may produce similar effects. Carbon monoxide poisoning can come about suddenly, from breathing automobile exhaust fumes in a suicide attempt or as a result of a faulty automobile exhaust system combined with poor ventilation of a car's interior. In current model cars in which ventilation depends on a system that brings air into the car when it is in motion and windows are closed, idling a motor when the car is stopped to provide heat or air conditioning is particularly hazardous. In addition, incomplete combustion of fuels, particularly coal, may cause toxic levels of carbon monoxide to be emitted into the air of a home.

Carbon monoxide causes anoxia by combining with blood hemoglobin to form a stable substance, carboxyhemoglobin. This condition prevents the uptake of oxygen by the hemoglobin. When severe or prolonged enough, carbon monoxide poisoning can cause death or permanent brain damage. The symptoms of confusion and a clouding of consciousness may be early indications of carbon monoxide poisoning. Mild cases may appear in persons working in such industries as auto repairing, in which a constant level of carbon monoxide results from motors being run in inadequately ventilated garages.

Several of the heavy metals—lead, mercury, and manganese—may cause brain dysfunction. Lead has received the greatest attention and may be the most commonly found of the heavy metals. The ingestion of lead by children has been greatly reduced as a result of government actions that ban the use of lead in paints, particularly in paints used on toys, children's furniture, and other items that young children may suck or chew on. The habit of pica, or the craving of unnatural foods such as plaster from walls, may still be a hazard to children, and occasionally to adults, who live in older dwellings in which lead paint remains on the walls.

In adults, lead poisoning is usually caused by inhalation associated with industrial activities. Workers in the construction industry are particularly vulnerable when they are dismantling or removing paint from older structures on which lead paints had been used over a period of time. Removal of lead paint from older houses by homeowners can also result in lead inhalation.

Lead intoxication may produce an acute delirious state, or it may result in chronic brain syndrome—particularly if treatment is delayed or ineffective. Lead produces a fragility of the red blood cell membrane, with subsequent destruction or hemolysis of the cell. Lead may be stored in the bones, which can lead to symptoms recurring as it is later released without further inhalation or ingestion (Luckmann and Sorensen, 1974).

A light metal, aluminum, is being investigated as a possible causitive agent in the presenile dementia, Alzheimer's disease (Roberts, 1982; Levick, 1980; Perl and Brody, 1980; Trapp et al., 1978). Victims of the disorder are found to have high levels of aluminum in their brains on autopsy. Dietary and environmental sources of the metal include many over-the-counter antacids, underarm deodorants (Roberts, 1982) and aluminum cookware (Levick, 1980). ''Dialysis dementia,'' a progressive dementia related to renal dyalisis, was traced to a high concentration of aluminum found in postmortem examination of victims of the syndrome. The large amounts of tap water used to flush out the blood stream were believed to be the source, since many municipalities rely on aluminum to remove impurities from the water supply (Tanne, 1983).

PHARMACOLOGICAL AGENTS

Many pharmaceuticals may cause an acute confusional state in some people. This side effect may occur in susceptible individuals at normal therapeutic dosage levels, as well as in high dosage levels and overdoses. Among the drugs that may cause such a response are anticholinergics, diuretics, digitalis, levodopa, hypnotics, sedatives, and some of the hormonal substances. Kolb (1973) points out that some children may develop delirium following a single application of atropine eye drops. The reason why some children are so affected is not known. The long-term use of major tranquilizers (such as Mellaril, Thorazine, and Haldol) which has been associated with the physical disorder *tardive dyskinesia** is now being related to a psychological counterpart, a serious mental and emotional disorder that is a side effect and something apart from the functional disorder. The syndrome has been termed *tardive dysmentia* (Herbert, 1983).

Other drugs may produce acute confusional states when taken in overdoses or in combination with other chemicals such as alcohol or other central nervous system depressants. A synergistic or potentiating effect takes place when such drugs are taken in combination. Baldessarini (1977) mentions the tricyclic antidepressants and lithium salts as drugs that cause delirium and other neurologic symptoms when they are taken in toxic levels. He

---

*See Chapter 21.

also notes that tricyclic drugs are increasingly being used in suicide attempts. Mild intake of alcohol, in combination with such drugs as phenothiazines, antidepressants, and barbiturates, may produce an acute intoxication and may even lead to coma and death as a result of depression of the respiratory centers.

Many therapeutic procedures may produce an acute confusional state. Diuretic therapy and low sodium diets, for example, unless carefully monitored, can produce fluid electrolyte imbalances that may lead to symptoms of delirium. Anesthesia and prolonged surgical procedures may also cause an acute brain dysfunction.

ALCOHOL AND DRUG WITHDRAWAL

There are two ways in which alcohol may produce an acute brain syndrome. First, excessive ingestion produces acute alcoholism. Second, for people who habitually consume large quantities of alcohol and who are physiologically addicted, the abrupt withdrawal of the substance may produce the symptom picture known as delirium tremens. This condition is often encountered in persons admitted to a general hospital for treatment of a physical illness or injury. Very often it is not known that the individual is physically addicted to alcohol until the symptoms appear. Withdrawal symptoms, including brain dysfunction, may also occur in individuals addicted to such drugs as opiates, meprobamates, and barbiturates.

NUTRITIONAL DEFICIENCIES

A deficiency in the B vitamins (particularly thiamine) is the most common nutritional deficiency associated with psychiatric and neurological disorders. The condition known as Wernicke's syndrome is caused by a deficiency of thiamine in the diet (Seltzer and Frazier, 1978). Because of the addition of the B vitamins to many foods, most people in the United States have an adequate intake of these essential substances. Deficiencies of B vitamins are seen most often in chronic alcoholics, because of the poor nutritional habits and the interference with intestinal absorption that are associat-

ed with chronic alcoholism. Thiamine deficiency may, however, occur in cases of hyperemesis gravidarum and pernicious anemia and in elderly persons who have inadequate nutritional intake. Delirium may be one of the early symptoms of the syndrome. Prolonged deficiency of thiamine may cause permanent neurological damage and chronic dysfunction. The chronic condition is known as Korsakoff's psychosis.

Severe dehydration may also produce delirium. Elderly people living alone may be especially vulnerable in hot summer weather because of inadequate fluid intake or excessive loss of fluids.

HEAD INJURIES

An acute confusional state is often associated with head injuries, particularly in instances involving a concussion and loss of consciousness. The delirium may result from neuronal injury from the concussion, but prolonged or recurring delirium may indicate hemorrhage and intracranial pressure (Kolb, 1977).

Chronic brain syndrome

Like acute brain dysfunction, chronic brain dysfunction may be secondary to many pathological processes. For example, Lehman (1983) states: "Great progress in the prevention of OBS [organic brain syndrome] in the aged would be made with the discovery of an effective prevention or cure for arteriosclerosis." In addition to the toxic, metabolic, and circulatory disorders that may underlie chronic brain dysfunction, examples of which have been noted, intracranial neoplasms and infections, normal-pressure hydrocephalus, and Huntington's chorea* (a genetic disorder) are among other causative factors.

---

*A group of investigators have found a marker near the Huntington's Disease gene that promises to pinpoint its exact location. Isolation of the gene seems imminent and may lead to means of preventing expression. Even now, this finding means that a large percentage of those at risk will be able to learn if they will, in fact, develop the syndrome (Kotala, 1983; Miller, 1983).

In the majority of cases, however, symptoms of chronic brain dysfunction cannot, in our present state of knowledge, be attributed to any such pathological processes. The disorders are, then, somewhat arbitrarily, as Seltzer and Frazier (1978) point out, considered to be primary and labeled presenile or senile dementia, depending on age of onset. When the onset occurs in the sixth decade of life or later, the condition is considered senile dementia. An earlier onset, often in the fourth decade of life, results in the condition being termed presenile dementia. Presenile dementia may be further classified as Alzheimer's disease or Pick's disease, after the physicians who first described these organic dysfunctions, which have their onset in midlife.

Alzheimer's disease is a disorder that is receiving a great deal of attention. Actually, there are two types—Alzheimer's disease (AD) and senile dementia of the Alzheimer's type (SDAT). The two disorders differ in age of onset and rate of progression, but are similar in terms of their pathology (Whitehouse et al., 1983). Some believe that these two types of Alzheimer's disease are the most common cause of dementia in middle and late life (Whitehouse et al., 1983). Both are characterized by progressive abnormalities of memory, behavior, and cognition. Brain changes include neurofibrilary tangles, neuritic plaques, and loss of specific populations of nerve cells (Coyle et al., 1983). Some work is being done relating brain changes in AD and SDAT to those in Down's syndrome (Sinex and Merril, 1982). Coyle et al. (1983, p. 1188) state: "Individuals with Down's syndrome, trisomy 21, often experience a progressive deterioration in their limited cognitive abilities beginning at approximately 30 to 35 years of age. Brains of affected patients show neuropathological changes virtually identical to those in AD."

Integration of theories

Organic brain dysfunction is not a disease entity in itself. The brain syndromes represent complex responses of the central nervous system to disturbances in neurophysiological processes that maintain normal functioning. Brain tissue is highly dependent on a constant supply of oxygen, glucose, and certain amino acids to maintain normal functioning. Any systemic or local condition that interferes with these essential elements or that inhibits or alters the normal metabolic processes can produce brain dysfunction of either an acute or a chronic nature. It should be noted that the present state of our knowledge of neurophysiology is not sufficient to explain all of the mechanisms through which systemic disorders affect brain function.

Organic brain disorders may occur at any age along the life span. When the causative agent results in chronic dysfunction early in life, the inhibition in learning ability often results in mental retardation. The highest incidence of organic brain disorders, however, is in the older age groups, in which there are often functional impairments in sensory, motor, and homeostatic mechanisms and in central nervous system integrative efficiency. Persons in this age group are also more susceptible to chronic metabolic or systemic disorders and to psychosocial problems related to changes in role and status that are contributory factors. The emotional responses of grief, anger, and depression may distort the degree of cognitive dysfunction; in older persons particularly, such symptoms are often mistaken for signs of an organic disorder.

TREATMENT MODALITIES

The treatment of acute brain dysfunction depends on the underlying medical condition with which the dysfunction is associated. Aspects of treatment will be discussed further in the section on nursing intervention.

Many of the chronic brain dysfunctions associated with underlying pathological disorders may be reversed or ameliorated through proper treatment during the early stages. In a few disorders, advances in the treatment of the acute stages have virtually eliminated the appearance of chronic brain disease. For example, early and effective treatment of syphilis with penicillin has prevented the general paresis associated with syphilis, which was at one time a common cause of dementia. Early diagnosis of Wernicke's syndrome and treatment with thiamine cure this acute organic disorder and prevent the development of a chronic dysfunction.

Increased knowledge and better diagnostic procedures have enhanced the possibility of recognition and treatment of underlying pathology. For many years a diagnosis of psychosis with cerebral arteriosclerosis was almost routinely made for persons older than 65 who were admitted to large state mental hospitals. At the present time this diagnosis is being increasingly questioned as a valid cause of chronic brain syndrome. As Seltzer and Sherwin point out, cerebral arteriosclerosis would be more apt to cause an acute condition such as a cerebral vascular accident. There is, however, a possibility of brain damage from multiple cerebral infarcts occurring over a period of time. Such a condition is associated with hypertension; if hypertension is recognized and treated early, such multiple infarctions could be prevented (Seltzer and Sherwin, 1978).

Normal-pressure hydrocephalus is another disorder that has received increased attention during the past decade. Normal-pressure hydrocephalus is characterized by a progressive dementia, accompanied by incontinence and a peculiar gait. As the name indicates, the cerebrospinal fluid pressure is normal in this condition. Diagnosis is made by pneumoencephalogram and other neurological diagnostic measures. A history of head trauma, infection, or another brain disease has been associated with the condition in some cases. A cerebrospinal shunt has been effective in reversing the symptoms in some patients (Seltzer and Sherwin, 1978).

The psychiatric treatment modalities used in therapy for clients with chronic organic brain dysfunction include individual, group, and family psychotherapy; occupational, recreational, and work therapies; activity therapies, including dance and movement therapies; crisis intervention; brief hospitalization; and administration of psychopharmaceuticals. Since most of these forms of treatment have been dealt with in earlier chapters, discussion in this chapter will be limited to aspects that are particularly relevant to clients who have organic insufficiency.

The use of individual and group psychotherapy in the treatment of clients with organic brain syndrome has been increasing since World War II. The extent to which these forms of therapy are available to such clients will depend on a variety of factors. Among those factors are the socioeconomic status of the individual, the availability and interest of psychotherapists, the willingness of the client to accept these forms of therapy, and so forth. Perhaps major inhibiting factors are attitudes toward chronic brain dysfunction and toward the elderly population, who make up the largest number of potential clients. Many professionals, including therapists and nurses, experience feelings of hopelessness and helplessness in response to chronic brain dysfunction and to elderly people. Such emotional responses inhibit the ability of the health professional to function or to maintain an interest in working with such clients. Goldfarb (1974) points out the importance of psychotherapy for the elderly person with organic brain dysfunction and the importance of setting realistic goals. Many such people suffer from anxiety, fear, depression, and anger, which in themselves can be disorganizing to the personality. Goldfarb (1974) notes that the therapeutic relationship can be made more effective if clients who feel dependent and helpless are offered an opportunity to achieve or feel that they have achieved mastery and gratification. Such mastery or feelings of mastery, Goldfarb points out, come about as a result of the need of the client to ally with a powerful person or parent surrogate, in this case, the therapist. The therapist, in Goldfarb's method, does not act out the powerful ascribed role, but accepts the client's perception by neither confirming nor denying it. In the ongoing therapeutic sessions, the interest, concern, and appropriate approval expressed by the therapist provide emotional support that meets the needs of the client. This form of therapy, like any other form of psychotherapy, should be used only by professionals who have adequate training and preparation.

Psychopharmaceuticals are widely employed in the treatment of people with organic dysfunction to control such symptoms as agitation, anxiety, and depression. In addition, many substances have been used and studied in relation to their effect on cognition. Among these are stimulants such as amphetamines, vasodilators, anticoagulants, hormones, vitamins, and procaine. The anticoagulants continue to be widely used in the geriatric population in the treatment of circulatory and cognitive disorders. The possibility of hemorrhage, from even a minor injury, when anticoagulants are used, requires close monitoring of blood levels and close health supervision. In the case of persons who have organic dysfunctions with memory defects, which may interfere with the ability to follow through prescribed treatment and medication instructions, monitoring by community health nurses is important. Some drugs have been used in an attempt to improve or affect cognitive function, but studies have not supported their effectiveness. The use of vitamins, particularly for clients whose nutritional intakes may not provide adequate amounts of vitamins, has shown some promise (Eisendorfer and Fridel, 1977).

The use of antipsychotic and antidepressant drugs in older people has a higher risk of toxic side effects than it does in younger people.* The absorption, metabolism, and excretion of many of these drugs are altered in the older age group. The side effects that may appear include confusion, disorientation, lethargy or agitation, and aggression. Since confusion and disorientation are common symptoms in organic brain dysfunction in both the acute and the chronic states, antipsychotic

or antidepressant drugs may exacerbate these symptoms. Although lower-than-average doses may prevent such side effects, it is important that nursing staff be alert to toxic side effects in assessing client behavior (Baldessarini, 1977).

NURSING INTERVENTION

PRIMARY PREVENTION

Primary prevention in organic brain dysfunction is a serious and multifaceted problem that involves many aspects of our complex social system. The importance of the prevention of a condition that in many instances is preventable and that often has a devastating effect upon the individual, the family, and the community cannot be overemphasized. The nurse, as a member of a health profession and as a citizen, has an opportunity and a responsibility to participate in the primary prevention of organic disorders.

Primary prevention in organic disorders focuses on individuals, families, and groups who may be at risk and on factors in the environment that contribute to the disease process. Because the etiology of organic disorders may lie in a broad range of factors and because the etiology is closely interrelated with other health problems, primary prevention activities will often be an integral part of general health promotion. The prevention of suicide through "hot lines," for example, or programs that enable nurses to prevent and intervene in alcohol and drug abuse may have an impact on the incidence of organic brain disorders.

Social and political action related to such community concerns as environmental pollution, consumer products safety, and highway and transportation safety may also be part of primary prevention of organic disorders. Although Ralph Nader has demonstrated that one committed individual

---

*For discussion of side effects of antipsychotic drugs, see Chapter 21; for side effects of antidepressant drugs, see Chapter 18.

can have an impact upon public safety, the most effective action has come about through persistent and informed group action.

The degree to which environmental pollution contributes to organic brain disease is not known. It is known, however, that certain chemicals—heavy metals and carbon monoxide, for example—play a very direct role. The ever-increasing number of reports in the news media of severe environmental pollution by industry is alarming. Reports of the long-term pollution of a town in Italy after a single emission of a toxic chemical from a factory and of buried chemicals seeping to the surface in the Love Canal in Niagara Falls, New York, and their destructive impact on the health of residents, are but two examples. Whether or not people have a right to pure drinking water is an issue that the United States Supreme Court may soon confront.

Professional nurses working in industry have long been involved in occupational health and safety. They have been effective in the early identification of health and safety hazards and in early diagnosis and treatment of health problems. Such nurses also have had an opportunity to work with environmental and safety engineers and with the Occupational Safety and Health Administration to identify and eliminate potential hazards to health in industry and to assist in the promotion of safety measures through health teaching and health supervision of workers.

Since brain dysfunction is often a secondary response to underlying metabolic or other systemic disorders, any advances in the prevention of such conditions would automatically have a preventive effect on the incidence of acute brain syndrome caused by them. Immunization against communicable diseases and treatment of primary and secondary stages of syphilis are examples of such prevention. Early diagnosis and effective treatment of many systemic disorders—treatment of pneumonia with antibiotics, for example—has also been important. Efforts to prevent alcohol abuse, drug abuse, and toxic substance use have been less than successful despite the expenditure of much effort

toward this end. Early identification of people at risk and the availability of community services for effective treatment are important aspects of these efforts. Public education, particularly of the younger population, can play a role. Research into the underlying causative factors may eventually lead to more effective preventive measures.

Primary prevention in chronic brain syndrome is more complex, since the etiology is not known in the majority of cases. Wells (1978) points out that the increasing interest in such conditions and the awareness that they are disease processes and not the normal concomitants of aging are hopeful signs for further research and treatment of these disorders. He further points out that the greatest advances to date have been in the fields of neuropathology and neurochemistry. Wells (1978), Seltzer and Sherwin (1978), and others have noted that a number of people, labeled as having chronic brain syndrome, have symptoms that represent an underlying disorder that in many instances can be alleviated or ameliorated through appropriate treatment. Improved diagnostic measures, including neurological evaluation, could lead to the institution of such treatment. Normal-pressure hydrocephalus, for example, is a neurological condition that is often mistaken for senile dementia when the diagnosis is based on the symptom picture alone, without an adequate neurological evaluation.

Depression in an older person is also often misdiagnosed as senile dementia. Goldfarb (1974) points out that ''many older people labeled as having chronic brain syndrome, are often angry, depressed and apathetic.'' Treatment for the depression alleviates the symptoms in such cases. The prevalence of such conditions in the elderly has become widely enough recognized to have spawned the term ''pseudodementia'' to describe them. McAllister (1983) suggests that there may be at least two categories of pseudodementia. He believes, based on the available data, that the cognitive impairment that can be associated with depression is more correctly viewed as ''depression-induced organic mental disorder.'' The prognosis for these individuals tends to be, with adequate psychiatric treatment, very hopeful. The prognosis for those people who have coexisting organic and functional illnesses is less hopeful and is determined by the extent to which the current deficit is being caused by the functional or psychiatric component of their illness (McAllister, 1983).

Professional nurses working in hospitals and communities can be effective in many aspects of primary prevention of chronic brain dysfunction. Early identification and treatment of physical and psychological health problems often rest with the community health nurse, who may be the first health professional to become aware of the existence of such health problems. Differentiating between symptoms of depression and chronic brain dysfunction may be more possible for a nurse, who frequently has greater contact with a client, than for a physician, who may see the person only briefly. Communication of such observations to other health professionals is important in obtaining appropriate treatment. Case finding among people living alone and somewhat isolated in a community and providing information about resources for recreation, crisis intervention, and social interaction are also appropriate nursing functions that may play a part in prevention.

The frequency with which many health problems coincide with some degree of organic brain dysfunction, particularly in elderly people, points up the need for and importance of ongoing health supervision and teaching for clients with these health problems. Many such people are receiving medical care and have had drugs prescribed for the treatment of the physical disorders. However, even a mild degree of organic dysfunction, and the memory deficit that accompanies it, often makes it difficult for a person to understand, remember, or carry out prescribed treatment. This situation can be complicated by anxiety, attitudes toward taking drugs, ethnic beliefs about illness, food preferences, and a variety of other factors.

Several aspects of health supervision and teaching are particularly relevant preventive measures in working with such clients. *Counseling* that is oriented toward helping people identify the concerns they may have about medications and other treatments, whether these be lack of understanding of purpose, ethnic beliefs about illness, or whatever, will provide a baseline of mutual understanding for nursing intervention and will serve to communicate interest in and concern for clients as individuals.

Frequently, prescribed medical treatment is not followed because a person does not understand or remember the purpose of the therapy or is confused by the variety of pills and capsules ordered by a physician. An understanding of the purpose of each medication and treatment usually overcomes such difficulties. Helping the person to devise an organized system for taking medication can help combat a medication error or omission resulting from a memory deficit. Adapting special diets to accommodate ethnic food preferences may provide a person the incentive necessary to maintain a prescribed dietary regimen. Consultation with family, friends, or people of the same ethnic background as a client can be used for a variety of purposes.

Acting in support of or on behalf of a client— client advocacy—has long been a part of professional nursing practice, and it is currently receiving renewed attention as a part of mental health practice. Client advocacy is particularly important when nurses are working with clients who may be at risk of developing organic brain dysfunction. The objective in both prevention and treatment is to help a person maintain an optimal level of independent functioning. Attempting to cope with the bureaucracies of social agencies, the isolation that confronts older people, and other aspects of our society often requires that a client have the support and assistance of a nurse or other health professionals.

Service as a client advocate can involve a variety of activities or actions carried out in cooperation with a client or, with permission, on the client's behalf. Maintaining contact and cooperation with a physician, clinic, or health agency serving a client can help the nurse to reinforce, clarify, or amplify prescribed medical or other treatment. Assisting a client to contact social, recreational, and other community services and to follow through on appointments are often important aspects of working with people with organic brain disorders. Seeking out social support systems in the community and helping clients to make use of them can help them to overcome isolation and loneliness.

In carrying out an advocacy role for a client, a nurse must protect the client's rights, and any actions must have the full support and approval of the client. Client advocacy may also be carried out in cooperation with or on behalf of a group, class, or community to achieve social goals, through social and political action.

SECONDARY PREVENTION

Secondary prevention in organic brain dysfunction is oriented toward early diagnosis and effective treatment so that a person may be restored to the optimal level of functioning. The professional nurse performs an important function in both aspects of this objective.

For a client in the acute confusional state, early recognition of symptoms of organic dysfunction and prompt treatment of the underlying pathological condition are often essential to preserving the integrity of the brain and, at times, the life of the client. Since the nurse is frequently the health professional in closest contact with the client, he or she may be the first to identify early signs of cognitive dysfunction and thus to take action (including communication of findings to medical and nursing staff) to initiate early treatment. Which treatment is appropriate will depend on the underlying pathology. But it is important to note that symptoms of cognitive dysfunction may, in some instances, be the first indications of systemic and other disorders. Shear and Sacks (1978) note that delirium may be the earliest manifestation of a toxic level of digitalis.

Nursing intervention in acute confusional states is based on the nurse's ability to use the nursing process in assessment and correlation of data and to protect the client and prevent chronicity. Kolb (1977) points out that delirium can be progressive.

Early symptoms include shifting levels of awareness, difficulty in focusing attention, and an inability to screen out irrelevant stimuli. These symptoms may be accompanied by clouding of consciousness or an inability to think clearly or to comprehend what is said. There may be a haziness or vagueness of perception. In later stages there is confusion and disorientation and evidence of memory impairment. In severe stages there may be loss of motor control. Kolb also notes that shifts in degrees of awareness and orientation and changes in emotional responses, from calmness to restlessness, fearfulness to apathy, or irritability to placidity, are always suggestive of delirium.

Nursing process

Nursing intervention in an acute confusional state often depends on the ability of the nurse to assess and interpret symptoms. The nursing history is an important part of the assessment process in delerious states. An understanding, obtained from the family or the client, of the person's functioning prior to the onset of the illness and of the ways in which the person coped with stress may be important in distinguishing chronic from acute brain syndrome and in identifying early symptoms of organic dysfunctions, particularly in the elderly. Pertinent information about many other factors that can contribute to delirium, such as medication, drug and alcohol use, and diet, may be a part of such a history. Correlation of the symptoms with the medical history, the diagnosis, and the laboratory data is also an important aspect of assessment. Communications of findings to other members of the health team, particularly the physician and the nursing staff, is essential to appropriate intervention.

ASSESSMENT

The assessment of a client who is coping with impaired brain function that has led to either an acute or chronic confusional state, should consider the following areas:

1. Presenting symptoms—defects in percep-

tion, attention, memory, and so on, that are creating problems for the client

2. Emotional state—such feelings as helplessness, anxiety or anger that are responses to a stimulus situation
3. Maladaptive coping behaviors—these tend to be regressive patterns (dependency, denial, projection) in attempts to satisfy needs and protect the self-system
4. Origin of maladaptive coping behaviors—identification of stressful experiences in the present that are helping to generate the maladaptive behavior
5. Stimulus situations—stressful life situations that are characterized by a threat to one's security and the frustration of one's attempts to satisfy needs and that can be exacerbated or engendered by losses in cognitive functioning: impaired memory and learning; diminished attention and concentration; distorted perceptions; loss of orientation
6. Holistic health status—physical, intellectual, emotional, sociocultural, and spiritual status of the client, factors that may either facilitate wellness (for example, a concerned and relatively large extended family system may be able to compensate for some of the client's impairment through the care the family members extend to the client) or may impede wellness (for example, the inadequate nutrition of an elderly and poor client may complicate the symptoms of chronic organic brain syndrome)

ANALYSIS OF DATA

As the presenting symptoms, emotional states, maladaptive coping behavior, and stimulus situations are fully assessed, some understanding of the client's (and often of the family's) situation will emerge. Using this understanding, appropriate nursing diagnoses can be made. The following section is concerned with the nursing diagnoses of *acute confusional state* and *chronic confusional state*. The nursing process as it applies to intervening with children and their families has been dis-

cussed in Chapter 15 and will not be repeated here. However, some discussion of important points to remember when intervening with children and their families is included.

Nursing diagnosis: Acute confusional state related to one or more of the following: systemic disorder; infectious disorder; pharmacological agents; alcohol and drug withdrawal; nutritional deficiency; head injury (behavior associated with DSM-III diagnoses under ICD-9-CM, sections 1 and 2, that are characterized by the terms "delirium," "intoxication," "withdrawal," "hallucinosis")

Planning: The nurse* will establish the following goals.

1. Long-term goals
   a. Prevent any chronicity of impaired brain functioning.
   b. Restore the client to normal (premorbid) levels of functioning in all areas.
2. Short-term goals
   a. Preserve the integrity of the brain.
   b. Protect the integrity of the organism as a whole (monitoring of nutrition, safety, and skin care; modulation of environment).
   c. Help to determine the specific cause of the syndrome.
   d. Differentiate between chronic and acute syndrome.
   e. Protect the self-esteem of the client.
   f. Provide support to family and significant others.
   g. Communicate any findings, assessment to other members of the health team (physician; nursing staff).

Implementation: Treatment of a person in an acute confusional state depends on the etiology. In view of the fact that such a state may be precipitated or caused by a broad range of medical problems, therapeutic measures may encompass a broad range of treatments. In some conditions, such as drug and alcohol withdrawal, chemical in-

---

*When a client is in an acute confusional state, the locus of decision making lies with the nurse.

toxication, head trauma, and intracranial neoplasms or infections, an acute confusional state may be an anticipated complication. In other conditions, an organic dysfunction is far less predictable. Some people may be more vulnerable to organic brain dysfunction than other people are. Older people, for example, may be more vulnerable to the toxic effects of prescribed medications or a fluid electrolyte imbalance. A low-grade fever in an elderly person may not be indicative of the degree of an inflammatory process, because the normal physiological responses to inflammation (elevated temperature, elevated white blood count, and so on) may be altered in older people. The temperature, for example, may be only slightly elevated in the presence of a severe inflammatory process. In such a situation, the severity of the disease process may go unrecognized.

Nursing intervention will, of course, include participation in the diagnostic and therapeutic measures employed to care for the client in each situation. A patient, careful, and ongoing explanation of these measures is an essential part of the nurse's participation. Ongoing assessment of the client's responses to the therapeutic measures employed is also an important component of intervention. Regardless of the etiology, some aspects of nursing intervention are applicable to any client with delirium, since they provide protection and aid the client in maintaining cognitive abilities to the extent possible. To achieve these objectives, nursing team planning, in an ongoing process, is essential. These aspects include the following:

1. The number of people providing direct care to the client should be limited; a group should consist of the smallest number possible to provide adequate care. Nurses and other members of the group should function as a team, sharing information and offering guidance and support to each other. A small number of people providing continuity of care will be less demanding of the client's cognitive abilities than a large number and will aid in maintaining orientation to people. Consistency in the staff caring for the client, which is implied in this team concept, will also promote the establishment of supportive relationships.

2. Close supervision of client by team members is important in order to protect safety.

3. The atmosphere should be as quiet as possible to limit distracting external stimuli. Placing a client in a room near the call box results in distraction, as does a room in which or near which there is a high level of activity.

4. Communication with clients in acute confusional states should be brief and clear, and abstractions should be avoided. Questioning should be limited to essential information, and it should be terminated if the client becomes more confused or appears frustrated. Staff members should call patients by name and should also identify themselves by name, avoiding asking if clients remember them.

5. Since clients in acute confusional states are often frightened or anxious, reassurance appropriate to the situation can help allay fears. When it is known that a condition is temporary and directly related to a physical condition, a simple explanation of this fact can be reassuring to a client. Often, the presence and understanding of the nurse are the most important factors in helping allay fears.

6. When possible, the presence of a familiar and caring family member can be a stabilizing factor. This is particularly important when ethnic and language differences exist between the client and the health staff.

7. Disorientation is often more severe during the night, when energy levels are lower and darkness increases the possibility of visual distortion. Keeping the room of a client with delirium well lighted at night may prevent the increase in cognitive dysfunction and development of illusions (visual misperceptions).

In addition to these forms of intervention, which are applicable to anyone experiencing an acute confusional state, there are some conditions in which particular kinds of intervention are indicated. For example, Kolb (1973) points out that in brain injuries, treatment should be started as soon as the individual has regained consciousness. He notes that such clients are often extremely fearful and suggestible. He recommends that an explanation of the injury be given the client and that providing an expectation of the outcome can reassure him. Because of the suggestibility of the client, Kolb (1977) recommends that questions concerning symptoms that the client has not raised should be avoided. He further suggests that, as soon as it is medically feasible, a carefully planned program of progressive physical activity should be instituted. Kolb cautions against overtaxing the client physically, intellectually, or emotionally.

Another condition to which special attention should be given is in intracranial neoplasm. Often, the earliest symptoms of brain tumor are symptoms of brain dysfunction. Acute, temporary disturbances in memory, levels of awareness, and ability to pursue a thought or line of communication may precede other symptoms. The affected person recognizes these disturbances in memory and level of consciousness and becomes terrified. "What is happening to me?" "What does it mean?" "When is it going to happen again?" Such thoughts run through the mind of the sufferer, arousing fear and even panic.

Complicating the picture is the fact that a diagnosis often cannot be made until the intracranial neoplasm is fairly well advanced, especially when the primary site of the neoplasm is in the brain. The prevalence of brain tumors may be far greater than demographic data suggest, and many such clients may be found among people in hospitals. Burgess and Lazare (1973) point out that brain tumors are found in 2% of all persons on whom autopsies are performed, regardless of the cause of death. Only a portion of these can be attributed to metastasis (15% to 20% of all brain tumors are metastatic).

Although nursing intervention is focused on the nursing, rather than the medical, diagnosis, an awareness of the symptom picture, particularly when it is persistent or progressive, can enable the nurse working in the community to make referrals to appropriate diagnostic resources. In addition, a supportive nurse-client relationship may provide an individual with needed emotional support.

Nursing diagnosis: Chronic confusional state related to one or more of the following: systemic disorder (toxic, metabolic, circulatory); genetic disorder; infectious disorder; pharmacological agents; nutritional deficiency; neoplasm; head injury (behavior associated with DSM-III diagnoses ICD-9-CM, sections 1 and 2, that are characterized by the term "dementia")

Planning: With assistance or guidance from the client* when possible, the nurse will establish goals.

1. Long-term goals
   a. Restore the client to highest possible level of functioning in all areas.
   b. Sustain the client and the family in their experiences.
2. Short-term goals
   a. Maintain ongoing assessment and monitoring of the client's status in all areas.
   b. Protect the integrity of the organism as a whole (monitoring of nutrition, safety, skin care; modulation of environment; health teaching and supervision).
   c. Promote the client's ability for independent functioning to the maximum degree possible.
   d. Protect the self-esteem of the client (see Chapter 18).
   e. Communicate any findings, assessment to the other members of the health team.

Implementation: The nature of secondary intervention in chronic brain syndrome depends on the identified needs and the circumstances of the particular client. Needs and circumstances may vary among persons with chronic organic dysfunction as much as they vary in any other group of people. People with chronic brain dysfunction have the

---

*Depending on the severity of the organic impairment, the sharing of the locus of decision making will vary.

same physical, psychological, social, cultural, and spiritual needs as everyone else. The degree to which a client is able to meet these needs depends, to some degree, on the extent of cognitive dysfunction, the state of physical and mental health, the availability of social support networks and community resources, and the individual's economic situation. Needs vary with the age of onset. Subjective reports are not always reliable in clients who are coping with impaired brain function. For this reason, continual ongoing assessment is an integral part of the implementation of any care plan. Ongoing, patient explanations of any diagnostic, medical, or nursing procedures that are being carried out is necessary to minimize any anxiety associated with them.

The major objective in secondary intervention in organic brain syndrome is to promote and sustain, to the maximum degree possible, a client's ability for independent functioning. The following services are essential to meeting this objective.

1. Adequate medical care and health supervision (Treatment and rehabilitation of existing physiological disorders or disabilities are essential. Preventive intervention through health supervision and teaching in such areas as nutrition and hygiene are particulary important for such clients.)
2. Early identification and treatment of emotional disorders such as depression, which can complicate organic dysfunction
3. Preventive measures to promote emotional security and comfort through use of such resources as family, friends, social, religious, and ethnic groups, and community agencies
4. Provision of economic security
5. Availability in the community of resources to provide such services as:
   a. Crisis intervention and emergency medical and psychiatric care
   b. Services to meet economic and social needs
6. Providing information to the client on the availability and location of health, social welfare, recreational, and other community services and serving as client advocate in securing and using these resources

As noted earlier in this chapter, stress and the emotional responses to it may increase the degree of cognitive dysfunction and the usual ability of an individual to cope with daily living. For this reason assessment in chronic brain disturbances must have a multiple focus in the collection and interpretation of data. That is, in addition to assessment of the cognitive functions of comprehension, memory, and orientation, there is also a need to assess mood or affect and the status of physical health and nutrition, as well as to be alert for the presence of psychosocial factors that may be serving as stressors.

For example, a person living alone who develops an abscessed tooth or suffers pain from ill-fitting dentures may become extremely anxious and depressed, lacking the means of transportation to a dentist or the necessary funds to pay for dental services. In addition, the pain and discomfort experienced may make it impossible to eat a normal diet, so that nutrition becomes inadequate. A failure to take into account all of these factors could easily lead to an erroneous impression of the degree of cognitive dysfunction.

A combination of social, economic, health, and other problems, and the fear, anxiety, helplessness, and depression that they often arouse may distort the symptoms of organic brain dysfunction, making a mild or moderate degree of disability appear more severe. Anxiety, for example, can be disorganizing to any personality. For the individual with some degree of organic dysfunction, there may be less ability to cope with the anxiety or with the stress factors that aroused it.

Identification of these variables and intervention to reduce psychosocial stress and provide treatment for physical health problems and emotional disorders can restore a person to an optimal level of functioning. In situations in which there has been an ongoing relationship with a nurse and other members of the health team, sudden changes in the person's ability to function may be readily apparent to those who know the client well. The stress factors that are contributing to the client's anxiety level may also be known to the health team. In other instances, a nurse working in the community, for example, may need to make an initial assessment of the degree of cognitive dysfunction of a new client. This assessment may have to be made in the home, where little information is available about such variables as psychosocial stress.

Goldfarb (1974) points out that two tests, when used in combination, are effective tools for measuring organic brain dysfunction: the ''Mental Status Questionnaire—Special Ten'' and the ''Face Hand Test.'' The Mental Status Questionnaire—Special Ten is a brief (ten questions) questionnaire designed to test orientation to time and place and recent and remote memory of personal and general information. The test is scored on the basis of number of errors given in the responses, to indicate the degree of dysfunction. The Face Hand Test assesses the ability of a client to identify double nonverbal stimuli (touch) when simultaneously touched on one cheek and one hand in an alternating pattern (left hand, right cheek, and so on).

Both tests have been well validated (Goldfarb, 1974); when given together and properly administered and interpreted, they may be useful in determining the degree of cognitive dysfunction in instances in which emotional problems are present. Since many factors in addition to organic disorders can influence responses to questions on a mental status examination, a discrepancy between the findings of the Mental Status Questionnaire and the Face Hand Test may be indicative of depression or other emotional factors. In such an instance, assessment of cognitive functioning may be more difficult.

Although these measurement tools are designed for medical use, familiarity with them could help a professional nurse in the community make an initial assessment of a client's cognitive dysfunction prior to referral or consultation.

Health teaching and supervision are important aspects of nursing intervention for persons with organic brain dysfunctions. Since the majority of such clients are in the older age groups, they are more vulnerable to the degenerative diseases that require close health supervision and adequate medical treatment of underlying physical disorders. A client's economic status may limit the availability of such services. This situation is often complicated by a lack of knowledge of the existence and location of community resources.

Maintaining adequate nutrition is often a problem for clients with organic dysfunction, whether they are treated in the home or in a community agency. Psychosocial factors such as poverty, ethnic background, and lack of transportation, as well as lack of knowledge of nutritional needs, may contribute to poor nutrition. Health teaching for such clients should incorporate an understanding of ethnic food preferences; nutritional teaching and planning should be adapted to these preferences, as well as to economic status.

EVALUATION

Whenever feasible the client and the client's family or significant others should be included in estimating the client's progress toward attainment of goals. Evaluation should encompass the following areas:

1. Estimation of the degree to which there has been improvement and/or stabilization in coping with impaired brain functioning and associated psychosocial losses. This would include *awareness* of conflicts and problem areas and beginning efforts toward working them through.
2. Estimation of the degree to which goals have been achieved and client functioning has improved or stabilized (demonstrated by decreased anxiety; decreased disorder in interpersonal relationships; increased ability to function in society; decreased tendency to use regressive coping mechanisms; reaching maximum potential for self-care; maintaining

an adequate level of safety in functioning through appropriate client-family participation)

3. Identification of goals that need to be modified or revised
4. Referral of the client and the client's family to support systems other than the nurse-client relationship
   a. People in the client's and the client's family's social network who are willing to serve as a support system
   b. Clinics or individuals for ongoing individual and group psychotherapy for client's family members, when indicated
   c. Community agencies that help clients learn to live with disorders that may never be completely eliminated (e.g., day hospital settings structured to meet the needs of organically impaired clients)
   d. Centers or organizations that provide support for families of organically impaired clients (e.g., support groups for families of individuals with Alzheimer's disease)

Children with impaired brain function*

Diagnostic labeling of children is at least as controversial as diagnostic labeling of adults. However, a significant number of children with behavior and learning difficulties are diagnosed as having minimal brain dysfunction. The term "hyperactive syndrome" is sometimes preferred. The terms are used interchangably. The incidence may be as high as 5% to 10% of children who have not reached the age of puberty (Cantwell, 1977). The symptoms that make up the minimal brain dysfunction or hyperactive syndrome include "hyperactivity, distractibility, excitability," and a shortened attention span (Cantwell, 1977).

Whether or not such behavioral manifestations are due to organic dysfunction is debatable. Such symptoms have, in the past, been attributed to a

*See Chapter 15.

variety of emotional disorders in children. Cantwell (1977) observes that we lack the ability to determine the degree of brain dysfunction in children. Others observe that we lack diagnostic criteria for assessing brain dysfunction in children. A major disadvantage of attributing these behavioral manifestations in children to organic dysfunction is the connotation of irreversibility that often accompanies such a diagnosis, and the possibility that less effort may, therefore, be expended in treatment.

Despite the controversy, we have included a brief discussion of secondary prevention for such children and their families in this chapter on organic dysfunction. It should be remembered that treatment measures and nursing functions are applicable whether or not the symptoms are regarded as evidence of brain dysfunction.

The major objectives in secondary intervention in cases involving children are to promote normal development, including education, of the children to the extent possible and to provide the supportive services to their families that are essential to achieving the goals for the children. These objectives are dependent on the availability of human services to meet the needs of the children and families. Among these services are the following.

SCHOOLS FOR SPECIAL EDUCATION

Schools for special education offer very small classes, with teachers who have special training in working with hyperactive children. An essential ingredient in schools providing special education is the availability, at least on a part-time basis, of a mental health team with special preparation in pediatric psychiatry. The availability of a psychiatrist, a psychologist, a social worker, and a child mental health nurse is important in planning, implementing, and evaluating the coordination of therapeutic and educational objectives for each child. The mental health team is also a resource for supportive measures with teachers, parents, and teacher assistants working with the children.

COMPREHENSIVE HEALTH SERVICES

In addition to providing health supervision and teaching, comprehensive health services can provide family counseling, crisis intervention, and group and family therapy to families of hyperactive children. The treatment objectives for the child are to reduce hyperactivity, to change disruptive behavioral patterns, and to promote mental health. Various therapeutic modalities are used in combination to achieve these objectives. Reducing the hyperactivity and excitability of a child is often essential to the promotion of health development and to the child's participation in the educational process. Medication is often prescribed to reduce hyperactivity. It is somewhat paradoxical that central nervous system stimulants are more effective in reducing hyperactivity in children than are sedative drugs. Cantwell (1977) recommends the use of methylphenidate (Ritalin) or d-amphetamine as the drugs of choice. Behavior therapy is often employed to change patterns of behavior that may be disruptive in the home and school. Play therapy and other forms of psychotherapy are employed in combination with the other therapies to promote normal development.

COMPREHENSIVE SOCIAL SERVICES

Maintaining a hyperactive or emotionally disturbed child in the home may cause social and economic problems for a family far beyond those involved in raising a normal child. Although it is generally agreed that home care for such a child is far superior to institutional care, government funding in many areas tends to favor the institutions. Providing social services to families to meet economic and other social problems is essential. Social and political action to achieve this goal is an important aspect of secondary prevention in meeting the needs of families with hyperactive children. Assisting families in the utilization of the resources that do exist is an important aspect of client advocacy.

Nursing intervention for hyperactive children may involve working with the children, their families, and often teachers and other members of the educational system involved with the children. Collaboration and cooperation between schools providing special educational services and facilities providing comprehensive health services is essential to meeting health and educational objectives. Coordination of these services is often a function of the community health nurse. Health supervision on the part of the school nurse–teacher or community health nurse offers an opportunity for case finding and referral of children in whom learning and behavioral difficulties may be indicative of organic dysfunction or hyperactive syndrome. Health supervision of children also includes identifying physical health problems that may only be expressed through such behavioral manifestations as increased hyperactivity and excitability.

Nursing intervention for families of hyperactive children might include group discussions with parents or groups of parents, with the objective being to assist the parents in identifying problems and developing strategies for coping with their hyperactive children. Participation, in the home, to help families to follow behavior therapy programs designed to shape behavior patterns in children is often an important nursing function. Close cooperation between the nurse and the behavior therapist is essential to this kind of endeavor. Crisis intervention and home visits to provide support for parents are additional nursing activities that can assist parents of hyperactive children.

The nurse working in a school serving hyperactive children has opportunities beyond those related to health supervision. Direct participation in the classroom with the teacher offers an opportunity for assessment of behavior, through observation in the class setting, and for participation with one or more children in meeting mental health and education objectives. Such a nurse may want to establish nurse-client relationships with individual children. Participation in group meetings with teachers and other staff members offers the opportunity to share experiences and insights and to plan strategies for meeting mental health and educational objectives.

TERTIARY PREVENTION

As noted earlier, some individuals cope to the cognitive impairment associated with organic brain dysfunction and are able to function adequately in their culture, except at times of crisis, when supportive services may be needed. In this respect, such individuals differ little from the general population, with the possible exception of a greater vulnerability to stress and a somewhat diminished capacity to cope with stress without assistance.

In other individuals the cognitive dysfunction and associated psychosocial factors may inhibit the ability to care for oneself and may become progressively incapacitating. Perception, memory, orientation, and judgment may be so impaired that an individual cannot be responsible for his or her own care. Such individuals require a fairly constant level of care and supervision by other people. They may be found living with families who are willing and able to care for them or in mental hospitals or other institutions. Whatever the decision of the family as far as institutionalization is concerned, the nurse can play an important role in providing information during the family's decision-making process and support of the family that combats destructive guilt and helps maximize their continuing involvement with the client.

Whether it is given in the home or in a community agency, care for such individuals has the following major objectives:

1. Promoting and maintaining the optimum level of functioning possible for the individual
2. Promoting a sense of dignity and worth
3. Maintaining physical health and well-being by means of adequate diagnostic measures so that treatment may be instituted for those conditions that may respond to treatment
4. Maintaining and promoting reality orientation

5. Encouraging independent functioning to the degree possible
6. Providing opportunity to meet psychosocial needs, such as recreation, intellectual stimulation, and socialization
7. Providing support when needed

Meeting such treatment objectives necessitates close cooperation between the health team members and, when possible, between the family and the health team. Since the nurse is often the health professional in the most direct and continuous contact with the client, some responsibility for promoting interdisciplinary team functioning often rests with nursing members of the health team. The role of liaison between the client and family and between members of the health team is an important function of the nurse, whether the client resides in an agency or at home.

A therapeutic environment is especially important in meeting objectives for providing protection, support, and rehabilitation for clients. The therapeutic milieu as a treatment modality that employs all aspects of the environment to promote health has been discussed in earlier chapters. Special emphasis in a milieu treating clients with brain dysfunction should be placed on providing physical and emotional support, encouraging independent functioning to the extent possible for the individual, and promoting reality orientation.

Maintaining orientation can be encouraged through the placement of large-faced clocks and calendars in prominent places and through individual and group discussions focused on events associated with daily living and affairs of interest in the broader community. Contact between the community and the hospital or agency unit may also be used to stimulate interest and interaction between clients and the broader environment. Use of community resources for recreation, health care, support systems, and so on is important in preventing the isolation of a client.

Recreational, occupational, and movement therapies are important in promoting mental and physical health. Such therapies should be adapted to the interests and physical abilities of clients.

Interpersonal therapies, both individual and group, are important modalities in maintaining emotional security. The nurse-client relationship, which has been discussed at length in earlier chapters, provides opportunity for emotional support.

CHAPTER SUMMARY

The organic brain disorders are a group of complex conditions that involve disturbances in cognition caused by disruptions in the normal neurophysiological processes essential to intellectual functioning. Behavioral manifestations of cognitive impairment include disturbances in levels of awareness, comprehension, memory, association, orientation, and judgment, which interfere with a person's ability to perceive, interpret, and respond effectively to the environment. The cognitive dysfunction may range from mild to severe, and it is often accompanied by emotional responses of fear, anger, feelings of helplessness, and depression.

Organic brain dysfunction may be acute and temporary, in which case the individual recovers completely in a relatively brief period of time with appropriate treatment and effective restorative processes. In other instances, the brain dysfunction may be chronic and irreversible because of a continuing disturbance in metabolic functioning or a diffuse destruction of brain tissue.

The etiology of organic brain dysfunction may lie in any systemic or central nervous system pathological condition, including metabolic disorders, systemic and central nervous system infections, trauma, and conditions caused by chemicals and drugs. In some chronic forms, the etiology is unknown, in which case the onset is often slow and insidious, rather than acute.

Therapeutic modalities in the treatment of acute organic brain dysfunction include the early diagnosis and treatment of the underlying pathological condition so that cognitive dysfunction may be reversed or ameliorated. In some acute disorders, early diagnosis may be essential to preventing progressive dysfunction, which can lead to coma and death. Which specific treatment is used depends on etiology. For the client with acute brain dysfunction, who is most often seen in a general hospital, nursing assessment of cognitive dysfunction may be very important to early diagnosis.

Treatment modalities in chronic brain dysfunction have the objective of promoting independent functioning to the maximum degree possible. They include adequate medical and nursing care for treatment and rehabilitation of physical and emotional disorders and preventive intervention through health teaching and supervision. Preventive measures to promote emotional security and comfort include client advocacy in the use of community resources to meet psychosocial needs and in the development and strengthening of social networks. In addition, a protective therapeutic environment, all of the forms of psychosocial therapy, and chemotherapy are employed. Treatment settings include general hospitals, private homes, foster homes, nursing homes, and mental hospitals.

Clients with organic brain dysfunction may be found in almost every area in which professional nurses practice. Nursing intervention spans both the preventive and the therapeutic aspects of organic brain disorders, although not every nurse will be involved in every area. Primary prevention encompasses the nurse's role both as a citizen and as a health professional. As a citizen, participation in social, political, and community action groups that seek to reduce environmental pollution, promote occupational safety, or provide community facilities to meet the needs of vulnerable individuals is an important preventive activity. Professional roles include health education, genetic counseling, case finding, and client advocacy in meeting health and psychosocial needs.

Secondary prevention and tertiary prevention include collaboration with the health team, participation in therapeutic modalities, health supervision and promotion, and participation in individual and group activities that promote the emotional comfort and the cognitive functioning of clients.

SENSITIVITY-AWARENESS EXERCISES

The purposes of the following exercises are:

- Develop awareness about the interrelationship of factors in the etiology of organic brain syndromes
- Develop awareness about the subjective experience of clients who are coping with impaired brain functioning
- Develop awareness about the subjective experience of the families of clients who are coping with impaired brain functioning
- Develop awareness about your own feelings and attitudes in working with clients who are coping with impaired brain functioning

1. Try to imagine that you are suffering with either an acute organic brain syndrome or a chronic organic brain syndrome.
2. Describe what you think that experience would entail. Describe some of your symptoms and how you might cope with them.
3. Describe what you think it would be like to be the family member of someone who is suffering from an organic brain syndrome. How would you cope with this situation? What are your thoughts and feelings about institutionalization if a family member of yours was coping with a chronic organic brain syndrome?
4. Develop a plan of care for assisting a family to cope with a client with impaired brain functioning:
   a. When the family has decided that it is necessary to institutionalize the client
   b. When the family has decided to care for the client at home

REFERENCES

Baldessarini, R.J.
   1977 Chemotherapy in Psychiatry. Cambridge, Mass: Harvard University Press.
Burgess, A., and A. Lazare
   1973 Psychiatric Nursing in the Hospital and the Community. Englewood Cliffs, N.J.: Prentice-Hall, Inc.
Butler, R.N.
   1975a "Psychiatry and the elderly: An overview." American Journal of Psychiatry 132(9):893-900.
   1975b Why Survive? Being Old in America. New York: Harper & Row, Publishers, Inc.

Cantwell, D.P.
   1977 "Drug treatment of the hyperactive syndrome in children." In Psychopharmacology in the Practice of Medicine. M.E. Jarvick (ed.). New York: Appleton-Century-Crofts.
Coyle, J., D. Price, and M. DeLong
   1983 "Alzheimer's disease: A disorder of cortical cholinergic innervation." Science 219:1184-1189.
Eisdorfer, C., and R.O. Friedel
   1977 "Psychotherapeutic drugs in aging." In Psychopharmacology in the Practice of Medicine. M.E. Jarvik (ed.). New York: Appleton-Century-Crofts.
Goldfarb, A.I.
   1974 "Minor maladjustments of the aged." In American Handbook of Psychiatry (ed. 2), Vol. 3. S. Arieti and E. Brody (eds.). S. Arieti (ed.-in-chief). New York: Basic Books, Inc., Publishers, Ch. 37.
Heller, S.S., and D.S. Kornfeld
   1974 "Delirium and related problems." In American Handbook of Psychiatry (ed. 2), Vol. 4. M.F. Reiser (ed.). S. Arieti (ed.-in-chief). New York: Basic Books, Inc., Publishers.
Herbert, W.
   1983 "Mental illness from psychiatric drugs?" Science News 124(14):214.
Kolb, L.C.
   1973 Modern Clinical Psychiatry (ed. 8). Philadelphia: W.B. Saunders Co.
   1977 Modern Clinical Psychiatry (ed. 9). Philadelphia: W.B. Saunders Co.
Kotala, G.
   1983 "Huntington's disease gene located." Science 222:913-915.
Lehman, H.
   1983 "Psychopharmacological approaches to the organic brain syndrome." Comprehensive Psychiatry, 24(5):412-430.
Leighton, A.H.
   1974 "Social disintegration and mental disorders." In American Handbook of Psychiatry (ed. 2), Vol. 2. G. Caplan (ed.). S. Arieti, (ed-in-chief). New York: Basic Books, Inc., Publishers, Ch. 28.
Levick, S.
   1980 "Dementia from aluminum pots?" New England Journal of Medicine 303(3):164.
Luckman, J., and K. Sorensen
   1974 Medical-Surgical Nursing: A Psychophysiologic Approach. Philadelphia: W.B. Saunders Co.
McAllister, T.
   1983 "Overview: Pseudodementia." American Journal of Psychiatry, 140(5):528-532.

Miller, J.

1983 "Venezuelan connection." Science News 124: 408-411.

Raskus, R.S., S. Lerner, and B.E. Kline

1979 "The elderly patient in a therapeutic community." Comprehensive Psychiatry 20:4.

Roberts, E.

1982 "Potential therapies in aging and senile dementias." In "Alzheimer's disease, Down's syndrome, and aging." Annals of the New York Academy of Sciences 396:175.

Seltzer, B., and S.H. Frazier

1978 "Organic mental disorders." In The Harvard Modern Guide to Psychiatry. Armand M. Nicholi, Jr. (ed.). Cambridge, Mass.: Belknap Press of Harvard University Press.

Seltzer, B., and I. Sherwin

1978 "Organic brain syndromes: An empirical study and critical review." American Journal of Psychiatry 135(1):13-21.

Shear, K.M., and M.H. Sacks

1978 "Digitalis delirium: Report of two cases." American Journal of Psychiatry 135(1):109-110.

Perl, D., and A. Brody

1980 "Alzheimer's disease: X-ray spectrometric evidence of aluminum accumulation in neurofibrillary tangle-bearing neurons." Science 208:297-299.

Spector, R.E.

1979 Cultural Diversity in Health and Illness. New York: Appleton-Century-Crofts.

Sinex, F., and C. Merril (eds.)

1982 "Alzheimer's disease, Down's syndrome, and aging." Annals of the New York Academy of Sciences, vol. 396.

Tanne, J.

1983 "Alzheimer's and aluminum: an element of suspicion." American Health 2(5):48-54.

Trapp, G., et al.

1978 "Aluminum levels in brain in Alzheimer's disease." Biological Psychiatry 13:709-718.

Tuerk, K., I. Fish, and J. Ransohoff

1974 "Head injury." In American Handbook of Psychiatry (ed. 2), Vol. 4. M.F. Reiser (ed.). S. Arieti (ed.-in-chief). New York: Basic Books, Inc., Publishers, Ch. 7.

Wells, C.E.

1978 "Chronic brain disease: An overview." American Journal of Psychiatry 135(1):1-12.

Wender, P.H., and L. Eisenberg

1974 "Minimal brain dysfunction in children." In American Handbook of Psychiatry (ed. 2), Vol. 2. G. Caplan (ed.). S. Arieti (ed.-in-chief). New York: Basic Books, Inc., Publishers, Ch. 8.

Whitehouse, P., et al.

1982 "Alzheimer's disease and senile dementia: Loss of neurons in the basal forebrain." Science 215:1237-1239.

ANNOTATED SUGGESTED READINGS

Davidhizar, R., and E. Gunden

1978 "Recognizing and caring for the delirious patient." Journal of Psychiatric Nursing and Mental Health Services 16(5):38-41.

This article focuses on nursing assessment and intervention in acute organic dysfunction. The importance of early intervention in this acute condition and the role of the nurse in early identification and treatment are stressed.

Goldfarb, A.I.

1974 "Minor maladjustments of the aged." In The American Handbook of Psychiatry (ed. 2), Vol. 3. S. Arieti and E.B. Brody (eds.). S. Arieti (ed.-in-chief). New York: Basic Books Inc., Publishers, Ch. 37.

The author, an expert in problems of the aging, takes a holistic view of the aging process and its impact on the individual. Particular emphasis is placed on recognizing and distinguishing between depression (or other psychiatric conditions) and organic brain dysfunction in the older person. The author includes measurement tools that have proved useful in distinguishing between organic brain syndrome and depression.

Lehamn, H.

1983 "Psychopharmacological approaches to the organic brain syndrome." Comprehensive Psychiatry 24(5): 412-430.

In addition to a discussion about advances in the pharmacological treatment of the organic brain syndromes, this excellent article gives an overview of definitions, epidemiology, treatment issues, and symptomatology. Differential diagnoses are also included.

McAllister, T.

1983 "Overview: Pseudodementia." American Journal of Psychiatry 140(5):528-533.

A review of the literature on the syndrome of pseudodementia. This disorder is particularly common in the elderly and it presents a diagnostic and therapeutic dilemma to the practitioner who must differentiate the cognitive impairment of depression from organically based dementia. The author suggests that there are actually at least two categories of pseudodementia: (1) pseudodementia without associated cerebral dysfunction and (2) pseudodementia with coexisting cerebral dysfunction. Prognosis for the first group is better than it is for the second. In addition to a review of the literature, some clinical case material is presented, as well as suggestions for future research in this area.

Pajk, M., B. Reisberg, and I. Beam
  1984 ''Continuing education: Alzheimer's disease.'' American Journal of Nursing, 84(2):215-232.
    Three separate articles comprise this continuing education presentation for credit units: ''Inpatient care'' by M. Pajk; ''Stages of cognitive decline'' by B. Reisberg; and ''Helping families survive'' by I. Beam. These articles represent a comprehensive approach to understanding the etiology, course, and treatment of Alzheimer's disease. Appropriate interventions for each level of cognitive impairment and for supportive care for the family are included.

Seltzer, B., and S.H. Frazier
  1978 ''Organic mental disorders.'' In The Harvard Modern Guide to Psychiatry. A.M. Nicoli, Jr. (ed.). Cambridge, Mass.: Belknap Press of Harvard University Press.
    The authors provide a background for understanding the neuropsychiatric disorders that are caused by diffuse impairment of brain tissue functioning. The entire range of organic dysfunction—from the acute confusional states to severe organic brain syndromes—is discussed in relation to newer developments in neurophysiology and brain function.

Wells, C.E.
  1978 ''Chronic brain disease: An overview.'' American Journal of Psychiatry 135:1.
    This article provides an overview of current thinking about organic brain disease of a chronic nature. The importance of adequate diagnostic and treatment measures is stressed, and the need for basic research in relation to organic brain disease is emphasized.

Glossary

accommodation—A Piagetian term referring to the identification and elimination of disequilibrium. As accommodation occurs, more accurate perceptions result.

acculturation—The process of reciprocal retentions, losses, and/or adaptations of culture patterns that results when members of two or more cultural groups interact

acute confusional state—Acute brain dysfunction caused by any interference with the complex biochemical or metabolic processes essential to brain functioning. Symptoms include disturbances in cognition, levels of awareness, memory, and orientation, accompanied by restlessness, apprehension, irritability, and apathy. SYNONYMS: delirium, acute delirious state, acute brain syndrome, toxic psychosis

adaptation—Adjusting one's responses in order to cope with internal or external stress

addictive personality—characterized by compulsive and habitual use of a substance or practice to cope with psychic pain engendered by conflict and anxiety.

affect—Mood, emotion, or feeling tone

agoraphobia—Irrational fear of open spaces or of entering public places alone, because of a psychic phenomenon in which internal fears or anxiety are projected onto an aspect of the environment

alienation—A failure in reciprocal connectedness between a person and significant others; estrangement of self from others

alternation rules—The rules that establish the options available to a person when he or she is speaking to someone else. Social categories such as kinship, sex, status, age, and type of interpersonal relationship influence the range of alternatives available to a speaker.

ambivalence—The simultaneous existence of strong feelings of both love and hate toward a person, an object, or a situation

amnesia—An emergency response to stress and anxiety in which a part or all of a person's past life is forgotten or forced out of awareness through repression

anal phase—In psychosexual development, the stage that encompasses ages 15 months to 3 years. Libidinal energy is shifted from the mouth as a source of gratification to the anus.

andropause—The return to the nonreproductive state of function of the male genitalia. Andropause occurs later than menopause, usually beginning in the middle to late fifties.

anger—A sense of intense tension or discomfort that arises when a goal is thwarted

anhedonia—An inability to find pleasure in situations that would normally be pleasurable

anomie—A state of alienation and disassociation from social values and beliefs; normlessness

anorexia nervosa—A condition characterized by excessive dieting, which is often carried to the point of severe malnutrition and emaciation and which, in some instances, leads to death through starvation

anticipatory planning—The identification of possible stressors in one's life—for example, pregnancy or change in job—and the initiation of the problem-solving process to reduce or eliminate a crisis situation before it occurs

antisocial personality—Characterized by impulsive and asocial behavior, poor judgment, irresponsibility, and lack of insight into the consequences of one's behavior

anxiety—A diffuse feeling of apprehension and of dread of being threatened or alienated. The threat may be real or perceived. Anxiety can maintain one's alertness, or it can immobilize an individual.

anxiety disorders—Conditions characterized by overt physiological and psychological manifestations of anxiety in which there are no stable defense mechanisms to enable the person to cope with the anxiety. This form of neurosis may be chronic, or it may occur in acute attacks. Generalized anxiety disorder, panic disorder, phobic disorders, and obsessive-compulsive disorders are types of anxiety disorders.

apathy—A blunting of affect; an absence of feeling from a psychological point of view

approximation—The movement of one individual toward another in the development of an interpersonal relationship

associative looseness—A thinking disorder in which relationships among ideas are autistically determined

assimilation—A Piagetian term referring to an individual's ability to comprehend and integrate new experiences

asthenic personality—Characterized by constant and extreme fatigue, listlessness, and indecisiveness. Asthenic personality is believed to be a precursor of neurasthenia.

attention deficit disorders—Disorders characterized by short attention span, clumsiness, lack of symmetry of hand movements, intellectual and memory faults, restlessness, and quarrelousness. Hyperactivity may or may not be present.

attitudes—Major integrative forces in the development of personality that give consistency to an individual's behavior. Attitudes are cognitive in nature, formed through interactions with the environment. Attitudes serve to direct an individual's commitments and responsibilities; they reflect innermost convictions about what is good or bad, right or wrong, desirable or undesirable.

authority—The right to use power to command behavior, enforce rules, and make decisions. Authority is often based on rank or position in a social hierarchy, and it may be either of two types: line authority or staff authority.

autism—Exclusive focus is on the self. Subjective, introspective thinking and a good deal of fantasy are prominent aspects of autism.

autistic phase—In Mahler's system of preoedipal development, the stage from birth to 1 month. This is termed *normal autism,* and it gradually changes as children become aware that they cannot satisfy their needs by themselves.

aversion therapy—A type of negative conditioning that uses learning theory to change behavior from maladaptive to adaptive

basic group identity—Shared social characteristics such as world view, language, and value and ideological systems. Basic group identity evolves from membership in an ethnic group.

biogenic—Motivated by physiological states

bipolar depressive response—An affective disorder that is characterized by symptoms of both depression and mania

blame placing—Process of placing responsibility for one's behavior, and especially misbehavior, on others

body image—An individual's conscious and unconscious perceptions of his or her body. Body image is an integral component of self-concept.

boundary maintenance mechanisms—Behavior and practices that exclude members of some groups from the customs and values of a particular group

bulimia—An eating disorder characterized by binge eating (often done in secret) and by self-induced purging

castration—Removal of the testes in a male or the ovaries in a female

catatonic schizophrenia—A type of schizophrenia. In the *catatonic stupor* form, prominent symptoms may include stupor, stereotypical behavior, cerea flexibilitas (waxy flexibility), and negativism. In the *catatonic excitement* form, there may be hyperkinesia, stereotypical behavior, bizarre mannerisms, and impulsivity.

catharsis—A therapeutic outpouring of repressed ideas or conflicts through verbalization and working through of conscious material. An appropriate emotional reaction accompanies catharsis.

cerea flexibilitas—Waxy flexibility—a symptom often seen in catatonic schizophrenia. The individual's muscular system is in a condition that permits the molding of arms and legs into any position where they will remain indefinitely.

change agent—A person who tries to influence the making and implementing of decisions in the direction of change

character neuroses—Character neuroses are personality organizations characterized by excessive anxiety and unconscious conflict in which the compromise solutions needed to maintain adjustment or adaptation result in rigidity of personality and inhibit interpersonal relations, although there are no overt clinical symptoms.

childhood-onset pervasive developmental disorders— Disturbances in thought, affect, social relatedness, and behavior that emerge between the ages of 30 months and 12 years

childhood triad—Three types of behavior (firesetting, bedwetting, and cruelty to animals) that when used in combination and consistently may predict emerging sociopathy

chronic, undifferentiated schizophrenia—The symptoms of more than one of the classic types of schizophrenia (simple, paranoid, catatonic, hebrephrenic) are demonstrated in this category.

circum-speech—Behavior characteristic of conversation. Instrumentals, markers, interactional behavior, demonstratives, and stress kinesics are types of circum-speech.

circumstantiality—A speech pattern in which there is difficulty in screening out irrelevant material in describing an event. The inclusion of many irrelevant details results in a lengthy and rambling account before the end point is reached. This speech pattern may be found in chronic brain dysfunction.

coalition across generational boundaries—A conspiracy or alliance between a parent and a child. Such a conspiracy is usually against the other parent.

coding—The process of categorizing information. Information is sorted and then stored in various types of memory codes.

cognition—The processing of information by the nervous system. This processing structures reality and gives meaning to human experience.

cognitive dissonance—A state of disequilibrium and tension produced when two or more sets of information are at variance with one another

cohesiveness, group—The quality of unity that characterizes a group. It results from all of the factors, evident and subtle, that interact to encourage close bonds among group members so that the group tends to stay together.

command hallucination—A hallucinated voice that an individual experiences as commanding him or her to perform a certain act. Command hallucinations may influence a person to engage in behavior that is dangerous to himself, herself, or others.

communication theme—A recurrent idea or concept that underlies and ties together communication. There are three types of communication themes: content theme (the idea that underlies or links together seemingly varied topics of discussion), mood theme (the affect or emotion an individual communicates), interaction theme (the idea or concept that best describes the dynamics between communicating participants).

community mental health—The prevention, early diagnosis, effective treatment, and rehabilitation of people with mental disorders and disabilities in geographically defined communities, through a network of collaborative health and social welfare systems, community organizations, and consumers

compulsion—A persistent, irrational need or urge to perform a particular act or acts. A compulsion, which often has the quality of a ritual, serves a defensive purpose by controlling anxiety, guilt, and other noxious feelings.

compuphobia—Irrational fear of working with computers, which may arise from anxiety engendered by a sense of inadequacy, helplessness, or loss of control

concrete thinking—Part of the thought disorder characteristic of schizophrenia. Concrete thinking is a primitive way of thinking in which an individual tends to take the literal meanings of ideas. It is indicative of a difficulty in abstracting.

conduct disorders—Disorders of childhood characterized by either socialized or unsocialized aggressive behaviors, such as stealing, lying, truancy, promiscuity, and cheating. The purpose of such behavior is to enhance self-esteem and provide courage in anxiety-producing situations.

conductor—A term used to describe a family therapist who uses his or her own dynamic personality to give direction to a family in therapy.

confabulation—An adaptive or defensive phenomenon in which a person with memory deficits fills in gaps in memory with relevant but imaginary information

conscience—The part of the superego system that monitors thoughts, feelings, and actions and measures them against internalized values and standards

conscious—The conscious level of experience includes those aspects of experience that are in awareness at any given time. Consciousness is a psychodynamic concept that embraces three levels of awareness, each of which influences behavior. These levels are the conscious, the preconscious, and the unconscious.

consensual validation—A term coined by Harry Stack

Sullivan that refers to a method for diminishing interpersonal and communication distortions. It involves a comparison of one's evaluations of experience with those of another person.

consolidation of individuality and emotional object constancy—The fourth and final subphase of the separation-individuation phase of preoedipal development (in Mahler's system). It begins toward the end of the second year, and it is seen as open ended. A degree of object constancy is accomplished, and separation of self and object representations is established.

consumer—An individual, group, or community that utilizes a product or service. In the area of mental health, consumerism refers to the utilization of all levels of mental health services (services designed for primary, secondary, and tertiary prevention of mental illness).

conversion—The transformation of unacceptable, anxiety-provoking impulses into sensorimotor symptoms such as paralysis or blindness. There is no organic basis for such impairment. Conversion is an emergency response to stress.

coping mechanisms—Measures utilized to reduce tension. These measures are often learned through early interactions with significant others in the environment.

coprolalia—Excessive use of profane language

countersociety—A society that runs counter to or against the established society in which it exists

countertransference—An emotional and often unconscious process in the helping person that is related to the client and that has an effect on the therapeutic interaction between therapist and client

crisis—A situation that cannot be readily resolved by an individual's normal repertoire of coping strategies. A crisis is precipitated by an actual or perceived threat to self-esteem or physical integrity.

crisis intervention—Provision of immediate treatment for individuals undergoing acute psychological distress

cultural event—The communication of meaning that takes place each time one member of a society interacts with another member

culturally specific—Unique to a particular culture and a function of that cultural context

culture—An ordered system of shared and socially transmitted symbols and meanings that structures world view and guides behavior

culture shock—A drastic change in the cultural environment that is both precipitated by and a response to cognitive dissonance

cyclothymic personality—Characterized by vacillation between depression and elation. Differentiation between cyclothymic personality and manic depressive psychosis is a matter of degree of symptomatology.

day hospital—A psychiatric facility where formerly hospitalized clients participate in a therapeutic program during the normal working hours

deinstitutionalization—The practice of discharging chronically mentally ill clients into the community

delirium—See *acute confusional state*

delusion—A false belief (other than a commonly believed myth or superstition of a culture)

dementia praecox—An outdated term used to describe schizophrenia. Dementia (insanity) praecox (youthful) was used to distinguish schizophrenia from the dementias of later life, such as senility.

demonstrative—A type of circum-speech that accompanies and illustrates speech

denial—Unconsciously motivated behavior that manifests itself as evasion or negation of objective reality

dependence—Reliance on others in the environment to meet needs for nurturance, security, love, shelter, and sustenance

dependent personality—Characterized by excessive or compulsive needs for attention, acceptance, and approval from other people in order to maintain security and self-esteem and to resolve neurotic conflict. Dependent personality is a concept of Karen Horney.

depersonalization—A state in which an individual feels a loss of personal identity. The feeling that the environment is also changed and unreal may also be present. This latter feeling is termed *derealization.*

depression—An extension of the grieving process that is considered abnormal. Depression can be described in terms of affect, mood disorder, and a cluster of clinical symptoms.

developmental crisis—A period of vulnerability encountered as one progresses from one developmental stage to the next

differentiation—The first subphase of the separation-individuation phase in Mahler's system of preoedipal development. It occurs from approximately 5 months to 9 months of age. This phase coincides with maturation of partial locomotor functioning and the differentiation of a primitive but distinct body image. At this time, the child begins tentative moves away from the mother and begins to view her as a separate being.

discreditable people—Refers to people who, if their socially deviant behavior were visible or known, would be devalued and condemned by society. For instance, "secret" alcoholics and prostitutes are discreditable people.

discredited people—Refers to people who, because their socially deviant behavior is visible or known, are devalued and condemned by society. For instance, known alcoholics and prostitutes are discredited people.

displacement—Unconscious transferal of strivings or feelings from the original object to a different object, activity, or situation

dissociative disorders—Characterized by psychiatric symptoms that represent a form of psychological flight from the self. A part or all of the personality is denied or dissociated from present reality. Psychogenic amnesia, psychogenic fugue, and multiple personality are types of dissociative disorders.

distance regulation—Behavior that marks off a quantum of space. Three types of distance are maintained: flight distance (distance that a wild animal will tolerate between itself and an enemy before fleeing), personal distance (the normal spacing maintained between animals of the same species), and social distance (maximal distance before a social animal begins to feel either psychologically threatened or physically and socially isolated from the group).

double-bind communication—A communication pattern that involves the giving of two conflicting messages at the same time. One message may be verbal and the other nonverbal, or both messages may be verbal. The conflicting nature of the messages serves to immobilize and confuse the listener.

dyad—A combination of two—for example, husband and wife, parent and child

dyspareunia—An abnormal condition in women, in which pain is experienced during sexual intercourse. The condition may be caused by inadequate lubrication of the vagina.

echolalia—Imitating and repeating the speech of another person. Echolalia is a pathological form of speech that is demonstrated by some schizophrenic individuals.

echopraxia—Imitating and repeating the body movements of another person. Echopraxia is a symptom demonstrated by some schizophrenic individuals.

educational therapy—Educational and vocational training programs designed to develop self-esteem, group identification, and school and occupational adjustment

ego—The part of the personality that is in interaction with the external environment and with somatic and psychic aspects of the internal environment. Ego functions, which encompass intellectual and social abilities, maintain an equilibrium between id and superego, as well as the integrity of the personality in coping with stress.

egocentricity—The tendency to view one's own thoughts and ideas as the best possible, without considering the views of others.

ego-dystonic—An adjective used to describe ideas, defenses, or behaviors that are unacceptable to a person and inconsistent with his or her total personality. SYNONYM: ego-alien

ego-syntonic—An adjective used to describe ideas, defenses, or behaviors that are acceptable to a person and consistent with his or her total personality

electroconvulsive therapy (ECT)—A somatic therapy in which electric current is applied to the brain through electrodes placed on the temporal areas of the skull. The desired generalized convulsion is precipitated by applying 70 to 130 volts for 0.1 to 0.5 seconds. The treatment is used in mania, depression, and certain cases of schizophrenia. SYNONYM: Electrostimulation therapy (EST), Electric shock therapy

emotional divorce—A schism that occurs when emotional investment between spouses is withdrawn

empathy—The ability to understand and share the emotions and thoughts of another person without losing one's objectivity

enculturation—The process of learning the conceptual and behavioral systems of one's culture

equilibration—The balancing and integrating of new experiences with those of the past as an individual progresses along a developmental course

Eros—According to Freud, the instinct for life

ethnic culture—The attitudinal, value, and behavioral patterns associated with an ethnic group

ethnic enclave—An area in a city, town, or village that is populated by a minority ethnic group

ethnic group—A collectivity of people organized around an assumption of common origin

ethnic heritage—The cultural history that is passed from generation to generation within an ethnic group

ethnic identification—Where a person places himself or herself on the "ethnic chart"

ethnic interaction—An interaction in which interpersonal relationships are based on ethnic affiliation

ethnocentrism—The attitude that one ethnic group's folkways are superior and right and those of other ethnic groups are inferior and wrong. Each ethnic group uses its culture as a standard for judging all other cultures.

euthymism—Normal mood responses

explosive personality—Characterized by episodes of uncontrollable rage and physical abusiveness in response to relatively minor pressures

experience—A person's reaction, consisting of perception, interpretation and response, to a situation or event

extended family—A family unit consisting of three or more generations

family—A group of people who are united by bonds of kinship, at least two of whom are conjugally related

family disorganization—Breakdown of the family system; associated with parental overburdening and/or loss of significant others who served as role models for children or support systems for family members. Such a breakdown of the family may contribute to the loss of social controls that families usually impose on their members.

family myths—A communication pattern involving the construction of myths that serve to deny the reality of family situations

family therapy—Simultaneous treatment of more than one family member in the same session. The family's communication patterns and their patterns of relating are considered the focus of the treatment.

feedback—A regulatory function of a system. It serves to monitor, reinforce, and/or correct the structure and conditions of a system. Positive feedback facilitates change within a system, while negative feedback promotes system stability.

fictive kin—Refers to peole who are not related by consanguinal or affinal bonds but who are regarded as "just like family." Fictive kinship binds people together in ties of affection, concern, obligation, and responsibility.

fixation—The concentration of libidinal energies in one psychosexual stage of development, because of over gratification or under gratification in that stage.

flight of ideas—Communication that is characterized by rapid movement from one idea to another. There is a connection between the ideas, but it is tenuous and often influenced by the immediate environment. This phenomenon is sometimes demonstrated in manic-depressive psychosis.

forensic psychiatry—A subspecialty in psychiatry that deals with the legal facets of mental illness

formation—A cluster of people that occupies, and thereby defines, a quantum of space

frame of reference—An individual's personal guidelines, taken as a whole. A person's frame of reference reflects his or her social situation, cultural norms, and ideas.

fugue—A dreamlike or trance state, during which a person may travel distances from home, act out impulsively, or engage in childish behavior. Fugue is an emergency response to stress and anxiety, and it may precede amnesia.

genogram—A diagram that depicts family relationships over at least three successive generations. It is useful as a tool for tapping into the process of a family system over time.

grief—A series of subjective responses that follow a significant loss—for example, loss of body function, a body part, status, or a relative.

guilt—Tension between ego and superego that occurs when one falls short of standards set for onself.

hallucination—A false sensory perception; a perception for which there is no apparent external stimulus. Any of the senses may be involved; individuals have experienced hallucinations that are auditory, visual, tactile, olfactory, gustatory, or kinesthetic.

hebephrenic schizophrenia—A type of schizophrenia that is characterized by severe thought and emotional disorders. Behavior is bizarre, silly, and inappropriate. *Regression* is the main defense mechanism that is used in an exaggerated form. Hallucinations and delusions are present. This form of schizophrenia is generally believed to have the poorest prognosis. The age of onset tends to be young—before the twenties. This term is no longer included in DSM-III.

helplesness—A state characterized by the existence of an unfulfilled need and the inability to meet that need. Helplessness can be a learned response.

holistic health—Refers to the view that people are organic wholes. Well-being evolves from the development and integration of the component dimensions of this organic whole: the physical, the intellectual, the psychological, the sociocultural, and the spiritual.

homeodynamics—Refers to a state of relative balance and flux in a system

homeostasis—Refers to the maintenance of equilibrium or to a steady state of balance in a system

homosexuality—The preference for a sexual partner of one's own sex.

hopelessness—A situation characterized by the belief that all efforts to alter one's life situation will be fruitless

hostility—The tendency of an organism to do something harmful to another organism or to itself. Hostility may be passively rather than actively expressed.

household—A group of people bound together by common residence, economic cooperation, and the task of child rearing. Members of a household may or may not be united by bonds of kinship. A household is not concerned with the function of procreation.

human ecosystem—Refers to the interaction between human beings and their environment, specifically their physical and social environment

humor—The culturally influenced concept of what is funny, whimsical, capricious, and/or ludicrous

hydrotherapy—The form of treatment for mental illness that involved the use of water at various temperatures. Hydrotherapy is mostly of historical interest; it included such measures as continuous tub baths, application of wet sheet packs, and use of shower sprays.

hypochondriasis—A morbid preoccupation with the state of one's health, usually accompanied by physical symptoms or the conviction that some disease process is present that cannot be substantiated by medical evidence

hypomania—A state of elation. A hypomanic individual has boundless energy; is witty and outgoing, and is considered the life of the party. Hypomanic behavior is purposeful and goal-directed.

hysterical neurosis—An emergency psychological response to overwhelming anxiety. Hysterical neurosis includes a variety of symptom formations, such as amnesia and fugue state.

hysterical personality—Characterized by extremely excitable, emotionally labile, and overly dramatic behavior

id—In psychoanalytical theory, one of three interacting systems of the personality. The id represents the early or archaic parts of the personality. Id functioning occurs on an unconscious level, the existence of which can only be inferred through dreams, impulsive acts, and such psychiatric symptoms as primitive or unacculturated drives, needs, and so forth.

idealized image—A person who has a compulsive craving for perfection and admiration may come to view himself or herself as unreal and to create instead a self-conception based on high and often unattainable goals. Such a person then tries to live up to this ideal conceptualization and to receive affirmation from others that the self and the ideal conceptualization are one and the same.

ideas of reference—Pathological belief system that the actions and speech of others have reference to oneself. For example, an individual who is experiencing ideas of reference may believe that what a television announcer is saying is actually a coded reference to him or her. Since ideas of reference can occur in degrees, this example might be termed a *delusion of reference*.

identification—The process whereby an individual imitates the desired qualities of a significant person in the environment

impotence—The inability of the male to achieve or maintain an erection

imu—A culturally patterned form of hysteria found among people in northern Japan. Although men occasionally exhibit *imu*, women are primarily affected.

inadequate personality—Characterized by faulty judgment and poor physical and emotional endurance

incest—A form of sexual abuse where generational boundaries are crossed. Sexual relations occur between people who ignore cultural prohibitions, such as mother and son, father and daughter, or between close family members.

infantile autism—A disorder characterized by profound disturbances of speech, perception, and neurological functioning in children under the age of 30 months

institutional think—Tendency of people who are fully indoctrinated into institutional ideology to believe and think along institutional lines. When institutional think occurs, people may so closely identify with the institution that an attack on the institution becomes an attack on them.

instrumental—A type of circum-speech that is task oriented. Walking, smoking, and eating, when carried on while a person is speaking, are examples of instrumentals.

insulin coma therapy—The production of a coma, with or without convulsions, through intramuscular administration of insulin. The treatment, introduced by Sakel, was once used with schizophrenic persons. It is now of historical interest only.

integrated drinking—Refers to the incorporation of drinking alcoholic beverages into the life style of a cultural group

intellectualization—A defense mechanism in which reasoning is used as a defense against the conscious realization of an unconscious conflict

interaction coaching—An attempt to modify disturbed mother-infant interactions. The goal is to improve the interactional "fit" between mother and child.

interactional behavior—A type of circum-speech that includes body shifts or movements that increase, decrease, or maintain space between interacting individuals

interactional model—A model of family therapy that views the family as a communication system comprised of interlocking subsystems (the individual family members). Family dysfunction is seen as occurring when the rules that govern family interaction become vague and ambiguous. The goal of family therapy is to help the family clarify the rules that govern family relationships.

intrapsychic—Taking place *within* the mind

introject—A mental image of someone or something that becomes incorporated into one's ego system. The process of introjection is opposite to that of projection. An introject becomes emotionally invested for the individual and is involved in the process of identification and superego development.

introjection—The incorporation of qualities of a loved or hated object or individual into one's own ego structure. Introjection is an unconscious mechanism.

involutional melancholia—A form of depression that occurs during the middle to later periods of life. One of its primary characteristics is agitation.

isolation—A state in which the linkage between facts and emotions has been broken. Facts are allowed into the individual's experience, yet the emotional component is excluded from awareness.

kinesics—The use of body movements to communicate meaning

latency—The stage of development, according to Freud and Erikson, that encompasses ages 6 to 12.

latah—A culturally patterned form of hysteria found among people in Southeast Asia and Indonesia. Although men occasionally exhibit *latah,* women are predominantly affected.

liaison nursing—Provision, by clinical specialists in psychiatric nursing, of consultation services for nursing colleagues and members of other disciplines working in medical-surgical, parent-child, and geriatric settings.

libido—According to Freud, one's sexual drive

limpia—A culturally prescribed ritual performed by Central American native healers to treat *susto.* The *limpia* ritual is a process for resolving the schism in a *susto* victim's extended family and for reincorporating the *susto* sufferer into the extended family.

lithium carbonate—Chemical compound utilized primarily for the treatment of manic-depressive psychosis

loss—The relinquishing of supportive objects, persons, functions, or status

mania—An extreme state of elation characterized by rapid motor activity, inappropriate dress, and illogical thought processes.

manic-depressive response—A cluster of behaviors characterized by mood swings, ranging from profound depression to euphoria, with periods of normalcy in between

manipulation—The habitual use of others to gratify one's own needs and desires

markers—A type of body movement that aids in communication. Markers act as punctuation points and indicators.

meditation theapy—A way of achieving relaxation and consciousness expansion by focusing on a mantra (a word, sound, or image)

menopause—The return to the nonreproductive state of function of the female genitalia; usually begins in the early to late forties

metacommunication—Communication that indicates how verbal communication should be interpreted. Metacommunication may support or contradict verbal communication.

Metrazol shock therapy—A form of convulsive therapy (introduced in 1934 but rarely used today) in which the seizure is produced through an intravenous injection of Metrazol

milieu therapy—Treatment of a hospitalized person that makes use of the entire hospital environment: workers, scheduled and unscheduled activities, the physical plant, and so on (see "therapeutic community")

monoamine oxidase (MAO) inhibitors—Substances that counteract the reduction of norepinephrine, epinephrine, and serotonin levels in the body. The reactivation of these hormones to normal levels has an antidepressant effect.

monopolization—Domination of the discussion within a group by one member of the group

morpheme—A group of minimal meaningful sounds that cannot be broken down into smaller meaningful sounds. Morphemes are a basic unit of the expressive system (sound system) of spoken language.

motivation—The reasons for one's actions, for what one experiences, and for the way one experiences one's actions. These reasons can be on a conscious, preconscious, or unconscious level.

mourning—The psychological processes or reactions

activated by an individual to assist him or her in overcoming a loss. The process is finally resolved when reinvestment in a new object relationship has occurred.

multifactorial—Having a variety of causes

multigenerational model—A model of family therapy that focuses on reciprocal role relationships over time and thus takes a longitudinal approach to family therapy. The family is viewed as an emotional system where patterns of interacting and coping, as well as unresolved issues, can be passed down from generation to generation and can cause stress to the family members on whom they are projected. Family dysfunction is viewed as the transmission of undifferentiation across generational lines. The goal of family therapy is to help family members attain a higher level of differentiation.

multiple personality—A disorder chasracterized by a primary personality that is usually shy and introverted and two or more alter or secondary pesonalities, each exhibiting values and behaviors and sometimes ages and sexual orientations that differ from each other and from the primary personality. Multiple personality usually develops as a means of coping with severe physical and/or sexual abuse in one's childhood.

mutism—Inability or unwillingness to speak

mutual cuing—A circular interaction process between mother and infant by which they empathically read one another's signs and signals and react to each other

mystification—An habitual communication process that may include vagueness, tangentiality, double-bind communication, and family myths. Mystification serves to maintain the equilibrium of a family system even while it confuses family members.

narcissism—self-love or self-admiration. Depending upon degree and consequential behavior, narcissism can be healthy or pathological.

neologism—An invented word that has an obscure and purely subjective meaning. Neologisms are very often symbolic for a person; they are sometimes demonstrated in the speech of schizophrenic individuals.

networking—A mechanism for providing support and sharing information among members of a group (e.g., a professional group such as one of the specialty area groups within the Council of Specialists in Psychiatric and Mental Health Nursing).

neuroses—A group of disorders characterized by excessive anxiety and unconscious conflict. Although there is no gross distortion of the personality, the compromise solutions and defense mechanisms needed to cope with anxiety and conflict can inhibit personality functioning and may result in pathological symptoms. The terms ''neuroses'' and ''psychoneuroses'' are used synonymously.

non-with spaces—Spaces in which interacting persons use body parts and regions to show that they have different spatial orientations and thus are unaffiliated with one another.

nuclear family—A family unit composed of a man, a woman, and their children

nursing process—A method of scientific inquiry used to explore and intervene in a client's experience. The steps in the nursing process are assessment, analysis of data, formulation of a plan of care, implementation of the care plan, and evaluation. The nursing process forms the cognitive framework for nursing practice.

object constancy—This occurs in the development of a child when the child is able to maintain mental and emotional representations of mother (as first object) within. This is an indication that the child has been able to synthesize ''good'' and ''bad'' object representations in order to be able to relate to a whole object (person).

obsession—A state in which a repetitive thought or thought pattern keeps recurring despite the individual's efforts to banish it or prevent it from recurring.

obsessive-compulsive personality—Characterized by orderly, methodical, ritualistic, inhibited, and frugal behavior

obsessive-compulsive disorder—A psychiatric disorder characterized by repetitious performance of ritualistic behavior and the presence of obsessive thoughts that cannot be banished

Oedipus complex—Direction of a child's erotic attachment toward the parent of the opposite sex, during the phallic stage of development. Concurrently, there is jealousy toward the parent of the same sex.

omigenous family—A family unit consisting of the family that is formed when parents divorce and remarry. A complex kinship system of relatives and steprelatives may develop. The omigenous family is also referred to as a ''blended'' family.

open charting—A charting system in which a client has access to his or her chart. The more progressive mental health facilities have open charting in varying degrees.

oral phase—The freudian developmental phase that encompasses approximately the first 15 months of life. This period is characterized by a concentration of libidinal energies in the oral zone, particularly the mouth and lips.

organic brain dysfunctions—Neuropsychiatric conditions caused by any disturbance in brain tissue functions and characterized by the following syndrome: disturbances in comprehension, memory, orientation, and judgment and lability of emotional responses. Brain dysfunctions may be either acute or chronic. SYNONYM Organic brain syndromes.

organic brain syndromes—See *organic brain dysfunctions.*

orgasmic dysfunction—The inability of the female to achieve orgasm. Women may be "preorgasmic," referring to those who have never achieved an orgasm.

orientation phase—The first stage of the nurse-client relationship. During this stage, the framework of the relationship is established, the client maps out areas of concern and the nurse begins the process of assessment.

outcome criteria—Criteria identified by the American Nurses' Association Division on Psychiatric and Mental Health Nursing Practice that focus on observable or measurable results of nursing activities and mental health services

overinclusiveness—An association disturbance seen in the thought disorder of schizophrenia. The individual is unable to think in a precise manner because of an inability to keep irrelevant elements outside of perceptual boundaries.

paranoid personality—Characterized by extremely sensitive, rigid, suspicious, and jealous behavior. An individual makes exaggerated use of projection in an attempt to cope with insecure and negative feelings.

paranoid schizophrenia—A form of schizophrenia in which the paramount symptoms include suspicion, hallucinations, and delusions. The delusions are often grandiose or persecutory.

parataxic mode—In Sullivanian theory, perception of the whole physical and social environment as being illogical, disjointed, and composed of inconsistent parts. This process is common during childhood and the juvenile period.

passive-aggressive personality—Characterized by both independent and hostile behavior. Aggressiveness is usually covertly expressed through obstinateness, procrastination, vacillation, and helplessness.

patient (client) government—An organization, composed of clients, through which clients have some influence in the running of a unit

perceptual deprivation/restriction—Absence of or decrease in the meaningful grouping of stimuli, caused, for example, by an ever-present hum or constant dim lighting

perceptual monotony—A state characterized by a lack of variety in the normal pattern of everyday stimuli. Perceptual monotony can result, for example, from having the television on all day.

pervasive developmental disorders—Those disorders of infancy and childhood characterized by severe impairment of relatedness and behavioral aberrations previously known as childhood psychoses. Infantile autism, childhood schizophrenia, and symbiotic psychosis are included in this category.

phobia—An irrational or illogical fear of some object or aspect of the environment, because of the externalization of inner fears or anxiety

phobic disorder—A psychiatric condition in which internal anxiety and conflict are displaced or externalized onto some object in the environment, which can then be avoided

phoneme—A minimal unit of sound that distinguishes one utterance from another. Phonemes are a basic unit of the expressive system (sound system) of spoken language.

piblotoq—A culturally patterned form of hysteria that is found among the Polar Eskimo in northern Greenland. Although men occasionally exhibit *piblotoq*, women are primarily affected.

planned change—Altering the status quo by means of a carefully formulated program or scheme. There are three basic types of planned change: collaborative, coercive, and emulative. Planned change is characterized by four phases: unfreezing the present level, establishing a change relationship, moving to a new level, and freezing at the new level.

point behavior—Orienting body parts in some direction within a quantum of space

polarization—Within a group, the concentration of members' interests, beliefs, and allegiances around two conflicting positions

political nursing—The use of knowledge about power processes and strategies to influence the nature and direction of health care and professional nursing. The constituency of political nursing is clients: communities, groups, and individuals, both diagnosed and potential.

political system—A network of ideas and interpersonal relationships that effectively influences people's thoughts, decisions, and behavior. Each political system contains ideologies, goals, loyalties, interests, norms, and rules that foster cohesion and differentiate it from other political systems.

politics—The process of achieving and using power for the purpose of influencing decisions and resolving disputes between factions

positional behavior—Orienting body regions in order to claim a quantum of space. Positional behavior involves four body regions: head and neck, upper torso, pelvis and thighs, and lower legs and feet.

power—The ability to act, to do, and/or to control others. Power may arise from various sources, and it may be of various types (for example, expert power, associative power, and legitimate power).

powerlessness—Inability to effect change in one's environment

practicing—The second subphase of the separation-individuation phase in Mahler's system of preoedipal development. In this subphase, the child is able to move away from mother and return to her. The child feels elation in response to this investigation of the environment and through practicing locomotor skills.

preconscious—Those areas of mental functioning in which information is not in immediate awareness but is subject to recall

prefrontal lobotomy—A psychosurgical procedure in which some of the connections between the prefrontal lobes of the brain and the thalamus are severed. The procedure was used as a treatment for long-standing schizophrenia involving uncontrollable, destructive behavior. After surgery, individuals were often apathetic, docile, and lacking in social graces. The procedure is rarely used today, and it is frowned upon by many mental health professionals. The operation is called a lobotomy if tissue is removed; if only white fibers are severed, the procedure is called prefrontal leucotomy.

premature ejaculation—A sexual dysfunction which is characterized by the ejaculation of semen before partners reach a state of mutual enjoyment

preoperational thought phase—According to Piaget, the phase of development during which the child focuses on the development of language as the tool to meet his or her needs. This period encompasses ages 2 to 7.

preschizophrenic state—The period before psychosis is evident. The individual deviates from normality but does not demonstrate grossly psychotic symptoms such as delusions, hallucinations, or stupor.

primary prevention—Health promotion with individuals, families, groups, and communities through the identification and alleviation of stress-producing factors

primary processes—Unconscious processes, originating in the id, that obey different laws from those of the ego (reality, logic, and the environment influence the ego). These processes are seen in the least disguised forms in infancy and in the dreams of the adult. Much of the distorted thinking of an acutely psychotic person is based on primary process thinking.

primary triad—In Beck's theory of depression, the three major cognitive patterns that force the individual to view self, environment, and future in a negativistic manner

primitive idealization—A primitive defense mechanism in which the individual tends to see another person as *all good* and powerful and a necessary help against *all bad* objects (including one's own bad parts)

privacy—A culturally specific concept defining the degree of one's personal responsibility to others and behaviors that are regarded as interpersonally intrusive

process criteria—Criteria identified by the American Nurses' Association Division on Psychiatric and Mental Health Nursing Practice that focus on nursing activities

process schizophrenia—In contrast to reactive schizophrenia, organic, inborn factors are seen as paramount. The premorbid adjustment is usually poor, and onset is early in life. The process develops gradually and progresses to irreversibility.

projection—An unconscious mechanism that involves the attributing of one's own unacceptable thoughts, wishes, fears, and actions to another person or object

projective identification—A more primitive level of the defense mechanism of projection. It is characterized by a tendency to experience impulses that are simultaneously projected onto another person. The individual using projective identification then fears the recipient of this projection and feels the need to control this now "dangerous" person.

prototaxic mode—According to Sullivanian theory, the mode, occurring in infancy, that is characterized by a lack of differentiation between the self and the environment.

proxemics—The use of space to communicate meaning

pseudodementia—Cognitive impairment associated with depression, particularly in the elderly. It may occur as (1) depression-induced organic mental disorder or (2) coexisting organic and functional disorder.

pseudomutuality—A term used in family therapy theory and practice. It denotes an atmosphere, maintained by family members, in which there is surface harmony and a high degree of agreement with one another. The atmosphere of agreement covers deep and destructive intrapsychic and interpersonal conflicts.

pseudoneurotic schizophrenia—A form of the schizophrenic syndrome characterized by defenses that are, at least superficially, neurotic. On closer investigation, a schizophrenic process becomes evident.

psychodrama—A type of group treatment in which an individual is encouraged to act out his or her conflicts and problems in a supervised setting. Other people in the group take on the roles of significant others in the person's life. Insight and/or catharsis may develop through the use of psychodrama as a therapy.

psychoneuroses—See *neuroses*.

psychosomatogenic—Causing or leading to the development of psychophysiological coping measures that are learned as responses to stressful situations. Minuchin describes the "psychosomatogenic family" as one in which a child receives positive reinforcement for symptoms.

psychotic insight—A stage in the development of psychosis that follows the initial experience of confusion, bizarreness, and apprehension. When the individual reaches the point of psychotic insight, everything begins to fit together and to become understandable. He or she then understands the external world in terms of this new system of thinking: the delusional system explains all of the things he or she had been confused by. The individual experiences this development as the attainment of exceptionally lucid thinking. The defensive nature of this phenomenon is obvious.

quality assurance—Activities designed to indicate the quality of health care or to improve the quality of health care

rape—Sexual intercourse without the partner's consent. It is an act of violence, not an act of passion.

rapprochement—The third subphase of the separation-individuation phase of Mahler's system of preoedipal development. This subphase occurs from approximately fourteen months to two years or more. This stage is characterized by a rediscovery of mother after the initial separation of the practicing subphase. The narcissistic inflation of the practicing subphase is replaced by a realization of separation and vulnerability.

The subphase of rapprochement is seen as extremely significant in the subsequent development of borderline personality pathology.

rationalization—The process of constructing plausible reasons to explain and justify one's behavior

reaction formation—The unconscious assumption of behavior patterns that are in direct opposition to what a person really feels or believes

reactive depression—Depression that is exogenous—in other words, depression that has a definite cause

reactive schizophrenia—In contrast to process schizophrenia, reactive schizophrenia is attributed more to environmental factors than to inborn factors. There is usually a fairly good premorbid adjustment, onset is rapid, and the psychotic episode is usually brief.

reactor—A term used to describe a family therapist who lets a family in therapy take the lead and then follows in that direction

reality—The culturally constructed world of preception, meaning, and behavior that members of any given culture regard as an absolute

reciprocal—A type of body movement that aids in communication. A reciprocal indicates affiliation between people.

reductionism—An approach that tries to explain a form of behavior or an event in terms of a particular category of phenomena (for example, biological, psychological, or cultural), negating the possibility of an interrelation of causal phenomena

reference group—A group with which a person identifies or to which he or she wishes to belong

regression—A return to an earlier stage of behavior, where modes of gratification had been more satisfying and needs had been met and where the ego had been acted upon rather than initiating the action

relationship therapy—Therapy that emerges out of the totality of a client-therapist relationship. The therapist *begins where the client is* and encourages the growth of self in the client. Relationship therapy is an experience in living that takes place within a relationship with another person.

relativism—An attitude or belief that all cultures are logically consistent and viable and can only be understood and examined in terms of their own standards, attitudes, values, and beliefs. Relativism is the opposite of ethnocentrism.

religiosity—A psychiatric symptom characterized by the demonstration of excessive or affected piety

remotivation group—A type of treatment group that is

often used to stimulate the interest, awareness, and communication of withdrawn and institutionalized clients

repression—A defense mechanism through which unpleasant thoughts, memories, and actions are pushed out of conscious awareness involuntarily. Repression is the cornerstone of defense mechanisms.

resistance—Conscious or unconscious reluctance to bring repressed ideas, thoughts, desires, or memories into awareness

retarded ejaculation—The inability of the male to ejaculate after having achieved an erection. This often accompanies the aging process.

retention procedure—A method established by state statute or mental health code for committing a person to a psychiatric institution. Most states recognize four types of retention: informal, voluntary, emergency, and involuntary.

role blurring—The tendency for professional roles to overlap and become indistinct

rules of co-occurrence—Mandate that a person use the same level of lexical and/or syntactic structure when speaking

saka—A culturally patterned form of hysteria found among the Wataita tribe of Kenya. Although men occasionally exhibit *saka,* women are primarily affected.

scapegoating—Projecting blame, hostility, suspicion, and so forth onto one member of a group by the other group members in order to avoid self-confrontation. This behavior may be demonstrated in groups or families.

schizoaffective schizophrenia—Schizophrenic illness in which affective symptoms (depression, elation, and excitement) are prominent.

schizoid personality—Characterized by eccentric, introverted, withdrawn, and aloof behavior. The differentiation between schizoid personality and schizophrenia is a matter of degree of symptomatology.

schizophrenogenic—Adjective used to describe behavior that is believed by some family therapy theorists to cause schizophrenia

school phobia—A disorder in children which is characterized by increased anxiety secondary to separation from parenting figure in relation to school. Parental fears of separation and uncertainty are transferred to the child.

scripting—A technique of family therapy involving the development of new family transactional patterns

sculpting—A technique of family therapy involving the construction of a live family portrait that depicts family alliances and conflicts

secondary prevention—Early diagnosis and treatment through the provision of referral services, the facilitation of the use of these services, and the rapid initiation of treatment

self-concept—A mental picture that includes an individual's identity—strengths, weaknesses, and self-perception—based on reflected appraisals from the environment

self-esteem—The amount of worth and competence an individual attributes to himself or herself, which acts as a protective mechanism against anxiety

self-fulfilling prophecy—A distortion of an event or situation that eventually leads an individual to behave as he or she is expected to behave by others in the social setting

sensorimotor phase—According to Piagetian theory, the developmental phase encompassing the period from birth to 2 years

sensory deprivation/restriction—The reduction of environmental stimuli to a minimum

sensory-perceptual overload—A state characterized by an increase in the intensity and amount of stimuli to the point that a person loses the ability to discriminate among varying incoming stimuli

separation-individuation phase—In Mahler's system of preoedipal development, this phase begins when the infant begins to ''hatch'' from the ''symbiotic orbit'' with the mother and to see itself as separate. This occurs in the period from approximately five months to two and one half years and it evolves through four distinct subphases (see: *differentiation, practicing, rapprochement,* and *consolidation of individuality* and *emotional object constancy*)

sexism—An attitude or belief that one sex is inferior or superior to the other

sex role—The expectations held by society about what constitutes appropriate or inappropriate behavior for each sex

sexual dysfunction—A psychophysiological disorder in which the experiencing of sexual pleasure is inhibited because of psychosocial factors and in some cases physical factors

sexuality—An integral part of the human condition. Sexuality integrates the physical, emotional, intellectual, sociocultural and spiritual dimensions of human beings. Sexuality continues throughout the life cycle and does not disappear as one ages.

sexually deviant personality—Characterized by sexual behavior that significantly differs from society's norms. Either the quality of sexual drives or the object of sexual drives is at variance with cultural norms for adults. While these forms of sexual behavior are considered deviant for adults, most of them are part of normal psychosexual growth and development.

significant other—A person in the environment who is considered by another as being special and as having an impact on that individual

simple schizophrenia—The form of schizophrenia in which impoverishment of emotions, intellect, and will is evident but in which secondary symptoms such as hallucinations and delusions are absent. The person is often viewed as eccentric, isolated, and dull.

single-parent family—A family unit consisting of a man or a woman and his or her children

site—The quantum of space occupied and defined by a cluster of people

situational crisis—A crisis that occurs when a person is confronted with a stressful event of such unusual or extreme intensity or duration that the habitual methods of coping are no longer effective. SYNONYM: Incidental crisis

social class—A grouping of persons who have similar values, interests, income, education, and occupations

social deviance—Behavior that violates social standards, engendering anger, resentment, and/or the desire for punishment in a significant segment of society

social mobility—The process of moving upward or downward in the social hierarchy

social network—An interconnected group of cooperating significant others, both relatives and non relatives, with whom a person interacts

social network therapy—The gathering together of client, family, and other social contacts into group sessions for the purpose of problem solving

social order—The way in which a society is organized and the rules and standards of behavior that maintain that organization

social sanctions—Measures used by a group to enforce acceptable behavior or to punish unacceptable behavior

sociogenic—Motivated by social values and constraints

sociolinguistics—The study of the relationship between language and the social context in which it occurs

somatoform disorders—Characterized by physical symptoms without organic basis. Somatoform disorders are a response to overwhelming anxiety. Such disorders as hypochondriasis and conversion disorder are types of somatoform disorders.

spatial zones—Spatioperceptual fields in which people interact. There are four spatial zones: intimate zone (distance of 18 or fewer inches), personal zone (1½ to 4 feet), social zone (4 to 12 feet), and public zone (12 to 25 feet or more).

splitting—A primitive defense mechanism that when overused, represents a developmental arrest. There is a failure to synthesize the positive and negative experiences and ideas one has of oneself, other people, situations or institutions.

spot—The small quantum of space that becomes the territorial object and extension of point behavior

stereotype—A generalization about a form of behavior, an individual, or a group

stereotypical behavior—A pattern of body movements that has autistic and symbolic meaning for an individual

stress kinesic—A type of circum-speech that serves to mark the flow of speech and that generally coincides with linguistic stress patterns

stress management—A series of techniques utilized by individuals to identify stressors and to implement strategies to reduce or alleviate potential and/or actual stressors. Such strategies include: progressive relaxation, guided imagery, biofeedback and active problem solving.

structural model—A model of family therapy that views the family as an open system and identifies subsystems within the family that carry out specific family functions. When faced with demands for change, individual family members, family subsystems or the family as a whole may respond with growth behaviors or with maladaptive behaviors. Family dysfunction is seen as occurring because these maladaptive behaviors are dysfunctional transactional patterns (scripts) for organizing family life and family relationships. The goal of family therapy is to help the family learn new scripts or transactional patterns.

stupor—A condition in which an individual's senses are blunted and in which the person is, to some degree, unaware of his or her environment

sublimation—The directing of unacceptable libidinal energies into socially acceptable channels

substance intoxication—A state that results when a person ingests toxic amounts of a substance—for example, alcohol or another drug.

suicide—The infliction of bodily harm on self that results in death

superego—In psychoanalytical theory, the system of the personality that represents the internalized ethical precepts and taboos of parents and others who are responsible for the enculturation of the child. The ego ideal and the conscience are aspects of the superego system.

susto (also known as *espanto*)—A culture-bound syndrome found among Central Americans. It is related to stress engendered by a self-perceived failure to fulfill sex-role expectations.

symbiotic phase—In Mahler's system of preoedipal development, the stage from 1 month to approximately 5 months of age. The child participates in a "symbiotic orbit" with the mother. All parts of mother (including voice, gestures, clothing, and space in which she moves) are joined with the infant.

symptom neuroses—Psychological disorders in which dysfunctional coping mechanisms appear as clinical symptoms that represent direct manifestations of anxiety or the unconscious defenses utilized to cope with anxiety

syntax—A property of language. Syntax refers to structural cues for the arrangement of words into phrases and sentences. In English, the usual order of a sentence is subject-verb-object.

syntaxic mode—In Sullivanian theory, the ability to perceive whole, logical, coherent pictures as they occur in reality

system—A set of component parts that are in dynamic interaction. A system is characterized by interrelatedness, flow of information, feedback, and boundaries. Feedback, boundary-maintenance mechanisms, and self-corrective mechanisms serve a regulatory function in maintaining order within a system.

taijin kyofu—A culturally patterned phobic fear of meeting people. *Taijin kyofu* is found among people in Japan.

tangentiality—An association disturbance characterized by the tendency to digress from one's original topic of conversation. Tangentiality can destroy or seriously hamper a person's ability to communicate effectively with other people.

tardive dysmentia—A syndrome of emotional disturbance associated with tardive dyskinesia. Both are believed to be related to the long-term use of phenothiazines. The syndrome is sometimes termed "iatrogenic schizophrenia."

termination phase—The last stage of the nurse-client relationship. During this stage, nurses and clients evaluate goals attained and outcomes achieved. During this stage, nurses may also help clients establish networks of support, other than the nurse-client relationship, that may be of assistance in coping with problems that might arise in the future.

territorial—A type of body movement that aids in communication. A territorial frames an interaction and defines a territory.

territory—An area or space over which an animal or human being maintains some degree of control. Both the claiming of space and acknowledgment of the claim are necessary for the establishment of a territory.

tertiary prevention—The rehabilitative process. Its goals are the reduction of the severity of a disability or dysfunction and the prevention of further disability.

Thanatos—According to Freud, the instinct for death

therapeutic community—The concept that every aspect of hospitalization should be used as treatment for a client. In a therapeutic community all staff members work together as a team, and the environment is structured to be of maximum benefit to clients. (see milieu therapy)

token economy—A therapeutic program that uses reward procedures (or positive reinforcement) in order to effect desirable behavioral change in individuals. This therapy is sometimes used in day hospitals, halfway houses, and wards for chronically ill persons in psychiatric hospitals.

touch—Tactile means of communicating such emotions as love, sympathy, hostility and fear. One's use of and response to touch is culturally influenced.

toxic psychosis—See *acute confusional state*.

transference—The displacement of feelings and attitudes originally experienced toward significant others in the past onto persons in the present

transitional object—An object used by a child to provide comfort and security while he or she is moving away from a secure base (such as mother or home)

triad—A combination of three—for example, two parents and a child

tricyclics—A group of medications that are effective in the treatment of depression

trust—A risk-taking process whereby an individual's situation depends upon the future behavior of another individual

unconscious—A psychodynamic concept that refers to

mental functioning that is out of awareness and cannot be recalled. Drives, wishes, ideas, and so forth that are in conflict with internalized standards and ideals are maintained in the unconscious level through repression and other mental mechanisms.

undoing—Performing a specific action that is intended to negate, in part, a previous action or communication. Undoing is related to the magical thinking of childhood.

unipolar depressive response—An affective disorder that is characterized by symptoms of depression only

vaginismus—The development of spasticity in the pelvic muscles surrounding the vagina, which results in decreased probability of penetration

vagueness—A communication pattern involving the use of global pronouns and loose associations that lead to ambiguity and confusion in communication

verbal language—A culturally organized system of vocal sounds that communicate meaning

violence—Refers to behavior that has the physical intent of inflicting harm on people or property. For violence to be considered criminal, the behavior must conform to the definition of violent behavior delineated by the society in which it occurs.

wellness—A dynamic condition of well-being that evolves from the development and integration of the five dimensions of a person: physical, intellectual, psychological, sociocultural and spiritual. Wellness is a process of ongoing growth toward self-actualization.

with spaces—Spaces in which interacting persons use body parts and regions to show that they share a similar spatial orientation and thus are affiliated.

word salad—A type of speech characterized by phrases that are confusing and apparently meaningless. A word salad may contain neologisms. Only the client can provide the meaning of such highly personal, coded communication.

working phase—The second stage of the nurse-client relationship. During this stage, clients explore their experiences. Nurses assist clients in this process of exploration by helping them to describe and clarify their experiences, to plan courses of action and try out the plans, and to begin to evaluate the effectiveness of their new behavior. Should new behavior prove ineffective, nurses may assist clients to revise their courses of action.

worthlessness—A component of low self-esteem; a feeling of uselessness and inability to contribute meaningfully to the well-being of others or to one's environment

DSM-III classification: axes I and II categories and codes*

The *Diagnostic and Statistical Manual of Mental Disorders* is published by the American Psychiatric Association and is periodically revised. The third edition (DSM-III) appeared in 1980.

The *Manual* categorizes and codifies psychiatric diagnoses. A description of diagnostic criteria accompanies each diagnosis. Categories and codes are used by physicians when they make diagnoses and by institutional personnel when they compile statistics and complete insurance forms.

All official DSM-III codes and terms are included in ICD-9-CM. However, in order to differentiate those DSM-III categories that use the same ICD-9-CM codes, unofficial non-ICD-9-CM codes are provided in parentheses for use when greater specificity is necessary.

The long dashes indicate the need for a fifth-digit subtype or other qualifying term.

DISORDERS USUALLY FIRST EVIDENT IN INFANCY, CHILDHOOD OR ADOLESCENCE

Mental retardation

Code in fifth digit: 1 = with other behavioral symptoms (requiring attention or treatment and that are not part of another disorder), 0 = without other behavioral symptoms.

317.0x Mild mental retardation, _____
318.0x Moderate mental retardation, _____
318.1x Severe mental retardation, _____
318.2x Profound mental retardation, _____
319.0x Unspecified mental retardation, _____

Attention deficit disorder

314.01 with hyperactivity
314.00 without hyperactivity
314.80 residual type

Conduct disorder

312.00 undersocialized, aggressive
312.10 undersocialized, nonaggressive
312.23 socialized, aggressive
312.21 socialized, nonaggressive
312.90 atypical

Anxiety disorders of childhood or adolescence

309.21 Separation anxiety disorder
313.21 Avoidant disorder of childhood or adolescence
313.00 Overanxious disorder

Other disorders of infancy, childhood or adolescence

313.89 Reactive attachment disorder of infancy
313.22 Schizoid disorder of childhood or adolescence
313.23 Elective mutism
313.81 Oppositional disorder
313.82 Identity disorder

Eating disorders

307.10 Anorexia nervosa
307.51 Bulimia
307.52 Pica
307.53 Rumination disorder of infancy
307.50 Atypical eating disorder

Stereotyped movement disorders

307.21 Transient tic disorder
307.22 Chronic motor tic disorder
307.23 Tourette's disorder
307.20 Atypical tic disorder
307.30 Atypical stereotyped movement disorder

Other disorders with physical manifestations

307.00 Stuttering
307.60 Functional enuresis
307.70 Functional encopresis
307.46 Sleepwalking disorder
307.46 Sleep terror disorder (307.49)

Pervasive developmental disorders

Code in fifth digit: 0 = full syndrome present. 1 = residual state.
299.0x Infantile autism, _____
299.9x Childhood onset pervasive developmental disorder, _____
      299.8x Atypical, _____

Specific developmental disorders

Note: These are coded on Axis II.

315.00 Developmental reading disorder
315.10 Developmental arithmetic disorder
315.31 Developmental language disorder
315.39 Developmental articulation disorder
315.50 Mixed specific developmental disorder
315.90 Atypical specific developmental disorder

ORGANIC MENTAL DISORDERS

Section 1. Organic mental disorders whose etiology or pathophysiological process is listed below (taken from the mental disorders section of ICD-9-CM).

Dementias arising in the senium and presenium

Primary degenerative dementia, senile onset

290.30 with delirium
290.20 with delusions
290.21 with depression
290.00 uncomplicated
    Code in fifth digit: 1 = with delirium, 2 = with delusions, 3 = with depression, 0 = uncomplicated.

290.1x Primary degenerative dementia, presenile onset, _____

290.4x Multi-infarct dementia, _____

Substance-induced

Alcohol

303.00 intoxication
291.40 idiosyncratic intoxication
291.80 withdrawal
291.00 withdrawl delirium
291.30 hallucinosis
291.10 amnestic disorder
    Code severity of dementia in fifth digit: 1 = mild, 2 = moderate, 3 = severe, 0 = unspecified.
291.2x Dementia associated with alcoholism, _____

Barbiturate or similarly acting sedative or hypnotic

305.40 intoxication (327.00)
292.90 withdrawal (327.01)
292.00 withdrawal delirium (327.02)
292.83 amnestic disorder (327.04)

Opioid

305.50 intoxication (327.10)
292.00 withdrawal (327.11)

Cocaine

305.60 intoxication (327.20)

Amphetamine or similarly acting sympathomimetic

305.70 intoxication (327.30)
292.81 delirium (327.32)
292.11 delusional disorder (327.35)
292.00 withdrawal (327.31)

Phencyclidine (PCP) or similarly acting arylcyclohexylamine

305.90 intoxication (327.40)
292.81 delirium (327.42)
292.90 mixed organic mental disorder (327.49)

Hallucinogen

305.30 hallucinosis (327.56)
292.11 delusional disorder (327.55)
292.84 affective disorder (327.57)

Cannabis

305.20 intoxication (327.60)
292.11 delusional disorder (327.65)

Tobacco

292.00 withdrawal (327.71)

Caffeine

305.90 intoxication (327.80)

Other or unspecified substance

305.90 intoxication (327.90)
292.00 withdrawal (327.91)
292.81 delirium (327.92)
292.82 dementia (327.93)
292.83 amnestic disorder (327.94)
292.11 delusional disorder (327.95)
292.12 hallucinosis (327.96)
292.84 affective disorder (327.97)
292.89 personality disorder (327.98)
292.90 atypical or mixed organic mental disorder (327.99)

Section 2. Organic brain syndromes whose etiology or pathophysiological process is either noted as an additional diagnosis from outside the mental disorders section of ICD-9-CM or is unknown.

293.00 Delirium
294.10 Dementia
294.00 Amnestic syndrome
293.81 Organic delusional syndrome
293.82 Organic hallucinosis
293.83 Organic affective syndrome
310.10 Organic personality syndrome
294.80 Atypical or mixed organic brain syndrome

SUBSTANCE USE DISORDERS

Code in fifth digit: 1 = continuous, 2 = episodic, 3 = in remission, 0 = unspecified.
305.0x Alcohol abuse, _____
303.9x Alcohol dependence (Alcoholism), _____
305.4x Barbiturate or similarly acting sedative or hypnotic abuse
304.1x Barbiturate or similarly acting sedative or hypnotic dependence, _____
305.5x Opioid abuse, _____
304.0x Opioid dependence, _____
305.6x Cocaine abuse, _____
305.7x Amphetamine or similarly acting sympathomimetic abuse, _____

304.4x Amphetamine or similarly acting sympathomimetic dependence, _____
305.9x Phencyclidine (PCP) or similarly acting arylcyclohexylamine abuse, _____ (328.4x)
305.3x Hallucinogen abuse, _____
305.2x Cannabis abuse, _____
304.3x Cannabis dependence, _____
305.1x Tobacco dependence, _____
305.9x Other, mixed or unspecified substance abuse, _____
304.6x Other specified substance dependence, _____
304.9x Unspecified substance dependence, _____
304.7x Dependence on combination of opioid and other nonalcoholic substance, _____
304.8x Dependence on combination of substances, excluding opiods and alcohol, _____

SCHIZOPHRENIC DISORDERS

Code in fifth digit: 1 = subchronic, 2 = chronic, 3 = subchronic with acute exacerbation, 4 = chronic with acute exacerbation, 5 = in remission, 0 = unspecified.

Schizophrenia

295.1x disorganized, _____
295.2x catatonic, _____
295.3x paranoid, _____
295.9x undifferentiated, _____
295.6x residual, _____

PARANOID DISORDERS

297.10 Paranoia
297.30 Shared paranoid disorder
298.30 Acute paranoid disorder
297.90 Atypical paranoid disorder

PSYCHOTIC DISORDERS NOT ELSEWHERE CLASSIFIED

295.40 Schizophreniform disorder
298.80 Brief reactive psychosis
295.70 Schizoaffective disorder
298.90 Atypical psychosis

NEUROTIC DISORDERS

These are included in affective, anxiety, somatoform, dissociative, and psychosexual disorders. In order to facilitate the identification of the categories that in DSM-II were grouped together in the class of neuroses, the DSM-II terms are included separately in parentheses after the corresponding categories.

These DSM-II terms are included in ICD-9-CM and therefore are acceptable as alternatives to the recommended DSM-III terms that precede them.

AFFECTIVE DISORDERS
Major affective disorders

Code major depressive episode in fifth digit: 6 = in remission, 4 = with psychotic features (the unofficial non-ICD-9-CM fifth digit 7 may be used instead to indicate that the psychotic features are mood-incongruent), 3 = with melancholia, 2 = without melancholia, 0 = unspecified.

Code manic episode in fifth digit: 6 = in remission, 4 = with psychotic features (the unofficial non-ICD-9-CM fifth digit 7 may be used instead to indicate that the psychotic features are mood-incongruent), 2 = without psychotic features, 0 = unspecified.

Bipolar disorder

296.6x mixed, _____
296.4x manic, _____
296.5x depressed, _____

Major depression

296.2x single episode, _____
296.3x recurrent, _____

Other specific affective disorders

301.13 Cyclothymic disorder
300.40 Dysthymic disorder (or Depressive neurosis)

Atypical affective disorders

296.70 Atypical bipolar disorder
296.82 Atypical depression

ANXIETY DISORDERS
Phobic disorders (or Phobic neuroses)

300.21 Agoraphobia with panic attacks
300.22 Agoraphobia without panic attacks
300.23 Social phobia
300.29 Simple phobia

Anxiety states (or Anxiety neuroses)

300.01 Panic disorder
300.02 Generalized anxiety disorder
300.30 Obsessive compulsive disorder (or Obsessive compulsive neurosis)

Post-traumatic stress disorder

308.30 acute
309.81 chronic or delayed
300.00 Atypical anxiety disorder

SOMATOFORM DISORDERS

300.81 Somatization disorder
300.11 Conversion disorder (or Hysterical neurosis, conversion type).
307.80 Psychogenic pain disorder
300.70 Hypochondriasis (or Hypochondriacal neurosis)
300.70 Atypical somatoform disorder (300.71)

DISSOCIATIVE DISORDERS (OR HYSTERICAL NEUROSES, DISSOCIATIVE TYPE)

300.12 Psychogenic amnesia
300.13 Psychogenic fugue
300.14 Multiple personality
300.60 Depersonalization disorder (or Depersonalization neurosis)
300.15 Atypical dissociative disorder

PSYCHOSEXUAL DISORDERS
Gender identity disorders

Indicate sexual history in the fifth digit of transsexualism code: 1 = asexual, 2 = homosexual, 3 = heterosexual, 0 = unspecified.
302.5x Transsexualism, _____
302.60 Gender identity disorder of childhood
302.85 Atypical gender identity disorder

Paraphilias

302.81 Fetishism
302.30 Transvestism
302.10 Zoophilia
302.20 Pedophilia
302.40 Exhibitionism
302.82 Voyeurism
302.83 Sexual masochism
302.84 Sexual sadism
302.90 Atypical paraphilia

Psychosexual dysfunctions

302.71 Inhibited sexual desire
302.72 Inhibited sexual excitement
302.73 Inhibited female orgasm
302.74 Inhibited male orgasm
302.75 Premature ejaculation

302.76 Functional dyspareunia
306.51 Functional vaginismus
302.70 Atypical psychosexual dysfunction

Other psychosexual disorders

302.00 Ego-dystonic homosexuality
302.89 Psychosexual disorder not elsewhere classified

FACTITIOUS DISORDERS

300.16 Factitious disorder with psychological symptoms
301.51 Chronic factitious disorder with physical symptoms
300.19 Atypical factitious disorder with physical symptoms

DISORDERS OF IMPULSE CONTROL NOT ELSEWHERE CLASSIFIED

312.31 Pathological gambling
312.32 Kleptomania
312.33 Pyromania
312.34 Intermittent explosive disorder
312.35 Isolated explosive disorder
312.39 Atypical impulse control disorder

ADJUSTMENT DISORDER

309.00 with depressed mood
309.24 with anxious mood
309.28 with mixed emotional features
309.30 with disturbance of conduct
309.40 with mixed disturbance of emotions and conduct
309.23 with work (or academic) inhibition
309.83 with withdrawal
309.90 with atypical features

PSYCHOLOGICAL FACTORS AFFECTING PHYSICAL CONDITION

Specify physical condition on Axis III.
316.00 Psychological factors affecting physical condition

PERSONALITY DISORDERS

Note: These are coded on Axis II.

301.00 Paranoid
301.20 Schizoid
301.22 Schizotypal
301.50 Histrionic
301.81 Narcissistic
301.70 Antisocial
301.83 Borderline
301.82 Avoidant
301.60 Dependent
301.40 Compulsive
301.84 Passive-Aggressive
301.89 Atypical, mixed or other personality disorder

V CODES FOR CONDITIONS NOT ATTRIBUTABLE TO A MENTAL DISORDER THAT ARE A FOCUS OF ATTENTION OR TREATMENT

V65.20 Malingering
V62.89 Borderline intellectual functioning (V62.88)
V71.01 Adult antisocial behavior
V71.02 Childhood or adolescent antisocial behavior
V62.30 Academic problem
V62.20 Occupational problem
V62.82 Uncomplicated bereavement
V15.81 Noncompliance with medical treatment
V62.89 Phase of life problem or other life circumstance problem
V61.10 Marital problem
V61.20 Parent-child problem
V61.80 Other specified family circumstances
V62.81 Other interpersonal problem

ADDITIONAL CODES

300.90 Unspecified mental disorder (nonpsychotic)
V71.09 No diagnosis or condition on Axis 1
799.90 Diagnosis or condition deferred on Axis I

V71.09 No diagnosis on Axis II
799.90 Diagnosis deferred on Axis II

ANA standards of psychiatric and mental health nursing practice

Standard I—Theory

The nurse applies appropriate theory that is scientifically sound as a basis for decisions regarding nursing practice.

Standard II—Data collection

The nurse continuously collects data that are comprehensive, accurate, and systematic.

Standard III—Diagnosis

The nurse utilizes *nursing diagnoses* and standard classification of mental disorders to express conclusions supported by recorded assessment data and current scientific premises.

Standard IV—Planning

The nurse develops a nursing care plan with specific goals and interventions delineating nursing actions unique to each client's needs.

Standard V—Intervention

The nurse intervenes as guided by the nursing care plan to implement nursing actions that promote, maintain, or restore physical and mental health, prevent illness, and effect rehabilitation.

Standard V-A—Psychotherapeutic interventions

The nurse (generalist) uses *psychotherapeutic interventions* to assist clients to regain or improve their previous coping abilities and to prevent further disability.

Standard V-B—Health teaching

The nurse assists clients, families, and groups to achieve satisfying and productive patterns of living through health teaching.

Standard V-C—Self-care activities

The nurse uses the activities of daily living in a goal-directed way to foster adequate self-care and physical and mental well-being of clients.

Standard V-D—Somatic therapies

The nurse uses knowledge of somatic therapies and applies related clinical skills in working with clients.

Standard V-E—Therapeutic environment

The nurse provides, structures, and maintains a therapeutic environment in collaboration with the client and other health care providers.

Reprinted with permission of the American Nurses' Association, Kansas City, Mo., 1982.

Standard V-F—Psychotherapy

The nurse (specialist) utilizes advanced clinical expertise in individual, group, and family psychotherapy, child psychotherapy, and other treatment modalities to function as a psychotherapist and recognizes professional accountability for nursing practice.

Standard VI—Evaluation

The nurse evaluates client responses to nursing actions in order to revise the data base, nursing diagnoses, and nursing care plan.

Standard VII—Peer review

The nurse participates in peer review and other means of evaluation to assure quality of nursing care provided for clients.

Standard VIII—Continuing education

The nurse assumes responsibility for continuing education and professional development and contributes to the professional growth of others.

Standard IX—Interdisciplinary collaboration

The nurse collaborates with interdisciplinary teams in assessing, planning, implementing, and evaluating programs and other mental health activities.

Standard X—Utilization of community health systems

The nurse (specialist) participates with other members of the community in assessing, planning, implementing, and evaluating mental health services and community systems that include the promotion of the broad continuum of primary, secondary, and tertiary prevention of mental illness.

Standard XI—Research

The nurse contributes to nursing and the mental health field through innovations in theory and practice and participation in research.

Index